APhA's Complete Review for Pharmacy

APhA's Complete Review for Pharmacy

Second Edition

Dick R. Gourley, PharmD
Editor-in-Chief
Dean and Professor
University of Tennessee College of Pharmacy
Memphis, Tennessee

James C. Eoff, PharmD
Associate Editor-in-Chief
Executive Associate Dean and Professor, Clinical Pharmacy
University of Tennessee College of Pharmacy
Memphis, Tennessee

American Pharmacists Association™
Improving medication use. Advancing patient care.

APhA

**Castle Connolly Graduate
Medical Publishing, Ltd.**
New York, New York

Published by
Castle Connolly Graduate Medical Publishing, Ltd.
17 Battery Place
New York, NY 10004
212-644-9696
http://www.ccgmp.com
info@ccgmp.com

Library of Congress Cataloging-in-Publication Data

APhA's complete review for pharmacy / Dick R. Gourley, editor-in-chief ;
James C. Eoff, editor-in-chief. – 2nd ed.
    p. cm.
Includes bibliographical references.
ISBN 0-9723076-4-8 (softcover)
1. Pharmacy—Outlines, syllabi, etc. 2. Pharmacy—Examinations,
questions, etc.
I. Gourley, D. R. (Dick R.), 1944- II. American Pharmacists Association. III. Title.
RS98.A64 2004
615'.4'076—dc22
                       2004022715

PRINTED IN THE UNITED STATES OF AMERICA

Contents

Preface

It is indeed an honor to have been asked to serve as Editor-in-Chief of *APhA's Complete Review for Pharmacy*. The faculty of the University of Tennessee College of Pharmacy and I appreciate the confidence that the American Pharmacists Association, Castle Connolly Graduate Medical Publishing, and Johnson & Johnson companies McNeil, Ortho Biotech, Janssen Pharmaceutica/Eisai, and Johnson & Johnson/Merck demonstrated by allowing us this opportunity to assist pharmacy students in preparing for the NAPLEX® Examination. This project is very important to pharmacy students across the United States, and I know they appreciate the support of APhA and the four Johnson & Johnson companies for this project.

As pharmacy students prepare to take the NAPLEX® examination, it is imperative that they have the most up-to-date and relevant information concerning the practice of pharmacy available to them. The information explosion is such that information changes daily, and approximately 30 new drugs are marketed each year. The amount of information that any student in pharmacy must master is significant and doubles every 2 to 3 years.

The board examination is the culmination of at least 6 years of university work; it is impossible to go back to the beginning and review all aspects of pharmacy education in order to prepare for it. Therefore, we have developed a comprehensive review of pharmacy for students preparing to take the NAPLEX® examination and for practitioners wanting to review a given area of practice.

This study guide has attempted to summarize the information in a user friendly manner. The information included has been deemed by our faculty, including a panel we convened of ten recent PharmD graduates, to be the most important. The review includes educational material (synthesizing the most salient points), key points (further delineation of the most important factors), references, and finally, self-study questions.

It is highly recommended that any student preparing for the NAPLEX® examination review the instructions on the NABP® web page (www.nabp.net). Students should also read the current literature in journals and review areas where they feel they have a weakness.

My thanks and appreciation go to my Associate Editor James C. Eoff, PharmD, Executive Associate Dean of the University of Tennessee College of Pharmacy, the faculty of the University of Tennessee College of Pharmacy who participated in preparing this comprehensive review, and to Karin Ingram, Administrative Assistant to the Dean, for her coordination of the preparation of the review book. I also wish to thank Michael D. Wolf, PhD at Castle Connolly Graduate Medical Publishing; James Appleby, RPh, Senior Vice President, Business Development at the American Pharmacists Association; and the Johnson & Johnson companies noted above for providing the unrestricted educational funding which made this project possible. The insight of APhA and Johnson & Johnson in recognizing the need of pharmacy students for this review book, and their willingness to provide this for all pharmacy graduates in the United States, is a true service to the profession of pharmacy.

Dick R. Gourley, PharmD
Professor and Dean
The University of Tennessee College of Pharmacy
Memphis, Tennessee
October, 2004

Study Guide to NAPLEX Review and Test-Taking Strategies

James C. Eoff III, Pharm.D.
University of Tennessee College of Pharmacy

Welcome to *APhA's Complete Review for Pharmacy.* With so many different academic backgrounds, such a variety of learning experiences, and the increasing volume of information taught at U.S. colleges of pharmacy, it is impossible to cover all materials from each course you have taken while in pharmacy school. Therefore the primary purpose of *APhA's Complete Review for Pharmacy* is to provide a summary of therapeutics as well as other basic pharmaceutical principles (dosage forms, math, biopharmaceutics, kinetics, basic and parenteral compounding, among others) which will be valuable in your preparation for the NAPLEX®, and also be a resource as you enter practice.

This review book is not an exhaustive discussion of the topics presented; it utilizes instead an abbreviated outline format to enable you to review and organize the material in an efficient manner for easy recall and recognition. The NAPLEX® is a difficult exam, and it covers a tremendous amount of material. In recent years, the NAPLEX® has become even more relevant to professional practice, with less emphasis on the basic sciences and more emphasis on drug therapy and pharmaceutical care.

Your success in pharmacy school has been due to diligence and hard work. You should have confidence that your pharmacy education has prepared you for the NAPLEX® and you should not have anxieties about the exam. However, your self-confidence should not prevent you from being meticulous about preparation for the NAPLEX®. Realizing that approximately 10% of students fail to achieve a passing score on their first attempt at the NAPLEX®, do not take this exam lightly.

The following are helpful hints that will improve your success on this examination:

1. ***Positive attitude:*** You are encouraged to approach preparation for the NAPLEX® with a positive attitude. Study to learn and understand concepts, not just memorize enough facts to pass the exam. Remember that in addition to being a minimum standard required for entry into pharmacy practice, an important benefit of taking the NAPLEX® is the comprehensive review, which will make you a better pharmacy practitioner. Without the NAPLEX®, few pharmacy graduates would spend the time and effort to review the entire discipline immediately prior to completing their studies. You should be confident that you have the knowledge to pass the exam if you have prepared diligently.

2. ***Plan ahead:*** Do not delay your review and preparation for the NAPLEX® until the last week before your scheduled exam date. While the total amount of time varies greatly from student to student, it is recommended that you start a serious review no less than 4-6 weeks before you plan to take the exam. However, if you have limited pharmacy work experience, you should start much earlier, especially learning generic and trade names. Be conscientious about scheduling specific times to prepare for the NAPLEX® over this time period. Cramming the last few days before the NAPLEX® will potentially increase your anxiety and could also confuse you with such a large volume of material. Read one or two chapters per day 4 or 5 days per week, and review the generic and trade names daily.

3. ***Generic and trade names:*** The first place to begin your preparation is to learn the generic and trade names for the top 200 drugs. The importance of this basic recommendation cannot be overemphasized. Without this base, you will experience tremendous difficulty on the NAPLEX®, which is traditionally over half trade names. In addition, you will also need to learn the generic and trade names for the unique drugs, which may not be among the top 200 drugs (eg, Cogentin® & Artane®, which are used to manage the extrapyramidal side effects of psychotherapeutic agents; Tofranil®, which is used to treat enuresis; Tapazole®, which is used to treat hyperthyroidism). Most of the patient medication profiles contain numerous drugs that may be listed either by the generic or trade name. Therefore knowledge of generic and trade names is essential to identify therapeutic duplication (eg, the patient who is prescribed Corgard® who is already taking the beta-blocker propranolol). You will also be expected to determine potential causes for adverse effects, as well as screen for drug interactions and drug-disease interactions, either from drugs on the profile or the new prescriptions. In some cases drugs will be listed by their generic names and in others by their trade names.

4. *Math:* Other than generic and trade names, pharmacy math is the most important single area to review. You should practice working several examples of each type of math problem to be sure you are comfortable and confident in your ability. While some therapeutic topics may not be covered extensively, the large number of math questions on the NAPLEX® makes this a high priority. Many students struggle with math on the NAPLEX®. Therefore it is recommended that you schedule several math study sessions. The metric system is emphasized, but you must know the other systems and be able to make conversions. While the apothecary system is used infrequently, the avoirdupois system (sometimes called the "household" system) is still used (eg, prepare one pound of ointment). When apothecary or avoirdupois measures are used, you should usually convert them to metric.

5. *Competencies:* You should review the areas of emphasis defined in the NAPLEX® competency statements that are available on the NABP® website: www.nabp.net. As you review the top 200 drugs you should ask yourself the following questions:

   * What is the therapeutic category of this drug?
   * What is the mechanism of action?
   * What type of patient counseling information should be provided?
   * What are the major adverse effects (side effects and toxic effects)?
   * What is the dosage schedule (frequency)?
   * What are the major drug interactions and dis-ease contraindications?

   These topics should also be the priority areas as you review each therapeutic class of agents.

6. *Dosage schedules:* Summary charts of the major categories of drugs are provided in each of the therapeutic chapters of this book. You will find the generic as well as trade names, along with commonly available dosage forms, dosage, and frequency of use. The frequency of use is emphasized more on the NAPLEX® than the specific dosages. The following therapeutic lists with multiple agents should also be emphasized in your studying: β-blockers, calcium channel blockers, ACE inhibitors, benzodiazepines, cephalosporins, quinolones, aminoglycosides, NSAIDs, H_2 blockers, protease inhibitors, oral antidiabetics, and statins. Be able to recognize the agents within these categories, and to know how to compare the differences within the category (eg, length of action, dosage schedules, side effects, and distinct advantages in patients with certain diseases).

7. *Appendices:* There are also many tables that can help you recall or recognize answers for NAPLEX® questions in the appendices, such as the major drug-drug interactions, the drugs that should not be crushed, and the top 200 OTC agents. There are also other important tables to study throughout the book, such as the table of common antidotes for poisons and overdosages in the toxicology chapter. By reviewing these therapeutic agents by categories and in tables, you will increase your recall of them on the exam.

8. *Chronic and common diseases:* The NAPLEX® emphasizes the more common and chronic diseases and their therapy. While it is a good idea to have a general knowledge of the disease process, remember that the NAPLEX® is heavily weighted toward drug therapy. Therefore you should not devote the majority of your study time on the disease process (eg, etiology, pathophysiology, diagnosis, and signs and symptoms) at the expense of the therapy (including nondrug therapy). While it is helpful to review your areas of strength, you should concentrate more on your areas of weakness. The less familiar you are with a topic, the more time the topic should be given in review.

9. *Priorities:* There are several areas that should *not* be emphasized in your review: (1) the manufacturer of the specific drug (eg, Zithromax® manufactured by Pfizer); (2) chemical structures; and (3) identification or physical descriptions (eg, color, shape, etc). These areas are covered only minimally on the NAPLEX®.

10. *Review questions:* Reviewing sample exam questions is very helpful. However, to make this a more effective learning experience, study the explanations along with their answers. Do not look only at the correct answer, but look at distractors and learn why they are incorrect. Therapeutics reference texts may also be helpful in your NAPLEX® review for their more detailed information and to assist with difficult or complex material. This will also reinforce learning points about material covered in your review.

11. ***Exam format:*** The NAPLEX® consist of 185 multiple-choice questions in a computer adaptive format that is individualized to each candidate's level of ability. The computer adapted test system selects your next questions based on your response to previous questions, and thus each question must be answered before you can proceed. The 150 questions that have been pre-tested for validity are the basis for your evaluation. In addition, 35 questions that are being evaluated for use in future exams are distributed throughout the exam.

12. ***Question format:*** You should log on to the NABP® website (www.napb.net) to review the format for exam questions and the patient profiles. NABP® also offers a "pre-NAPLEX®" test for a fee, that will allow you to practice with the computerized format. This will help allay your anxiety and be especially beneficial if you are not comfortable with exams given in a computer format.

All questions have 5 choices with only *one* "best" answer. You may not continue the exam until you have answered the question. You may not skip the question and come back. Therefore you will be unable to leave any question blank. The question is superimposed at the bottom of the screen below the patient medication record. After deciding on the best answer you will:

1. Highlight the answer.
2. Request the next question.
3. Confirm that you want the next question, which will finalize your answer.

You cannot go back to change an answer after step 3.

There are two types of multiple-choice questions:

1. The traditional single-answer type as in the example below:

   The agent of choice for the initial treatment of contact dermatitis, whether irritant or allergic, is a:

   A. topical antihistamine
   B. oral antihistamine
   C. topical corticosteroid
   D. local anesthetic
   E. coal tar product

   and

2. The combined-response ("K" type) question with 1, 2, or 3 components listed, as in the example below:

   The most common side effects of isotretinoin include which of the following?

   I. Cheilitis
   II. Acute depression
   III. Decreased night vision

   A. I only
   B. II only
   C. III only
   D. I and II
   E. I, II, and III

13. ***Patient medication record:*** The patient medication record is usually followed by 10-15 questions. You must refer to the patient profile for many of the questions. However, some questions may be answered as presented or "stand alone." You will ***not*** be able to see the entire profile on the top of the screen without scrolling down to review the whole profile. You may want to write down the significant points from the profile, such as allergies, age of the patient, and preexisting diseases, on scrap paper. Note carefully if the patient has multiple diseases, and for females, look for pregnancy or nursing, or likely to become pregnant. Some prefer to read the questions prior to reviewing the profile, but you could miss an important fact like a drug allergy, a drug-disease contraindication, or an adverse effect being treated currently that resulted from a previously prescribed drug, and answer the question without all of the necessary information. Therefore always conduct a quick review of the profile prior to answering the questions.

14. ***Testing center location:*** If you are not familiar with the exact location of the testing center, locate it no later than the day before the exam. Arrive at the testing site at least 30 minutes prior to the scheduled time in order to be as calm as you can. You do not want to be caught in traffic or get lost trying to find the testing center and panic immediately prior to taking the exam.

15. ***The night before the exam:*** Do not study the night before the exam; last minute cramming will only add to your anxiety and will not improve your test score. I recommend that you

take a night off from study the evening before the exam. Go out for a relaxing dinner and/or a movie. Be sure to get to bed early, especially if you are scheduled for a morning exam, so your ability to reason, recognize, and recall information is sharp.

16. *Afternoon exam:* If your exam is scheduled in the afternoon, fatigue can dull your test-taking abilities. Be on guard against this by having a light lunch, preferably with coffee, tea, or some caffeine-containing beverage to be sure that you stay sharp for the afternoon session.

Taking the Exam

1. Read all directions carefully. Read each question a minimum of two times to determine the nature of the question and the point of asking the question. Note any modifying terms like always, all, never, most, usually, double negatives, and anything else that may change the meaning of the question. Modifiers like "always" and "never" mean what they say.

2. Read all the choices thoroughly before you answer the question. Attempt to eliminate the distractor choices or incorrect answers. Two or three answers can usually be eliminated for one reason or another, and the final choice is between two answers. The more distractors you identify and eliminate, the more you increase your probability of obtaining the best answer. Then select the *single best answer*. Your first instinct is generally the best choice. Be cautious about not reading multiple possibilities into questions; the questions are straightforward and are not designed to trick you.

3. If you are positive that you do not know the answer, eliminate any distractors and guess intelligently, making the best choice you can of the remaining answers. If you can limit your guess to two possible correct answers, your score will be much better than if you try to guess the correct answer from five possible choices. Proceeding in this fashion over the course of the exam, you can increase your success if you guess consistently. While blind guessing is not recommended, after narrowing possibilities, intelligent guessing is definitely recommended.

4. Pace yourself, but do not rush through the exam. The 4 hours 15 minutes scheduled for the

NAPLEX® is more than adequate, and the majority of students have plenty of time to complete the exam. You need to proceed at a reasonable pace and need to answer approximately 45-50 questions per hour to finish comfortably in the time available. There is a timer visible at the corner of the screen with your remaining exam time. If you notice that you have only completed 40 questions in the first hour, you should increase your speed.

5. Some of the math questions may be weighted more heavily and some will take several minutes to answer. Take the time to answer the math questions correctly. Incorrect answers may lead to additional math questions (eg, missing the first milliequivalent question could lead to more milliequivalent questions on your exam). Use the scrap paper provided for your calculations. Be sure to include units as you complete the math questions on your scrap paper.

6. It is important that you remember that you cannot return to a previous question after you have confirmed an answer. There is no need to get upset over a previous question you realize you have missed as you proceed through the exam. Do not get nervous during the exam or panic or you may lose your ability to recall or recognize common information. Remain calm and do the best you can. Best of luck with the test!

James C. Eoff III, PharmD
Executive Associate Dean
University of Tennessee College of Pharmacy
847 Monroe Avenue
Memphis, Tennessee 38163
Email: jeoff@utmem.edu

NAPLEX® is a federally registered trademark owned by the National Association of Boards of Pharmacy® (NABP®). This review course is in no way authorized or sponsored by the NABP®. Please check the NABP® webwite, www.nabp.net, for more complete information.

Dear Colleague:

It is with great pleasure that we take this opportunity to congratulate you on completing your final year of pharmacy training. As you prepare to take the North American Pharmacist Licensure Exam™, Janssen Pharmaceutica-Eisai, Johnson & Johnson-Merck, McNeil Consumer & Specialty Pharmaceuticals, and Ortho-Biotech would like to assist you in studying for this examination. We are proud to bring to you the 2nd Edition of *APhA's Complete Review for Pharmacy*, and excited to once again have Dick R. Gourley, Pharm.D., from the University of Tennessee College of Pharmacy, as editor of this educational manual which reviews the many important aspects of pharmacy.

This review is intended to assist you in synthesizing much of the materials you have learned through your years of training. The thirty-eight chapters in the manual were updated for this second edition by leaders in the field, and will help you assess the extent of your knowledge in various aspects of pharmacy, provide information on the latest developments, and act as a clear guide for NAPLEX preparation.

On behalf of our companies, the APhA, and the contributors to *APhA's Complete Review for Pharmacy*, we are pleased to assist you in your preparation and wish you much success in your future pharmacy practice. We hope this manual will make your preparation for the board exam just a little bit easier.

Cordially yours,

Tiziana M. Fox

Tiziana M. Fox, Pharm.D.
Senior Director, Medical Information & Communications
Medical and Regulatory Affairs
McNeil Consumer & Specialty Pharmaceuticals

McNeil Consumer & Specialty Pharmaceuticals • Division of McNeil - PPC, Inc. • 7050 Camp Hill Road, Fort Washington, PA 19034-2299 • 215-273-7000

ORTHO BIOTECH

William C. Pearson
Vice President
Oncology Franchise and Strategic Customer Group

ORTHO BIOTECH PRODUCTS, L.P.
430 Route 22 East
Bridgewater, New Jersey 08807-0914

(908) 541-4501   Phone
(908) 253-6055   Fax
wpearson@obius.jnj.com

Dear Colleague:

Congratulations on completing your final year of residency training. As you prepare for the North American Pharmacist Licensure Exam, Ortho Biotech Products, L.P. is pleased to provide you with an important resource to support you in launching your career. We are very excited to provide you with this valuable educational manual, along with the help of APhA, Dick R. Gourley, PharmD, from the University of Tennessee College of Pharmacy, and other Johnson & Johnson companies.

On behalf of Ortho Biotech Products, L.P., please accept our best wishes as you prepare for the NAPLEX and for continued professional success and personal fulfillment.

Best wishes,

William C Pearson

William C. Pearson
Vice President, Oncology Franchise
Ortho Biotech Products, L.P.

JANSSEN MEDICAL AFFAIRS, L.L.C.

Dear Colleagues:

Congratulations on completing your final year of pharmacy education and training! Janssen Pharmaceutica in partnership with APhA and other Johnson and Johnson companies is pleased to provide you with an important educational resource to help you prepare for the North America Pharmacist Licensure Exam.

On behalf of Janssen Pharmaceutica, we are pleased to assist you in your preparation for NAPLEX® and wish you professional success and personal success in your future career in pharmacy.

Best wishes,

Dave Domann, MS, RPh.
Executive Director, Medical Services
Janssen Medical Affairs, LLC

Your Guide to APhA Resources

American Pharmacists Association

Providing information, education, and advocacy to help all pharmacists improve medication use and advance patient care.

As you embark on your career as a pharmacist, APhA is here to help you. APhA provides members with information about new medications and therapies, continuing education, professional development opportunities, and career options. In addition, APhA promotes the interests of pharmacists to the federal government and maintains an active public relations program designed to help consumers learn about the contributions that pharmacists make to patient health and well-being.

APhA membership costs just pennies a day—and recent graduates, postgraduates, and residents benefit from special discount dues rates. In addition to providing value in the form of exceptional professional information and education, your dues help support APhA's advocacy efforts on behalf of all pharmacists.

Your Guide to APhA Resources provides at-a-glance information on APhA's offerings—information, education, and advocacy. No matter where you are in your career or which practice setting you choose, you can benefit from APhA's many resources.

APhA—Your Professional Information Home

Rely on APhA to deliver the information you need for your busy practice. As a leader in bringing professional information for pharmacists, APhA provides current news, drug information, the latest in patient-focused practice, and numerous career resources.

Pharmacy Today, the profession's newspaper, provides the latest news on new drug products, drug therapy,

developments in pharmacy practice, trends in health care that affect pharmacists, and legal and regulatory developments. Published monthly, *Pharmacy Today* also offers APhA's point of view on the many challenges facing the profession today.

APhA DrugInfoLine, published monthly, offers timely clinical and drug information useful in day-to-day practice. Providing at-a-glance information, the articles are published in summary format and focus on drug therapy developments and major therapeutic areas. Our top-flight pharmacist-experts give you the information to provide "key points," "what you need to know" and "what your patients need to know." Exclusively for APhA members. Available in print and online. See www.pharmacist.com for current and past issues of *APhA DrugInfoLine.*

The *Journal of the American Pharmacists Association (JAPhA),* the official peer-reviewed journal of APhA, publishes research on pharmacy practice as well as in-depth features, columns, and informed opinion. *JAPhA* is now available on the Web at www.japha.org, where APhA members can see the latest issue or search past issues.

Books and Electronic Products—APhA offers print, online, and PDA-based resources for pharmacists, student pharmacists, and pharmacy technicians. From respected text and in-depth reference works, to quick-search handbooks and PDA-based drug information databases, you'll find the resources you need in self-care, pharmacotherapy, drug interactions, and other topics—all at special discount prices for APhA members.

Transitions—exclusively for pharmacist members in the first five years after graduation, *Transitions* is the quarterly newsletter containing information that focuses on your life outside of pharmacy practice and provides guidance in various areas of professional and practice development.

Career Solutions—whether it's career advice you need or current trends in pharmacy management, look to APhA as your career information source. We help take the guesswork out of finding a new job, give you access to pharmacists when you need to fill a position, and offer resources when you want to develop and strengthen your management expertise. Search the Career Center online at www.pharmacist.com for a wide variety of positions available and the tools you need to take control of your career!

APhA Professional Education

Your education doesn't end when you graduate. As a practitioner, you'll need ongoing professional development and continuing education to further your career. APhA is your one-stop resource for professional development and education. Whether you need quick CE to fulfill your requirements for relicensure, comprehensive certificate training programs to learn new clinical skills, live educational programming, or training in advanced practice or management, APhA offers professional development programs to help you succeed.

Continuing Education, in print and online—Convenient and accessible, the CE Center at pharmacist.com offers a large library of nearly 100 valuable and relevant continuing education programs developed by APhA. You'll also find information on state relicensure requirements; progress tracking capability; instant statements of credit; and an online personal transcript storage that automatically maintains a record of your CE. And for APhA members, the CE Center features are entirely free of charge!

APhA's Annual Meeting & Exposition—the nation's only education-based conference for pharmacists in all practice settings. Held annually in the spring, participants can select from numerous programs geared toward the latest drug therapies and innovations in patient-centered pharmacy practice, make or renew professional relationships, and explore career opportunities. Members benefit from discounted registration rates, and for pharmacist members, a credit of up to $50 to apply to the registration fee.

Certificate Training Programs—These intensive and interactive educational programs are designed to help pharmacists develop the skills needed to become confident, successful disease state managers. Thousands of pharmacists have benefited from APhA's Certificate Training Programs. Whether you're ready to develop the advanced skills needed to improve patient care, explore the possibilities with regard to disease management, or are interested in in-depth education in management of asthma, diabetes, dyslipidemias, or immunizations, APhA's Certificate Training Programs are right for you.

Executive Management Program for Pharmacy Leaders—APhA, in partnership with Glaxo-SmithKline, the Leonard Davis Institute of Health Economics, and the University of Pennsylvania's Wharton School offers the Executive Management Program for Pharmacy Leaders (EMPPL). This seven-day program provides the management tools necessary to lead health care businesses and organizations in a period of dynamic change. Interactive and experiential learning activities, including small group workshops, case studies, and computer simulations, form an essential part of the program. To learn more about this program and the application process, contact Elizabeth Keyes, RPh, Senior Director, Strategic Alliances (email: ekeyes@aphanet.org).

The APhA Foundation Advanced Practice Institute (API)—API is a multi-day program designed for practitioners to hone their communication and drug therapy management skills, and offers advanced learning for pharmacists practicing in ambulatory care settings. This three-day program focuses on developing a pharmacist's knowledge and skill to implement an advanced, patient-focused practice that is directed toward building collaborative practices; managing disease states, including intervention documentation that targets specific therapeutic outcomes; using technology to facilitate pharmaceutical care; obtaining reimbursement for services; and using basic research techniques to participate in clinical studies, to market pharmaceutical services, and to improve the participant's practice. To learn more about the Advanced Practice Institute, contact the APhA Foundation at info@aphafoundation.org. *Advanced Practice Institute: Diabetes is made possible through an unrestricted educational grant from Takeda Pharmaceuticals North America.*

Advocacy

For more than 150 years, the American Pharmacists Association has served as the representative voice of pharmacists and is the only organization representing pharmacists in ALL practice settings. When you join APhA, your membership dues help support APhA's advocacy program, efforts to defend and expand the scope of pharmacy practice, outreach to improve understanding of the value pharmacists provide to the nation's health care system, and support of APhA's work to enhance the role of pharmacy technicians to support pharmacists as patient-care providers. APhA works to see that pharmacists are recognized for their health care expertise as drug therapy managers—to ensure that your patients, the medical community, the government, and third-party payors better understand the profession and your role.

As an APhA member, our Legislative Action Center gives you access to your Representative or Senators on Capitol Hill. You'll learn about changes that can affect your practice and APhA's position on these issues. For additional information on APhA's advocacy priorities and the issues of the day, visit *www.aphanet.org*, or read *Pharmacy Today*. And for members, subscribe to APhA's *Legislative & Regulatory Update*, a bi-weekly e-newsletter covering legislative activities that impact your daily practice.

Take advantage of APhA's unparalleled professional resources. Support your profession and invest in the future of pharmacy by joining APhA!

American Pharmacists Association
2215 Constitution Ave., N.W.
Washington, DC 20037-2985

Phone: 800-237-APhA (2742)

For additional information about APhA, visit www.aphanet.org.

For the latest pharmacy news, drug information, career information, and continuing education, or to shop the APhA store, go to www.pharmacist.com, the nation's premier Web site for practicing pharmacists.

1. Pharmacy Math

George E. Bass, PhD
Associate Professor of Pharmaceutical Sciences
University of Tennessee College of Pharmacy

1. Units of Measure

Calculations in pharmacy may involve four different systems of measure: metric, apothecaries, avoirdupois and household.

Metric System

The metric system fundamental units are the gram, the liter, and the meter. Prefixes are used extensively to express quantities much greater and much less than the fundamental units. Some of the most commonly used prefixes are provided in Table 1.

Apothecaries' System

While the metric system is the official system of measure for pharmacy today, the apothecaries' system is the traditional system and some elements might sometimes be found in prescriptions. Units of the apothecaries system are presented in Table 2.

Avoirdupois System

The avoirdupois system measure of weight is employed in ordinary commerce. Here, the ounce corresponds to 437.5 grains. The avoirdupois grain unit is equal to the apothecaries' grain. Sixteen ounces (7000 grains) corresponds to 1 pound. Note that the avoirdupois ounce (473.5 grains) and pound (7000 grains)

Table 1.

Metric system prefixes

mega-	one million times the base unit (10^6)
kilo-	one thousand times the base unit (10^3)
deci-	one-tenth the base unit (10^{-1})
centi-	one-hundredth the base unit (10^{-2})
milli-	one-thousandth the base unit (10^{-3})
micro-	one-millionth the base unit (10^{-6})
nano-	one billionth the base unit (10^{-9})
pico-	one-trillionth the base unit (10^{-12})

Table 2.

Apothecaries' system of measure

Weight
20 grains = 1 scruple
3 scruples = 1 dram
8 drams = 1 ounce
12 ounces = 1 pound

Volume
60 minims = 1 fluidram
8 fluidrams = 1 fluidounce
16 fluidounces = 1 pint
2 pints = 1 quart
4 quarts = 1 gallon

measures are not equal to the apothecaries' ounce (480 grains) and pound (5760 grains) measures.

Household Measures

A tablespoon is equivalent to 15 mL and a teaspoon is equivalent to 5 mL.

Conversion Factors

A short list of convenient conversion factors is provided below.

Convenient Conversion Factors

1 inch = 2.54 cm
1 fluidounce = 30 milliliters
1 gram = 15.4 grains
1 kilogram = 2.20 pounds (avoir.)
1 pound (avoir.) = 454 grams
1 gallon, US = 3785 mL

2. Significant Figures

All measured quantities are approximations. The accuracy of a given measurement is conveyed by the number of figures that are recorded. The number of significant figures in a measurement includes the first approximate figure. The last recorded digit to the right of a measured quantity is taken to be an approximation. For example, the weight 13.24 g has four significant figures where the final digit, 4, is approximate. Calculations should be conducted so as to carry the correct numbers of significant figures.

It frequently happens in a given calculation that the different quantities in the calculation have different numbers of significant figures. When this occurs, follow the rules below.

Addition and Subtraction

When adding or subtracting decimal numbers, round all measurements to have the same number of decimal places as the least in the set. For example, 13.78 mL and 53.5 mL would be added as 13.8 + 53.5 = 67.3 mL, using and retaining only one decimal place.

Multiplication and Division

When multiplying or dividing decimal numbers, round the measurements to include the number of significant figures contained in the least accurate number. For example, 25.678 mL multiplied by 1.24 g/mL would be handled as 25.7 mL times 1.24 g/mL = 31.9 g, using and retaining three significant figures.

Handling Zero

Whether or not the digit zero is counted as a significant figure depends on where it appears in the measured number. If zero occurs at an interior position in the number (eg, as in 3052 and 2.031) it is significant. If zero occurs as the last digit to the right of the decimal (eg, 44.50), it is significant. If zero occurs as the first digit to the right of the decimal in a number that is less than one, it is not significant. For example, in 0.078 there are only two significant figures. If zero occurs as the last digit, or digits, in a whole number (ie, no decimal is expressed), its significance is unknown without further information. For example, 3500 might have two, three, or four significant figures.

3. Ratios and Proportions

The most frequently encountered calculations in pharmacy will employ ratios and proportions. In mathematics, a ratio is the quotient of one quantity divided by another of the same kind, and a proportion is an equality between ratios. Thus a proportion involves a relationship between four quantities. You can always solve for one of these when the other three are known. If the ratio x/y is equal to the ratio a/b, one has the proportion $x/y = a/b$, and can obtain by algebraic manipulation: $x = ay/b$, etc. Such problems are frequently encountered when adjusting dosages.

One common source of error in proportion problems involves writing one of the ratios upside down, eg, writing $x/y = b/a$ when it should be $x/y = a/b$. A disciplined approach to setting up such problems can help. For example, you might follow the rule to express each ratio as the quotient of like quantities. Then, when you equate the two ratios, if the numerator of one ratio is smaller (or larger) than its denominator, the same should be true of the other ratio as well. Another source of error involves using mixed units, eg, using one number expressed in grams and the other in milligrams. To guard against this kind of error, always write the units into the equation along with the numbers. All unit expressions should cancel except those required for the quantity being solved for (dimensional analysis).

Example: If 250 mg of drug are contained in 300 mL of a preparation, what weight (x) would be contained in 1800 mL of the preparation?
Equate the ratios x:250 mg and 1800 mL:300 mL to solve for x:

$$\text{ie, } x/250 \text{ mg} = 1800 \text{ mL}/300 \text{ mL}$$
$$x = 250 \text{ mg} \times 1800 \text{ mL}/300 \text{ mL} = 1500 \text{ mg}$$

(Note that since the new volume is six times greater, the new weight should be six times greater as well.)

4. Specific Gravity and Density

At times you will be required to convert a volume measure to a weight measure or vice versa. To accomplish this, you will need to employ either the specific gravity or the density of the material. The specific gravity (SpGr) is a ratio of the weight of the material to the weight of the same volume of a standard material. For liquids, the standard material is water, which has a density of 1 g/mL. Specific gravity is unit-less. Density is the quotient of any measure of the weight of a sample of the material divided by any measure of the volume of the sample. The units must be explicitly expressed (eg, grams per milliliter, pounds per gallon, etc). When density is expressed in g/mL, it is numerically equal to specific gravity. Algebraically, it is easier to work with density (d = wt/vol) than the corresponding expression for specific gravity.

Example: What is the weight of 750 mL of concentrated hydrochloric acid (SpGr = 1.20)?
From the specific gravity definition and using the volume of 750 mL,

$$\text{SpGr (HCl)} = \frac{\text{wt of 750 mL HCl}}{\text{wt of 750 mL H}_2\text{O}}$$

Rearranging and noting that the density of H_2O is 1 g/mL,

$$\text{wt of 750 mL HCl} = (\text{SpGr}) \times (\text{wt of 750 mL H}_2\text{O}) = 1.20 \times 750 \text{ g} = 900 \text{ g}$$

Alternatively, specific gravity is numerically equal to density expressed in g/mL. Thus,

$$d = 1.20 = \text{wt HCl/Vol HCl};$$
$$\text{or, wt HCl} = d \times \text{vol HCl} =$$
$$1.20 \text{ g/mL} \times 750 \text{ mL} = 900 \text{ g}$$

5. Percentage Error

Associated with the fact that all measurements are approximations is the need to characterize the extent of the error involved. Percentage of error is such a quantity and is defined as:

$$\% \text{ error} = (\text{error} \times 100\%)/(\text{quantity desired})$$

The term *error* in the numerator is taken as the maximum potential error in the measurement, while the term *quantity desired* in the denominator represents the total amount measured. Percentage error may be calculated for either a weight or a volume measurement.

Example: Suppose a given quantity of material weighed 5.810 g on a prescription balance. Using a much more accurate analytical balance, the quantity was found to weigh 5.893 g. What is the percentage error for the original weighing?

$$\text{error} = 5.893 \text{ g} - 5.810 \text{ g} = 0.083 \text{ g}$$

The desired quantity is 5.810 g. Thus,

$$\% \text{ error} = 0.083 \text{ g} \times 100/5.810 = 1.4\%$$

6. Minimum Measurable Quantity

By regulation, weighings by a pharmacist cannot exceed a percentage error of greater than 5%. This requires that the sensitivity of the balance be known and limits the smallest quantity that can be weighed. Balance sensitivity is defined in terms of the *sensitivity requirement (SR)*, the weight that will move the indicator one marked unit on the index plate of the balance. For a class A prescription balance, SR = 6 mg. The minimum weighable quantity for a given balance can be calculated using the percentage error formula by replacing the "error" term with the SR (eg, 6 mg), the percentage error term with 5%, and the "desired quantity" term with "minimum weighable quantity." Thus, one would have:

minimum weighable quantity = SR x 100/5.

Example: What is the minimum weighable quantity for a balance that has a sensitivity requirement of 4 mg to assure an error no greater than 2%?

% error = error x 100/desired quantity
= SR x 100/minimum weighable quantity
minimum weighable quantity = SR x 100/% error
= 4 mg x 100/2 = 200 mg

7. Patient-Specific Dosage Calculations

Drugs with a narrow therapeutic range often are dosed based on patient weight or body surface area. For patients with renal impairment, some drugs are dosed based on creatinine clearance.

Dosing Based on Body Weight

Weight-based dosing might involve using the patient's actual body weight (ABW), ideal body weight (IBW), or perhaps an adjusted ideal body weight that is a function of IBW and ABW. These weights are invariably expressed in kilograms.

Example: A patient weighing 180 lb is to receive 0.25 mg/kg per day amphotericin B (reconstituted and diluted to 0.100 mg/mL) by IV infusion. What volume of solution is required to deliver the daily dose?

patient weight = 180 lb/2.20 = 82 kg
daily dose = 82 kg x 0.25 mg/kg = 20.5 mg
x mL/1 mL = 20.5 mg/0.100 mg
x = 1 mL x 20.5 mL/0.100 mg = 205 mL

A commonly used equation for calculating IBW is:

IBW = (gender factor) + 2.3 x (each inch >5 ft) kg,

where the gender factor for males is 50 kg and for females is 45.5 kg.

Example: The recommended adult daily dosage for patients with normal renal function for tobramycin is 3 mg/kg IBW given in three evenly divided doses. What would each injection be for a male patient who weighs 185 lb and is 5 ft 9 in. tall?

IBW = 50 kg + 2.3 x 9 kg = 50 kg + 21 kg = 71 kg
(ignore ABW of 84 kg)
daily dose (tid) = 71 kg x 3 mg/kg
= 213 mg (per day)

Thus each injection = 213 mg/3 = 71 mg.

In the absence of other information, the usual drug doses are considered generally suitable for 70-kg individuals. Thus in the absence of more specific information, an adjusted dosage for a notably larger or smaller individual may be obtained by multiplying the usual dose by the ratio of patient weight to 70 kg (Clark's rule).

Example: If the adult dose of a drug is 100 mg and no child-specific dosing information is available, what would be the weight-adjusted dose for a child who weighs 40 kg?

$$\text{child dose} = 100 \text{ mg} \times 40 \text{ kg}/70 \text{ kg} = 57 \text{ mg}$$

Dosing Based on Body Surface Area

Dosing based on body surface area requires an estimation of the patient's body surface area, BSA, expressed in square meters (m^2). This parameter might be estimated from a nomogram using height and weight, or for adults, by using one of several equations such as:

$$BSA = [(\text{height in centimeters})(\text{weight in kilograms})/3600]^{1/2} \ m^2$$

Example: What is the computed BSA for an adult who weighs 88 kg and is 5 ft 10 in. tall?

$$\text{height} = 70 \text{ in.} \times 2.54 \text{ cm/in.} = 178 \text{ cm}$$
$$BSA = [178 \text{ cm} \times 88 \text{ kg}/3600]^{1/2} \ m^2 = 2.09 \ m^2$$

The average adult BSA is taken to be 1.73 m^2. This value can be used to obtain an approximate child's dose given the usual dose for an adult and the child's estimated BSA.

Example: If the adult dose of a drug is 50 mg, what would be the BSA-adjusted dose for a child having an estimated BSA of 0.55 m^2?

$$\text{child dose} = 50 \text{ mg} \times 0.55 \ m^2/1.73 \ m^2 = 16 \text{ mg}$$

Dosing Based on Creatinine Clearance

For many drugs, the rate of elimination is dependent on kidney function. Creatinine clearance (CrCl) is a measure of the volume of blood plasma that is cleared of creatinine by kidney filtration per minute and is expressed in mL/min. It can be calculated using the Cockcroft and Gault equation as a function of patient gender, age, body weight, and serum creatinine. For males:

$$CrCl \ (mL/min) = (140 - \text{age in years}) \times (\text{body wt in kg})/(72 \times \text{serum creatinine in mg/dL})$$

For females:

$$CrCl = 0.85 \times CrCl \text{ for males}$$

Example: Calculate the creatinine clearance rate for a 76-year-old female weighing 65 kg and having a serum creatinine of 0.52 mg/dL using the Crockcroft and Gault equation.

$$CrCl = 0.85 \times (140 - 76 \ y) \times 65 \text{ kg}/(72 \times 0.52 \text{ mg/dL})$$
$$= 94 \text{ mL/min}$$

Alternatively, creatinine clearance may be estimated using the Jelliffe equations. For males:

$$CrCl = [98 - 0.8 \times (\text{patient age in years} - 20)]/\text{serum creatinine in mg/dL}]$$

For females:

$$CrCl = 0.9 \times CrCl \text{ for males}$$

The normal value for creatinine clearance is taken to be 100 mL/min. It is sometimes advisable to adjust CrCl to the patient's BSA. This is calculated thus:

$$\text{adjusted } CrCl = CrCl \times BSA/1.73$$

The maintenance dose for some drugs is based on ideal body weight (IBW) and CrCl. See the chapter on pharmacokinetics, drug metabolism and drug disposition for more detailed coverage.

8. Using Batch Preparation Formulas

The relative amounts of ingredients in a pharmaceutical product are specified in a *formula*. A pharmacist may be required to reduce or enlarge the formula to prepare a lesser or greater amount of product. A given formula might specify either the actual amount (weight or volume) of each ingredient for a specified total amount of product or just the relative amounts (parts) of each ingredient. In the latter case, the ingredients must all be of the same measure (eg, weight in grams).

Example: From the following formula, calculate the quantity of triethanolamine required to make 200 mL of the lotion.

Triethanolamine	10 mL
Oleic acid	25 mL
Benzyl benzoate	250 mL
Water to make	1000 mL

$$x{:}10 \text{ mL} = 200 \text{ mL}{:}1000 \text{ mL}$$
$$x = 10 \text{ mL} \times 200 \text{ mL}/1000 \text{ mL} = 2.0 \text{ mL}$$

Example: From the following formula, calculate the quantity of chlorpheniramine maleate required to make 500 g of the product.

Chlorpheniramine maleate	6 parts
Phenindamine	20 parts
Phenylpropanolamine HCl	55 parts

Note that the formula will give a total of 81 parts, which will correspond to the desired quantity of 500 g. Then,

$$x{:}500 \text{ g} = 6 \text{ parts}{:}81 \text{ parts}$$
$$x = 500 \text{ g} \times 6 \text{ parts}/81 \text{ parts} = 37 \text{ g}$$

9. Conventions in Expression of Concentration

A diversity of conventions for expressing drug concentrations are encountered in pharmacy. One must be prepared to calculate these directly from their definitions and to inter-convert among them.

Percentage Strength

Percentage, strictly speaking, specifies the number of parts per 100 parts. In pharmacy, this comes in three varieties:

- Percent weight-in-weight = %(w/w) = grams of ingredient in 100 grams of product. Assumed for mixtures of solids and semisolids.
- Percent volume-in-volume = %(v/v) = milliliters of ingredient in 100 milliliters of product. Assumed for solutions or mixtures of liquids.
- Percent weight-in-volume = %(w/v) = grams of ingredient in 100 milliliters of product. Assumed for solutions of solids in liquids.

Example: What is the concentration in %(w/v) for a preparation containing 250 mg of drug in 50 mL of solution? Note that %(w/v) is defined as g/100 mL. So:

$$\text{concentration} = 0.250 \text{ g} \times 100/50 \text{ mL} = 0.50 \text{ \%(w/v)}$$

Parts (Ratio Strength)

Concentrations may be expressed in "parts" or ratio strength, when the active ingredient is highly diluted. Assumptions concerning (w/w), (v/v), and (w/v) are identical to those above for percentages.

Example: What is the concentration in %(v/v) of a solution that has a ratio strength of 1:2500 (v/v)?

$$x \text{ mL}{:}1 \text{ mL} = 100 \text{ mL}{:}2500 \text{ mL}$$
$$x = 100 \text{ mL} \times 1 \text{ mL}/2500 \text{ mL} = 0.040 \text{ \%(v/v)}$$

Millimoles

By definition, a 1 molar solution contains 1 gram molecular weight (1 GMW = 1 mole = weight in grams of Avogadro's number of particles) per liter of solution. The molarity expresses the number of moles per liter. The millimolarity (millimoles/liter) is 1000 times the molarity of a solution.

Example: What is the millimolar concentration of a solution consisting of 0.90 g of sodium chloride (GMW = 58.5) in 100 mL of water? The quantity of 0.9 g in 100 mL corresponds to 9.0 g in 1000 mL.

$$\text{molarity} = \text{moles}/1000 \text{ mL} = (9.0 \text{ g}/58.5 \text{ g/mole})$$
$$= 0.154$$
$$\text{millimolarity} = 1000 \times \text{molarity} = 154$$

Milliequivalents

By definition, the equivalent weight of an ion is the atomic or formula weight of the ion divided by the absolute value of its valence. Thus the equivalent weight of ferric ion, Fe^{3+} (atomic weight 55.9, valence 3) is 18.6. A milliequivalent is one-thousandth of an equivalent weight, ie, there are 1000 milliequivalent weights in 1 equivalent weight. For a molecule, the equivalent weight is obtained as the gram molecular weight (formula weight) divided by the total cation OR the total anion charge. For example, the equivalent weight of $MgCl_2$ (Mg^{2+}, atomic weight 24.3, valence +2; Cl^{1-}, atomic weight 35.5, valence −1) is $(24.3 + 2 \times 35.5)/2 = 47.7$ g. Its milliequivalent weight is 0.0477 g, or 47.7 mg. In the case of a nondissociating (nonionizing) molecule, eg, dextrose or tobramycin, the equivalent weight is equal to the formula weight.

Example: What is the concentration, in milliequivalents per liter, of a solution containing 14.9 g of potassium chloride (GMW = 74.5 g) in one liter? Note that the valence of potassium is 1+, so the equivalent wt. = molecular wt. Accordingly,

$$\text{mEq/L of KCl} = \text{mEq/L of } K^+ = \text{mEq/L of } Cl^-$$
$$= 1000 \times (14.9 \text{ g/L})/(74.5 \text{ g/Eq}) = 200 \text{ mEq/L}$$

Example: What weight of $MgSO_4$, GMW = 120, is required to prepare 1 liter of a solution that is 25.0 mEq/L in Mg^{2+}? To obtain 25.0 mEq of Mg requires 25.0 mEq of $MgSO_4$. Since the valence of Mg (and total positive charge) is 2+, the equivalent weight of $MgSO_4$ is 120/2 = 60 g. Accordingly, 60 mg corresponds to 1 mEq of $MgSO_4$. Then,

$$x{:}60 \text{ mg} = 25 \text{ mEq}{:}1 \text{ mEq}$$
$$x = 60 \text{ mg} \times 25 \text{ mEq}/1 \text{ mEq} = 1500 \text{ mg} = 1.50 \text{ g}$$

Example: How many milliequivalents of Ca^{2+} are contained in 100 mL of a solution that is 5.0 %(w/v) in $CaCl_2$ (GMW $CaCl_2$ = 111, atomic wt. Ca^{2+} = 40, atomic wt. Cl^- = 35.5)? Note that the valence of calcium is 2+. The solution contains 5.0 g $CaCl_2$ per 100 mL. This corresponds to $(5.0 \text{ g}/111) \times 2 = 0.090$

equivalents of $CaCl_2$, as well as Ca^{2+}. Accordingly, 100 mL of the solution contains 90 mEq of Ca^{2+}.

Milliosmoles

Osmotic concentration is a measure of the total number of particles in solution and is expressed in milliosmoles (mOsm). Thus the number of milliosmoles is based on the total number of cations AND total number of anions. The milliosmolarity of a solution is the number of milliosmoles per liter of solution (mOsm/L), where

$$\text{mOsm/L} = (\text{moles/L}) \times \text{number of species}$$
$$\times 1000 \text{ moles} = \text{wt/molecular weight}$$
$$\text{number of species} = \text{number of ionic species}$$
$$\text{on complete dissociation}$$
(eg, dextrose, 1 specie; NaCl, 2 species; $MgCl_2$, 3 species, etc)

The (total) osmolarity of a solution is the sum of the osmolarities of the solute components of the solution. When calculating osmolarities, in the absence of other information, assume that salts (eg, NaCl, etc) dissociate completely (referred to as the "ideal" osmolarity). You should be aware of the distinction between the terms milliosmolarity (milliosmoles per liter of solution) and milliosmolality (milliosmoles per kilogram of solution).

Example: What is the concentration, in mOsm/L of a solution that contains 224 mg of KCl (GMW = 74.6 g) and 234 mg of NaCl (GMW = 58.5) in 500 mL? What is the mOsm/L of K^+ alone?

$$\text{mOsm KCl}/500 \text{ mL} = (0.224 \text{ g}/74.6) \times 2 \times 1000$$
$$= 6.0 \text{ for } 500 \text{ mL}$$
$$\text{mOsm NaCl}/500 \text{ mL} = (0.234 \text{ g}/58.5) \times 2 \times 1000$$
$$= 8.0 \text{ for } 500 \text{ mL}$$
$$\text{total mOsm/L} = 2 \times (6.0 \text{ mOsm KCl} +$$
$$8.0 \text{ mOsm NaCl}) = 28.0 \text{ mOsm/L}$$
$$\text{mOsm/L of } K^+ = \text{mOsm/L of KCl}/2 = 12.0/2 = 6.0$$

Mg%; Mg/dL

Traditionally, some lab test values are reported as the number of milligrams per 100 milliliters (mg%) or equivalently, milligrams per deciliter (mg/dL).

Example: What is the %(w/v) concentration of glucose in a patient with a blood glucose reading of 230 mg/dL? Note that 1 dL = 100 mL and that 230 mg = 0.230 g. Then,

$$\text{glucose concentration} = 0.230 \text{ g}/100 \text{ mL}$$
$$= 0.230 \text{ \%(w/v)}$$

"Units" and µg/mg

The concentrations for some drugs whose production involves incomplete isolation from natural sources might be expressed in terms of "units" of activity or µg/mg as determined by a standardized bioassay.

Example: A preparation of penicillin G sodium contains 2.2 mEq of sodium (atomic wt. = 23, valence = 1+) per 1 million units of penicillin. How many milligrams of sodium are contained in an IV infusion of 5 million units? The 5 million unit dose will contain 5 x 2.2 mEq = 11.0 mEq.

$$\text{mEq weight of sodium} = 23 \text{ mg}$$
$$\text{wt. sodium} = (23 \text{ mg/mEq}) \times 11.0 \text{ mEq} = 253 \text{ mg}$$

Parts Per Million and Parts Per Billion

Very low concentrations often are expressed in terms of parts per million (ppm), the number of parts of ingredient per million parts of mixture or solution, or parts per billion (ppb), the number of parts of ingredient per billion parts of mixture or solution. Thus ppm and ppb are special cases of ratio strength concentrations.

Example: Re-express 1:25,000 in terms of parts per million.

$$x \text{ parts:1 part} = 1,000,000 \text{ parts:25,000 parts}$$
$$x = 1,000,000 \times 1/25,000 = 40 \text{ parts,}$$
$$\text{ie, the concentration is 40 ppm}$$

10. Dilutions and Concentrations

Simple Dilutions

In simple dilutions, a desired drug concentration is obtained by adding more solvent (or diluent) to an existing solution or mixture. Mathematically, the key feature of this process is that the initial and final amount of drug present remains unchanged. The amount of drug in any solution is proportional to the concentration times the quantity of the solution. Thus, taking the initial concentration as C_1, the initial quantity of solution as Q_1, the final concentration as C_2, and the final quantity of solution as Q_2, one has the relationship: $C_1 \times Q_1 = C_2 \times Q_2$. When provided values for any three of these variables, the fourth variable can be calculated. (Because this equation can be rearranged to $C_1/C_2 = Q_2/Q_1$, it is sometimes referred to as an "inverse proportionality.")

Example: How much water should be added to 250 mL of a solution of 0.20 %(w/v) benzalkonium chloride to make a 0.050 %(w/v) solution?

$$C_1 = 0.20 \text{ \%(w/v)} \quad Q_1 = 250 \text{ mL}$$
$$C_2 = 0.05\text{\%(w/v)} \quad Q_2 = ? \quad x = Q_2 - 250 \text{ mL}$$
$$C_1 \times Q_1 = C_2 \times Q_2$$
$$Q_2 = C_1 \times Q_1/C_2 = 0.20\% \times 250 \text{ mL}/0.050\%$$
$$= 1000 \text{ mL}$$
$$x = Q_2 - 250 \text{ mL} = 1000 \text{ mL} - 250 \text{ mL}$$
$$= 750 \text{ mL of water to be added}$$

Alcohol Solutions

The preceding treatment of dilutions assumes that solution and solvent volumes are reasonably additive. For dilutions of concentrated ethyl alcohol in water, this is not the case; a contraction in volume occurs on mixing. Consequently, you cannot extend the calculation to determine the exact volume of water to add to the initial alcohol solution. That is, the volume of water to be added cannot be obtained simply as $Q_2 - Q_1$. Rather, you can only specify that sufficient water be added to the initial concentrated alcohol solution (Q_1) to reach the specified or calculated final volume (Q_2) of the diluted alcohol solution.

Example: How much water should be added to 100 mL of 95%(v/v) ethanol to make 50%(v/v) ethanol?

$$C_1 = 95\% \quad Q_1 = 100 \text{ mL} \quad C_2 = 50\% \quad Q_2 = ?$$
$$C_1 \times Q_1 = C_2 \times Q_2$$
$$Q_2 = C_1 \times Q_1/C_2 = 95\% \times 100 \text{ mL}/50\%$$
$$= 190 \text{ mL (this is the final total volume)}$$

Thus, to the 100 mL of 95% add sufficient water to make 190 mL. This quantity will be more than 90 mL because of the contraction that occurs when concentrated alcohol is mixed with water.

Concentrated Acids

Concentrated mineral acids (hydrochloric, sulfuric, nitric, phosphoric) are manufactured by bubbling the pure acid gas into water to produce a saturated solution. The manufacturer specifies the concentration as a %(w/w). However, when preparing diluted acids for compounding, the pharmacist must express the concentration as a %(w/v). This requires utilization of the specific gravity of the concentrated acid.

Example: What volume of 35% (w/w) concentrated HCl, specific gravity 1.20, is required to make 500 mL of 5% (w/v) solution?

First, determine the weight of HCl required for the dilute solution. Since the dilute solution is 5%(w/v), it will contain 5 g in each 100 mL, or 25 g in 500 mL.

Next, one must determine what weight, x, of the 35%(w/w) solution contains 25 g of HCl. By proportion,

$$x{:}100 \text{ g} = 25 \text{ g}{:}35 \text{ g} \quad x = 100 \text{ g} \times 25 \text{ g}/35 \text{ g}$$
$$= 71.4 \text{ g of the concentrated solution}$$

Finally, use the SpGr of the concentrated solution to convert the weight to volume. Here, recall that SpGr is numerically equal to the density when the latter is expressed in g/mL. Thus, density = 1.20 g/mL = Wt/Vol. Rearranging,

$$\text{vol} = \text{wt/density} = 71.4 \text{ g}/1.20 \text{ g/mL} = 59.5 \text{ mL}.$$

Triturations

Triturations (used as a noun) are simply 10%(w/w) finely powdered (triturated) mixtures of a drug in an inert substance.

Example: What weight of colchicine trituration is required to prepare 30 doses of 0.25 mg each of colchicine?

For the trituration, 10 mg of the mixture contains 1 mg of drug. Thus,

$$x \text{ mg of trituration}{:}10 \text{ mg of trituration} =$$
$$(30 \times 0.25 \text{ mg drug}){:}1 \text{ mg drug}$$
$$x = 10 \text{ mg trituration} \times (30 \times 0.25 \text{ mg drug})/$$
$$1 \text{ mg drug} = 75 \text{ mg trituration}$$

Alligation Alternate

There are times when a drug concentration is required that is intermediate between those of two (or more) stock solutions (or available drug products). In this event, the alligation alternate method may be employed to quickly obtain the relative parts of each of the stock solutions needed to yield the desired concentration. If stock solutions of concentrations A% and B% (A% > B%) are to be used to make a solution of concentration C%, one sets up the diagram below to obtain the relative parts of solutions A and B.

A%		(C% − B%) parts of A
	C%	
B%		(A% − C%) parts of B

Example: In what proportion should 20% (w/v) dextrose be mixed with 5% (w/v) dextrose to obtain 15% (w/v) dextrose? How much of each is required to make 75 mL of 15% (w/v) solution?

20%		10 parts of 20%
	15%	
5%		5 parts of 5%

Thus, combine in the ratio of 10 parts of 20%:5 parts of 5%, ie, 2:1. Accordingly, to make 75 mL of 15% solution, mix 50 mL of 20% solution with 25 mL of 5% solution.

Alligation Medial

There may be times when one needs to know the final concentration of a solution obtained by mixing specified volumes of two or more stock solutions. In this event, the alligation medial method may be employed.

Example: What is the concentration of a solution prepared by combining 100 mL of a 10% solution, 200 mL of a 20% solution and 300 mL of a 30% solution? Proceed as illustrated below:

10%	×	100 mL	=	1000 %mL
20%	×	200 mL	=	4000 %mL
30%	×	300 mL	=	9000 %mL
		600 mL		14,000 %mL

Mixture concentration = 14000 %mL/600 mL = 23.3%

11. Isotonic Solutions

The preparation of many solutions used in pharmacy requires attention to osmotic pressure, a colligative property that is especially relevant for membrane transport. Other colligative properties include freezing point depression and boiling point elevation. These properties are a function of the total number of particles dissolved in the solution, regardless of the identity of the particles. Here, the term "particles" corresponds to cations, anions, and neutral undissociated molecules. A solution that has the same osmotic pressure as bodily fluids (blood, tears) is said to be *isotonic* (and *isosmotic*). As points of reference, 5.0% (w/v) dextrose, a nondissociating molecule, and 0.9% (w/v) sodium chloride, a dissociating molecule, are isotonic.

Dissociating Solutes

Preparation of solutions of specific tonicities requires knowledge of the dissociation properties of the solutes involved. One must know if the solute in question dissociates, and if so, to what extent and into how many particles. For example, in weak solutions sodium chloride dissociates about 80% into two particles, yielding a solution containing Na^+ ions, Cl^- ions and undissociated NaCl molecules. A measure of the extent of dissociation is provided by the dissociation factor, i, defined as the ratio of the total number of particles following dissociation to the number of molecules prior to dissociation. For example, 100 molecules of sodium chloride (prior to dissociation) will dissociate 80% to produce 80 particles of Na^+, 80 particles of Cl^- and 20 particles of NaCl, or 180 particles in all. The dissociation factor (i) for NaCl then is 180/100 = 1.8. A nondissociating molecule (like dextrose or tobramycin) is assigned a dissociation constant of 1.0. If measured dissociation information is not available, one can assume approximately 80% dissociation for weak solutions of salts. In this event, salts (including drugs) which dissociate into 2 ions will have a dissociation factor of 1.8 (like NaCl and ephedrine hydrochloride); 3 ions (like ephedrine sulfate), 2.6; 4 ions (like sodium citrate), 3.4; and 5 ions, 4.2 (ie, 0.9 per ion).

Example: What is the dissociation factor (i) for a compound which dissociates 60% into 3 ions?

For each 100 undissolved molecules, one will obtain on dissolution:

60 x 3 = 180 particles of ions plus 40 particles of undissociated molecules for a total of 220 particles.

Thus the dissociation factor = i = 220/100 = 2.2.

Example: What is the dissociation factor for dextrose, a nondissociating compound?

For each 100 undissolved molecules, one will obtain on dissolution:

zero particles of ions and 100 particles of undissociated molecules for a total of 100 particles.

Thus the dissociation factor = i = 100/100 = 1.0.

Sodium Chloride Equivalents

When preparing isotonic drug solutions, it is necessary to take into consideration the tonicity contribution of the drug. This can be accomplished by using the *sodium chloride equivalent* for the drug, defined as the number of grams of sodium chloride that would produce the same tonicity effect as 1 gram of the drug. If the value of the sodium chloride equivalent is not provided, it can be calculated using the molecular weights and dissociation factors of sodium chloride and the drug in question:

sodium chloride equivalent = (MW of NaCl) x (drug dissociation factor)/(MW of drug) x (sodium chloride dissociation factor) = (58.5)(i)/(MW of drug)(1.8)

Example: What is the sodium chloride equivalent of demecarium bromide (GMW = 717, i = 2.6)?

sodium chloride equivalent = (58.5 x 2.6)/ (717 x 1.8) = 0.12

Thus each gram of demecarium bromide is equivalent to 0.12 g of NaCl.

So how does one proceed to prepare a drug solution that must be made isotonic? Using the total volume of isotonic solution to be prepared, first calculate the hypothetical weight, x, of NaCl (alone) that would be required to make that volume of water isotonic (0.9%). Next, using the weight of drug to be incorporated in the solution and its sodium chloride equivalent, calculate the weight of NaCl, y, that would correspond to the weight of the drug. Then calculate the true weight of NaCl, z, to be added to the preparation as $z = x - y$.

Example: What weight of sodium chloride would be required to prepare 50 mL of an isotonic solution containing 500 mg of pilocarpine nitrate (sodium chloride equivalent = 0.23)?

Since isotonic saline requires 0.9 g/100 mL, 50 mL of isotonic saline will require 0.45 g, ie, $x = 0.45$ g.

The 500 mg of pilocarpine nitrate will correspond to 500 mg x 0.23 = 115 mg of NaCl, ie, $y = 0.12$ g.

Sodium chloride to add to make isotonic = $z = x - y = $ 0.45 g – 0.12 g = 0.33 g

12. Intravenous Infusion Flow Rates

The physician may specify the rate of flow of IV fluids in drops per minute, amount of drug per hour, or the duration of time of administration of the total volume of the infusion. It may then be necessary to calculate the infusion rate in per-minute or per-hour increments in order to program an infusion pump to give the medication at the correct rate.

Example: If 250 mg of a drug is added to a 500-mL D_5W bag, what should be the flow rate, in milliliters per hour, to deliver 50 mg of drug per hour?

$$x \text{ mL/h}:500 \text{ mL/h} = 50 \text{ mg/h}:250 \text{ mg/h}$$
$$x = (500 \text{ mL/h}) \times (50 \text{ mg/h})/(250 \text{ mg/h}) = 100 \text{ mL/h}$$

Example: If an infusion flow rate is at 100 mL/h and the infusion set delivers 15 drops/mL, what is the rate of flow in drops per minute?

$$15 \text{ drops/mL} \times 100 \text{ mL/h} = 1500 \text{ drops/h}$$
$$= 25 \text{ drops/min}$$

13. Buffers

Buffer solutions are employed to reduce pH fluctuations associated with introduction of small amounts of strong acids or bases. Typical buffer solutions are composed of a weak acid or weak base plus a salt of the acid or base. Solution pH in the presence of a buffer can be calculated using the Henderson-Hasselbalch equations.

For weak acids, $pH = pK_a + \log(\text{salt}/\text{acid})$.
For weak bases, $pH = pK_w - pK_b + \log(\text{base}/\text{salt})$,
where $pK_w = 14$.

Example: What is the pH of a buffer solution prepared to be 0.50 M in sodium acetate and 0.050 M in acetic acid (pK_a of acetic acid = 4.76)?

For weak acids, $pH = pK_a + \log(\text{salt}/\text{acid})$.
Thus $pH = 4.76 + \log(0.50/0.050) = 4.76 + \log(10)$
$= 4.76 + 1 = 5.76$.

14. Temperature

Frequently, one must convert temperatures from Fahrenheit (F) to Centigrade (C), and conversely. The following formula can be used : $9C = 5F - 160$.

Example: A patient has an oral temperature of 100°F. What is this temperature in °C?

$$9C = 5F - 160$$
$$C = (5F - 160)/9 = (5 \times 100 - 160)/9 = 37.8$$

15. Practice Problems

1. If 100 capsules contain 340 mg of active ingredient, what would be the weight of active ingredient contained in 75 capsules?

   A. 453 mg
   B. 340 mg
   C. 255 mg
   D. 128 mg
   E. 75 mg

2. What is the weight of 500 mL of a liquid whose specific gravity is 1.13?

   A. 442 mg
   B. 565 g
   C. 442 g
   D. 885 mg
   E. 221 g

3. Suppose a pharmacist weighs out 325 mg of a substance on her class A prescription balance. When she subsequently checked this weight on a more sensitive analytical balance, she found it to be only 312 mg. What was the percentage error in the original weighing?

   A. 4%
   B. 5%
   C. 6%
   D. 10%
   E. 12%

4. What is the minimum weighable quantity for a maximum of 5% error using a balance with a sensitivity requirement of 6 mg?

   A. 80 µg
   B. 100 mg
   C. 120 mg
   D. 150 mg
   E. 240 mg

5. A patient weighing 175 lb is to receive an initial daily IM dosage of procainamide HCl (500 mg/mL vial) of 50 mg/kg (ABW) to be given in divided doses every 3 hours. How many mL should each injection contain?

   A. 3.98 mL
   B. 0.49 mL
   C. 8.23 mL
   D. 1.87 mL

   E. 0.99 mL

6. What is the ideal body weight of a female patient whose height is 5 ft 8 in.?

   A. 68 kg
   B. 64 kg
   C. 150 lb
   D. 121 lb
   E. 53 kg

7. What is the approximate BSA of an adult patient who weighs 154 lb and is 6 ft tall?

   A. 1.73 m^2
   B. 3.15 m^2
   C. 1.89 m^2
   D. 0.70 m^2
   E. 2.67 m^2

8. If the adult dose of a drug is 125 mg, what would be the dose for a child whose BSA is estimated to be 0.68 m^2?

   A. 485 µg
   B. 318 mg
   C. 85 mg
   D. 49 mg
   E. 33 mg

9. What is the creatinine clearance for a 65-year-old female patient who weighs 50 kg and has a serum creatinine level of 1.3 mg/dL?

   A. 34 mL/min
   B. 40 mL/min
   C. 26 mL/min
   D. 82 mL/min
   E. 100 mL/min

10. Using the formula below, how much zinc oxide would be required to make 750 g of the mixture?

Zinc Oxide	150 g
Starch	250 g
Petrolatum	550 g
Coal Tar	50 g

    A. 200 g
    B. 188 g
    C. 413 g
    D. 113 g
    E. 38 g

11. Using the formula below, what weight of kaolin would be required to produce 500 g of the mixture?

Kaolin	12 parts
Magnesium oxide	3 parts
Bismuth subcarbonate	5 parts

A. 83 g
B. 300 g
C. 208 g
D. 333 g
E. 250 g

12. How much dextrose is required to prepare 500 mL of an aqueous 10% solution?

A. 250 mg
B. 500 mg
C. 10 g
D. 25 g
E. 50 g

13. What weight of hexachlorophene should be used in compounding 20 g of an ointment containing hexachlorophene at a concentration of 1:400?

A. 25 µg
B. 50 µg
C. 50 mg
D. 80 mg
E. 5 g

14. What weight of magnesium chloride ($MgCl_2$, formula weight = 95.3) is require to prepare 200 mL of a solution which is 5.0 millimolar?

A. 191 mg
B. 95.3 mg
C. 19.1 mg
D. 477 µg
E. 95 g

15. What weight of magnesium chloride ($MgCl_2$, formula weight = 95.3; Mg^{2+} atomic wt. = 24.3; Cl^{1-}, atomic wt. = 35.5) is require to prepare 1000 mL of a solution which contains 5.0 milliequivalents of magnesium?

A. 238 mg
B. 4.76 g
C. 1.19 g
D. 60.7 mg
E. 476 µg

16. What is the milliosmolarity (ideal) of normal saline (NaCl formula weight = 58.5)?

A. 100 mOsm/L
B. 154 mOsm/L
C. 254 mOsm/L
D. 287 mOsm/L
E. 308 mOsm/L

17. How much water for injection should be added to 250 mL of 20% dextrose to obtain 15% dextrose?
A. 333 mL
B. 83 mL
C. 250 mL
D. 166 mL
E. 58 mL

18. What volume of a 5% dextrose solution should be mixed with 200 mL of a 20% dextrose solution to prepare 300 mL of a 15% dextrose solution?

A. 150 mL
B. 200 mL
C. 100 mL
D. 50 mL
E. 250 mL

19. What is the final concentration obtained by mixing 200 mL of 20% dextrose with 100 mL of 5% dextrose?

A. 10%
B. 15%
C. 7.5%
D. 12.5%
E. 17.5%

20. Magnesium chloride ($MgCl_2$) is a 3-ion electrolyte that dissociates 80% at the relevant concentration. Calculate its dissociation factor (i).

A. 1.8
B. 2.2
C. 2.4
D. 2.6
E. 3.2

21. Tobramycin (formula weight = 468) has a dissociation factor of 1.0. What is its sodium chloride equivalent?

A. 0.069
B. 0.0092

C. 0.117
D. 0.286
E. 0.782

22. What weight of sodium chloride should be used in compounding the following prescription for ephedrine sulfate (formula weight = 429, dissociation factor = 2.6, sodium chloride equivalent = 0.23)?

Rx Ephedrine sulfate	0.25 g
Sodium chloride	qs
Purified water ad	30 mL
Make isoton. sol.	

A. 1.22 g
B. 784 μg
C. 212 mg
D. 527 μg
E. 429 mg

23. A patient is to receive an infusion of 2 g of lidocaine in 500 mL D_5W at a rate of 2 mg/min. What is the flow rate in mL/h?

A. 2.0 mL/h
B. 6.5 mL/h
C. 15 mL/h
D. 30 mL/h
E. 150 mL/h

24. What is the pH of a buffer solution prepared with 0.05 M disodium phosphate and 0.05 M sodium acid phosphate (pK_a = 7.21)?

A. 4.55
B. 5.23
C. 6.18
D. 7.05
E. 7.21

25. Convert 104°F to centigrade.

A. 22° C
B. 34° C
C. 40° C
D. 46° C
E. 54° C

Answers

1. **C.**

$$x \text{ mg:}340 \text{ mg} = 75 \text{ cap:}100 \text{ cap}$$
$$x = 340 \text{ mg} \times 75 \text{ cap/}100 \text{ cap} = 255 \text{ mg}$$

2. **B.**

A specific gravity of 1.13 corresponds to a density of 1.13 g/mL.

$$\text{density} = \text{weight/volume, thus,}$$
$$\text{weight} = \text{density} \times \text{volume} = 1.13 \text{ g/mL} \times 500 \text{ mL}$$
$$= 565 \text{ g}$$

3. **A.**

$$\text{\% error} = (\text{error} \times 100)/\text{desired quantity}$$
$$= (325 - 312) \times 100/325 = 4\%$$

4. **C.**

$$\text{minimum weighable quantity} = SR \times 100/5$$
$$= 6 \text{ mg} \times 100/5 = 120 \text{ mg}$$

5. **E.**

$$\text{daily dosage} = 50 \text{ mg/kg} \times 175 \text{ lb/2.2 lb/kg} = 3977 \text{ mg}$$
$$\text{single IM injection} = (3977/8) \text{ mg} \times 1/500 \text{ mg/mL}$$
$$= 0.99 \text{ mL}$$

6. **B.**

$$IBW = 45.5 + 2.3 \times 8 = 64 \text{ kg}$$

7. **C.**

$$\text{wt} = 154 \text{ lb/2.2 lb/kg} = 70 \text{ kg; ht}$$
$$= 6 \text{ ft} \times 12 \text{ in./ft} \times 2.54 \text{ cm/in.} = 183 \text{ cm}$$
$$BSA = \text{square root } [70 \times 183/3600]$$
$$= \text{square root } [3.56] = 1.89 \text{ m}^2$$

8. **D.**

$$\text{child dose} = \text{adult dose} \times \text{child BSA/1.73}$$
$$= 125 \text{ mg} \times 0.68 \text{ m}^2/1.73 \text{ m}^2 = 49 \text{ mg}$$

9. **A.**

$$CrCl = 0.85 \times (140 - 65) \times 50/(72 \times 1.3) = 34 \text{ mL/min}$$

10. **D.**
Note that the formula is designed to produce a total of 1000 g of the mixture. Then, by proportions,

$$x \text{ g ZnO:}150 \text{ g ZnO} = 750 \text{ g mix:}1000 \text{ g}$$
$$x = 150 \text{ g} \times 750 \text{ g/}1000 \text{ g} = 113 \text{ g}$$

11. **B.**
Note that the formula will produce a total of 20 parts of the mixture. Then, by proportions,

x g kaolin:500 g mix = 12 parts kaolin:20 parts mix
$x = 500$ g **x** 12 parts/20 parts = 300 g

12. E.
Note that this will be a solution of a solid in a liquid and thus the concentration will be %(w/v).

$$10\%(w/v) = x \text{ g dextrose } \textbf{x } 100/500$$
$$x = 10 \textbf{ x } 500/100 = 50 \text{ g}$$

13. C.
By proportions,

x g hexachlorophene:20 g ung. = 1 part hexachlorophene:400 parts ung.
$x = 20$ g **x** 1 part/400 parts = 0.050 g = 50 mg

14. B.
A 1.0 molar solution will contain 95.3 g in 1000 mL. A 5.0 molar solution will contain 95.3 **x** 5 = 477 g in 1000 mL. A 5.0 millimolar solution will contain 477 mg in 1000 mL. Thus, 200 mL of a 5 millimolar solution will contain 477/5 = 95.3 mg in 200 mL.

15. A.
Because magnesium has a valence of 2, a formula weight of $MgCl_2$ will contain two equivalent weights of magnesium (and chloride for that matter). Thus, 5 equivalents of Mg is contained in 5 **x** 95.3/2 g = 238 g of $MgCl_2$. Accordingly, 5 milliequivalents of Mg is contained in 238 mg of $MgCl_2$.

16. E.
Normal saline is 0.90%(w/v), or 0.90 g/100 mL = 9.0 g/1000 mL.

mOsmolarity = (9 g/58.5) **x** 2 **x** 1000 = 308 mOsm/L

17. B.

$$C_1 = 20\%, Q_1 = 250 \text{ mL}, C_2 = 15\%, Q_2 = ?$$
$$C_1 \textbf{ x } Q_1 = C_2 \textbf{ x } Q_2$$
$$Q_2 = C1 \textbf{ x } Q_1/C_2 = 20\% \textbf{ x } 250 \text{ mL}/15\% = 333 \text{ mL}$$
added water = 333 mL – 250 mL = 83 mL

18. C.

20% (conc of stock A)   15 – 5 = 10 = parts of A

15% (desired conc)

5% (conc of stock B)   20 - 15 = 5 = parts of B

Relative volumes are 10:5, or, 2:1. Thus, 200 mL of 20% solution (A) will require 100 mL of 5% solution (B) to produce 300 mL of 15% dextrose.

19. B.

20 %	x	200 mL =	4000 %mL
5%	x	100 mL =	500 %mL
		300 mL	4500 %mL

Mixture concentration = 4500 %mL/300 mL = 15%.

20. D.
Each 100 molecules will provide:

80 Mg ions
160 Cl ions
20 undissociated molecules
260 particles total

Thus the dissociation factor = 260/100 = 2.6 .

21. A.

sodium chloride equivalent = (58.5)(1.0)/(468)(1.8)
= 0.069

22. C.
Since 900 mg of sodium chloride in 100 mL is isotonic,

$$x:900 \text{ mg} = 30 \text{ mL}:100 \text{ mL and}$$
$$x = 900 \textbf{ x } 30/100 = 270 \text{ mg},$$

the amount of NaCl alone to make 30 mL isotonic. But 1 g of ephedrine sulfate is equivalent to 0.23 g of sodium, thus

$$y = 0.25 \text{ g } \textbf{x } 0.23 = 0.058 \text{ g}$$
$$= 58 \text{ mg of sodium chloride}$$

Accordingly, the amount of sodium chloride to add ($z = x - y$) is (270 mg – 58 mg) = 212 mg.

23. D.
The bag contains 2000 mg in 500 mL, thus 4 mg/mL. A rate of 2 mg/min then corresponds to 0.5 mL/min, that in turn corresponds to 30 mL/h.

24. E.

pH = pK_a + log(salt/acid) = 7.21 + log(0.05/0.05)
= 7.21 + log(1) = 7.21

25. C.

$$9C = 5F - 160$$
$$9C = 5 \textbf{ x } 104 - 160 = 520 - 160 = 360$$
$$C = 360/9 = 40$$

16. References

Ansel HC, Stoklosa MJ. *Pharmaceutical Calculations*, 11th ed. Philadelphia: Lippincott Williams & Wilkins; 2001.

O'Sullivan TA. *Understanding Pharmacy Calculations*, Washington: American Pharmaceutical Association; 2002.

Khan MA, Reddy IK. *Pharmaceutical and Clinical Calculations*, 2nd ed. Lancaster, PA: Technomic Publishing Co; 2000.

2. Federal Pharmacy Law

Walter L. Fitzgerald, Jr, BSPharm, MS, JD
Professor, Department of Pharmacy
University of Tennessee College of Pharmacy

Contents

Introduction

This study guide was developed for the purpose of assisting candidates for the National Association of Boards of Pharmacy® (NABP®) Multistate Pharmacy Jurisprudence Examination™ (MPJE®). It is recognized that candidates will have been exposed, through the academic pharmacy degree program, to the federal and state laws subject to inquiry on the MPJE®. Upon this recognition, this study guide is not intended to be a comprehensive collection or compilation of the text of these laws. Rather, it is a general overview of the relevant federal laws with which the candidate should be familiar.

1. Resources to Assist in Preparing for the MPJE®

Information from NABP®

The first resource the MPJE® candidate should review is the information about the MPJE® located on the NABP® website at www.nabp.org. When the NABP® homepage appears, scroll down to locate the section entitled "Examinations." Here you will find information about the MPJE® and a downloadable MPJE® Candidate's Review Guide.

Another resource available from NABP® that may be of benefit to the MPJE® candidate in relation to state law is the publication entitled *Survey of Pharmacy Law*. This annually revised publication reports summary data for each state on a variety of pharmacy practice and pharmacy law topics. The publication is provided at no charge to all final-year pharmacy students through a grant from Wyeth-Ayerst Global Pharmaceuticals.

If the candidate does not have the publication, it can be ordered from NABP® at a cost of twenty dollars ($20.00). To access additional information about this publication, again go to the NABP® website, and just below the section entitled "Examinations," look for a section entitled "Pharmacy Law." Select the active link "General Information" and when the webpage appears the candidate will see information about the *Survey of Pharmacy Law* and the active link "Publications" from which you can order the publication.

Information from Electronic Databases of Federal Law

Of great assistance to the MPJE® candidate is a wealth of databases of federal law available via the Internet at no cost. The candidate is encouraged to utilize these electronic databases as necessary during the review process. One of the greatest advantages of these electronic databases is the ability, through active links contained in the databases, to quickly retrieve and review cross-references to individual sections of the laws, as well as to other relevant laws.

Accessing the Federal Food, Drug, and Cosmetic Act and the Federal Controlled Substances Act

Go to the U.S. Code Collection maintained by the Legal Information Institute of the Cornell Law School. The website address for this collection is:

http://www4.law.cornell.edu/uscode/

When the webpage appears, scroll down and select Title 21. From the webpage that will next appear you can access both the Federal Food, Drug, and Cosmetic Act and the Federal Controlled Substances Act.

Federal Food, Drug, and Cosmetic Act

On the webpage select Chapter 9, which is titled Federal Food, Drug, and Cosmetic Act. When the next webpage appears you will see all nine Subchapters that comprise the Federal Food, Drug, and Cosmetic Act. When you select a subchapter, you will then see on the next webpage the individual sections of the Act contained in that subchapter, or in some cases, the individual parts contained in that subchapter. Where the subchapter contains individual parts, when you select a part you will then see on the next webpage the individual sections of the Act in that part.

Federal Controlled Substances Act

On the webpage select Chapter 13, which is titled Drug Abuse Prevention and Control, in which you will find the Federal Controlled Substances Act. Upon selecting Chapter 13, you will find subchapters and parts, as described immediately above for the Federal Food, Drug, and Cosmetic Act.

Accessing the regulations of the U.S. Food and Drug Administration and the U.S. Drug Enforcement Administration
Go to the electronic Code of Federal Regulations (CFR) maintained by the Government Printing Office (GPO). The website address for this collection is:

http://www.gpoaccess.gov

When the webpage appears, look for the heading "GPO Access Resources by Branch" and under "Executive Resources" select "Code of Federal Regulations." When the next webpage appears look for the heading "Most Current Data (2003-2002)" and under that heading select "Browse and/or search the CFR." When the next webpage appears, scroll down until you find Title 21, and then select the box to the right with the most current date, and then scroll down to the bottom of the webpage and click "Continue." When the next webpage appears, you will see a listing of the individual Parts of Title 21. Parts 1-99 through 800-1299 contain the regulations of the U.S. Food and Drug Administration (FDA). Beginning at Parts 1300-1399 you will find the regulations of the U.S. Drug Enforcement Administration (DEA).

The FDA regulations
The scope and length of the FDA regulations is significantly large, constituting literally thousands of pages. Rather than include the sections of FDA regulations in this guide, the MPJE® candidate should go to the GPO's CFR website as described immediately above for review.

As to what to review, the FDA regulations governing drugs begin at Part 200, which is found on the website at Parts 200-299. Thus the candidate should select Parts 200-299 in the column with the heading "Browse Parts." When the next webpage appears, the individual parts will appear, and upon selecting any of the parts, the individual sections in that part will appear on the next webpage. FDA's regulations governing drugs continue into the next set of parts, specifically, Parts 300-499. The next set of parts (500-599) contain FDA's regulations governing animal drugs, and should be reviewed. The next set of parts (600-799) concern two items, biologicals and cosmetics, and also should be reviewed. The final set of parts (800-1299) contain FDA's regulations governing medical devices, and should be reviewed.

An important note is that by use of the word "review" in the above paragraph it is not meant that the candidate should read each and every word of every FDA regulation. To do so would require an unreasonable and unnecessary time commitment. It is anticipated that the candidate can look at the caption for each section within each part and recognize whether the candidate needs to review the text of that section, or whether the candidate is sufficiently knowledgeable as to the subject matter of that section that he or she can move on to the next section. Also, from the NABP® Candidate's Review Guide for the MPJE® the candidate should be able to identify those sections that contain text not subject to inquiry on the MPJE®.

The MPJE® candidate can begin by opening Part 200 of the FDA regulations as directed above, and open the first section of Part 200. Then the candidate should recognize from the section title whether this is (1) information about which the candidate is knowledgeable and does not require review or (2) information that is not subject to inquiry on the MPJE®. In the presence of either of these, the candidate should move forward to the next section.

The DEA regulations
As with the FDA regulations, the scope of the DEA regulations is quite extensive, but fortunately is more manageable than the FDA regulations. In addition, if the candidate has worked in pharmacy practice to any degree, the DEA regulations likely will be more famil-

iar to the candidate than the FDA regulations, since the FDA regulations are not as directly related to daily pharmacy practice as are the DEA regulations. The MPJE® candidate can review each section of the relevant DEA regulations using the process described above for the FDA regulations, beginning by opening Part 1300 and then each individual section in each part.

Information from Electronic Databases of State Law

It is anticipated that candidates for the MPJE® will have at least two resources for their study of relevant state law. The first of these is the textbook or other compilation of state law that was utilized in the pharmacy law course taught in the academic degree program. This first resource will, of course, be of value only if the candidate is taking the MPJE® and seeking licensure as a pharmacist in the same state where the candidate completed the academic degree program. The second is what is commonly referred to as the "state board of pharmacy law book." In many states, upon submission of an application for examination for licensure as a pharmacist, the applicant will be provided a copy of the state board's pharmacy law book. The candidate may also have a third resource, that being the *Survey of Pharmacy Law* described above in the section on resources available from NABP®.

But in addition to these resources, like with federal law, there are a number of free electronic databases for accessing state law. The candidate should first look to his or her state's Internet homepage for resources on state law. While it is not possible to describe here for each state how to find relevant state law on the state homepage, the candidate will likely be able to successfully navigate through the homepage. But as an example, the candidate can search to see if the state's secretary of state has an individual homepage, and if it does, look on that homepage for a link to state agency rules and regulations, such as those of the state board of pharmacy.

Beyond the state homepage, there are legal resource websites that the candidate can use for accessing state law, again at no cost. The following websites may be useful to the candidate seeking additional information not only on state law, but also federal and other law:

http://www.romingerlegal.com/

http://www.findlaw.com/

http://www.law.com

http://www.alllaw.com/

http://www.100.com/Top/Law

http://www.paralegals.org/LegalResources/home.html

http://gsulaw.gsu.edu/metaindex

Publications

At many colleges and schools of pharmacy a textbook, or other compilation of federal and state drug and pharmacy law, may have been used in the pharmacy law course. Thus the MPJE® candidate may already have a publication that covers the laws subject to inquiry on the MPJE®. If not, there are publications that may be of assistance, including the two publications listed below that provide a practical, easy-to-understand explanation of the federal law subject to inquiry on the MPJE®. Additionally, these publications contain sample questions for the MPJE® candidate to use in gaining experience in answering questions related to federal law, as well as to obtain a measure of knowledge prior to the MPJE®.

References

Reiss, Barry S. and Hall, Gary D. *Guide to Federal Pharmacy Law*, 3rd ed. Apothecary Press. Contact information: (888) 609-2665 or www.apothecary-press.com.

Strauss, Steven. *Strauss's Federal Drug Laws and Examination Review*, 5th ed. CRC Press. Contact information: (800) 272-7737 or www.crcpress.com.

2. The Comprehensive Drug Abuse Prevention and Control Act of 1970 and Regulations of the U.S. Drug Enforcement Administration (DEA)

The Comprehensive Drug Abuse Prevention and Control Act, enacted by Congress in 1970, has as its primary purpose preventing illicit manufacture, distribution, and use of controlled substances. This purpose is achieved through numerous requirements in the Act and DEA regulations.

Introduction

The Comprehensive Drug Abuse Prevention and Control Act, more commonly known as the Controlled Substances Act (CSA), establishes a "closed system" for distribution of drugs that are "controlled substances." Reference is made to a closed system because controlled substances can only be distributed by and between persons registered with the DEA. The DEA is a unit within the U.S. Department of Justice, and was established in July 1973 by an executive reorganization plan and replaced the former Bureau of Narcotics and Dangerous Drugs (BNDD). But it must be noted that the U.S. Food and Drug Administration (FDA) has also promulgated regulations that affect the distribution of controlled substances. One example is treatment programs for narcotic addicts, where the FDA regulations contain medical guidelines for a program and the DEA regulations contain requirements for dispensing and record-keeping activities for a program.

It is important to recognize that in 1988 Congress amended existing federal laws, including the CSA, with enactment of the Chemical Diversion and Trafficking Act. This Act establishes record-keeping and reporting requirements for persons who manufacture, distribute, import or export a listed precursor or essential chemical and tableting and encapsulating machines. When the MPJE® candidate studies the CSA and DEA regulations, the text added as a result of this 1988 Act is generally easily recognized. For example, the DEA regulation at 21 CFR 1300.02 is entitled "definitions relating to listed chemicals." The MPJE® candidate needs to be attentive to how the CSA and DEA regulations address commercially available controlled substances versus chemicals. Finally, the CSA and DEA regulations are quite complex and technical, with significant effect on pharmacy practice, and demand thorough study by the MPJE® candidate.

Key Provisions of the CSA

The CSA is located at Chapter 13 of Title 21 of the United States Code. There are 2 subchapters in Chapter 13, as follows:

I.   Control and Enforcement
II. Import and Export

The MPJE® candidate should be familiar with both subchapters, and particularly the following provisions from Subchapter I of the CSA. But in addition, the MPJE® candidate should review the sections in Subchapter II on import and export, using the instructions for reviewing the United States Code provided at the beginning.

Subchapter I. Control and Enforcement

. . .

Part A—Introductory Provisions
§ 801. Congressional findings and declarations: controlled substances
This section sets forth the reasons why Congress enacted the CSA. The MPJE® candidate should be generally familiar with these findings and declarations.

§ 801a. Congressional findings and declarations: psychotropic substances
This section recognizes the international treaty—the Convention on Psychotropic Substances—that the U.S. entered into in 1971 and sets forth the reasons why Congress implemented the Convention. The MPJE® candidate should be generally familiar with these findings and declarations.

§ 802. Definitions
The MPJE® candidate should be familiar with all terms defined in this section of the CSA, which will aid in understanding the language of the sections that follow. Note the limitation in dispensing that results from the relationship between the definition of "dispense" and the definition of "ultimate user." Note also that some of the definitions contain important substantive content, such as the definition of a regulated transaction and it's placing of "thresholds" on the retail sale of ephedrine, pseudoephedrine and phenylpropanolamine.

. . .

Part B—Authority to Control; Standards and Schedules

§ 811. Authority and criteria for classification of substances

This section gives the U.S. Attorney General the authority to add a drug to a schedule, transfer a drug between schedules, and remove a drug from a schedule. This section also contains the factors to be considered when determining whether a drug should be placed in or removed from a schedule. This section also allows for exclusion of a non-narcotic substance from a schedule if the substance may be lawfully sold, under the FDCA, without a prescription. Finally, this section provides that dextromethorphan shall not be included in any schedule by reason of enactment of the CSA unless controlled after October 27, 1970 based on the factors in this section.

§ 812. Schedules of controlled substances

This section establishes the five schedules (I-V) of controlled substances and the findings required for each schedule. The MPJE® candidate should be familiar with these findings, such as that a Schedule I controlled substance "has no currently accepted medical use in treatment."

§ 813. Treatment of controlled substance analogues

This section provides that a controlled substance analogue, to the extent intended for human use, shall be treated as a controlled substance in Schedule I.

§ 814. Removal of exemption of certain drugs

This section, among other things, allows the Attorney General to remove from exemption [see definition (39)(A)(iv) at section 802 concerning ephedrine, pseudoephedrine, and phenylpropanolamine] a drug or group of drugs that is being diverted to obtain a listed chemical for use in illicit production of controlled substances.

Part C—Registration of Manufacturers, Distributors, and Dispensers of Controlled Substances

§821. Rules and regulations

This section authorizes the U.S. Attorney General to promulgate rules and regulations and to charge reasonable fees relating to the registration and control of regulated persons and transactions.

§822. Persons required to register

This section sets forth the registration requirements for persons who handle controlled substances. The MPJE® candidate should understand who is and who is not required to obtain a registration, and recognize that a separate registration is required for separate locations and that an inspection may be conducted prior to granting a registration.

§ 823. Registration requirements

This section provides specific detail regarding registration of practitioners, including pharmacies but not pharmacists, and the factors to be considered in determining whether to grant a registration.

§ 824. Denial, revocation, or suspension of registration

This section lists the grounds for denying, suspending, or revoking a registration. Note that a suspension or revocation may be limited to a particular schedule or schedules, and that the registration can be revoked simultaneously with initiation of proceedings (issuing an "order to show cause") if there is an imminent danger to the public health or safety.

§ 825. Labeling and packaging

This section establishes the labeling requirements for commercial containers of controlled substances.

§ 826. Production quotas for controlled substances

This section authorizes the Attorney General to determine and establish production quotas for Schedule I and II controlled substances to be manufactured each calendar year to provide for the estimated medical, scientific, research, and industrial needs of the U.S., for lawful export requirements, and for establishing and maintaining reserve stocks.

§ 827. Records and reports of registrants

This section establishes requirements for the biennial inventory (in relation to May 1, 1971) and adding any newly scheduled drug to the existing inventory. This section requires every registrant to maintain a complete and accurate record of each controlled substance received, sold, delivered or otherwise disposed of, but this section does not require a perpetual inventory. The MPJE® candidate should recognize the exceptions to the inventory requirement.

§ 828. Order forms

This section establishes the requirement that distribution of Schedule I and II controlled substances occur only pursuant to a form issued by the Attorney General (the DEA 222 Form), and record-keeping requirements for the form.

§ 829. Prescriptions

This section sets forth the prescription requirements for each schedule of controlled substances, and notes that Schedule V controlled substances, when not dispensed pursuant to a prescription, may only be sold for a medical purpose.

§ 830. Regulation of listed chemicals and certain machines
This section establishes the record-keeping and reporting requirements for those engaged in activities related to listed chemicals and tableting and encapsulating machines.

Part D—Offenses and Penalties
§841. Prohibited acts A
This section and the next two sections list unlawful acts and the penalties associated with these acts. It is important for the MPJE® candidate to recognize that some of the listed unlawful acts apply to all persons, while others only apply to registrants. The MPJE® candidate should recognize what acts are unlawful and generally be familiar with the associated penalties.

§ 842. Prohibited acts B
See note to section 841.

§ 843. Prohibited acts C
See note to section 841.

§ 844. Penalties for simple possession
This section makes possession, for any person or a registrant, of a controlled substance or listed chemical unlawful unless allowed under the CSA, establishes penalties for unlawful possession and defines what is meant by a "drug, narcotic, or chemical offense."

§ 844a. Civil penalty for possession of small amounts of certain controlled substances
This section provides penalties, for any person or a registrant, for unlawful possession of "personal use amounts" as specified by the U.S. Attorney General by regulation.

...

§ 846. Attempt and conspiracy
This section provides that persons who "attempt" or "conspire" to commit a controlled substance offense are subject to the same penalties as prescribed for the offense.

§ 847. Additional penalties
This section provides that any criminal penalties imposed for violation of the CSA do not preclude other civil and administrative penalties, such as monetary fines under the federal Civil Monetary Penalties Law or suspension or revocation of a DEA Certificate of Registration.

§ 848. Continuing criminal enterprise
This section defines a "continuing criminal enterprise" and imposes very severe penalties—including life imprisonment and the death penalty—for those convicted of engaging in a continuing criminal enterprise. The MPJE® candidate should also recognize that the text of this section also includes other offenses that are not a continuing criminal enterprise. For example, this section provides that any person, during the commission of, in furtherance of, or while attempting to avoid apprehension, prosecution or service of a prison sentence for, a felony violation of the CSA who intentionally kills or counsels, commands, induces, procures, or causes the intentional killing of any federal, state, or local law enforcement officer engaged in, or on account of, the performance of such officer's official duties and such killing results, shall be sentenced to any term of imprisonment, which shall not be less than 20 years, and which may be up to life imprisonment, or may be sentenced to death.

§ 849. Transportation safety offenses
This section doubles the penalty for the first conviction, and triples the penalty for subsequent convictions, of certain controlled substance offenses in a "rest area" or "truck stop" as these terms are defined in this section.

§ 850. Information for sentencing
This section, unless provided otherwise in another federal law, establishes that no limitation be placed on the information concerning the background, character, and conduct of a person convicted of a controlled substance offense that may be received and considered for purposes of imposing an appropriate sentence.

§ 851. Proceedings to establish prior convictions
This section sets forth the process for establishing that a person has prior convictions of a controlled substance offense or offenses.

§ 852. Application of treaties and other international agreements
This section provides that no treaties and other international agreements entered into by the U.S. shall limit the provision of treatment, education, or rehabilitation as alternatives to conviction or criminal penalty for offenses involving any drug or other substance subject to a treaty or agreement.

§ 853. Criminal forfeitures
This section provides that persons convicted of controlled substance offenses shall forfeit to the U.S. all real and personal property constituting or derived from, any proceeds the person obtained, directly or indirectly, as the result of the offense; and any of the

person's property used, or intended to be used, in any manner or part, to commit, or to facilitate the commission of the offense.

. . .

§ 854. Investment of illicit drug profits

This section makes it unlawful for a person to use or invest in certain "enterprises" as defined in this section any income derived, directly or indirectly, from a violation of the CSA punishable by imprisonment for more than one year if the person participated as a principal in the violation, and provides penalties for making such investments.

§ 855. Alternative fine

This section provides that in lieu of a fine otherwise authorized by Part D, a defendant who derives profits or other proceeds from an offense may be fined not more than twice the gross profits or other proceeds.

§ 856. Establishment of manufacturing operations

This section makes it unlawful to knowingly open or maintain any place for the purpose of manufacturing, distributing, or using any controlled substance, as well as to manage or control any building, room, or enclosure, either as an owner, lessee, agent, employee, or mortgagee, and knowingly and intentionally rent, lease, or make available for use, with or without compensation, the building, room, or enclosure for the purpose of unlawfully manufacturing, storing, distributing, or using a controlled substance, and establishes penalties for a violation.

. . .

§ 858. Endangering human life while illegally manufacturing controlled substance

This section provides that whoever, while unlawfully manufacturing a controlled substance, or attempting to do so, or transporting or causing to be transported materials, including chemicals, to do so, creates a substantial risk of harm to human life shall be subject to a fine and imprisonment.

§ 859. Distribution to persons under age twenty-one

This section provides enhanced penalties for first and second offenses of a person who is at least 18 years of age unlawfully distributing a controlled substance to a person under 21 years of age.

§ 860. Distribution or manufacturing in or near schools and colleges

This section provides enhanced penalties for first and second offenses of any person who is unlawfully distributing, possessing with intent to distribute, or manu-

facturing a controlled substance in or on, or within one thousand feet of, the real property comprising a public or private elementary, vocational, or secondary school or a public or private college, junior college, or university, or a playground, or housing facility owned by a public housing authority, or within 100 feet of a public or private youth center, public swimming pool, or video arcade facility. This section also makes it an offense for any person at least 21 years of age to knowingly and intentionally employ, hire, use, persuade, induce, entice, or coerce a person under 18 years of age to violate this section; or employ, hire, use, persuade, induce, entice, or coerce a person under 18 years of age to assist in avoiding detection or apprehension for any offense under this section by any federal, state, or local law enforcement official.

§ 861. Employment or use of persons under 18 years of age in drug operations

This section makes it unlawful for any person at least 18 years of age to knowingly and intentionally employ, hire, use, persuade, induce, entice, or coerce, a person under eighteen years of age to violate any provision of the CSA; or employ, hire, use, persuade, induce, entice, or coerce, a person under eighteen years of age to assist in avoiding detection or apprehension for any offense of the CSA by any federal, state, or local law enforcement official; or receive a controlled substance from a person under 18 years of age, other than an immediate family member, in violation of the CSA. This section also establishes penalties for first and subsequent violations of this section. This section also makes it unlawful to knowingly provide or distribute a controlled substance or a controlled substance analogue to a person under 18 years of age or to a pregnant person.

§ 862. Denial of federal benefits to drug traffickers and possessors

This section provides for denial of federal benefits, with differences in denial based upon whether the person is a drug trafficker or drug possessor.

§ 862a. Denial of assistance and benefits for certain drug-related convictions

This section provides for denial of federal benefits and assistance to an individual convicted under federal or state law of any offense which is classified as a felony by the law of the jurisdiction involved and which has as an element the possession, use, or distribution of a controlled substance.

§ 862b. Sanctioning for testing positive for controlled substances

This section provides that states shall not be prohibited by the federal government from testing welfare recipients for use of controlled substances nor from sanctioning welfare recipients who test positive for use of controlled substances.

§ 863. Drug paraphernalia

This section makes unlawful a number of activities with respect to drug paraphernalia, establishes penalties for violations, and defines drug paraphernalia.

§ 864. Anhydrous ammonia

This section makes it unlawful to steal anhydrous ammonia, or to transport stolen anhydrous ammonia across state lines, knowing, intending, or having reasonable cause to believe that such anhydrous ammonia will be used to manufacture a controlled substance in violation of this part.

The last two parts of Subchapter I contain a variety of sections, many of which are not of interest to the MPJE® candidate. As directed in the explanation to the study guide, the candidate should open each part, and from the titles of the sections in each part, determine those that the MPJE® candidate should review.

Subchapter II. Import and Export

This subchapter of the Controlled Substances Act contains several sections governing the importation and exportation of controlled substances, including requirements for registration of importers and exporters. These sections should be reviewed in general fashion by the MPJE® candidate.

Regulations of the U.S. Drug Enforcement Administration (DEA)

The DEA regulations may be found in Title 21 of the Code of Federal Regulations (CFR). The body of DEA regulations is divided into 17 "Parts."

The MPJE® candidate should review relevant DEA regulations on the electronic database as described in the explanation to this study guide. Following is a very basic summary of the content of each part.

Part 1300—Definitions

The DEA regulations begin at Part 1300 of Title 21 of the Code of Federal Regulations (CFR). Part 1300 has two sections, both of which contain definitions of terms related to controlled substances and to listed chemicals. Because there are many definitions, they are not included here, but as noted above for definitions contained in the CSA, the MPJE® candidate should retrieve and review all of the definitions from the following two sections of the DEA regulations. Some of these definitions are quite extensive and contain very important information for the MPJE® candidate. For example, restrictions related to the sale of ephedrine, pseudoephedrine, and phenylpropanolamine will be found in the definition of "regulated transaction" at 21 CFR 1300.02.

21 CFR 1300.01—Definitions relating to controlled substances

21 CFR 1300.02—Definitions relating to listed chemicals

Part 1301—Registration of manufacturers, distributors, and dispensers of controlled substances

Part 1301 governs the many aspects of registration with the DEA. This part includes the sections related to who is required to register, applying for registration, exemptions to registration, and allowances for importation for personal use. Also included are specific details about the DEA Certificate of Registration and the number assignment, procedure for suspension or revocation of a registration, and modification or termination of a registration. Very importantly, requirements for security, including the prohibition on employing certain individuals, are included in this part. The MPJE® candidate should study this part in detail. While not included specifically here, the method for determining the legitimacy of a DEA registration number is important for the MPJE® candidate, and thus is included below.

Prior to 1 October 1985, DEA Certificate of Registration Numbers for practitioners began with the letter "A." Since that date, the DEA Certificate of Registration Numbers for practitioners begins with the letter "B." Further, a DEA Certificate of Registration Number issued to a mid-level practitioner begins with the letter "M." Following the first letter is a second letter, and this letter is the first letter of the registrant's last name. Following the two letters is a seven-digit computer-generated sequential number. The number is constructed in a way that it can be tested for verification, using the following formula.

Step 1: Determine the sum of the first, third, and fifth digits added together.
Step 2: Determine the sum of the second, fourth, and sixth digits added together, and then multiply the sum by two.
Step 3: Determine the sum of the two numbers determined in Step 1 and Step 2.
Step 4: The last digit of this third sum should be the same as the last digit of the seven-digit DEA Certificate of Registration Number.

Part 1302—Labeling and packaging requirements for controlled substances

Part 1302 contains the requirements for labeling of the "commercial container" of a controlled substance. The MPJE® candidate should be generally familiar with these requirements.

Part 1303—Quotas

Part 1303 contains the sections related to the establishment of production and procurement quotas for controlled substances for the estimated medical, scientific, research and industrial needs. The MPJE® candidate should be generally familiar with the sections in this part.

Part 1304—Records and reports of registrants

Part 1304 contains the many requirements associated with record-keeping in relation to the various aspects of handling controlled substances by practitioners, and also including narcotic treatment programs. Also included in this part are the requirements associated with inventories of controlled substances, including the "biennial inventory." The MPJE® candidate should be very familiar with the sections in this part.

Part 1305—Order forms

Part 1305 includes the sections describing the DEA Form 222 for ordering Schedule II controlled substances. Also included in this part are the details associated with the granting of a power of attorney in association with order forms. The MPJE® candidate should be very familiar with the sections in this part.

Part 1306—Prescriptions

Part 1306 contains the sections concerning the many details of issuing, dispensing, and labeling of prescriptions for controlled substances. Also included in this part in relation to prescriptions are the requirements for electronic record-keeping of prescription refills and for transfer of prescriptions between pharmacies. Finally, this part includes the requirements for the sale of controlled substances which are not "prescription drugs." The MPJE® candidate should be very familiar with the sections in this part.

Part 1307—Miscellaneous

Part 1307 contains a few sections of interest to the MPJE® candidate. Of particular note are the sections on "distribution" by dispensers and disposal of controlled substances.

Part 1308—Schedules of controlled substances

Part 1308 describes the "Administration Controlled Substances Number" and its uses, and lists controlled substances in their respective schedules. Part 1308 also provides for "exempt" and "excluded" substances, control of immediate precursors, and emergency scheduling. The MPJE® candidate should be generally familiar with controlled substances and the schedule into which they have been placed, and those products that are exempt and excluded as described in Part 1308.

Part 1309—Registration of manufacturers, distributors, importers, and exporters of List I chemicals

Part 1309 includes several provisions related to those engaged in activities with List I chemicals. While the practice of pharmacy is not generally affected by Part 1309, the MPJE® candidate should review these sections for familiarity.

Part 1310—Records and reports of listed chemicals and certain machines

While the comment about Part 1309 immediately above also applies to some sections of Part 1310, it is noted that some sections in Part 1310 relate to ephedrine, and thus this part deserves review by the MPJE® candidate.

. . .

Part 1312—Importation and exportation of controlled substances

Part 1312 includes several provisions related to those engaged in importing and exporting controlled substances. While the practice of pharmacy is not generally affected by this part, the MPJE® candidate should review these sections for familiarity.

Part 1313—Importation and exportation of precursors and essential chemicals
Part 1313 includes several provisions related to those engaged in importing and exporting precursors and essential chemicals. While the practice of pharmacy is not generally affected by this part, the MPJE® candidate should review these sections for familiarity.

. . .

Part 1316—Administrative functions, practices, and procedures
Part 1316 contains several sections that address inspections, probable cause, and other issues related to warrants, matters related to research, procedures for hearings, burden of proof, and miscellaneous other matters. The MPJE® candidate should be generally familiar with these matters.

3. The Food, Drug, and Cosmetic Act of 1938 and Regulations of the U.S. Food and Drug Administration (FDA)

The Food, Drug, and Cosmetic Act (FDCA), enacted by Congress in 1938, has as its primary purpose preventing interstate distribution of foods, drugs, cosmetics, and devices that are adulterated or misbranded. This purpose is achieved through numerous requirements in the Act and FDA regulations.

Introduction

The MPJE® candidate should be familiar with the historical development of the Food, Drug, and Cosmetic Act of 1938 (FDCA), and its predecessor, the Pure Food and Drug Act of 1906. And the candidate should also be familiar with amendments to the FDCA since 1938, including the following:

> Durham-Humphrey Amendment of 1951
> Kefauver-Harris Amendment of 1962
> Medical Device Amendment of 1976
> Orphan Drug Act of 1983
> Drug Price Competition and Patent Term
>   Restoration Act of 1984
> Prescription Drug Marketing Act of 1987
> Safe Medical Devices Act of 1990
> Dietary Supplement Health and Education Act
>   of 1994
> Food and Drug Administration Modernization
>   Act of 1997

Key Provisions of the FDCA

The FDCA is located at Chapter 9 of Title 21 of the United States Code. There are 9 subchapters in Chapter 9, as follows:

> I.   Short Title
> II.   Definitions
> III. Prohibited Acts and Penalties
> IV.   Food
> V.   Drugs and Devices
> VI.   Cosmetics
> VII. General Authority
> VIII. Imports and Exports
> IX.   Miscellaneous

The MPJE® candidate should be particularly familiar with Subchapters II, III, V (which is divided into Subparts A through E), and VI, and particularly the following sections within the subchapters of the FDCA.

Subchapter I. Short title

. . .

Subchapter II. Definitions

§ 321. Definitions; generally

The MPJE® candidate should be familiar with all terms defined in this section of the FDCA, which will aid in understanding the language of the sections that follow. The candidate also should be able to distinguish between terms such as "drug," "counterfeit drug," "new drug," "device," "dietary supplement," "food," and "cosmetic."

. . .

Subchapter III. Prohibited acts and penalties

§ 331. Prohibited acts

The MPJE® candidate should be familiar with conduct that is prohibited by the FDCA, as set forth in this section.

§ 332. Injunction proceedings

This section provides that the U.S. district courts and all courts exercising jurisdiction in U.S. territories have jurisdiction to enjoin violations of section 331, with some exception as set forth in this section. Further, an alleged violation of an injunction or restraining order shall, upon demand of the accused, be tried before a jury.

§ 333. Penalties

The penalties for violation of the FDCA range from not very severe to very severe. The MPJE® candidate should be familiar with the penalties, and particularly those related to the prescription drug marketing violations (ie, drug samples) and distribution of human growth hormone. Notice the use of the term "knowingly," as defined in Section 321.

. . .

§ 334. Seizure

This section describes the process related to seizure and disposition of adulterated and misbranded foods, drugs, and cosmetics, a process with which the MPJE® candidate should be familiar.

§ 335. Hearing before report of criminal violation

This section provides that before any violation of this chapter is reported to a U.S. attorney for criminal proceedings, the person against whom the proceeding is contemplated shall be given appropriate notice and an opportunity to present his views, either orally or in writing.

§ 335a. Debarment, temporary denial of approval, and suspension

This section describes the "debarment" from submitting or assisting in the submission of applications for drug approvals of businesses and individuals based on prior misconduct related to the drug approval process. The MPJE® candidate should be able to distinguish the various characteristics of mandatory and permissive debarments.

§ 335b. Civil penalties

This section continues the matter of misconduct in the drug approval process. The MPJE® candidate should be familiar with the conduct prohibited and the associated penalties, together with the provision concerning informants.

§ 335c. Authority to withdraw approval of abbreviated drug applications

This section authorizes the withdrawal of approval of abbreviated drug applications where the approval was obtained, expedited, or otherwise facilitated through bribery, payment of an illegal gratuity, or fraud or material false statement, and further, if the manufacturer has repeatedly demonstrated a lack of ability to produce the drug for which the application was submitted in accordance with the formulations and manufacturing processes set forth in the application and has introduced, or attempted to introduce, such adulterated or misbranded drug into commerce. This section also provides procedures for withdrawals.

§ 336. Report of minor violations

This section provides that the HHS Secretary is not required to report for prosecution, or for the institution of libel or injunction proceedings, minor violations of this chapter whenever he believes that the public interest will be adequately served by a suitable written notice or warning.

§ 337. Proceedings in the name of United States; provision as to subpoenas

This section requires that legal proceedings for enforcement or restraining of violations be in the name of the U.S. However, this section also allows states to bring actions under the Act, but only upon notice being given to the HHS Secretary as set forth in this section.

Subchapter IV. Food

Although this subchapter is entitled "Food" the MPJE® candidate should review select sections of this subchapter as they contain requirements related to dietary supplements. The MPJE® candidate should review the portions addressing dietary supplements in the following sections: 341, 342, 343, 343-1, 343-2, and 350-b.

In addition, the MPJE® candidate should review section 350 on vitamins and minerals.

Subchapter V. Drugs and devices
Part A—Drugs and devices
§ 351. Adulterated drugs and devices
A drug or device can be "adulterated" for several reasons, as listed in this section. The MPJE® candidate should be familiar with these reasons.

§ 352. Misbranded drugs and devices
A drug or device can be "misbranded" for several reasons, as listed in this section. The MPJE® candidate should be familiar with these reasons.

§ 353. Exemptions and consideration for certain drugs, devices, and biological products
A very key section of the FDCA, it is this section that, among other things, exempts legend drugs from the general labeling requirements of the FDCA, including when sold upon a prescription. (Note the label requirement of the "Rx Only symbol" which replaces the labeling requirement of "Caution: Federal law prohibits dispensing without a prescription," a change created by the Food and Drug Administration Modernization Act of 1997.) Also included in this section are the sales restrictions imposed by the Prescription Drug Marketing Act of 1987 with respect to legend drug samples and coupons for legend drugs, together with the wholesaler licensing requirements. Finally, veterinary use drugs are addressed in this section.

§ 353a. Pharmacy compounding
This section was added to the FDCA by the Food and Drug Administration Modernization Act of 1997. However, in an April 29, 2002 opinion, the U.S. Supreme Court ruled the section unconstitutional in the case of *Thompson et al. v. Western States Medical Center et al.*, Case No. 01-344. However, it is important to realize that other sections of the FDCA also address pharmacy compounding. The MPJE® candidate should be very familiar with the federal law on pharmacy compounding. A good source for the Supreme Court opinion and other materials, particularly the FDA Compliance Policy Guidance on pharmacy compounding, is the FDA's Center for Drug Evaluation and Research at www.fda.gov/cder/pharmcomp/default.htm.

§ 354. Veterinary feed directive drugs
This section defines what is meant by a veterinary feed directive drug, and sets forth requirements in relation to use and labeling of such drugs.

§ 355. New drugs
This quite lengthy section sets forth the requirements and process for approval of a "new drug" through filing of a new drug application or abbreviated new drug application. The MPJE® candidate should be familiar with the process for approval of drugs, and note particularly in this section the definition and use of the terms "bioavailability" and "bioequivalent." The references listed in the introduction to this review provide a good overview of the drug approval process.

§ 355a. Pediatric studies of drugs
This section authorizes the HHS Secretary to request pediatric studies, which are defined in this section, from the holder of an approved application for a new or previously approved drug, where the drug may produce health benefits in the pediatric population. If the holder of the approved application completes the studies, the holder will be granted additional "market exclusivity," through extension of patent life for the periods described in this section, for the drug. Finally, this section establishes requirements relative to the conducting of pediatric studies.

§ 356. Fast track products
This section authorizes the HHS Secretary, at the request of the sponsor of a new drug, to facilitate the development and expedite the review of such drug if it is intended for the treatment of a serious or life-threatening condition and it demonstrates the potential to address unmet medical needs for such a condition, which serves as the definition of a "fast track product."

§ 356a. Manufacturing changes
This section describes "manufacturing changes" and sets forth those changes that require filing of a supplemental application and those that do not.

§ 356b. Reports of postmarketing studies
This section establishes the requirements for postmarketing studies where the sponsor of a drug has entered into an agreement with the HHS Secretary to conduct such a study.

§ 356c. Discontinuance of life saving drug
This section creates the requirement that the sole manufacturer of a drug, that has an approved application and that was not originally derived from human tissue and was replaced with recombinant product, and that is life-supporting, life-sustaining, or intended for use in the prevention of a debilitating disease or condition, notify the HHS Secretary of discontinuance of manufacture of the product at least six months prior to the discontinuance date. Reduction in the six-month notice requirement is authorized in certain circumstances, as described in this section.

...

§ 358. Authority to designate official names

This section authorizes the HHS Secretary to designate an official name for a drug or device, except where the official name infringes a valid trademark. It also contains a requirement that the HHS Secretary review official names in the United States Pharmacopoeia, the Homoeopathic Pharmacopoeia, and the National Formulary to determine whether revision of those names is necessary or desirable. Finally, in such reviews the HHS Secretary is required to make determinations, in relation to the designation of an official name, based upon complexity, usefulness, multiplicity, or lack of a name.

§ 359. Nonapplicability of subchapter to cosmetics

As the title of this section states, nothing in this Subchapter applies to cosmetics, unless the cosmetic is also a drug or device or component of a drug or device.

§ 360. Registration of producers of drugs or devices

This section establishes the registration and drug listing/National Drug Code requirements for drug manufacturers. The MPJE® candidate should be familiar with the National Drug Code system. And significantly, this section, at (g)(1), exempts pharmacies and certain others from the registration and drug listing requirements.

...

§ 360b. New animal drugs

As with drugs for human use, the MPJE® candidate should be familiar with new animal drugs under the FDCA, as described in this lengthy section.

§ 360c. Classification of devices intended for human use

The MPJE® candidate should be familiar with the FDCA provisions related to devices. This section establishes three classes of devices, as follows.

Class I   General Controls
Class II   Special Controls
Class III   Premarket Approval

This section also sets forth the standards for determination of the safety and effectiveness of a device and provides for classification panel organization and operation.

§ 360d. Performance standards

This section establishes performance standards for Class II, and in some cases Class III, devices, and the procedures for establishing and recognizing the standards.

§ 360e. Premarket approval

This section establishes the requirements and procedures for an application for premarket approval of a Class III device.

§ 360f. Banned devices

This section authorizes the HHS Secretary to promulgate regulations to ban certain devices, as described in this section.

§ 360g. Judicial review

This section sets forth the procedures for judicial review of decisions of the HHS Secretary with regard to devices.

§ 360h. Notification and other remedies

This section provides that when a device presents an unreasonable risk of substantial harm and notification is necessary to eliminate the risk of harm, the HHS Secretary may issue an order to assure that adequate notification is provided in an appropriate form, by the persons and means best suited under the circumstances involved, to all health professionals who prescribe or use the device, and to any other person (including manufacturers, importers, distributors, retailers, and device users) who should properly receive such notification in order to eliminate such risk. This section also authorizes the HHS Secretary to order the manufacturer of a device to make repair, replacement, or refund in relation to the device. Finally, this section gives the HHS Secretary authority to order a recall of a device.

§ 360i. Records and reports on devices

This section requires reports, as described in the section, from device manufacturers and device user facilities, such as hospitals. It also authorizes the HHS Secretary to order a device manufacturer to adopt a method for tracking certain Class II and III devices.

§ 360j. General provisions respecting control of devices intended for human use

This section contains a variety of requirements, including provisions for custom devices, restricted devices, good manufacturing practice requirements, and exemption of devices for investigational use.

§ 360k. State and local requirements respecting devices

This section establishes the relationship between the FDCA provisions on devices and any state laws that may exist in relation to devices.

§ 360l. Postmarketing surveillance
This section authorizes the HHS Secretary to impose upon manufacturers of certain devices various post-marketing surveillance requirements related to devices.

§ 360m. Accredited persons
This section requires the HHS Secretary to establish an "accreditation program" as described in the section, for persons who review reports related to devices.

Part B—Drugs for rare diseases or conditions
§ 360aa. Recommendations for investigations of drugs for rare diseases or conditions
This section provides that a sponsor of a drug for a disease or condition which is rare may request the HHS Secretary to provide written recommendations for the nonclinical and clinical investigations that must be conducted with the drug before it may be approved for such disease or condition, or, if the drug is a biological product, before it may be licensed for such disease or condition.

§ 360bb. Designation of drugs for rare diseases or conditions
This section allows a manufacturer or sponsor of a drug to request, prior to submission of an application for approval, the HHS Secretary to designate the drug as a drug for a rare disease or condition. This section defines a "rare disease or condition" as any disease or condition that affects fewer than 200,000 persons in the U.S. or affects more than 200,000 in the U.S. and for which there is no reasonable expectation that the cost of developing and making available in the U.S. a drug for such disease or condition will be recovered from sales in the U.S. It also contains a requirement for notice to the HHS Secretary for discontinuance of production of the drug.

§ 360cc. Protection for drugs for rare diseases or conditions
This section provides that if the HHS Secretary approves an application for a drug designated for a rare disease or condition, the HHS Secretary may not approve another application for such drug for such disease or condition for a person who is not the holder of such approved application until the expiration of seven years from the date of approval, except where the holder of the approved application cannot assure the availability of sufficient quantities of the drug to meet the needs of persons with the disease or condition for which the drug was designated, or such holder provides the HHS Secretary written consent for the approval of other applications before the expiration of such seven-year period.

§ 360dd. Open protocols for investigations of drugs for rare diseases or conditions
This section provides, under certain circumstances, for the HHS Secretary to encourage the sponsor of a drug designated for a rare disease or condition to design protocols for clinical investigations of the drug that may be conducted to permit the addition to the investigations of persons with the disease or condition who need the drug to treat the disease or condition, and who cannot be satisfactorily treated by available alternative drugs.

§ 360ee. Grants and contracts for development of drugs for rare diseases and conditions
This section authorizes the HHS Secretary to make grants to and enter into contracts with public and private entities and individuals to assist in defraying the costs of qualified testing expenses incurred in connection with the development of drugs for rare diseases and conditions, defraying the costs of developing medical devices for rare diseases or conditions, and defraying the costs of developing medical foods (a food formulated to be consumed or administered enterally under the supervision of a physician) for rare diseases or conditions.

Part C—Electronic product radiation control

. . .

Part D—Dissemination of treatment information
§ 360aaa. Requirements for dissemination of treatment information on drugs or devices
This section allows a manufacturer to disseminate written information concerning the safety, effectiveness, or benefit of a use not described in the approved labeling of a drug or device if the manufacturer meets certain requirements. Those parties to whom a manufacturer may disseminate such information are a health care practitioner; a pharmacy benefit manager; a health insurance issuer; a group health plan; and a federal or state governmental agency. Among the requirements are that the manufacturer must submit the information to the HHS Secretary at least 60 days prior to dissemination and the information must contain a prominently displayed statement that discloses very specific language as set forth in this section.

§ 360aaa-1. Information authorized to be disseminated
This section describes what information may be disseminated, such as reprints of peer-reviewed articles and reference publications, but both of which must meet standards set by this section.

§ 360aaa-2. Establishment of a list of articles and publications disseminated and a list of providers that received articles and reference publications

This section requires a manufacturer that disseminates information to biannually provide to the HHS Secretary a list containing the titles of all articles and reference publications that were disseminated, and a list of the categories of providers that received the articles and reference publications. The manufacturer must also keep records that may be used to take corrective action in relation to any information that was disseminated.

§ 360aaa-3. Requirement regarding submission of supplemental application for new use; exemption from requirement

This section generally requires that a manufacturer that disseminates information submit to the HHS Secretary a supplemental application for such use, subject to a number of conditions and exemptions as described in this section.

§ 360aaa-4. Corrective actions; cessation of dissemination

This section authorizes the HHS Secretary to take a variety of actions in relation to a manufacturer's dissemination of information, including order that the manufacturer cease dissemination of the information, and possibly requiring the manufacturer to correct the information that was disseminated. Grounds for ordering that dissemination be ceased are set forth in the section. It also imposes a duty on manufacturers to notify the HHS Secretary of any additional knowledge of the manufacturer on clinical research or other data that relate to the safety or effectiveness of the new use.

§ 360aaa-5. Definitions

This section defines a number of terms, such as "health care practitioner" and "new use" that are essential to understanding the sections related to manufacturer dissemination of information. The MPJE® candidate should be familiar with these terms and their definitions.

§ 360aaa-6. Rules of construction

This section contains a number of what are referred to as "rules of construction." Examples from the section include that section 360aaa shall not be "construed" as prohibiting a manufacturer from disseminating information in response to an unsolicited request from a health care practitioner. The MPJE® candidate should be familiar with the content of this section.

Part E—General provisions relating to drugs and devices

§ 360bbb. Expanded access to unapproved therapies and diagnostics

This section authorizes the HHS Secretary to allow shipment of investigational drugs or investigational devices for the diagnosis, monitoring, or treatment of a serious disease or condition in emergency situations. Further, an individual patient, acting through a physician, may request from a manufacturer or distributor an investigational drug or investigational device for the diagnosis, monitoring, or treatment of a serious disease or condition if a number of conditions as set forth in this section are fulfilled.

§ 360bbb-1. Dispute resolution

This section requires the HHS Secretary to establish a procedure for a sponsor, applicant, or manufacturer to obtain a review, including by a scientific advisory panel, in situations in which there is a scientific controversy with the HHS Secretary.

§ 360bbb-2. Classification of products

This section provides that a person submitting an application for a product may submit a request to the HHS Secretary with respect to the classification of the product as a drug, biological product, device, or a combination, or with respect to the component of the Food and Drug Administration that will regulate the product. In submitting the request, the person shall recommend a classification for the product, or a component to regulate the product, as appropriate. Also provides what action the HHS Secretary shall take in response to such a request being filed.

Subchapter VI. Cosmetics

The MPJE® candidate should review the three sections (361 through 363) contained in this subchapter on cosmetics.

The last three subchapters of Chapter 9 contain a variety of sections, many of which are not of interest to the MPJE® candidate. As directed in the explanation to the study guide, the candidate should open each subchapter, and from the titles of the parts and sections, determine those that the MPJE® candidate should review.

Regulations of the U.S. Food and Drug Administration (FDA)

The FDA regulations may be found in Title 21 of the Code of Federal Regulations (CFR). The body of FDA regulations is divided into "Subchapters" as follows.

Subchapter A   General (21 CFR Parts 1 to 99)

Subchapter B   Food for Human Consumption
(21 CFR Parts 100 to 199)

Subchapter C   Drugs: General (21 CFR 200 to 299)

Subchapter D   Drugs for Human Use (21 CFR Parts
300 to 499)

Subchapter E   Animal Drugs, Feeds, and Related
Products (21 CFR Parts 500 to 599)

Subchapter F   Biologics (21 CFR Parts 600 to 699)

Subchapter G   Cosmetics (21 CFR Parts 700 to 799)

Subchapter H   Medical Devices (21 CFR
Parts 800 to 899)

Subchapter I   Mammography Quality Standards Act
(21 CFR Parts 900 to 999)

Subchapter J   Radiological Health (21 CFR
Parts 1000 to 1099)

Subchapter K   Reserved

Subchapter L   Regulations Under Certain Other
Acts (21 CFR Parts 1200 to 1299)

The MPJE® candidate should review relevant FDA regulations on the electronic database as described in the explanation to this study guide.

4. The Poison Prevention Packaging Act of 1970 and Regulations of the U.S. Consumer Product Safety Commission (CPSC)

The Poison Prevention Packaging Act (PPPA), enacted by Congress in 1970, has as its purpose preventing poisonings in children under five years of age. This purpose is achieved through numerous requirements in the Act and CPSC regulations.

Introduction

The Poison Prevention Packaging Act of 1970 (PPPA) establishes packaging requirements for certain household products. Included among these products are both prescription and nonprescription drug products.

Key provisions of the PPPA
The MPJE® candidate should be familiar with the packaging requirements contained in the PPPA and the regulations of the Consumer Product Safety Commission (CPSC). The PPPA is located at Chapter 39A of Title 15 of the United States Code. The MPJE® candidate should retrieve and the review the sections contained in Chapter 39A as described in the explanation to this study guide.

Regulations of the U.S. Consumer Product Safety Commission (CPSC)
The CPSC regulations may be found at Part 1700 of Title 16 of the Code of Federal Regulations (CFR). The MPJE® candidate should retrieve and the review the sections contained in Part 1700 as described in the explanation to this study guide.

5. Miscellaneous Federal Laws

Omnibus Budget Reconciliation Act of 1990

This act, more commonly referred to as OBRA '90, required the states to enact laws to require patient profiling, prospective drug utilization review, and patient counseling by pharmacies. While the federal mandate applied only to the provision of pharmacy services to Medicaid beneficiaries, the states extended application of the requirements to all pharmacy patients. While the MPJE® candidate should review state law on these requirements, the federal regulations may be found beginning at section 45 CFR 456.700.

Anti-Tampering Act of 1982

This Act makes it a federal offense to tamper with consumer products, and was passed as a result of a series of incidents of intentional contamination of Tylenol® capsules while held for sale in retail establishments. Regulatory authority resides with the Federal Bureau of Investigation, U.S. Department of Agriculture, and FDA. Regulations for specific types of products may be retrieved (as described in the explanation to this study guide) and reviewed as follows:

Over-the-counter drug products (21 CFR 211.132)
Medical devices (21 CFR 800.12)
Cosmetics (21 CFR 700.25)

Federal Law on Medicinal Use of Alcohol

Under federal law, retailers that sell alcohol are subject to an annual tax, and in order to handle any type of alcohol, a license from the U.S. Bureau of Alcohol, Tobacco, and Firearms (ATF) is required. Retailers selling take-home liquors are required to obtain a federal retail liquor dealer's stamp. In a community pharmacy, if the alcohol is sold only for medicinal purposes, a federal medicinal spirits dealer's stamp may be obtained instead of the retail liquor dealer's stamp.

Through use of Form ATF-11, pharmacies may purchase 190-proof grain alcohol (95% ethanol). Some pharmacies require much larger volumes (usually obtained in 10- or 55-gallon drums) of alcohol, and it can be purchased tax-free by using Form ATF-1447. However, the use of tax-free alcohol is subject to a number of federal law restrictions.

- The alcohol must be used for medicinal or scientific purposes, or patient treatment.
- The alcohol must not be sold or loaned to other pharmacies or other practitioners.

- The alcohol, whether in pure form or in combination with other substances, must not be sold to outpatients, with the exception of nonprofit clinics so long as the patient is not charged.
- The alcohol must be kept in a secure, fire-resistant room.
- A perpetual inventory of the alcohol stock must be maintained.

For additional information, the MPJE® candidate can review the sections beginning at 27 CFR 22.1 as described in the explanation to this study guide.

3. Dosage Forms and Drug Delivery Systems

Ram I. Mahato, PhD
Assistant Professor, Department of Pharmaceutical Sciences
University of Tennessee College of Pharmacy

Contents

1. Introduction

Pharmaceutical dosage forms are drug delivery systems. Some common examples are tablets, suppositories, injections, and transdermal patches. To achieve an optimum response from any dosage form, a drug should be delivered to its site of action at a rate and concentration that both minimize its side effects and maximize its therapeutic effects. The development of safe and effective drug dosage forms and delivery systems requires a thorough understanding of *physicochemical principles* that allow a drug to be formulated into a pharmaceutical dosage form. Design of the appropriate dosage form or delivery system depends on the:

- Physicochemical properties of the drug, such as solubility, oil-to-water partition coefficient ($K_{o/w}$), pK_a value, and molecular weight

- Dose of the drug

- Route of administration

- Type of drug delivery systems desired

- Pathologic condition to be treated

- Desired therapeutic effect

- Drug release from the delivery system

- Bioavailability of the drug at the absorption site

- Pharmacokinetics and pharmacodynamics of the drug

How Drug Molecules Move Across Barriers in the Body

Most drugs are absorbed from the site of their application by simple diffusion. Drug diffusion through a barrier may occur by simple molecular permeation known as *molecular diffusion* or by movement through pores and channels known as *pore-diffusion*. In pore-diffusion, drug release rate is affected by degree of crystallinity and crystal size, degree of swelling, porous structure, and tortuosity of polymers.

With passive molecular diffusion, a drug travels by *passive transport* (does not require an external energy source) from a region of high concentration to a region of low concentration. However, other transport processes occur in the body as well. For example, *active transport* of drugs can proceed from regions of low concentration to regions of high concentration

through the pumping action of one or more biologic transport systems. These active transport systems require an energy source such as an enzyme or biochemical carrier to ferry the drug across the membrane.

For passive molecular diffusion, Fick's first law of diffusion states that the amount of material (M) flowing through a unit cross-section (S) of a barrier in unit time (t), which is known as the flux (J), is proportional to the concentration gradient (dc/dx).

$$J = \frac{dM}{S \cdot dt}$$

J = flux in $g/cm^2 s$
S = cross section of barrier in cm^2
dM/dt = rate of diffusion in g/s
(M = mass in g; t = time in sec)

The flux is proportional to the concentration gradient, dC/dx:

$$J = -D \frac{dC}{dx}$$

D = diffusion coefficient of a penetrant in cm^2/s
C = concentration in g/cm^3 or g/mL
x = distance in centimeters of movement perpendicular to the surface of the barrier

The diffusion coefficient, D, is a physical chemical property of the drug molecule. It is not constant and can vary with changes in concentration, temperature, pressure, solvent properties, and chemical nature of the diffusant.

Fick's first law of diffusion describes the diffusion process under the condition of *steady state* when the concentration gradient (dc/dx) does not change with time. Figure 1 shows the diaphragm of thickness "h" and cross-sectional area "S" which separates the two compartments of the diffusion cell. Equating both equations for flux, Fick's first law of diffusion may be written as:

$$J = \frac{dM}{S \cdot dt} = \frac{D(C_1 - C_2)}{h}$$

In which $(C_1 - C_2)/h$ approximates dC/dx. Concentrations C_1 and C_2 within the membrane can be replaced by the partition coefficient multiplied by the concentration C_d in the donor compartment or C_r in the receptor compartment. The *partition coefficient*, K, is given by $K = C_1/C_d = C_2/C_r$
Hence,

$$\frac{dM}{dt} = \frac{DSK(C_d - C_r)}{h}$$

Under sink conditions, the drug concentration in the receptor compartment is much lower than the drug

Figure 1.

Concentration gradient of diffusant across a diaphragm of a diffusion cell.

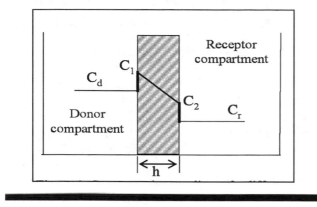

concentration in the donor compartment. Therefore $Cr \rightarrow 0$. The above equation can be simplified as:

$$\frac{dM}{dt} = \frac{DSKC_d}{h} = PSC_d$$

where D is the diffusion coefficient (cm²/s), S is the surface area of the cross section of the barrier (cm²), K is the partition coefficient, C_d is the concentration of drug in the donor compartment (g/mL), h is the barrier thickness (cm), and P is the permeability coefficient (cm/s), where $P = DK/h$.

Drug transport and absorption

A drug travels by *passive transport* from a region of high concentration to a region of low concentration. In contrast, *active transport* of drugs requires an energy source such as an enzyme or biochemical carrier to ferry the drug across the membrane. Active transport can proceed from regions of low concentration to regions of high concentration through the pumping action of these biologic transport systems.

Transport of a drug by diffusion across a membrane such as the gastrointestinal mucosa is represented by Fick's law:

$$-\frac{dM}{dt} = \frac{DmSK}{h}(C_g - C_p)$$

where M is the amount of drug in the gut compartment at time t, D_m is drug diffusivity in intestinal membrane, S is the surface area of GI membrane available for absorption, K is the partition coefficient between the membrane and aqueous medium in the intestine, h is the thickness of the GI membrane, C_g is the drug

concentration in the intestinal compartment, and C_p is the drug concentration in the plasma compartment.

Since the gut compartment usually has a high drug concentration compared to the plasma compartment, C_p may be omitted. Therefore, the above equation then becomes

$$-\frac{dM}{dt} = \frac{DmSK \cdot C_g}{h}$$

This suggests that the rate of gastrointestinal absorption of a drug by passive diffusion depends on the surface area of the membrane available for drug absorption. The small intestine is the major site for drug absorption due to the presence of villi and microvilli, which provide an enormous surface area for absorption.

pH-Partition Theory and Its Limitation

The pH-Partition Theory states that drugs are absorbed from the biological membranes by passive diffusion, depending on the fraction of un-ionized form of the drug at the pH of the fluids close to that biological membrane. The degree of ionization of the drug depends on both the pK_a and the pH of the drug solution. The gastrointestinal tract acts as a lipophilic barrier and thus ionized drugs, compared to un-ionized ones, are more hydrophilic and have minimal membrane transport. The solution pH affects the overall partition coefficient of an ionizable substance. The pK_a of the molecule is the pH at which there is a 50:50 mixture of conjugate acid-base forms. The conjugate acid form predominates at a pH lower than the pK_a, and the conjugate base form is present at a pH higher than that of the pK_a. The extent of ionization of a drug molecule, given by the following **Henderson-Hasselbalch equations**, describe a relationship between ionized and non-ionized species of a weak electrolyte:

Weakly Acidic Drugs	**Weakly Basic Drugs**
$pH = pKa + \log\dfrac{[A-]}{[HA]}$	$pH = pKa + \log\dfrac{[B-]}{[BH^+]}$

Although pH-partition theory is useful, it often does not hold true for certain experimental observations. For example, most weak acids are well-absorbed from the small intestine, which is contrary to the prediction of the pH-partition hypothesis. Similarly, quaternary ammonium compounds are ionized at all pHs, but are readily absorbed from the GI tract. These discrepancies arise because *pH-partition theory does not take into consideration the following (this list is not exhaustive):*

- Large epithelial surface areas of small intestine compensates for ionization effects

- Long residence time in the small intestine also compensates for ionization effects

- Charged drugs, such as quaternary ammonium compounds and tetracyclines, may interact with opposite charged organic ions, resulting in a neutral species, which is absorbable

- Some drugs are absorbed via active transport

The Noyes-Whitney Equation of Dissolution

The rate at which a solid drug of limited water solubility dissolves in a solvent can be determined using the **Noyes-Whitney equation**:

$$\frac{dM}{dt} = k \cdot S \cdot (C_s - C)$$

where dM/dt is the rate of dissolution (mass/time), k is the dissolution rate constant (cm/s) (k = D/h), S is the surface area of exposed solid (cm^2), D is the diffusion coefficient of solute in solution (cm^2/s), h is the thickness of diffusion layer (cm), C_s is the drug solubility (g/mL), and C is the drug concentration in bulk solution at time t (g/mL).

Under *sink conditions* when C is much less than C_s, Noyes-Whitney equation can be simplified as:

$$\frac{dM}{dt} = k\,S\,C_s \quad \text{or} \quad \frac{dC}{dt} = \frac{kSC_s}{V}$$

where dC/dt is the dissolution rate (conc/time) and V is the volume of the dissolution medium (mL)

Factors influencing dissolution rate
- The dissolution rate of a drug may be influenced by the physicochemical conditions in the GI tract. For example, the presence of foods that increase the viscosity of GI fluids decreases the diffusion coefficient, D, of a drug and its dissolution rate.

- The thickness of the diffusion layer, h, is influenced by the degree of agitation experienced by each drug particle in the GI tract. Hence an increase in gastric and/or intestinal motility may increase the dissolution rate of poorly soluble drugs.

- The removal rate of dissolved drugs due to absorption through the GI blood barrier and the GI fluid volume affects drug concentration in the GI tract and thus also affects the dissolution rate.

- The dissolution rate of a weakly acidic drug in GI fluids is influenced by the drug solubility in the diffusion layer surrounding each dissolving drug particle. The pH of the diffusion layer has significant effect on the solubility of a weak electrolyte drug and its subsequent dissolution rate. The dissolution rate of a weakly acidic drug in GI fluid (pH 1-3) is relatively low because of its low solubility in the diffusion layer. If the pH in the diffusion layer could be increased, the solubility (C_s) exhibited by the weak acidic drug in this layer (and hence the dissolution rate of the drug in GI fluids) could be increased. The potassium or sodium salt form of the weakly acidic drug has a relatively high solubility at the elevated pH in the diffusion layer. Thus the dissolution of the drug particles takes place at a faster rate.

- Particle size and the surface area of the drug have significant influence on the drug dissolution rate. An increase in the total effective surface area of drug in contact with GI fluids causes an increase in its dissolution rate. The smaller the particle size, the greater the effective surface area exhibited by a given mass of drug and the higher the dissolution rate. However, particle size reduction is not always helpful and may fail to increase the bioavailability of a drug. In case of certain hydrophobic drugs, excessive particle size reduction tends to cause re-aggregation into larger particles. To prevent the formation of aggregates, small drug particles are dispersed in polyethylene glycol (PEG), polyvinylpyrrolidone (PVP), dextrose, or other agents. For example, a dispersion of griseofulvin in PEG 4000 enhances its dissolution rate and bioavailability. Certain drugs such as penicillin G and erythromycin are unstable in gastric fluids and do not dissolve readily in them. Regarding such drugs, particle size reduction yields an increased rate of drug dissolution in gastric fluid and also increases the extent of drug degradation.

- *Amorphous* or noncrystalline forms of a drug may have faster dissolution rates than crystalline forms.

- Temperature also affects solubility. An increase in temperature will increase the solubility of a solid with a positive heat of solution. The solid will therefore dissolve at a more rapid rate on heating the system.

- Surface active agents will increase the dissolution rates by lowering the interfacial tension, which allows better wetting and penetration by the solvent.

Interfacial Electrical Properties

Most dispersed substances in a solvent such as water acquire a surface electric charge by *ionization, ion adsorption,* and *ion dissolution.*

Ionization
- Surface charge arising from ionization on the particles is the function of the pH of the environment and the pK_a of the drug. Proteins acquire charge through the ionization of carboxyl and amino groups to obtain COO^- and NH_3^+ ions. Ionization of these groups, and the net molecular charge, depends on the pH of the medium. At pH below its isoelectric point (PI), a protein molecule is positively charged, $-NH_2 \rightarrow NH_3^+$, and at pH above its PI, the protein is negatively charged, $-COOH \rightarrow COO^-$. At the isoelectric point of a protein, the total number of positive charges equals the total number of negative charges and the net charge is zero. This may be represented as follows:

$R\text{-}NH_2\text{-}COO^-$	Alkaline solution
$\Updownarrow$	
$R\text{-}NH_3^+\text{-}COO^-$	Isoelectric point (Zwitterion)
$\Updownarrow$	
$R\text{-}NH_3^+\text{-}COOH$	Acidic solution

Often a protein is least soluble at its isoelectric point and is readily precipitated by water-soluble salts such as ammonium sulfate.

Ion adsorption
- A net surface charge can result from the unequal adsorption of oppositely charged ions. Surfaces that are already charged usually show a tendency to adsorb counter-ions. It is possible for counter-ion adsorption to cause a reversal of charge. Surfactants strongly adsorb by hydrophobic effect and thus will determine the surface charge when adsorbed.

Ion dissolution
- Ionic substances can acquire a surface charge by virtue of unequal dissolution of the oppositely charged ions of which they are composed. For example, in a solution of silver iodide with excess $[I^-]$, the silver iodide particles carry a negative charge; however, the charge is positive if excess $[Ag^+]$ is present. The silver and iodide ions are referred to as potential-determining ions since their concentrations determine the electric potential at the particle surface.

Adsorption at solid interfaces
Adsorption of materials at solid interfaces may take place from either an adjacent liquid or gas phase. *Adsorption* is different from *absorption*, since the process of absorption implies the penetration of an entity through the organ and tissues. The degree of adsorption depends on the chemical nature of the adsorbent (a material that is being absorbed onto a substrate, called adsorbate), the chemical nature of the adsorbate, the surface area of the adsorbent, the temperature and the partial pressure of the adsorbed gas. Adsorption can be physical or chemical in nature.

Physical adsorption
- Physical adsorption is rapid, nonspecific, and relatively weak. Furthermore, it is associated with van der Waals attractive forces and is reversible. Removal of the adsorbate from the adsorbent is known as *desorption.* A physically adsorbed gas may be desorbed from a solid by increasing the temperature and reducing the pressure.

Chemical adsorption
- Chemical adsorption or chemisorption is an irreversible process in which the adsorbent is attached to the adsorbsate by primary chemical bonds. Chemisorption is specific, and may require an activation energy; therefore the process is slow and only a monomolecular chemisorbed layer is possible.

Factors affecting adsorption from solution

- *Solubility of adsorbate:* The extent of adsorption of a solute is inversely proportional to its solubility in the solvent from which adsorption occurs.

- *Solute concentration:* An increase in the solute concentration causes an increase in the amount of adsorption that occurs at equilibrium until a limiting value is reached.

- *Temperature:* An increase in temperature leads to decreased adsorption.

- *pH:* The influence of pH is through a change in the ionization and solubility of the adsorbate drug molecule. For many simple small molecules, adsorption increases as the ionization of the drug is suppressed, ie, the extent of adsorption reaches a maximum when the drug is completely un-ionized. For amphoteric compounds, adsorption is at a maximum at the isoelectric point. pH and solubility effects act in concert since the un-ionized form of most drugs in aqueous solution has a low solubility.

- *Surface area of adsorbent:* An increased surface area, achieved by a reduction in particle size or the use of a porous adsorbing material, increases the extent of adsorption.

Rheology

Rheology is *the study of flow properties* of liquids and deformation of solids. The flow of simple liquids can be described by viscosity, an expression of the resistance to flow; however, other complex dispersions cannot be simply expressed by viscosity.

According to *Newton's law of flow,* the rate of flow (D) is directly proportional to the applied stress (τ). That is, $\tau = \eta \cdot D$, where η is the viscosity. Fluids that obey Newton's law of flow are referred to as *Newtonian fluids* and fluids which deviate are known as *non-Newtonian fluids.* The force per unit area (F′/A)

shearing stress gives a straight line (Figure 2A), thus η is a constant. In the case of Newtonian fluids, viscosity does not change with increasing shear rate. Various types of water and pharmaceutical dosage forms that contain a high percentage of water are examples of liquid dosage forms that have Newtonian flow properties.

Most pharmaceutical fluids (including colloidal dispersions, emulsions, and liquid suspensions) do not follow Newton's law of flow, and the viscosity of the fluid varies with the rate of shear. There are three types of non-Newtonian flow: *plastic, pseudoplastic,* and *dilatant* (Figure 2B, C, and D).

Plastic flow
Substances that undergo plastic flow are called *Bingham bodies,* which are defined as substances that

Figure 2.

Plots of rate of shear as a function of shearing stress for (A) Newtonian, (B) plastic, (C) pseudoplastic, (D) dilatant, and (E) thixotropic flow.

required to bring about flow is called the shearing stress (F):

$$F = \frac{F'}{A} = \eta \frac{dv}{dr}$$

where η is the viscosity, dv/dr is the rate of shear = G (s^{-1}), and F′/A units are in dynes per cm.^{2} For simple Newtonian fluids, a plot of the rate of shear against

exhibit a yield value (Figure 2B). Plastic flow is associated with the presence of flocculated particles in concentrated suspensions.

- Plastic flow does not begin until a shearing stress, corresponding to a *yield value*, f, is exceeded.

- The curve intersects the shearing stress axis but does not cross through the origin.

- The materials are said to be "elastic" at shear stresses below the yield value.

- Viscosity decreases with increasing shear rate at shear stress below the yield value.

Flocculated solids

Flocculated solids are light, fluffy conglomerates of adjacent particles held together by weak van der Waals forces. The yield value exists because a certain shearing stress must be exceeded in order to break up van der Waals forces. A plastic system resembles a Newtonian system at shear stresses above the yield value. Yield value, f, is an indicator of flocculation (higher yield value, greater degree of flocculation).

Pseudoplastic flow

Pseudoplastic flow is exhibited by polymers in solution. A large of number of pharmaceutical products, including natural and synthetic gums (eg, liquid dispersions of tragacanth, sodium alginate, methyl cellulose, and sodium carboxymethylcellulose) exhibit *pseudoplastic flow properties.*

- Pseudoplastic substances begin flow when a shearing stress is applied, ie, there is no yield value (it does cross the origin).

- Viscosity of a pseudoplastic substance decreases with increasing shear rate.

- With increasing shearing stress, the rate of shear increases; these materials are called *shear-thinning* systems.

- Shear thinning occurs when molecules (polymers) align themselves along their long axes and slip and slide past each other.

Dilatant flow

Certain suspensions with a high percentage of dispersed solids exhibit an increase in resistance to flow with increasing rates of shear. This type of behavior may be exhibited by dispersions containing a high percentage ($\geq$50%) of small, deflocculated particles.

- Dilatant materials *increase in volume* when sheared.

- They are also known as *shear-thickening* systems (opposite of pseudoplastic systems).

- When the stress is removed, the dilatant system returns to its original state of fluidity.

- Viscosity increases with increasing shear rate.

- Dilatant materials may solidify under conditions of high shear.

Thixotropy

Thixotropy is a nonchemical isothermal gel-sol-gel transformation. If a thixotropic gel is sheared (by simple shaking), the weak bonds are broken and a lyophobic solution is formed. On standing the particles collide, flocculation occurs, and the gel is reformed. The advantage that thixotropic preparations have is that the particles remain in suspension during storage, but when required for use, the pastes are readily made fluid by tapping or shaking. The shearing force on the injection as it is pushed through the needle ensures that it is fluid when injected; however, the rapid resumption of the gel structure prevents excessive spreading in the tissues, and consequently a more compact depot is produced than with nonthixotropic suspensions. Flow curves (rheograms) for thixotropic materials are highly dependent on the rate at which shear is increased or decreased and the length of time a sample is subjected to any one rate of shear.

Negative thixotropy

Negative thixotropy is also known as antithixotropy, which represents an increase rather than a decrease in consistency on the down-curve (an increase in thickness or resistance to flow with an increased time of shear). It may result from an increased collision frequency of dispersed particles (or polymer molecules) in suspension, which causes increased interparticle bonding with time.

Shelf-life Stability of a Drug Product

The shelf life of a drug in a dosage form is the amount of time that the product can be stored before it becomes unfit for use because of chemical decomposition and/or physical deterioration. Shelf-life stability of a dosage form can be determined by the Arrhenius equation given below:

$$k = A\, e^{\,Ev/RT}, \text{ which can rewritten as}$$

$$\log \frac{k_2}{k_1} = \frac{Ea(T_2 - T_1)}{2.303 R T_2 T_1}$$

where k_2 and k_1 are the reaction rates at the absolute temperatures T_2 and T_1, respectively, R is gas constant (1.987 cal/Kmol), E_v is the activation energy (cal/mol), and A is the constant (based on molecular weight and molar volume of liquid).

2. Surfactants and Micelles

Surface active agents or surfactants have two distinct regions in one chemical structure. One area is hydrophilic ("water-liking"); another is hydrophobic ("water-hating"). The existence of two such moieties in a molecule is known as amphipathy and the molecules are consequently referred to as amphipathic molecules or amphiphiles. Depending on the number and nature of the polar and nonpolar groups present, the amphiphile may be predominantly hydrophilic, lipophilic, or somewhere in between. For example, straight chain alcohols, amines, and acids are amphiphiles that change from being predominantly hydrophilic to lipophilic as the number of carbon atoms in the alkyl chain is increased. The hydrophobic portions are usually saturated or unsaturated hydrocarbon chains, or, less commonly, heterocyclic or aromatic ring systems.

Surfactants are classified according to the nature of the hydrophilic or hydrophobic groups. In addition, some surfactants possess both positively and negatively charged groups, and can exist as either anionic or cationic, depending on the pH of the solution. These surfactants are known as *ampholytic* compounds.

At low concentrations in solutions, amphiphiles exist as monomers. As the concentration is increased, aggregation occurs over a narrow concentration range. These aggregates, which may contain 50 or more monomers, are called *micelles.* Therefore, micelles are small spherical structures composed of both hydrophilic and hydrophobic regions. The micelles are in dynamic equilibrium with free molecules (monomers) in solution, ie, the micelles are continuously breaking down and reforming. The concentration of monomer at which micelles are formed is called the *critical micellization concentration,* or *CMC.* Surface tension decreases up to the CMC, but remains constant above the CMC. The longer the hydrophobic chain or the lower the polarity of the polar group, the greater the tendency for monomers to "escape" from the water to form micelles and hence lower the CMC.

Types of Micelles

In the case of amphiphiles in water, in dilute solution (still above but close to the CMC) the micelles are considered to be *spherical* in shape. At higher concentrations they become more asymmetric and eventually assume *cylindrical* or *lamellar* structures. More oil-soluble surfactants have a tendency to self-associate into "*reverse micelles*" in nonpolar solvents, with their polar groups oriented away from the solvent.

Factors Affecting CMC and Micellar Size

- Structure of hydrophobic group

- Nature of hydrophilic group: an increase in chain length increases hydrophilicity and the CMC

- Nature of counter ions: $Cl^- < Br^- < I^-$ for cationic surfactants and $Na^+ < K^+$ for anionic surfactants

- Addition of electrolytes to ionic surfactants decreases the CMC and increases the micellar size. In contrast, micellar properties of nonionic surfactants are only minimally affected by the addition of electrolytes.

- Effect of temperature

HLB (Hydrophile-Lipophile Balance) Systems

Griffin's method of selecting emulsifying agents is based on the balance between the hydrophilic and lipophilic portions of the emulsifying agent; this is now widely known as the hydrophile-lipophile balance (HLB) system. The higher the HLB value of an emulsifying agent, the more hydrophilic it is. The emulsifying agents with lower HLB values are less polar and more lipophilic. The Spans, ie, sorbitan esters, are lipophilic and have low HLB values (1.8-8.6); the Tweens, polyoxyethylene derivatives of the Spans, are hydrophilic and have high HLB values (9.6-16.7). Surfactants with the proper balance of hydrophilic and lipophilic affinities are effective emulsifying agents since they concentrate at the oil-water interface. The type of an emulsion that is produced depends primarily on the property of the emulsifying agent. The HLB of an emulsifier or a combination of emulsifiers determines whether an o/w or w/o emulsion results. In general, o/w emulsions are formed when the HLB of the emulsifier is within the range of about 9-12; w/o emulsions are formed when the range is about 3-6. The type of emulsion is a function of the relative solubility of the supernatant. An emulsifying agent with high HLB is preferentially soluble in water and results in the formation of an o/w emulsion. The reverse situation is true with surfactants of low HLB value, which tend to form w/o emulsions.

3. Dispersed Systems

Dispersed systems consist of particulate matter, known as the *dispersed phase*, distributed throughout a *continuous* or *dispersion* medium. The particulate matter, or dispersed phase, consists of particles that range from 1 nm to 0.5 mm (10^{-9} m to 5×10^{-7} m). Dispersed systems are classified as follows:

- *Molecular dispersions:* <1 nm, invisible under electron microscopy (EM). Examples are oxygen molecules, ions, and glucose.

- *Colloidal dispersions:* 1 nm to 0.5 mm, visible under EM. Examples are colloidal silver sols and natural and synthetic polymers.

- *Coarse dispersions:* larger than 0.5 mm, visible under light microscopy. Examples are grains of sand, emulsions, suspensions, and red blood cells.

Types of Colloidal Systems

Colloidal systems are classified as lyophilic or lyophobic. Their association is based on the interaction of the particles or molecules of the dispersed phase with the molecules of the dispersion medium.

Lyophilic colloids
Systems containing colloidal particles that interact with the dispersion medium are referred to as *lyophilic colloids*. Because of their affinity for the dispersion medium, such materials form colloidal dispersions with relative ease. For example, the dissolution of acacia or gelatin in water or celluloid in amyl acetate leads to the formation of a solution. Most lyophilic colloids are polymers (eg, gelatin, acacia, povidone, albumin, rubber, and polystyrene).

Lyophobic colloids
Lyophobic colloids, or inorganic particles dispersed in water, are composed of materials that have little attraction, if any, for the dispersion medium. Lyophobic colloids are intrinsically unstable and irreversible.

Association colloids
Association (referring to amphiphilic colloids) *colloids* are formed by the grouping or association of amphiphiles, ie, molecules that exhibit both lyophilic and lyophobic properties. At low concentrations, amphiphiles exist separately and do not form a colloid. At higher concentrations, aggregation occurs at around 50 or more monomers, which induces micelle formation. As with lyophilic colloids, formation of association colloids is spontaneous, provided that the concentration of the amphiphile in solution exceeds the CMC.

Zeta Potential and Its Effect on Colloidal Stability

Zeta (ζ) potential is defined as the difference in potential between the surface of the tightly bound layer (shear plane) and the electroneutral region of the solution. The ζ potential governs the degree of repulsion between adjacent, similarly charged, dispersed particles. If ζ potential is reduced below a certain value, the attractive forces exceed the repulsive forces, and the particles come together. This phenomenon is known as flocculation.

Stabilization is accomplished by providing the dispersed particles with an electric charge and a protective solvent sheath surrounding each particle to prevent mutual adherence due to collision. This second effect is significant only in the case of lyophilic colloids. Lyophilic and association colloids are thermodynamically stable and exist in a true solution so that the system constitutes a single phase. In contrast, lyophobic colloids are thermodynamically unstable, but can be stabilized by preventing aggregation/coagulation by providing the dispersed particles with an electric charge, which can prevent coagulation by repulsion of like particles.

4. Pharmaceutical Ingredients

To turn a drug substance into a pharmaceutical dosage form or a drug delivery system, pharmaceutical ingredients are required. For example, in the preparation of tablets, *diluents* or *fillers* are commonly added to increase the bulk of the formulation. *Binders* are added to promote adhesion of the powdered drug to other ingredients. *Lubricants* assist the smooth tabletting process. *Disintegrants* promote tablet break-up after administration. *Coatings* improve stability, control disintegration, or enhance appearance. Similarly, in the preparation of pharmaceutical solutions, *preservatives* are added to prevent microbial growth, *stabilizers* are added to prevent drug decomposition, and *colorants* and *flavorants* are added to ensure product

appeal. Thus for each dosage form, the pharmaceutical ingredients establish the primary features of the product and control the physicochemical properties, drug release profiles, and bioavailability of the product. Table 1 lists some typical pharmaceutical ingredients used in different dosage forms.

Table 1

Typical Pharmaceutical Ingredients

Ingredient type	Definition	Examples
Antifungal preservatives	Used in liquid and semisolid formulations to prevent growth of fungi	Anti-fungal: benzoic acid, butylparaben, ethylparaben, sodium benzoate, sodium propionate
Antimicrobial preservatives	Used in liquid and semi-solid formulations to prevent growth of microorganisms	Benzalkonium chloride, benzyl alcohol, cetylpyridinium chloride, phenyl ethyl alcohol
Antioxidant	Used to prevent oxidation	Ascorbic acid, ascorbyl palmitate, sodium ascorbate, sodium bisulfate, sodium metabisulfite
Emulsifying agent	Used to promote and maintain dispersion of finely divided droplets of a liquid in a vehicle in which it is immiscible	Acacia, cetyl alcohol, glyceryl monostearate, sorbitan monostearate
Surfactant	Used to reduce surface or interfacial tension	Polysorbate 80, sodium lauryl sulfate, sorbitan monopalmitate
Plasticizer	Used to enhance coat spread over tablets, beads and granules	Glycerin, diethyl palmitate
Suspending agent	Used to reduce sedimentation rate of drug particles dispersed throughout a vehicle in; they are not soluble	Carbopol, hydroxymethylcellulose, hydroxypropyl cellulose, methylcellulose, tragacanth
Binders	Used to cause adhesion of powder particles in tablet granulations	Acacia, alginic acid, ethylcellulose, starch, povidone
Diluent	Used as fillers to create desired bulk, flow properties, and compression characteristics in tablet and capsule preparations	Kaolin, lactose, mannitol, cellulose, sorbitol, starch
Disintegrant	Used to promote disruption of solid mass into small particles	Microcrystalline cellulose, carboxymethylcellulose calcium, sodium alginate, sodium starch glycollate, alginic acid
Glidant	Used to improve flow properties of powder mixture	Colloidal silica, cornstarch, talc
Lubricant	Used to reduce friction during tablet compression and facilitate ejection of tablets from the die cavity	Calcium stearate, magnesium stearate, mineral oil, stearic acid, zinc stearate
Humectant	Used for prevention of dryness of ointments and creams	Glycerin, propylene glycol, sorbitol

5. Types of Commonly Used Dosage Forms

Solutions, Syrups, and Elixirs

Solutions are homogeneous mixtures of one or more solutes dispersed in a dissolving medium (solvent). Aqueous solutions containing a sugar or sugar substitute with or without added flavoring agents and drugs are classified as *syrups*. Sweetened hydroalcoholic (combinations of water and ethanol) solutions are termed *elixirs*. Hydroalcoholic solutions of aromatic materials are termed *spirits*. Solutions intended for oral administration usually contain flavorants and colorants to make the medication more attractive and palatable to the patient. They may contain stabilizers to maintain the physicochemical stability of the drug and preservatives to prevent the growth of microorganisms in the solution. A drug dissolved in an aqueous solution is in the most bioavailable form. Since the drug is already in solution, no dissolution step is necessary before systemic absorption occurs. Solutions that are prepared to be sterile, pyrogen-free, and intended for parenteral administration are classified as *injectables*.

Some drugs, particularly certain antibiotics, have insufficient stability in aqueous solution to withstand long shelf-lives. These drugs, formulated as dry powder or granule dosage forms, are reconstituted with purified water immediately before dispensing to the patient. The dry powder mixture contains all of the formulation components (ie, drug, flavorant, colorant, buffers, and others, except for the solvent). Examples of dry powder mixtures intended for reconstitution to make oral solutions include cloxacillin sodium, nafcillin sodium, oxacillin sodium, penicillin V potassium, and potassium chloride.

Sucrose is the sugar most frequently employed in syrups; in special circumstances it may be replaced in whole or in part by other sugars (eg, dextrose) or nonsugars (eg, sorbitol, glycerin, and propylene glycol). Most syrups consist of between 60 and 80% sucrose. Sucrose not only provides sweetness and viscosity to the solution; it renders the solution inherently stable (unlike dilute sucrose solutions, which are unstable).

Elixirs are usually less sweet and less viscous than syrups. Since elixirs contain a lower proportion of sugar, they are consequently less effective than syrups in masking the taste of drugs. In contrast to aqueous syrups, elixirs are better able to maintain both water-soluble and alcohol-soluble components in solution due to their hydroalcoholic properties. These stable characteristics often make elixirs preferable to syrups.

All elixirs contain flavoring and coloring agents to enhance their palatability and appearance. Elixirs containing over 10-12% alcohol are usually self-preserving and do not require the addition of antimicrobial agents for preservation. Alcohols precipitate tragacanth, acacia, agar, and inorganic salts from aqueous solutions; therefore such substances should either be absent from the aqueous phase or present in such low concentrations so as not to promote precipitation on standing. Examples of some commonly used elixirs include dexamethasone elixir USP, pentobarbital elixir USP, diphenhydramine HCl elixir, and digoxin elixir.

Tablets

Depending on the physicochemical properties of the drug, site and extent of drug absorption in the gastrointestinal (GI) tract, stability to heat or moisture, biocompatibility with other ingredients, solubility, and dose, the following types of tablets are commonly formulated.

- *Tablets that are swallowed whole*

- *Effervescent tablets* that need to be dissolved in water prior to administration

- *Chewable tablets* are used when a faster rate of dissolution and/or buccal absorption is desired. Chewable tablets consist of a mild effervescent drug complex dispersed throughout a gum base. The drug is released from the dosage form by physical disruption associated with chewing, chemical disruption caused by the interaction with the fluids in the oral cavity, and the presence of effervescent material. For example, antacid tablets should be chewed to obtain quick indigestion relief.

- *Buccal and sublingual tablets* dissolve slowly in the mouth, cheek pouch (buccal), or under the tongue (sublingual). Buccal or sublingual absorption is often desirable for drugs subject to extensive hepatic metabolism, often referred to as the *first-pass effect*. Examples are isoprenaline sulfate (bronchodilator), glyceryl trinitrate (vasodilator), nitroglycerin, and testosterone tablets. These tablets do not contain a disintegrant and are compressed lightly to produce a fairly soft tablet.

- *Controlled-release tablets* are used to improve patient compliance and to reduce side effects. Some water-soluble drugs are formulated as sustained-release tablets so that their release and dissolution is controlled over a long period. A hydrophobic matrix composed of carnauba wax and partially hydrogenated cottonseed oil were used to prepare sustained-release tablets of a highly water-soluble drug, ABT-089, a cholinergic channel modulator for the treatment of cognitive disorders. Theo-Dur® is a controlled-release tablet of theophylline and consists of two components: a matrix of compressed theophylline crystals and coated theophylline granules embedded in the matrix. In contact with fluid, theophylline diffuses slowly through the wall of the free granules, which dissolves with time. After oral administration of Theo-Dur 300 mg tablets to human subjects, serum theophylline concentrations over 1 mg/mL were maintained over 24 hours. To provide a zero-order release of ibuprofen, core-in-cup tablets were developed by compressing the mixture of ethyl cellulose and carnauba wax, followed by compression with core tablets containing ibuprofen. Drugs with unpleasant flavors that irritate the stomach walls are formulated inside the tablets so as to be bound to ion-exchange resins and coated with a water-insoluble polymer membrane made of ethylcellulose or a similar substance. These drugs include codeine, dextromethorphan, acetaminophen, ephedrine, and chlorpheniramine. Aspirin has been shown to produce less gastric bleeding when formulated as a sustained-release formulation than conventional tablets. The combination of high- and low-viscosity grades of hydroxypropylmethylcellulose (HPMC) was used as the matrix base to prepare diclofenac sodium and zileuton sustained-release tablets. A ternary polymeric matrix system composed of protein, HPMC, and highly water-soluble drugs such as diltiazem HCl was developed by the direct compression method. Xanthan gum was used for a hydrophilic matrix for sustained release ibuprofen tablets. Sustained-release tablets can also be prepared by formulating inert polymers like polyvinyl chloride, polyvinyl acetate, and methyl methacrylate. These polymers protect the tablet from disintegration and also reduce the dissolution rate of the drug inside the tablet. Examples of commonly used sustained-release drug delivery products are listed in Table 2.

- **Coated tablets.** There are several types of coated tablets: film coated, sugar coated, gelatin coated (gel caps), or **enteric-coated tablets.** Enteric coatings are resistant to gastric juices, but readily dissolve in the small intestine. These enteric coatings can protect drugs against decomposition in the acid environment of the stomach. Commonly used polymers for enteric coating are acid-impermeable polymers, such as cellulose acetate trimellitate (CAT), hydroxypropylmethylcellulosephthalate (HPMCP), polyvinyl acetate phthalate (PVAP), cellulose acetate phthalate (CAP) and Eudragit®. Aspirin has been shown to produce less gastric bleeding when formu-

lated as enteric-coated sustained-release tablets than conventional aspirin preparations. Film-coated tablets are compressed tablets that are coated with a thin layer of a water insoluble or water soluble polymer, such as HPMC, ethylcellulose, povidone or polyethylene glycol. Abacavir™ is a capsule-shaped film-coated tablet containing a nucleoside reverse transcriptase inhibitor, which is a potent antiviral agent for the treatment of HIV infection.

Tablet formulation

In addition to the drug, the following materials are added to make the powder system compatible with tablet formulation by the compression or granulation methods:

- **Diluents.** A tablet should weigh at least 50 mg and therefore very low-dose drugs invariably require a diluent or bulking agent to bring overall table weight to at least 50 mg. Commonly used diluents are lactose, dicalcium phosphate, starches, microcrystalline cellulose (MCC), dextrose, sucrose, mannitol, and sodium chloride. Dicalcium phosphate absorbs less moisture than lactose and is therefore used with hygroscopic drugs such as pethidine hydrochloride.

- **Adsorbents** are substances capable of holding quantities of fluids in an apparently dry state. Oil-soluble drugs or fluid extracts can be mixed with adsorbents and then granulated and compressed into tablets. Examples are fumed silica, microcrystalline cellulose, magnesium carbonate, kaolin, and bentonite.

- **Moistening agents** are liquids that are used for wet granulation. Examples include water, industrial methylated spirits, and isopropanol.

- **Binding agents (adhesives)** bind powders together in the wet granulation process. They also help bind granules together during compression. Examples include starch, gelatin, polyvinylpyrrolidone, alginic acid derivatives, cellulose derivatives, glucose, and sucrose. Choice of binders affects the dissolution rate. For example, the tablet formulation of furosemide with PVP as the binder has t_{50} (time required for 50% of the drug to be released during an in vitro dissolution study) of 3.65 minutes, but with starch mucilage as the binder, the t_{50} of the tablets was 117 minutes.

- **Glidants** are added to tablet formulations to improve the flow properties of the granulations. They act by reducing interparticulate friction. Commonly used glidants are fumed (colloidal) silica, starch, and talc.

Table 2

Examples of Sustained-Release Drug Delivery Products

Dosage forms	Manufacturer	Active ingredients	Indications
Controlled-release tablets			
Theo-Dur™	ALZA Corp.	Theophylline	Asthma
Abacavir™ (Ziagen)	GlaxoWellcome Inc	Nucleoside reverse transcriptase inhibitor	HIV-1 infection
Sinemet®	Bristol Myers Squibb	Carbidopa + levodopa	Parkinson's disease
Volmax®	ALZA Corp.	Albuterol	Bronchospasm
Voltaren®	Novartis	Diclofenac sodium	Osteoarthritis and rheumatoid arthritis
Efidac 24®	ALZA Corp.	Chlorpheniramine	Allergy symptom and nasal congestion
DynaCirc® CR	ALZA Corp.	Isradipine	Hypertension
Capsules			
Dexedrine Spansules®	SmithKline Beecham	Dextroamphetamine	Narcolepsy
Adderal XL®	Shire Pharmaceuticals	Amphetamine + dextroamphetamine	Attention deficit hyperactivity disorder (ADHD)
Ritalin LA®	Novartis	Methylphenidate hydrochloride	ADHD
VIDEX® EC	Bristol Myers Squibb	Didanosine	HIV-1 infection
Aerosols			
Ventolin HFA	GlaxoSmithKline	Albuterol sulfate	Bronchodilator
Azmacort®	Adventis	Triamcinolone acetonide	Asthma
Serevent®	GlaxoSmithKline	Salmeterol	Bronchodilator
Osmotic system			
Oros® System	ALZA Corp.	Oral delivery of different drugs	
Ditropan XL®	ALZA Corp.	Oxybutynin chloride	Overreacting bladder
Covera-HS®	ALZA Corp.	Verapamil	Antihypertensive
Concerta®	ALZA Corp.	Methylphenidate HCl	Attention deficit hyperactivity disorder (ADHD)
DURO® implant systems			
Viadur®	ALZA Corp.	Leuprolide	Prostate cancer
Inserts			
Pilocarpine Occusert™	ALZA Corp.	Pilocarpine	Glaucoma
Lacrisert™	ALZA Corp.	Hydroxypropyl cellulose	Ophthalmic moisturizer
Progestasert®	ALZA Corp.	Progesterone	Contraceptive
Atridox™	ALZA Corp.	Doxycycline	Periodontal disease
Transdermal patches			
Alora®	Watson Pharmaceuticals, Inc.	Estradiol	Menopausal symptoms
CambiPatch™	Novartis	Estradiol/norethindrone acetate	Vasomotor symptoms associated with menopause
Androderm®	Watson Pharmaceuticals, Inc.	Testosterone	Testosterone deficiency
Nicotine transdermal system	Watson Pharmaceuticals, Inc.	Nicotine	Smoking cessation
PEGylated proteins			
PEG-Intron™	Schering-Plough	PEGylated interferon	Hepatitis C
Pegasys™	Roche	PEGylated interferon + ribavirin	Hepatitis B, hepatitis C
Liposomes			
DoxilTM	ALZA Corp.	Doxorubicin HCl	Kaposi's sarcoma
DaunoXome®	NeXstar Pharmaceuticals	Daunorubicin	Kaposi's sarcoma
PLGA/PLA microspheres			
Lupron Depot®	TAP Pharmaceuticals	Luteinizing hormone-releasing hormone agonist	Prostate cancer, endometriosis
Zoladex Depot®	AstraZeneca	Goserelin acetate	Prostate cancer, endometriosis
Nutropin Depot®	Genentech	Recombinant human growth hormone	Growth deficiencies

- *Lubricants* are required to prevent adherence of the granules to the punch faces and dies. They also ensure smooth ejection of the tablet from the die. Many lubricants also enhance the flow properties of the granules. Commonly used lubricants are magnesium stearate, talc, stearic acid and its derivatives, PEG, paraffin, and sodium or magnesium lauryl sulfate. Among these, magnesium stearate is the most popular lubricant, as it is effective as both a die and punch lubricant. However, for many drugs, magnesium stearate is chemically incompatible (eg, aspirin) and therefore talc or stearic acid is often used.

- *Disintegrating agents* are added to the tablets to promote breakup of the tablets when placed in the aqueous environment. This increases the effective surface area of drug particles to the GI fluid and promotes rapid release of the drug. Disintegrants act by either bursting open the tablet and/or by promoting the rapid ingress of water into the center of the tablet or capsule. Examples include starch, cationic exchange resins, cross-linked polyvinylpyrrolidone, celluloses, modified starches, alginic acid and alginates, magnesium aluminum silicate, and cross-linked sodium carboxymethylcellulose. Among them, starch is the most popular disintegrant, as it has a great affinity for water and swells when moistened, thus facilitating the rupture of the tablet matrix.

Disintegration, dissolution, and absorption

Following oral administration, a tablet or other solid dosage form disintegrates into granules, and these granules deaggregate in turn into fine particles. Disintegration, deaggregation, and dissolution may occur simultaneously with the release of a drug from the tablet. The effectiveness of a tablet in releasing its drug for systemic absorption depends on the rate of disintegration of the dosage forms and deaggregation of the granules. A solid drug product has to disintegrate into small particles and release the drug before absorption can take place. However, tablets that are intended for chewing or sustained release do not have to undergo disintegration. The various excipients for tablet formulation affect the rates of disintegration, dissolution, and absorption. Systemic absorption of most products consists of a succession of rate processes, such as

- disintegration of the drug product and subsequent release of drug,

- dissolution of the drug in an aqueous environment, and

- absorption across cell membranes into the systemic circulation.

Rate-limiting step for absorption

In the process of tablet disintegration, dissolution, and absorption, the rate at which drug reaches the circulatory system is determined by the slowest step in the sequence. Disintegration of a tablet is usually more rapid than drug dissolution and absorption. For the drug that has poor aqueous solubility, the rate at which the drug dissolves (dissolution) is often the slowest step, and therefore exerts a rate-limiting effect on drug bioavailability. In contrast, for the drug that has a high aqueous solubility, the dissolution rate is rapid and the rate at which the drug crosses or permeates cell membranes is the slowest or rate-limiting step.

Capsules

Capsules are solid dosage forms in which the drug substance is enclosed in either a hard or soft, water-soluble container or shell of gelatin. *Coating* of capsule shell or drug particles within the capsule can affect bioavailability. There are two types of capsules: hard and soft capsules; however, hard gelatin capsules are more versatile for controlled drug delivery.

Hard gelatin capsules

A hard gelatin capsule consists of two pieces, a cap and a body, that fit one inside the other. They are produced empty and are then filled in a separate operation. Hard gelatin capsules are usually filled with powders, granules, or pellets containing the drug. After ingestion, the gelatin shell softens, swells, and begins to dissolve in the gastrointestinal tract. Encapsulated drugs are released rapidly and dispersed easily, leading to high bioavailability. Capsules are supplied in a variety of sizes, and high-speed filling machinery capable of filling ~1500 capsules per minute is available. The hard gelatin empty capsules are numbered from 000, the largest size, to 5, which is the smallest. The approximate filling capacity of capsules ranges from 6000 to 30 mg, depending on the types and bulk densities of powdered drug materials.

Formulation of hard gelatin capsules

Powder formulations for encapsulation into hard gelatin capsules require a careful consideration of the filling process, such as lubricity, compactibility, and fluidity. Additives present in the capsule formulations, such as amount and choice of fillers and lubricants, inclusion of disintegrants and surfactants, and the degree of plug compaction, can influence drug release from the capsule. Formulation factors influencing drug release and bioavailability are as follows:

- *Fillers (or diluents).* Active ingredient is mixed with a sufficient volume of a diluent, usually lactose, mannitol, starch, and dicalcium phosphate, to yield the desired amount of the drug in the capsule when the base is filled with the powder mixture.

- *Glidants.* The flow properties of the powder blend should be adequate to assure a uniform flow rate from the hopper. Glidants such as silica, starch, talc, and magnesium stearate are used to improve the fluidity. The optimal concentration of the glidant used to improve the flow of a powder mixture is generally less than 1%.

- *Lubricants* ease the ejection of plugs by reducing adhesion of powder to metal surfaces and friction between sliding surfaces in contact with powder. Typical lubricants for capsule formulations include magnesium stearate and stearic acid.

- *Surfactants* may be included in capsule formulations to increase wetting of the powder mass and enhance drug dissolution. The most commonly used surfactants in capsule formulations are 0.1-0.5% of sodium lauryl sulfate and sodium docusate.

- *Hydrophilization.* Another approach for improving the wettability of poorly soluble drugs is to treat the drug with a hydrophilic polymer solution. Powder wettability and dissolution rate of several drugs including hexobarbital and phenytoin from hard gelatin capsules have been shown to be enhanced if the drug is treated with methylcellulose or hydroxyethylcellulose.

Vancomycin HCl is highly hygroscopic antibiotic. To achieve acceptable stability, Eli Lilly has developed a hard gelatin capsule filled with a PEG 6000 matrix of vancomycin HCl, which produces plasma and urine levels of the antibiotic similar to those obtained with the solution of vancomycin HCl. Controlled-release beads and minitablets are often filled into gelatin capsules for convenient administration of an oral controlled-release dosage form. For example, sustained-release antihistamines, antitussives, and analgesics are first preformulated into extended-release microcapsules or microspheres and then placed inside a gelatin capsule. Another example is enteric-coated lipase minitablets that are placed in a gelatin capsule for more effective protection and dosing of these enzymes.

Soft gelatin capsules

Soft gelatin capsules are prepared from plasticized gelatin by a rotary die process in which they are formed, filled, and sealed in a single operation. Soft gelatin capsules may contain a nonaqueous solution, a powder, or a drug suspension, none of which solubilize the gelatin shell. In contrast to hard gelatin capsules, soft gelatin capsules contain ~30% glycerol as a plasticizer in addition to gelatin and water. The moisture uptake of soft gelatin capsules plasticized with glycerol is considerably higher than that of hard gelatin capsules. Therefore oxygen-sensitive drugs should not be inserted into soft gelatin capsules; nor should emulsions, since they are unstable and crack the shell of the capsule when the water is lost in the manufacturing process. Extreme acidic and basic pH must also be avoided, since a pH below 2.5 hydrolyzes gelatin, while a pH above 9 has a tanning effect on the gelatin. Insoluble drugs should be dispersed with an agent such as beeswax, paraffin, or ethylcellulose. Surfactants are also often added to promote wetting of the ingredients. Drugs that are commercially prepared in soft capsules include declomycin, chlorotrianisene, digoxin, vitamin A, vitamin E, and chloral hydrate.

Formulation of soft gelatin capsules
Formulation of soft gelatin capsules involves liquid, rather than powder, technology. It requires careful consideration of the composition of the gelatin shell and filling materials. The composition of the soft capsule shell consists of two main ingredients: gelatin and a plasticizer. Water is used to form the capsule and other additives are often added as described below:

- *Gelatin.* Properties of gelatin shells are controlled by choice of gelatin grade and by adjusting the concentration of plasticizer in the shell.

- *Plasticizers.* The main plasticizer used for soft gelatin capsules is glycerol. Sorbitol and polypropylene glycol are also used in combination with glycerol. Compared to hard gelatin capsules and tablet film coatings, a relatively large amount (~30%) of plasticizers are added in soft gelatin capsule formulation to ensure adequate flexibility.

- *Water.* The desirable water content of the gelatin solution used to produce a soft gelatin capsule shell depends on the viscosity of gelatin used and ranges between 0.7 and 1.3 parts of water to each part of dry gelatin.

- *Other additives.* Preservatives are added to prevent mold growth in the gelatin shell. Potassium sorbate, and methyl, ethyl, and propyl hydroxybenzoate are commonly used as preservatives.

Emulsions

An emulsion is a thermodynamically unstable system consisting of at least two immiscible liquid phases, one of which is dispersed as globules (*dispersed phase*) in the other liquid phase (*continuous phase*), stabilized by the presence of an emulsifying agent. Emulsified systems range from *lotions* of relatively low viscosity, to *ointments* and creams, which are semisolid in nature.

Types of emulsions
One liquid phase in an emulsion is essentially polar (eg, aqueous), while the other is relatively nonpolar (eg, an oil).

- *Oil-in-water (o/w) emulsion:* When the oil phase is dispersed as globules throughout an aqueous continuous phase, the system is referred to as an oil-in-water (o/w) emulsion.

- *Water-in-oil (w/o) emulsion:* When the oil phase serves as the continuous phase, the emulsion is termed an water-in-oil (w/o) emulsion.

- *Multiple (w/o/w or o/w/o) emulsions:* These are emulsions whose dispersed phase contains droplets of another phase. Multiple emulsions are of interest as delayed-action drug delivery systems.

- *Microemulsions:* These consist of homogeneous transparent systems of low viscosity which contain a high percentage of both oil and water and high concentrations of emulsifier mixture. Microemulsions form spontaneously when the components are mixed in the appropriate ratios and are thermodynamically stable.

Externally applied emulsions may be o/w or w/o. The o/w emulsions employ the following *emulsifiers:* Sodium lauryl sulfate, triethanolamine stearate, sodium oleate, and glyceryl monostearate. The w/o emulsions are used mainly for external applications and may contain one or several of the following emulsifiers: calcium palmitate, sorbitan esters (Spans), cholesterol, and wool fats.

Interfacial free energy and emulsification
Two immiscible liquids in emulsions often fail to remain mixed due to the greater cohesive force between the molecules of each separate liquid than the adhesive force between the two liquids. This leads to phase separation, which is the state of minimum surface free energy. When one liquid is broken into small particles, the interfacial area of the globules constitutes a surface that is enormous compared with the surface area of the original liquid. The adsorption of a surfactant or other emulsifying agent at the globule interface lowers the oil-to-water or water-to-oil interfacial tension. In addition, the process of emulsification is made easier and the drug's stability may be enhanced.

Emulsifying agents
To prevent coalescence, it is necessary to introduce an emulsifying agent that forms a film around the dispersed globules. Emulsifying agents may be divided into three groups:

- *Surface active agents.* Surfactants are adsorbed at oil-water interfaces to form *monomolecular films* and reduce interfacial tensions. Unless the interfacial tension is zero, there is a natural tendency for the oil droplets to coalesce to reduce the area of oil-water contact, but the presence of the surfactant monolayer at the surface of the droplet reduces the possibility of collisions leading to coalescence. To retain a high surface area for the dispersed phase, surface active agents must be used to decrease the surface free energy. Often a mixture of surfactants is used: one with hydrophilic character and the other with hydrophobic character. A hydrophilic emulsifying agent is needed for the aqueous phase, and a hydrophobic emulsifying agent is needed for the oil phase. A complex film results, which produces an excellent emulsion. Nonionic surfactants are widely used in the production of stable emulsions. They are less toxic than ionic surfactants and are less sensitive to electrolytes and pH variation. Examples include sorbitan esters, polysorbates, and others.

- *Hydrophilic colloids.* A number of hydrophilic colloids are used as emulsifying agents. These include gelatin, casein, acacia, cellulose derivatives, and alginates. These materials adsorb at the oil-water interface and form multilayer films around the dispersed droplets of oil in an o/w emulsion. Hydrated lyophilic colloids differ from surfactants since they do not cause an appreciable lowering in interfacial tension. Their action is due to the fact that multimolecular films are strong and resist coalescence. Additionally, they increase the viscosity of the dispersion medium. Hydrophilic colloids are used for formation of o/w emulsions since the films are hydrophilic. Most cellulose derivatives are not charged, but can sterically stabilize the systems.

- *Finely divided solid particles* are adsorbed at the interface between two immiscible liquid phases and form a film of particles around the dispersed globules. Finely divided solid particles that are wetted to some degree by both oil and water can act as emulsifying agents. They are concentrated at the interface where they produce a film of particles around the dispersed droplets so as to prevent coalescence. Finely divided solid particles that are wetted by water form o/w emulsions; those that are wetted by oil form w/o emulsions.

Emulsion stability

The stability of an emulsion is characterized by the absence of coalescence of the internal phase, the absence of creaming, and maintenance of elegance with respect to appearance, odor, color, and other physical properties. An emulsion becomes unstable due to creaming, breaking, coalescence, phase inversion, and some other factors.

1. ***Creaming and sedimentation.*** Creaming is the upward movement of dispersed droplets relative to the continuous phase, while sedimentation, the reverse process, is the downward movement of particles. These processes take place due to the density differences in the two phases and can be reversed by shaking. However, creaming is undesirable, because a creamed emulsion increases the likelihood of coalescence due to the close proximity of the globules in the cream. Factors which influence the rate of creaming are similar to those involved in the sedimentation rate of suspension particles and are indicated by Stokes Law as follows:

$$v = \frac{d^2(\rho_s - \rho_0)g}{18\eta_o}$$

where v is the velocity of creaming, d is the globule diameter, ρ_s and ρ_0 are the densities of dispersed phase and dispersion medium respectively, η_o is the viscosity of the dispersion medium (poise), and g is the acceleration of gravity (981 cm/sec^2). According to this equation, the rate of creaming is decreased by:

- a reduction in the globule size,

- a decrease in the density difference between the two phases, and

- an increase in the viscosity of the continuous phase.

This may be achieved by homogenizing the emulsion to reduce the globule size and increasing the viscosity of the continuous phase by the use of thickening agents such as tragacanth or methylcellulose.

2. ***Breaking, coalescence and aggregation.*** Creaming is different from breaking, since creaming is a reversible process, whereas breaking is irreversible. When breaking occurs, simple mixing fails to resuspend the globules in a stable emulsified form, since the film surrounding the particles has been destroyed and the oil tends to coalesce. Coalescence is the process by which emulsified particles merge with each other to form large particles. The major factor preventing coalescence is the mechanical strength of the interfacial barrier. Formation of a thick interfacial film is essential for minimal coalescence. In aggregation, the dispersed droplets come together but do not fuse. Aggregation is to some extent reversible.

3. ***Phase inversion.*** An emulsion is said to invert when it changes from an o/w to a w/o emulsion or vice versa. Inversion can occur by the addition of an electrolyte or by changing the phase:volume ratio. For example, an o/w emulsion stabilized with sodium stearate can be inverted to an w/o emulsion by adding calcium chloride to form calcium stearate.

4. ***Preservation of emulsions.*** Growth of microorganisms in an emulsion can cause physical separation of the phases. Bacteria can degrade nonionic and anionic emulsifying agents and therefore preservatives must be added in adequate concentrations to the product.

Suspensions

Suspensions are dispersions of finely divided solid particles of a drug in a liquid medium in which the drug is not readily soluble. ***Suspending agents*** are often hydrophilic colloids (eg, cellulose derivatives, acacia, or xanthan gum) added to suspensions to increase viscosity, inhibit agglomeration, and decrease sedimentation. Highly viscous suspensions may prolong gastric emptying time, slow drug dissolution, and decrease the absorption rate. A suspension that is ***thixotropic*** as well as ***pseudoplastic*** should prove to be useful since it forms a gel on standing and becomes fluid when disturbed.

Suspended material should not settle rapidly. The particles that do settle on the bottom should not form a ***hard cake,*** but should be readily redispersed into a uniform mixture when shaken. ***Aggregation*** can be prevented if the particles have a similar electrical charge.

Flocculation

The large surface area of the particles is associated with a surface free energy that makes the system thermodynamically unstable. This makes particles highly energetic and tend to regroup, resulting in the decrease in total surface area and surface free energy. The particles in a liquid suspension, therefore, tend to ***flocculate. Flocculation*** is the formation of light, fluffy conglomerates held together by weak van der Waals forces. *Aggregation* occurs in a compact cake situation (growth and fusing together of crystals in the precipitates to form a solid aggregate). *Flocculating agents* can prevent caking, whereas *deflocculating agents* increase the tendency to cake. Surfactants can reduce interfacial tension, but it cannot be made equal to zero, so suspensions of insoluble particles tend to have a positive finite interfacial tension, and particles tend to flocculate.

Forces at the surface of a particle affect the degree of flocculation and agglomeration in a suspension. *Forces of attraction* are of the London van der Waals type, whereas the *repulsive forces* arise from the interaction of the electric double layers surrounding each particle. When the repulsion energy is high, collision of the particles is opposed; the system remains deflocculated and when sedimentation is complete, the particles form a close-packed arrangement with the smaller particles filling the void between the larger ones. Those particles lowest in the sediment are gradually pressed together by the weight of the ones above; the energy barrier is thus overcome, allowing the particles to come into close contact with each other. To resuspend and redisperse these particles, it is necessary to overcome the high energy barrier. Since this is not easily achieved by agitation, the particles tend to remain strongly attracted to each other and form a hard cake. When the particles are flocculated, the energy barrier is still too large to be surmounted, and so the approaching particles in the second energy minimum, which is at a distance of separation of perhaps 1000 to 2000 Å, is sufficient to form the loosely structural flocs.

Properties of deflocculated (dispersed) particles
- They have a high zeta potential.

- Their repulsive forces exceed attractive (London) forces.

- They settle slowly.

- They have a pleasing appearance; the supernatant remains cloudy.

- They eventually form a sediment in which aggregation occurs (caking).

- They are difficult to resuspend once caked.

Properties of flocculated particles
- They have a lower zeta potential.

- Their forces of attraction predominate over the repulsive forces.

- They are weakly bonded.

- They settle rapidly.

- They have an unsightly appearance; the supernatant is clear.

- They do not form a cake.

- They are easily resuspended.

Sedimentation of flocculated particles
"*Flocs*" tend to fall together, producing a distinct boundary between the sediment and the supernatant liquid. The liquid above the sediment is clear because even the small particles present in the system are associated with flocs. In contrast to this are deflocculated systems with variable particle sizes; the large particles here settle more rapidly than the smaller particles, and no clear boundary is formed. The supernatant remains turbid for a longer period of time.

Formulation of suspensions
There are two ways of formulating physically stable suspensions:

- The use of a structured vehicle to maintain deflocculated particles in suspension. However, the major disadvantage of deflocculated systems is that when the particles eventually settle, they form a compact cake.

- Production of flocs, which may settle rapidly, but are easily resuspended with a minimum of agitation. Optimum physical stability is obtained when the suspension is formulated with flocculated particles in a structured vehicle of hydrophilic colloid type.

Ointments

Ointments are semisolid preparations intended for external application. Ointments are typically used as:

- *Emollients* to make the skin more pliable

- *Protective barriers* to prevent harmful substances from coming in contact with the skin

- *Vehicles* in which to incorporate medication

Ointment bases are classified into four general groups: (1) hydrocarbon bases, (2) absorption bases, (3) water-removable bases, and (4) water-soluble bases.

1. *Hydrocarbon (oleaginous) bases* are anhydrous

and insoluble in water. They cannot absorb or contain water and are not washable in water.

- *Petrolatum* is a good base for oil-insoluble ingredients. It forms an occlusive film on the skin and absorbs less than 5% water under normal conditions. Wax can be incorporated to stiffen the base.

- *Synthetic esters* are used as constituents of oleaginous bases. These esters include glycerol monostearate, isopropyl myristate, isopropyl palmitate, butyl stearate, and butyl palmitate.

2. *Absorption bases* may be of two types: (1) those that permit the incorporation of aqueous solutions, resulting in the formation of water-in-oil (w/o) emulsions (eg, hydrophilic petrolatum and anhydrous lanolin), and (2) those that are already w/o emulsions (emulsion bases), that permit the incorporation of small additional quantities of aqueous solutions (eg, lanolin and cold cream). These bases are useful as emollients although they do not provide the degree of occlusion afforded by the oleaginous bases. Absorption bases are also not easily removed from the skin with water. An aqueous solution may be first incorporated into the absorption base, and then this mixture added to the oleaginous base.

3. *Emulsion bases,* water washable or water removable bases commonly referred to as creams, represent the most commonly used type of ointment base. The majority of dermatologic drug products are formulated in an emulsion or cream base. Emulsion bases are washable and removed easily from skin or clothing. An emulsion base can be subdivided into three component parts, designated the oil phase, the emulsifier, and the aqueous phase. Drugs can be included in one of these phases or added to the formed emulsion. The oil phase, also known as the internal phase, is typically made up of petrolatum and/or liquid petrolatum together with cetyl or stearyl alcohol. Types of emulsion bases include:

- *Hydrophilic ointment* is an o/w emulsion that uses sodium lauryl sulfate as an emulsifying agent. It is readily miscible with water and is removed from the skin easily. The aqueous phase of an emulsion base contains the preservative(s) that are included to control microbial growth. The preservatives in the emulsion include methylparaben, propylparaben, benzyl alcohol, sorbic acid, or quaternary ammonium compounds. The aqueous phase also contains the water-soluble components of the emulsion system, together with any additional stabilizers, antioxidants, and buffers that may be necessary for stability and pH control.

- *Cold cream* is a semisolid white w/o emulsion prepared with cetyl ester wax, white wax, mineral oil, sodium borate, and purified water. Sodium borate combines with free fatty acids present in the waxes to form sodium soaps that act as the emulsifiers. Cold cream is employed as an emollient and ointment base. Eucerin® cream is a w/o emulsion of petrolatum, mineral oil, mineral wax, wool wax, alcohol, and bronopol. It is frequently prescribed as a vehicle for delivery of lactic acid and glycerin to treat dry skin.

- *Lanolin* is a w/o emulsion that contains approximately 25% water and acts as an emollient and occlusive film on the skin, effectively preventing epidermal water loss.

- *Vanishing cream* is an o/w emulsion that contains a large percentage of water as well as a humectant (eg, glycerin or propylene glycol) that retards surface evaporation. An excess of stearic acid in the formula helps to form a thin film when the water evaporates.

4. *Water-soluble bases* may be anhydrous or may contain some water. They are washable in water and absorb water to the point of solubility. Polyethylene glycol (PEG) ointment is a blend of water-soluble PEG that forms a semisolid base. This base can solubilize water-soluble drugs and some water-insoluble drugs. It is compatible with a wide variety of drugs. This base contains 40% PEG 4000 and 60% PEG 400. Another water-soluble base is the ointment prepared with propylene glycol and ethanol, which form a clear gel when mixed with 2% hydroxypropyl cellulose. This base is a commonly used dermatologic vehicle.

Incorporation of drugs into an ointment

Drugs may be incorporated into an ointment base by levigation and fusion. Normally, drug substances are in fine powered forms before being dispersed in the vehicle. Levigation of powders into a small portion of base is facilitated by the use of a melted base or a small quantity of compatible levigation aid, such as mineral oil or glycerin. Water-soluble salts are incorporated by dissolving them in a small volume of water and incorporating the aqueous solution into a compatible base. Fusion method is used when the base contains solids that have higher melting points (eg, waxes, cetyl alcohol, or glyceryl monostearate).

Inserts, Implants, and Devices

Inserts, implants, and *devices* are used to control drug delivery for localized or systemic drug effects. In these systems, drugs are embedded into biodegradable or nonbiodegradable materials to allow slow release of the drug. The inserts, implants, and devices are inserted into a variety of cavities (eg, vagina, buccal cavity, cul de sac of the eye, or subcutaneous tissue).

A number of degradable and nondegradable inserts are currently available for ophthalmic delivery. These ophthalmic inserts can be insoluble, soluble, or bioerodible. Insoluble inserts are further classified as diffusional, osmotic, and contact lens (Figure 4).

Diffusional and osmotic systems contain a reservoir that is in contact with the inner surface of a controller to which it supplies the drug. The reservoir contains a liquid, a gel, a colloid, a semisolid, a solid matrix, or a carrier containing drug. Carriers consist of hydrophilic or hydrophobic polymers. Degradable inserts consist of polyvinyl alcohol, hydroxypropylcellulose, polyvinylpyrrolidone, and hyaluronic acid. Nondegradable inserts are prepared from insoluble materials such as ethylene vinyl acetate copolymers and styrene-isoprene-styrene block copolymers. The initial use of contact lenses was for vision correction; however, they are becoming more useful as potential drug delivery devices by presoaking them in drug solutions. The use of contact lenses can simultaneously correct vision and release drug.

Figure 4.

Different types of ophthalmic inserts.

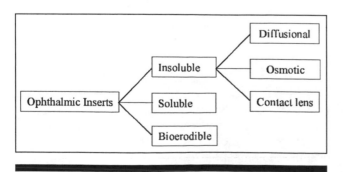

Ocular inserts are no more affected by nasolacrimal drainage and tear flow than conventional dosage forms, and instead can provide slow drug release and longer residence times in the conjunctival cul-de-sac. *Occusert®* is an interesting device consisting of a drug reservoir (eg, pilocarpine HCl in an alginate gel) enclosed by two release-controlling membranes made of ethylene-vinyl acetate copolymer and enclosed by a white ring, allowing positioning of the system in the eye. Pilocarpine Occusert has demonstrated slow release of pilocarpine which can effectively control the increased intraocular pressure in glaucoma. Other inserts (eg, medicated contact lenses, collagen shields, and minidiscs) have been shown to diminish the systemic absorption of ocularly applied drugs as a result of decreased drainage into nasal cavity. *Lacrisert®* is a soluble insert composed of hydroxypropylcellulose (HPC) and is useful in the treatment of dry eye syndrome. The device is placed in the lower fornix where it slowly dissolves over 6-8 hours to stabilize and thicken the tear film.

In addition to ophthalmic delivery, inserts are also used for localized delivery of drugs to various other tissues. For example, the *Progestasert®* device is designed for implantation into the uterine cavity, where it releases 65 mg progesterone per day to provide contraception for 1 year. Similarly, *Transderm®* relies on the rate-limiting polymeric membranes to control drug release. *ATRIDOX™* is a FDA-approved product designed for controlled-release delivery of the antibiotic doxycycline for the treatment of periodontal disease. When injected into the periodontal cavity, the formulation sets, forming a drug delivery depot that delivers the antibiotic to the cavity.

The ALZA Corporation developed *DURO®* implants for continuous therapy for up to 1 year. The nondegradable, osmotically driven system is intended to enable delivery of small drugs, peptides, proteins, and DNA for systemic or tissue-specific therapy. *Viadur®* is a once-yearly implant for the palliative treatment of advanced prostate cancer.

One of the more commonly used devices is the *oral osmotic pump,* composed of a core tablet and a semipermeable coating with a 0.3- to 4-mm diameter hole produced by a laser beam for drug exit. This system requires only osmotic pressure to be effective, but the drug release rate is dependent on the surface area, nature of the membrane, and the diameter of the hole. When the dosage form comes in contact with water, water is imbibed because of the resultant osmotic pressure of the core and the drug is released from the orifice at a controlled rate.

Transdermal Patches

Transdermal patches deliver drugs directly through the skin and into the bloodstream. In general, patches are composed of three key compartments: a protective seal that forms the external surface and protects it from damage, a compartment that holds the medication itself and has an adhesive backing to hold the entire patch on the skin surface, and a release liner that protects the adhesive layer during storage and is removed just prior to application. Watson Pharmaceuticals, Inc. has developed *Alora*® (estradiol) and *Androderm*® (testosterone) transdermal patches for the treatment of menopausal symptoms and endogenous testosterone deficiency, respectively.

Aerosol Products

Aerosols are pressurized dosage forms designed to deliver drugs with the aid of a liquefied or propelled gas (propellant). Aerosol products consist of a pressurizable container, a valve that allows the pressurized product to be expelled from the container when the actuator is pressed, and a dip tube that conveys the formulation from the bottom of the container to the valve assembly. Inhalation devices broadly fall into three categories: pressurized metered-dose inhalers (MDIs), nebulizers, and dry-powder inhalers (DPIs). The most commonly used inhalers on the market are MDIs. They contain active ingredient as a solution or as a suspension of fine particles in a liquefied propellant held under high pressure. MDIs use special metering valves to regulate the amount of formulation that is dispensed with each dose. Nebulizers do not require propellants and can generate large quantities of small droplets capable of penetrating into the lung. Sustained release of drugs, such as bronchodilators and corticosteroids for the treatment of asthma and chronic obstructive pulmonary diseases, involves encapsulation of the drugs in slowly degrading particles that can be inhaled. For accumulation in the alveolar zone of the lungs, which has very large surface area, inhaled liquid or dry-powder aerosols should have particle sizes in the range of 1-5 µm. Inhaled drugs play a very prominent role in the treatment of asthma, because this route has significant advantages over oral or parenteral administration. *Azmacort*® (triamcinolone acetamide), *Ventolin*® *HFA* (albuterol sulfate), and *Serevent*® (salmeterol) are examples of commercially available aerosols for the treatment of asthma.

6. Targeted Drug Delivery Systems

Targeted drug delivery systems are drug carrier systems that deliver the drug to the target or receptor site in a manner that provides maximum therapeutic activity, prevents degradation or inactivation during transit to the target sites, and protects the body from adverse reactions because of inappropriate disposition. Design of an effective delivery system requires a thorough understanding of the drug, the disease, and the target site (Figure 5). Examples include macromolecular drug carriers (protein drug carriers), particulate drug delivery systems (eg, microspheres, nanospheres, and liposomes), monoclonal antibodies, and cells. Plasma clearance kinetics, tissue distribution, metabolism, and cellular interactions of a drug can be controlled by the use of a site-specific delivery system. Targeting of drugs to specific sites in the body can be achieved by linking particulate systems or macromolecular carriers to monoclonal antibodies or to cell-specific ligands (eg, asialofetuin, glycoproteins, or immunoglobulins), or by alterations in the surface characteristics so that they are not recognized by the reticuloendothelial systems (RES).

Macromolecular Carrier Systems

Both natural and synthetic water-soluble polymers have been used as macromolecular drug carriers. The drug can be attached to the polymer chain either directly or via a spacer. Attachment of polyethylene glycol (PEG) to proteins can protect them from rapid hydrolysis or degradation within the body, and increase blood circulation time and lower the immunogenicity of proteins. PEGylated forms of interferons, *PEG-Intron*™ and *Pegasys*™ (for treatment of hepatitis C, to reduce dosing frequency from daily injections to

Figure 5.

Essential components of drug delivery.

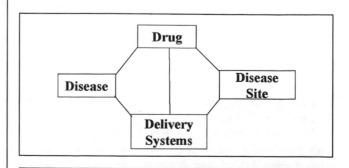

once-a-week injection dosing), adenosine deaminase, and L-asparaginase are currently on the market. PEGylation improves macromole solubility and stability by minimizing the uptake by the cells of the reticuloendothelial systems (RES). Since PEG drug conjugates are not well absorbed from the gut, they are mainly used as injectables. The drug-polymer conjugate may also contain a receptor-specific ligand to achieve selective access to, and interaction with, the target cells.

Particulate Drug Delivery Systems

Liposomes
Liposomes are microscopic phospholipid vesicles composed of uni- or multilamellar lipid bilayers surrounding compartments. Multilamellar vesicles (MLVs) have diameters in the range of 1-5 μm. Sonication of MLVs results in the production of small unilamellar vesicles (SUVs) with diameters in the range of 0.02-0.08 μm. Large unilamellar vesicles (LUVs) can also be made by evaporation under reduced pressure, resulting in liposomes with a diameter of 0.1-1 μm. The bilayer-forming lipid is the essential part of the lamellar structure, while the other compounds are added to impart certain characteristics to the vesicles. Water-soluble drugs can be entrapped in liposomes by intercalation in the aqueous bilayers, while lipid-soluble drugs can be entrapped within the hydrocarbon interiors of the lipid bilayers. Liposomes can encapsulate small-molecular-weight drugs, proteins, peptides, oligonucleotides, and genes. The use of the antifungal agent amphotericin B formulated in liposomes has been approved by the FDA. Since conventional liposomes are recognized by the immune systems as foreign bodies, the ALZA Corporation developed *STEALTH*™ liposomes, which evade recognition by the immune system because of their unique polyethylene glycol (PEG) coating. *Doxil*™ is a STEALTH liposome formulation of doxorubicin used for the treatment of AIDS-related Kaposi's sarcoma.

Microencapsulation
Microencapsulation is a technique that involves the encapsulation of small particles or solution of drugs in a polymer film or coat. Different methods of microencapsulation result in either microcapsules or microspheres. For example, interfacial polymerization of a monomer almost always produces microcapsules, whereas solvent evaporation may result in microspheres or microcapsules, depending on the amount of drug loading. A microcapsule has drug located centrally within the particle, whereas a microsphere has its drug dispersed throughout the particle. Microcapsules usually release their drug at a constant rate (zero-order

release), whereas microspheres typically give a first-order release of drugs. Small-molecular-weight drugs, proteins, oligonucleotides, and genes can be encapsulated into microparticles to provide their sustained release at disease sites.

The most commonly used method of microencapsulation is *coacervation*, which involves addition of a hydrophilic substance to a colloidal drug dispersion. The hydrophilic substance, which acts as a coating material, may be selected from a variety of natural and synthetic polymers, including shellacs, waxes, gelatin, starches, cellulose acetate phthalate, ethylcellulose, and others. Following dissolution of the coating materials, the drug inside the microcapsule is available for dissolution and absorption.

Biodegradable polylactide (PLA) and its copolymers with glycolide (polylactide-co-glycolide; PLGA) are commonly used for preparation of microparticles from which the drug can be released slowly over a period of a month or so. Microspheres can be used in a wide variety of dosage forms, including tablets, capsules, and suspensions. *Lupron Depot*® from TAP Pharmaceuticals is a FDA-approved preparation of PLGA microspheres for sustained release of a small peptide luteinizing hormone-releasing hormone (LHRH) agonist. More recently, PLGA microspheres of recombinant human growth hormone have been developed and marked successfully by Genentech, Inc. under the trade name of *Nutropin Depot*®.

7. Key Points

- Fick's first law of diffusion describes the diffusion process under the steady-state conditions when the drug concentration gradient does not change with time.

- Drug absorption depends not only on the fraction of un-ionized form of the drug, but also on the surface area available for absorption.

- The Noyes-Whitney equation can be used for determination of the dissolution rate of a drug from its dosage form, while the Arrhenius equation can be used for the determination of the shelf life of a drug dosage form.

- Surfactants consist of hydrophilic and hydrophobic groups and can be used as emulsifying agents to reduce the interfacial tensions.

- The pharmaceutical dosage form contains the active drug ingredient in association with nondrug (usually inert) ingredients (excipients). Together they comprise the vehicle, or formulation matrix.

- Water-soluble drugs are often formulated as sustained-release tablets so that their release and dissolution rates can controlled, while enteric-coated tablets are used to protect drugs from gastric degradation.

- Capsules are solid dosage forms with hard or soft gelatin shells that contain drugs and excipients.

- Aerosols are pressurized dosage forms designed to deliver drugs to pulmonary tissues with the aid of a liquefied or propelled gas.

- Inserts, implants, and devices allow slow release of the drug into a variety of cavities (eg, vagina, buccal cavity, cul de sac of the eye, and skin).

- Transdermal patches deliver drugs directly through the skin and into the bloodstream.

- The drug delivery system deals with the pharmaceutical formulation and the dynamic interactions among the drug, its formulation matrix, its container, and the physiologic milieu of the patient. These dynamic interactions are the subject of pharmaceutics.

- Macromolecular drug carriers, such as protein-polymer conjugates, and particulate delivery systems such as microspheres and liposomes, are commonly used for delivery of drugs with small molecular size such as peptides and proteins to different disease targets.

- Targeted (or site-specific) drug delivery systems are used for drug delivery to the target or receptor site in a manner that provides maximum therapeutic activity, by preventing degradation during transit to the target site while avoiding delivery to nontarget sites.

8. Questions and Answers

1. Which of the following is true for Fick's first law of diffusion?

   A. Refers to the non–steady-state flow
   B. The amount of material flowing through a unit cross section of a barrier in unit time is known as the concentration gradient
   C. Flux of material is proportional to the concentration gradient
   D. Diffusion occurs in the direction of increasing concentration
   E. All of the above

2. Which equation describes the rate of drug dissolution from a tablet?

   A. Fick's law
   B. Henderson-Hasselbalch equation
   C. Michaelis-Menten equation
   D. Noyes-Whitney equation
   E. All of the above

3. The pH of a buffer system can be calculated with

   A. the Henderson-Hasselbalch equation
   B. the Noyes-Whitney equation
   C. the Michaelis-Menten equation
   D. Yong's equation
   E. All of the above

4. Which of the following is NOT true for gas adsorption on a solid?

   A. Chemical adsorption is reversible
   B. Physical adsorption is based on weak van der Waals forces
   C. Chemical adsorption may require activation energy
   D. Chemical adsorption is specific to the substrate
   E. All of the above

5. What is bioavailability?

   A. Bioavailability is the measurement of the rate and extent of active drug that reaches the systemic circulation.
   B. It is the relationship between the physical and chemical properties of a drug and its systemic absorption.
   C. It is the movement of the drug into body tissues over time.

   D. It is dissolution of the drug in the gastrointestinal tract.
   E. All of the above

6. Which of the following may be used to assess the relative bioavailability of two chemically equivalent drug products in a crossover study?

   A. Dissolution test
   B. Peak concentration
   C. Time-to-peak concentration
   D. Area under the plasma level time curve
   E. All of the above

7. What condition usually increases the rate of drug dissolution for a tablet?

   A. Increase in the particle size of the drug
   B. Decrease in the surface area of the drug
   C. Use of the ionized, or salt, form of the drug
   D. Use of the free acid or free base form of the drug
   E. Use of sugar coating around the tablet

8. The characteristics of an active transport process include all of the following EXCEPT:

   A. Active transport moves drug molecules against a concentration gradient
   B. Active transport follows Fick's law of diffusion
   C. Active transport is a carrier-mediated transport system
   D. Active transport requires energy
   E. Active transport of drug molecules may be saturated at high drug concentrations

9. Which of the following dosage forms may utilize surface active agents in their formulations?

   A. Emulsions
   B. Suspensions
   C. Colloidal dosage forms
   D. Creams
   E. All of the above

10. Which of the following statements about lyophilic colloidal dispersions is true?

    A. They tend to be more sensitive to the addition of electrolytes than lyophobic systems
    B. They tend to be more viscous than lyophobic systems
    C. They can be precipitated by prolonged dialysis
    D. They separate rapidly

E. All of the above

11. Which of the following is NOT true for tablet formulations?

   A. A disintegrating agent promotes granule flow
   B. Lubricants prevent adherence of granules to the punch faces of the tabletting machine
   C. Glidants promote flow of the granules
   D. Binding agents are used for adhesion of powder into granules
   E. All of the above

12. The absorption rate of a drug is most rapid when the drug is formulated as

   A. Controlled-release product
   B. Hard gelatin capsule
   C. Compressed tablet
   D. Solution
   E. Suspension

13. The passage of drug molecules from a region of high drug concentration to a region of low drug concentration is known as

   A. Active transport
   B. Simple diffusion or passive transport
   C. Pinocytosis
   D. Bioavailability
   E. Biopharmaceutics

14. Which equation is used to predict the stability of a drug product at room temperature from experiments at increased temperatures?

   A. Stokes equation
   B. Arrhenius equation
   C. Michaelis-Menten equation
   D. Fick's equation
   E. Noyes-Whitney equation

15. Choose which of the following statements is true.

   A. Flocculation is desirable for pharmaceutical suspensions.
   B. The diffusion rate of molecules of a smaller particle size is less than that of a larger particle size.
   C. Particle size of molecular dispersions is larger than a coarse dispersion.
   D. Pseudoplastic flow is shear thickening type and dilatant is shear thinning type.
   E. All of the above are true statements.

16. Choose which of the following statements is false.

   A. The Henderson-Hasselbalch equation describes the effect of physical parameters on the stability of pharmaceutical suspensions.
   B. The passive diffusion rate of hydrophobic drugs across biological membranes is higher than that of hydrophilic compounds.
   C. When the dispersed phase in an emulsion formulation is heavier than the dispersion medium, creaming can still occur.
   D. Targeted drug delivery systems deliver the drug to the target or receptor site in a manner that provides maximum therapeutic activity.
   E. All of the above are false statements.

17. Which of the following is an emulsifying agent?
   A. Sorbitan monooleate (Span 80)
   B. Polyoxyethylene sorbitan mono-oleate (Tween 80)
   C. Sodium lauryl sulfate
   D. Gum acacia
   E. All of the above

18. Which of the following surfactants is incompatible with bile salts?

   A. Polysorbate 80
   B. Potassium stearate
   C. Sodium lauryl sulfate
   D. Benzalkonium chloride
   E. All of the above

19. Which of the following statements is false?

   A. The partition coefficient is the ratio of drug solubility in n-octanol to that in water.
   B. Absorption of a weak electrolyte drug does not depend on the extent to which the drug exists in its un-ionized form at the absorption site.
   C. The drug dissolution rate can be determined using the Noyes-Whitney equation.
   D. Amorphous forms of drug have faster dissolution rates than crystalline forms.
   E. All of the above are false.

20. Which of the following statements is true?

   A. Most substances acquire a surface charge by ionization, ion adsorption, and ion dissolution.
   B. The term "surface tension" is used for liquid-vapor and solid-vapor tensions.

C. At the isoelectric point, the total number of positive charges is equal to the total number of negative charges.

D. All of the above are true.

E. None of the above are true.

21. Agents that may be used in the enteric coating of tablets include

A. Hydroxypropyl methylcellulose

B. Carboxymethylcellulose

C. Cellulose acetate phthalate

D. All of the above

E. None of the above

Answers

1. **C.** Fick's first law of diffusion states that the amount of material flow through a unit cross-section of a barrier in unit time, which is known as the flux, is proportional to the concentration gradient. Fick's first law of diffusion describes the diffusion process under steady-state conditions when the concentration gradient does not change with time.

2. **D.** The Noyes-Whitney equation describes the rate of drug dissolution from a tablet. Fick's first law of diffusion is similar to the Noyes-Whitney equation in that both equations describe drug movement due to a concentration gradient. The Michaelis-Menten equation involves enzyme kinetics, whereas Henderson-Hasselbalch equations are used for determination of pH of the buffer and the extent of ionization of a drug molecule.

3. **A.** The Henderson-Hasselbalch equation for a weak acid and its salt is represented as: $pH = pK_a + \log [salt]/[acid]$, where pK_a is the negative log of the dissolution constant of a weak acid, as [salt]/[acid] is the ratio of the molar concentration of salt and acid used to prepare a buffer.

4. **A.** Chemical absorption is an irreversible process, which is specific and may require activation energy, while physical adsorption is reversible and associated with van der Waals forces.

5. **A.** Bioavailability is the measurement of the rate and extent of systemic circulation of an active drug.

6. **C.** The plasma drug concentration versus time curve measures the bioavailability of a drug from a product. The peak plasma drug concentration (C_{max}) relates to the intensity of the pharmacologic response, while the time for peak plasma drug concentration (T_{max}) relates to the rate of systemic absorption.

7. **C.** The ionized, or salt, form of a drug is generally more water soluble and therefore dissolves more rapidly than the non-ionized (free acid or free base) form of the drug. According to the Noyes-Whitney equation, the dissolution rate is directly proportional to the surface area and inversely proportional to the particle size. Therefore an increase in the particle size or a decrease in the surface area slows the dissolution rate.

8. **B.** In passive transport, a drug travels from a high concentration to a low concentration, while active transport moves drug molecules against a concentration gradient and requires energy.

9. **E.** Surface active agents facilitate emulsion formation by lowering the interfacial tension between the oil and water phases. Adsorption of surfactants on insoluble particles enables these particles to be dispersed in the form of a suspension.

10. **E.** Most lyophilic colloids are organic molecules (including gelatin and acacia), they spontaneously form colloidal solution, and tend to be viscous. Dispersion of lyophilic colloids is stable in the presence of electrolytes.

11. **A.** Disintegrating agents are added to the tablets to promote breakup of the tablets when placed in the aqueous environment. Lubricants are required to prevent adherence of the granules to the punch faces and dies. Binding agents are added to bind powders together in the granulation process. Glidants are added to tablet formulations to improve the flow properties of the granulations.

12. **D.** For a drug in solution, no dissolution is required before absorption. Consequently, compared with other drug formulations, a drug in aqueous solution has the highest bioavailability rate, and is often used as the reference preparation for other formulations.

13. **B.** In simple diffusion or passive transport, a drug travels from a high concentration to a low concentration, while active transport moves drug molecules against a concentration gradient and

requires energy. Pinocytosis is a vesicular transport process of engulfment of small particles or fluid volumes.

14. **B.** Stability at room temperature can be predicted from accelerated testing data by the Arrhenius equation: $\log (k_2/k_1) = E_a (T_2 - T_1)/(2.303 \ RT_2T_1)$, where k_2 and k_1 are the rate constants at the absolute temperatures T_2 and T_1, respectively; R is the gas constant; and E_a is the energy of activation. Stokes equation is used to determine the sedimentation rate of a suspension, while the Noyes-Whitney equation is used to determine the dissolution rate.

15. **A.** Flocculation is the formation of light, fluffy conglomerates held together by weak van der Waals forces and is a reversible process. Pseudoplastic flow is a shear thinning process, while dilatant is a shear thickening type process.

16. **A.** The Henderson-Hasselbalch equation describes the relationship between ionized and non-ionized species of a weak electrolyte.

17. **E.** Surfactants such as sorbitan mono-oleate (Span 80), polyoxyethylene sorbitan mono-oleate (Tween 80), sodium lauryl sulfate, and gum acacia are surfactants used as emulsifiers.

18. **D.** Benzalkonium chloride is a cationic surfactant and can interact with bile salts.

19. **B.** According to pH partition theory, absorption of a weak electrolyte drug depends on the extent to which the drug exists in its un-ionized form at the absorption site. However, pH partition theory often does not hold true, as most weakly acidic drugs are well absorbed from the small intestine, possibly due to the large epithelial surface areas of the organ.

20. **D.** Most substances acquire a surface charge by ionization, ion adsorption, and ion dissolution. At the isoelectric point, the total number of positive charges is equal to the total number of negative charges.

21. **C.** An enteric-coated tablet has a coating that remains intact in the stomach, but dissolves in the intestine when the pH exceeds 6. Other enteric-coating materials include cellulose acetate trimellitate, polyvinyl acetate phthalate, and hydroxypropyl methylcellulose phthalate.

9. References

Ansel HC, Popovich NG, Allen LV, eds. *Pharmaceutical Dosage Forms and Drug Delivery Systems,* 6th ed. Malvern, PA: Williams & Wilkins; 1995.

Aulton ME, ed. *Pharmaceutics: The Science of Dosage Form Design.* New York: Churchill Livingstone; 1988.

Block LH, Yu ABC. Pharmaceutical principles and drug dosage forms. In: Shargel L, Mutnick AH, Souney PH, Swanson LN, eds. *Comprehensive Pharmacy Review.* New York: Lippincott Williams & Wilkins; 2001:28-77.

Block LH, Collins CC. Biopharmaceutics and drug delivery systems. In: Shargel L, Mutnick AH, Souney PH, Swanson LN, eds. *Comprehensive Pharmacy Review.* New York: Lippincott Williams & Wilkins; 2001:78-91.

Hillery AM. Advanced drug delivery and targeting: An introduction. In: Hillery AM, Lloyd AW, Swarbrick J, eds. *Drug Delivery and Targeting: For Pharmacists and Pharmaceutical Scientists.* New York: Taylor & Francis; 2001:63-82.

Martin A. *Physical Pharmacy,* 4th ed. Baltimore: Lippincott Williams & Wilkins; 1993.

Gennaro AR, Gennaro AL, eds. *Remington: The Science and Practice of Pharmacy.* Baltimore: Lippincott, Williams & Wilkins, 2000.

Mathiowitz E, Kretz MR, Bannon-Peppas L. Microencapsulation. In: *Encyclopedia of Controlled Drug Delivery.* New York: John Wiley & Sons; 1999:493-546.

Florence AT, Attwood D. *Physicochemical Principles of Pharmacy,* 3rd ed. Palgrave, New York: MacMillan; 1998.

Banker GS, Rhodes CT, eds. *Modern Pharmaceutics,* 3rd ed. New York: Marcel Dekker; 1995.

Washington N, Washington C, Wilson CG. *Physiological Pharmaceutics: Barriers to Drug Absorption,* 2nd ed. New York: Taylor & Francis; 2001.

4. Compounding

Charles N. May, BSPh, MSHP
Assistant Professor, Department of Pharmaceutical Sciences
University of Tennessee College of Pharmacy

Contents

1. Introduction

Pharmacists extemporaneously compound medications to provide patients and prescribers more options for treatment and therapy than are provided by commercially available products. There are many reasons patients need individualized custom-prepared medications, and these include (1) some therapeutic agents are not commercially manufactured, (2) some therapeutic agents are not manufactured in the form or size needed, (3) some manufactured therapeutic agents contain offending ingredients such as dyes, preservatives, fillers, binders, etc, (4) some manufactured therapeutic agents contain offending flavors, fragrances, or colors and (5) some patients do not fit into the standard categories that manufactured products treat. In addition, from time to time commercially manufactured products are unavailable for a variety of reasons, such as (1) drug recalls, (2) the manufacturing facility is closed down, (3) strikes or disasters, (4) the product is no longer commercially profitable, or (5) for other corporate reasons the manufacturer no longer supplies the product. There are several segments of the population that are not properly served by pharmaceutical manufacturers and these include pediatric patients, geriatric patients, veterinary patients, and patients with rare and/or very complicated disease states. Prescribers and pharmacists working very closely with patients improve the quality of life for those patients as no other practice can do.

2. Philosophy of Compounding

- Extemporaneous per patient

- Fulfills needs for unique dosage forms and sizes

- Works as part of three-member team: the patient, the pharmacist, and the prescriber, to satisfy a patient's unique needs that cannot be satisfied by commercially available products

- Follows-up with patient and/or prescriber to determine if compounded preparation needs further adjustment or refinement to completely satisfy the patient's needs

3. Compounding versus Manufacturing

Compounding

- Patient-specific in conjunction with the prescriber

- Regulated by state board of pharmacy

- Compounded preparations are not advertised

- Compounded preparations have "beyond use dates"

- Compounded preparations are not prepared in advance except in the case of documented usage or demand

- Compounded preparations have no NDC number

Manufacturing

- Products subject to an approved NDA

- Products subject to FDA-approved labeling

- Products are manufactured in FDA-approved plants in accordance with Good Manufacturing Practices

- Products may be advertised

- Products carry an expiration date

- Products carry an NDC number

- Regulated by the FDA

4. Guidelines for Compounding

The following are published guidelines pharmacists utilize in designing and carrying out their compounding activities. Pharmacists' compounding practices are regulated by the laws of the state board of pharmacy of the state in which the pharmacist practices.

Pharmacy Compounding: Chapter 795. *U.S. Pharmacopoeia 26/National Formulary 21*, Rockville, MD: U.S. Pharmacopoeia Convention, Inc.; 2003:2197-2201.

Allen Jr LV. Extemporaneous prescription compounding: Chapter 98. *Remington: The Science and Practice of Pharmacy*, 20th ed. Baltimore: Lippincott, Williams & Wilkins; 2000:1706-1715.

Compliance Policy Guide, Compliance Policy Guidance for FDA Staff and Industry, Chapter 4, Sub Chapter 460, Sec. 460.200. *Pharmacy Compounding*, Washington: U.S. Food and Drug Administration; June, 2002.

Good Compounding Practices Applicable to State Licensed Pharmacies. Park Ridge, IL: The National Association of Boards of Pharmacy; 1993.

5. Requirements

Pharmacy

Space
- Appropriate amount: dedicated area is ideal

- Properly arranged and maintained: ingredients and equipment close at hand

- Controlled atmosphere: limited traffic flow, air flow away from operator

- Separate areas for sterile and nonsterile compounding

- Source of potable water and purified water: sink readily available

- Constructed of materials that are nonporous and seamless as possible: light, bright fixtures, walls, and floors give a clean, professional appearance

Equipment

- Appropriate measuring devices: eg, graduated cylinders, pharmacy graduates, pipettes, etc

- Appropriate balances for weighing: eg, electronic balance or class A prescription balance

- Appropriate mixing devices: eg, Wedgewood, porcelain and glass mortars and pestles, blenders, etc

- Appropriate counters and shelves: eg, sufficient countertop space must be available so compounding will not be cramped and shelving must be sufficient and appropriately located so ingredients can be convenient and properly stored

- Appropriate processing equipment: eg, hot plates and magnetic stirrers, ointment mills, electronic mortar and pestle, tablet pulverizers, etc

- Appropriate safety equipment: eg, rubber gloves, face masks, hair covers, etc, for personnel; devices that gently exhaust the air from the work area to keep the air free of contamination with ingredients; and containment areas in which to work when personnel are working with light, fine, fluffy ingredients or ingredients that are irritating or foul-smelling

- Appropriate packaging equipment: eg, capsule filling machines, tube sealing equipment, calibrated measuring and filling devices, etc

- Appropriate computer equipment: eg, for processing labels, profiles, formulas, and maintaining required records regarding ingredients

Other

Formulas
Ingredient classification and quality
- USP/NF (United States Pharmacopoeia/National Formulary) (ingredients meet official standards and are suitable for human use)

- FCC (Food Chemicals Codex) (Food Grade)

- ACS (American Chemical Society) (Reagent Grade)

- AR (Analytical Reagent) (High Purity)

- CP (Chemically Pure) (Uncertain Quality)

- Tech (Technical) (Industrial Quality)

Supplies
- Weigh boats, weighing paper (parchment and glassine), filter paper, ointment paper, spatulas (stainless steel and hard rubber), stirring rods (glass and polypropylene), rubber scrapers, beakers, flasks, funnels, casseroles, etc, and containers of all types and sizes to properly package all the unique dosage forms and sizes patients require. These include all sizes of prescription bottles, powder jars, capsule vials and ointment jars as well as ointment tubes, troche molds, plastic suppository molds, powder paper boxes, suppository boxes, "ride-up" tubes, etc

Records
- An exact record of each compounded prescription must be made and maintained. A chronological record of each day's compounding activity should be made and kept for future reference and use.

Policies and procedures including
- Standard Operating Procedures (SOPs)

- Material Safety Data Sheets (MSDSs)

- Certificates of Analysis (COAs)

- Quality Assurance Checks, etc

The Pharmacist

- *Interest:* a distinct interest in being creative, solving difficult patient problems, working closely with prescribers and patients, and formulating and compounding special customized medications is very important.

- *Education:* the emphasis on compounding varies among the colleges of pharmacy. Even graduates of programs which require students to compound a wide variety of formulations may find they need more training.

- *Training:* Additional training is often obtained through CE courses, seminars, professional development programs, or professional associations.

- *Experience:* Experience in compounding is perhaps the key to how effective a pharmacist can be in creating special formulations that make a significant difference in a patient's life when everything else up to that point has failed.

- Experience enables the pharmacist to suggest to the prescriber a therapeutic agent in a unique dosage form that has an better chance of solving the patient's problem. Conversely, a pharmacist with less-than-optimal experience and interest may compound a medication that is not effective, and thereby not satisfy the patient's need, and perhaps even undermine the prescriber's confidence in all compounded medications.

- *Compounding support:* compounding pharmacists should join professional organizations that support compounding such as the International Academy of Compounding Pharmacists; they should subscribe to journals that focus on compounding such as the *International Journal of Pharmaceutical Compounding*, the *U.S. Pharmacist*, etc; and they should utilize the professional resources of the companies that fulfill their compounding needs.

Professional considerations
- Is there a commercially available product in the exact dosage, size, form and package required?

- Is there an alternative product that will completely satisfy the patient's needs?

- Can I do the required pharmaceutical calculations to make and package the product?

Quality Control Requirements

- Accurate calculations

- Accurate weights

- Accurate measurements

- Proper processing techniques

- Proper packaging

- Proper records

- Proper labeling including "beyond use date"

Beyond use dates
- Pharmacists assign beyond use dates to compounded preparations to provide patients guidance in the proper use of the preparation.

- The goal is to provide a beyond use date that will allow the patient enough time to fully utilize the amount of preparation dispensed, but not enough time to allow the preparation to degrade and/or lose potency or be stored for future use.

- If the pharmacist does not have a reference on stability of the specific dosage form or if experience with it is insufficient, the USP guidelines are followed.

6. Compounded Preparations

Solutions

- **Definition:** chemically and physically homogenous mixtures of two or more substances

- **Types:** syrups, elixirs, aromatic waters, tinctures, spirits, nonaqueous, etc

- **Properties:** hypertonic, isotonic, hypotonic, osmolar, osmolal, etc

- Stability enhanced by adjusting pH or adding preservatives, antioxidants, etc

- Rate of solution enhanced by stirring, heat, particle size reduction, etc

- Beyond use dates: aqueous solutions have short beyond use dates

- Testing: organoleptic, pH, etc

An example of an isotonic *aqueous* solution:

Ephedrine sulfate	1%
Sodium chloride	qs
Purified water qs ad	30 mL
M.Ft. isotonic solution	

Steps in compounding:
1. Calculate the required quantity of each ingredient (NaCl equivalent of ephedrine sulfate is 0.2).
2. Accurately weigh or measure each ingredient.
3. Dissolve the solid ingredients in about 25 mL of purified water.
4. Add sufficient purified water to measure 30 mL.

The following is an example of a *nonaqueous* solution:

Urea	10 g
Salicylic acid	5 g
Coal tar solution	5 mL
Propylene glycol qs ad	100 mL

Steps in compounding:
1. Accurately weigh or measure each ingredient
2. Dissolve the urea and salicylic acid in about 75 mL of propylene glycol
3. Add the coal tar solution and mix well
4. Add sufficient propylene glycol to measure 100 mL

Note: If using a mechanical stirrer, it may take significant time to dissolve the urea and salicylic acid.

Suspensions

- **Definition:** a two-phased system containing a finely divided solid in a vehicle

- **Requirement:** drug is uniformly dispersed throughout vehicle

- **Suspending agents** are typically used in a concentration of 0.5-6%

Categories of suspending agents
- * Natural hydrocolloids: acacia, alginic acid, gelatin, guar gum, sodium alginate, tragacanth, xanthan gum
- * Semisynthetic hydrocolloids: ethylcellulose, methylcellulose, sodium carboxymethylcellulose
- * Synthetic hydrocolloids: carbomers (carbopol), poloxamers (pluronic), polyvinyl alcohol, polyvinylpyrolidone
- * Clays: bentonite, magnesium aluminum silicate (veegum)

- Vehicle: has viscosity to keep drug particles suspended separately

- Active ingredient: insoluble in vehicle

Tip: Wet insoluble powder with vehicle-miscible liquid.

- Advantage: allows the preparation of a liquid form of an insoluble drug

- Stability is enhanced by adding preservative

- Testing: organoleptic

An example of an oral suspension:

Progesterone, micronized	2.4 g
Glycerin	3 mL
Methylcellulose 2 % soln	30 mL
Flavored syrup qs ad	60 mL

Steps in compounding:
1. Accurately weigh or measure each ingredient.
2. In a glass mortar, wet the progesterone with the glycerin making a thick paste.
3. Slowly add the methylcellulose solution while triturating.
4. When mixed thoroughly, pour into a graduate.

5. Add small amounts of syrup in mortar, mix and add to graduate until the desired volume is reached.

Emulsions

- *Definition:* a two-phase system of two immiscible liquids, one of which is dispersed throughout the other as small droplets

- *Components:* a dispersion medium or external or continuous phase, an internal or discontinuous or dispersed phase, and an emulsifying agent

- *Type:* oil-in-water (o/w) or water-in-oil (w/o), based on which is the internal and external phase

Emulsifying agents
  * Natural gums: acacia, agar, chondrus, pectin, tragacanth
  * Hydrophilic/lipophilic agents: the esters of sorbitan
    - Lipophilic: trade named Arlacel® and Span®
    - Hydrophilic: trade named Myrj® and Tween®

- A lower hydrophilic-lipophilic balance (HLB) value favors a w/o emulsion; a higher HLB value favors an o/w emulsion.

- Agents with an HLB value of 1 through 9 are considered to be lipophilic; agents with an HLB value of 10 and above are considered to be hydrophilic.

- Other agents include bentonite, cholesterol, gelatin, lecithin, methylcellulose, soaps of fatty acids, sodium docusate, sodium lauryl sulfate, triethanolamine, etc

- Equipment: mortar and pestle, homogenizers, colloid mill, mechanical mixers, agitators, ultrasonic vibrators, etc

- Solid ingredients should be dissolved before they are incorporated into the emulsion, or if a sizeable quantity is added, a levigating or wetting agent may be needed.

- Flavors should be incorporated into the external phase.

- Preservatives should be added in aqueous phase; may also be added to oily phase if needed.

- Stability: either cream or crack (coalesce)

- The Continental or dry gum method of preparing an emulsion nucleus involves using the oil:water:dry gum emulsifier in a 4:2:1 ratio.

- Advantages of an emulsion as a vehicle: mask taste, improve palatability, increase absorption, enhance bioavailability, etc

An example of preparing an emulsion by the Continental or dry gum or 4-2-1 method:

Cod liver oil	50 mL
Acacia	12.5 g
Syrup	10 mL
Flavor oil	0.4 mL
Purified water, qs ad	100 mL

Steps in compounding:
1. Accurately weigh or measure each ingredient.
2. Place the cod liver oil in a dry mortar.
3. Add the acacia and give it a very quick mix.
4. Add 25 mL of purified water and immediately triturate rapidly to form the thick, white, homogenous emulsion nucleus.
5. Add the flavor and mix thoroughly.
6. Add the syrup and mix thoroughly.
7. Add sufficient purified water to measure 100 mL.

Capsules

- *Definition:* a dosage form incorporating ingredients into a shell called a capsule

- *Procedure:* triturate powders to reduce particle size, mix powders by geometric dilution, incorporate diluent by geometric dilution, calculate total weight to fit a certain size capsule, clean the outside of filled capsules

- *Advantages:* mask unpleasant taste; mix ingredients that could not be mixed in other vehicles; alter the release rate of ingredients; incorporate several ingredients into one dosage form; provide an accurate dosage size for liquids, semisolids, and powders; provide a dosage form that is easier to swallow and more acceptable to the patient

- Method of filling: hand punch from powder on pill tile; use capsule filling machine

- Sizing: determining the size capsule to use for your dosage size involves assessing the density/fluffiness of your powder, comparing it to known weights of various reference powders with published capsule size capacities, then actually weighing your capsule.

If the requested dosage doesn't fill a specific size capsule, a filler should be added to fill the capsule.

An example of an altered-release capsule:

Progesterone, micronized	25 mg
Methocel E4M®	50%
Lactose, qs ad	
M.Ft. capsules	dtd #15

Steps in compounding:
1. Select capsule size and calculate the required quantity of each ingredient.
2. Accurately weigh each ingredient.
3. If necessary, reduce particle size and mix thoroughly.
4. Fill capsules.
5. Weigh capsules, calculate average weight, and determine percentage of error.

Tablet Triturates (Sublingual or Molded Tablets)

- **Definition:** a small tablet made in a mold and intended for sublingual administration, usually weighing about 30 to 250 mg

- **Advantages:** rapidly dissolves under tongue, rapidly absorbed, avoids first pass through liver, provides rapid therapeutic response

- **Components:** active ingredient and base, which may consist of lactose, sucrose, dextrose, mannitol, etc

- **Formulation:** based on size of mold cavities, mix active ingredient with base, which often consists of 4 parts of lactose and 1 part of sucrose. Thoroughly triturate powders and mix by geometric dilution, then moisten with soluton containing 4 parts alcohol and 1 part purified water until powder mixture is adhesive. Press into mold.

Tip: Tablets may be flavored and colored by adding flavor and color to the wetting solution.

An example of a tablet triturate:

Testosterone	3 mg
Base, qs ad	
M.Ft. tabs	

Steps in compounding:
1. The base may consist of a 1:4 mixture of sucrose and lactose.
2. The wetting solution may consist of a 1:4 mixture of water and alcohol.

3. Based on the size mold you will use and the number of tablets it makes, calculate the required quantity of each ingredient.
4. Accurately weigh or measure each ingredient.
5. Reduce particle size and mix ingredients by geometric dilution.
6. In a glass mortar gradually moisten the powder mixture until it becomes adhesive.
   Note: Drop the wetting solution onto the powder a few drops at a time and triturate after each addition until powder becomes moist and adhesive.
7. Press moist powder evenly into all holes in tablet triturate mold plate.
8. Place mold plate on base plate and press down until tablets rest on top of pegs.
9. Let tablets air dry.
10. Very gently remove dried tablets from pegs.

Troches, Lozenges, Lollipops (Suckers)

- **Definition:** solid dosage forms intended to be slowly dissolved in the mouth for local or systemic effects

- **Formulation:** active ingredient and base that may consist of sugar and other carbohydrates that produce a hard candy troche, or the polyethylene glycols with other ingredients that produce a softer troche or a glycerin-gelatin combination that produces a chewable troche

- Formulations made in a sucker mold complete with sticks are called lollipops or suckers.

- Formulations must be calculated to fit the size mold that will be utilized.

- Flavors and colors are added just before the molds are filled.

- **Advantages:** easy to administer, convenient for patients who cannot swallow oral dosage forms, maintain a constant level of drug in the oral cavity and throat, pleasant tasting, etc

An example of a troche:

Gelatin	4.68 g
Glycerin	16.70 mL
Purified water	2.30 mL
Acacia	0.50 g
Bentonite	0.50 g
Benzocaine	0.30 g
Citric acid	0.66 g
Saccharin sodium	0.17 g
Flavor and color	qs

Steps in compounding:
1. Based on the size mold to be used and the number of troches to be made, calculate the required quantity of each ingredient.
2. Accurately weigh or measure each ingredient.
3. Heat the glycerin in a boiling water bath several minutes.
4. Add the water and heat a few more minutes.
5. While stirring, VERY SLOWLY add the gelatin. *Note:* Gelatin must be lump-free; mixture must be homogenous.
6. Triturate and thoroughly mix the powders.
7. Add the powders to the warm liquid and mix thoroughly.
8. Add flavor and color, mix, and pour into mold and let cool.

Transdermal Gels

- *Definition:* gels that move medications through the skin in quantities sufficient to produce a therapeutic effect

Components
  * Active ingredient(s)
  * Gelling agents: the carbomers (eg, Carbopol 934P®), methylcellulose, the poloxamers (eg, Pluronic F-127®), sodium carboxymethylcellulose, etc
  * Wetting/levigating agents: propylene glycol, glycerin, etc
  * Penetration-enhancing agents: water, alcohol, lecithin, dimethyl sulfoxide, isopropyl myristate, isopropyl palmitate, propylene glycol, polyethylene glycol, etc
  * Suspending/dispersing agents: bentonite, silica gel, etc

- *Advantages:* convenient, effective, avoids problems other dosage forms have such as GI irritation from oral dosages, pain from injections, undesirability of suppositories, and has great acceptability by patients.

- Formulation: use proper techniques for creating the gel, adjust the pH for carbomer gels, respect the temperature for poloxamer gels, use small amounts of nonaqueous solvents, and if possible keep electrolyte ingredients to a minimum.

Tip: Do not use transdermal gels for the systemic use of antibiotics, and do not try to get large molecules such as proteins through the skin via transdermal gels.

An example of a transdermal gel using carbomer as the base:

Ketoprofen	5%
Carbomer 934P	2%
Alcohol	qs
Trolamine	2 mL
Purified Water, qs ad	30 mL

Steps in compounding:
1. Calculate the required quantity of each ingredient.
2. Accurately weigh or measure each ingredient.
3. Triturate the carbomer 934P in a glass mortar.
4. While triturating, gradually add about 18 mL of purified water.
5. Be sure the carbomer and water are thoroughly mixed and the mixture is homogenous.
6. Dissolve the ketoprofen in about 10 mL of alcohol.
7. While triturating, add this to the carbomer/water mixture and mix thoroughly.
8. If necessary, add purified water to make about 28 mL and pour into ointment jar.
9. Add trolamine and stir quickly with stirring rod until the gel is thoroughly formed.

Note: A trade name for carbomer 934P is Carbopol 934P®.

An example of a transdermal gel using organogel (PLO) as the base:

Ketoprofen	5%
Propylene glycol	10%
Lecithin isopropyl palmitate liq.	20%
Poloxamer 407 20% gel qs ad	100 mL

Steps in compounding:
1. Calculate the required quantity of each ingredient.
2. Accurately weigh or measure each ingredient.
3. In a glass mortar triturate the ketoprofen with the propylene glycol.
4. Make a smooth uniform paste.
5. Add the lecithin isopropyl palmitate liquid and mix well.
6. Add sufficient poloxamer 407 20% gel to measure 100 mL.
7. Triturate until a high quality gel is produced.
8. Package in a light resistant container.

Note: The lecithin isopropyl palmitate liquid and the poloxamer 407 20% gel should be prepared ahead of time so they are ready for use.

The lecithin isopropyl palmitate liquid may be prepared as follows:

Soy lecithin, granular	10 g
Isopropyl palmitate	10 g
Sorbic acid	0.2 g

1. Accurately weigh or measure each ingredient.
2. Add the soy lecithin granules and the sorbic acid to the isopropyl palmitate, mix well, and allow to set overnight at room temperature.
3. The next morning, very gently stir to assure complete mixing.

Note: Isopropyl myristate may be used in place of isopropyl palmitate.

The poloxamer 407 20% gel may be prepared as follows:

Poloxamer 407	20 g
Potassium sorbate	0.2 g
Purified water, qs ad	100 mL

1. Accurately weigh or measure each ingredient.
2. Add the poloxamer 407 and the potassium sorbate to a portion of the purified water, mix well and add purified water to 100 mL.
3. Mix thoroughly ensuring the poloxamer 407 is completely wet.
4. Allow to set overnight in the refrigerator.
5. The next morning, stir slowly to be sure mixing is complete.
6. Store in the refrigerator.

Note: A trade name for poloxamer 407 is Pluronic F-127®.

Suppositories

- *Definition:* solid dosage forms for insertion into the rectum, vagina, or urethra to provide localized therapy or systemic therapy.

- *Sizes:* rectal, approx 2 g; vaginal, 3-5 g; urethral, 2 g female, 4 g male (urethral suppositories formerly called bougies)

- *Formulation:* usually made by fusion with either a fatty or water miscible base (can also be hand molded or made by compression)

- Usually made in a metal or plastic mold

- Active ingredients in powder from should be triturated (comminuted) to reduce particle size and should be levigated with a levigating or wetting agent before incorporation into the melted base.

- The melted formulation should be poured continuously into the mold to prevent layering.

- Calculations: the capacity in grams of the suppository mold must be known to determine the quantity of base needed (if this capacity is not known, the capacity must be determined by filling the mold with the suppository base and weighing the resulting suppositories). The space in the suppository occupied by the active ingredient(s) must calculated using the density factor of each active ingredient (if the density factor is not known, it can be calculated by making a suppository containing a known amount of the active ingredient).

- Advantages: delivers medication for local or systemic effects (the systemically absorbed medication avoids the first pass through the liver), delivers medication systemically when patients cannot take it orally or by injection

An example of a rectal suppository:

Progesterone, micronized	25 mg
Polyethylene glycol base	qs
M.Ft. supp	dtd #12

Steps in compounding:
Use the following formula for the polyethylene glycol base:

Polyethylene glycol 300	50%
Polyethylene glycol 6000	50%

1. Based on the size of your mold, calculate the required amount of each ingredient.
2. Accurately weigh or measure each ingredient.
3. Carefully heat the PEG 6000 until it melts.
4. Add the PEG 300 and mix well.
5. Very slowly add the micronized progesterone and mix thoroughly.
6. Pour into suppository mold.

Note: When using the plastic molds (shells), the liquid mixture must not be too hot.

Powders

- *Definition:* fine particles that result from the comminution of dry substances. Particle sizes are usually determined by the size sieve they will pass through, and may be described as very coarse, coarse, moderately coarse, fine, and very fine.

- Mixtures of powders should have the same or similar size particles and mixing should be accomplished by geometric dilution.

- **Preparation:** comminution is the process of reducing particle size in powders and is accomplished manually by trituration, levigation, and/or pulverization by intervention, and mechanically by grinders and various types of mills.

- **Uses:** powders are taken by mouth and may provide systemic effects; powders are applied topically for local effects; powders are insufflated into body cavities; powders that contain mucoadhesive ingredients will adhere to moist body surfaces.

- Advantages: since they are dry, they often have greater stability, they may not react with ingredients with which they are otherwise incompatible (except explosive mixtures), once in the GI tract they are ready to be absorbed, and they tend to have longer beyond use dates.

An example of a powder for external use:

Calamine	
Zinc oxide, aa	8%
Red mercuric oxide	1%
Magnesium oxide, heavy, qs ad	60 g
M.Ft. powder	

Steps in compounding:
1. Calculate the required amount of each ingredient.
2. Accurately weigh each ingredient.
3. Thoroughly mix the powders by geometric dilution.
4. If using a mortar and pestle, use a porcelain mortar and begin with the ingredient having the smallest weight.
5. Use the "spread test" to determine when mixture is totally homogenous.

Powder Papers (Charts)

- **Definition:** powders or mixtures of powders enfolded in paper and containing one dose and dispensed in an appropriate box or container

- **Preparation:** powders are finely subdivided (comminuted) and mixed by geometric dilution and the appropriate size dose is placed on a powder paper and properly folded. The appropriate size dose can be obtained by weighing. An alternate method is to place all the powder on a pill tile and "blocking and dividing" the powder into the proper number of doses and placing one dose on each powder paper.

- **Advantages:** for patients who cannot swallow, for patients who have difficulty swallowing certain tablets or capsules, and for patients who have nasogastric tubes indwelling, powder papers provide an ideal dosage form. Several medications can be given as one dose. The medication is in powder form and ready to be absorbed once in the gastrointestinal tract. For patients who have many medications to take each day, they may be combined into a smaller number of powder papers. Powder papers have longer beyond use dates than many other compounded dosage forms.

An example of a powder paper (chart):

Aspirin	3.5 g
Acetaminophen	2.5 g
Caffeine	0.5 g
M.Ft. chart	dtd #12

Steps in compounding:
1. Calculate the required quantity of each ingredient.
2. Accurately weigh each ingredient.
3. Triturate each ingredient separately to reduce particle size.
4. Thoroughly mix ingredients by geometric dilution.
5. Weigh the correct amount for each chart on a separate paper.
6. Properly fold each paper and place in powder box.

Ointments and Creams

- **Definition:** semisolid dosage forms for external application

- Properties are typically characteristic of the base selected (eg, white petrolatum, hydrophilic petrolatum, cold cream, hydrophilic ointment, polyethylene glycol ointment). Ointments and creams protect the skin and mucous membranes, moisturize the skin, and provide a vehicle for various types of medications.

Types and classifications of ointment bases

Oleaginous/hydrocarbon ointment bases

Characteristics	Examples
Occlusive	White petrolatum
Greasy	White ointment
Emollient	Vegetable shortening
Not water washable	
Will not absorb water	
Insoluble in water	

Absorption ointment bases

Characteristics	Examples
Occlusive	Hydrophilic petrolatum
Greasy	Lanolin, USP (anhydrous)
Emollient	Aquaphor®
Not water washable	Aquabase®
Can absorb water	
Insoluble in water	

Emulsion, water/oil ointment bases

Characteristic	Examples
Occlusive	Cold cream
Greasy	Rose water ointment
Emollient	Eucerin®
Not water washable	Hydrous lanolin
Will absorb water	Hydrocream
Insoluble in water	Nivea®

Emulsion, oil/water ointment bases

Characteristics	Examples
Nonocclusive	Hydrophilic ointment
Nongreasy	Acid mantle cream
Water washable	Cetaphil®
Will absorb water	Dermabase®
Insoluble in water	Keri® lotion
	Lubriderm®
	Neobase®
	Unibase®
	Vanishing cream
	Velvachol®

Water soluble ointment bases

Characteristics	Examples
Nonocclusive	Polyethylene glycol ointment
Nongreasy	Polybase®
Water washable	
Will absorb water	
Water soluble	

- *Preparation:* typically by fusion or levigation. Powders should be comminuted to fine particles; some powders may be dissolved.

- If using the fusion method, only enough heat should be used to melt the ingredient having the highest melting point.

- If using the levigation method, an ointment slab and metal spatula usually work well. Levigating agents should be carefully selected considering both the ingredient(s) to be incorporated and the base. The following list shows commonly used levigating agents grouped by type and matched with the appropriate group of ointment base classifications:

Aqueous agents	Ointment base classifications
Glycerin	Oil in water emulsion
Propylene glycol	Water soluble
Polyethylene glycol 400	Water washable

Oily agents	Ointment base classifications
Mineral oil	Oleaginous/hydrocarbon
Castor oil	Absorption
Cottonseed oil	Water in oil emulsion

Note: Other agents may be useful for certain preparations such as Tween 80® for incorporating coal tar. Castor oil is useful for incorporating ichthammol and peru balsam.

- Uses: an effective dosage for treating skin and mucous membranes. On occasion an ointment or cream will move sufficient quantities of medication through the skin to produce a systemic effect. Some formulations provide effective protection for the skin and mucous membranes.

- Packaging: typically ointments and creams are packaged in ointment jars. The tube is often an ideal alternative package because it protects the product until it is squeezed out and used.

An example of a nongreasy ointment:

Benzoyl peroxide	10%
Sulfur	1%
Polyethylene glycol base qs ad	30 g

Steps in compounding:
1. Calculate the required quantity of each ingredient.
   Note: Benzoyl peroxide, hydrous, USP contains about 26% water.
   Note: The polyethylene glycol base consists of:
   Polyethylene glycol 400   65%
   Polyethylene glycol 3350   35%
2. Accurately weigh or measure each ingredient.
3. Triturate each powder to a fine particle size.
4. Melt the polyethylene glycol 3350 and remove from heat source.
5. Add the polyethylene glycol 400 and mix thoroughly.
6. Add the powders and mix thoroughly.
7. Before the preparation begins to harden, stir thoroughly and pour into ointment jar.

An example of a greasy ointment:

Salicylic acid	3%
White petrolatum, qs ad	30 g

Steps in compounding:
1. Calculate the required quantity of each ingredient.
2. Accurately weigh each ingredient.
3. Triturate the salicylic acid to reduce particle size.
4. Levigate with a small quantity of mineral oil.
5. By geometric dilution, incorporate the levigated salicylic acid into the white petrolatum.

The following is an example of a cream:

Almond oil	56 g
White wax	12 g
Light mineral oil	10 g
Cetyl esters wax	2.5 g
Sodium borate	0.5 g
Purified water	19 g
Total	100 g

M.Ft. cream, S.A.

Steps in compounding:
1. Accurately weigh or measure each ingredient.
2. Melt the white wax.
3. Add the cetyl esters wax, almond oil, and light mineral oil.
4. Bring to a temperature of 70°C.
5. Dissolve the sodium borate in the purified water.
6. Bring to a temperature of 70°C.
7. With both liquids at 70°C, mix and stir.
8. Stir until cream is completely formed.
9. Package in tube or jar.

Sticks

- *Definition:* a topical dosage form made in the shape of a rod or stick or variation thereof packaged in a container that allows it to be advanced upward as it is used/consumed.

- *Advantages:* an effective, convenient method of applying a topical agent exactly in the location desired. Can deliver a variety of agents such as therapeutic, protective, cosmetic, etc. Very portable.

- Preparation: select a semisolid vehicle from a variety of polyethylene glycols, waxes, and oils that will produce the consistency desired. Triturate solid ingredients and wet them with an appropriate wetting/levigating agent and add them along with any liquid ingredients to the melted vehicle. Mix thoroughly. Pour into an appropriate "ride-up" container.

Tip: Sticks can usually be considered a stable dosage form and assigned a corresponding beyond use date.

An example of a stick:

Menthol	1%
Camphor	0.5%
Phenol	0.25%
Flavor	qs
Color	qs
Polyethylene glycol 400	7 g
Polyethylene glycol 4500	3 g

Steps in compounding:
1. Calculate the required quantity of each ingredient.
2. Accurately weigh or measure each ingredient.
3. Melt the polyethylene glycol 4500.
4. Remove from heat source.
5. Add the polyethylene glycol 400 and mix thoroughly.
6. Mix the menthol, camphor, and phenol together; they will liquefy forming a eutectic mixture.
7. Add the eutectic mixture and the other ingredients and mix thoroughly.
8. Pour into a "ride-up" lip balm tube and let cool.

7. Key Points

- Each extemporaneously compounded prescription is for a specific patient.

- Three parties are involved in extemporaneous compounding: the prescriber, the patient, and the pharmacist.

- A thorough knowledge of pharmacy math is required for extemporaneous compounding of prescriptions.

- The sensitivity of the pharmacy balance must be determined and the minimum weighable quantity calculated for that particular balance.

- All weighing and measuring must be accurate and within USP guidelines which allow for a variance up to 5%.

- Trituration is utilized to reduce the particle size of powders so a greater surface area will be available; to uniformly mix powders using geometric dilution; and to dissolve solutes in solvents.

- Levigation is the process of mixing or triturating a powder with a liquid in which it is insoluble to reduce particle size and aid in incorporating it into the ointment base.

- The pharmacist must choose a levigating agent that is miscible with the ointment base.

- Mineral oil is an appropriate levigating agent for a hydrophobic ointment base such as white petrolatum.

- Up to 5% levigating agent is usually sufficient unless the amount of powder is large.

- Heat should be used sparingly in compounding, using only enough heat to melt ingredients, effect solution, enhance a reaction, etc—never any extra.

- Use of a water bath normally prevents overheating ingredients when compounding.

- Care must be taken to never lose or waste any ingredients in the preparation process since this can alter the concentration of active ingredients in the finished preparation and produce a sub-potent or super-potent preparation.

- To promote accuracy in the compounding process, place all unused stock containers on the left side of the work station; as each one is used, place it on the right side.

- The dry gum (or Continental) method of preparing an emulsion uses the oil, purified water, and gum (eg, acacia) in a ratio of 4:2:1, respectively.

- The extemporaneously compounded preparation has no NDC number.

8. Questions and Answers

1. When water is an ingredient in a nonsterile compounded preparation and the type of water is not specified, the pharmacist is correct to use

   A. Tap water
   B. Potable water
   C. Purified water
   D. Water for injection
   E. Sterile water for injection

2. When alcohol is an ingredient in a nonsterile compounded preparation and the type and percent alcohol is not specified, the pharmacist is correct to use

   A. Ethyl alcohol 100%
   B. Ethyl alcohol 95%
   C. Ethyl alcohol 70%
   D. Ethyl alcohol 50%
   E. Isopropyl alcohol 70%

3. Ingredients that soften the skin and make it more flexible when applied topically are called

   A. Keratolytics
   B. Emollients
   C. Rubefacients
   D. Counterirritants
   E. Astringents

4. To increase the stability of potassium iodide oral solution (SSKI), _____ may be used as an antioxidant to prevent the release of free iodine.

   A. Sodium alginate
   B. Sodium borate
   C. Sodium glycinate
   D. Sodium succinate
   E. Sodium thiosulfate

5. In preparing diluted hydrochloric acid, a temperature change is noted. The reaction is called
   A. Hypothermic
   B. Hyperthermic
   C. Endothermic
   D. Exothermic
   E. Isothermic

6. Ingredients that tend to tighten or shrink tissues when applied topically are called

   A. Astringents

B. Emollients
C. Keratolytic agents
D. Occlusive agents
E. Suspending agent

7. A solution expressed as 35% w/w has the following:

   A. 35 mg of solute dissolved in 100 mL of solution
   B. 35 g of solute dissolved in 100 g of solvent
   C. 35 mg of solute dissolved in 100 g of solvent
   D. 35 g of solute dissolved in 100 g of solution
   E. 35 mL of solute dissolved in 100 mL of solution

8. When dissolving potassium iodide in purified water, a temperature change is noted. The reaction is called

   A. Hypothermic
   B. Hyperthermic
   C. Endothermic
   D. Exothermic
   E. Isothermic

9. A solution expressed as 35% w/v has the following:

   A. 35 mg of solute dissolved in 100 mL of solvent
   B. 35 g of solute dissolved in 100 mL of solution
   C. 35 mg of solute dissolved in 100 mL of solution
   D. 35 g of solute dissolved in 100 mL of solvent
   E. 35 mL of solute dissolved in 100 g of solution

10. Hydrophilic ointment, USP is an o/w type ointment base, therefore it possesses the property of being

    A. Emollient
    B. Greasy
    C. Occlusive
    D. Water washable
    E. Anhydrous

11. When compounding an emulsion that contains a flavoring agent, the flavoring agent should be in

    A. the continuous (external) phase
    B. the discontinuous (internal) phase
    C. the aqueous phase
    D. the oil phase

E. the emulsifier

The next four questions pertain to the following compounded prescription.

Mineral oil	60 mL
Acacia	qs
Syrup	12 mL
Flavor	qs
Purified water, qs ad	120 mL

M.Ft. emulsion using dry gum method

12. Mineral oil is in the

I. Internal phase
II. External phase
III. Discontinuous phase

   A. I only
   B. II only
   C. I and III only
   D. II and III only
   E. I, II, and III

13. Acacia is the

   A. Primary active ingredient
   B. Preservative
   C. Emulsifying agent
   D. Wetting agent
   E. Coloring agent

14. How much acacia is needed for this preparation?

   A. 5 g
   B. 10 g
   C. 15 g
   D. 30 g
   E. 35 g

15. How much purified water is needed to make the initial emulsion?

   A. 5 mL
   B. 10 mL
   C. 15 mL
   D. 30 mL
   E. 48 mL

16. When cocoa butter is used as a suppository base, its melting point can pose a problem. To overcome this problem, the compounding pharmacist can replace _____ of the cocoa butter with white wax.

   A. 5%

B. 10%
C. 15%
D. 20-25%
E. 30%

17. When cocoa butter is used as a suppository base, its melting point can pose a problem. To overcome this problem, the compounding pharmacist can replace _____ of the cocoa butter with cetyl esters wax.

   A. 5%
   B. 10%
   C. 15%
   D. 20-25%
   E. 30%

18. Hydrophilic petrolatum, USP is used as an ointment base. It possesses the characteristic(s) of being

I. Emollient
II. Occlusive
III. Greasy

   A. I only
   B. II only
   C. I and III only
   D. II and III only
   E. I, II, and III

19. When lime water and olive oil are processed together to form an emulsion, a reaction occurs that produces the emulsifying agent which is

   A. Lime oil
   B. Lime oxide
   C. Calcium oxide
   D. Calcium oleate
   E. Olive oxide

20. The advantage(s) of sublingual tablets as a dosage form is/are

I. Quick absorption into the bloodstream
II. Rapid onset of action
III. Avoids the first pass through the liver

   A. I only
   B. II only
   C. I and III only
   D. II and III only
   E. I, II, and III

Compounded Rx

Camphor	1%
Menthol	1%
Thymol	0.5%
White petrolatum, qs ad	30 g

M.Ft. oint

21. To prepare this compounded prescription, the pharmacist should

   A. Dissolve the camphor, menthol, and thymol in alcohol and incorporate into the white petrolatum by geometric dilution

   B. Dissolve the camphor, menthol, and thymol in glycerin and incorporate into the white petrolatum by geometric dilution

   C. Dissolve the camphor, menthol, and thymol in propylene glycol and incorporate into the white petrolatum

   D. Form a eutectic mixture and incorporate it into the white petrolatum by geometric dilution

   E. Alter the formula to avoid incompatibilities

22. The advantage(s) of capsules as a dosage form is/are

  I. Provides an accurate dose
  II. Masks unpleasant tastes
  III. Provides an immediate therapeutic response

   A. I only
   B. II only
   C. I and II only
   D. II and III only
   E. I, II, and III

Compounded Rx

Salicylic acid	5%
White petrolatum, qs ad	30 g

23. The pharmacist has on hand 2% salicylic acid ointment to use in preparing this prescription. When using it, the pharmacist should

   A. Weigh 0.5 g of salicylic acid powder and qs to 30 g with 2% salicylic acid ointment, incorporating the salicylic acid powder by geometric dilution

   B. Weigh 0.5 g of salicylic acid powder, levigate it with 5 mL of alcohol and qs to 30 g with 2% salicylic acid ointment, incorporating the salicylic acid by geometric dilution

   C. Weigh 1.5 g of salicylic acid powder, levigate

it with 6 mL of mineral oil and qs to 30 g with 2% salicylic acid ointment, incorporating the salicylic acid by geometric dilution

   D. Weigh 1.5 g of salicylic acid powder and qs to 30 g with 2% salicylic acid ointment, incorporating the salicylic acid powder by geometric dilution

   E. Weigh 1 g of salicylic acid powder, levigate it with 4.5 mL of mineral oil (SpGr 0.89) and incorporate it into 25 g of 2% salicylic acid ointment by geometric dilution

24. The advantage(s) of a transdermal gel as a dosage form is/are

  I. Convenience of administration/application
  II. Quick therapeutic response
  III. Patient acceptance

   A. I only
   B. II only
   C. I and II only
   D. II and III only
   E. I, II, and III

25. One gram of iodine is soluble in 3000 mL of water. In Lugol's solution (strong iodine solution) 1 g of iodine is dissolved in 20 mL of solution. Lugol's solution contains 5% iodine and 10% potassium iodide. The phenomenon by which the KI increases the solubility of iodine is known as

   A. Alligation
   B. Coalescence
   C. Comminution
   D. Complexation
   E. Diffusion

Answers

  1. **C.** For nonsterile compounding, the USP specifies that purified water be used.

  2. **B.** When type or percentage of alcohol is not specified, alcohol, USP is used and it is 95% ethyl alcohol.

  3. **B.** Ingredients that make the skin soft and pliable when applied locally are called emollients.

  4. **E.** Sodium thiosulfate is the antioxidant that prevents the iodide ion from oxidizing to form free iodine.

5.   **D.** When diluted hydrochloric acid is prepared, heat is generated and the reaction is called exothermic.

6.   **A.** Ingredients that shrink or tighten the skin when applied locally are called astringents.

7.   **D.** W/w means weight in weight, consequently 35 g of solute must be contained in 100 g of solution to have a 35% w/w solution.

8.   **C.** When potassium iodide is dissolved in purified water, the solution becomes distinctively cold and the reaction is called endothermic.

9.   **B.** W/v means weight in volume, consequently 35 g of solute must be contained in 100 mL of solution to have a 35% w/v solution.

10.   **D.** Hydrophilic ointment is water washable, but does not possess the other properties listed.

11.   **A.** For the flavoring agent to be tasted, it must be in the external or continuous phase.

12.   **C.** Mineral oil is in the internal or discontinuous phase and should not be tasted.

13.   **C.** Acacia is the emulsifying agent forming an oil-in-water emulsion.

14.   **C.** Using the 4:2:1 ratio, the 1 part or 15 g is the acacia.

15.   **D.** Using the 4:2:1 ratio, the 2 parts or 30 mL is the water for the initial emulsion.

16.   **A.** Five percent cocoa butter replaced by white wax will overcome the low melting point problem.

17.   **D.** Twenty to twenty-five percent cocoa butter replaced by cetyl esters wax will overcome the low melting point problem.

18.   **E.** Hydrophilic petrolatum is greasy, occlusive, and emollient.

19.   **D.** The lime water is calcium hydroxide solution and the olive oil contains oleic acid. The two react together to form calcium oleate, which is the emulsifying agent that forms a water-in-oil emulsion.

20.   **E.** All three items are advantages of sublingual tablets as dosage forms.

21.   **D.** The camphor, menthol, and thymol are three ingredients which when mixed together will liquefy, forming what is called a eutectic mixture. This liquid mixture is then gradually incorporated into the white petrolatum by geometric dilution.

22.   **C.** Capsules do not provide an immediate therapeutic response; the other two choices are correct.

23.   **E.** Your compounded preparation must contain 1.5 g of salicylic acid. Twenty-five grams of your 2% ointment contains 500 mg. You must weigh out 1 g of salicylic acid powder. The remaining ingredients must not contain any salicylic acid. The remaining weight can be made up with the levigating agent or a combination of the levigating agent and white petrolatum.

24.   **E.** All three choices are correct.

25.   **D.** In solution KI ionizes into potassium and the iodide ion. The iodide ion complexes with elemental iodine to form the soluble I^3 complex.

9. References

The following are references that should be available in the compounding pharmacy to provide assistance as the pharmacist formulates the variety of dosage forms of customized medications patients require.

Allen Jr LV. *The Art, Science and Technology of Pharmaceutical Compounding*, 2nd ed. Washington: American Pharmaceutical Association; 2002.

Ansel HC, Alen LV, Popovich NG. *Pharmaceutical Dosage Forms and Drug Delivery Systems*, 7th ed. Baltimore: Lippincott, Williams & Wilkins; 1999.

Ansel HC, Stoklosa MJ. *Pharmaceutical Calculations*, 11th ed. Baltimore: Lippincott, Williams & Wilkins; 2001.

Bodavari S, ed. *The Merck Index*, 13th ed. Whitehouse Station, NJ: Merck & Co.; 2001.

Gennaro AR ed. *Remington: The Science and Practice of Pharmacy*, 20th ed. Baltimore: Lippincott, Williams & Wilkins; 2000.

Parfitt K, ed. *Martindale: The Complete Drug Reference*, 32nd ed. London: Pharmaceutical Press; 1999.

Shrewsbury R. *Applied Pharmaceutics in Contemporary Compounding*, Englewood, CO: Morton Publishing; 2001

Thompson JE. *A Practical Guide to Contemporary Pharmacy Practice*, Baltimore: Williams & Wilkins; 1998.

Trissel LA. *Stability of Compounded Formulations*, 2nd ed. Washington: American Pharmaceutical Association; 2000.

U.S. Pharmacopeia 26/National Formulary 21. Rockville, MD: U.S. Pharmacopoeia Convention, Inc.; 2003.

5. Sterile Products

Laura A. Thoma, PharmD
Director/Associate Professor,
  Department of Pharmaceutical Sciences
Parenteral Medications Lab
University of Tennessee College of Pharmacy

Contents

1. Parenteral Products

Parenteral products are products that are administered by injection and therefore bypass the gastrointestinal (GI) tract. Parenteral products must be sterile and free of pyrogens and particulate matter. Drugs that are destroyed, inactivated in the GI tract, or poorly absorbed can be given by a parenteral route. Parenteral routes of administration may also be used when the patient being treated is uncooperative, unconscious, or unable to swallow. This route is also used when rapid drug absorption is essential, such as in emergency situations.

Parenteral Routes of Administration

Intravenous route
An intravenous (IV) medication is administered directly into the vein. The IV route gives a rapid effect with a predictable response. The IV route is used for irritating medications because the medication is rapidly diluted. This route does not have as much volume restriction as other parenteral routes.

A *bolus* means the drug is injected into the vein over a short period of time. A bolus is used to administer a relatively small volume and is often written as "IV push" (IVP).

An *infusion* refers to the introduction of larger volumes of solution given over a longer period of time. A continuous infusion is used to administer a large volume of solution at a constant rate. Intermittent infusions are used to administer a relatively small volume of solution over a specified amount of time at specific intervals.

Intramuscular route
An intramuscular medication (IM) is injected deep into a large muscle mass, such as the upper arm, thigh, or buttocks. The medication is absorbed from the muscle tissue, acting more quickly than when given by the oral route, but not as quickly as a medication given by the IV route. Up to 2 mL may be administered intramuscularly as a solution or suspension given in the upper arm, and 5 mL may be given in the gluteal medial muscle of each buttock. A sustained-release–type action can be achieved with certain drugs that have low solubility as they are released from muscle tissue at a slow rate. IM injections are often painful, and reversing adverse effects from medications given by this route is very difficult. Antibiotics are often given by this route.

Subcutaneous route
Subcutaneous (SC or SQ) injections of solution or suspension are given beneath the surface of the skin. Medications administered by this route are not absorbed as well and have a slower onset of action than medication given by the IV or IM route. The volume of solution or suspension that can be injected subcutaneously is 2 mL or less. Drugs often given by this route include epinephrine, insulin, heparin, and vaccines.

Intradermal route
An intradermal (ID) injection is injected into the top layer of the skin. The injection is not as deep as a SQ injection. Medications used for diagnostic purposes such as a tuberculin (TB) test or an allergy test are often administered by this route. The volume of solution that can be administered intradermally is limited to 0.1 mL. The onset of action and the rate of absorption of medication from this route is slow.

Intra-arterial
An intra-arterial injection is injected directly into an artery. It delivers a high drug concentration to the target site with little dilution by the circulation. Generally, this route is used only for radiopaque materials and some antineoplastic agents.

Other routes
1. *Intracardiac:* an injection directly into the heart

2. *Intra-articular:* administration by injection into a joint space. Corticosteroids are often administered by this route for the treatment of arthritis.

3. *Intrathecal:* injection into the lumbar intraspinal fluid sacs. Local anesthetics are frequently administered via this route during surgical procedures. Preservative-free drugs should be used for intrathecal administration.

2. Definitions for Sterile Product Compounding

admixture: when parenteral dosage forms are combined for administration as a single entity.

aseptic processing: when product components, containers, and closures, and the product itself, are sterilized separately and then brought together and assembled in an aseptic environment. The primary objective of aseptic processing is to create a product that is sterile.

aseptic technique: carrying out a procedure or procedures under controlled conditions in a manner that will minimize the chance of contamination. Contaminants can be introduced from the environment, equipment and supplies, or personnel.

class 100 area: the air in the area has a count of no more than 100 particles that are 0.5 micron or larger per cubic foot of air. This is the quality of air required for sterile product preparation.

class 10,000 area: the air in the area has a count of no more than 10,000 particles that are 0.5 micron or larger per cubic foot of air.

class 100,000 area: the air in the area has a count of no more than 100,000 particles that are 0.5 micron or larger per cubic foot of air.

controlled area (buffer area): the area the laminar flow workbench is in.

critical site: any opening or surface that can provide a pathway between the sterile product and the environment.

hypertonic: a solution which contains a higher concentration of dissolved substances than the red blood cell, which causes the red blood cell to shrink.

hypotonic: a solution which contains a lower concentration of dissolved substances than the red blood cell, causing the red blood cell to swell and possibly burst.

isotonic: a solution that is isotonic has an osmotic pressure close to that of body fluids. This minimizes patient discomfort and damage to red blood cells. Dextrose 5% in water and sodium chloride 0.9% solutions are approximately isotonic.

sterilizing filter: a filter which, when challenged with the microorganism *Brevundimonas diminuta*, at a minimum concentration of 10^7 organisms per cm^2 of filter surface, will produce a sterile effluent. A sterilizing filter has a pore size rating of 0.2 or 0.22 micron.

tonicity: refers to osmotic pressure exerted by a solution from the solutes or dissolved solids present.

validation: establishing documented evidence that provides a high degree of assurance that a specific process will consistently produce a product meeting its predetermined specifications and quality attributes.

3. Sterile Product Preparation Area

Horizontal Laminar Flow Workbench (HLFW)

The horizontal laminar flow workbench works by drawing air in through the pre-filter. The prefiltered air is pressurized in the plenum for consistent distribution of air to the HEPA (high-efficiency particulate air) filter (Figure 1).

The pre-filter protects the HEPA filter from prematurely clogging. Pre-filters should be checked regularly and changed as needed. A record of these checks and changes of the pre-filter must be kept.

The plenum of the hood is the space between the pre-filter and the HEPA filter. Air is pressurized here and distributed over the HEPA filter.

Laminar flow is defined as air in a confined space moving with uniform velocity along parallel lines. Inside the laminar flow workbench is a class 100 area.

Vertical Laminar Flow Workbench (VLFW)

The vertical laminar flow workbench (VLFW) works just like a HLFW in that the air is drawn in through the pre-filter, and pressurized in the plenum to distribute it over the HEPA filter. However, the air is blown down from the top of the workstation onto the work surface, not across it (Figure 2).

Working in vertical laminar flow (VLF) requires different techniques than working in horizontal laminar flow (HLF). In VLF, the hands of the operator or any object must not be above an object in the hood. In HLF, the hands of the operator or any object must not be in back of another object. The hands of the operator must never come between the HEPA filter and the object.

The High-Efficiency Particulate Air (HEPA) Filter

The HEPA filter consists of a bank of filter media separated by corrugated pleats of aluminum. These pleats act as baffles to direct the air into laminar sheets. The HEPA filter is 99.97% efficient at removing particles 0.3 micron and larger.

Certification of the HEPA filter

The velocity of air from the HEPA filter is checked with a velometer or hot wire anemometer. Federal Standard 209E recommends that the average air velocity should be 90 linear feet per minute, plus or minus 20%.

Integrity of the HEPA filter (DOP test)

The integrity of the HEPA filter is checked by introducing a high concentration of aerosolized Emery

Figure 1.

Horizontal laminar flow workbench.

Illustration courtesy of the University of Tennessee Parenteral Medications Lab.

Figure 2.

Vertical laminar flow workbench.

Illustration courtesy of the University of Tennessee Parenteral Medications Lab.

3004 (a synthetic hydrocarbon) upstream of the filter on a continuous basis, while monitoring the penetration on the downstream side of the HEPA filter.

The aerosol has an average particle size of 0.3 micron. An aerosol photometer is used to check for leaks by passing the wand slowly over the filter and the gasket. None of the surfaces should yield greater than 0.01% of the upstream smoke concentration. Any value greater than 0.01% indicates a serious leak is present and it must be sealed. All repaired areas must be retested for compliance. At one time DOP (dioctyl phalate) was used to generate the aerosol. However, since DOP is a carcinogen, Emery 3004 is now used. An electronic particle counter cannot be used to certify the integrity of the HEPA filter. The particle counter is used to determine room classification.

Buffer Area (Controlled Area)

The laminar flow workstation is your most clean area. You have a class 100 area inside the LFW. The LFW must be located in a controlled environment, away from excess traffic, doors, air vents, or anything that could produce air currents greater than the velocity of the airflow from the HEPA filter. Air currents greater than the velocity of the airflow from the HEPA filter may introduce contaminants into the hood. It is very easy to overcome air flowing at 90 feet per minute.

The buffer area should be enclosed from other pharmacy operations. Floors, walls, ceiling, shelving, counters, and cabinets of the controlled area must be of nonshedding, smooth, and nonporous material to allow for easy cleaning and disinfecting. All surfaces should be resistant to sanitizing agents. Cracks, crevices, and seams should be avoided, as should ledges or other places that could collect dust. The floor of the buffer area should be smooth and seamless with sealed edges.

The walls of the buffer area can be sealed panels, or if drywall, painted with epoxy paint, which is nonshedding. The corner of the ceiling and the walls should be sealed to avoid cracks. A solid ceiling may be painted with epoxy paint, or nonshedding washable ceiling tiles that are caulked into place may be used.

Light fixtures should be mounted flush with the ceiling and sealed. All penetration through the ceiling or walls should be sealed.

Air entering the room should be fresh, HEPA filtered, and air-conditioned, and the room must be maintained in positive pressure in relation to the adjoining rooms or corridors (air flow should be out from the room, not in). There should be at least 10 air changes per hour.

People entering the buffer area should be properly scrubbed and gowned. Access to the buffer area should be restricted only to qualified personnel. Controlling the traffic in the buffer area is a critical factor in keeping the area clean. Only items required to perform compounding should be brought into the buffer room. These items must be cleaned and sanitized before being taken into the buffer area. Items may be stored in the buffer room for a limited time. However, try and keep the number of items stored in the buffer room to a minimum. All equipment used in the buffer room should remain in the room except for calibration or repair.

These items should not be in the controlled area: Refrigerators and freezers should be kept out of the buffer area as they can harbor many organisms. Sinks or floor drains should not be in the buffer area for the same reason. If you have a sink or floor drain in the buffer area, disinfectants must be poured down the drain on a regular basis. Computers and printers should be located outside of the buffer area since they generate many particles. Cardboard boxes should also not be stored in the buffer area. However, vials stored in laminated cardboard may be stored in the buffer area.

Preparation of Operators

The operator must be properly scrubbed before entering the controlled area. This is critical to the maintenance of asepsis. The greatest source of contamination in a clean room is the people in the area. A seated person releases an average of 100,000 particles per minute. The garb is designed to help contain the particles that are being shed.

The operator should scrub from elbows to hands for an appropriate length of time using an antimicrobial skin cleanser. After scrubbing, the operator should don a hair cover, shoe covers, and a clean knee-length nonshedding gown and sterile latex gloves. Once the gloves are out of the package they are no longer sterile. Frequent rinsing with sterile 70% isopropyl alcohol is essential to keep the gloves sanitized. Before working in the hood the operator should put on a facemask. All facial hair must be covered at all times.

Validation of the Operator

A *media fill* or *media transfer* is when media is used instead of the drug product, and all the normal compounding manipulations are done. Usually the medium used is soybean casein digest, which is also called trypticase soy broth (TSB). This medium will support the growth of many organisms, including some fungi and mold. A media fill can be used to check an operator's aseptic technique or to validate a compounding process.

Initially, before an operator can compound sterile injectable products, they must successfully complete three media fills. This means no growth in any of the units. The operator should revalidate quarterly by completing one media fill. Ideally, the media fills should be designed to mimic techniques the operator will use during a normal day. Once the operator has successfully completed the initial qualification with no growth in any of the media containers, they may participate in the validation of each high-risk operation they will be doing. An example of a high-risk operation is the compounding of a sterile product from nonsterile drug powder. Validation for high-risk compounding focuses on making sure the process, along with the operator, is capable of producing a sterile product with all its purported quality attributes.

4. Working in the Laminar Flow Workbench

Items not in a protective overwrap should be wiped with a lint-free wipe soaked with sterile 70% isopropyl alcohol (IPA) before being placed in the hood. Check containers for cracks, tears, and particles. Items in a protective overwrap, such as syringes and bags, should be taken from the overwrap at the edge of the hood (within the first 6 inches of the hood), and placed in the hood with the injection port facing the HEPA filter. The overwrap should not be placed in the hood, as this would introduce particles and organisms into the hood.

When working in the HLFW, supplies should be arranged to the left or right of the critical work area. The critical site must be in uninterrupted laminar airflow at all times. The operator must be careful not to place an object or their hand in between the HEPA filter and the critical site. To do so would interrupt the airflow to the critical site and potentially cause particles to be washed from the hand or object onto the critical site.

All work done in the HLFW must be done at least 6 inches inside the hood. The laminar air flow is blowing toward the operator. The body acts as a barrier to the laminar airflow, causing it to pass around the person and create backflow. This turbulence can cause room air to be carried into the front of the hood.

Items placed in the HFLW disturb the laminar flow. The laminar airflow is disturbed downstream of the item for approximately three times the diameter of the object. If the item is placed next to the sidewall of the hood, the airflow is disturbed approximately six times the diameter of the object. Air downstream from the nonsterile objects also becomes contaminated with particles. For these reasons, it is very important that a direct path exists between the HEPA filter and the area where the manipulations will occur.

With the VLFH, supplies in the hood should be placed so that the operator may work without placing a hand or object above the critical site. It is possible to place many more items in the VLFH and still work without compromising the laminar flow. It must be kept in mind that within 1 inch of the work surface you will have turbulent air. The air is coming from the HEPA filter and strikes the work surface. It then has to change directions and move horizontally across the work surface. All work in the VLFW should be done at least 1 inch above the work surface.

When compounding sterile products it is important

that all movements in and out of the hood be minimized, to decrease the risk of carrying contaminants into the critical site. This can be achieved by introducing all items needed for the aseptic manipulation into the work area at one time, by dropping discarded items over the edge of the hood, or leaving the items within the first 6 inches until the manipulations are complete.

5. Needles, Syringes, Ampuls, and Vials

The Syringe

The basic parts of the syringe are the barrel, plunger, collar, the rubber tip of the plunger, and the tip of the syringe. The syringes are sterile, pyrogen-free, and packaged either in paper or in a rigid plastic container. It is important that the syringe packages be inspected to make sure the wrap is intact to ensure that the syringe is still sterile. Syringes have either a Luer-Lok tip, in which case the needle is screwed tightly onto the threaded tip, or a slip tip, in which case the needle is held on by friction (Figure 3). Syringes are supplied with and without needles attached, and are available in a variety of sizes. Some syringes are packaged with a protective tip on them to keep the syringe sterile until the needle is attached. Other syringes do not have the protective tip, so care must be taken not to lay the syringe down under the hood until the needle has been attached.

There are calibration marks on the barrel of the syringe. These marks are accurate to one-half the interval marked on the syringe. The critical sites on the syringe are the tip of the syringe and the ribs of the plunger. This is because the ribs of the plunger go back inside the syringe upon injection of the fluid from the syringe and could potentially contaminate the syringe.

Figure 3.

Types of syringes.

Illustration courtesy of the University of Tennessee Parenteral Medications Lab.

The Needle

The basic parts of a needle include the hub, needle shaft, bevel, bevel heel, and the tip of the needle (Figure 4).

Needles are sterile and come wrapped in plastic with a twist-off top or wrapped in paper. This wrap must be inspected for integrity before using the needle. The *gauge* of the needle refers to the outer diameter of the needle. The larger the number, the smaller the bore of the needle. The smallest is 27 gauge and the largest is 13 gauge. The length of the needle is measured in inches, and the most common lengths are 1-1$^1/_2$ inches.

The critical sites on the needle are the hub of the needle, the needle shaft, and the tip of the needle.

Ampuls

Ampuls are single-dose containers. Once ampuls are broken, they are an open-system container, and air can pass freely in and out of the ampul. Any solution taken from an ampul must be filtered with a 5-micron filter needle, because glass particles fall into the ampul when it is broken. Before breaking the ampul, the neck of the ampul should be wiped with a sterile alcohol prep pad.

Vials

A vial is a molded glass or plastic container with a rubber closure secured in place with an aluminum seal. They may contain sterile solutions, dry-filled powders, lyophilized drugs, or may be an empty evacuated container. Vials may be single-dose or multiple-dose containers.

A single-dose container usually contains no preservative system to prevent the growth of microorganisms if they are accidentally introduced into the container. The standard of practice is that the single-dose vial can be used for 24 hours after the initial entry into the vial, provided it is never removed from the laminar flow hood. When the vial is first used, it should be labeled with the date, time, and initials of the person using the vial so the length of time the vial has been in the hood can be determined.

A multi-dose vial contains preservatives, and these vials can be entered more than once. The pharmaceutical manufacturer has done studies to prove the preservative system will remain effective and the closure will reseal after penetration by the needle.

Figure 4.

Needle.

Illustration courtesy of the University of Tennessee Parenteral Medications Lab.

6. Biological Safety Cabinets

A class II biological safety cabinet (BSC) should be used to prepare cytotoxic and other hazardous drugs. All BSCs are vertical flow hoods, but not all vertical flow hoods are BSCs. There are four different types of class II BSCs. The most often used is a class II type A cabinet, which has approximately 70% of the air recirculated and 30% of the air exhausted through a HEPA filter into the room. Intake of the make-up air is through the front grill of the workbench.

Preparation of Cytotoxic Drugs

When working with cytotoxic drugs it is imperative that positive pressure is not allowed to build up in the vial. It is recommended that some type of air venting device be used, such as a Chemo Dispensing Pin®. The 0.2-micron hydrophobic filter on this device allows air to pass in and out of the vial, but prevents the passage of aerosolized drug (Figure 5). If this type of device is not available, care must be taken to keep the vial at negative pressure to prevent spewing of drug into the BSC.

When preparing cytotoxic drugs it is recommended the operator wear a gown with a closed front, that is nonshedding and nonabsorptive, with elastic or knit cuffs. Surgical gloves should be worn, and the operator should double-glove. The first set of gloves should be put under the cuff of the gown and the second pair should be pulled up over the cuff of the gown.

When compounding, syringes and IV sets with Luer-Lok fittings should be used. Use a large enough syringe so the plunger does not separate from the barrel of the syringe when filled with solution. When possible, attach IV sets and prime them before adding the hazardous drug. Wipe the outside of the bag or bottle to remove any inadvertent contamination. The use of nonshedding plastic-backed absorbent pads is also conducive to keeping the BSC as clean as possible.

Figure 5.

Chemo Dispensing Pin.

Illustration courtesy of the University of Tennessee Parenteral Medications Lab.

7. Overview of Standards of Practice Related to Sterile Products

American Society of Health-System Pharmacists (ASHP)

The ASHP published the Technical Assistance Bulletin on Quality Assurance for Pharmacy-Prepared Sterile Products in September 1993. This document has been revised and is now called the ASHP Guidelines on Quality Assurance for Pharmacy-Prepared Sterile Products.

This document groups sterile products into three risk levels based on the risk to the patient posed by the compounded product. Level I products have the least risk and level III products have the greatest risk for the patient. Some factors can increase the risk of microbial contamination of the product, such as increased complexity of compounding steps, lengthy exposure of the critical site, increased storage time, and the temperature of the prepared injectable product. The document provides a method to match quality assurance/quality control (QA/QC) activities with the potential risk of the product to the patient. Information is provided on QA/QC activities that should be in place.

For risk levels I and II the product is prepared using sterile equipment, ingredients, solutions, and sterile contact surfaces for the final product.

A level I product exhibits a, b, and c, below:
- a. Stored at room temperature and administered within 28 hours, or refrigerated under USP conditions for ≤7 days, or frozen for ≤30 days prior to complete administration to a patient over a period not to exceed 24 hours.
- b. A product prepared for one patient that is unpreserved or a batch product compounded for multiple patients that contains a preservative.
- c. A product prepared by closed-system aseptic transfer of sterile product to sterile final container.

If the compounded product exhibits a, b, or c, below, it is considered a level II product:
- a. Stored beyond 7 days in the refrigerator or greater than 30 days in the freezer, or administered beyond 28 hours from preparation time at room temperature.
- b. Sterile batch preparation made without preservatives, intended for use by more than one patient.
- c. Product compounded by combining multiple sterile ingredients, obtained from a licensed manufacturer using closed-system aseptic transfer, before subdivision into multiple units to be dispensed to patients.

Any compounded parenteral product that exhibits a or b, below, is a level III product:
- a. Sterile products made from nonsterile ingredients or using nonsterile components or equipment.
- b. Prepared by combining multiple ingredients, sterile or nonsterile, by using open-system transfer or open reservoir before terminal sterilization or subdivision into multiple dispensing units.

The United States Pharmacopeia 25/ National Formulary 20

USP25/NF20 currently has chapter <1206> Sterile Drug Products for Home Use. This chapter is currently under revision with the proposed chapter number changing to <797> and the title changing to Pharmaceutical Compounding—Sterile Preparations. This proposed change of chapter number is very important. Chapters numbered <1> to <999> contain general requirements. Chapters numbered from <1000> to <1999> are informational only. Chapter <1206> also has three risk levels of compounded sterile products. The risk levels are determined based on the potential for the introduction of microorganisms into the product. The chapter covers such topics as validation of sterilization and of the aseptic process, environmental control and monitoring, end-product testing, bacterial endotoxins, training, and a quality assurance program.

Compounding is classified as low-risk when all of the following conditions prevail:
1. Commercially available sterile products are used in compounding.
2. Compounding involves few aseptic manipulations.
3. Closed-system transfers are used. Withdrawal from an open ampul is classified as a closed system.

High-risk compounding is divided into categories 1 and 2.

High-risk category 1 pertains to products compounded from commercially prepared sterile components meeting one or more of the following conditions:
1. Compounding involves pooling of additives.
2. Compounding involves complex manipulations performed over a long period of time.

3. The finished product is administered as a multi-day infusion.

High-risk category 2 compounding is compounding that involves either of the following:
1. A sterile product compounded from a nonsterile product.
2. Open-system transfers are used. Ingredients are combined in a nonsterile tank or the solution is put into an unsealed container.

8. Sterilization Methods

Filtration

Filtration works by a combination of sieving, adsorption, and entrapment. When deciding which filter to use to sterilize the product, care must be taken to choose the correct filter. Membrane filters generally are compatible with most pharmaceutical solutions, but interactions do occur. This is often due to sorption or leaching. Sorption is the binding of drug or other formulation component to the filter. This can occur with peptide or protein formulations. There are filters that have little or no affinity for peptides or proteins. Leaching is the extracting of components of the filter into the solution. Often surfactants are added to the filter to make it hydrophilic, and these may leach into the product. Large-molecular-weight peptides may be affected by filtration. The passage through a filter with a small pore size may cause shear stress and alter the three-dimensional structure of peptide. Filters may also be affected by solvents in the parenteral formulation. All filter manufacturers have compatibility data on their membrane type and are a great source of information when choosing a membrane.

Choosing a Filter

Choose the appropriate size and configuration of filtration device that will accommodate the volume being filtered to permit complete filtration without clogging of the membrane. A 25-mm syringe disk filter should filter no more than 100 mL of solution. If the solution you are filtering has a heavy particulate load, a 5-micron filter should be used before the 0.2-micron filter to decrease the particulate load to the 0.2-micron filter. The filter membrane and housing must be physically and chemically compatible with the product to be filtered and capable of withstanding the temperature, pressures, and hydrostatic stress imposed on the system.

A pharmacy may rely on the certificate of quality provided by the vendor. Certification should include microbial retention testing with *Brevundimonas diminuta* at a minimum concentration of 10^7 organisms per cm^2, as well as testing for membrane and housing integrity, nonpyrogenicity, and extractables.

Hydrophobic and Hydrophilic Filters

Hydrophilic membranes wet spontaneously with water. They are used for filtration of aqueous solutions and aqueous solutions containing water miscible solvents. *Hydrophobic filters* do not wet spontaneously with water. They are used for filtering gases and solvents.

Filter Integrity

A sterilizing filter assembly should be tested for integrity after filtration has occurred. The *bubble point* is a simple, nondestructive check of the integrity of the filtration assembly, including the filter membrane. The test is based on the fact that liquid is held in the capillary structure of the membrane by surface tension. The minimum pressure required to force the liquid out of the capillary space is a measure of the largest pore in the membrane.

A bubble point test is performed by wetting the filter with water, increasing the pressure of air upstream of the filter, and watching for air bubbles downstream, to indicate passage of air through the filter capillaries. The typical water bubble point pressure of a sterilizing filter with a pore size rating of 0.2 micron is 54 pounds per square inch gauge (psig). As pore size decreases, the bubble point increases. Keep in mind that the bubble point given on the certificate of quality from the filter manufacturer is usually the water bubble point. Many drug formulations have a lower surface tension than water and will have a lower bubble point. Bubble points are also often given for 70% IPA and water. If you have a hydrophobic filter, you should use the alcohol test.

After filtration of your solution, the filter membrane should be flushed with water to wash the product solution off the membrane as much as possible before performing the filter integrity test.

Heat Sterilization

Moist-heat sterilization (autoclave)
Moist-heat sterilization is one of the most widely used methods of sterilization. Saturation of steam at high pressure is the foundation for the effectiveness of moist heat sterilization. When steam makes contact with a cooler object, it condenses and loses latent heat to the object. The amount of energy released is ~524 kcal/g at 121°C. Most sterilization cycles are at 121°C at 15 psig for a minimum of 15 minutes. Moist heat sterilization is quicker and does not require as high a temperature as dry heat.

Dry-heat sterilization
Dry-heat sterilization is usually done as a batch process in an oven designed for sterilization. It is designed to provide heated filtered air that is evenly distributed throughout the chamber by a blower. The oven is equipped with a system to control the temperature and exposure period. Dry-heat sterilization requires higher temperatures and longer exposure times than moist-heat sterilization. Typical sterilization cycles are 120-180 minutes at 160°C or 90-120 minutes at 170°C. Dry heat is also used to depyrogenate equipment.

9. Stability

Each compounded sterile product must have a label that specifies the product's storage requirements and the expiration date. Stability refers to physical, chemical, and microbial stability. Any product that is not meant for immediate use should be refrigerated at a temperature no higher than 4°C, as this is the temperature that will inhibit microbial growth. If the sterile product is intended for multi-day administration, the infusion should be started as soon as possible after preparation. There are several good references available on drug stability, such as *Trissel's Handbook on Injectable Drugs*. When compounding sterile products for home use, there is often a need to push the envelope on expiration dating. When setting the expiration date, consideration must be given to the concentration of the product, the temperature at which the product will be administered, and the duration of administration. For example, if the product will be in an implantable infusion device where it will be exposed to body temperature for several days, the stability data referenced must take into account the increased temperature and the increase in concentration that is required for this dosing regimen. The most accurate way to determine stability is to do a product-specific experiment.

Instability usually refers to chemical reactions that are incessant, irreversible, and result in distinctly different chemical entities. These new chemical entities can be both therapeutically inactive and possibly exhibit greater toxicity.

Incompatibility usually refers to physicochemical phenomena such as concentration-dependent precipitation and acid-base reactions, that occur when one drug is mixed with others to produce a product unsuitable for administration to the patient. An incompatibility could cause the patient not to receive the full therapeutic effect, or toxic decomposition products could form. A precipitated incompatibility may irritate the vein or cause occlusion of vessels.

There are three categories of incompatibilities: *therapeutic incompatibility*, *physical incompatibility*, and *chemical incompatibility*.

Therapeutic Incompatibility

This results when two or more drugs administered at the same time result in undesirable antagonistic or synergistic pharmacologic action.

Physical Incompatibility

This is the combination of two or more drugs in solution, resulting in a change in the appearance of the solution, a change in color, formation of turbidity or a precipitate, or the evolution of a gas. Physical incompatibilities are related to solubility changes or container interactions rather than to molecular change to the drug entity itself.

Six major areas of concern about physical incompatibility:

1. *The compatibility or incompatibility of two or more drugs mixed in the same syringe.*
   For example, preoperative medications: a combination of a narcotic, an analgesic, an antiemetic, an anticholinergic. These drugs are mixed in the same syringe to save the patient from multiple IM injections.

2. *The compatibility of two or more drugs given through the same IV administration line.*
   This is common in intensive care units where patients are on a number of IV meds and could also be fluid restricted.
   An example: dopamine HCl 800 mg in 500 mL D_5W. The nurse wants to push 2 amps of sodium bicarbonate through the IV line.
   pH of dopamine: 3.0-4.5
   pH of $NAHCO_3$: ~8
   If this is done a color change occurs due to decomposition of the product. The pH of the bicarb is too high for dopamine stability.

3. *Compatibility of two or more drugs placed in the same bottle or bag of IV fluid.*
   KCl, the most common additive, is a neutral salt composed of monovalent ions which are not likely to produce compatibility problems. Therefore if a drug is compatible in NS it is probably compatible in KCl.

   Parenteral nutrition solutions can especially difficult. The number of components, the long duration of contact time, and exposure to ambient temperature and light enhance the potential for an adverse compatibility interaction to occur. The interaction of Ca and PO_4 to form $CaPO_4$, which appears as fine white particles that create a milky solution, is a problem.

   Ways to decrease the risk of injury:
   a. Calculate the solubility of the added calcium from the volume at the time when calcium is added. Flush the line between addition of any potentially incompatible components.

b. Add the calcium before the lipid emulsion, so if a precipitate forms, the lipid will not obscure its presence.

c. Periodically agitate the admixture and check for precipitates. Train patients and caregivers to visually inspect for signs of precipitation and to stop the infusion if precipitation is noted.

The following factors enhance formation of precipitate of calcium and phosphate:
* High concentrations of calcium and phosphate
* Increases in solution pH
* Decreases in amino acid concentrations
* Increases in temperature
* Addition of calcium before phosphate
* Lengthy time delay or slow infusion rates
* Use of the chloride salt of calcium

Do not exceed 15 mEq of calcium with up to 15 mL PO_4 per 1000 mL of solution.

4. ***Compatibility of the additive with the composition of the IV container itself.***
Nitroglycerin readily migrates into many plastics, especially PVC.
Insulin adsorbs to both glass and plastic containers, IV tubing, and filters.

5. ***Compatibility of the additive with the additional equipment used to prepare or administer the IV admixture.***
Cisplatin interacts with aluminum by forming a black precipitate when coming in contact with it.

6. ***Stability of the drug after admixture.***
Ampicillin sodium is stable for 72 hours refrigerated and 24 hours at room temperature in normal saline. However, if it is added to D_5W, it is stable for only 4 hours refrigerated and 2 hours at room temperature.

Other potential sources of physical incompatibilities:
Concentration
A drug will remain in aqueous solution as long as its concentration is less than its saturation solubility.

Cosolvent system
Drugs that are poorly water soluble are often formulated using water-miscible cosolvents. Examples of water miscible cosolvents are ethanol, propylene glycol, and polyethylene glycol. Dilution of drugs that are in a cosolvent system often causes precipitation of the drug. A good example is diazepam injection. Dilution of the drug results in precipitation in some concentra-

tions, but sufficient dilution to a point below diazepam's saturation solubility results in a physically stable admixture.

pH
The greatest single factor in causing an incompatibility is a change in acid-base environment. Solubility of drugs that are weak acids or bases is a direct function of solution pH. The drug's dissociation constant and pH controls the portion of drug in its ionized form and the solubility of the un-ionized form. A drug that is a weak acid may be formulated at a pH sufficient to yield the desired solubility. Sodium salts of barbiturates, phenytoin, and methotrexate are formulated at high pH values to achieve adequate solubility.

Sodium salts of weak acids precipitate as free acids when added to IV fluids having an acidic pH. If the pH of these drugs is lowered, the drug's solubility at the final pH may be exceeded, resulting in possible precipitation. Drugs that are salts of weak bases may precipitate in an alkaline solution.

Ionic interactions
Large organic anions and cations may also form precipitates. An examples of this is the precipitation that occurs when heparin (anionic) and aminoglycoside antibiotics (cationic) are mixed. These heparin salts of the cationic drug are relatively insoluble in water.

Sorption phenomena
The intact drug is lost from the solution by adsorption to the surface or absorption into the matrix of container material, administration set, or filter.

Adsorption to the surface can result from interactions of functional groups within the drug's molecule to binding sites on the surfaces.

Absorption of lipid-soluble drug into the matrix of plastic containers and administration sets, especially those made from polyvinyl chloride (PVC), does occur. The substantial amount of phthalate plasticizer used to make the PVC bag pliable and flexible allows the lipid-soluble drugs to diffuse from the solution into the plasticizer in the plastic matrix. Plastics such as polyethylene and polypropylene, which contain little or no phthalate plasticizer, do not readily absorb lipid-soluble drug into the polymer core. Leaching of the phthalate plasticizer into the solution may also occur, especially if surface-active agents or large amount of organic cosolvent are present in the formulation.

Chemical Incompatibility

Chemical incompatibilities are interactions resulting in

molecular changes or rearrangements to different chemical entities. Most chemical interactions are not visibly observable.

Chemical degradation pathways

Hydrolysis is a common mode of chemical decomposition. Water attacks labile bonds in dissolved drug molecules. Functional groups labile to hydrolysis are carboxylic acid and phosphate esters, amides, lactams, and imines.

Oxidation is an electron loss, causing a positive increase in valence. Many drugs are in the reduced form and oxygen creates stability problems. Steroids, epinephrine, and tricyclic compounds are sensitive to oxygen. To control the stability problem, oxygen can be excluded, pH can be adjusted, and chelating agents or antioxidants can be added.

Reduction is when an electron is gained, causing a decrease in valence and the addition of halogen or hydrogen to the double bond. Beta-lactam antibiotics can produce reducing aldehydes upon hydrolysis.

Photolysis is the catalysis by light of degradation reactions such as oxidation or hydrolysis. Examples of drugs that are light sensitive are amphotericin B, furosemide, and sodium nitroprusside. The reaction rate depends on the intensity and wavelength of light. Sodium nitroprusside in D_5W has a faint brownish cast, but exposure to light causes deterioration, which is evident by a change to a blue color due to the reduction of the ferric to ferrous ion.

Extreme pH can be a catalysis of drug degradation. Drug reaction rates are generally less at intermediate pH values than at high or low ranges. Many times a buffer system is used to ensure the maintenance of the proper pH.

Effects of temperature. Usually, but not always, an elevation in temperature may increase reaction rates.

An increase in drug concentration will usually increase the degradation rate exponentially. Again, this rule does not always apply. Some drugs appear to have a lower rate of decomposition at high concentration. An example of this is the reduced hydrolysis of nafcillin in the presence of aminophylline. Greater buffer concentration at higher nafcillin concentrations protects the drug from aminophylline's high pH and slows the hydrolysis.

Expiration dates and removal of IV bag overwrap. The overwrap protects against evaporation of the solution, desiccation of the container, drug oxidation, and photochemical inactivation of the drug. Substantial moisture loss may occur, increasing drug concentration. With ready-to-use dopamine or dobutamine injections, removal of the overwrap can allow oxygen to enter the container, reducing drug stability. After removal of the overwrap the expiration date should be changed at once.

10. Sterile Products Compounded from Nonsterile Drugs

When compounding a sterile drug product from a nonsterile component several concerns arise: how to sterilize the drug and/or the container and closure; and how to ensure the drug and components are sterile. All sterilization processes must be validated, whether it is terminal sterilization of the product in the final container or aseptic processing of the product. End-product testing must be done on all compounded sterile injectable drug products. When compounding a sterile product from a nonsterile drug, end-product testing must include the sterility test and the bacterial endotoxin test. The product should not be dispensed from the pharmacy until the results of the bacterial endotoxin test are known. Because the USP sterility test takes 14 days, the sterile product is usually dispensed before the results are known. However, a method must be in place to track the product in case it does not meet the requirement of the sterility test.

Sterility Testing

All products that are made from a nonsterile component or components should undergo sterility testing. A sample from each lot of product compounded should be tested. There are two methods of sterility testing: direct inoculation and membrane filtration. The USP states that when possible, membrane filtration should be performed, and two culture media are required: fluid thioglycollate medium (FTM) and trypticase soy broth (TSB), also called soybean casein digest medium.

Media suitability test

Before beginning the test it must be confirmed that the media being used is sterile, and it will support the growth of micro-organisms.

Sterility

Confirm the sterility of each sterilized batch of medium by incubating a portion of the batch at the specified incubation temperatures (TSB 20-25°C, FTM 30-35°C) for not less than 14 days, or by incubating uninoculated containers as negative controls during a sterility test procedure. When purchasing a new batch of sterile media from a vendor, it is advisable to incubate a portion for several days to make sure it did not become contaminated during shipment.

Growth promotion test (GP)

A lot of dehydrated medium bearing the manufacturer's lot number must be tested for its growth-promoting qualities. Separately inoculate, in duplicate, containers of each medium with fewer than 100 viable micro-organisms of each of the strains listed below. If visual evidence of growth appears in all inoculated media containers within 5 days of incubation, the test media is satisfactory. The test may be conducted simultaneously with testing of the media for sterility.

The organisms to be used for the growth promotion test of fluid thioglycollate media are *Staphylococcus aureus* (*Bacillus subtilis* may be used instead), *Pseudomonas aeruginosa* (*Micrococcus luteus* may be used instead), and *Clostridium sporogenes* (*Bacteroides vulgatus* may be used instead). The test organisms for soybean casein digest media are *Bacillus subtilis*, *Candida albicans,* and *Asperigllus niger*. Soybean casein digest media is incubated at 20-25°C, and fluid thioglycollate media is incubated at 30-35°C, both under aerobic conditions.

Bacteriostasis/fungistasis test (B&F)

The B&F must be done on each product to determine if the product itself will inhibit the growth of microorganisms. This test only needs to be done one time for each product tested. The organisms used are the same as for growth promotion. The test uses two sets of containers. One set is inoculated with the drug product and microorganisms. The other set is inoculated with just the microorganisms. Both sets will be incubated at the appropriate temperature for no more than 7 days. The same amount of growth should be seen in both sets.

Number of articles to test

Below is the minimum number of articles to be tested in relation to the number of articles in the batch:
* For up to 100 articles, test 10% or 4 articles, whichever is greater.
* For more than 100 but not more than 500, test 10 articles.

Interpretation of results

No growth

At days 3, 5, 7, and 14, examine the media visually for growth. If microbial growth is not observed, the article tested meets the requirements of the sterility test. No growth does not prove that all units in the lot are sterile.

Growth observed

When microbial growth is observed and confirmed microscopically, the article does not meet the requirements of the test for sterility. If there is no doubt that the microbial growth can be ascribed to faulty aseptic techniques or materials used in conducting the testing procedure, the test is invalid and must be repeated.

An investigation must take place, and the organism must be identified down to the species. All records must be reviewed, including all employee training procedures and records, aseptic gowning practices, equipment maintenance records, component sterilization data, and environmental monitoring data.

Visual inspection
Every unit compounded in the pharmacy should be subjected to a physical inspection against a white background and a black background.

Any container whose contents show evidence of contamination with visible foreign material must be rejected.

Pyrogens
When compounding a sterile injectable product from nonsterile components there is concern about endotoxin contamination. An endotoxin is a type of pyrogen. A pyrogen is a substance that produces fever.

Gram-negative bacteria produce more potent endotoxins than gram-positive bacteria and fungi. The lipopolysaccharide (LPS) portion of the cell wall causes the pyrogenic response. The LPS can be sloughed off and the bacteria do not have to be living for the LPS to be pyrogenic.

Some of the effects caused by pyrogens in the body are an increase in body temperature, chills, cutaneous vasoconstriction, a decrease in respiration, an increase in arterial blood pressure, nausea and malaise, and severe diarrhea.

The official endotoxin limits are 5 endotoxin units (EU)/kg/h or 350 EU/total body/h for drugs and biologicals. Drugs for intrathecal use have a much lower endotoxin limit of 0.2 EU/kg.

Water is the number one source of pyrogens. This is because *Pseudomonas*, a gram-negative bacterium, grows readily in water. Other sources of endotoxins or pyrogens are raw material, equipment, processing, and human contamination. It is very important to use good quality raw materials, and request a certificate of analysis with each lot of material when compounding. Endotoxins can be destroyed by dry heat. Three hours at 200°C will depyrogenate glass vials and beakers. The endotoxin concentration can be reduced by rinsing with water for injection, or sterile water for injection. When compounding a sterile product from a nonsterile product, anything that can withstand the heat of 200°C should be depyrogenated. If an article is depyrogenated it is also sterile. Endotoxins are not completely

removed by filtration, and steam sterilization only reduces endotoxin levels by a small amount.

Pyrogen test (rabbit test)
The pyrogen test is designed to limit to an acceptable level the risk of febrile reaction in the patient to the administration, by injection, of the product concerned. The test involves measuring the rise in the temperature of rabbits following the intravenous injection of a test solution, and is designed for products that can be tolerated by the test rabbit in a dose, not to exceed 10 mL/kg, injected intravenously within a period of no more than 10 minutes.

The rabbit test has several limitations. It is a in-vivo method, it is expensive and time-consuming, and is not a very sensitive test. Drugs which have pyretic side effects, or which are antipyretics, cannot be tested by the rabbit test. It is not quantitative, and the pyrogenic response is dose-dependent, not concentration-dependent.

Bacterial endotoxin test (limulus amebocyte lysate test; LAL)
The bacterial endotoxin test (BET) provides a method for estimating the concentration of bacterial endotoxins that may be present in or on the sample of the article to which the test is applied using LAL reagent. The blood cells of the horseshoe crab are sensitive to endotoxin and form a gel in its presence. LAL reagent is made from the lysate of amebocytes from the horseshoe crab.

There are two types of techniques for this test. The gel-clot technique, which is based on the formation of the gel, and the photometric technique, which is based on either the development of turbidity or the development of color in the test sample.

The routine gel clot test requires 0.1 mL of test sample to be mixed with 0.1 mL of LAL reagent. This mixture is incubated for 1 hour at 37°C. A positive reaction is confirmed by formation of a firm gel that remains intact when the tube is inverted 180 degrees.

The BET is 5-50 times more sensitive, more simple and rapid, and less expensive than the pyrogen test. However, the clotting enzyme is heat sensitive, pH sensitive and chemically related to trypsin. It is only dependable for detection of pyrogens originating from gram-negative bacteria. Also, some drugs can inhibit the reaction, while other drugs can enhance the reaction. The BET does not determine the fever-producing potential of the bacterial endotoxins.

The photometric technique requires the establishment of a standard regression curve. The endotoxin content of the test material is determined by interpolation from the curve. The test can either be an endpoint determination, with the reading made immediately at the end of the incubation period, or a kinetic test, in which the absorbance is measured throughout the reaction period and the rate values.

11. Key Points

- A sterilizing filter (0.2 micron) is required to filter sterilize a drug product. The filter must be integrity tested before the product may be released. The test is often referred to as the "bubble point test."

- The HEPA (High-efficiency particulate air) filter is 99.97% efficient at filtering out particles 0.3 microns and larger. Certification of the HEPA filter involves testing the velocity of airflow from the filter and the integrity of the filter.

- The air in a class 100 area has no more that 100 particles 0.5 microns and larger per cubic foot of air. The laminar flow workbench provides a class 100 area.

- The critical site is any opening or pathway between the product and the environment. The larger the critical site and the longer it is exposed to the environment, the greater the risk of contamination of the product.

- The bacterial endotoxin test is designed to detect the level of bacterial endotoxin from gram-negative organisms in the drug product. All bacterial endotoxins are pyrogens, but not all pyrogens are bacterial endotoxins.

- The sterility test and the bacterial endotoxin test should be done on all sterile products compounded from nonsterile products. The bacterial endotoxin test must be done before the product can be dispensed.

- Any pharmacist preparing sterile products must have training in aseptic technique. One way to validate aseptic technique is by performing media fills. The growth media which is most often used is trypticase soy broth, also called soybean casein digest in the USP.

- The laminar airflow in a horizontal laminar flow workbench (HLFW) flows toward the operator. The pharmacist must never put their hands in back of an object, between the HEPA filter and the critical site.

- The laminar airflow in a vertical laminar flow workbench (VLFW) flows down onto the work surface.

- A biological safety cabinet should always be used for preparing cytotoxic drugs. All biological safety cabinets have vertical laminar flow.

- The hot air oven is used to depyrogenate items used in compounding.

- Moist-heat sterilization is a common way to sterilize equipment used in the compounding process. Only items that can be moistened by steam can be sterilized by autoclaving.

12. Questions and Answers

1. A sterile injection prepared from a nonsterile component must undergo all of these tests except one before release to a patient. Choose the test that does **not** have to be completed before release of the product.

    A. Bacterial endotoxin test
    B. Visual inspection
    C. Sterility test
    D. Verification of the filter integrity
    E. LAL test

2. Choose the **most correct** answer concerning certification of a laminar flow workbench.

    A. The particles introduced into the plenum of the hood must be approximately 0.5 microns in size.
    B. Air flow from the HEPA filter must be 120 fpm.
    C. A leak of 0.01% of the upstream smoke concentration through the filter is considered a serious leak.
    D. A total particle counter can be used to check the integrity of the HEPA filter.
    E. If a HEPA filter leaks it cannot be patched, but must be replaced.

3. Please choose the **most correct** answer. The bacterial endotoxin test is used to determine:

    A. The amount of pyrogens.
    B. The level of pyrogens from gram-negative bacteria.
    C. The fever-producing potential of bacterial endotoxins from gram-negative bacteria.
    D. The level of bacterial endotoxin from gram-positive bacteria.
    E. The amount of live bacteria present in the drug solution.

4. Please choose the **best answer** concerning USP media transfers.

    A. An operator must complete one media fill before compounding any sterile products.
    B. An operator who passes two consecutive media fills may compound sterile products.
    C. An operator who has passed 3 consecutive media fills qualifying their aseptic technique for low-risk compounding may compound high-risk category II products.

D. Once an operator successfully completes three consecutive media fills for low-risk compounding, they need to revalidate quarterly by completing one media fill.

E. Fluid thioglycollate media is used for media transfers.

5. Choose the *most correct* answer. When transferring product into the controlled area:

A. Bottles, bags, and syringes must be removed from brown cardboard boxes before being brought into the buffer area.

B. Vials stored in laminated cardboard may not be brought into the controlled area.

C. Stainless steel carts may be used to transfer items into the controlled area directly from the storage area.

D. Large-volume parenteral bags of IV solution must be removed from their protective overwrap before being brought into the controlled area.

E. The refrigerator should be placed next to the laminar flow hood for easy access.

6. Choose the *most correct* answer concerning a vertical laminar flow hood:

A. A VLFH is always a biological safety cabinet.

B. In vertical laminar flow the hands of the operator must not be behind an object.

C. A VLFH has turbulent airflow within 1 inch of the work surface.

D. A VLFH has the laminar flow air blowing at the operator.

E. The operator works in a vertical flow hood and a horizontal flow hood in the same manner.

7. Certain factors may increase the risk of microbial contamination of a sterile product. Please choose the item that would *not* be a risk factor.

A. Very complex compounding steps

B. Lengthy exposure of a critical site during compounding

C. Using appropriate aseptic technique

D. Batch compounding for multiple patients without preservatives

E. Preparing a sterile product from nonsterile powders

8. Choose the *true* statement concerning the ASHP risk levels of compounded sterile products.

A. Products intended for administration over 3 days would be classified as risk level I.

B. A sterile product that is stored in the refrigerator for 6 days would be classified as a risk level II product.

C. A sterile product that is unpreserved and compounded for one patient is classified as a risk level II product.

D. An intrathecal injection compounded from nonsterile powder would be classified as a risk level III product.

E. A batch of unpreserved product prepared for multiple patients is at risk level I.

9. Choose the *correct* statement.

A. When working in a horizontal laminar flow workbench, arrange items in the hood such that when you work your hand never is between the HEPA filter and an object.

B. When working in a horizontal laminar flow workbench, vials that are not being used should be stacked up along the side of the hood to increase workspace in the hood.

C. 70% isopropyl alcohol is used to sterilize the laminar flow workbench before each shift.

D. An object placed in the HLFW disturbs the airflow downstream of the object equal to two times the diameter of the object.

E. Syringes and IV bags are placed in the hood in their protective overwrap.

10. Operators in the buffer area must be properly gowned. Choose the *most* correct statement.

A. Operators gown because they shed particles and the nonshedding gowns keep the operator sterile.

B. Sterile gloves are used so if the operator accidentally touches a critical site during compounding of the sterile product it will not become contaminated.

C. Frequent sanitization with sterile 70% isopropyl alcohol is essential to keep your hands sterile during the compounding process.

D. Nonshedding garb and sterile gloves help to contain the particles shed from the operator.

E. Operators must gown before working at the laminar flow workbench, but not before entering the buffer area.

11. Concerning placement of items in the laminar flow workstation and working in the laminar flow workstation, choose the *most correct* answer.

A. Items should be placed in a horizontal flow hood to the right or left of the work area.

B. Items in a vertical laminar flow hood should be placed so that when working in the hood your hand never goes over the top of a critical site.

C. An object placed in a horizontal flow hood disturbs the airflow three times the diameter of the object behind the object.

D. When working in a horizontal laminar flow workstation, all work must be done at least 6 inches inside the hood.

E. All of the above are correct.

12. Which parts of the syringe are considered critical sites?

I. The ribs of the plunger
II. The collar of the syringe
III. The tip of the syringe

A. I only
B. II only
C. I and III only
D. II and III only
E. I, II, and III

13. Which parts of the needle are considered critical sites?

I. The hub
II. The needle shaft
III. The bevel and bevel tip of the needle

A. I only
B. II only
C. I and III only
D. II and III only
E. I, II, and III

14. Which of the following statements are true concerning ampuls?

I. Ampuls are single-dose containers.
II. Ampuls must have the neck wiped with a sterile alcohol pad before breaking.
III. Ampuls can be left in the hood and used for several days once opened.

A. II only
B. I and III only
C. I and II only
D. I, II, and III

15. When working with cytotoxic agents, several steps are taken to protect the operator. Which of the statements below are true?

I. Preparation of cytotoxic drugs must occur in a biological safety cabinet.
II. Syringes with Luer-lock tips should be used when compounding cytotoxic sterile products.
III. It is very important that positive pressure is not allowed to build up inside the vial when working with cytotoxic drugs.

A. I only
B. II only
C. I and III only
D. II and III only
E. I, II, and III.

16. Choose the **most correct** statement.

A. Filter integrity testing of the filter membrane is done to determine at what pressure the filter will break.

B. The manufacturer of the filter membrane determines the bubble point of the membrane. This value is always the same, no matter what solution has been filtered.

C. As the pore size of the filter membrane decreases, the pressure at which the air can be pushed from the largest pore increases.

D. The bubble point test is a destructive test.

E. It is not necessary to perform the bubble point test if you have a certificate of quality from the filter manufacturer.

17. When choosing a sterilizing filter there are several items that must be considered. Choose the **incorrect** statement.

A. The volume of product to be filtered.

B. The compatibility of the membrane with the product to be filtered.

C. The number of times the filter will be reused.

D. Whether the solution to be filtered is hydrophobic or hydrophilic.

E. The compatibility of the filter housing with the product to be filtered.

18. Please choose the **most correct** statement concerning the USP sterility test.

A. The bacteriostasis and fungistasis tests must be done on each product to determine if the article to be tested does not adversely affect the reliability of the test.

B. The growth promotion test does not require that the test organisms listed in the USP be used.

C. After inoculation the media must be incubated for 14 days or less at the appropriate temperature.

D. No growth on the sterility test proves that the aseptically produced product is sterile.

E. Trypticase soy broth is incubated at 30-35°C and fluid thioglycollate is incubated at 20-25°C.

19. Choose the *most correct* answer from the following statements.

   A. Gram-negative bacteria must be alive to cause a pyrogenic response.

   B. The lipopolysaccharide portion of a gram-negative bacteria's cell wall causes the pyrogenic response.

   C. Endotoxin can be removed by a 0.2 micron filter.

   D. Steam sterilization will depyrogenate the object just as well as the hot air oven.

   E. An article that is depyrogenated is not necessarily sterile.

20. Choose the *most correct* answer from the following statements.

   A. The rabbit test and the LAL test are the same test.

   B. LAL reagent will determine the fever-producing potential of the pyrogens.

   C. There are two types of techniques for the bacterial endotoxin test: the gel clot technique and the photometric technique.

   D. The drug product being tested has no effect on the test.

   E. All drug products may be tested by the rabbit test.

21. Choose the *most correct* statement.

   A. The rabbit test is the most sensitive test because it can detect pyrogens from all sources.

   B. The rabbit test is an in-vitro test.

   C. Some drugs may inhibit the formation of a gel in the bacterial endotoxin test.

   D. No drug will enhance the formation of the gel in the bacterial endotoxin test.

   E. The pyrogen test is a quantitative test.

22. Please choose the *most correct* statement. The plenum in a laminar flow workbench is:

   A. Where the air is prefiltered.

   B. The area where air is pressurized for distribution over the HEPA filter.

   C. The area where compounding takes place.

   D. An area that serves no purpose.

   E. An area directly above the HEPA filter in a horizontal laminar flow hood.

23. Calcium and phosphate can interact to form a precipitate in parenteral nutrition solutions. Listed below are some situations that could enhance precipitate formation. Please choose the one that would *not*.

   A. High concentration of calcium and phosphate.

   B. Increase in solution pH.

   C. Decrease in temperature.

   D. The use of the chloride salt of calcium.

   E. A slow infusion rate.

24. Listed below are some potential sources of physical or chemical incompatibilities. Please choose the one that is *not*.

   A. Dilution of a drug in a cosolvent system into an aqueous system.

   B. Addition of a drug solution with a high pH into a solution with a low pH.

   C. Adsorption of a lipid-soluble drug into the matrix of a polypropylene container.

   D. A photosensitive drug such as sodium nitroprusside in dextrose 5% in water exposed to light.

   E. Leaching of phthalate plasticizer into the solution from a polyvinyl chloride container.

Answers

1. **C.** The bacterial endotoxin test, LAL, visual inspectiontest, and bubble point test should all be completed before product is dispensed. Because the sterility test takes 14 days, the product may be dispensed before the results are known. However, a system to recall the product must be in place in case the product does not meet the requirement of the test.

2. **C.** Any leak greater than 0.01% of upstream smoke concentration is a serious leak. The HEPA filter can be patched. The smoke particles are 0.3 micron in size. The air flow from the HEPA filter should be 90 fpm plus or minus 20%. A total particle counter is used to classify the environment, not certify the integrity of the HEPA filter.

3. **B.** The BET determines the level of bacterial endotoxin only from gram-negative bacteria. The BET cannot determine fever-producing potential of the endotoxins. The gram-negative bacteria do not have to be alive for the endotoxin to produce an effect.

4. **D.** The operator must complete three consecutive media fills for low-risk compounding. Once validated for low-risk compounding, the operator must perform three additional media fills specific for each high-risk compounding task they will do. Once validated, a media fill should be done quarterly for low-risk compounding. Trypticase soy broth is the medium most often used in media fills.

5. **A.** Cardboard must be kept out of the buffer area. Vials in laminated cardboard may be stored in the buffer area. No items should be brought into the buffer area without being sanitized. LVP bags should be removed from their overwrap just before being used. The refrigerator should not be in the buffer room. It is a source of contamination.

6. **C.** There are several types of vertical flow hoods, of which the biological safety cabinet is one. The operator must never work over the top of items in the hood and all work should be above one inch of the work surface.

7. **A.** Using good aseptic technique is one way to ensure a good product.

8. **D.** Any sterile product that is made from nonsterile ingredients is a risk level III product. A product that is at room temperature for longer than 28 hours is a risk level II product. A batch of unpreserved product intended for use by one patient is a risk level I product. If this batch is intended for multiple patients it is a Risk Level II product.

9. **A.** In HLF you never put your hand behind an object, whereas in VLF you never put your hand above an object. A vial disturbs the laminar air flow three times the diameter of the object when in HLF. If the vial is next to the side wall, the air flow is disturbed six times the diameter of the object. Syringes and IV bags should be taken from their overwrap at the edge of the hood.

10. **D.** Operators in the buffer area should wear clean nonshedding gowns and gloves to help contain the particles that they shed. The sterile gloves that are worn are not sterile once they are out of the package. Proper aseptic technique must always be used.

11. **E.** All of the following are true statements concerning placement of items in the laminar flow workstation and working in the laminar flow workstation: a. Items should be placed in a horizontal flow hood to the right or left of the work area; b. Items in a vertical laminar flow hood should be placed so that when working in the hood your hand never goes over the top of a critical site; c. An object placed in a horizontal flow hood disturbs the airflow three times the diameter of the object behind the object; d. When working in a horizontal laminar flow workstation all work must be done at least 6 inches inside the hood.

12. **C.** The ribs of the plunger and the tip of the syringe are considered critical sites of the syringe.

13. **E.** The hub, the needle shaft, the bevel, and bevel tip of the needle are all considered critical sites.

14. **C.** Once an ampul is opened it must be used immediately.

15. **E.** When working with cytotoxic agents the following steps are taken to protect the operator: 1. Preparation must occur in a biological safety cabinet: 2. Syringes with Luer-lock tips should be used; 3. Positive pressure is not allowed to build up inside the vial.

16. **C.** The bubble point test is not a destructive test, and the value is dependent on the solution being filtered. When filter sterilizing a product, the bubble point test must be done before the product may be dispensed.

17. **C.** When using presterilized disposable filters it is not appropriate to reuse the device.

18. **A.** The B&F must be completed one time for each product. The growth promotion organisms listed in the USP are used for the B&F test and for the growth promotion test.

19. **B.** Endotoxin will pass through a 0.2 micron filter. Steam sterilization will not depyrogenate an article. Bacteria do not have to be alive to be pyrogenic.

20. **C.** The pyrogen test is also known as the rabbit test, which determines the fever-producing potential of the pyrogens. The bacterial endotoxin test is also known as the LAL test. The drug product can inhibit or enhance the gel formation in the BET test.

21. **C.** The pyrogen (rabbit) test, an in-vivo test, is not as sensitive as the BET test. It is not a quantitative test.

22. **B.** The plenum is the area behind the HEPA filter, which allows air to be pressurized for even distribution over the filter.

23. **C.** An increase in temperature could enhance precipitate formation.

24. **C.** Absorption of lipid-soluble drug into the matrix of polyvinyl chloride containers does occur. Polypropylene and polyethylene contain little or no phthalate plasticizer.

13. References

Akers MJ. *Parenteral Quality Control*. New York: Marcel Dekker; 1994.

American Society of Health-System Pharmacists. ASHP Guidelines on Quality Assurance for Pharmacy-Prepared Sterile Products. *Am J Hosp Pharm*. 2000;57:1150-1169.

Anderson RA. The status of environmental control. Practical approaches to the safe handling of anticancer products. Proceeding of a Symposium in Mayaguez, Puerto Rico, November 2-5, 1983.

Bacterial endotoxin test. In: *United States Pharmacopeia*, 25th rev.: national formulary, 20th ed. Rockville, MD: United States Pharmacopeial Conventions; 2001:1889-1893.

Buchanan C, McKinnon B, Scheckelhoff D, Schneider P. *Principles of Sterile Product Preparation*. Bethesda, MD: American Society of Health-System Pharmacists; 2002:50.

Commission, Federal Supply Service, General Services Administration. Federal Standard 209e. Clean room and work station requirements, controlled environments. Washington: U.S. Government Printing Office; 1992.

McKinnon B, Avis K. Membrane filtration of pharmaceutical solutions. *Am J Hosp Pharm*. 1993;50:1021-1036.

Pyrogen test. In: *United States Pharmacopeia*, 25th rev.: national formulary, 20th ed. Rockville, MD: United States Pharmacopeial Convention; 2001:1914-1915.

Sterile drug products for home use. In: *United States Pharmacopeia*, 25th rev: national formulary, 20th ed. Rockville, MD: United States Pharmacopeial Convention; 2001:2234-2247.

Sterility Tests. In: *United States Pharmacopeia*, 25th rev: national formulary, 20th ed. Rockville, MD: United States Pharmacopeial Convention; 2001:1878-1883.

Trissel LA. *Handbook on Injectable Drugs*, 11th ed. Bethesda, MD: American Society of Health-System Pharmacists; 2001.

6. Pharmacokinetics, Drug Metabolism, and Drug Disposition

Charles R. Yates, PharmD, PhD
Assistant Professor, Department of Pharmaceutical Sciences

Bernd Meibohm, PhD, FCP
Associate Professor of Pharmaceutical Sciences
University of Tennessee College of Pharmacy

Contents

1. **Pharmacokinetics**

2. **Absorption and Disposition**

3. **Bioavailability**

4. **Constant Rate Regimens**

5. **Multiple Dosing**

6. **Volumes of Distribution and Protein Binding**

7. **Elimination and Clearance Concepts**

8. **Renal Clearance**

9. **Hepatic Clearance**

10. **Clinical Examples**

11. **Key Points**

12. **Questions and Answers**

1. Pharmacokinetics

Pharmacokinetics is the science of a drug's fate in the body. A drug's therapeutic potential is intimately linked to its pharmacokinetic profile. For example, a drug's pharmacologic response may be severely diminished as a result of poor absorption and/or rapid elimination from the body. The most important factors contributing to drug disposition include absorption, distribution, metabolism, and excretion (ADME).

Absorption

The rate and extent of drug absorption is referred to as bioavailability. The fraction of drug absorbed (f_a), an important determinant of the extent of bioavailability, is affected not only by its physicochemical properties, but also by physiologic barriers at the site of absorption. For example, intestinal expression of the drug efflux transporter P-glycoprotein is known to limit the oral drug absorption.

Distribution

Many drugs circulate in the body and are bound to plasma proteins (eg, human serum albumin). The fraction of drug not bound to protein (f_{up}) is responsible for the pharmacologic effect. A drug may also bind significantly to tissue proteins resulting in a small unbound fraction of drug in the tissue (f_{ut}). Drugs with a large f_{up}:f_{ut} ratio have a large volume of distribution, whereas drugs with a small f_{up}:f_{ut} ratio are largely confined to the vascular space. Volume of distribution is directly related to half-life ($t_{1/2}$), the time required to eliminate half the drug from the body.

Metabolism

Approximately 50% of drugs undergo some form of hepatic metabolism. The cytochrome P450 (CYP450) family of drug metabolizing enzymes is primarily responsible for drug inactivation in the liver. Hepatic clearance is dependent on liver blood flow and the extraction ratio. The hepatic extraction ratio can be used to estimate fraction of drug escaping first-pass metabolism (F*), an important determinant of oral bioavailability. Intestinal inactivation of drugs by CYP450 enzymes in the gut is responsible for reduced F of a number of drugs.

Excretion

The primary purpose of hepatic metabolism is to increase a drug's water solubility to facilitate its renal elimination. The kidneys also serve as the primary eliminating organ for drugs that do not undergo hepatic metabolism. Renal clearance comprises three main physiologic processes: glomerular filtration, reabsorption, and secretion. Filtration clearance is the product of f_{up} and glomerular filtration rate (a physiologic parameter that diminishes with age). Renal reabsorption is a predominantly passive process dependent upon physicochemical drug properties and urine drug concentration and pH, whereas secretion is an active process facilitated by various transport mechanisms. The net of filtration, reabsorption, and secretion determine a drug's total renal clearance.

Variability in drug response can be partially explained by inter-individual differences in drug pharmacokinetics. Thus a thorough understanding of the physiologic processes affecting drug disposition is essential to drug individualization and optimization.

2. Absorption and Disposition

Drug Input

Drugs are administered to the body by one of two routes, intravascular or extravascular. For intravascular administration, drugs are usually administered via intravenous infusion (continuous, short-term, or bolus). The concentration C is given by the following expressions:

IV bolus

$$C = \frac{Dose}{V} * e^{-K*t}$$

$\frac{dC}{dt}$ (Rate of change in plasma concentration) = Rate of drug elimination (output rate)

K – Elimination rate constant = CL/V

Clearance = Dose/AUC

IV infusion

For drugs that are administered extravascularly (PO, IM, SC) and act systemically, absorption must occur.

First-order absorption

$$C = \frac{k_a * F * Dose}{V * (k_a - K)} * \left(e^{-K*t} - e^{-k_a*t} \right)$$

k_a = First-order rate constant for drug absorption
Absorption half-life = $0.693/k_a$
K = First-order rate constant for drug elimination (CL/V)
CL = F * Dose/AUC
Oral Clearance = CL/F = Dose/AUC
F = bioavailability; fraction of drug absorbed.

3. Bioavailability

Bioavailability refers to the rate and extent of absorption. The extent of absorption can be expressed as absolute or relative bioavailability.

Absolute Bioavailability

Fraction (or percentage) of a dose administered nonintravenously (or extravascularly) that is systemically available (compared to an intravenous dose). If given orally, absolute bioavailability (F) is:

$$F = \frac{D_{IV}}{D_{PO}} * \frac{AUC_{PO}}{AUC_{IV}}$$

Relative Bioavailability

Fraction of a dose administered as a test formulation that is systemically available as compared to a reference formulation:

$$F = \frac{AUC_{test\,formulation}}{AUC_{reference}} * \frac{D_{reference}}{D_{test\,formulation}}$$

Determinants of the Plasma Concentration-Time Curve After an Extravascular Dose

Four pharmacokinetic parameters determine the plasma concentration-time profile after an extravascular dose: k_a, F, CL, and V.

$$\frac{dC}{dt} = (\text{Rate in}) - (\text{Rate out})$$

$$\frac{dC}{dt} = (\text{Rate of drug absorption}) - (\text{Rate of drug elimination})$$

$$\frac{dC}{dt} = \frac{k_a * F * Dose}{V} - K * C$$

Time to peak (t_{max})
The maximum plasma concentration occurs when dC/dt = 0.

The equation below can be derived to determine the factors that affect t_{max}.

$$t_{max} = \frac{\ln\left(\frac{k_a}{K}\right)}{k_a - K}$$

Maximum plasma concentration (C_{max})

The maximum plasma concentration occurs at tmax. The following equation for Cmax can be used to determine which factors affect Cmax.

$$C_{max} = \frac{k_a * F * Dose}{V * (k_a - K)} * \left(e^{-K * t_{max}} - e^{-k_a * t_{max}} \right)$$

Area under the plasma concentration-time curve (AUC)

$$AUC = \frac{F * Dose}{CL} = \frac{F * Dose}{V * K}$$

Terminal half-life ($t_{1/2}$)

$$t_{1/2} = \frac{0.693 * V}{CL}$$

4. Constant Rate Regimens

Introduction

For many drugs to be therapeutically effective, drug concentrations of a certain level have to be maintained at the site of action for a prolonged period of time (eg, β-lactam antibiotics, antiarrhythmic medications), while for others, alternating plasma concentrations are more preferable (eg, aminoglycoside antibiotics like gentamicin).

To continuously maintain drug concentrations in a certain therapeutic range over a prolonged period of time, two basic approaches to administer the drug can be applied:

1. Drug administration at a constant input rate
2. Sequential administration of discrete single doses (multiple dosing)

Drug Administration as Constant Rate Regimens

At any time during the infusion, the rate of change in drug concentration is the difference between the input rate (infusion rate R_0 / Volume of distribution V) and the output rate (elimination rate constant K * concentration C):

Rate of change = Input rate – Output rate

In concentrations:

$$\frac{dC}{dt} = \frac{R_0}{V} - K * C$$

In amounts:

$$V * \frac{dC}{dt} = R_0 - CL * C$$

R_0 = Infusion rate (in amount/time [eg, mg/h])
V = Volume of distribution
CL = Clearance
K = First-order rate constant for drug elimination (CL/V)
As

$$\frac{dC}{dt} = 0 \qquad \frac{R_0}{V} = K * C_{ss} \quad \text{or} \quad R_0 = CL * C_{ss}$$

Hence, the steady-state concentration C_{ss} is only determined by the infusion rate R_0 and the clearance CL.

Drug concentration at steady-state:

$$C_{ss} = \frac{R_0}{CL}$$

Drug concentration before steady-state:

$$C = \frac{R_0}{CL} * \left(1 - e^{-K*t}\right)$$

Time to Reach Steady-State

For therapeutic purposes, it is often of critical importance to know how long it will take after initiation of an infusion to finally reach the targeted steady-state concentration C_{ss}.

Concentration during an infusion:

before steady-state $C = \dfrac{R_0}{CL} * \left(1 - e^{-K*t}\right)$

steady-state $C_{ss} = \dfrac{R_0}{CL}$

the fraction of steady-state f is then

$$f = \frac{C}{C_{ss}} = \left(1 - e^{-K*t}\right)$$

After a duration of infusion of:
1 $t_{1/2}$ → 50% of steady-state is reached
2 $t_{1/2}$ → 75% of steady-state is reached
3 $t_{1/2}$ → 87.5% of steady-state is reached
3.3 $t_{1/2}$ → 90% of steady-state is reached
4 $t_{1/2}$ → 93.8% of steady-state is reached
5 $t_{1/2}$ → 96.9% of steady-state is reached

The following conclusions can be drawn:
1. The approach to the steady-state concentration C_{ss} is exponential in nature and is controlled by the elimination process (elimination rate constant K), *not* the infusion rate R_0.
2. Only the value of the steady-state concentration C_{ss} is controlled by the infusion rate R_0 (and of course by the clearance CL).
3. Assuming for clinical purposes that a concentration of >95% of steady-state is therapeutically equivalent to the final steady-state concentration C_{ss}, it takes approximately *five elimination half-lives $t_{1/2}$* to reach steady-state after initiation of an infusion.

Concentration-Time Profiles Postinfusion

The postinfusion plasma concentration cannot be distinguished from readings following administration of an intravenous bolus dose. As the drug input has been discontinued, the rate of change in drug concentration is only determined by the output rate. If the drug follows one-compartment characteristics, then the plasma concentration profile can be described by

$$C = C' * e^{-K*t_{pi}}$$

where C' = concentration at the end of the infusion, and t_{pi} = time post infusion (ie, time after the infusion has stopped)

Thus, a general expression can be used to calculate the plasma concentration during and after a constant rate infusion:

$$C = \frac{R_0}{CL} * \left(1 - e^{-K*t}\right) * e^{-K*t_{pi}}$$

where t = is the elapsed time after the beginning of the infusion
t_{pi} = the postinfusion time, ie, the difference between the duration of the infusion (infusion time T_{inf}) and t: $t_{pi} = t - T_{inf}$
For describing concentrations during the infusion, t_{pi} is set to zero.
For describing concentrations postinfusion, t is set to T_{inf}.

Four different cases can be distinguished:
1. ***During the infusion, but before steady-state is reached:***

$$t = t, t_{pi} = 0 \Rightarrow \quad C = \frac{R_0}{CL} * \left(1 - e^{-K*t}\right)$$

2. ***During the infusion at steady-state:***

$$t \to \infty, t_{pi} = 0 \Rightarrow \quad C = \frac{R_0}{CL}$$

3. ***After cessation of the infusion before steady-state:***

$$t = T_{inf}, t_{pi} = t - T_{inf} \Rightarrow C = \frac{R_0}{CL} * \left(1 - e^{-K*T_{inf}}\right) * e^{-K*\left(t - T_{inf}\right)}$$

4. ***After cessation of the infusion at steady-state:***

$$t \to \infty, t_{pi} = t - T_{inf} \Rightarrow \quad C = \frac{R_0}{CL} * e^{-K*\left(t - T_{inf}\right)}$$

Determination of Pharmacokinetic Parameters

- The elimination rate constant K, and the elimination half-life $t_{1/2}$ can be determined from:
  a) the terminal slope after the infusion has been stopped
  b) the time to reach half of C_{ss}
  c) the slope of the relationship of $\ln (C_{ss} - C)$ versus t, based on

  $$C = C_{ss} * \left(1 - e^{-K * t}\right)$$

and the resulting $\quad \ln \left(C_{ss} - C\right) = \ln C_{ss} - K * t$

- The clearance CL can be determined from the relationship:

  $$CL = \frac{R_0}{C_{ss}}$$

- The volume of distribution can be determined from the relationship:

  $$V = \frac{CL}{K}$$

Loading Dose and Maintenance Dose

- The loading dose (LD) is supposed to immediately (t = 0) reach the desired target concentration C_{target}. It is administered as an IV bolus injection, or more frequently as a short-term infusion.

- The maintenance dose (MD) is intended to sustain C_{target}. It is administered as a constant rate infusion.

Loading dose (LD)
Target concentration calculated for a drug with one-compartment characteristics:

$$C_{target} = \frac{LD}{V} \quad \rightarrow LD = C_{target} * V$$

Maintenance dose (MD)
The maintenance dose is the infusion rate necessary to sustain the target concentration:

$$C_{target} = \frac{MD}{CL} \quad \rightarrow MD = R_0 = C_{target} * CL$$

5. Multiple Dosing

Introduction

Continuous drug concentrations for prolonged therapy can be maintained either by drug administration at a constant input rate or by sequential administration of discrete single doses. The latter is the more frequently used approach and can be applied to extravascular as well as intravascular routes of administration.

Multiple dose regimens are defined by two components, the *dose D* that is administered at each dosing occasion, and the *dosing interval τ*, the time period between the administration of two subsequent doses. Dose and dosing interval can be summarized in the *dosing rate DR*:

$$DR = \frac{D}{\tau}$$

Concentration-Time Profiles During Multiple Dosing

The *multiple dose function MDF* can be used for calculating drug concentrations before steady-state (during a multiple dose regimen) has been reached:

$$MDF = \frac{1 - e^{-n * K * \tau}}{1 - e^{-K * \tau}}$$

where K is the respective rate constant of the drug, τ the dosing interval, and n the number of the dose.

Once steady-state has been reached, n approaches infinity and the MDF simplifies to the *accumulation factor AF:*

$$AF = \frac{1}{1 - e^{-K * \tau}}$$

Multiple Dosing Regimens: Instantaneous Input (IV Bolus)

For an IV bolus multiple dose regimen, the concentrations during the first dosing interval, the nth dosing interval, and at steady-state are described by the following relationships:

Dose number	Equation	Maximum or peak concentration	Minimum or trough concentration at the end of the dosing interval
1	$C = \dfrac{D}{V} * e^{-K*t}$	$C_{1,max} = \dfrac{D}{V}$	$C_{1,min} = \dfrac{D}{V} * e^{-K*\tau}$
n	$C = \dfrac{D}{V} * e^{-K*t} * \dfrac{1 - e^{-n*K*\tau}}{1 - e^{-K*\tau}}$	$C_{n,max} = \dfrac{D}{V} * \dfrac{1 - e^{-n*K*\tau}}{1 - e^{-K*\tau}}$	$C_{n,min} = \dfrac{D}{V} * e^{-K*\tau} * \dfrac{1 - e^{-n*K*\tau}}{1 - e^{-K*\tau}}$
Steady-state	$C = \dfrac{D}{V} * \dfrac{e^{-K*t}}{1 - e^{-K*\tau}}$	$C_{ss,max} = \dfrac{D}{V} * \dfrac{1}{1 - e^{-K*\tau}}$	$C_{ss,min} = \dfrac{D}{V} * \dfrac{e^{-K*\tau}}{1 - e^{-K*\tau}}$

The peak and trough concentrations at steady-state can thus be expressed as the peak and trough after the first dose multiplied by the accumulation factor AF:

$$C_{ss,max} = \frac{C_{1,max}}{1 - e^{-K*\tau}}$$

$$C_{ss,min} = \frac{C_{1,min}}{1 - e^{-K*\tau}} = \frac{C_{1,max} * e^{-K*\tau}}{1 - e^{-K*\tau}}$$

Average Steady-State Concentration

By definition, the average drug input rate is equal to the average drug output rate at steady-state. While the average input rate is the drug amount entering the systemic circulation per dosing interval, the average output rate is equal to the product of clearance CL and the average plasma concentration within one dosing interval $C_{ss,av}$.

$$\frac{D}{\tau} = CL * C_{ss,av}$$

Thus, the average steady-state concentration $C_{ss,av}$ during multiple dosing is only determined by the dose, the dosing interval τ (or both together as dosing rate DR = D/τ) and the clearance CL:

$$C_{ss,av} = \frac{D}{\tau * CL}$$

The area under the curve resulting from administration of a single dose AUC_{single} is equal to the area under the curve during one dosing interval at steady-state AUC_{ss}, if the same dose is given per dosing interval τ:

$$C_{ss,av} = \frac{AUC_{ss}}{\tau} = \frac{D}{\tau * CL} = \frac{AUC_{single}}{\tau}$$

Thus:

$$AUC_{single} = AUC_{ss}$$

Extent of Accumulation

The extent of accumulation during multiple dosing at steady-state is determined by the dosing interval τ and the half-life of the drug $t_{1/2}$ (or the elimination rate constant K):

$$AF = \frac{1}{1 - e^{-k*\tau}}$$

Thus, the extent of accumulation is not only dependent on the pharmacokinetic properties of a drug, but also on the multiple dosing regimen chosen.

Fluctuation

The degree of fluctuation between peak and trough concentrations during one dosing interval, ie, $C_{ss,max}$ and $C_{ss,min}$, is determined by the relationship between elimination half-life $t_{1/2}$ and dosing interval τ.

$$Fluctuation = \frac{C_{ss,max} - C_{ss,min}}{C_{ss,min}}$$

Multiple Dosing Regimens: First-Order Input (Oral Dosing)

The average steady-state concentration $C_{ss,av}$ is now determined by the bioavailable fraction F of the dose

(D) administered per dosing interval τ and the clearance (CL):

$$C_{ss,av} = \frac{F * D}{\tau * CL}$$

As the concentration-time profile after a single oral dose is given by

$$C = \frac{F * D * k_a}{V * (k_a - K)} * \left(e^{-K*t} - e^{-k_a*t}\right),$$

the concentration at any time within a dosing interval during multiple dosing at steady-state is determined by

$$C = \frac{F * D * k_a}{V * (k_a - K)} * \left(\frac{e^{-K*\tau}}{1 - e^{-K*\tau}} - \frac{e^{-k_a*t}}{1 - e^{-k_a*\tau}}\right)$$

Thus, the trough concentration is readily available assuming that the absorption is completed:

$$C_{ss,min} = \frac{F * D * k_a}{V * (k_a - K)} * \left(\frac{e^{-K*\tau}}{1 - e^{-K*\tau}}\right)$$

The peak concentration is assessable via the time-to-peak t_{max}, which is dependent on the rate of absorption and has to be determined via:

$$t_{max} = \frac{\ln\left(\frac{k_a * (1 - e^{-k_e*\tau})}{K * (1 - e^{-K*\tau})}\right)}{(k_a - K)}$$

6. Volumes of Distribution and Protein Binding

Introduction

Drug distribution means the reversible transfer of drug from one location to another within the body.

Once a drug has entered the vascular system, it becomes distributed throughout the various tissues and body fluids. However, most drugs do not distribute uniformly and in a similar manner throughout the body. This is reflected by the difference in their volumes of distribution. Thus in the following, we will focus on the factors and processes determining the rate and extent of distribution and the resulting consequences for pharmacotherapy.

Factors affecting distribution:
- Binding to blood or tissue elements

- Blood flow (ie, the delivery of drug to the tissues)

- Ability to cross biomembranes

- Physicochemical properties of the drug (lipophilicity, extent of ionization) that determine partitioning into tissues

Protein Binding

The fraction unbound in plasma varies widely among drugs. Drugs are classified as

- Highly protein bound:
  $f_{up} \leq 0.1$ ($\leq$10% unbound, $\geq$90% bound)

- Moderately protein bound:
  $f_{up} = 0.1\text{-}0.4$ (10-40% unbound, 60-90% bound)

- Low protein binding:
  $f_{up} \geq 0.4$ ($\geq$40% unbound, $\leq$60% bound)

Factors Determining the Degree of Protein Binding

The reversible binding of a drug to proteins obeys the law of mass action,

$$[Drug] + [Protein] \underset{k_2}{\overset{k_1}{\rightleftharpoons}} [Drug\text{-}Protein\text{-}Complex]$$

where the expressions in parentheses represent the molar concentrations of the components. k_1 and k_2 are rate constants for the forward and reverse reactions, respectively. The equilibrium association constant K_a is defined as k_1/k_2.

This results in the following relationship for the fraction unbound:

$$f_{up} = \cfrac{1}{1 + \cfrac{N}{(1/K_a) + C_u}}$$

where N is the number of available binding sites and C_u is the unbound concentration.

Binding Proteins

Human plasma contains over 60 proteins. Of these, three proteins account for the binding of most drugs. *Albumin,* which comprises approximately 60% of total plasma protein, fully accounts for the plasma binding of most anionic drugs and many endogenous anions (*high-capacity, low-affinity binding site*). Many cationic and neutral drugs bind appreciably to α_1-*acid glycoprotein (AAG)* (high-affinity, low-capacity binding site) and/or *lipoproteins* in addition to albumin. Other proteins, such as transcortin, thyroid-binding globulin, and certain antibodies have specific affinities for a small number of drugs.

Volumes of Distribution

Volume of distribution at steady-state V_{ss}

The volume of distribution at steady-state is by definition the sum of the pharmacokinetic volumes of distribution for the different pharmacokinetic compartments. Theoretically:

$$V_{ss} = V_p + \frac{f_u}{f_{u,t}} * V_t$$

where V_p is the volume of plasma (3 L), V_t is the volume of tissue water (total body water minus plasma volume: $42 - 3 = 39$ L based on a "standard" person). f_{up} and f_{ut} are the fraction unbound for the drug in plasma and tissue, respectively.

The relationship for V_{ss} shows that the extent of distribution is (besides physicochemical properties of the drug) largely determined by the differences in protein binding in plasma and tissue, respectively:

$$V_{ss} = 3\,L + \frac{f_u}{f_{u,t}} * 39\,L$$

Unbound steady-state concentrations

The average steady-state concentration during a multiple dose regimen or during a constant rate infusion is determined by

$$C_{ss} = \frac{Dose\ rate}{CL} = \frac{Dose\ rate}{f_{up} * CL_u}$$

The free steady-state concentration Css,u is given by

$$C_{ss,u} = f_{up} * C_{ss}$$

Thus, the unbound steady-state concentration $C_{ss,u}$ is determined by

$$\frac{C_{ss,u}}{f_{up}} = \frac{Dose\ rate}{f_{up} * CL_u} \Rightarrow C_{ss,u} = \frac{Dose\ rate}{CL}$$

7. Elimination and Clearance Concepts

Clearance (CL) is defined as the irreversible removal of drug from the body by an organ of elimination. Since the units of CL are flow per time (eg, mL/min or L/h), CL is often defined as the volume of blood irreversibly cleared of drug per unit of time.

CL by the eliminating organ (CL_{organ}) is defined as the product of (blood flow to the organ) and (the extraction ratio of that organ).

$$CL_{organ} = Q * ER$$
Organ clearance = Blood flow * Extraction ratio

Individual organ clearances are additive. For the majority of drugs we use clinically, the liver is the major, and sometimes only, site of metabolism; the kidneys are the major site of excretion for drugs and metabolites. Thus the equation for total clearance can be written to include renal clearance (CL_R) and hepatic clearance (CL_H):

$$CL = CL_R + CL_H$$

The fraction of drug excreted unchanged by the kidneys (f_e) tells us what fraction of the drug we administered will be excreted into the urine.

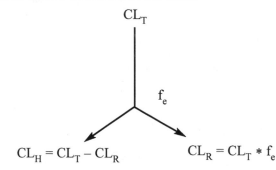

$$CL_T$$

$$f_e$$

$$CL_H = CL_T - CL_R \qquad CL_R = CL_T * f_e$$

8. Renal Clearance

Drugs may undergo three processes in the kidney, two of which act to remove drug from the body—filtration and secretion—while the other acts to return the drug to the body—reabsorption. Thus we may express renal clearance of a drug as:

$$CL_R = [CL_{filtration} + CL_{secretion}] * (1 - f_{reabsorbed})$$

Calculating Filtration Clearance of Creatinine (CL_{cr})

Normal serum concentrations of creatinine are:
  0.8-1.3 mg/dL for men
  0.6-1.0 mg/dL for women.

Creatinine is a useful marker of renal function since it is an endogenous by-product of muscle breakdown. Creatinine is eliminated by the kidney at a rate approximately equal to GFR. A number of formulas have been developed which allow us to estimate creatinine clearance (CL_{cr}) from serum creatinine concentrations. The most widely used clinically is the *Cockroft-Gault equation:*

$$CL_{cr} = \frac{(140 - age) * IBW}{S_{cr} * 72}$$

(multiply result by 0.85 if patient is female)

where S_{cr} is the serum creatinine concentration in mg/dL, and IBW is the ideal body weight.

IBW_{males} (kg) = 50 + (2.3 * height in inches >5 ft)
$IBW_{females}$ (kg) = 45.5 + (2.3 * height in inches >5 ft)

Secretion Clearance

Drug in blood may also be secreted into the kidney tubule. This occurs *against* a concentration gradient (concentration of drug in kidney tubule is very high because of water reabsorption) and therefore is *an active process.*

Cellular processes (eg, presence of active transporters) exist to facilitate tubular secretion. The two most well characterized include transporters responsible for the secretion of *basic* (anionic) and *acidic* (anionic) drugs.

Reabsorption

Passive reabsorption of many drugs also occurs in the kidneys. Since reabsorption is a passive process (ie, diffusion), reabsorption will depend on the physicochemical properties of the drug (eg, molecular weight, polarity, and pKa).

Weak bases: $B + H \leftrightarrow BH^+$

Low urine pH = **more ionized, less reabsorption**
High urine pH = **less ionized, more reabsorption**

Thus, only weak bases with pKa between 6 and 12 show changes in the extent of reabsorption (and thus CL_R) with changes in urine pH.

Weak acids: $HA \leftrightarrow A^- + H^+$

Low urine pH = **less ionized, more reabsorption**
High urine pH = **more ionized, less reabsorption**

Thus, only weak acids with pKa in the range of 3-7.5 show changes in the extent of reabsorption (and thus CL_R) with changes in urine pH.

All drugs which are not bound to plasma proteins are filtered, therefore filtration clearance is:

$$CL_{filtration} = f_{up} * GFR = f_{up} * 125 \text{ mL/min}$$

Some drugs are secreted or reabsorbed, or both. We can determine the net process a drug undergoes by calculating the excretion ratio (**Eratio**):

$$\text{Eratio} = \frac{CL_R}{CL_{filtration}} = \frac{CL_R}{f_{up} * 125 \text{ mL/min}}$$

9. Hepatic Clearance

Relation of Hepatic Extraction Ratio and Bioavailability

The fraction of drug escaping first-pass metabolism (F^*) can be described in terms of the hepatic extraction ratio (ER).

$$F^* = 1 - ER$$

The overall oral bioavailability (F) of a drug is dependent on the fraction absorbed (f_a), the fraction escaping metabolism in the intestinal wall (f_g), and the fraction escaping hepatic first-pass metabolism (F^*).

$$F = f_a * f_g * F^*$$

Venous Equilibrium Model for Hepatic Clearance

The venous equilibrium model relates hepatic extraction ratio (ER) to f_{up}, intrinsic clearance (CL_{int}), and liver blood flow (Q) as follows (from Wilkinson et al, 1975):

$$ER = \frac{f_{up} * CL_{int}}{Q + f_{up} * CL_{int}}$$

and (remembering that $CL_H = Q_H * ER_H$),

$$CL_H = \frac{Q * f_{up} * CL_{int}}{Q + f_{up} * CL_{int}}$$

The fraction of drug escaping hepatic first-pass metabolism using the venous equilibrium model.

$$F^* = \frac{Q}{Q + f_{up} * CL_{int}}$$

Drugs undergoing hepatic metabolism can be broadly divided into three categories:

1. Low-extraction drugs: ER <0.3 and thus F^* >0.7

2. Intermediate-extraction drugs: $0.3 < ER < 0.7$ and thus $0.3 < F^* < 0.7$

3. High-extraction drugs: ER >0.7 and thus F^* <0.3

Determinants of Hepatic Clearance

The determinants of hepatic extraction ratio, hepatic clearance, and the fraction escaping hepatic first-pass metabolism are Q, f_{up}, and CL_{int}.

1. Liver blood flow (Q)

2. Protein binding (f_{up})

   ER < f_{up}. For some drugs, hepatic clearance is limited or restricted to the unbound or free drug. This is known as *restrictive clearance.* Because clearance is limited to unbound drug, changes in protein binding will alter the concentration of drug that is available for elimination.

   ER > f_{up}. Some drugs defy this principle such that the hepatic extraction ratio (ER) is greater than the fraction of drug unbound in plasma (f_{up}). When this occurs, it suggests that drug clearance is not restricted to unbound drug. Drugs behaving in this manner are said to undergo *nonrestrictive clearance.* Because non-restrictive clearance is not limited to the fraction unbound in plasma, changes in protein binding will not alter the concentration of drug that is available for elimination (ie, all drug is available for elimination regardless of whether it is bound or unbound).

3. Intrinsic clearance (CL_{int})

   Intrinsic clearance (CL_{int}) is defined as the intrinsic ability of the hepatic enzymes to elimi-nate drug when there are no limitations due to blood flow or protein binding.

   CL_{int} is a measure of the capacity and affinity of drug-metabolizing enzymes (eg, cytochrome P450s) for the drug. The determinants of CL_{int} can be explained using the Michaelis-Menten equation:

   $$v = \frac{V_{max} * C_u}{K_m + C_u} \text{ and } CL_u = \frac{V_{max}}{K_m + C_u}$$

   where v is the rate of drug metabolism (amount/time), V_{max} is the maximal rate of metabolism for a given metabolic pathway (amount/time), K_m is the concentration of the drug at which the rate of metabolism is half-maximal (amount/volume), and C_u is the unbound drug concentration (amount/volume).

   Physiologically, V_{max} describes the quantity (capacity) of a drug-metabolizing enzyme to metabolize drug. K_m describes the interaction between the drug-metabolizing enzyme and the drug.

Factors that affect CL_{int}

a. *Enzyme induction:* this refers to an increased number (capacity) of drug-metabolizing enzymes, which results in an increase in clear-ance. An increased number (capacity) of drug-metabolizing enzymes results in an increase in V_{max} and Cl_{int}.

b. *Enzyme inhibitors:* this is competitive inhibition of the drug-metabolizing enzyme by another drug. The apparent K_m is increased in this situa-tion (ie, a higher concentration of drug will be required to achieve a half-maximal rate of metabolism). Increase in apparent K_m results in a decrease in CL_{int}.

An extensive list of potential P450 inducers and inhibitors can be found at:
www.drug-interactions.com

10. Clinical Examples

Clinical Example #1

A patient (age 55, weight 73 kg) was started on a multiple-dose regimen with gentamicin 80 mg q8h given as IV short-term infusion over 30 minutes. As his infection was serious, it was decided to set the target for a peak concentration of 10 mg/L and a trough concentration of 1 mg/L. Three blood samples were drawn 30 minutes prior to the third dose, and 30 minutes and 7 hours after the end of the infusion of the third dose, respectively. The measured plasma concentrations were 1.73, 5.96, and 1.80 mg/L, respectively.

Optimize the gentamicin dosing regimen based on the individual pharmacokinetic parameters of the patient to achieve the therapeutically-targeted concentrations.

Step 1: Calculate the elimination rate constant K

$$K = \frac{\ln\left(\frac{C^*_{max}}{C^*_{min}}\right)}{\Delta t} = \frac{\ln\left(\frac{5.96}{1.80}\right)}{(8 - 1 - 0.5)h} = 0.184 \text{ h}^{-1}$$

Step 2: Calculate volume of distribution V

$$C_{max} = \frac{C^*_{max}}{e^{-K*t}} = \frac{5.96 \text{ mg/L}}{e^{-0.184 \text{ h}^{-1} *0.5 \text{ h}}} = 6.53 \text{ mg/L}$$

$$C_{min} = C^*_{min} * e^{-K*t^*} = 1.73 \text{ mg/L} * e^{-0.184 \text{ h}^{-1} *0.5 \text{ h}} = 1.58 \text{ mg/L}$$

$$V = \frac{R_0}{K} * \frac{1 - e^{-K*T_{inf}}}{C_{max} - C_{min} * e^{-K*T_{inf}}} =$$

$$\frac{80 \text{ mg}}{0.184 \text{ h}^{-1} * 0.5 \text{ h}} * \frac{1 - e^{-0.184 \text{ h}^{-1} *0.5 \text{ h}}}{6.53 \text{ mg/L} - 1.58 * e^{-0.184 \text{ h}^{-1} *0.5 \text{ h}}} = 15.0 \text{ L}$$

Step 3: Calculate recommended dosing interval t

$$\tau = \frac{\ln\left(\frac{C_{ss,max(desired)}}{C_{ss,min(desired)}}\right)}{K} + T_{inf} \quad \frac{\ln\left(\frac{10}{1}\right)}{0.184 \text{ h}^{-1}} + 0.5 \text{ h} = 13.0 \text{ h}$$

Practically reasonable, recommended dosing interval: 12 hours

Step 4: Calculate recommended dose D

$$D = C_{ss,max(desired)} * K * V * T_{inf} * \frac{1 - e^{-K*\tau}}{1 - e^{-K*T_{inf}}}$$

$$D = 10 \text{ mg/L} * 0.184 \text{ h}^{-1} * 15 \text{ L} * 0.5 \text{ h} * \frac{1 - e^{-0.184 \text{ h}^{-1} *12 \text{ h}}}{1 - e^{-0.184 \text{ h}^{-1} *0.5 \text{ h}}}$$

$$= 139.7 \text{ mg}$$

Recommended dosing regimen: 140 mg every 12 hours

Step 5: Check expected peak $C_{ss,max}$ and trough $C_{ss,min}$

$$C_{ss,max} = \frac{R_0}{K*V} * \frac{1 - e^{-K*T_{inf}}}{1 - e^{-K*\tau}} * \frac{140 \text{ mg}}{0.184 \text{ h}^{-1} * 15 \text{ L} * 0.5 \text{ h}} *$$

$$\frac{1 - e^{-0.184 \text{ h}^{-1} *0.5 \text{ h}}}{1 - e^{-0.184 \text{ h}^{-1} *12 \text{ h}}} = 10.0 \text{ mg/L}$$

$$C_{ss,min} = C_{ss,max} * e^{-K*(\tau - T_{inf})} = 10.0 \text{ mg/L} * e^{-0.184 \text{ h}^{-1} *(12 \text{ h} - 0.5 \text{ h})}$$

$$= 1.21 \text{ mg/L}$$

Clinical Example #2

A 70-year-old white male who weighs 95 pounds and is 5 feet tall has a serum creatinine of 1.1 mg/dL. He is admitted to the hospital complaining of shortness of breath; he denies chest pain. Digoxin is prescribed for him. You are asked to design a dosage regimen using tablets for him to achieve and maintain a $C_{target,ss}$ of 1 ng/mL. The PK parameters for digoxin are as follows: CL = 2.7 mL/min/kg (TBW) ; f_e = 0.68; V_{ss} = 6.7 L/kg (IBW); F of tablet = 0.75.

1. Estimate CL, CL_{cr}, RF, and CL* (clearance in renally impaired patient) of digoxin in this patient. IBW = 45.5 kg; TBW = 43 kg. Therefore use TBW for all calculations.

CL for a normal 43-kg patient = 116 mL/min

CL_{cr} and RF are:

$$CL_{cr} = \frac{(140 - 70) * 43}{1.1 * 72} = 38 \text{ mL/min}$$

$$RF = \frac{38 \text{ mL/min}}{125 \text{ mL/min}} = 0.304$$

2. Estimate CL, clearance of digoxin, in this patient with renal impairment.

CL* = 116 mL/min * [1 − .68 * (1− .304)] = 61.1 mL/min

3. Calculate dose rate.

$$\text{Dose rate} = \frac{1 \text{ ng/mL} * 61.1 \text{ mL/min}}{0.75} = 81.5 \text{ ng/min}$$

4. Determine dosing interval τ^*: estimate half-life of digoxin.

$$\tau^*_{1/2} = \frac{0.693 * V_{ss}}{CL^*}$$

V_{ss} (V_d) for digoxin from PK tables is 6.7 L/kg, or 289 L in this patient. Thus,

$$\tau^*_{1/2} = \frac{0.693 * 289 \text{ L}}{0.061 \text{ L/min}} = 3283 \text{ minutes} \cong 55 \text{ hours}$$

We normally administer digoxin every 24 hours ($\tau = 24$ h); we could administer 0.25 mg every 48 hours ($\tau = 48$ h). However, I would not change the dosing interval here because 24 hours is very convenient, and the resultant peak:trough ratio would be lower with a $\tau = 24$ compared to $\tau = 48$ hours.

Clinical Example #3:

A.M. is a 6'0", 195-pound, 61-year-old white male with a diagnosis of pneumonia. His serum creatinine is 2.3 mg/dL. Design a dosage regimen of gentamicin to achieve C_{peak} and C_{trough} values of 8 and 1 mg/L, respectively. $Vd = 0.2$ L/kg IBW

1. CL of gentamicin and f_e in normal adults.
   CL of gentamicin is 85 mL/min and $f_e = 1.0$

2. Degree of renal impairment.

$$CL = CL_{cr} = \frac{(140 - 61) * 77.6}{2.3(72)}$$

$$RF = \frac{37 \text{ mL/min}}{125 \text{ mL/min}} = .296$$

3. CL of gentamicin in this patient.

$$CL^* = 85 \text{ mL/min} * [1 - 1 (1 - .296)] = 25.2 \text{ mL/min} = 1.5 \text{ L/h}$$

4. Elimination rate constant in this patient.

$$k = \frac{CL}{V_{ss}} = \frac{1.5 \text{ L/h}}{0.2 \text{ L/kg} * 77.6 \text{ kg}} = 0.097 \text{ h}^{-1}$$

5. Infusion rate and dosing interval.

$$\tau = \frac{\ln\left(\dfrac{C_{ss,\max(desired)}}{C_{ss,\min(desired)}}\right)}{K} + T_{inf} = \frac{\ln\left(\dfrac{8 \text{ mg/L}}{1 \text{ mg/L}}\right)}{0.097 \text{ h}^{-1}} + 0.5 \text{ h} = 22 \text{ h} \cong 24 \text{ h}$$

$$D = C_{ss,\max} * K * V * T_{inf} * \frac{1 - e^{-K*\tau}}{1 - e^{-K*T_{inf}}} = 8 \text{ mg/L} * .097 \text{ h}^{-1}$$

$$* (.2 * 77.6) * 0.5 * \frac{1 - e^{-.097 \text{ h}^{-1} *24}}{1 - e^{-.097 \text{ h}^{-1} *0.5}} = 115 \text{ mg} \cong 120 \text{ mg}$$

Clinical Example #4

Patient D.M. is a 50-year-old white male (74.1 kg) who is being treated with phenytoin (Vd = 0.6 L/kg), 300 mg/d (using the capsule formulation) for seizure control. He has been taking phenytoin for 2 weeks. He experienced a seizure on day 14 of treatment. His blood level was 5.2 mg/L. His dose rate was increased to 400 mg/d of the capsule formulation. Three weeks later his level was 11.8 mg/L.

Phenytoin capsules and parenteral solution = sodium phenytoin
Phenytoin tablets and suspension = phenytoin acid
100 mg phenytoin sodium = 92 mg phenytoin acid

a. The V_{max} (mg phenytoin per day) for phenytoin in patient DM is:
   a. 491
   b. 499
   c. 542
   d. 590
   e. 614

Since D.M. is using capsules, we need to multiply the R_{in} by 0.92.

DR (mg/day)	C_{ss} (mg/L)	DR/C_{ss} (L/day)
300 * 0.92 = 276	5.2	53.08
400 * 0.92 = 368	11.8	31.19

$$\mathbf{DR = V_{max}} - \left(\frac{\mathbf{DR}}{\mathbf{C_{ss}}}\right) * \mathbf{K_m}$$

$$\mathbf{Y = intercept + X * (- slope)} \quad \text{Plot DR vs DR/C}_{ss}.$$

Y-intercept = V_{max} = 499 mg phenytoin/day,
slope = $-K_m$ = -4.20 mg/L, therefore, K_m = 4.2 mg/L

b. What dosage regimen would you recommend to achieve an average steady state phenytoin concentration of 15 mg/L in patient D.M. using the capsule formulation?

   a. 100 mg q6h
   b. 100 mg q8h
   c. 200 mg q6h
   d. 200 mg q8h

$$DR = CL * C_{ss,target} = \frac{V_{max} * C_{ss,target}}{K_m + C_{ss,target}} = \frac{499 \text{ mg/d} * 15 \text{ mg/L}}{4.2 \text{ mg/L} + 15 \text{ mg/L}}$$

$$= 390 \text{ mg phenytoin/d}$$

390 mg/d phenytoin = 424 mg/d sodium phenytoin
Would recommend 400 mg Dilantin Kapseals® in three or four divided doses (eg, 100 mg q6h).

c. Estimate the time required to achieve steady-state levels of phenytoin in patient DM at the dosage regimen if he were changed to a dosage regimen of a 100-mg capsule q6h.
   a. 1 day
   b. 5 days
   c. 9 days
   d. 13 days
   e. 17 days

$$t_{90} = \frac{K_m * V_{ss}}{(V_{max} - DR)^2} * (2.3 * V_{max} - 0.9 * DR)$$

$$t_{90} = \frac{4.2 \text{ mg phenytoin/L} * 0.6 \text{ L/kg} * 74.1 \text{ kg}}{(499 \text{ mg phenytoin/d} - 368 \text{ mg phenytoin/d})^2}$$

$$* (2.3 * 499 \text{ mg phenytoin/d} - 0.9 * 368 \text{ mg phenytoin/d})$$

$$t_{90} = 8.9 \text{ days}$$

About 9 days to reach 90% of new steady state plasma concentration

d. Calculate the loading dose of phenytoin in this patient that would be needed to achieve a phenytoin blood level of 12 mg/L (assume that blood levels of phenytoin = 0 at time of administration of LD).

   a. 491 mg
   b. 535 mg
   c. 580 mg
   d. 603 mg

$LD = C_{ss,\,target} * V_{ss}$ = 12 mg phenytoin/L * 0.6 L/kg * 74.1 kg = 534 mg of phenytoin = 580 mg of phenytoin sodium (parenteral)

Clinical Example #5

In order to treat her asthma exacerbation, L.Y. (55 kg, 68 years of age) has received a continuous infusion of aminophylline (infusion rate 0.45 mg/kg/h) for 5 days. This morning, she suffers from theophylline toxicity indicated by tachycardia, headache, and dizziness. A blood sample is drawn and the theophylline plasma concentration is 24.3 mg/L. The therapeutic range is 10-20 mg/L, the population average of the volume of distribution is 0.5 L/kg.

a. What is the theophylline clearance in this patient under the assumption that steady-state had already been reached at the time the blood sample was obtained?

   a. 0.81 L/h
   b. 0.95 L/h
   c. 1.35 L/h
   d. 2.15 L/h
   e. 2.80 L/h

$$CL = \frac{R_0}{C_{ss}} = \frac{0.45 \text{ mg/kg/h} * 0.8 * 55 \text{ kg}}{24.3 \text{ mg/L}} = 0.81 \text{ L/h}$$

b. To what aminophylline infusion rate should the infusion be reduced to achieve a steady-state concentration in the middle of the therapeutic range, ie, 15 mg/L?

a. 0.17 mg/kg/h
b. 0.18 mg/kg/h
c. 0.20 mg/kg/h
d. 0.22 mg/kg/h
e. 0.28 mg/kg/h

$MD = C_{target} * CL = 15 \text{ mg/L} * 0.81 \text{ L/h}$
$= 12.15 \text{ mg/h theophylline}$
$= 15.2 \text{ mg/h aminophylline}$
BW 55 kg: $MD = 0.28 \text{ mg/kg/h}$

c. Approximately how long does it take to achieve the new steady-state after the infusion rate has been changed?
   a. 26 h
   b. 68 h
   c. 118 h
   d. 156 h
   e. 192 h

Estimated $V = 55 \text{ kg} * 0.5 \text{ L/kg} = 27.5 \text{ L}$

$$t_{1/2} = \frac{\ln 2}{K} = \frac{\ln 2 * V}{CL} = \frac{0.693 * 27.5 \text{ L}}{0.81 \text{ L/h}} = 23.5 \text{ h}$$

Time to new steady-state is approximately $5 \, t_{1/2}$ ≈ 118 hours

d. The pharmacist suggests that the new target concentration can be achieved faster if the first infusion with the higher infusion rate is completely stopped and the second infusion with the lower infusion rate is not initiated until the plasma concentration has decreased to 15 mg/L, the target concentration. Calculate the period of time the therapy has to pause (ie, the time one waits after cessation of the first infusion before the second infusion is started).

   a. 14.7 h
   b. 16.4 h
   c. 20.7 h
   d. 36.1 h
   e. 55.1 h

$C_{target} = C_{ss,old} * e^{-K * t_{pause}}$

$$t_{pause} = \frac{\ln\left(\dfrac{C_{target}}{C_{ss,old}}\right)}{-K} = \frac{\ln\left(\dfrac{15 \text{ mg/L}}{24.3 \text{ mg/L}}\right) * 27.5 \text{ L}}{-0.81 \text{ L/h}} = 16.4 \text{ h}$$

11. Key Points

- The clearance CL can be determined from the relationship

$$CL = \frac{DR}{C_{ss,avg}} \quad \text{or} \quad CL = \frac{D}{AUC}$$

- The volume of distribution can be determined from the relationship

$$V = \frac{CL}{K}$$

- The average steady-state concentration $C_{ss,av}$ during multiple dosing is only determined by the dose, the dosing interval τ (or both together as dosing rate DR $= D/\tau$), and the clearance CL:

$$C_{ss,av} = \frac{D}{\tau * CL}$$

- The area under the curve resulting from administration of a single dose AUC_{single} is equal to the area under the curve during one dosing interval at steady-state AUC_{ss}, if the same dose is given per dosing interval τ.

$$C_{ss,av} = \frac{AUC_{ss}}{\tau} = \frac{D}{\tau * CL} = \frac{AUC_{single}}{\tau}$$

- The volume of distribution at steady-state is by definition the sum of the pharmacokinetic volumes of distribution for the different pharmacokinetic compartments. It is the theoretical:

$$V_{ss} = V_p + \frac{f_u}{f_{u,t}} * V_t$$

where V_p is the volume of plasma (3 L), V_t is the volume of tissue water (total body water minus plasma volume: $42 - 3 = 39$ L based on a "standard" person). f_{up} and f_{ut} are the fraction unbound for the drug in plasma and tissue, respectively.

- Clearance (CL) is defined as the irreversible removal of drug from the body by an organ of elimination. CL by the eliminating organ (CL_{organ}) is defined as the product of blood flow to the organ (Q) and the extraction ratio of that organ (ER). The fraction of drug escaping first-pass metabolism (F*) can be described in terms of the hepatic ER ($F* = 1 - ER$).

- The venous equilibrium model relates hepatic ER to hepatic blood flow (Q), unbound drug fraction (f_{up}), and the intrinsic clearance (CL_{int}):

$$CL_H = \frac{Q * f_{up} * CL_{int}}{Q + f_{up} * CL_{int}}$$

- The venous equilibrium model can be simplified for drugs with low ER (<0.3) and high ER (>0.7). For low ER drugs, $CL_H \approx f_{up} * CL_{int}$. For high ER drugs, $CL_H \approx Q$.

- The absolute bioavailability is the fraction (or percentage) of a dose administered non-intravenously (or extravascularly) which is systemically available as compared to an intravenous dose. The overall oral bioavailability (F) of a drug is dependent on the fraction absorbed (f_a), the fraction escaping metabolism in the intestinal wall (f_g), and the fraction escaping hepatic first-pass metabolism (F*).

- Drugs may undergo three processes in the kidney. Two of these act to remove drug from the body: filtration and secretion. The other, reabsorption, acts to return the drug to the body. We can determine the net process a drug undergoes by calculating the excretion ratio (E_{ratio}) using total renal clearance (CL_R) and filtration clearance (CL_F):

$$E_{ratio} = \frac{CL_R}{CL_F} = \frac{CL_R}{f_{up} * 125 \text{ mL/min}}$$

12. Questions and Answers

1. A pediatric patient receives an immunosuppressive therapy with oral cyclosporine solution. His concentration-adjusted dosing regimen is 85 mg every 12 hours. Due to a recent change in his insurance coverage, he needs to be switched from the drug product he is currently using to a generic solution dosage form of cyclosporine that is covered by his insurance. The bioavailability of the dosage form he previously used is 43%, and the bioavailability of the generic dosage form is 28%. What is the appropriate dosage regimen for the generic dosage form in order to maintain the same systemic exposure as obtained from the previously used dosage form?

   A. 25 mg every 12 hours
   B. 55 mg every 12 hours
   C. 184 mg every 12 hours
   D. 130 mg every 12 hours
   E. 305 mg every 12 hours

2. A drug is administered via continuous infusion at a rate of 60 mg/h, resulting in a steady-state plasma concentration of 5 µg/mL. If the plasma concentration is intended to be doubled to 10 µg/mL, the infusion rate must be

   A. Left the same
   B. Increased by 30 mg/h
   C. Increased by 60 mg/h
   D. Increased by 120 mg/h
   E. Decreased by 30 mg/h

3. Jonathan R. (72 kg, 23 years of age) has been admitted to the emergency room with acute asthma symptoms. He shall be started on a continuous infusion of aminophylline with a target theophylline concentration of 12 mg/L (therapeutic range 10-20 mg/L). To achieve the target concentration more rapidly, an additional loading dose shall be administered as a short-term infusion over 30 min. The population mean values for clearance and volume of distribution of theophylline are 2.7 L/h and 34 L, respectively. What aminophylline loading and maintenance dose should be given? (Select practical and useful doses and remember that aminophylline contains 80% theophylline.)

3a. Loading dose:
   A. 400 mg
   B. 450 mg
   C. 500 mg

D. 550 mg
E. 600 mg

3b. Maintenance dose:
A. 35 mg/h
B. 40 mg/h
C. 45 mg/h
D. 50 mg/h
E. 55 mg/h

4. Lidocaine shall be given as a constant rate infusion for the treatment of ventricular arrhythmia. A plasma concentration of 3 µg/mL was decided as therapeutic target concentration. The concentration of the infusion solution is 20 mg/mL lidocaine. The average volume of distribution of lidocaine is 90 L, the elimination half-life is 1.1 hours. What infusion rate (in mL/min) has to be set on the infusion pump in order to achieve the desired target concentration?

A. 5 mL/h
B. 8.5 mL/h
C. 14 mL/h
D. 23.5 mL/h
E. 194 mL/h

5. After termination of an intravenous constant rate infusion, the plasma concentration of a drug declines monoexponentially ($C = C * e^{-k*t}$). Concentrations measured at 2 hours and 12 hours after the end of the infusion are 12.9 µg/mL and 6.0 µg/mL, respectively. Calculate the initial concentration at the end of the infusion, and predict the concentration 24 hours after termination of the infusion.

A. 13.5 and 2.9 µg/mL
B. 16.5 and 3.8 µg/mL
C. 16.5 and 1.3 µg/mL
D. 15 and 2.4 µg/mL
E. 15 and 1.3 µg/mL

6. Margaret Q. (100 kg, 26 years of age) presents to the emergency room with acute symptoms of asthma. She recently started smoking again and has been taking oral theophylline for several years. The immediate determination of her theophylline plasma concentration results in a level of 4 mg/L. Theophylline population pharmacokinetic parameters: CL 0.04 L/h/kg, V 0.5 L/kg Therapeutic range: 10-20 mg/L. The appropriate intravenous loading dose of aminophylline for Margaret to achieve a target concentration of 12 mg/L is:

A. 300 mg
B. 400 mg
C. 500 mg
D. 600 mg
E. 750 mg

7. For a drug product in clinical drug development, an oral dosing regimen needs to be established for a Phase III study that maintains an average steady-state concentration of 50 ng/mL. In single dose studies, an oral dose of 80 mg resulted in an AUC of 962 ng/h/mL and an elimination half-life of 10.3 hours. What dosing regimen should be used?

A. 35 mg every 12 hours
B. 50 mg every 12 hours
C. 72 mg every 12 hours
D. 95 mg every 12 hours
E. 125 mg every 12 hours

8. Mary D. (47 years of age, 68 kg) has recently received her first 0.25-mg dose of digoxin. Plasma digoxin concentrations 12 and 24 hours following oral administration of this dose are 0.72 and 0.33 µg/L, respectively. The therapeutic plasma concentration range is 0.8-2.0 µg/L. Predict Mary's digoxin trough concentration at steady-state, assuming that oral digoxin therapy is continued at a dose rate of 0.25 mg once daily.

A. 0.62 µg/L
B. 0.93 µg/L
C. 1.32 µg/L
D. 1.57 µg/L
E. 1.95 µg/L

9. The population average values for the clearance and volume of distribution of nifedipine have been reported as 0.41 L/h/kg and 1.2 L/kg. What would be the maximum dosing interval you can use for a multiple-dose regimen with an immediate-release oral dosage form of nifedipine if peak-to-trough fluctuation should not exceed 100%?

A. 2 hours
B. 4 hours
C. 6 hours
D. 8 hours
E. 12 hours

10. Beth R. (63 years of age, 58 kg) is suffering from symptomatic ventricular arrhythmia. She will be started on an oral multiple-dose regimen with the antiarrhythmic mexiletine. The population average values of mexiletine for clearance and volume of distribution are CL = 0.5 L/h/kg and V = 6 L/kg, respectively. Although a therapeutic range of 0.5-2.0 mg/L has been described, it is recommended to avoid large peak-to-trough fluctuations. The available oral dosage forms are 150-, 200-, and 250-mg capsules with an oral bioavailability of F = 0.9. Design an appropriate and practically reasonable oral dosing regimen that keeps the plasma concentrations at an average concentration of approximately 1 mg/L, with a peak-to-trough fluctuation of 100% (ie, with concentrations within the limits of 0.75 and 1.5 mg/L).

A. 150 mg q6h
B. 200 mg q6h
C. 200 mg q8h
D. 250 mg q8h
E. 375 mg q12h

11. Edgar W. (20 years old, 58 kg) is receiving 80 mg of gentamicin as an IV infusion over a 30-minute period q8h. Two plasma samples are obtained to monitor serum gentamicin concentrations as follows: one sample 30 minutes after the end of the short-term infusion and one sample 30 minutes before the administration of the next dose. The serum gentamicin concentrations at these times are 4.9 and 1.7 mg/L, respectively. Assume steady-state. Develop a practically reasonable dosing regimen that will produce peak-and-trough concentrations of approximately 8 and 1 mg/L, respectively.

A. 120 mg q8h
B. 160 mg q8h
C. 140 mg q12h
D. 180 mg q12h
E. 280 mg q24h

12. A patient who is receiving chronic phenytoin therapy is hospitalized for an elective surgical procedure. On admission labs, it is noted that the patient has a phenytoin concentration of 8 µg/mL (therapeutic range: 10-20 µg/mL) and an albumin concentration of 3.0 g/dL.
Phenytoin: F= 0.2-0.9, CL variable, <1% excreted unchanged in the urine, 88-93% bound to plasma proteins (primarily albumin)
Based on this information, and the therapeutic range of phenytoin, you would recommend that the physician:

A. Decrease the dose of phenytoin, because high E drugs (eg, phenytoin) exhibit increased unbound concentrations with increases in fraction unbound in the plasma.
B. Increase the dose rate of phenytoin, because low E drugs (eg, phenytoin) exhibit increased CL with increases in fraction unbound in the plasma.
C. Not change the dose rate of phenytoin because low E drugs (eg, phenytoin) do not exhibit changes in unbound concentrations with increases in fraction unbound in the plasma.
D. Not change the dose rate of phenytoin because low E drugs (eg, phenytoin) exhibit equal and offsetting changes in CL and F with increases in fraction unbound in plasma.

13. The conditions that indicate the possibility of renal clearance of a weakly acidic drug being sensitive to changes in urine pH are that:

I. It is secreted and not reabsorbed
II. It has a pKa value of 5.0
III. It has a small volume of distribution
IV. All of the drug is excreted unchanged by the kidneys (ie, $f_e = 1$)

A. Only item I is correct
B. Only item II is correct
C. Only item III is correct
D. Items II and III are correct
E. Items II and IV are correct

14. A young man (age 28 years, 73 kg, creatinine clearance 124 mL/min) receives a single 200-mg oral dose of an antibiotic. The following pharmacokinetic parameters of the antibiotic are reported in the literature:
F: 90%; Vd: 0.31 L/kg; $t_{1/2}$: 2.1 h; f_{up}: 0.77.
67% of the antibiotic's absorbed dose is excreted unchanged in the urine. Determine the renal clearance of the antibiotic. What is the probable mechanism for renal clearance of this drug?

A. 84 mL/min; glomerular filtration and tubular reabsorption
B. 98 mL/min; glomerular filtration and tubular reabsorption
C. 112 mL/min; glomerular filtration
D. 167 mL/min; glomerular filtration and tubular reabsorption
E. 236 mL/min; glomerular filtration and tubular secretion

15a. The pharmacokinetic parameters for captopril in healthy adults are:
Clearance: 800 mL/min; $f_e = 0.5$; V_{ss}: 0.81 L/kg.
Plasma protein binding: 75%
Captopril is a weakly basic drug used in the treatment of hypertension. Assume a glomerular filtration rate of 125 mL/min. The mechanism(s) for renal clearance of captopril is:

A. Filtration only
B. Reabsorption only
C. Secretion only
D. Filtration and net secretion
E. Filtration and net reabsorption

15b. When cimetidine (a highly lipid-soluble weak base that is highly secreted in the renal proximal tubules) and captopril are co-administered, the renal clearance of captopril is reduced to approximately 125 mL/min. What is the most likely mechanism to account for this reduction in renal clearance?

A. Cimetidine reduces the filtration clearance of captopril
B. Cimetidine enhances the reabsorption of captopril
C. Cimetidine increases the unbound fraction of captopril
D. Cimetidine blocks the renal secretion of captopril

16. One of the most severe drug interactions is that between digoxin and quinidine. Administration of quinidine to patients taking digoxin results in a two- to threefold increase in digoxin C_{ss} and AUC after oral and intravenous administration of digoxin. Digoxin and quinidine are substrates for the multidrug resistance transporter P-glyco-protein. Based on the following pharmacokinetic data for digoxin, what is the most likely mechanism to explain this drug/drug interaction?
CL: 125 mL/min; V_{ss}: 1.2 L/kg (IBW)
f_e: >0.99; f_{up}: 0.25

A. Quinidine reduces digoxin fraction escaping first-pass metabolism.
B. Quinidine inhibits renal secretion of digoxin by blocking P-glycoprotein.
C. Quinidine decreases digoxin fraction reabsorbed in the kidney tubule.
D. Quinidine reduces the fraction of digoxin absorbed.

17. The drug transporter P-glycoprotein (Pgp) is involved in numerous processes in drug disposi-

tion. Pgp activity is directly responsible for the following processes:

I. Glomerular filtration
II. Transport of drug from hepatocytes into the bile
III. Transport of drug from the small intestine into the systemic circulation (ie, bloodstream)
IV. Degradation of drug in the lumen of the duodenum
V. Maintenance of the integrity of the blood-brain barrier by transport of drug out of the brain

A. Only V
B. II and V
C. II and III
D. I, II, and V
E. All of the above

18. A 59-year-old white female is hospitalized for a ruptured duodenal diverticulum. She is 5' 6", weighs 65 kg, and has a serum creatinine of 1.5 mg/dL. Design a dosage regimen to achieve C_{peak} and C_{trough} values of 8 and 0.5 mg/L, respectively, with an infusion time of 30 minutes. Assume Vd of gentamicin of 0.2 L/kg IBW in this patient. The typical population value of CL for gentamicin is 85 mL/min/70 kg. Which of the following dosage regimens would you recommend for this patient?

A. 100 mg q8h
B. 100 mg q18h
C. 100 mg q24h
D. 160 mg q12h
E. 160 mg q24h

19. J.D. is a 47-year-old white male who has been prescribed codeine for lower back pain. The pharmacist dispensing the medication remembers reading a study in which patients who took codeine with grapefruit juice experienced an enhanced analgesic effect. The study found that grapefruit juice enhanced oral bioavailability (F) of codeine. Interestingly, there was no effect on codeine hepatic clearance or volume of distribution. Thus the pharmacist counseled the patient not to take his codeine with grapefruit juice. Based on the pharmacokinetic data for codeine listed below, what is the most likely explanation for the enhanced oral bioavailability (F) of codeine?
CL: 1350 mL/min; f_e: 0.10; Vss: 3.3 L/kg.
Plasma protein binding: 35%

A. Grapefruit juice increases the absorption (f_a) of codeine.

B. Grapefruit juice decreases the fraction escaping first-pass metabolism (F*).

C. Grapefruit juice increases renal secretion of codeine.

D. Grapefruit juice increases the fraction escaping first-pass metabolism (F*).

20. The pharmacokinetic parameters for codeine in healthy adults are:
Oral F: 50%; f_e <0.01; Vss: 2.6 L/kg.
Plasma protein binding: 7%
Codeine is well absorbed ($f_a = 1$, $f_g = 0.8$). You may assume that hepatic blood flow in a 70-kg adult is 1350 mL/min. The hepatic clearance of codeine is:

A. 851 mL/min
B. 1350 mL/min
C. 500 mL/min
D. 675 mL/min

Answers

1. **D.** The systemic exposure or average steady-state concentration for an oral dosing regimen is given by

$$C_{ss,av} = \frac{F * DR}{CL}$$

where DR is the dose rate and F the oral bioavailability of the respective dosing regimens.
If $C_{ss,av}$ should be maintained constant, if follows that

$$C_{ss,av} = \frac{F_1 * DR_1}{CL} = \frac{F_2 * DR_2}{CL} \text{ or } F_1 * DR = F_2 * DR$$

where the subscript denotes the different dosing regimens.
Thus DR_2, the dose rate for the generic dosage form, can be calculated as

$$DR_2 = \frac{F_1 * DR_1}{F_2} = \frac{43\% * 85 \text{ mg/12 h}}{28\%} = 130.5 \text{ mg/12 h}$$

2. **C.** Steady-state plasma concentration of a constant rate infusion is directly proportional to the infusion rate R_0 via

$$C_{ss} = \frac{R_0}{CL}$$

Thus R_0 has to be doubled from 60 mg/h to 120 mg/h in order to increase C_{ss} from 5 to 10 µg/mL, ie, an increase of infusion rate by 60 mg/h.

3a. **C.** 500 mg for the loading dose.

3b. **B.** 40 mg/h for the maintenance dose.

Loading dose (LD) and maintenance dose (MD) can be calculated from target concentration and volume of distribution or clearance:

LD = C_{target} * V = 12 mg/L * 34 L
= 408 mg theophylline
= 510 mg aminophylline

MD = C_{target} * CL = 12 mg/L * 2.7 L/h
= 32.4 mg/h theophylline
= 40.5 mg/hr aminophylline

4. **B.** The infusion rate R_0 or maintenance dose MD needed to achieve and maintain a steady-state concentration of 3 µg/mL is given by

$$MD = R_0 = C_{ss} * CL = C_{ss} * V * \frac{0.693}{t_{1/2}}$$

$$= 3 \text{ µg/mL} * 90 \text{ L} * \frac{0.693}{1.1 \text{ h}} = 170 \text{ mg/h}$$

The infusion pump setting can then be calculated as

$$Infusion \ volume/time = \frac{170 \text{ mg/h}}{20 \text{ mg/mL}} - 8.5 \text{ mL/h}$$

5. **D.** The first step is to calculate the elimination rate constant k from the measured plasma concentrations:

$$k = \frac{\ln\left(\frac{C_{12h}}{C_{2h}}\right)}{12 \text{ h} - 2 \text{ h}} = \frac{\ln\left(\frac{12.9 \text{ µg/mL}}{6.0 \text{ µg/L}}\right)}{12 \text{ h} - 2 \text{ h}} = 0.077 \text{ h}^{-1}$$

The initial concentration C_0 at the end of the infusion can than be back-extrapolated by solving the following relationship for C_0:

$$C = C_0 * e^{-k*t}$$

$$C_0 = \frac{12.9 \text{ µg/mL}}{e^{-0.077 \text{ h}^{-1} * 2 \text{ h}}} = 15 \text{ µg/mL}$$

The concentration 24 hours after termination of the infusion can be predicted by

$$C_{24h} = 15 \text{ µg/mL} * e^{-0.077 \text{ h}^{-1} * 24 \text{ h}} = 2.4 \text{ µg/mL}$$

6. **C.** The loading dose can be determined based on the target concentration to be achieved and the volume of distribution. The predose level of 4 mg/L needs to be subtracted from the target concentration, since the loading dose only has to account for the concentration difference. The

calculated theophylline dose needs to be converted to aminophylline:

$$LD = (C_{target} - C_{predose}) * Vd = (12 - 4) \text{ mg/L} * 0.5 \text{ L/kg} * 100 \text{ kg} = 400 \text{ mg theophylline}$$

A loading dose of 400 mg theophylline is equivalent to 500 mg aminophylline.

7. **B.** The maintenance dose MD required to achieve an average steady-state concentration of 50 ng/mL for an oral dosing regimen is given by

$$MD = C_{ss,av} * CL/F$$

The oral clearance CL/F can be determined from the relationship between dose and area under the plasma concentration-time curve AUC:

$$CL/F = \frac{D}{AUC}$$

Thus the required MD can be calculated as

$$MD = C_{ss,av} * \frac{D}{AUC} = 50 \text{ ng/mL} * \frac{80 \text{ mg}}{962 \text{ ng/h/mL}} = 4.16 \text{ mg/h}$$

This corresponds to a dosing regimen of 50 mg (4.16 mg/h × 12 h) given every 12 hours.

8. **D.** Since trough concentrations after the first dose are known (0.33 µg/L), trough concentrations during multiple doses at steady state can be predicted by multiplying the trough after the first dose with the accumulation factor:

$$C_{ss,min} = C_{ss,1} * \frac{1}{e^{-k*\tau}}$$

The dosing interval τ is 24 hours, k can be calculated from

$$k = \frac{\ln\left(\frac{C_1}{C_2}\right)}{\Delta t} = \frac{\ln\left(\frac{0.72}{0.33}\right)}{(24 - 12) \text{ h}} = 0.065 \text{ h}^{-1}$$

Thus,

$$C_{ss,min} = 0.33 \text{ µg/L} * \frac{1}{e^{-0.065 \text{ h}^{-1}*24 \text{ h}}} = 1.57 \text{ µ/L}$$

9. **A.** For immediate-release formulations, upper limits for peak concentrations ($C_{ss,max}$) and lower limits for trough concentrations ($C_{ss,min}$) can be estimated by assuming immediate drug absorption. If fluctuation is equal to 100%, $C_{ss,min}$ is exactly one half of $C_{ss,max}$. This is the case when the dosing interval τ is equal to the elimination half-life $t_{1/2}$ of the drug. A population average half-life for nifedipine can be calculated as

$$k = \frac{CL}{V} = \frac{0.41 \text{ L/h/kg}}{1.21 \text{ L/kg}} = 0.34 \text{ h}^{-1}$$

$$t_{1/2} = \frac{0.693}{0.34 \text{ h}^{-1}} = \frac{0.41 \text{ L/h/kg}}{1.21 \text{ L/kg}} = 2.03 \text{ h}$$

Thus τ has to be smaller than 2.03 hours in order to avoid peak-to-trough fluctuation exceeding 100%.

10. **D.** Calculate necessary dose rate DR to maintain $C_{ss,avg}$ = 1 mg/L:

$$DR_{necessary} = \frac{D}{\tau} = \frac{C_{ss,av} * CL}{F} = \frac{1 \text{ mg/L} * 0.5 \text{ L/h/kg} * 58 \text{ g}}{0.90}$$

$$= 32.22 \text{ mg/h} = 773.3 \text{ mg/d}$$

Determine the maximum dosing interval:

$$\tau_{max} = \frac{\ln\left(\frac{C_{ss,max}}{C_{ss,min}}\right)}{K} = \frac{\ln\left(\frac{C_{ss,max}}{C_{ss,min}}\right) * V}{CL} = \frac{\ln\left(\frac{1.5}{0.75}\right) * 6 \text{ L/kg}}{0.5 \text{ L/h/kg}}$$

$$= 8.3 \text{ h}$$

Reasonable dosing regimen:
Practical dosing interval: 8 hours

$$D = DR_{necessary} * \tau = 32.22 \text{ mg/h} * 8 \text{ h} = 257.8 \text{ mg}$$

Recommended dosing regimen: 250 mg every 8 hours

11. **C.** Calculate the elimination rate constant k:

$$k = \frac{\ln\left(\frac{C_1}{C_2}\right)}{\Delta t} = \frac{\ln\left(\frac{4.9}{1.7}\right)}{6.5 \text{ h}} = 0.163 \text{ h}^{-1}$$

Calculate volume of distribution assuming steady-state:

$$C_{ss,max} = \frac{C_{measured peak}}{e^{-k*t}} = \frac{4.9 \text{ mg/L}}{e^{-0.163 \text{ h}^{-1}*0.5 \text{ h}}} = 5.32 \text{ mg/L}$$

$$C_{ss,min} = C_{measured trough} * e^{-k*t} = 1.7 \text{ mg/L} * e^{-0.163 \text{ h}^{-1}*0.5 \text{ h}}$$
$$= 1.57 \text{ mg/h}$$

$$V = \frac{R_0}{k} * \frac{1 - e^{-k*T_{inf}}}{C_{max} - C_{min} * e^{-k*T_{inf}}} = \frac{80 \text{ mg}}{0.163 \text{ h}^{-1} * 0.5 \text{ h}} *$$

$$\frac{1 - e^{-0.163 \text{ h}^{-1}*0.5 \text{ h}}}{5.32 \text{ mg/h} - 1.57 \text{ mg/h} * e^{-0.163 \text{ h}^{-1}*0.5 \text{ h}}} = 19.8 \text{ L}$$

Calculate recommended dosing interval:

$$\tau = \frac{\ln\left(\dfrac{C_{ss,\max(desired)}}{C_{ss,\min(desired)}}\right)}{k} + T_{inf} = \frac{\ln\left(\dfrac{8}{1}\right)}{0.163\ h} + .5\ h = 13.3\ h$$

Recommend dosing interval: 12 hours
Calculate recommended dose:

$$D = C_{ss,\max(desired)} * K * V * T_{inf} * \frac{1 - e^{-K*\tau}}{1 - e^{-K*T_{inf}}} =$$

$$= 8\ mg/L * 0.163\ h^{-1} * 19.8\ L * 0.5\ h * \frac{1 - e^{-0.163\ h^{-1}*12\ h}}{1 - e^{-0.163\ h^{-1}*0.5\ h}}$$

$D = 142\ mg$
Recommended dosing regimen: 140 mg
every 12 hours

12. **C.** Phenytoin has to be a low-extraction drug since its bioavailability is as high as 90%. The large range in F is due to variability in the absorption of the drug. You know it is not high E because if it was, you could never get an F of 90%. Assume ER <0.1, f_{up} = 0.07 to 0.12. Low-extraction drug and restrictively cleared (all low extraction drugs are assumed to be restrictively cleared). Normal albumin range: 3.5-5 g/dL. Thus the patient probably has increased f_{up} because of decreased albumin. f_{up} (based on the equation below) would be 0.14 (slightly elevated).

$$f_{up} = \frac{1}{1 + 2.1 * albumin}$$

It is a low-E drug, therefore CL is dependent on f_{up} and CL_{int}. Increased f_{up} would lead to increased CL and decreased total plasma concentrations (thus Cp of 8, which is below the therapeutic range). However, unbound concentrations would be predicted to be normal (therapeutic) even though total concentration is low. You would not recommend an increase in the patient's phenytoin dose as it may result in toxic concentrations. If available from the hospital's lab, it may be reasonable to obtain a free phenytoin plasma concentration to document therapeutic concentrations.

13. **B.** Only item II is correct.

Item I is incorrect. No pH sensitivity in CL_R is expected unless the drug is reabsorbed (ie, E_{ratio} <<1).

Item II is possible. Weakly acidic drugs with pKa values between 3 and 7.5 can be highly un-ionized in the range of urine pH (5-8) and thus undergo significant reabsorption if the un-ionized form is nonpolar.

Item III is incorrect. Cl and V have nothing to do with a drug's likelihood of being affected by changes in urine pH.

Item IV is also incorrect. The fraction excreted unchanged tells us nothing about the mechanisms of renal elimination. However, it is important to note that for drugs with high f_e values that are susceptible to changes in urine pH, large changes in the PK of the drug (ie, CLR) may be observed.

14. **A.** The antibiotic's total clearance can be determined from the reported Vd and $t_{1/2}$:

$$CL = Vd * \frac{\ln 2}{t_{1/2}} = 0.31\ L/kg * 73\ kg * \frac{0.693}{2.1\ h} = 7.47\ L/h$$

Renal clearance CL_R is then given by total clearance and the fraction excreted f_e:

$$CL_R = f_e * CL = 0.67 * 7.47\ L/h = 5.00\ L/h = 83.3\ mL/min$$

The predominant renal clearance mechanism can be estimated by determining the E_{ratio}:

$$E_{ratio} = \frac{CL_R}{f_{up} * GFR} = \frac{83.3\ mL/min}{0.77 * 124\ mL/min} = 0.87$$

The E_{ratio} <1 indicates that glomerular filtration and net reabsorption are the probable renal clearance mechanisms.

15a. **D.** The excretion ratio for captopril is significantly greater than 1, indicating captopril undergoes filtration and net secretion.

$$CL_R = CL_T * f_e$$

$$CL_R = 800\ mL/min * 0.5 = 400\ mL/min$$

$$E_{ratio} = \frac{CL_R}{f_{up} * GFR} = \frac{400\ mL/min}{0.25 * 125\ mL/min}$$

$$= 12.8 = filtration\ and\ net\ secretion$$

15b. **D.** The most likely mechanism to account for this reduction in renal clearance is that the cimetidine blocks the renal secretion of captopril.

16. **B.** Digoxin undergoes net secretion via active transport processes (eg, P-glycoprotein). Quinidine is a potent inhibitor of P-glycoprotein. Therefore, P-glycoprotein inhibition by quinidine results in a reduced renal clearance of digoxin.

$$CL_R = CL_T * f_e$$

$$CL_R = 125 \text{ mL/min} * 1.0 = 125 \text{ mL/min}$$

$$E_{ratio} = \frac{CL_R}{f_{up} * GFR} = \frac{125 \text{ mL/min}}{0.25 * 125 \text{ mL/min}}$$

$$= 4.0 = \text{filtration and net secretion}$$

17. **B.** The drug transporter P-glycoprotein (Pgp) is directly responsible for the transport of drug from hepatocytes into the bile and maintenance of the integrity of the blood-brain barrier by transport of drug out of the brain.

18. **C.** Calculation of CL: IBW = 59.3 kg

$$CL_{cr} = \frac{(140 - \text{age}) * \text{IBW}}{72 * S_{cr}} = \frac{(140 - 59) * 59.3}{72 * 1.5}$$

$$* 0.85 = 37.8 \text{ mL/min}$$

RF = 37.8/125 = 0.30. CL of gentamicin is 85 mL/min/70 kg TBW (1.2 mL/min/kg). CL of gentamicin in this patient if she did not have renal impairment would be:

$$CL = 1.21 \text{ mL/min/kg} * 65 \text{ kg} = 79 \text{ mL/min}$$

$$CL^* = CL * [1 - f_e * (1 - RF)]$$
$$= 79 * [1 - 1 * (1 - 0.30)] = 23.7 \text{ mL/min}$$
$$= 1.42 \text{ L/h}$$

$$K^* = \frac{CL^*}{V_{ss}} = \frac{1.42 \text{ L/h}}{0.2 \text{ L/kg} * 59.3 \text{ kg}} = 0.12 \text{ h}^{-1}$$

Calculate the dosing interval (τ) that you would recommend:

$$\tau = \frac{\ln\left(\frac{8}{0.5}\right)}{0.12 \text{ h}^{-1}} + 0.5 \text{ h} = 23.1 \text{ h}$$

Calculate the dose of gentamicin that will maintain C_{peak} and C_{trough} of 8 and 0.5 mg/L, respectively:

$$\text{Dose} = C_{ss,max} * K * V * t_{inf} * \frac{1 - e^{-K*\tau}}{1 - e^{-K*t_{inf}}}$$

$$\text{Dose} = 8 \text{ mg/L} * 0.12 \text{ h}^{-1} * 11.86 \text{ L} * 0.5 \text{ h} * \frac{1 - e^{-0.12*24}}{1 - e^{-0.12*0.5}}$$
$$= 92.3 \text{ mg}$$

Administration of 100 mg of gentamicin infused over 30 minutes given every 24 hours will provide C_{peak} and C_{trough} of approximately 8 and 0.5 mg/L, respectively.

19. **A.**

$$CL_H = 1350 * 0.9 = 1215 \text{ mL/min}$$

$$ER = \frac{1215 \text{ mL/min}}{1350 \text{ mL/min}} \approx 1$$

$$F = f_a * f_g * F^*$$

No effect on CL_H. No effect on F^*.

20. **C.**

$$F = f_a * f_g * F^*$$

$$F = \frac{F}{fa * fg} = \frac{0.5}{1 * 0.8} = 0.63$$

$$ER = 1 - F^* = 1 - 0.63 = 0.37$$

$$CL_H = Q * ER = 1350 \text{ mL/min} * 0.37$$
$$= 500 \text{ mL/min}$$

13. References

Atkinson A, Daniels C, Dedrick R, Grudzinskas C, Markey S. *Principles of Clinical Pharmacology.* San Diego, CA: Academic Press; 2001.

Ensom MH, Davis GA, Cropp CD, Ensom RJ. Clinical pharmacokinetics in the 21st century. Does the evidence support definitive outcomes? *Clin Pharmacokinet.* 1998;34:265-279.

Levy RH, Bauer LA: Basic pharmacokinetics. *Ther Drug Monit.* 1986;8:47-58.

Meibohm B, Derendorf H. Basic concepts of pharmacokinetic/pharmacodynamic (PK/PD) modelling. *Int J Clin Pharmacol Ther.* 1997;35:401-413.

Rolan PE. Plasma protein binding displacement interactions—why are they still regarded as clinically important? *Br J Clin Pharmacol.* 1994;37:125-128.

Rowland M, Tozer T. *Clinical Pharmacokinetics,* 3rd ed. Media, PA: Williams & Wilkins; 1995.

Saitoh A, Jinbayashi H, Saitoh AK, et al. Parameter estimation and dosage adjustment in the treatment with vancomycin of methicillin-resistant *Staphylococcus aureus* ocular infections. *Ophthalmologica.* 1997;211:232-235.

Sawchuck RJ, Zaske DE, Cipolle RJ, Wargin WA, Strate RG. Kinetic model for gentamicin dosing with the use of individual patient parameters. *Clin Pharmacol Ther.* 1977;21:362-369.

Tod MM, Padoin C, Petitjean O. Individualising aminoglycoside dosage regimens after therapeutic drug monitoring: simple or complex pharmacokinetic methods? *Clin Pharmacokinet.* 2001;40:803-814.

Wilkinson GR, Shand DG. Commentary: a physiological approach to hepatic drug clearance. *Clin Pharmacol Ther.* 1975;18:377-390.

7. Biotechnology and Pharmacogenomics

P. David Rogers, PharmD, PhD
Assistant Professor, Department of Pharmacy
University of Tennessee College of Pharmacy

Contents

1. **Introduction to Biotechnology and Pharmacogenomics**

2. **Key Points**

3. **Questions and Answers**

4. **References**

1. Introduction to Biotechnology and Pharmacogenomics

Since the discovery of the DNA double helix half a century ago, man has made significant use of biotechnology for the improvement of human health (Table 1). Accompanying these advances are a number of biological products with therapeutic applications. With the arrival of the post-genomic era, the field of pharmacogenomics has emerged and shows great promise to revolutionize the way in which pharmacy and medicine is practiced. This chapter highlights key concepts relevant to the practicing pharmacist in the areas of biotechnology and pharmacogenomics.

Biotechnology has revolutionized the pharmaceutical industry by imparting the ability to mass produce safe and pure versions of chemicals produced naturally in the body. A multitude of disease states have been impacted by therapeutic agents derived through biotechnology, including AIDS, anemia, cancer, cystic fibrosis, congestive heart failure, diabetes, hemophilia, hepatitis B and C, growth hormone deficiency, and multiple sclerosis, to name a few.

Biotechnology is defined by the United States Food and Drug Administration as "the use of recombinant DNA (or RNA) technology; direct DNA transfer technology; nucleic acid amplification technology; hybridoma technology; cell fusion; molecular modification of cellular receptors; or the application of cells, tissues, or their components such that their potential biological activity has been modified."

Key Terms

antibody (immunoglobulin): a protein produced by β-lymphocytes in response to antigen molecules determined to be non-self. Antibodies recognize and bind to antigens, resulting in their inactivation or opsonization for phagocytosis or complement-mediated destruction. A number of immunoglobulin (Ig) G products have been developed for therapeutic use in various immune disorders.

antigen: a molecule that elicits an antibody-mediated immune response.

bioinformatics: the application of computer sciences and information technology to the management and analysis of biological information.

biotherapy: any treatment involving the administration of a microorganism or other biologic material.

clotting factor (blood factor): chemical blood constituents that interact to cause blood coagulation.

combinatorial chemistry: a drug development strategy that utilizes nucleic acids and amino acids in various combinations to synthesize vast libraries of oligonucleotide or peptide compounds for high-throughput lead compound screening.

cytokine: an extracellular signaling protein that mediates communication between cells.

DNA (deoxyribonucleic acid): a polynucleotide molecule consisting of covalently linked nucleic acids. DNA serves as the genetic material.

enzyme: a protein that catalyzes a chemical reaction.

gene: a region of DNA that encodes a specific RNA or protein responsible for a specific hereditary characteristic.

gene therapy: therapeutic technologies that directly target human genes responsible for disease.

genome: the complete set of genetic information for a given organism.

Table 1

Milestones in Biotechnology

Event	Year
Identification of DNA as the genetic material	1940
Discovery of DNA double helix by James Watson and Francis Crick	1953
Elucidation of the genetic code (64 nucleic acid triplets, or codons, encode 20 amino acids)	1961
Cloning of DNA and the production of the first recombinant DNA derived protein	1973
Introduction of monoclonal antibodies	1975
Production of the first human protein (somatostatin) from recombinant DNA technology	1977
Cloning of the human insulin gene	1978
Human insulin derived from recombinant DNA technology licensed in the U.S.	1982
Conception of the polymerase chain reaction (PCR) for amplification of DNA	1983
Initiation of the Human Genome Project	1990
Sequencing of the human genome	2001

genomics: the scientific discipline of mapping, sequencing, and analyzing genomes. It encompasses structural genomics, functional genomics, and pharmacogenomics.

hormone: a chemical substance that imparts specific cellular effects that is transmitted by the bloodstream to cells distant from its physiologic source.

hybridoma: a cell line generated by the fusion of antibody-producing β-lymphocytes with lymphocyte tumor cells for the production of monoclonal antibodies.

interferon: a member of a group of cytokines that prevents viral replication and slows the growth and replication of cancer cells.

interleukin: a member of a group of cytokines involved in orchestration and regulation of the immune response.

liposome: a microscopic, sphere-like lipid droplet that functions as a therapeutic carrier.

monoclonal antibody: an antibody derived from a hybridoma cell line.

pharmacogenomics: the scientific discipline of using genome-wide approaches to understand the inherited basis of differences between individuals in the response to drugs. This is an expansion of the field of pharmacogenetics, which traditionally considered such inherited differences on a gene-by-gene basis.

plasmid: a small, circular, extrachromosomal DNA molecule capable of replication independent of that of the genome.

polymerase chain reaction (PCR): a molecular biologic technique for amplification of specific DNA molecules.

protein: a functional product of a specific gene consisting of amino acids linked together through peptide bonds in a specific sequence.

proteomics: the scientific field of the study of sequencing and analyzing the expression, modification, and function of proteins on a genome-wide or global scale.

recombinant DNA (rDNA) technology: the application of DNA molecules derived by joining two DNA molecules from different sources.

restriction endonucleases: an enzyme capable of cleaving a DNA molecule in a site-specific manner.

ribozymes: RNA molecules with intrinsic enzymatic activity.

RNA (ribonucleic acid): a polynucleotide molecule consisting of covalently linked ribonucleic acids. Messenger RNA serves as the template for protein synthesis. Transfer RNA serves as the adaptor molecules between amino acids and mRNA during protein synthesis. Ribosomal RNA serves as a component of the ribosome and participates in protein synthesis.

small molecule chemistry: the field of drug development focusing on small organic nucleotide or peptide-based molecules derived through either combinatorial chemistry or rational drug design.

single nucleotide polymorphism: Common DNA sequence variations among individuals involving a single nucleotide substitution.

vaccine: A preparation of antigenic material administered to stimulate the development of antibodies conferring active immunity against a particular pathogen or disease.

Biological Products

There are many FDA-approved biological products currently on the market, including blood factors, cytokines, enzymes, growth factors, hormones, interferons, monoclonal antibodies, and vaccines. A list of such biological products is provided in Table 2.

Gene Expression and Protein Synthesis

Proteins are the major macromolecular component of the cell and are responsible for conducting most of a cell's biological activity. Proteins consist of a linear polymer of amino acids linked together in a specific sequence. This specific sequence is responsible for a protein's structure and function. The initial code for the synthesis of a given protein is stored in a gene on a sequence of DNA that is part of a chromosome within the nucleus of a cell.

• The central dogma of molecular biology is that DNA encodes RNA, which in turn encodes protein.

• A given amino acid within a protein is encoded by a triplet of nucleic acid base pairs within the gene encoding the protein. This triplet is called a *codon*.

Table 2

FDA-Approved Biological Products

Generic name	Brand name (manufacturer)	Indications
Blood factors		
Factor VII	NovoSeven® (Novo Nordisk)	Hemophilia
Factor VIII	Bioclate™, Recombinate™ (Baxter); Kogenate®; Helixate (Bayer) ReFacto® (Genetics Institute)	Hemophilia A
Factor IX	BeneFIX® (Genetics Institute	Hemophilia B
Cytokines		
Aldesleukin (IL-2)	Proleukin® (Chiron)	Metastatic renal cell carcinoma and melanoma
Denileukin diftitox	Ontak™ (Ligand)	Cutaneous T-cell lymphoma
Interferon alfacon-1	Infergen® (Amgen)	Hepatitis C
Interferon alfa-n1	Wellferon™ (GlaxoSK)	Chronic hepatitis C
Interferon alfa-2a	Roferon-A® (Roche)	Hairy cell leukemia; AIDS-related Kaposi's sarcoma; CML
Interferon alfa-2b	Intron-A® (Schering)	Hairy cell leukemia; AIDS-related Kaposi's sarcoma; chronic hepatitis B and C; condylomata acuminata; malignant melanoma
Interferon alfa-n3	Alferon-N® (InterMune)	Condylomata acuminata
Interferon beta-1b	Betaseron® (Berlex)	Acute relapsing-remitting multiple sclerosis
Interferon beta-1a	Avonex® (Biogen); Rebif® (Serono)	Acute relapsing-remitting multiple sclerosis
Interferon gamma-1b	Actimmune® (InterMune)	Chronic granulomatous disease; osteoporosis
Oprelvekin (IL-11)	Neumega® (Genetics Institute)	Thrombocytopenia from chemotherapy
Enzymes		
Alteplase	Activase® (Genentech)	Acute myocardial infarction; pulmonary embolism; stroke
Bivalirudin	Angiomax® (Medicines Co.)	Coronary angioplasty (PTCA); unstable angina
Dornase alfa	Pulmozyme® (Genentech)	Respiratory complication from cystic fibrosis
Eptifibatide	Integrelin® (Cor/Schering)	Acute coronary syndromes; angioplasties
Imiglucerase	Carezyme® (Genzyme)	Type 1 Gaucher's disease
Lepirudin	Refludan® (Aventis)	Coronary angioplasty (PTCA); unstable angina
Reteplase	Retavase® (Centocor/J&J)	Acute myocardial infarction
Tenecteplase	TNKase™ (Genentech)	Acute myocardial infarction
Tirobifan	Aggrastat® (Merck)	Acute coronary syndromes
Growth factors		
Becaplermin (PDGF)	Regranex® (Ortho-McNeil)	Diabetic foot ulcer
Darbepoetin alfa	Aranesp™ (Amgen)	Anemia associated with end-stage renal disease and chronic renal insufficiency
Epoetin alfa	Epogen® (Amgen); Procrit® (Ortho Biotech)	Anemia due to chronic renal disease; zidovudine-induced anemia; cancer; anemia due to chemotherapy; surgery patients
Filgrastim	Neupogen® (Amgen)	Neutropenia due to myelosuppressive chemotherapy; myeloid reconstitution after BMT; severe chronic neutropenia; peripheral blood progenitor cell transplant; induction and consolidation therapy in AML
Pegfilgrastim	Neulasta™ (Amgen)	Neutropenia and infection due to myelosuppressive chemotherapy
Sargramostim	Leukine® (Schering)	Myeloid reconstitution after BMT; BMT failure; adjunct to chemotherapy in AML; peripheral blood progenitor cell transplant
Hormones		
Choriogonadotropin alfa	Ovidrel® (Serono)	Fertility
Follitropin alpha	Follistim® (Organon)	Ovulatory failure
Follitropin beta	Gonal-F® (Serono)	Ovulatory failure

Table 2

FDA-Approved Biological Products (continued)

Generic name	Brand name (manufacturer)	Indications
Hormones (cont.)		
Human insulin	Humulin®; Humalog® (Eli Lilly); Novolin® (Novo Nordisk); Lantus® (Aventis)	Insulin-dependent diabetes mellitus
Human growth hormone	Protopin®, Nutropin® (Genentech)	Growth hormone deficiency in pediatric patients;
	Humatrope® (Eli Lilly)	Growth retardation in chronic renal disease
	Saizen®, Serostim® (Serono)	AIDS wasting
	Norditropin® (Novo Nordisk)	Turner's syndrome
	Genotropin® (Pharmacia); Biotropin® (Sol Source Technologies)	Growth hormone deficiency in adults
Ganirelix	Antagon™ (Organon)	LH surge during fertility therapy
Glucagon	Glucagen™ (Nova Nordisk)	Hypoglycemia
Growth hormone-releasing hormone	Geref® (Serono)	GH deficiency in pediatric patients
Thyrotropin	Thyrogen® (Genzyme)	Thyroid cancer
Monoclonal antibodies		
Abciximab	ReoPro® (Centocor/Eli Lilly)	Prevention of blood clots post PTCA; unstable angina prior to PTCA
Alemtuzumab	Campath® (Ilex/Millennium)	Chronic lymphocytic leukemia
Basiliximab	Simulect® (Ligand/Novartis)	Acute organ transplant rejection
Daclizumab	Zenapax® (PDL/Roche)	Kidney transplant, acute rejection
Gemtuzumab (ozogamicin)	Mylotarg® (Wyeth/PDL)	Acute myeloid leukemia (CD33+)
Ibritumomab (tiuxetan)	Zevalin® (IDEC)	B-cell non-Hodgkin's lymphoma
Infliximab	Remicade® (Centocor)	Crohn's disease; rheumatoid arthritis
Palivizumab	Synagis® (MedImmune/PDL)	Prevention of RSV and fatal pneumonia in pediatrics
Rituximab	Rituxan® (IDEC/Genentech)	Low-grade non-Hodgkin's lymphoma
Trastuzumab	Herceptin® (Genentech/PDL)	Metastatic breast cancer (Her 2 Neu+)
Vaccines		
Haemophilus b/ hepatitis B	Comvax® (Merck)	Prevention of *H influenzae* and hepatitis B
Hepatitis B vaccine	Engerix-B® (GlaxoSK); Recombivax HB® (Merck)	Prevention of hepatitis B
Others		
Anakinra	Kineret™ (Amgen)	Rheumatoid arthritis
BCNU-polymer	Gliadel® (Guilford)	Recurrent glioblastoma multiforme
Daunorubicin-liposomal	DaunoXome® (Giliad)	Kaposi's sarcoma
Doxorubicin-liposomal	DOXIL® (Alza)	Kaposi's sarcoma; ovarian cancer
Drotrecogin alfa	Xigris™ (Eli Lilly)	Sepsis
Etanercept	Enbrel® (Amgen)	Rheumatoid arthritis; poriatic arthritis
Fomivirsen	Vitravene® (Isis)	CMV retinitis
Glatiramer	Copaxone® (Teva)	Relapsing multiple sclerosis
Lipid-based amphotericin B	Abelcet® (Elan)	Aspergillosis
	Amphotec® (Sequus)	Cryptococcal meningitis in HIV
	AmBisome (Fujisawa/Gilead)	Systemic fungal infections
Nesiritide	Natrecor® (Scios/Innovex)	Congestive heart failure

AIDS, acquired immunodeficiency syndrome; AML, acute myelogenous leukemia; BMT, bone marrow transplant; CML, chronic myelogenous leukemia; CMV, cytomegalovirus; GH, growth hormone; HIV, human immunodeficiency virus; IL, interleukin; LH, luteinizing hormone; PDGF, platelet-derived growth factor, PTCA, percutaneous transluminal coronary angioplasty; RSV, respiratory syncytial virus.

- There are 64 codons encoding 20 different amino acids as dictated by the genetic code.

- An overview of transcription, translation, and post-translational modification is shown in Figure 1.

Recombinant DNA Technology

- Recombinant DNA (rDNA) technology uses several molecular biological tools to insert a desired DNA fragment with a specific purpose in proximity to other DNA fragments within a DNA molecule. Most often, a gene encoding a desired protein is isolated through screening the genomic library or by utiliza-tion of the viral enzyme reverse transcriptase to generate cDNA from the mRNA transcript of the gene. Enzymes called restriction endonucleases allow the cleavage of DNA in the plasmid at very specific locations. The gene is then ligated into a vector such as a plasmid for gene cloning or to control the expression of the encoded protein.

- An *expression vector* is a plasmid designed to allow inducible expression of the inserted gene within a host cell (such as the bacterium *Escherichia coli* or the yeast *Saccharomyces cerevisiae*). This mechanism permits production of large quantities of the desired protein. The protein must then be isolated

Figure 1.

Gene expression: The synthesis of proteins.

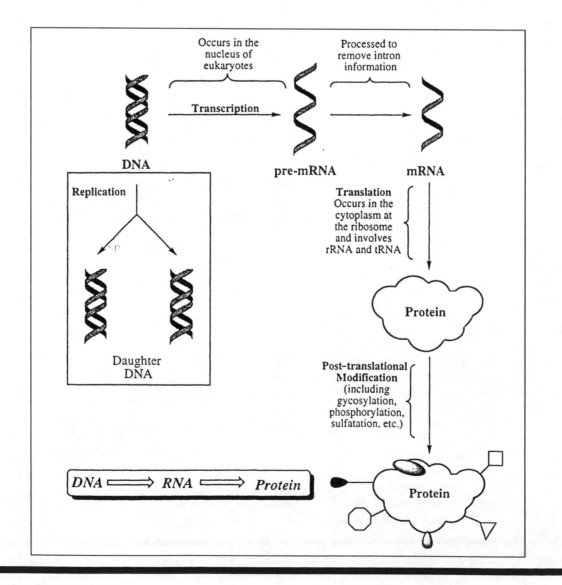

Reproduced from Sindelar, 2002.

and purified for further use. Such techniques, used on an industrial scale, mass-produce therapeutically useful biological products such as cytokines, enzymes, hormones, blood factors, and vaccines (Figure 2).

• Cytokines (ie, molecules secreted by cells) orchestrate the immune response and activate immune cells such as lymphocytes, monocytes, macrophages, and neutrophils. Therapeutically useful recombinant cytokines include interferons, interleukins, and colony-stimulating factors. Examples of these include interferon beta-1b (Betaseron®), which is used to treat acute relapsing-remitting multiple sclerosis; aldesleukin (IL-2) (Proleukin®), which aids in the management of metastatic renal cell carcinoma

Figure 2.

Summary of typical rDNA production of a protein from either genomic DNA or cDNA.

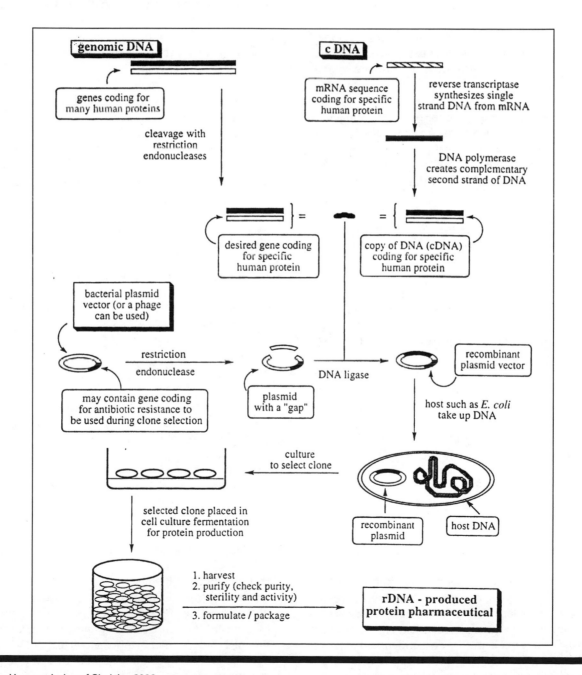

Reprinted by permission of Sindelar, 2002.

and melanoma; and oprelvekin (IL-11) (Neumega®), which treats thrombocytopenia caused by chemotherapy.

- An enzyme is a protein that catalyzes a specific chemical reaction. A number of different enzymes with therapeutic use have been produced using recombinant DNA technology. Alteplase (Activase®), for example, treats acute myocardial infarction, pulmonary embolism, and stroke. Dornase alfa (Pulmozyme®) treats respiratory complications that develop in cystic fibrosis. Eptifibatide (Integrelin®) is used to treat acute coronary syndromes.

- Hormones, chemical substances transmitted via the bloodstream, are designed to impart specific cellular effects to cells distant from their physiologic source. Since the introduction and success of recombinant human insulin in 1982, many other recombinant hormones have been developed, for example, human growth hormone, which treats growth hormone deficiency in pediatric patients, and follitropin alpha and beta (Gonal-F® and Follistim®, respectively), which are used to remedy ovulatory failure.

- Clotting or blood factors are chemical blood constituents that interact to cause blood coagulation. Patients suffering from hemophilia A (due to factor VIII deficiency) and hemophilia B (due to factor IX deficiency) have benefited greatly from recombinant DNA technology. Factors VIII, IX, and factor VII are available in recombinant forms for clinical use.

- Vaccines, preparations of antigenic material administered to stimulate the development of antibodies, confer active immunity against a particular pathogen or disease. Vaccine development has also benefited from advances is rDNA technology. Traditional vaccine production used killed or nonvirulent organisms, microbial toxins, or actual microbial components to elicit long-term immune protection. Safer and more specific vaccine antigens have been devised as recombinant proteins. This technology has led to the very successful recombinant hepatitis B vaccine.

Monoclonal Antibodies

- Antibodies, proteins produced by the immune system's B lymphocytes, use specific methods to recognize foreign molecules within the body. Subsets of B lymphocyte clones produce identical antibodies that recognize the same antigen. These identical antibodies are said to be *monoclonal*. Fusing B lymphocytes with lymphocyte tumor cells produces a hybridoma. This fused cell type is immortal and can be cultured in large quantities for the mass production of a given monoclonal antibody.

- Monoclonal antibodies that bind to and inactivate their targets can be developed and have great therapeutic utility (Figure 3). Nomenclature of monoclonal antibodies is highly structured. The first component of the name is product-specific, the second component indicates its therapeutic use: *ci* denotes cardiovascular use; *li* for use in inflammation; and *tu* for use in cancer. The third component indicates the type of monoclonal antibody: *mo* for murine; *xi* for chimeric; and *zu* for humanized. The fourth component, *mab* represents "monoclonal antibody." An example of a monoclonal antibody used clinically is abciximab (ReoPro®), which prevents blood clots post-PTCA and prevents unstable angina prior to PTCA. Another example, inflixima (Remicade®), is used to treat Crohn's disease and rheumatoid arthritis.

Gene Therapy

- Gene therapy is an excellent example of the therapeutic application of biotechnology. This technology holds promise for the treatment of inherited disorders as well as acquired illnesses such as infectious diseases and cancer.

- The molecular goal of gene therapy is to repair or correct a dysfunctional gene by selectively introducing recombinant DNA into cells or tissues, thereby allowing the expression of a functional gene product.

- Novel drug delivery strategies must be used to introduce exogenous DNA into the cell to treat retroviruses, lentiviruses, and adeno-associated virus. These novel drug delivery strategies have applications for nonviral delivery systems as well (eg, liposomes or uncomplexed plasmid DNA).

- Alternative approaches using ribozymes (eg, RNA repair) may prove effective. The enzymatic activity of these RNA molecules can be used to repair defective mRNAs.

- Chimeric RNA/DNA oligonucleotides make use of the cell's "DNA mismatch repair apparatus" to correct mutations at the genomic level. Clinical utility has been proven useful in employing antisense oligonucleotides for gene inactivation. Fomivirsen (Vitravene®), an antisense oligonucleotide, targets the mRNA of human cytomegalovirus (CMV). This agent is indicated for the treatment of CMV retinitis in patients with AIDS.

Figure 3.

Production of monoclonal antibodies.

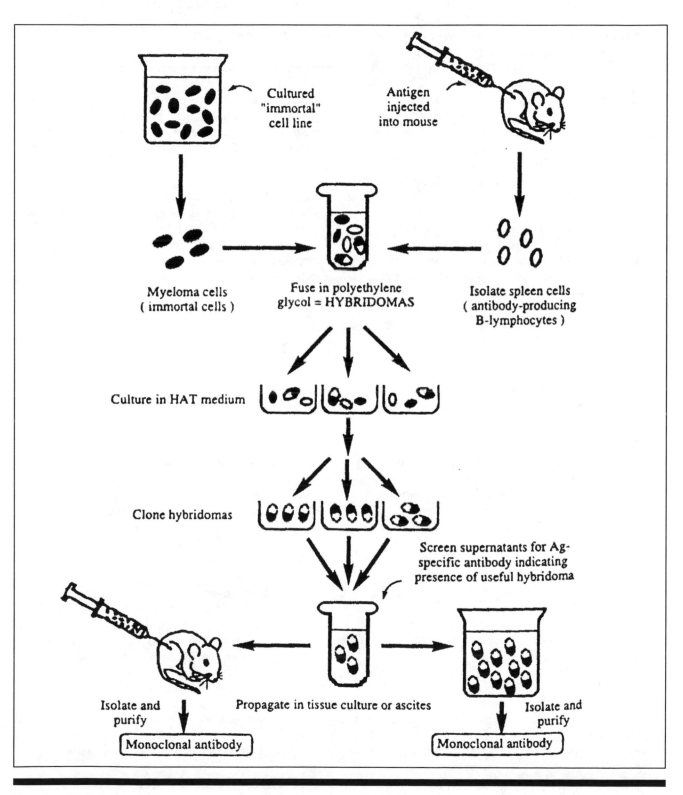

Drug Delivery

- Biotechnology has facilitated the development of novel drug delivery strategies.

- The use of liposomes has had a positive impact on drug delivery. Drugs can be formulated into liposomes, ie, microscopic spherical lipid droplets. The outer membrane of the liposome fuses with the membrane of the target cell, thereby facilitating highly targeted drug delivery. Such technology has greatly improved the therapeutic index of the antifungal drug amphotericin B. Lipid-based formulations now allow greater quantities of the drug to be delivered with substantially less toxicity to the patient.

- Another promising approach is the use of immunotoxins. These delivery agents combine a monoclonal antibody with a toxin such as an anticancer or antimicrobial agent, thereby allowing targeted drug delivery with minimal toxicity.

- Another novel strategy is the use of pegylation, ie, the addition of polyethylene glycol to therapeutic proteins to minimize the deleterious immune response to an individual protein.

Pharmacogenomics

- *Pharmacogenomics* is the scientific discipline of using genome-wide approaches to understand the inherited basis of differences between individuals in the response to drugs. This is an expansion of the field of pharmacogenetics, which traditionally considered such inherited differences on a gene-by-gene basis.

- Genetic differences in drug metabolism, drug disposition, and drug targets have a large impact on efficacy and toxicity. Comprehension of the relationships between specific genetic factors and drug response can be used to predict drug response and optimize drug therapy in any given individual.

Table 3

Genetic Polymorphisms in Drug Target Genes That Can Influence Drug Response[1]

Gene or gene product	Medication	Drug effect associated with polymorphism
Angiotensin-converting enzyme (ACE)	ACE inhibitors (eg, enalapril)	Renoprotective effects; blood pressure reduction; reduction in left ventricular mass; endothelial function
	Fluvastatin	Lipid changes (reductions in low-density lipoprotein cholesterol and apolipoprotein B); progression or regression in coronary atherosclerosis
Arachidonate 5-lipoxygenase	Leukotriene inhibitors	Improvement of FEV_1
β_2-adrenergic receptor	β_2-Agonists	Bronchodilatation; susceptibility to agonist-induced desensitization; cardiovascular effects
Bradykinin B_2 receptor	ACE inhibitors	ACE inhibitor–induced cough
Dopamine receptors (D_2, D_3, D_4)	Antipsychotics (eg, haloperidol, clozapine)	Antipsychotic response (D_2, D_3, D_4); antipsychotic-induced tardive dyskinesia (D_3); antipsychotic-induced acute akathisia (D_3)
Estrogen receptor-α	Conjugated estrogens	Increase in bone mineral density
	Hormone replacement therapy	Increase in high-density lipoprotein cholesterol
Glycoprotein IIIa subunit of glycoprotein IIb/IIIa	Aspirin or glycoprotein IIb/IIIa inhibitors	Antiplatelet effect
Serotonin (5-hydroxytryptamine transporter)	Antidepressants (eg, clomipramine, fluoxetine, paroxetine)	Serotonin neurotransmission; antidepressant response

FEV_1, forced expiratory volume in 1 second.

[1]The examples shown are illustrative and not representative of all published studies.

Reprinted by permission from Evans et al, 2003.

Table 4

Genetic Polymorphisms in Disease-Modifying or Treatment-Modifying Genes That Can Influence Drug Response[1]

Gene or gene product	Disease or response association	Medication	Influence of polymorphism on drug effect or toxicity
Adducin	Hypertension	Diuretics	Myocardial infarction or strokes
Apolipoprotein E (APOE)	Progression of atherosclerosis; ischemic cardiovascular events	Statins (eg, simvastatin)	Enhanced survival
	Alzheimer's disease	Tacrine	Clinical improvement
Human leukocyte antigen (HLA)	Toxicity	Abacavir	Hypersensitivity reaction
Cholesterol ester transfer protein (CETP)	Progression of atherosclerosis	Statins (eg, pravastatin)	Slowing of progression of atherosclerosis
Ion channels (HERG, KvLQT1, Mink, MiRP1)	Congenital long-QT syndrome	Erythromycin; terfenadine; cisapride; clarithromycin; quinidine	Increased risk of drug-induced torsade de pointes
Methylguanine methyltransferase (MGMT)	Glioma	Carmustine	Response of glioma to carmustine
Parkin	Parkinson's disease	Levodopa	Clinical improvement and levodopa-induced dyskinesias
Prothrombin and factor V	Deep-vein thrombosis and cerebral-vein thrombosis	Oral contraceptives	Increased risk of deep-vein thrombosis and cerebral-vein thrombosis with oral contraceptives
Stromelysin-1	Atherosclerosis progression	Statins (eg, pravastatin	Reduction in cardiovascular events by pravastatin (death, myocardial infarction, stroke, angina, and others); deduction in risk of repeated angioplasty

[1]The examples shown are illustrative and not representative of all published studies.
Reproduced with permission from Evans et al, 2003.

- Of particular significance are single nucleotide polymorphisms (SNPs). SNPs are differences in a single nucleotide base that occur at a significant frequency (usually >5%) within the population. An SNP may or may not promote change in the encoded amino acid of a codon. It may change the encoded amino acid, but yield no change in the function of the encoded protein. When an SNP causes amino acid substitution, a phenotypic difference that carries clinical relevance may result . Even when the SNP results in no change in the encoded amino acid, it may be associated with a phenotypic change, thereby serving as a predictive marker of that change.

- Examples of significant genetic polymorphisms that can influence drug response are shown in Tables 3 and 4.

- Examples of significant genetic polymorphisms in drug-metabolizing enzymes are shown in Tables 5 and 6.

Table 5

Pharmacogenomics of Phase I Drug Metabolism[1]

Drug-metabolizing enzyme	Frequency of variant poor-metabolism phenotype	Representative drugs metabolized	Effect of polymorphism
Cytochrome P-450 2D6 (CYP2D6)	6.8% in Sweden	Debrisoquin	Enhanced drug effect
	1% in China	Sparteine	Enhanced drug effect
		Nortriptyline	Enhanced drug effect
		Codeine	Decreased drug effect
Cytochrome P-450 2C9 (CYP2C9)	Approximately 3% in England (those homozygous for the *2 and *3 alleles)	Warfarin	Enhanced drug effect
		Phenytoin	Enhanced drug effect
Cytochrome P-450 2C19 (CYP2C19)	2.7% among white Americans 3.3% in Sweden 14.6% in China 18% in Japan	Omeprazole	Enhanced drug effect
Dihydropyrimidine dehydrogenase	Approximately 1% of population is heterozygous	Fluorouracil	Enhanced drug effect
Butyrylcholinesterase (pseudocholinesterase)	Approximately 1 in 3500 Europeans	Succinylcholine	Enhanced drug effect

[1]Examples of genetically polymorphic phase I enzymes are listed that catalyze drug metabolism, including selected examples of drugs that have clinically relevant variations in their effect.
Reproduced with permission from Weinshilboum, 2003.

Table 6

Pharmacogenetics of Phase II Drug Metabolism[1]

Drug-metabolizing enzyme	Frequency of variant poor-metabolism phenotype	Representative drugs metabolized	Effect of polymorphism
N-Acetyltransferase 2	52% among white Americans	Isoniazid	Enhanced drug effect
	17% of Japanese	Hydralazine	Enhanced drug effect
Uridine diphosphate-glucurono- syltransferase 1A1 (TATA box polymorphism)	10.9% among whites	Procainamide	Enhanced drug effect
	4% of Chinese	Irinotecan	Enhanced drug effect
	1% of Japanese	Bilirubin	Gilbert's syndrome
Thiopurine S-methyltransferase	Approximately 1 in 300 whites	Mercaptopurine	Enhanced drug effect (toxicity)
	Approximately 1 in 2500 Asians	Azathioprine	Enhanced drug effect (toxicity)
Catechol O-methyltransferase	Approximately 25% of whites	Levodopa	Enhanced drug effect

[1]Examples of genetically polymorphic phase II (conjugating) enzymes are listed that catalyze drug metabolism, including selected examples of drugs that have clinically relevant variations in their effects.
Reproduced with permission from Weinshilboum, 2003.

2. Key Points

- Biotechnology, as defined by the United States Food and Drug Administration, is "the use of recombinant DNA (or RNA) technology; direct DNA transfer technology; nucleic acid amplification technology; hybridoma technology; cell fusion; molecular modification of cellular receptors; or the application of cells, tissues, or their components such that their potential biological activity has been modified."

- The central dogma of molecular biology is that DNA encodes RNA, which in turn encodes protein.

- Recombinant DNA (rDNA) technology makes use of several molecular biological tools that allow for the placement of a desired DNA fragment in proximity to other DNA fragments within a DNA molecule for a specific purpose.

- Cytokines are molecules secreted by cells that orchestrate the immune response. They activate immune cells such as lymphocytes, monocytes, macrophages, and neutrophils.

- An enzyme is a protein that catalyzes a specific chemical reaction.

- Hormones are chemical substances transmitted by the bloodstream to cells distant from their physiologic source that impart specific cellular effects.

- Clotting or blood factors are chemical blood constituents that interact to cause blood coagulation.

- Vaccines are preparations of antigenic material administered to stimulate the development of antibodies for the purpose of conferring active immunity against a particular pathogen or disease.

- Subsets of B lymphocyte clones produce identical antibodies that recognize the same antigen. These identical antibodies are said to be monoclonal. Fusing B lymphocytes with lymphocyte tumor cells produces a hybridoma that can be cultured in large quantities for the mass production of a given monoclonal antibody.

- Gene therapy, an application of biotechnology, has great potential therapeutic benefit.

- Biotechnology has facilitated the development of novel drug delivery strategies, including liposomal technology, immunotoxins, and pegylation.

- Pharmacogenomics is the scientific discipline of using genome-wide approaches to understand the inherited basis of differences between individual responses to drugs.

- SNPs are differences in a single nucleotide base occurring at a significant frequency (usually >5%) within the population. They may result in no change in the encoded amino acid of a codon or a change in the encoded amino acid with no change in the function of the encoded protein. However, when the amino acid substitution due to a SNP results in a phenotypic difference, it may carry clinical relevance.

3. Questions and Answers

1. The process whereby the ribosome in the cytoplasm reads mRNA codons and matches them with the appropriate tRNAs (which in turn carry amino acids responsible for protein synthesis) is referred to as

   A. Transcription
   B. Translation
   C. Transformation
   D. Transfection
   E. Transduction

2. How many nucleotide triplets (or codons) exist for the encoding of the 20 possible amino acids specified by the genetic code?

   A. 4
   B. 12
   C. 20
   D. 61
   E. 64

3. A plasmid designed to allow for the expression of an inserted gene within a host cell for the production of the specified protein is referred to as which of the following?

   A. Cloning vector
   B. Expression vector
   C. Transcription factor
   D. Translation initiation factor
   E. Transposable genetic element

4. An example of a recombinant DNA-generated cytokine used for the management of acute relapsing-remitting multiple sclerosis is which of the following?

   A. Interferon beta-1b (Betaseron)
   B. Aldesleukin (IL-2) (Proleukin)
   C. Eptifibatide (Integrelin)
   D. Bivalirudin (Angiomax)
   E. Abciximab (ReoPro)

5. Alteplase (Activase) is a recombinant DNA protein of which of the following types?

   A. Hormone
   B. Enzyme
   C. Clotting factor
   D. Chemokine
   E. Cytokine

6. Which of the following biological agents is indicated for treatment of ovulatory failure?

   A. Ganirelix (Antagon)
   B. Glucagon (Glucagen)
   C. Follitropin alpha (Gonal-F)
   D. Eptifibatide (Integrelin)
   E. Thyrotropin (Thyrogen)

7. Which of the following recombinant blood factors is available in recombinant form for clinical therapeutic use?

   A. Factor III
   B. Factor V
   C. Factor VI
   D. Factor VII
   E. Factor X

8. Recombinant DNA technology has led to the development of vaccines for which of the following diseases?

   A. Hepatitis B
   B. Hepatitis A
   C. Disease from *Haemophilus influenzae* type B
   D. Malaria
   E. AIDS

9. As dictated by the nomenclature for monoclonal antibodies, which of the following is a chimeric monoclonal antibody therapeutically used for inflammatory disease?

   A. Abciximab
   B. Infliximab
   C. Palivizumab
   D. Rituximab
   E. Trastuzumab

10. The repair or correction of a dysfunctional gene by selectively introducing recombinant DNA into cells or tissues (ultimately leading to the expression of a functional gene product) best describes which of the following?

    A. Monoclonal antibody therapy
    B. Gene therapy
    C. Antiviral therapy
    D. Cell therapy
    E. Recombinant DNA therapy

11. Fomivirsen (Vitravene) is an example of which of the following biological products?

    A. A liposomal formulation

B. An antisense oligonucleotide
C. An siRNA molecule
D. A recombinant DNA produced protein
E. A monoclonal antibody

12. The use of liposomal technology has favorably impacted the therapeutic index of which of the following drugs?

   A. Cyclosporine
   B. Itraconazole
   C. Amphotericin B
   D. Cisplatin
   E. Propofol

13. The scientific discipline of using genome-wide approaches to understand the inherited basis of differences between individuals in the response to drugs best describes which of the following?

   A. Pharmacogenomics
   B. Functional genomics
   C. Comparative genomics
   D. Pharmacodynamics
   E. Molecular genetics

14. A single nucleotide polymorphism (SNP) always results in a change in which of the following?

   A. The nucleotide sequence in the genome
   B. The nucleotide sequence of a codon
   C. The encoded amino acid of the codon
   D. The encoded amino acid of the codon with no change in function of the encoded protein
   E. The encoded amino acid of the codon with a clinically relevant change in the function of the encoded protein

15. "The use of recombinant DNA (or RNA) technology; direct DNA transfer technology; nucleic acid amplification technology; hybridoma technology; cell fusion; molecular modification of cellular receptors; or the application of cells, tissues, or their components such that their potential biological activity has been modified" best describes which of the following?

   A. Biology
   B. Biotechnology
   C. Biotherapy
   D. Bioinformatics
   E. Nanotechnology

16. A drug discovery strategy that utilizes nucleic acids and amino acids in various combinations to synthesize vast libraries of oligonucleotide or peptide compounds for high throughput lead compound screening is which of the following?

   A. Whole cell screening
   B. Natural product screening
   C. Gene therapy
   D. Combinatorial chemistry
   E. rDNA technology

17. The application of computer sciences and information technology to the management and analysis of biological information best defines which of the following?

   A. Biometrics
   B. Biotherapy
   C. Bioinformatics
   D. Biostatistics
   E. Biotechnology

18. Which of the following best outlines the central dogma of molecular biology?

   A. RNA→DNA→Protein
   B. DNA→RNA→Protein
   C. Protein→RNA→DNA
   D. DNA→Protein→RNA
   E. Protein→DNA→RNA

19. Which of the following biotechnology agents is indicated for treating anemia caused by chronic renal disease?

   A. Epoetin alpha
   B. Becaplermin
   C. Filgrastim
   D. Alemtuzumab
   E. Sargramostin

20. Which of the following products is indicated for prevention of blood clots post PTCA?

   A. Abciximab
   B. Basiliximab
   C. Infliximab
   D. Trastuzumab
   E. Becaplermin

Answers

1. **B.** Transcription is the process by which RNA polymerase copies a strand of DNA into complementary RNA. Transformation refers to the alteration of the heritable properties of a eukaryotic cell. Transfection is the introduction

of foreign DNA into a eukaryotic cell. Transduction can refer to the transfer of DNA from one bacterium to another via a bacteriophage.

2. **D.** There is degeneracy in the genetic code. Some amino acids may be encoded by as many as six codons, whereas others may be encoded by only one. Of the 64 possible codons, three are stop codons (UAA, UGA, and UAG).

3. **B.** A cloning vector is used to carry a fragment of DNA into a cell for cloning. A transcription factor is a protein that regulates transcription in eukaryotic cells. A translation initiation factor, as its name implies, is involved in the initiation of translation. A transposable genetic element, or transposon, is a portion of DNA that can move from one part of the genome to another.

4. **A.** Aldesleukin (IL-2) (Proleukin) is a recombinant cytokine indicated for the treatment of metastatic renal cell carcinoma and melanoma. Eptifibatide (Integrelin) is a recombinant enzyme indicated for treatment of acute coronary syndromes. Bivalirudin (Angiomax) is an enzyme indicated for use in coronary angioplasty and unstable angina. Abciximab (ReoPro) is a monoclonal antibody indicated for prevention of blood clots post-PTCA and unstable angina prior to PTCA.

5. **B.** Alteplase (Activase) is a recombinant DNA protein of the enzyme type.

6. **C.** Ganirelix (Antagon) is a recombinant hormone indicated for the treatment of LH surge during fertility therapy. Glucagon (Glucagen) is a recombinant hormone indicated for treatment of hypoglycemia. Eptifibatide (Integrelin) is a recombinant enzyme indicated for the treatment of acute coronary syndromes. Thyrotropin (Thyrogen) is a recombinant hormone indicated for the treatment of thyroid cancer.

7. **D.** The other factors listed are not clinically available in recombinant form.

8. **A.** While promising, this technology has not yet yielded vaccines for hepatitis A, malaria, AIDS, or diseases caused by *H influenzae* type B.

9. **B.** Nomenclature of monoclonal antibodies is highly structured. The first component of the name is product specific, the second component indicates its therapeutic use (*ci* for

cardiovascular, *li* for inflammation, *tu* for cancer), the third component indicates the type of monoclonal antibody (*mo* for murine, *xi* for chimeric, *zu* for humanized), and the fourth component (*mab*) represents "monoclonal antibody."

10. **B.** The repair or correction of a dysfunctional gene by selectively introducing recombinant DNA into cells or tissues, ultimately leading to the expression of a functional gene product is called gene therapy.

11. **B.** Fomivirsen (Vitravene) is the first product based on this technology to come to market.

12. **C.** Formulation of this antifungal agent as a liposomal preparation (Ambisome) has significantly reduced the nephrotoxicity and other adverse effects associated with this drug.

13. **A.** The scientific discipline of using genome-wide approaches to understand the inherited basis of differences between individuals in the response to drugs best describes pharmacogenomics.

14. **A.** A SNP may occur outside of an open reading frame (coding region), it may induce a mutation where no change in encoded amino acid occurs, and it may or may not cause a functional change in an encoded protein.

15. **B.** "The use of recombinant DNA (or RNA) technology; direct DNA transfer technology; nucleic acid amplification technology; hybridoma technology; cell fusion; molecular modification of cellular receptors; or the application of cells, tissues, or their components such that their potential biological activity has been modified" best describes biotechnology.

16. **D.** A drug discovery strategy that utilizes nucleic acids and amino acids in various combinations to synthesize vast libraries of oligonucleotide or peptide compounds for high throughput lead compound screening is called combinatorial chemistry.

17. **C.** The application of computer sciences and information technology to the management and analysis of biological information best defines bioinformatics.

18. **B.** DNA is transcribed into mRNA, which is translated ultimately to protein.

19. **A.** Becaplermin is indicated for the management of diabetic foot ulcers. Filgrastim is indicated for treatment of neutropenia. Alemtuzumab is indicated for treatment of chronic lymphocytic leukemia. Sargramostin is indicated for myeloid reconstitution after BMT, BMT failure, as an adjunct to chemotherapy in AML, and in peripheral blood progenitor cell transplant.

20. **A.** Basiliximab is indicated for management of acute organ transplant rejection. Infliximab is indicated for the treatment of Crohn's disease and rheumatoid arthritis. Trastuzumab is indicated for management of metastatic breast cancer. Becaplermin is indicated for the treatment of diabetic foot ulcer.

4. References

Adams VR, Karlix JL. Monoclonal antibodies. In: *Concepts in Immunology and Immunotherapeutics,* 3rd ed. Bethesda, MD: American Society of Health-System Pharmacists' Production Office; 1997:269-299.

Alberts B, Bray D, Lewis J, et al, eds. *Molecular Biology of the Cell,* 3rd ed. New York, NY: Garland Publishing; 1994.

Carrico JM. Human Genome Project and pharmacogenomics—implications for pharmacy. *J Am Pharmaceut Assoc.* 2000;40:115-116.

Evans WE, McLeod HL. Pharmacogenomics—drug disposition, drug targets, and side effects. *N Engl J Med.* 2003;348:538-549.

Glick BR, Pasternak JJ, eds. *Molecular Biotechnology: Principles & Applications of Recombinant DNA,* 2nd ed. Washington: ASM Press; 1998.

Hollinger P, Hoogenboom H. Antibodies come back from the brink. *Nature Biotech* 1998;16:1015-1016.

Regan JW. Biotechnology and drug discovery. In: Delgado JN, Remers WA, eds. *Textbook of Organic Medicinal and Pharmaceutical Chemistry,* 10th ed. Philadelphia: Lippincott-Raven; 1998:139-152.

Rogers CS, Sullenger BA, George AL Jr. Gene therapy. In: Hardman JG, Limbird LE, eds. *Goodman & Gilman's The Pharmacological Basis of Therapeutics,* 10th ed. New York: McGraw-Hill; 2001:81-112.

Sindelar RD. Pharmaceutical biotechnology. In: Williams DA, Lemke TL, eds. *Foye's Principles of Medicinal Chemistry,* 5th ed. Philadelphia: Lippincott Williams & Wilkins; 2002:982-1015.

U.S. Food and Drug Administration (FDA). Center for Biologics Evaluation and Research webpage: http://www.fda.gov/cber

U.S. Food and Drug Administration (FDA). Center for Drug Evaluation and Research webpage: http://www.fda.gov/cder/

Vaughan TJ, Osbourn JK, Tempest PR. Human antibodies by design. *Nature Biotech.* 1998;16:535-539.

Weinshilboum R. Inheritance and drug response. *N Engl J Med.* 2003;348:529-537.

8. Hypertension

L. Brian Cross, PharmD, CDE
Assistant Professor, Department of Pharmacy
University of Tennessee College of Pharmacy

Contents

1. Disease Overview

- Hypertension is defined as a systolic blood pressure >140 mm Hg, a diastolic blood pressure >90 mm Hg, or any patient requiring antihypertensive therapy.

- 50 million Americans are affected by hypertension.
  * Approximately 3 of every 4 hypertensive Americans are not well controlled (Table 1).

- Increased incidence with increasing age

- Onset most common in third to fifth decades of life

- Prevalence differs by ethnic group, socioeconomic group, and by geographical region (Table 2).

Classification

- Classification of hypertension is based on the Sixth Report of the Joint National Committee on Detection, Evaluation, and Treatment of High Blood Pressure (JNC-VI) (see Table 3).

Clinical Presentation and Complications

Cardiovascular effects
- Left ventricular hypertrophy (LVH).

- Congestive heart failure (CHF).

- Peripheral arterial disease

- Angina pectoris

- Myocardial infarction

- Sudden death

Table 2

Prevalence of Hypertension by Ethnic Group for Adults Aged 20-74

	Male	Female
Caucasians	24%	19%
African-Americans	35%	34%
Mexican-Americans	25%	22%
Asian-Americans	13%	13%

Table 1

Trends in Awareness, Treatment, and Control of High Blood Pressure in Adults Ages 18-74

	NATIONAL HEALTH AND NUTRITION EXAMINATION SURVEY, PERCENT			
	II (1976–80)	III (PHASE 1) 1988–91	III (PHASE 2) 1991–94)	1999–2000
Awareness	51	73	68	70
Treatment	31	55	54	59
Control†	10	29	27	34

High blood pressure is systolic blood pressure (SBP) ≥140 mmHg or diastolic blood pressure (DBP) ≥90 mmHg or taking antihypertensive medication.
† SBP <140 mmHg and DBP <90 mmHg.

Sources: Unpublished data for 1999–2000 computed by M. Wolz, National Heart, Lung, and Blood Institute; JNC 6.

Adapted from JNC-7 Express. Source: National Heart, Lung, and Blood Institute.

Renal effects
- Nephropathy

- Renal failure

- Requirements for dialysis

Cerebrovascular effects
- Transient ischemic attacks (TIAs)

- Stroke

Ophthalmologic effects
- Retinal hemorrhage

- Retinopathy

- Blindness

Pathophysiology and Etiology

- Blood pressure = (stroke volume x heart rate) x peripheral resistance (Figure 1)

Sympathetic nervous system activation
Central activation
1. Presynaptic α_2 stimulation is negative feedback mechanism, leading to decreased norepinephrine release.
2. Presynaptic β stimulation leads to increased norepinephrine release.

Peripheral activation
1. β_1 Stimulation leads to increased heart rate and contractility, causing increased cardiac output.

Figure 1.

Sympathetic nervous system activation.

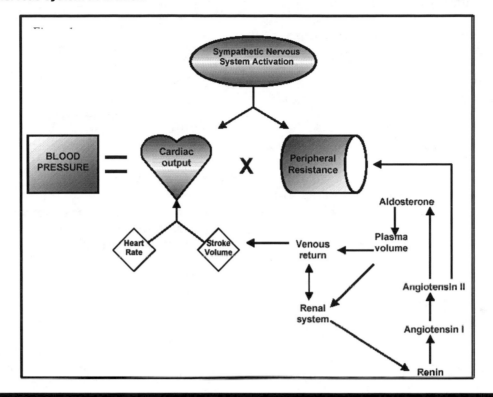

Table 3

Classification and Management of Blood Pressure for Adults

BP CLASSIFICATION	SBP* MMHG	DBP* MMHG	LIFESTYLE MODIFICATION	INITIAL DRUG THERAPY	
				WITHOUT COMPELLING INDICATION	WITH COMPELLING INDICATIONS (SEE TABLE 8)
NORMAL	<120	and <80	Encourage		
PREHYPERTENSION	120–139	or 80–89	Yes	No antihypertensive drug indicated.	Drug(s) for compelling indications.‡
STAGE 1 HYPERTENSION	140–159	or 90–99	Yes	Thiazide-type diuretics for most. May consider ACEI, ARB, BB, CCB, or combination.	Drug(s) for the compelling indications.‡ Other antihypertensive drugs (diuretics, ACEI, ARB, BB, CCB) as needed.
STAGE 2 HYPERTENSION	≥160	or ≥100	Yes	Two-drug combination for most† (usually thiazide-type diuretic and ACEI or ARB or BB or CCB).	

DBP, diastolic blood pressure; SBP, systolic blood pressure.

Drug abbreviations: ACEI, angiotensin converting enzyme inhibitor; ARB, angiotensin receptor blocker; BB, beta-blocker; CCB, calcium channel blocker.

* Treatment determined by highest BP category.

† Initial combined therapy should be used cautiously in those at risk for orthostatic hypotension.

‡ Treat patients with chronic kidney disease or diabetes to BP goal of <130/80 mmHg.

Adapted from JNC-7 Express. Source: National Heart, Lung, and Blood Institute.

2. β_2 Stimulation leads to arterial vasodilatation.
  * β Stimulation also causes increased renin release, causing increased angiotensin II production.
3. α_1 Stimulation leads to arterial and venous vasoconstriction.

Renin-angiotensin-aldosterone system
- Decreased renal perfusion pressure causes increases in renin levels.

- Renin reacts with angiotensinogen to produce angiotensin I (AT-I).

- Angiotensin converting enzyme (ACE) causes AT-I to become AT-II.

- Angiotensin II (AT-II) is a potent vasoconstrictor and stimulates aldosterone release, which increases sodium and fluid retention.

Water and sodium retention
- Acutely: increased fluid volume causes increased cardiac output, which causes increased BP.

- Chronically: excess intracellular sodium causes vascular hypertrophy, which increases vascular resistance and response to vasoconstriction, which increases BP.

Etiology
Primary (essential) hypertension
- Unknown cause

- 85-95% of all hypertension cases

Secondary hypertension
- *Renovascular disease* (suggested by increased blood urea nitrogen [BUN] and creatinine, and abdominal bruits)

- *Primary aldosteronism* (suggested by unprovoked hypokalemia)

- *Cushing's syndrome* (suggested by unprovoked hypokalemia and truncal obesity with purple striae)

- *Pheochromocytoma* (suggested by increased urinary catecholamine excretion (ie, vanillylmandelic acid and metanephrine, accompanied by headache, palpitations, and perspiration)

- *Aortic coarctation* (suggested by delayed or absent femoral pulses and decreased blood pressure in the lower extremities)

- *Drug-induced*
  * Steroids and estrogens (including oral contraceptives)
  * Alcohol
  * Cocaine
  * Cyclosporine and tacrolimus
  * Sympathomimetics
  * Erythropoietin
  * Licorice (in chewing tobacco)
  * Monoamine oxidase (MAO) inhibitors
  * Tricyclic antidepressants
  * NSAIDs

Diagnostic Criteria

- Diagnosis and treatment begin with proper blood pressure measurements (Table 4):
  1. Patient should avoid smoking or caffeine for 30 minutes prior to BP measurement.
  2. Patient should be resting for 5 minutes before measuring BP.
  3. Position arm (brachial artery) at heart level.
  4. Uncover arm; do not put cuff over clothes.
  5. Determine proper size cuff:

Table 4

Recommendations for Follow-Up Based on Initial Blood Pressure Measurements for Adults

Initial blood pressure (mm Hg)[1]		Recommended follow-up[2]
Systolic	Diastolic	
<130	<85	Recheck in 2 years
130-139	85-89	Recheck in 1 year[3]
140-159	90-99	Confirm within 2 months[3]
160-179	100-109	Evaluate or refer to source of care within 1 month
≥180	≥110	Evaluate or refer to source of care immediately or within 1 week depending on clinical situation

[1]If systolic and diastolic readings are different, follow recommendations for shorter time follow-up (eg, 160/86 mm Hg should be evaluated or referred to source of care within 1 month).
[2]Modify the scheduling of follow-up according to reliable information about past blood pressure measurements, other cardiovascular risk factors, or target organ disease.
[3]Provide advice about lifestyle modifications.
Adapted from JNC-7 Express. Source: National Heart, Lung, and Blood Institute.

Upper arm circumference	*Cuff size required*
16-22.5 cm	pediatric cuff
22.6-30 cm	regular adult cuff
30.1-37.5 cm	large adult cuff
37.6-43.7 cm	thigh cuff

6. Position cuff 1 inch above antecubital crease.
7. Ask patient about previous readings.
8. Place stethoscope over brachial artery (medial to the center).
9. Inflate cuff rapidly to approximately 30 mm Hg above previous readings.
10. Deflate cuff slowly.
11. Remember to deflate cuff completely when done.
12. Wait 1-2 minutes before repeating.
13. Take pressure in both arms.
14. If suspect orthostatic hypotension, take BP sitting, standing, and supine.
15. Two readings separated by at least 2 minutes should be averaged.
16. If readings differ by >5 mm Hg, additional readings should be taken.

• Patient's overall risk for cardiovascular disease is assessed and treatment goals are based on these measurements (Table 5 and Figure 2).

Risk group A
• BP >130/85 mm Hg

• No clinical CV disease or target organ damage

• No risk factors

Risk group B
• BP >130/85 mm Hg

• No clinical CV disease or target organ damage

• One or more risk factors (excluding diabetes)

Risk group C
• BP >130/85 mm Hg

• Clinical CV disease or target organ damage (including diabetes)

• With or without other risk factors

Treatment Principles and Goals

Goals of therapy (Figure 3A and B)
• Reduce end-organ damage

Figure 2.

Cardiovascular risk factors

MAJOR RISK FACTORS

Hypertension*
Cigarette smoking
Obesity* (body mass index ≥30 kg/m²)
Physical inactivity
Dyslipidemia*
Diabetes mellitus*
Microalbuminuria or estimated GFR <60 mL/min
Age (older than 55 for men, 65 for women)
Family history of premature cardiovascular disease
  (men under age 55 or women under age 65)

TARGET ORGAN DAMAGE

Heart
• Left ventricular hypertrophy
• Angina or prior myocardial infarction
• Prior coronary revascularization
• Heart failure
Brain
• Stroke or transient ischemic attack
Chronic kidney disease
Peripheral arterial disease
Retinopathy

GFR, glomerular filtration rate.
* Components of the metabolic syndrome.

Adapted from JNC-7 Express. Source: National Heart, Lung, and Blood Institute.

• Minimize or control other risk factors for cardiovascular disease

• Maintain blood pressure, with minimal side effects, at or below that for the patient's risk:
  * 140/90 with uncomplicated hypertension
  * 140/90 with target organ damage or CV disease
  * <130/85 with diabetes
  * <125/75 with proteinuria >1 g/24 h

Monitoring and Evaluation

Goals of initial evaluation of patients with hypertension
• Identify known causes of high blood pressure.

Table 5

Risk Stratification and Treatment of Hypertension[1]

Blood pressure stages (mm Hg)	Risk group A (no risk factors; no TOD/CCD)	Risk group B (at least one risk factor, not including diabetes; no TOD/CCD)	Risk group C (TOD/CCD and/or diabetes, with or without other risk factors)
High-normal (130-139/85-89)	Lifestyle modification	Lifestyle modification	Drug therapy[3]
Stage 1 (140-159/90-99)	Lifestyle modification (up to 12 months)	Lifestyle modification[2] (up to 6 months)	Drug therapy
Stages 2 and 3 (≥160/≥100)	Drug therapy	Drug therapy	Drug therapy

For example, a patient with diabetes and a blood pressure of 142/94 mm Hg plus left ventricular hypertrophy should be classified as having stage 1 hypertension with target organ disease (left ventricular hypertrophy) and with another major risk factor (diabetes). This patient would be categorized as stage 1, risk group C, and recommended for immediate initiation of pharmacologic treatment.

TOD/CCD, target organ disease/clinical cardiovascular disease.
[1]Lifestyle modification should be adjunctive therapy for all patients recommended for pharmacologic therapy.
[2]For patients with multiple risk factors, clinicians should consider drugs as initial therapy plus lifestyle modifications.
[3]For those with heart failure, renal insufficiency, or diabetes.

- Assess presence or absence of target organ damage and CV disease, extent of the disease, and the response to therapies.

- Identify other CV risk factors or concomitant disorders that may define prognosis and guide therapy.

Initial evaluation
History
- Duration and levels of elevated blood pressure

- History or symptoms of CHD, heart failure, cerebrovascular disease, pulmonary vascular disease, diabetes mellitus, renal disease, dyslipidemia

- Family history of hypertension, premature CHD, stroke, diabetes, dyslipidemias, or renal disease

- Symptoms suggesting cause of hypertension

- Recent weight changes, physical activity levels, smoking or other tobacco use

- Dietary assessment: intake of sodium, alcohol, saturated fat, and caffeine

- Complete medication history including prescription, over-the-counter, and herbal/natural products that may increase blood pressure or decrease effectiveness of antihypertensive agents

- Results and adverse effects of previous antihypertensive therapy

- Psychosocial/environmental factors that may influence hypertension control

Examination
- Two or more blood pressure measurements separated by at least 2 minutes

- Measurement of height, weight, and waist circumference

- Funduscopic exam for hypertensive retinopathy

- Exam of neck for carotid bruits, distended veins, or an enlarged thyroid gland

- Exam of heart for abnormalities in rate and rhythm, increased size, precordial heave, clicks, murmurs, and third and fourth heart sounds

- Exam of lungs for rales and evidence of bronchospasm

- Exam of abdomen for bruits, enlarged kidneys, masses, and abnormal aortic pulsation

- Exam of extremities for decreased or absent peripheral arterial pulsations, bruits, and edema

Figure 3A.

Algorithm for the treatment of hypertension.

LIFESTYLE MODIFICATIONS

Not at Goal Blood Pressure (<140/90 mmHg)
(<130/80 mmHg for patients with diabetes or chronic kidney disease)

INITIAL DRUG CHOICES

Without Compelling Indications

With Compelling Indications

Stage 1 Hypertension
(SBP 140–159 or DBP 90–99 mmHg)

Thiazide-type diuretics for most. May consider ACEI, ARB, BB, CCB, or combination.

Stage 2 Hypertension
(SBP ≥160 or DBP ≥100 mmHg)

Two-drug combination for most (usually thiazide-type diuretic and ACEI, or ARB, or BB, or CCB).

Drug(s) for the compelling indications (see below)

Other antihypertensive drugs (diuretics, ACEI, ARB, BB, CCB) as needed.

NOT AT GOAL BLOOD PRESSURE

Optimize dosages or add additional drugs until goal blood pressure is achieved. Consider consultation with hypertension specialist.

DBP, diastolic blood pressure; SBP, systolic blood pressure.
Drug abbreviations: ACEI, angiotensin converting enzyme inhibitor; ARB, angiotensin receptor blocker; BB, beta-blocker; CCB, calcium channel blocker.

Figure 3B.

Clinical trial and guideline basis for compelling indications for individual drug classes.

COMPELLING INDICATION*	RECOMMENDED DRUGS†						CLINICAL TRIAL BASIS‡
	DIURETIC	BB	ACEI	ARB	CCB	Aldo ANT	
Heart failure	•	•	•	•		•	ACC/AHA Heart Failure Guideline, MERIT-HF, COPERNICUS, CIBIS, SOLVD, AIRE, TRACE, ValHEFT, RALES
Postmyocardial infarction		•	•			•	ACC/AHA Post-MI Guideline, BHAT, SAVE, Capricorn, EPHESUS
High coronary disease risk	•	•	•		•		ALLHAT, HOPE, ANBP2, LIFE, CONVINCE
Diabetes	•	•	•	•	•		NKF-ADA Guideline, UKPDS, ALLHAT
Chronic kidney disease			•	•			NKF Guideline, Captopril Trial, RENAAL, IDNT, REIN, AASK
Recurrent stroke prevention	•		•				PROGRESS

* Compelling indications for antihypertensive drugs are based on benefits from outcome studies or existing clinical guidelines; the compelling indication is managed in parallel with the BP.

† Drug abbreviations: ACEI, angiotensin converting enzyme inhibitor; ARB, angiotensin receptor blocker; Aldo ANT, aldosterone antagonist; BB, beta-blocker; CCB, calcium channel blocker.

‡ Conditions for which clinical trials demonstrate benefit of specific classes of antihypertensive drugs.

Figure 3A and B adapted from JNC-7 Express. Source: National Heart, Lung, and Blood Institute.

- Neurologic assessment

Laboratory
Routine tests
- Urinalysis

- Complete blood count

- Blood chemistries (sodium, potassium, creatinine, BUN, glucose)

- Fasting lipid profile (total cholesterol, triglycerides, HDL, LDL)

- ECG

Optional tests
- Creatinine clearance

- Microalbuminuria

- 24-Hour urinary protein

- Blood calcium

- Uric acid

- Glycosylated hemoglobin

- Thyroid-stimulating hormone

- Limited echocardiography

- Ankle-brachial index (ABI)

- Plasma renin activity/urinary sodium determination

Follow-up evaluation
- Follow-up evaluation includes any of the previous exams completed during the initial evaluation as required to monitor both response to and possible adverse effects from prescribed antihypertensive therapies, in addition to assessment of any new symptoms of target organ damage and the assessment of patient adherence to therapy (Figure 4).

Figure 4.

General guidelines to improve patient adherence to antihypertensive therapy.

- Be aware of signs of patient nonadherence to antihypertensive therapy.
- Establish the goal of therapy: to reduce blood pressure to nonhypertensive levels with minimal or no adverse effects.
- Educate patients about the disease, and involve them and their families in its treatment. Have them measure blood pressure at home.
- Maintain contact with patients; consider telecommunication.
- Keep care inexpensive and simple.
- Encourage lifestyle modifications.
- Integrate pill-taking into routine activities of daily living.
- Prescribe medications according to pharmacologic principles, favoring long-acting formulations.
- Be willing to stop unsuccessful therapy and try a different approach.
- Anticipate adverse effects, and adjust therapy to prevent, minimize, or ameliorate side effects.
- Continue to add effective and tolerated drugs, stepwise, in sufficient doses to achieve the goal of therapy.
- Encourage a positive attitude about achieving therapeutic goals.
- Consider using nurse case management.

Adapted from JNC-7 Express. Source: National Heart, Lung, and Blood Institute.

2. Nondrug Therapy

- Lifestyle modifications are recommended both to improve blood pressure and overall cardiovascular health (Figure 5).

- Research has shown that diets rich in fruits, vegetables, and low-fat dairy foods, and with reduced saturated and total fats, significantly lowers blood pressure (Figures 6 and 7).

3. Drug Therapy

- All patient factors (severity of blood pressure elevation, presence of target organ damage, presence of CV disease or other risk factors) must be considered when initiating therapy.

Initial Therapy

- Candidates for therapy (Table 5)

- Use of lifestyle modifications should continue to be stressed to patients after the decision to initiate drug therapy has been made (Figure 5) to further decrease the risk of complications from cardiovascular disease.

Figure 5.

Lifestyle modifications to manage hypertension.

MODIFICATION	RECOMMENDATION	APPROXIMATE SBP REDUCTION (RANGE)
Weight reduction	Maintain normal body weight (body mass index 18.5–24.9 kg/m²).	5–20 mmHg/10 kg weight loss
Adopt DASH eating plan	Consume a diet rich in fruits, vegetables, and lowfat dairy products with a reduced content of saturated and total fat.	8–14 mmHg
Dietary sodium reduction	Reduce dietary sodium intake to no more than 100 mmol per day (2.4 g sodium or 6 g sodium chloride).	2–8 mmHg
Physical activity	Engage in regular aerobic physical activity such as brisk walking (at least 30 min per day, most days of the week).	4–9 mmHg
Moderation of alcohol consumption	Limit consumption to no more than 2 drinks (1 oz or 30 mL ethanol; e.g., 24 oz beer, 10 oz wine, or 3 oz 80-proof whiskey) per day in most men and to no more than 1 drink per day in women and lighter weight persons.	2–4 mmHg[30]

DASH, Dietary Approaches to Stop Hypertension.
   For overall cardiovascular risk reduction, stop smoking.
   The effects of implementing these modifications are dose and time dependent, and could be greater for some individuals.

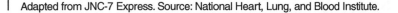

Adapted from JNC-7 Express. Source: National Heart, Lung, and Blood Institute.

- β-Blockers and diuretics are considered the initial agents for treatment of hypertension by JNC-VI unless compelling indications for the use of other medication classes exist or the patient has comorbid conditions that would suggest the use of classes other than β-blockers and diuretics (Figure 3 and Table 6).

- Recent data suggest that angiotensin-converting enzyme inhibitors (ACEIs), calcium channel blockers (CCBs), and possibly angiotensin II receptor blockers (ARBs) might also be considered as initial agents for treatment of hypertension.

- If patient requires a second agent for treatment of hypertension, it is strongly recommended to be a diuretic if one is not chosen as the initial agent.

- All causes for inadequate response should be addressed before additional agents are added to a patient's antihypertensive regimen (Figure 8).

- Vasodilators, α_1-receptor antagonists, α_2-receptor agonists, and postganglionic adrenergic neuron blockers should be avoided as initial agents for hypertension.

Diuretics

Thiazide and thiazide-like diuretics (Table 7)
Mechanism of action
- Direct arteriole dilation

- Reduction of total fluid volume through the inhibition of sodium reabsorption in the distal tubules, which causes increased excretion of sodium, water, potassium, and hydrogen.

Figure 6.

Dietary suggestions for hypertensive patients.

Food group	Daily servings	Serving sizes	Examples and notes	Significance of each food group to the DASH diet pattern
Grains and grain products	7-8	1 slice bread; $1/2$ c dry cereal; $1/2$ c cooked rice, pasta, or cereal	Whole wheat bread, english muffins, pita bread, bagel, cereals, grits, oatmeal	Major sources of energy and fiber
Vegetables	4-5	1 c raw leafy vegetable; $1/2$ c cooked vegetable; 6 oz. vegetable juice	Tomatoes, potatoes, carrots, peas, squash, broccoli, turnip greens, collards, kale, spinach, artichokes, beans, sweet potatoes	Rich sources of potassium, magnesium. and fiber
Fruits	4-5	6 oz. fruit juice; 1 medium fruit; $1/4$ c dried fruit; $1/4$ c fresh, frozen or canned fruit	Apricots, bananas, dates, grapes, oranges, orange juice, grapefruit, grapefruit juice, mangoes, melons, peaches, pineapple, prunes, raisins. Strawberries, tangerines	Important sources of potassium, magnesium, and fiber
Low-fat or nonfat dairy foods	2-3	8 oz. milk; 1 c yogurt; 1.5 oz. cheese	Skim or 1% milk, skim or low-fat buttermilk, nonfat or low-fat yogurt, part-skim mozzarella cheese, nonfat cheese	Major sources of calcium and protein
Meats, poultry, and fish	2 or less	3 oz. cooked meats, poultry, or fish	Select only lean; trim away visible fats; broil, roast, or boil, instead of frying; remove skin from poultry	Rich sources of protein and magnesium
Nuts, seeds, and legumes	4-5 per week	1.5 oz. or $1/3$ c nuts; $1/2$ oz. or 2 T. seeds; $1/2$ c cooked legumes	Almonds, filberts, mixed nuts, peanuts, walnuts, sunflower seeds, kidney beans, lentils	Rich sources of energy, magnesium, potassium, protein, and fiber

Adapted from JNC-7 Express. Source: National Heart, Lung, and Blood Institute.

Figure 7.

The DASH diet sample menu based on 2000 calories/day.

Food	Amount	Servings provided
Breakfast		
Orange juice	6 oz	1 fruit
1% Lowfat milk	8 oz (1 c)	1 dairy
Cornflakes (with 1 t sugar)	1 c	2 grains
Banana	1 medium	1 fruit
Whole wheat bread (with 1 T jelly)	1 slice	1 grain
Soft margarine	1 t	1 fat
Lunch		
Chicken salad	$^3/_4$ c	1 poultry
Pita bread	$^1/_2$ large	1 grain
Raw vegetable medley:		
Carrot and celery sticks	3-4 sticks each	
Radishes	2	1 vegetable
Loose-leaf lettuce	2 leaves	
Part-skim mozzarella cheese	1.5 slice (1.5 oz)	1 dairy
1% lowfat milk	8 oz (1 c)	1 dairy
Fruit cocktail in light syrup	$^1/_2$ c	1 fruit
Dinner		
Herbed baked cod	3 oz	1 fish
Scallion rice	1 c	2 grains
Steamed broccoli	$^1/_2$ c	1 vegetable
Stewed tomatoes	$^1/_2$ c	1 vegetable
Spinach salad:		
Raw spinach	$^1/_2$ c	
Cherry tomatoes	2	1 vegetable
Cucumber	2 slices	
Light Italian salad dressing	1 T	$^1/_2$ fat
Whole wheat dinner roll	1 small	1 grain
Soft margarine	1 t.	1 fat
Melon balls	$^1/_2$ c	1 fruit
Snacks		
Dried apricots	1 oz ($^1/_4$ c)	1 fruit
Minipretzels	1 oz ($^3/_4$ c)	1 grain
Mixed nuts	1.5 oz ($^1/_3$ c)	1 nuts
Diet ginger ale	12 oz.	0

Total number of servings in 2000-calorie-per-day menu

Food group	Servings
Grains	= 8
Vegetables	= 4
Fruits	= 5
Dairy foods	= 3
Meats, poultry, and fish	= 2
Nuts seeds, and legumes	= 1
Fats and oils	= 2.5

Tips on eating the DASH way

- Start small. Make gradual changes in your eating habits
- Center your meal around carbohydrates, such as pasta, rice, beans, or vegetables.
- Treat meat as one part of the whole meal, instead of the focus.
- Use fruits or low-fat, low calorie foods such as sugar-free gelatin for desserts and snacks.

REMEMBER! If you use the DASH diet to help prevent or control high blood pressure, make it part of a lifestyle that includes choosing foods lower in salt and sodium, keeping a healthy weight, being physically active, and, if you drink alcohol, doing so in moderation.

Adapted from JNC-7 Express. Source: National Heart, Lung, and Blood Institute.

Table 6

Considerations for Individualizing Antihypertensive Drug Therapy[1]

Indication	Drug therapy
Compelling indications unless contraindicated	
Diabetes mellitus (type 1) with proteinuria	ACE I
Heart failure	ACE I, diuretics
Isolated systolic hypertension (older patients)	Diuretics (preferred), calcium antagonists (long-acting DHP)
Myocardial infarction	β-Blockers (non ISA), ACE I (with systolic dysfunction)
May have favorable effects on comorbid conditions[2]	
Angina	β-Blockers, calcium antagonists
Atrial tachycardia and fibrillation	β-Blockers, calcium antagonists (non-DHP)
Cyclosporine-induced hypertension (caution with the dose of cyclosporine)	Calcium antagonists
Diabetes mellitus (types 1 and 2) with proteinuria	ACE I (preferred), calcium antagonists
Diabetes mellitus (type 2)	Low-dose diuretics
Dyslipidemia	α-Blockers
Essential tremor	β-Blockers (non-CS)
Heart failure	Carvedilol, losartan potassium
Hyperthyroidism	β-Blockers
Migraine	β-Blockers (non-CS), calcium antagonists (non-DHP)
Myocardial infarction	Diltiazem hydrochloride, verapamil hydrochloride
Osteoporosis	Thiazides
Preoperative hypertension	β-Blockers
Prostatism (benign prostatic hyperplasia)	α-Blockers
Renal insufficiency (caution in renovascular hypertension and creatinine ≥265.2 umoi/L [3 mg/dL])	ACEI
May have unfavorable effects on comorbid conditions[2,3]	
Bronchospastic disease	β-Blockers[4]
Depression	β-Blockers, central alpha-agonist, reserpine[4]
Diabetes mellitus (types 1 and 2)	β-Blockers, high-dose diuretics
Dyslipidemia	β-Blockers (non-ISA), diuretics (high-dose)
Gout	Diuretics
Second- or third-degree heart block	β-Blockers,[4] calcium antagonists (non-DHP)[4]
Heart failure	β-Blockers (except carvedilol), calcium antagonists (except amlodipine besylate, felodipine)
Liver disease	Labetalol hydrochloride, methyldopa[4]
Peripheral vascular disease	β-Blockers
Pregnancy	ACE I,[4] angiotensin II receptor blockers[4]
Renal insufficiency	Potassium-sparing agents
Renovascular disease	ACE I, angiotensin II receptor blockers

ACEI, angiotensin-converting enzyme inhibitors; DHP, dihydropyridine; ISA, intrinsic sympathomimetic activity; non-CS, noncardioselective.

[1] For initial drug therapy recommendations, see Figure 8.

[2] Conditions and drugs are listed in alphabetical order.

[3] These drugs may be used with special monitoring unless contraindicated.

[4] Contraindicated.

Adapted from JNC-7 Express. Source: National Heart, Lung, and Blood Institute.

Figure 8.

Causes of inadequate responsiveness to therapy.

Pseudoresistance
  "White-coat hypertension" or office elevations
  Pseudohypertension in older patients
  Use of regular cuff on very obese arm

Nonadherence to therapy

Volume overload
  Excess salt intake
  Progressive renal damage (nephrosclerosis)
  Fluid retention from reduction of blood pressure
  Inadequate diuretic therapy

Drug-related causes
  Doses too low
  Wrong type of diuretic
  Inappropriate combinations
  Rapid inactivation (eg, hydralazine)
  Drug actions and interactions
    Sympathomimetics
    Nasal decongestants
    Appetite suppressants
    Cocaine and other illicit drugs
    Caffeine
    Oral contraceptives
    Adrenal steroids
    Licorice (as may be found in chewing tobacco)
    Cyclosporine, tacrolimus
    Erythropoietin
    Antidepressants
    Nonsteroidal anti-inflammatory drugs

Associated conditions
  Smoking
  Increasing obesity
  Sleep apnea
  Insulin resistance/hyperinsulinemia
  Ethanol intake of more than 1 oz (30 mL) per day
  Anxiety-induced hyperventilation or panic attacks
  Chronic pain
  Intense vasoconstriction (arteritis)
  Organic brain syndrome (eg, memory deficit)

Identifiable causes of hypertension

Adapted from JNC-7 Express. Source: National Heart, Lung, and Blood Institute.

- Increase the effectiveness of other antihypertensive agents by preventing re-expansion of plasma volume
- Significant decrease in efficacy in renal failure (serum creatinine >2 mg/dL or GFR <30 mL/min)

Adverse drug events (Table 7)

Patient instructions and counseling
- Can be taken with food or milk

- Take early in the day to avoid nocturia.

- Patients may become more sensitive to sunlight; consider using sunscreen with SPF >15.

- May increase blood glucose in diabetics

- Report problems with muscle cramps which may indicate decreased potassium level.

Drug-drug and drug-disease interactions
- Steroids: cause salt retention and antagonize thiazide action

- NSAIDs: blunt thiazide response

- Antiarrhythmics (that prolong QT interval) → class IA or III → torsades de pointes may be precipitated with diuretic-induced hypokalemia.

- Probenecid and lithium: block thiazide effects by interfering with thiazide excretion into the urine

- Lithium: thiazides decrease lithium renal clearance and increase risk of lithium toxicity

Parameters to monitor
- Blood pressure

- Weight

- Serum electrolytes and uric acid

- BUN and creatinine

- Cholesterol levels

Loop diuretics (Table 7)
Mechanism of action
- Reduction of total fluid volume through the inhibition of sodium and chloride reabsorption in the ascending loop of Henle, which causes increased excretion of water, sodium, chloride, magnesium, and calcium

Table 7

Thiazide Diuretics, Thiazide-Like Diuretics, Loop Diuretics, Potassium-Sparing Agents, and Aldosterone-Receptor Blocker

Drug	Trade name	Usual dose range, total mg/d (frequency per day)	Adverse events and comments[1]
Thiazide diuretics			
Bendroflumethiazide	Naturetin®	2.5-5 (1)	**Short-term:** increased cholesterol and glucose
Benzthiazide	Aquatag®, Exna®	12.5-50 (1)	**Biochemical:** decreased potassium, sodium, and
Chlorothiazide	Diuril®	125-500 (1)	magnesium; increased uric acid and calcium
Chlorthalidone	Hygroton®, Hylidone®	12.5-25 (1)	**Rare:** blood dyscrasias, photosensitivity, pancreatitis,
Hydrochlorothiazide	HydroDIURIL®, Microzide®	12.5-50 (1)	hyponatremia, sulfonamide-type immune reactions
Hydroflumethiazide	Saluron®, Diucardin®	25-50 (1)	**Other:** impotence, fatigue, headache, rash, vertigo
Methyclothiazide		2.5-5 (1)	
Polythiazide	Renese®	2-4 (1)	
Trichlormethiazide	Metahydrin®, Naqua®	2-4 (1)	
Thiazide-like diuretics			
Metolazone	Mykrox®	2.5-10 (1)	(Less or no hypercholesterolemia compared to other
Metolazone	Zaroxolyn®	2.5-5 (1)	thiazides; decreased microalbuminuria in diabetes)
Indapamide	Lozol®	2.5-5 (1)	
Loop diuretics			
Bumetanide	Bumex®	0.5-2 (2)	Ototoxicity at high doses
Furosemide	Lasix®	20-80 (2)	(Short duration, no hypercalcemia)
Torsemide	Demadex®	2.5-10 (1)	(Short duration, no hypercalcemia)
Potassium-sparing agents[2]			
Amiloride	Midamor®	5-10 (1-2)	Hyperkalemia
Triamterene	Dyrenium®	50-100 (1-2)	(Avoid with history of kidney stones or hepatic disease)
Aldosterone-receptor blocker			
Spironolactone	Aldactone®	25-50 (1-2)	

[1]Side effects listed are for the class of drugs except where noted for individual drugs (in parentheses).
[2]See Table 8 for combination products.
Adapted from JNC-7 Express. Source: National Heart, Lung, and Blood Institute.

- Are more effective than thiazides in patients with renal failure (serum creatinine >2 mg/dL or GFR <30 mL/min)

Adverse drug events (Table 7)

Patient instructions and counseling
- Can be taken with food or milk

- Take early in day to avoid nocturia

- May become more sensitive to sunlight; consider using sunscreen with SPF >15.

- May increase blood glucose in diabetics

- Report problems with muscle cramps which may indicate decreased potassium level.

- Rise slowly from a lying or sitting position.

Table 8

Combination Drugs for Hypertension

COMBINATION TYPE*	FIXED-DOSE COMBINATION, mg†	TRADE NAME
ACEIs and CCBs	Amlodipine/benazepril hydrochloride (2.5/10, 5/10, 5/20, 10/20)	Lotrel
	Enalapril maleate/felodipine (5/5)	Lexxel
	Trandolapril/verapamil (2/180, 1/240, 2/240, 4/240)	Tarka
ACEIs and diuretics	Benazepril/hydrochlorothiazide (5/6.25, 10/12.5, 20/12.5, 20/25)	Lotensin HCT
	Captopril/hydrochlorothiazide (25/15, 25/25, 50/15, 50/25)	Capozide
	Enalapril maleate/hydrochlorothiazide (5/12.5, 10/25)	Vaseretic
	Lisinopril/hydrochlorothiazide (10/12.5, 20/12.5, 20/25)	Prinzide
	Moexipril HCl/hydrochlorothiazide (7.5/12.5, 15/25)	Uniretic
	Quinapril HCl/hydrochlorothiazide (10/12.5, 20/12.5, 20/25)	Accuretic
ARBs and diuretics	Candesartan cilexetil/hydrochlorothiazide (16/12.5, 32/12.5)	Atacand HCT
	Eprosartan mesylate/hydrochlorothiazide (600/12.5, 600/25)	Teveten/HCT
	Irbesartan/hydrochlorothiazide (150/12.5, 300/12.5)	Avalide
	Losartan potassium/hydrochlorothiazide (50/12.5, 100/25)	Hyzaar
	Telmisartan/hydrochlorothiazide (40/12.5, 80/12.5)	Micardis/HCT
	Valsartan/hydrochlorothiazide (80/12.5, 160/12.5)	Diovan/HCT
BBs and diuretics	Atenolol/chlorthalidone (50/25, 100/25)	Tenoretic
	Bisoprolol fumarate/hydrochlorothiazide (2.5/6.25, 5/6.25, 10/6.25)	Ziac
	Propranolol LA/hydrochlorothiazide (40/25, 80/25)	Inderide
	Metoprolol tartrate/hydrochlorothiazide (50/25, 100/25)	Lopressor HCT
	Nadolol/bendrofluthiazide (40/5, 80/5)	Corzide
	Timolol maleate/hydrochlorothiazide (10/25)	Timolide
Centrally acting drug and diuretic	Methyldopa/hydrochlorothiazide (250/15, 250/25, 500/30, 500/50)	Aldoril
	Reserpine/chlorothiazide (0.125/250, 0.25/500)	Diupres
	Reserpine/hydrochlorothiazide (0.125/25, 0.125/50)	Hydropres
Diuretic and diuretic	Amiloride HCl/hydrochlorothiazide (5/50)	Moduretic
	Spironolactone/hydrochlorothiazide (25/25, 50/50)	Aldactone
	Triamterene/hydrochlorothiazide (37.5/25, 50/25, 75/50)	Dyazide, Maxzide

* Drug abbreviations: ACEI, angiotensin converting enzyme inhibitor; ARB, angiotensin receptor blocker; BB, beta-blocker; CCB, calcium channel blocker.

† Some drug combinations are available in multiple fixed doses. Each drug dose is reported in milligrams.

Adapted from JNC-7 Express. Source: National Heart, Lung, and Blood Institute.

Drug-drug and drug-disease interactions

- Aminoglycosides: combined with loop diuretics can precipitate ototoxicity

- NSAIDs: blunt diuretic response

- Antiarrhythmics (that prolong QT interval) → class IA or III → may precipitate torsades de pointes with diuretic-induced hypokalemia.

- Probenecid: blocks loop diuretic effects by interfering with excretion into the urine

Parameters to monitor
• Weight

• Serum electrolytes

• BUN and creatinine

• Uric acid

• Hearing (in high doses)

Potassium-sparing diuretics (Table 7)
Mechanism of action
• Interferes with potassium/sodium exchange in the distal tubule; decreases calcium excretion, increases magnesium loss

Adverse drug events (Table 7)

Patient instructions and counseling
• Take early in day to avoid nocturia.

• Take after meals.

• Avoid excessive ingestion of foods high in potassium and use of salt substitutes.

• May increase blood glucose in diabetics

• Report problems with muscle cramps which may indicate decreased potassium levels.

• Sexual dysfunction

Drug-drug and drug-disease interactions
• ACE inhibitors: may increase risk of hyperkalemia

• Indomethacin: combination with triamterene can cause decrease in renal function

• Cimetidine: increase bioavailability and decrease clearance of triamterene

Parameters to monitor
• Weight

• Serum electrolytes (especially potassium)

• BUN and creatinine

Adrenergic Inhibitors

Postganglionic adrenergic neuron blockers (Table 9)
• *This medication class is best avoided unless necessary to treat refractory hypertension unresponsive to all other agents, as they are poorly tolerated.*

Mechanism of action
• Causes presynaptic inhibition of the release of neurotransmitter from peripheral neurons by agonistic activity on the α_2 receptor

Adverse drug events (Table 9)

Patient instructions and counseling
• Report symptoms of dizziness or hypotension.

• Don't take OTC cold productions without first asking doctor or pharmacist

• Rise slowly from a lying or sitting position.

• Report new fluid retention.

Table 9

Postganglionic Adrenergic Neuron Blockers

Drug	Trade name	Usual dose range, total mg/d (frequency per day)	Adverse events and comments
Guanadrel	Hylorel®	10-75 (2)	Postural hypotension, diarrhea
Guanethidine monosulfate	Ismelin®	10-150 (1)	Postural hypotension, diarrhea
Reserpine[1]	Serpasil®	0.05-0.25 (1)	Nasal congestion, sedation, depression, activation of peptic ulcer, dizziness, lethargy, memory impairment, sleep disturbances, weight gain

[1]Also acts centrally.
Adapted from JNC-7 Express. Source: National Heart, Lung, and Blood Institute.

- Sexual dysfunction

Drug-drug and drug-disease interactions
- OTC sympathomimetics: may potentiate an acute hypertensive effect

- Tricyclic antidepressants/chlorpromazine: antagonize therapeutic effects of guanethidine

- Pheochromocytoma is a contraindication to this class of medications.

- Should be avoided in patients with CHF, angina, and cerebrovascular disease

Parameters to monitor
- History of depression (reserpine)

- Sleep disturbances, drowsiness, lethargy (reserpine)

- Symptoms of peptic ulcer (reserpine)

Centrally active α-agonists (Table 10)
Mechanism of action
- Causes decreased sympathetic outflow to the cardio-vascular system by agonistic activity on central a_2 receptors

Patient instructions and counseling
- Report symptoms of dizziness or hypotension

- Sedation precautions

- Fever and flu-like symptoms may represent hepatic dysfunction (methyldopa)

- Report new fluid retention

- Sexual dysfunction

Drug-drug and drug-disease interactions
- Use cautiously with other sedating medications.

- Use cautiously in patients with angina, recent MI, CVA, and hepatic or renal disease (guanabenz and guanfacine).

Parameters to monitor
- CBC, positive Coomb's test in 25%, less than 1% develop hemolytic anemia (methyldopa)

- Sleep disturbances, drowsiness, dry mouth

- Symptoms of depression

- Impotence

Table 10

Centrally Active α_2-Agonists

Drug	Trade name	Usual dose range, total mg/d (frequency per day)	Adverse events and comments[1]
Clonidine HCl[2]	Catapres®	0.1-0.8 (2)	Sedation, dry mouth, bradycardia, withdrawal hypertension, orthostatic hypotension, depression, impotence, sleep disturbances (More withdrawal)
Guanabenz acetate	Wytensin®	8-32 (2)	
Guanfacine HCl	Tenex®	1-3 (1)	(Less withdrawal)
Methyldopa	Aldomet®	250-1000 (2)	(Hepatic and "autoimmune" disorders)

[1]Side effects listed are for the class of drugs except where noted for individual drugs (in parentheses).
[2]Also available as a once-weekly transdermal patch.
Adapted from JNC-7 Express. Source: National Heart, Lung, and Blood Institute.

- Pulse

- Rebound hypertension

Peripherally acting α-adrenergic blockers (Table 11)
Mechanism of action
- Blocks peripheral α_1 postsynaptic receptors, which causes vasodilation of both arteries and veins (indirect vasodilators)

- Causes less reflex tachycardia than direct vasodilators (hydralazine/minoxidil)

Adverse drug events (Table 11)

Patient instructions and counseling
- Take first dose of no more than 1 mg of any agent and take at bedtime.

- Rise slowly from a lying or sitting position.

- May cause dizziness

- Priapism

Drug-drug and drug-disease interactions
- NSAIDs: decreased antihypertensive effects of α_1 blockers

- Increased antihypertensive effects with diuretics and β-blockers

Parameters to monitor
- Blood pressure and pulse

- Peripheral edema

β-Blockers (Table 12)
Mechanism of action
- Competitively blocks response to β-adrenergic stimulation:
  * Blocked secretion of renin
  * Decreased cardiac contractility, thereby decreases cardiac output
  * Decreased central sympathetic output
  * Decreased heart rate, thereby decreasing cardiac output

Adverse drug events (Table 12)

Patient instructions and counseling
- Report symptoms of dizziness or hypotension.

- Sedation precautions (with lipid-soluble compounds)

- Abrupt withdrawal of the drug should be avoided.

- Sexual dysfunction

Drug-drug and drug-disease interactions
- Use with caution in patients with diabetes.

- Use with caution in patients with Raynaud's phenomenon or peripheral vascular disease.

Table 11

Peripherally Acting α_1-Blockers

Drug	Trade name	Usual dose range, total mg/d (frequency per day)	Adverse events and comments
			Postural hypotension, syncopal episode with first dose, postural hypotension, diarrhea, weight gain, peripheral edema, dry mouth, urinary urgency, constipation, priapism, nausea, dizziness, headache, palpitations, and sweating; no effects on glucose or cholesterol
Doxazosin mesylate	Cardura®	1-16 (1)	
Prazosin HCl	Minipress®	2-20 (2-3)	
Terazosin HCl	Hytrin®	1-20 (1-2)	

Reprinted with permission from JNC-VI.

Table 12

β-Blockers and Combination α- and β-Blockers

Generic name (trade name)	Lipid solubility/primary (secondary) routes of elimination	Usual dose range, total mg/d (frequency per day)	Adverse events and comments[3]
			Bronchospasm, bradycardia, heart failure, may mask insulin-induced hypoglycemia; *less serious*: impaired peripheral circulation, insomnia, fatigue, decreased exercise tolerance, hypertriglyceridemia (except agents with intrinsic sympathomimetic activity)
β-Blockers			
Acebutolol (Sectral®)[1,2]	low/H (R)	200-800 (1)	
Atenolol (Tenormin®)[1]	low/R (H)	25-100 (1)	
Betaxolol (Kerlone®)[1]	low/H (R)	5-20 (1)	
Bisoprolol fumarate (Zebeta®)[1]	low/R (H)	2.5-10 (1)	
Carteolol HCl (Cartrol®)[2]	low/R	2.5-10 (1)	
Metoprolol tartrate[1] (Lopressor®)	moderate/H (R)	50-100 (2)	
Metoprolol succinate[1] (Toprol-XL®)	moderate/H (R)	50-100 (1)	
Nadolol (Corgard®)	low/R	40-120 (1)	
Penbutolol sulfate (Levatol®)[2]	high/H (R)	10-20 (1)	
Pindolol (Visken®)[2]	moderate/H (R)	10-60 (2)	
Propranolol HCl (Inderal®)	high/H	40-160 (2)	
(Inderal LA®)		60-180 (1)	
Timolol maleate (Blocadren®)	low-moderate/H (R)	20-40 (2)	
Combined α- and β-blockers			Postural hypotension, bronchospasm
Carvedilol (Coreg®)	moderate/bile into feces	12.5-50 (2)	
Labetalol (Normodyne,® Trandate®)	moderate/R (H)	200-800 (2)	

H, hepatic; R, renal.

[1]Cardioselective.

[2]Intrinsic sympathomimetic activity.

[3]Side effects listed are for the class of drugs except where noted for individual drugs (in parentheses).

Reprinted with permission from JNC-VI.

- Sulfonylureas: β-blockers may decrease effectiveness of sulfonylureas.

- Nondihydropyridines: may increase effect/toxicity of β-blockers

Parameters to monitor
- ECG

- Rebound hypertension

- Cholesterol levels

- Pulse (apical and radial)

- Glucose levels

Direct Vasodilators

- *This medication class is best avoided (second-line agents) unless necessary to treat refractory hypertension unresponsive to all other agents.*

- *These agents should NOT be used alone secondary to increases in plasma renin activity, cardiac output, and heart rate, and should therefore be used only when β-blockers and diuretics are part of the antihypertensive regimen.*

Mechanism of action
- These agents cause direct relaxation of peripheral arterial smooth muscle and thereby significantly decrease peripheral resistance.

Adverse drug events (Table 13)

Patient instructions and counseling
- Report symptoms of dizziness or hypotension.

- Hirsutism (minoxidil)

- Report any new symptoms of fatigue, malaise, low-grade fever, and joint aches.

- Report: rapid weight gain (>5 lb), unusual swelling, increased pulse >20 beats/min above normal

- Rise slowly from a lying or sitting position.

Drug-drug and drug-disease interactions
- Use with caution in patients pulmonary hypertension.

- Use with caution in patients with significant renal failure or CHF.

- Use with caution in patients with CAD or a recent MI.

Parameters to monitor
- Weight (fluid status)

- Blood pressure and pulse

- CBC with ANA (hydralazine)

Calcium Antagonists

- Low-renin hypertensive, black, and elderly patients respond well to this class of medications.

Mechanism of action
- Inhibit the influx of calcium ions through slow channels in vascular smooth muscle and cause relaxation of both coronary and peripheral arteries

- Sinoatrial (SA) and atrioventricular (AV) nodal depression and decrease in myocardial contractility (nondihydropyridines)

Adverse drug events (Table 14)

Patient instructions and counseling
- Report symptoms of dizziness or hypotension.

- Constipation (verapamil)

- Report any new symptoms of shortness of breath, fatigue, or increased swelling of the extremities.

- Rise slowly from a lying or sitting position.

Drug-drug and drug-disease interactions
- Use with caution in patients on β-blockers (nondihydropyridines) which may increase CHF and bradycardia; this combination can also cause conduction abnormalities to the AV node.

- Use with extreme caution in patients with conduction disturbances in the SA or AV nodes.

- Grapefruit juice may increase the levels of some dihydropyridines.

Table 13

Direct Vasodilators

Drug	Trade name	Usual dose range, total mg/d (frequency per day)	Adverse events and comments[1]
			Headaches, fluid retention, tachycardia, peripheral neuropathy, postural hypotension
Hydralazine HCl	Apresoline®	25-100 (2)	(Lupus syndrome)
Minoxidil	Loniten®	2.5-80 (1-2)	(Hirsutism)

[1]Side effects listed are for the class of drugs except where noted for individual drugs (in parentheses).
Adapted from JNC-7 Express. Source: National Heart, Lung, and Blood Institute.

Table 14

Calcium Antagonists

Drug	Trade name	Usual dose range, total mg/d (frequency per day)	Adverse events and comments[1]
Nondihydropyridines			Conduction defects, worsening of systolic dysfunction, gingival hyperplasia
Diltiazem HCl	Cardizem SR®, Cardizem CD®, Dilacor XR®, Tiazac®	180-420 (1) 120-360 (1)	(Nausea, headache)
Verapamil immediate-release	Calan®, Isoptin®	80-320 (2)	
Verapamil long-acting	Calan SR®, Isoptin SR®	120-360 (1-2)	(Constipation)
Verapamil—Coer	Covera HS®, Verelan PM®	120-360 (1)	
Dihydropyridines			Edema of the ankle, flushing, headache, gingival hyperplasia
Amlodipine besylate	Norvasc®	2.5-10 (1)	
Felodipine	Plendil®	2.5-20 (1)	
Isradipine	DynaCirc®	2.5-10 (2)	
	DynaCirc CR®	5-20 (1)	
Nicardipine	Cardene SR®	60-120 (1)	
Nifedipine	Procardia XL®, Adalat CC®	30-60 (1)	
Nisoldipine	Sular®	10-40 (1)	

[1]Side effects listed are for the class of drugs except where noted for individual drugs (in parentheses).
Adapted from JNC-7 Express. Source: National Heart, Lung, and Blood Institute.

Parameters to monitor
• ECG
• Peripheral edema
• Blood pressure and pulse
• Bowel habits
• Symptoms of conduction disturbances

Angiotensin-Converting Enzyme Inhibitors (ACEIs) and Angiotensin II Receptor Blockers (ARBs)

• *Ethnic differences in the response to these classes of medications exist. These agents are relatively ineffective as monotherapy in black patients. However, the addition of diuretic therapy has been shown to sensitize black patients to these agents to obtain similar responses as in nonblack patients.*

Mechanism of action
ACEIs
• Inhibit the conversion of angiotensin I to angiotensin II (a potent vasoconstrictor; see Figure 1)

• Indirectly inhibit fluid volume increases by inhibiting angiotensin II–stimulated release of aldosterone

ARBs
• Inhibit the binding of angiotensin II to the angiotensin II receptor, thereby inhibiting the vasoconstrictive properties of angiotensin II as well its ability to stimulate release of aldosterone

• Currently considered as alternative therapy in patients not able to tolerate ACEIs due to cough

Adverse drug events (Table 15)

Patient instructions and counseling
• Report symptoms of dizziness of hypotension.

• Symptoms of swelling of the lips, mouth, or face should be considered an emergency, and patient should immediately report to MD's office or emergency room.

• Report new rashes (especially captopril)

• Do not use salt substitutes containing potassium, and do not take OTC potassium supplements.

Table 15

Angiotensin-Converting Enzyme Inhibitors (ACEIs) and Angiotensin II Receptor Blockers (ARBs)

Drug	Trade name	Usual dose range, total mg/d (frequency per day)	Adverse events and comments
ACEIs			
Benazepril HCl	Lotensin®	10-40 (1-2)	**Common:** cough
Captopril	Capoten®	25-100 (2-3)	**Rare:** angioedema, hyperkalemia, rash, loss of
Enalapril maleate	Vasotec®	2.5-40 (1-2)	taste, leukopenia
Fosinopril	Monopril®	10-40 (1-2)	**Other:** vertigo; headache; fatigue; first-dose
Lisinopril	Prinivil®, Zestril®	10-40 (1)	hypotension; minor GI disturbances; acute
Moexipril	Univasc®	7.5-30 (1)	renal insufficiency in patients with
Perindopril	Aceon®	4-8 (1-2)	predisposing factors such as renal stenosis
Quinapril HCl	Accupril®	10-40 (1-2)	and coadministration with thiazide diuretics;
Ramipril	Altace®	1.25-20 (1)	proteinuria (especially in patients with history
Trandolapril	Mavik®	1-4 (1)	of renal disease)
Angiotensin II receptor blockers (ARBs)			
Candesartan	Atacand®	8-32 (1)	Angioedema, hyperkalemia
Eprosartan	Teveten®	400-800 (1-2)	
Irbesartan	Avapro®	150-300 (1)	
Losartan	Cozaar®	25-100 (1-2)	
Telmisartan	Micardis®	40-80 (1)	
Valsartan	Diovan®	80-320 (1)	

Reprinted with permission from JNC-VI.

- Rise slowly from a lying or sitting position.

Drug-drug and drug-disease interactions
- NSAIDs will decrease the effectiveness of ACEIs and ARBs.

- Potassium-sparing diuretics, potassium supplements, and salt substitutes will increase the risk of hyperkalemia when used in combination with ACEIs and ARBs.

- ACEIs and ARBs should be avoided in patients with bilateral renal artery stenosis or stenosis in a single kidney.

- ACEIs and ARBs should be avoided in pregnant patients.

Parameters to monitor
- Serum electrolytes (especially creatinine and potassium)

- Symptoms of angioedema

- Blood pressure

- Symptoms of hypotension

- CBC (especially with captopril and enalapril) for neutropenia, which is more common in patients with preexisting renal impairment

- Cough

- Urinary proteins

4. Hypertensive Urgencies and Emergencies

- The classification of hypertensive urgencies and emergencies is determined by the presence or absence of acute target organ damage and **not** of blood pressure, which will determine the appropriate treatment approach.

- The relative rise and rate of increase in blood pressure is more important than the actual blood pressure.

Hypertensive Emergencies

- Acute elevations of blood pressure (>200 mm Hg systolic or >140 mm Hg diastolic) with the presence of acute or ongoing target organ damage constitutes a hypertensive emergency (Table 16).

- This requires immediate lowering of blood pressure to prevent or minimize target organ damage

Treatment (Table 17)

- Initial goal: reduce mean arterial pressure (MAP) by no more than 25% within minutes to hours; reach 160/100 mm Hg within 2-6 hours.

Table 16

Clinical Findings of Target Organ Damage

Target organ damage:
Hypertensive encephalopathy
Intracranial hemorrhage
Unstable angina
Acute myocardial infarction
Acute left ventricular failure with pulmonary edema
Dissecting aortic aneurysm
Eclampsia

Clinical findings:
Funduscopic: papilledema, hemorrhage, exudates
Neurologic: somnolence, confusion, seizures, coma, visual deficits or blindness
Cardiac: S_4 gallop, ischemic changes on ECG, chest x-ray consistent with pulmonary edema, chest pain
Renal: oliguria, progressive azotemia, hematuria, proteinuria
Other: dyspnea

Reprinted with permission from JNC-VI.

- Measure BP every 5-10 minutes until goal MAP is reached and life-threatening target organ damage resolves.

- Maintain goal BP for 1-2 days, further reduce BP toward normal over several weeks.

- Excessive falls in BP may precipitate renal, cerebral, or coronary ischemia.

- IV agents are preferred due to the ability to titrate dosages based on BP response; however, specific agents should be chosen based on patient findings (Table 18).

Hypertensive Urgencies

- Accelerated, malignant, or perioperative elevations in blood pressure in the absence of new or progressive target organ damage, therefore immediate lowering of BP not required.

- Patients are treated the same as patients with stage 3 hypertension (Table 3).

Treatment (Table 19)

- There is no agent of choice; medications should be selected based on patient characteristics.

- Oral therapy is preferred.

- Onset of action should be in 15-30 minutes, and peak effects seen in 2-3 hours.

- Check BP every 15-30 minutes to ensure response.

- Use of immediate-release nifedipine is inappropriate to lower blood pressure in patients with hypertensive urgencies.

Table 17

Parenteral Drugs for Treatment of Hypertensive Emergencies[1]

Drug	Dose[2]	Onset of action	Duration of action	Adverse effects[3]	Special indications
Vasodilators					
Sodium nitroprusside	0.25-10 µg/kg per min as IV infusion[4] (maximal dose for 10 min only)	Immediate	1-2 min	Nausea, vomiting, muscle twitching, sweating, thiocyanate and cyanide intoxication	Most hypertensive emergencies: caution with high intracranial pressure or azotemia
Nicardipine hydrochloride	5-15 mg/h IV	5-10 min	1-4 h	Tachycardia, headache, flushing, local phlebitis	Most hypertensive emergencies except acute heart failure; caution with coronary ischemia
Fenoldopam mesylate	0.1-0.3 µg/kg per min IV infusion	<5 min	30 min	Tachycardia, headache, nausea, flushing	
Nitroglycerin	5-100 µg/min as IV infusion[4]	2-5 min	3-5 min	Headache, vomiting, methemoglobinemia, tolerance with prolonged use	Coronary ischemia
Enalaprilat	1.25-5 mg every 6 h IV	15-30 min	6 h	Precipitous fall in pressure in high-renin states; response variable	Acute left ventricular failure; avoid in acute myocardial infarction
Hydralazine hydrochloride	10-20 mg IV; 10-50 mg IM	10-20 min; 20-30 min	3-8 h	Tachycardia, flushing, headache, vomiting, aggravation of angina	Eclampsia
Diazoxide	50-100 mg IV bolus repeated, or 15-30 mg/min infusion	2-4 min	6-12 h	Nausea, flushing, tachycardia, chest pain	Now obsolete; when no intensive monitoring available
Adrenergic inhibitors					
Labetalol hydrochloride	20-80 mg IV bolus every 10 min; 0.5-2.0 mg/min IV infusion	5-10 min	3-6 h	Vomiting, scalp tingling, burning in throat, dizziness, nausea, heart block, orthostatic hypotension	Most hypertensive emergencies except acute heart failure
Esmolol hydrochloride	250-500 µg/kg/min for 1 min, then 50-100 µg/kg/min for 4 min; may repeat sequence	1-2 min	10-20 min	Hypotension, nausea	Aortic dissection, perioperative
Phentolamine	5-15 mg IV	1-2 min	3-10 min	Tachycardia, flushing, headache	Catecholamine excess

[1]These doses may vary from this in the *Physicians Desk Reference* (51st ed.).
[2]IV indicates intravenous; IM, intramuscular.
[3]Hypotension may occur with all agents.
[4]Requires special delivery system.
Reprinted with permission from JNC-VI.

Table 18

Selected Agents for Specific Hypertensive Emergencies

Emergency	Recommended therapy	Comments
Encephalopathy	Labetalol; nicardipine; nitroprusside	*Avoid:* methyldopa (sedation); diazoxide (reduces cerebral blood flow); reserpine (sedation); hydralazine (increases intracranial pressure)
Myocardial infarction (MI)/ unstable angina	Nitroglycerin; esmolol	Reduce BP until pain is relieved, use in conjunction with conventional therapy for MI/angina. *Avoid:* Diazoxide and hydralazine (increases oxygen demand); dihydropyridines (may worsen angina); nitroprusside (coronary steal)
Congestive heart failure	Nitroprusside; nitroglycerin; enalaprilat	*Avoid:* labetalol, esmolol, other β-blockers (reduces cardiac output)
Subarachnoid hemorrhage, Intracerebral hemorrhage, stroke	Nitroprusside	BP reduction is controversial as it may cause hypoperfusion; generally recommended for severe hypertension (systolic >220 or diastolic >120 mm Hg)
Dissecting aortic aneurysm	Trimethaphan; esmolol; nitroprusside	*Avoid:* diazoxide and hydralazine (increase shear force)
Pheochromocytoma, cocaine overdose	Phentolamine; labetalol	Anecdotal reports of increased BP with labetalol; unopposed β blockade may worsen crisis
Renal insufficiency	Nitroprusside; calcium channel blocker; labetalol	Monitor cyanide and thiocyanate levels
Postoperative hypertension	Nitroprusside; nicardipine; labetalol	

Table 19

Agents Used to Treat Hypertensive Urgencies

Drug	Dose	Onset	Duration	Adverse effects
Captopril	25 mg, repeat in 1-2 hours as needed	5-15 minutes	4-6 hours	Hypotension, acute renal failure, angioedema
Clonidine	0.1-0.2 mg, repeat in 1-2 hours as needed (up to 0.6 mg)	5-15 minutes	6-12 hours	Hypotension, drowsiness, sedation, dry mouth
Labetalol	100-400 mg, repeat in 2-3 hours as needed	15-30 minutes	4-6 hours	Hypotension, heart block, bronchoconstriction

5. Key Points

- Hypertension is defined as a systolic blood pressure >140 mm Hg, a diastolic blood pressure >90 mm Hg, or any patient requiring antihypertensive therapy.

- Treatment goals of hypertension are stratified based on presence of cardiovascular disease or target organ damage and/or risk factors for cardiovascular disease, including smoking, dyslipidemia, diabetes mellitus, age >60 years, male sex, and family history of premature cardiovascular disease.

- Secondary causes of hypertension include: renovascular disease, primary aldosteronism, Cushing's syndrome, pheochromocytoma, aortic coarctation, and drug-induced (steroids/estrogens, alcohol, cocaine, cyclosporine/tacrolimus, sympathomimetics, erythropoietin, licorice, MAO inhibitors, TCA antidepressants, NSAIDs).

- Recommended lifestyle modifications both to improve blood pressure and overall cardiovascular health include: lose weight; limit alcohol intake; increase aerobic physical activity; reduce sodium intake; maintain adequate dietary intake of potassium, magnesium, and calcium; stop smoking; and reduce dietary cholesterol and saturated fat intake.

- β-Blockers and diuretics are considered initial agents for treatment of hypertension by JNC-VI unless compelling indications for the use of other medication classes exist or the patient has comorbid conditions that would suggest the use of classes other than β-blockers and diuretics.

- Recent data suggest that angiotensin-converting enzyme inhibitors (ACEIs), calcium channel blockers (CCBs), and possibly angiotensin II receptor blockers (ARBs) might be considered as initial agents for treatment of hypertension.

- Vasodilators, α_1-receptor antagonists, α_2-receptor agonists, and postganglionic adrenergic neuron blockers should be avoided as initial agents for hypertension.

- Antihypertensive drug therapy should be individualized, and there are classifications of recommendations from JNC-VI based on the level of evidence, which include: compelling indication unless contraindicated, may have favorable effects on comorbid conditions, and may have unfavorable effects on comorbid conditions.

- The classification and treatment of hypertensive urgencies and emergencies is determined by the presence or absence of acute target organ damage and **not** on blood pressure.

- All causes for inadequate response should be addressed before additional agents are added to a patient's antihypertensive regimen (ie, pseudo-resistance, nonadherence, volume overload, drug-related causes, associated conditions, and secondary causes of hypertension).

6. Questions and Answers

1. All of the following agents are suitable as initial therapy for the treatment of uncomplicated hypertension according to the Sixth Report of the Joint National Committee on Detection, Evaluation, and Treatment of High Blood Pressure (JNC-IV) EXCEPT:

    A. Esidrex
    B. Chlorthalidone
    C. Lozol
    D. Apresoline
    E. Tenormin

2. Hyperkalemia is a possible adverse effect of all the following medications EXCEPT:

    A. Mavik
    B. Teveten
    C. Doxazosin
    D. Amiloride
    E. Captopril

3. A 48-year-old patient presents with a new diagnosis of hypertension. The patient is also noted to have congestive heart failure (CHF) with an ejection fraction of 28%. Which agent would be an appropriate choice as initial therapy in this patient based on JNC-IV?

    A. Catapres
    B. Guanethidine
    C. Diltiazem
    D. Aceon
    E. Sular

4. A 62-year-old patient with a history of hypertension and gout presents to begin pharmacotherapy for hypertension. Which agent is the most appropriate choice as initial therapy based on JNC-IV?

    A. Diuril
    B. Demedex
    C. Tenormin
    D. Hygroton
    E. Metolazone

5. All of the following medications can cause bradycardia EXCEPT:

    A. Hytrin
    B. Isoptin
    C. Tiazac

D. Ziac
E. Catapres

6. A patient requires a cardioselective β-blocker in their outpatient medication regimen after recent discharge from the hospital with a new myocardial infarction. You suggest:

   A. Labetalol
   B. Esmolol
   C. Propranolol
   D. Atenolol
   F. Carvedilol

7. A patient presents to your ambulatory clinic with a blood pressure of 210/125. PMH is significant for type 2 diabetes, CHF, and renal insufficiency. Which of the following would cause the patient to be classified as a hypertensive emergency?

   A. Blood glucose levels >300, which increases the patient's risk for acute renal failure
   B. A serum creatinine of 3 mg/dL
   C. Nausea, vomiting, and diarrhea for 3 days
   D. S_4 gallop and a chest x-ray consistent with pulmonary edema
   E. Polyuria combined with polydipsia

8. What are the treatment goals for the patient with hypertensive emergency described in the Question 7?

   A. Systolic pressure should be reduced to 120 mm Hg within the first hour of treatment to reduce the risk of further end organ damage
   B. Diastolic pressure should be reduced to 80 mm Hg within the first hour of treatment to reduce the risk of further end organ damage
   C. Reduce blood pressure to 160/100 in the first 2-6 hours of therapy
   D. Reduce mean arterial pressure by at least 50% within the first minutes to hours of therapy
   E. Reduce blood pressure to no lower than 180/110 in the first hour, as excessive falls in blood pressure may precipitate coronary ischemia

9. What would be the recommended treatment for the patient with hypertensive emergency in Question 7?

   A. Clonidine PO 0.1-0.2 mg, repeat in 1-2 hours as needed (up to 0.6 mg)

   B. Labetalol PO 100-400 mg, repeat in 2-3 hours as needed
   C. Nifedipine SL 10 mg, repeat in 0.5-1 hours as needed (up to 60 mg)
   D. Labetalol IV 20-80 mg bolus, followed by 0.5-2 mg/min infusion
   E. Enalaprilat IV 1.25-5 mg every 6 hours

10. Which of the following antihypertensive agents can cause first-dose syncope, palpitations, peripheral edema, and priapism?

    A. Hydralazine
    B. Nitroprusside
    C. Prazosin
    D. Verelan
    E. Univasc

11. Which of the following antihypertensive agents is most likely to cause lupus syndrome, postural hypotension, and peripheral neuropathy?

    A. Tenormin
    B. Apresoline
    C. Tenex
    D. Mibefradil
    E. Nitroprusside

12. Which of the following medications is ***not*** associated with drug-induced hypertension?

    A. Prednisone
    B. Indomethacin
    C. Rosiglitazone
    D. Cocaine
    E. Cyclosporine

13. What is the best recommendation for antihypertensive medication in a patient who has atrial fibrillation, CAD with angina, and hyperthyroidism?

    A. Loniten
    B. Kerlone
    C. Micardis
    D. Cardene
    E. Midamor

14. What antihypertensive agent should ***not*** be used in a patient with essential hypertension and a history of depression with suicidal ideation?

    A. Captopril
    B. Minipress
    C. Diulo
    D. Serpasil

E. Amlodipine

15. All of the following are secondary causes of hypertension EXCEPT:

   A. Renovascular disease
   B. Pheochromocytoma
   C. Systemic lupus erythematosus
   D. Primary aldosteronism
   E. Aortic coarctation

Answer Questions 16-20 based on the patient medication profile provided below.

   A. I only is correct
   B. III only is correct
   C. I and II are both correct
   D. II and III are both correct
   E. I, II, and III are correct

16. Possible complications that the patient is at risk to develop secondary to uncontrolled hypertension include:

   I. Hyperaldosteronism
   II. Myocardial infarction

III. Blindness

17. Education regarding lifestyle modification issues in this patient should include:

   I. Limit smoking to $1/2$ pack per day and alcohol intake to no more than 2 drinks per day
   II. Maintain adequate intake of dietary magnesium, calcium, and sodium
   III. Increase aerobic physical activity, lose weight, and limit dietary saturated fat and cholesterol

18. Possible reasons for the patient's blood pressure being uncontrolled include:

   I. Use of NSAIDs causes decreased effectiveness of ACE inhibitor therapy
   II. Possible problems with adherence to antihypertensive therapy
   III. Lack of blood pressure response to ACE inhibitor therapy, which should not be used in combination with diuretics in an African-American patient

19. The appropriate initial antihypertensive agent in this patient could be:

DATE: 04/12/03

PATIENT MEDICATION PROFILE

PATIENT'S NAME ___Buddy Manwich___

ADDRESS ___61 Heavenly Highway___

Phone No. ___555-8181___

Date of Birth ___4/14/44___

Known diseases: _DM (15 yrs), HTN (20 yrs),_

Obstructive Sleep Apnea (5yrs), Osteoarthritis

Allergies/Sensitivities __NKDA__

NOTES: _+ tobacco – 1 ½ ppd,_

___4-5 cups of coffee / day___

___ETOH - 2 drinks / week___

Race: ___African American___

Ht: _5'11"_

Wt: _248 lbs_

OTC use: Aleve, Actron

DATE	Rx#	MEDICATION/ STRENGTH	ROUTE	QUANTITY	REGIMEN	REFILLS	PHARMACIST	PRESCRIBER
1/15/03	001	Glipizide 5mg	PO	30	1 qd	5	BCE	NTE
1/15/03	002	Lisinopril 5mg	PO	30	1 qd	5	BCE	NTE
1/15/03	003	Hydrodiuril 12.5mg	PO	30	1 qd	5	BBC	NPR
1/20/03	004	Ibuprofen 800mg	PO	90	1 tid	5	REM	FTD
2/11/03	001-RF	Glipizide 5mg	PO	30	1 qd	4	BCE	NTE
2/11/03	003-RF	Hydrodiuril 12.5mg	PO	30	1 qd	4	BBC	NPR
2/11/03	004-RF	Ibuprofen 800mg	PO	90	1 tid	4	REM	FTD
3/13/03	001-RF	Glipizide 5mg	PO	30	1 qd	3	BCE	NTE
3/13/03	002-RF	Lisinopril 5mg	PO	30	1 qd	3	BCE	NTE
3/13/03	004-RF	Ibuprofen 800mg	PO	90	1 tid	3	REM	FTD

I. Lotensin
II. Hytrin
III. Loniten

20. If the patient is not able to tolerate lisinopril due to adverse effects such as cough, an appropriate alternative agent would be:

I. Micardis
II. Trandate
III. Wytensin

Answers

1. **D.** Appropriate choices for initial agents in the treatment of uncomplicated hypertension include β-blockers and diuretics. Apresoline (hydralazine) is a direct vasodilator, which would never be considered a first-line agent in the treatment of hypertension.

2. **C.** Hyperkalemia is a possible side effect with angiotensin-converting enzyme inhibitors, angiotensin II receptor antagonists, and potassium-sparing diuretics. Doxazosin is a peripherally acting α_1 blocker, which does not cause hyperkalemia.

3. **D.** For patients who have hypertension and congestive heart failure, JNC-VI recommends the use of ACE inhibitors and diuretics (see Table 6). The only listed ACE inhibitor is Aceon (perindopril).

4. **C.** For patients who have hypertension and gout, JNC-VI recommends **not** using diuretic therapy, which increases the risk of gouty attacks (see Table 6). The only medication listed that is not a diuretic is Tenormin (atenolol) which is a β-blocker.

5. **A.** Isoptin (verapamil) and Tiazac (diltiazem) are nondihydropyridine calcium channel blockers; Ziac (bisoprolol/hydrochlorothiazide) is a β-blocker; and Catapres (clonidine) is a centrally acting α_2 agonist, and all these have negative inotropic effects on the myocardium. Hytrin (terazosin) is a peripherally acting α_1 blocker, which does not cause bradycardia.

6. **D.** Labetolol, propranolol, and carvedilol are all nonselective β-blockers. Esmolol is a cardio-selective agent only available in injectable form, and therefore would not be for outpatient use. Atenolol (Tenormin) is a cardioselective β-

blocker that is available as an oral tablet, and therefore can be used for outpatient dosing.

7. **D.** The classification of hypertensive urgencies and emergencies is determined by the presence or absence of acute target organ damage and ***not*** by the actual blood pressure measurement. Presence of an S_4 gallop and a chest x-ray consistent with pulmonary edema suggest acute left ventricular failure with pulmonary edema, which represents defined target organ damage, which means this patient should be classified as a hypertensive emergency.

8. **C.** According to JNC-VI, the initial goal of blood pressure lowering in patients with hypertensive emergencies is a drop in mean arterial pressure (MAP) of no more than 25% within minutes to hours, and to 160/100 mm Hg within 2-6 hours.

9. **E.** In a patient with CHF and a hypertensive emergency, recommended treatments include nitroglycerin, nitroprusside, and enalaprilat (Table 18). Clonidine and labetalol (PO) are incorrect choices because the patient requires IV therapy. Nifedipine SL is not indicated for immediate reduction of blood pressure. Labetalol IV is not an appropriate choice in this patient with CHF, which could decrease cardiac output.

10. **C.** Possible side effects of peripherally acting α_1 blockers (prazosin, Minpress) include first-dose syncope, palpitations, peripheral edema, and priapism (Table 11).

11. **B.** Possible side effects of direct vasodilators (Apresoline, hydralazine) include postural hypotension and peripheral neuropathy. However, lupus syndrome is unique to hydralazine and does not occur with minoxidil (Table 13).

12. **C.** All agents listed are possible causes of drug-induced hypertension through multiple mechanisms except rosiglitazone (Figure 8).

13. **B.** The diagnoses of atrial fibrillation, CAD with angina, and hyperthyroidism are all considered comorbid conditions with hypertension in which the use of β-blockers may have favorable effects.

14. **D.** Because of its possible increased risk of depression, Serpasil (reserpine) should not be

used in patients in whom the risk for depression and/or suicide already exists.

15. **C.** All listed diseases are possible causes of secondary hypertension through various mechanisms, except systemic lupus erythematosus.

16. **D.** Uncontrolled hypertension causes multiple organ system problems, including cardiovascular (CHF, MI, PAD), ophthalmologic (retinopathy, blindness), cerebrovascular (TIA, CVA), and renovascular (nephropathy, renal failure, dialysis). Therefore this patient is at risk for MI and blindness, not hyperaldosteronism.

17. **B.** Lifestyle modification issues to be considered in hypertensive patients include weight loss; limit of alcohol intake; increased aerobic activity; reduced sodium intake; maintenance of adequate dietary potassium, calcium, and magnesium intake; and smoking cessation.

18. **C.** Possible causes for inadequate responsiveness to therapy are listed in Figure 8.

19. **A.** In patients with hypertension and comorbid conditions of CHF and diabetes, the initial agent should be an ACE inhibitor (Table 6).

20. **A.** In patients who cannot tolerate ACE inhibitor therapy secondary to the adverse effect of cough, angiotensin II receptor antagonists are considered good alternative agents.

7. References

Carter BL, Saseen JL. Hypertension. In: DiPiro JT, ed. *Pharmacotherapy: A Pathophysiologic Approach*. New York: McGraw-Hill; 2002:157-183.

Joint National Committee on Prevention, Detection, Evaluation, and Treatment of High Blood Pressure (JNC-VI). The sixth report of the Joint National Committee on Prevention, Detection, Evaluation, and Treatment of High Blood Pressure. *Arch Intern Med.* 1997;157:2413-2446.

Joint National Committee on Prevention, Detection, Evaluation, and Treatment of High Blood Pressure (JNC-7) Express. NIH Pub. No. 03-5233, May 2003. Available at http://www.nhlbi.gov/guidelines/hypertension/express.pdf.

9. Heart Failure

Robert B. Parker, PharmD
Associate Professor, Department of Pharmacy
University of Tennessee College of Pharmacy

Contents

1. Overview

Heart failure is a clinical syndrome resulting from a variety of cardiac disorders that impair the ability of the ventricle to fill with or eject blood in which the heart is unable to pump blood at a sufficient rate to meet the metabolic demands of the body.

- Nearly 5 million people in the U.S. have heart failure with 500,000 new patients diagnosed each year.

- Only major cardiovascular disease that is increasing in prevalence.

- Approximately 300,000 patients die from heart failure each year. At the time of heart failure diagnosis, the 5-year mortality is nearly 50%.

- Most common hospital discharge diagnosis for Medicare patients. More Medicare dollars spent for diagnosis and treatment of heart failure than for any other disorder.

Classification

- The New York Heart Association Functional Classification has been widely used for many years. It primarily reflects the severity of symptoms based on a subjective assessment by the provider. It can change frequently over a short period and treatments do not differ significantly across classes.
  - * Functional class I: patients with cardiac disease but without limitations of physical activity. Ordinary physical activity does not cause undue fatigue, dyspnea, or palpitations.
  - * Functional class II: patients with cardiac disease that results in slight limitations of physical activity. Ordinary physical activity results in fatigue, palpitation, dyspnea, or angina.
  - * Functional class III: patients with cardiac disease that results in marked limitation of physical activity. Although patients are comfortable at rest, less than ordinary activity will lead to symptoms.
  - * Functional class IV: patients with cardiac disease that results in an inability to carry on physical activity without discomfort. Symptoms of heart failure are present even at rest. With any physical activity, increased discomfort is experienced.

- The most recent guidelines for evaluation and management of heart failure from the American College of Cardiology (ACC)/American Heart Association (AHA) recommend an additional classification scheme that emphasizes both the evolution and progression of the disease. It more objectively identifies patients within the course of the disease and links to treatments that are appropriate for each stage.
  - * Stage A: patients at high risk of developing heart failure because of the presence of conditions that are strongly associated with heart failure. These patients have no known cardiac abnormalities and no heart failure signs or symptoms. Examples include patients with hypertension, coronary artery disease, and diabetes mellitus.
  - * Stage B: patients who have developed structural heart disease that is strongly associated with the development of heart failure but who have never shown signs or symptoms of heart failure. Some examples include previous myocardial infarction and left ventricular hypertrophy.
  - * Stage C: patients who have current or prior symptoms of heart failure associated with underlying structural heart disease. Examples include patients with dyspnea or fatigue due to left ventricular systolic dysfunction and asymptomatic patients who are undergoing treatment for prior symptoms of heart failure.
  - * Stage D: patients with advanced structural heart disease and marked symptoms of heart failure at rest despite maximal medical therapy and who require specialized interventions. Examples include patients who are frequently hospitalized for heart failure and cannot be safely discharged from the hospital, patients in the hospital awaiting heart transplantation, and patients supported with a mechanical circulatory assist device.

Advanced or decompensated heart failure
- Patients that have persistent limiting symptoms despite therapy with drugs of proven efficacy and/or require hospitalization for exacerbation of previously stable symptoms.

- Causes include medication and dietary noncompliance, atrial fibrillation, myocardial ischemia, and progression of heart failure.

- Assignment to one of four hemodynamic profiles assists in determining approach to therapy.
  - * Warm and dry: adequate perfusion (ie, cardiac output) and no signs or symptoms of volume overload
  - * Warm and wet: adequate perfusion but signs or symptoms of volume overload
  - * Cold and dry: inadequate perfusion and no signs or symptoms of volume overload

* Cold and wet: inadequate perfusion and signs or symptoms of volume overload

• Most patients (about 70%) present with the warm and wet classification.

Clinical Presentation

• The primary manifestations of heart failure are dyspnea and fatigue, which may limit exercise tolerance, and fluid retention, which may lead to pulmonary and peripheral edema. Both abnormalities can limit a patient's functional capacity and quality of life, but do not necessarily occur at the same time. Some patients may have marked exercise intolerance but little evidence of fluid retention, whereas others have prominent edema with few symptoms of dyspnea or fatigue.

• Other symptoms may include paroxysmal nocturnal dyspnea, orthopnea, tachypnea, cough, ascites, and nocturia.

• Other signs include jugular venous distension, hepatojugular reflux, hepatomegaly, bibasilar rales, pleural effusion, tachycardia, pallor, and S_3 gallop.

• Symptoms in advanced heart failure are similar but may be more severe.

Pathophysiology

• Heart failure can result from any disorder (see below) that impairs the heart's systolic (ie, pumping ability) or diastolic (impaired cardiac relaxation) function. Many patients have manifestations of both abnormalities. In either case, a decrease in cardiac output is the initiating event in heart failure. The reduction in cardiac output results in activation of a number of compensatory mechanisms that attempt to maintain an adequate cardiac output.

• The beneficial effects of ACE inhibitors, β-blockers, and aldosterone antagonists on reducing mortality and slowing heart failure progression resulted in the neurohormonal model of heart failure pathophysiology.
   * The decrease in cardiac output leads to activation of systems that release a number of neurohormones including angiotensin II, norepinephrine, aldosterone, proinflammatory cytokines, and vasopressin. These neurohormones can increase renal sodium and water retention, vasoconstriction, tachycardia, and ventricular hypertrophy and remodeling.

* Activation of the compensatory systems results in a systemic disorder that is not just confined to the heart, whose progression is largely mediated by these neurohormones.

Specific Causes of Heart Failure

• Coronary artery disease is the cause of heart failure in about 65% of patients with left ventricular systolic dysfunction. Other causes include nonischemic cardiomyopathy (eg, due to hypertension, thyroid disease, or valvular disease). Most of these patients have a reduced left ventricular ejection fraction (usually <40%).

• Approximately 20-40% of patients have heart failure secondary to diastolic dysfunction although many patients who present with heart failure and normal systolic function do not have any identifiable myocardial disease.

• A number of drugs can precipitate or worsen heart failure

Drugs with negative inotropic effects
   * Antiarrhythmics: disopyramide, flecainide, propafenone
   * β-Blockers
   * Calcium channel blockers: verapamil and diltiazem

• Cardiotoxic drugs
   * Doxorubicin
   * Daunorubicin
   * Cyclophosphamide
   * Oral antifungals: itraconazole and terbinafine
   * Alcohol

• Sodium and water retention
   * NSAIDs (including the COX-2 inhibitors): also can attenuate the efficacy and increase the toxicity of diuretics and ACE inhibitors
   * Glucocorticoids
   * Rosiglitazone and pioglitazone

Diagnostic Criteria

• There is no single diagnostic test for heart failure; it is a clinical diagnosis based on history, signs and symptoms, and physical examination.

• The echocardiogram is one of the most useful diagnostic tests in patients with heart failure.

- Patients with a left ventricular ejection fraction less than 40% are generally considered to have systolic dysfunction.

- Note that in general there is a poor correlation between the ejection fraction and symptoms.

Treatment Principles and Goals of Therapy

- Goals of therapy are to improve the patient's quality of life, reduce symptoms, reduce hospitalizations for heart failure exacerbations, slow progression of the disease, and improve survival.

- ACC/AHA guidelines for heart failure treatment according to stage are shown in Figure 1. Therapy in stages A and B is primarily targeted toward prevention of heart failure development, whereas stages C and D focus on treatment of patients with symptomatic heart failure.

- An algorithm for treatment of patients with advanced/decompensated heart failure is shown in Figure 2.

2. Drug Therapy of Heart Failure

- The following section on drug therapy focuses on treatment of stage C heart failure patients (ie, patients with left ventricular dysfunction with current or prior symptoms). This is also commonly referred to as outpatient treatment of patients with heart failure. These patients should be routinely managed with a combination of four drugs: a diuretic, an ACE inhibitor, a β-blocker, and digoxin. Drug therapies that can be considered in selected patients include angiotensin receptor blockers (ARBs), aldosterone antagonists, and hydralazine/isosorbide dinitrate.

Loop Diuretics

- Most heart failure patients require use of the more potent loop diuretics versus thiazide diuretics (Table 1).

Mechanism of action
- Reduce the sodium retention associated with heart failure by inhibiting reabsorption of sodium or chloride in the loop of Henle

Patient instructions and counseling
- Patients allergic to sulfa-containing medications may also be allergic to these medications.

- Take once a day in the morning, or if taking twice daily, take in the morning and afternoon.

- Can cause frequent urination

- Patients should weigh themselves daily (best in the morning after urinating). Patients that gain more than 1 pound per day for several consecutive days or 3-5 pounds in a week should contact their health care provider.

Table 1

Loop Diuretics

Generic name (trade name)	Dosage form	Dosage range and frequency
Furosemide (Lasix®)	Oral tablet	20-160 mg 1-2 qd-bid
Bumetanide (Bumex®)	Oral tablet	0.5-5 mg qd-bid
Torsemide (Demadex®)	Oral tablet	10-100 mg qd-bid

Figure 1.

Stages in the evolution of heart failure and recommended therapy by stage.

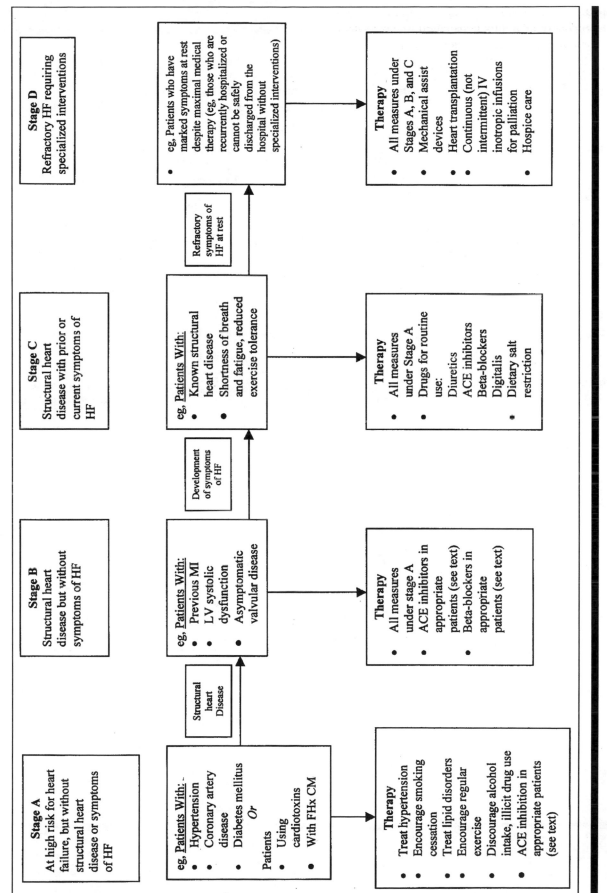

FHx CM indicates family history of cardiomyopathy; MI, myocardial infarction; LV, left ventricular.
Adapted from Hunt et al, 2001.

Figure 2.

Advanced or decompensated heart failure.

**After optimizing (ACE inhibitors [ACEIs],
β-blockers, digoxin, diuretics)
Class I-IV**

From Johnson et al, 2002.

- Report muscle cramps, dizziness, excessive thirst, weakness, or confusion as these may be signs of overdiuresis.

- Photosensitivity: patients should use sunscreen and/or avoid sun exposure.

Adverse drug events
- Electrolyte depletion: hypokalemia and hypo-magnesemia

- Hypotension

- Renal insufficiency

Drug-drug and drug-disease interactions
- Furosemide bioavailability and its diuretic effect is decreased by food and it should be taken on an empty stomach. Food does not affect torsemide absorption.

- NSAIDs may diminish the diuretic effect.

- Potassium supplementation may not be required in patients also receiving ACE inhibitors.

Parameters to monitor
- Serum sodium, potassium, magnesium, creatinine, and BUN

- Patient weight: loss of 0.5-1.0 kg daily is desired until the patient achieves their dry weight

- Urine output

- Blood pressure

- Improvement in heart failure symptoms: dyspnea, peripheral edema

Kinetics
- Bioavailability of torsemide is less variable than furosemide and is not affected by food.

Angiotensin-Converting Enzyme Inhibitors (ACE Inhibitors)

- Cornerstone of therapy in heart failure patients (Table 2). Clinical trials in over 7000 patients consistently demonstrate ACE inhibitors alleviate symptoms, improve clinical status and quality of life, and improve mortality. Current guidelines recommend that all patients with heart failure due to left ventricular systolic dysfunction should receive an ACE inhibitor unless contraindicated.

Table 2

Angiotensin-converting enzyme inhibitors

Generic name (trade name)	Dosage form	Dosage range and frequency
Captopril (Capoten®)	Oral tablet	6.25-50 mg tid
Enalapril (Vasotec®)	Oral tablet	2.5-20 mg bid
Fosinopril (Monopril®)	Oral tablet	5-40 mg qd
Lisinopril (Zestril®, Prinivil®)	Oral tablet	2.5-40 mg qd
Quinapril (Accupril®)	Oral tablet	10-40 mg bid
Ramipril (Altace®)	Oral capsule	1.25-10 mg qd

Mechanism of action
- Interfere with the renin-angiotensin system by inhibiting angiotensin-converting enzyme that is responsible for the conversion of angiotensin I to the potent vasoconstrictor angiotensin II. This results in a decrease in plasma angiotensin II and aldosterone concentrations, thus reducing the adverse effects of these neurohormones. Inhibition of angiotensin-converting enzyme also prevents the breakdown of the endogenous vasodilator bradykinin.

- Improve hemodynamics by increasing cardiac output and reducing left ventricular filling pressures, systemic vascular resistance, blood pressure, and heart rate.

- Improve heart failure symptoms and reduce hospitalizations for heart failure.

- Reduce mortality by 20-30%

Patient instructions and counseling
- Patients that are pregnant or breast-feeding should not take ACE inhibitors. If they become pregnant while taking an ACE inhibitor, they should contact their physician immediately.

- Captopril should be taken on an empty stomach, 1 hour before or 2 hours after meals.

- Use salt substitutes that contain potassium cautiously.

- Call your doctor immediately if you experience swelling of the face, eyes, lips, tongue, arms, or legs, or if you have difficulty breathing or swallowing.

- May cause cough

Adverse drug events

- Hypotension

- Dizziness

- Renal insufficiency

- Cough

- Angioedema

- Hyperkalemia

- Rash

- Taste disturbances

Drug-drug and drug-disease interactions

- NSAIDs (including the COX-2 inhibitors) can increase the risk of renal insufficiency and attenuate the beneficial hemodynamic effects of ACE inhibitors.

- Use potassium supplements or potassium-sparing diuretics with caution in patients receiving ACE inhibitors.

- Cyclosporine and tacrolimus may increase the risk of nephrotoxicity and hyperkalemia.

- Diuretics: increase risk of hypotension

Parameters to monitor

- Blood pressure

- Renal function (ie, serum BUN and creatinine)

- Serum potassium

- Heart failure symptoms

- Dose: therapy should be initiated at low doses followed by gradual increases if lower doses are well tolerated.

Other

- Pregnancy category C (first trimester) and D (second and third trimesters). Can cause fetal and neonatal morbidity and death when administered to pregnant women.

Beta-Blockers

- Because of their negative inotropic effects, β-blockers were classically considered to be contraindicated in patients with heart failure. However, these agents, by inhibiting the deleterious effects of long-term activation of the sympathetic nervous system in heart failure, have been repeatedly shown to provide hemodynamic, symptomatic, and survival benefits. Metoprolol succinate (extended-release metoprolol), bisoprolol, and carvedilol have all been shown to be effective in heart failure (Table 3).

Mechanism of action

- Blockade of β receptors by these agents antagonizes the increase in sympathetic nervous system activity that is responsible for progression of heart failure. Bisoprolol and metoprolol succinate are β_1-selective blockers, whereas carvedilol blocks β_1-, β_2-, and α_1-receptors. There is currently no evidence that these differences in pharmacologic actions have any important effects on outcomes in patients with heart failure.

- Treatment with β-blockers reduces symptoms, improves the clinical status, and decreases the risk of death and hospitalization.

- β-Blockers should be used in all patients with stable heart failure due to left ventricular systolic dysfunction unless they have a contraindication or have been shown not to tolerate them.

- In general, should be used in combination with ACE inhibitors.

Patient instructions and counseling

- May cause fluid retention or worsening of heart failure with initiation or an increase in dose. Report any cases of body or leg swelling or increased shortness of breath. Patients should weigh themselves daily and if they gain more than 1 pound per day for several consecutive days or 3-5 pounds in a week, they should contact their health care provider.

Table 3

Beta-Blockers

Generic name (trade name)	Dosage form	Dosage range and frequency
Bisoprolol (Zebeta®)	Oral tablet	1.25-10 mg 1-2 qd
Carvedilol (Coreg®)	Oral tablet	3.125-50 mg bid
Metoprolol succinate extended-release (Toprol-XL®)	Oral tablet	12.5-200 mg qd

- Fatigue or weakness may occur in the first few weeks of treatment, but will usually resolve spontaneously.

- Report any cases of dizziness, lightheadedness, or blurred vision. These may be caused by blood pressure being too low or from bradycardia or heart block.

- Take carvedilol with food.

- It is important not to miss doses or abruptly stop taking these medications.

- If patients have diabetes, β-blockers may cause their blood sugar to rise and mask the signs of hypoglycemia except for sweating.

Adverse drug events
- The adverse events listed below are the most common observed in heart failure patients receiving β-blockers. For other adverse effects of β-blockers, see the chapters on hypertension and ischemic heart disease.
    * Fluid retention and worsening heart failure
    * Fatigue
    * Bradycardia and heart block
    * Hypotension
    * Abrupt withdrawal can lead to hypertension, tachycardia, or myocardial ischemia.

Drug-drug and drug-disease interactions
- Amiodarone and calcium channel blockers (verapamil and diltiazem): increased risk of bradycardia, heart block, hypotension

- Quinidine, fluoxetine, paroxetine, and other inhibitors of cytochrome P450 2D6: inhibit hepatic metabolism of metoprolol and carvedilol and may result in increased plasma concentrations and enhanced effects.

- Ophthalmic β-blockers increase risk of bradycardia, heart block, and hypotension.

- May cause bronchoconstriction in patients with asthma or COPD.

- Should not use in patients with symptomatic bradycardia or heart block unless a pacemaker is present.

- May worsen blood glucose control in diabetics and mask the signs of hypoglycemia.

Parameters to monitor
- Blood pressure and heart rate

- Heart failure symptoms

- Weigh daily

Kinetics
- Bisoprolol is eliminated about 50% by the kidneys, so dosage adjustment may be required in patients with renal insufficiency.

- Both metoprolol and carvedilol are metabolized by the liver.

Other
- Patients must be stable (ie, minimal evidence of fluid overload or volume retention) before β-blocker treatment is initiated.

- Treatment should be initiated with low doses and titrated slowly upward until the target dose is reached. Doses are usually increased no more frequently than every 2 weeks with close monitoring of symptoms required during this titration period.

- Fluid accumulation during dose titration can usually be managed by adjusting diuretic doses.

- Staggering the schedule of other heart failure medications that lower blood pressure (eg, ACE inhibitors and diuretics) may help reduce risk of hypotension.

Digoxin

- Unlike ACE inhibitors or β-blockers, digoxin does not improve mortality, but does appear to produce symptomatic benefits (Table 4).

Table 4

Digoxin

Generic name (trade name)	Dosage form	Dosage range and frequency
Digoxin (Lanoxin®)	Oral tablet, IV, elixir	0.125-0.25 mg qd
Digoxin (Lanoxicaps®)	Oral capsule	0.1-0.2 qd

Mechanism of action

- Inhibits the Na^+-K^+ ATPase pump, which results in an increase in intracellular calcium, that in turn causes a positive inotropic effect.

- Recent evidence indicates that digoxin reduces sympathetic outflow from the central nervous system, thus blunting the excessive sympathetic activation that occurs in heart failure. These effects occur at low plasma concentrations where little positive inotropic effect is seen.

Patient instructions and counseling

- The patient should report to their health care provide if any of the following occur:
    * Dizziness, lightheadedness, fatigue
    * Changes in vision (blurred or yellow vision)
    * Irregular heartbeat
    * Loss of appetite
    * Nausea, vomiting, or diarrhea

Adverse drug events

- Major adverse effects involve three systems:
    * Cardiovascular: cardiac arrhythmias, bradycardia, and heart block
    * Gastrointestinal: anorexia, abdominal pain, nausea, and vomiting
    * Neurological: visual disturbances, disorientation, confusion, fatigue

- Toxicity is more commonly associated with serum digoxin concentrations >2 ng/mL but may occur at lower levels if patients have hypokalemia, hypomagnesemia, and in the elderly.

Drug-drug and drug-disease interactions

- Drugs that increase serum digoxin concentrations:
    * Quinidine, verapamil, amiodarone: the dose of digoxin should be decreased by 50% if these medications are added
    * Propafenone
    * Flecainide
    * Macrolide antibiotics: erythromycin and clarithromycin
    * Itraconazole
    * Spironolactone
    * Cyclosporine

- Drugs that decrease serum digoxin concentrations:
    * Antacids
    * Cholestyramine, colestipol
    * Kaolin-pectin
    * Metoclopramide

- Diuretics: increase risk of digoxin toxicity in the presence of hypokalemia or hypomagnesemia

- Digoxin clearance reduced in patients with renal insufficiency (see section on kinetics)

Parameters to monitor

- Digoxin serum concentration
    * Little relationship between serum digoxin concentration and therapeutic effects in heart failure
    * Current guidelines suggest a target range of 0.5-1.0 ng/mL.

- Heart rate

- Serum potassium and magnesium

- Renal function: serum BUN and creatinine

- Heart failure symptoms

Kinetics (Table 5)

- Approximately 60-80% of the dose is eliminated unchanged in the kidney. Dosage adjustment is required in patients with renal insufficiency.

- Lower doses (0.125 mg daily or every other day) should be used in the elderly or patients with a low lean body mass.

- No loading dose is needed in the treatment of heart failure.

- Because of the long distribution phase after either oral or intravenous digoxin administration, blood samples for determination of serum digoxin concentrations should be collected at least 6 and preferably 12 hours or more after the last dose.

Table 5

Digoxin Pharmacokinetics

Oral bioavailability	
Tablets	0.5-0.9 (average 0.65)
Elixir	0.75-0.85 (average 0.80)
Capsules	0.9-1.0 (average 0.95)

Elimination half-life	
Normal renal function	36 hours
Anuric patients	5 days
Volume of disribution	7 L/kg
Fraction excreted unchanged in urine	0.65-0.70

Angiotensin Receptor Blockers (ARBs)

- ARBs offer an alternative to ACE inhibitors for inhibiting the actions of angiotensin II. Their precise role in the pharmacotherapy of heart failure remains to be defined (for more information on ARBs, see the chapter on hypertension). They should not be considered equivalent or superior to ACE inhibitors, be used in patients who have not used ACE inhibitors before, or be substituted for ACE inhibitors in patients who are tolerating ACE inhibitors. They can be considered as alternatives to ACE inhibitors in patients who are intolerant of ACE inhibitors due to intractable cough or angioedema. ARBs are as likely as ACE inhibitors to cause hypotension, hyperkalemia, and renal insufficiency. There is no evidence that an ARB is of additional benefit when added to an adequate dose of an ACE inhibitor. Valsartan is approved for the treatment of heart failure in patients who cannot tolerate ACE inhibitors; it is the only ARB approved for this indication.

Aldosterone Antagonists

- Elevated plasma aldosterone plays an important detrimental role in the pathophysiology and progression of heart failure. Although short-term treatment with ACE inhibitors lowers circulating aldosterone concentrations, this suppression is not sustained with long-term therapy. In low doses, the aldosterone antagonist spironolactone reduces the risk of death and hospitalization in patients with moderate to severe heart failure. Current guidelines recommend the addition of low-dose spironolactone in patients with recent or recurrent symptoms at rest despite the use of digoxin, diuretics, ACE inhibitors, and (usually) a β-blocker.

Mechanism of action
- Antagonism of aldosterone results in reduced renal potassium excretion.

Patient instructions and counseling
- Avoid potassium-containing salt substitutes.

- Call physician immediately for muscle weakness or cramps; numbness or tingling in hands, feet, or lips; or slow or irregular heartbeat

- May cause swollen or painful breasts in men

Adverse drug events
- Hyperkalemia

- Gynecomastia

- Irregular menses

Drug-drug and drug-disease interactions
- ACE inhibitors and ARBs can increase risk of hyperkalemia.

- Can increase digoxin plasma concentrations

- Potassium supplements

Parameters to monitor
- Serum creatinine: should be <2.5 mg/dL before therapy is initiated

- Serum potassium: should be <5.0 mEq/L before therapy is initiated

Hydralazine-Isosorbide Dinitrate

- Initially combined because of complementary hemodynamic actions. An early clinical trial reported reduced mortality compared to placebo with this combination. A comparison with an ACE inhibitor showed that the ACE inhibitorr was superior to hydralazine-isosorbide. Adverse effects with the combination are common (primarily headache and gastrointestinal complaints), and result in many patients discontinuing therapy. Can be considered a therapeutic option in patients who experience cough, hypotension, or renal insufficiency while taking ACE inhibitors.

Table 6

Aldosterone Antagonist

Generic name (trade name)	Dosage form	Dosage range and frequency
Spironolactone (Aldactone®)	Oral tablet	25-50 mg qd or qod

3. Drug Therapy of Advanced or Decompensated Heart Failure

- Patients with advanced or decompensated heart failure are usually admitted to the hospital for aggressive treatment with IV diuretics, vasodilators, and positive inotropic drugs. Treatment goals are to reduce volume overload and improve cardiac output. The approach to treatment is dictated by the patient's hemodynamic profile.

Warm and dry
- No specific therapy is needed.

Warm and wet
- Goal is to reduce volume overload and minimize congestive symptoms

- IV loop diuretics are often used. For patients unresponsive to loop diuretics, addition of supplemental thiazide diuretics (eg, metolazone) may be helpful.

- Addition of IV vasodilators (nitroglycerin, nitroprusside, and nesiritide) can also reduce symptoms.

- Inotropic therapy is usually not necessary.

Cold and dry
- May be clinically stable and often don't present with acute symptoms

- Need to rule out volume depletion from over diuresis as the cause of decreased cardiac output.

- Gradual introduction of β-blockers may be helpful.

Cold and wet
- Improve cardiac output first (ie, before removing excess volume).

- Cardiac output can be increased by IV vasodilators and/or inotropes.

- Relative roles of vasodilators and inotropes in this patient population is controversial.

Vasodilators
- See Table 7.

Inotropes
- See Table 8.

Table 7

Vasodilators

Generic name (brand name)	Mechanism of action	Dose[1]	Adverse effects and comments
Nitroprusside (Nipride®)	Arterial and venous dilator	Initial dose 0.1-0.25 µg/kg per min and titrate to response	Hypotension, headache, tachycardia, cyanide and thiocyanate toxicity, myocardial ischemia
Nitroglycerin (Nitro-Bid®, Nitrostat®)	Venous dilator but also an arterial dilator at higher doses	Initial dose 5-10 µg/min and titrate to response	Hypotension, headache, tachycardia, tolerance to hemodynamic effects
Nesiritide (Natrecor®)	B-type natriuretic peptide that increases diuresis and is an arterial and venous dilator	Initially 2 µg/kg bolus followed by 0.01 µg/kg per min infusion; can increase to 0.03 µg/kg per min	Hypotension, headache when used in combination with diuretics

[1]All are given by continuous IV infusion.

Table 8

Inotropes

Generic name (brand name)	Mechanism of action	Dose[1]	Adverse effects and comments
Dopamine (Intropin®)	Dose-dependent agonist of dopamine and β and α_1 receptors	0-3 μg/kg per min: stimulates dopamine receptors (may improve urine output) 3-10 μg/kg per min: stimulates β_1 and β_2 receptors to increase cardiac output >10 μg/kg per min: stimulates α_1 receptors to increase blood pressure	Increases heart rate, contractility, myocardial oxygen demand, myocardial ischemia, arrhythmias, and systemic vascular resistance; should only be used in patients with marked systemic hypotension or cardiogenic shock
Dobutamine (Dobutrex®)	β_1- and β_2-receptor agonist and weak α_1 agonist; increases cardiac output and vasodilates	2.5-20 μg/kg per min	Increases heart rate, contractility, myocardial oxygen demand, myocardial ischemia, arrhythmias; not useful to increase blood pressure in hypotensive patients
Milrinone (Primacor®)	Inhibits phosphodiesterase III, resulting in positive inotropic and vasodilating effects	50 μg/kg loading dose over 10 mins, followed by 0.375 μg/kg per min; can titrate to 0.75 μg/kg per min based on response	Arrhythmias, hypotension, headache; alternative to patients not responding to dobutamine or dopamine; may be useful in patients receiving β-blockers since its positive inotropic effects are not mediated by β receptors; adjust dose in patients with renal insufficiency; preferred over amrinone because of decreased risk of thrombocytopenia

[1]All are given by continuous IV infusion.

4. Nondrug therapy

Intra-aortic balloon pump

Left ventricular assist devices

Biventricular pacing

Cardiac transplantation

5. Key Points

- Heart failure is a clinical syndrome caused by the inability of the heart to pump sufficient blood to meet the needs of the body.

- Although there are many causes of heart failure, the most common are coronary artery disease and hypertension.

- A number of compensatory mechanisms are activated to help maintain adequate cardiac output and activation of these systems is responsible for heart failure symptoms and contribute to disease progression. Medications that improve patient outcomes antagonize these compensatory mechanisms.

- Drugs that can precipitate or worsen heart failure should be avoided (eg, NSAIDs, verapamil, diltiazem).

- All patients with stage C (symptomatic) heart failure should be treated with diuretics, ACE inhibitors, β-blockers, and digoxin.

- The goal of treatment with diuretics is to eliminate signs of fluid retention, thus minimizing symptoms.

- ACE inhibitors are an integral part of heart failure pharmacotherapy. They improve survival and slow disease progression.

- β-Blockers are recommended for all patients with systolic dysfunction and mild to moderate symptoms. They improve survival, decrease hospitalizations, and slow disease progression. The agents with proven benefits are bisoprolol, carvedilol, and metoprolol extended release. They should be started at low doses with slow upward titration to the target dose.

- Digoxin does not improve survival in patients with heart failure but does provide symptomatic benefits. The goal plasma concentration is 0.5-1.0 ng/mL.

- Spironolactone improves survival in patients with moderate to severe heart failure.

- Patients with advanced or decompensated heart failure often require hospitalization and aggressive therapy with IV diuretics, vasodilators, and positive inotropic drugs.

6. **Questions and Answers**

1. Which of the following combinations represents optimal pharmacotherapy of heart failure?

   A. Furosemide, clonidine, hydrochlorothiazide, and propranolol
   B. Furosemide, lisinopril, digoxin, and carvedilol
   C. Carvedilol, verapamil, amlodipine, and nesiritide
   D. Diltiazem, hydrochlorothiazide, digoxin, and furosemide
   E. Dobutamine, milrinone, furosemide, and nitroglycerin

2. Which of the following mechanisms most likely contributes to the benefits of β-blockers in the treatment of heart failure?

   A. Stimulation of β_2 receptors
   B. Increased heart rate and decreased blood pressure
   C. Increased plasma norepinephrine
   D. Blockade of increased sympathetic nervous system activity
   E. Blockade of angiotensin II receptors

3. Appropriate monitoring parameters for enalapril therapy of heart failure include

   I. Serum creatinine
   II. Serum potassium
   III. Serum calcium

   A. I only
   B. III only
   C. I and II only
   D. II and III only
   E. I, II, and III

4. Patients taking spironolactone for heart failure should avoid taking

   A. Potassium supplements
   B. ACE inhibitors
   C. β-blockers
   D. Furosemide
   E. Calcium supplements

5. All of the following are adverse effects of digoxin EXCEPT

   A. Nausea
   B. Anorexia

C. Confusion
D. Arrhythmias
E. Hypotension

6. Heart failure may be exacerbated by which of the following medications?

I. Naprosyn
II. Glucotrol
III. Zocor

A. I only
B. III only
C. I and II only
D. II and III only
E. I, II, and III

7. Cough is an adverse effect associated with which of the following medications?

A. Vasotec
B. Diovan
C. Coreg
D. Torsemide
E. Aldactone

8. Which of the following ACE inhibitors has the shortest duration of action?

A. Ramipril
B. Capoten
C. Prinivil
D. Monopril
E. Fosinopril

9. Valsartan can be used for treating heart failure in patients intolerant to

A. Inocor
B. Demadex
C. Vasotec
D. Toprol-XL
E. Zebeta

10. A significant interaction can occur if digoxin is administered with

A. Clarithromycin
B. Fosinopril
C. Glyburide
D. Pravastatin
E. Warfarin

11. All of the following medications can cause bradycardia EXCEPT

A. Coreg
B. Amiodarone
C. Digoxin
D. Calan
E. Dobutamine

12. Which of the following is contraindicated in patients with a history of Prinivil-induced angioedema?

A. Vasotec
B. Bumex
C. Spironolactone
D. Milrinone
E. Aspirin

13. Natrecor would be indicated in

A. Patients with asymptomatic left ventricular dysfunction
B. Patients with acute decompensated heart failure not responsive to iv diuretics
C. Patients with stage B heart failure
D. Patients with type 2 diabetes
E. Patients intolerant to digoxin

14. All of the following are true about the use of furosemide in heart failure EXCEPT

A. The drug reduces mortality and slows heart failure progression
B. Hypokalemia is a common adverse effect
C. Response can be evaluated by monitoring patient weight
D. Oral absorption is slowed in patients with advanced or decompensated heart failure
E. The bioavailability is reduced by food

15. Which of the following is an important consideration when using β-blockers for treating heart failure?

A. They are only effective in post-MI patients
B. Cardioselective agents are more effective than nonselective agents
C. Therapy should be initiated at the target dose
D. Patients with fluid overload are the optimal candidates for initiating therapy
E. Therapy should be initiated at low doses and titrated upward slowly

16. The dose of which of the following medications should be reduced in patients with renal insufficiency?

A. Toprol-XL

B. Carvedilol
C. Lanoxin
D. Nitroglycerin
E. Dobutrex

17. The plasma concentration of digoxin is NOT affected by

   A. Renal function
   B. Amiodarone
   C. Quinidine
   D. Coreg
   E. Kaopectate

18. Which of the following β-blockers also blocks α_1 receptors and is effective for treating heart failure?

   A. Toprol-XL
   B. Coreg
   C. Zebeta
   D. Inderal
   E. Tenormin

19. Patients with heart failure that experience fluid retention after β-blocker initiation should have

   A. The β-blocker dose increased
   B. The digoxin dose increased
   C. The β-blocker discontinued
   D. Their ACE inhibitor discontinued
   E. Adjustment of their diuretic dose

20. Which of the following agents should be used in patients with advanced or decompensated heart failure and hypotension?

   A. Dopamine
   B. Milrinone
   C. Nitroprusside
   D. Dobutamine
   E. Hydralazine

Use Patient Profile #1 to answer Questions 21 and 22.

21. Which of the following medications should be added to Mr. Johnson's regimen?

Patient Profile #1

Patient Name	William Johnson		
Age	64	Height	5'11"
Sex	Male	Weight	185 lbs
Allergies	NKA		

DIAGNOSIS	Myocardial infarction 1999
	Hypertension
	Heart failure
	Hyperlipidemia

LABORATORY AND DIAGNOSTIC TESTS

Echocardiogram in 12/02 showed LV ejection fraction 30%

Blood pressure on 4/1/03: 145/90 mm Hg

Heart rate on 4/1/03: 88 bpm

Lipid profile on 4/1/03:

Total cholesterol 160 mg/dL

LDL cholesterol 95 mg/dL

HDL cholesterol 50 mg/dL

Triglycerides 100 mg/dL

Serum potassium 2.0 mg/dL

MEDICATION RECORD

Date	Rx #	Physician	Drug/Strength	Quantity	Sig	Refills
4/1	1000	Smith	Lanoxin 0.125 mg	90	1 tab qd	2
4/1	1001	Smith	Lasix 40 mg	60	1 tab q AM	3
4/1	1002	Smith	KCl 20 mEq	90	1 tab q AM	1
4/1	1003	Smith	Zocor 40 mg	90	1 tab qhs	3
4/1	1004	Smith	EC aspirin 325 mg	90	1 tab q AM	2

A. Lisinopril and Toprol-XL
B. Valsartan and prazosin
C. Demadex and Norvasc
D. Isoptin and Lopid
E. Clonidine and hydrochlorothiazide

22. Mr. Johnson's serum potassium level of 2.0 mEq/L (normal 4.0-5.0 mEq/L) could

   A. Increase the risk of Lanoxin toxicity
   B. Be treated by increasing the dose of Lasix
   C. Be considered a side effect of therapy with EC aspirin
   D. Be caused by an interaction between Zocor and Lanoxin
   E. Increase his blood pressure

Use Hospital Inpatient Profile #2 to answer Questions 23 and 24.

23. Based on her profile, the recent worsening of Mrs. Jones's heart failure is most likely related to

   A. Zestril
   B. Ibuprofen
   C. Subtherapeutic serum digoxin concentration
   D. Furosemide.

E. Drug interaction between Zestril and furosemide

24. Toprol-XL is an agent that

   A. Is contraindicated in heart failure
   B. Blocks β_1, β_2, and α_1 receptors
   C. Blocks only β_1 receptors
   D. Should not be used in combination with Zestril
   E. Increases the serum digoxin concentration

Answers

1. **B.** Furosemide, lisinopril (an ACE inhibitor), digoxin, and carvedilol (a β-blocker) in combination should routinely be used in patients with heart failure.

2. **D.** Activation of the sympathetic nervous system plays an important role in the initiation and progression of heart failure. The benefits of β-blockers are thought to be due to blockade of this increased activity of the sympathetic nervous system.

3. **C.** Enalapril, as well as other ACE inhibitors, can cause renal insufficiency and an increase in

Hospital Inpatient Profile #2

Patient Name	Ellen Smith		
Age	71	Height	5'4"
Sex	Female	Weight	150 lbs
Allergies	NKA		

DIAGNOSIS   Heart failure exacerbation with 20-lb weight gain over last 3-4 weeks
Hypertension
Osteoarthritis

LABORATORY AND DIAGNOSTIC TESTS
Echocardiogram in 2/03 showed LV ejection fraction 25%
Blood pressure on 4/1/03: 130/85 mm Hg
Heart rate on 4/1/03: 80 bpm
Serum digoxin concentration on 4/1/03: 0.8 ng/mL

MEDICATION RECORD

Date	Rx #	Physician	Drug/Strength	Quantity	Sig	Refills
2/1	100	Jones	Lanoxin 0.125 mg	90	1 tab qd	2
3/1	101	Jones	Furosemide 80 mg	60	1 tab q AM	3
1/1	102	Jones	Zestril 20 mEq	90	1 tab q AM	1
1/1	103	Jones	Toprol-XL 50 mg	90	1 tab qd	3
3/1	1004	Nelson	Ibuprofen 600 mg	90	1 tab qid with food	3

serum potassium. Thus serum creatinine and potassium should be monitored.

4. **A.** Use of spironolactone is associated with renal potassium retention. Concomitant use of potassium supplements significantly increases the risk of hyperkalemia.

5. **E.** Nausea, anorexia, confusion, and arrhythmias are all common signs and symptoms of digoxin toxicity. Digoxin does not affect blood pressure.

6. **A.** Naprosyn, an NSAID, can worsen heart failure by increasing renal sodium and water retention and by attenuating the efficacy and enhancing the toxicity of ACE inhibitors and diuretics. Neither Glucotrol or Zocor affect heart failure.

7. **A.** Cough is a frequently encountered adverse effect of ACE inhibitors.

8. **B.** Capoten must be given three times daily in patients with heart failure. The other agents can be given once daily.

9. **C.** The angiotensin receptor blocker valsartan is an alternative agent for patients intolerant to ACE inhibitors.

10. **A.** The macrolide antibiotic clarithromycin is associated with a 50-100% increase in serum digoxin concentrations.

11. **E.** Dobutamine is a β-receptor agonist and is associated with an increase in heart rate. The other choices all slow heart rate through various mechanisms.

12. **A.** Prinivil (lisinopril) is an ACE inhibitor and angioedema is a known adverse effect of all agents in this class. Thus Vasotec (enalapril), which is also an ACE inhibitor, should not be used in this situation.

13. B. Natrecor (nesiritide) is only indicated for use in patients with severe or decompensated heart failure. It can only be given intravenously.

14. **A.** Although furosemide plays an important role in patients with heart failure by interfering with sodium and water retention, they only provide symptomatic benefit. Neither furosemide nor other diuretics improve survival or affect heart failure progression.

15. **E.** When used in heart failure, β-blocker therapy should be started at low doses and gradually titrated upward to the target dose that was established in clinical trials to improve survival. Starting at the target dose or initiating treatment in patients with fluid overload increases the risk of worsening heart failure.

16. **C.** Only Lanoxin (digoxin) is eliminated by the kidneys.

17. **D.** Renal insufficiency reduces digoxin clearance and results in increased plasma concentrations. Amiodarone and quinidine both increase digoxin concentrations by 50-100%. Kaopectate can reduce digoxin concentrations by binding it in the gut, thus reducing absorption.

18. **B.** Only Coreg (carvedilol) blocks α receptors and has been shown to be effective in patients with heart failure.

19. **E.** Some patients with heart failure may experience increases in fluid retention after initiation of β-blocker therapy. This can usually be best managed by adjustment of the diuretic dose and close monitoring of patient weight.

20. **A.** Dopamine is a β- and α-receptor agonist and is useful in patients with severe heart failure and hypotension. The other agents listed all have vasodilatory effects and are not useful for increasing blood pressure.

21. **A.** An ACE inhibitor and β-blocker are indicated in this patient with heart failure to improve survival and slow disease progression.

22. **A.** Hypokalemia increases the risk of digoxin toxicity.

23. **B.** The addition of the NSAID ibuprofen ~3-4 weeks before admission is the likely cause of this episode of decompensated heart failure. NSAIDs can increase sodium and water retention and negate the effects of diuretics and ACE inhibitors.

24. **C.** Toprol-XL (metoprolol succinate) is a cardioselective β-blocker. It blocks only the β_1 receptor at usual therapeutic doses.

7. References

Brater DC. Diuretic therapy. *N Engl J Med.* 1998;339:387-395.

Cohn JN, Tognoni G, for the Valsartan Heart Failure Trial Investigators. A randomized trial of the angiotensin receptor blocker valsartan in chronic heart failure. *N Engl J Med.* 2001;345:1667-1675.

Effect of metoprolol CR/XL in chronic heart failure: Metoprolol CR/XL Randomised Intervention Trial in Congestive Heart Failure (MERIT-HF). *Lancet.* 1999;353:2001-2007.

Flather MD, Yusuf S, Kober L, et al. for the ACE-Inhibitor Myocardial Infarction Collaborative Group. Long term ACE-inhibitor therapy in patients with heart failure or left-ventricular dysfunction: A systematic overview of data from individual patients. *Lancet.* 2000;355:1575-1581.

Goldstein S. Benefits of beta-blocker therapy in heart failure. Weighing the evidence. *Arch Intern Med.* 2002;162:641-648.

Hunt SA, Baker DW, Chin MH, et al. ACC/AHA guidelines for the evaluation and management of chronic heart failure in the adult: a report of the American College of Cardiology/American Heart Association Task Force on Practice Guidelines (Committee to revise the 1995 guidelines for the evaluation and management of heart failure), 2001. Available at http://www.acc.org/clinical/guidelines/failure/hf_index.htm.

Johnson JA, Parker RB, Patterson JH. Heart failure. In: DiPiro JT, Talbert RL, Yee GC, et al, eds. *Pharmacotherapy: A Pathophysiologic Approach,* 5th ed. New York: McGraw-Hill; 2002:185-218.

Nohria A, Lewis E, Stevenson LW. Medical management of advanced heart failure. *JAMA.* 2002;287:628-640.

Packer M, Bristow MR, Cohn JN, et al. The effect of carvedilol on morbidity and mortality in patients with chronic heart failure. U.S. Carvedilol Heart Failure Study Group. *N Engl J Med.* 1996;334:1349-1355.

Pitt B, Zannad F, Remme WJ, et al. The effect of spironolactone on morbidity and mortality in patients with severe heart failure. Randomized Aldactone Evaluation Study Investigators. *N Engl J Med.* 1999;341:709-717.

Reuning RH, Geraets DR, Rocci ML, Vlasses PH. Digoxin. In: Evans WE, Schentag JJ, Jusko WJ, eds. *Applied Pharmacokinetics: Principles of Therapeutic Drug Monitoring.* Spokane, WA: Applied Therapeutics, Inc.; 1992:20-1 to 20-48.

The Digitalis Investigation Group. The effect of digoxin on mortality and morbidity in patients with heart failure. *N Engl J Med.* 1997;336:525-533.

10. Cardiac Arrhythmias

Scott D. Hanes, PharmD
Assistant Professor, Department of Pharmacy
University of Tennessee College of Pharmacy

Contents

1. **Overview**

2. **Drug and Nondrug Therapy**

3. **Key Points**

4. **Questions and Answers**

5. **References**

1. Overview

- Cardiac arrhythmias are abnormal heart rhythms resulting from alterations in impulse formation and conduction.

Electrophysiology

Impulse generation (automaticity) and conduction
- Initiation and propagation of the electrical impulse in cardiac cells is dependent on regulation of the action potential.

- Conduction velocity is determined by regulation of action potential, specifically the refractory period.

- The *absolute refractory period* is the time during which cardiac cells cannot conduct or propagate an action potential (Figure 1 and Table 1).

- The *relative refractory period* is the time during which cardiac cells may conduct and propagate action potentials secondary to strong electrical stimulus.

Normal conduction system
- The sinoatrial (SA) node initiates an impulse, which:
    * Stimulates the left atrium and atrioventricular (AV) node, which
    * Stimulates the left and right bundle branches via the bundle of His, which then
    * Stimulates Purkinje fibers and causes ventricular contraction.

Figure 1.

Action potential for atrial and ventricular tissue.

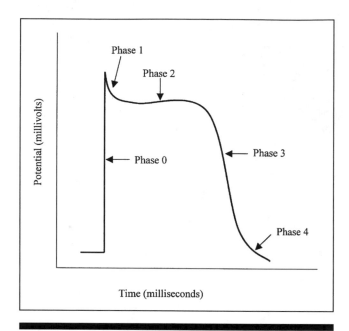

Mechanisms of Arrhythmia

- Cardiac arrhythmias arise secondary to disorders of:
    * Automaticity (impulse generation)
    * Latent pacemaker (non–SA node pacemaker)
    * Triggered automaticity (early or late after-depolarizations)
    * Reentry
    * Conduction
    * Automaticity and conduction

Table 1

Phases of Atrial and Ventricular Tissue Action Potential

Phase	Process	Ion flow	Corresponding ECG
0	Depolarization	Na^+ fast channel opens, Na^+ enters cell	Atrial: p wave; ventricular: QRS
1	Initial repolarization	Na^+ channel closes; passive Cl^- influx	
2	Prolongs depolarized state	Predominantly Ca^{2+} enters cell	ST segment
3	Repolarization	Rapid efflux of K^+ out of cell	T wave
4	Repolarization	Na^+ leaks into cell, K^+ pumped out of cell	

Clinical Manifestations

Symptoms

- Except for ventricular tachycardia and ventricular fibrillation, the patient may be asymptomatic.

- Symptoms generally related to poor cardiac output include dizziness, syncope, chest pain, fatigue, confusion, and exacerbation of heart failure.

- Patients with tachyarrhythmias may report palpitations.

- With atrial fibrillation/flutter, patients also experience signs and symptoms of transient ischemic attack (TIA) or stroke.

Signs

- Electrocardiogram (ECG) abnormalities

- Ventricular rate can be assessed by documenting the heart rate from the radial artery or carotid palpation.

Diagnostic Criteria and Therapy According to Arrhythmia Classification

Arrhythmias are defined by:
- Anatomic location
    * Supraventricular: these arise from abnormalities in the SA node, atrial tissue, the AV node, or bundle of His.
    * Ventricular: these are impulses originating from below the bundle of His.

- Ventricular rate:
    * Bradycardia: heart rate <60 bpm
    * Tachycardia: heart rate >100 bpm

Supraventricular Arrhythmias

Bradyarrhythmias
Sinus bradycardia
Diagnostic criteria and characteristics
* HR <60 bpm; otherwise normal ECG

Mechanism of arrhythmia
* Decreased SA node automaticity

Clinical etiology
* Acute myocardial infarction, hypothyroidism, drug-induced (β-blockers, digoxin, calcium channel blockers, cholinergic agents), hyperkalemia

Treatment goals
* Restore normal sinus rhythm if patient is clinically symptomatic.

Drug and nondrug therapy
* Intermittent episodes: atropine 0.5-1 mg IV repeated up to maximum dose of 3 mg. In denervated heart, use isoproterenol.
* For persistent episodes or if atropine nonresponsive: place transvenous or transcutaneous pacemaker.

Atrioventricular (AV) block
Diagnostic criteria and characteristics
* *First-degree*: prolonged PR interval >0.20 seconds, 1:1 atrioventricular conduction
* *Second-degree Mobitz type I*: gradual prolongation of PR interval followed by p wave without ventricular conduction
* *Second-degree Mobitz type II*: constant PR interval with intermittent p wave without ventricular contraction; often widened QRS complex
* *Third-degree*: HR 30-60 bpm; no temporal relation between atrial and ventricular contraction; ventricular contraction initiated by AV junction or ventricular tissue.

Mechanism of arrhythmia
* Prolonged conduction

Clinical etiology
* AV nodal disease, acute myocardial infarction, myocarditis, increased vagal tone, drug-induced (b-blockers, digoxin, calcium channel blockers, cholinergic agents), hyperkalemia

Treatment goals
* Restore sinus rhythm if patient is symptomatic

Drug and nondrug therapy
* If cause is reversible: temporary pacemaker or intermittent atropine; if chronic, implant permanent pacemaker.

Tachyarrhythmias
Atrial fibrillation and atrial flutter
Diagnostic criteria and characteristics
* Fibrillation: no p waves, irregularly, irregular QRS pattern
* Flutter: saw-tooth p wave pattern; regular QRS pattern

Mechanism of arrhythmia
* Enhanced automaticity and reentrant circuits

Clinical etiology
* Rheumatic heart disease, heart failure, ischemic heart disease, pericarditis, cardiomyopathy, mitral valve prolapse, cardiac surgery, infection, alcohol abuse, hyperthyroidism, chronic obstructive pulmonary disease, pulmonary embolism, idiopathic (lone atrial fibrillation)

Specific treatment goals for atrial fibrillation (Figure 2)
* Control ventricular rate.
  * Digoxin (slow-onset, poor control in hyper-adrenergic-induced AF)

Figure 2.

Treatment algorithm for atrial fibrillation.

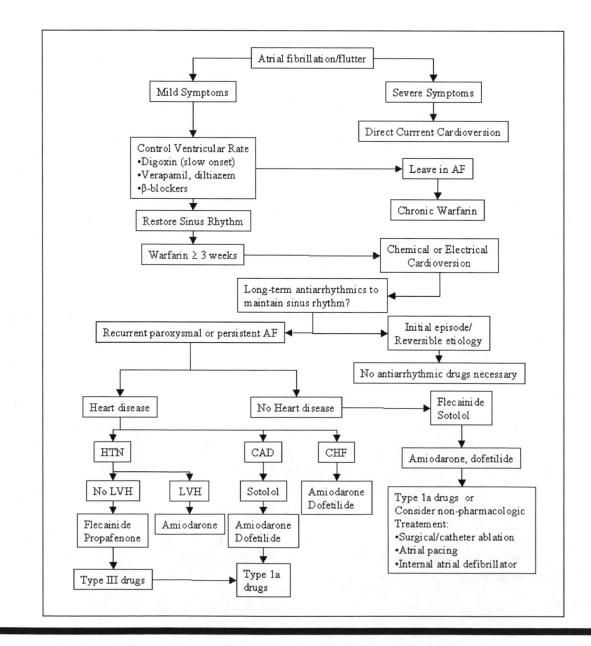

CAD, coronary artery disease; CHF, congestive heart failure; HTN, hypertension; LVH, left ventricular hypertrophy.

* β-Blockers (esmolol, metoprolol, propranolol, others)
* Calcium channel blockers (diltiazem, verapamil)
* Digoxin, calcium channel blockers, and β-blockers do not restore sinus rhythm

Restore and maintain sinus rhythm
* Chronic antiarrhythmic therapy reserved for recurrent, symptomatic episodes.

Prevent thromboembolism
* Pharmacologic or direct-current (DC) cardioversion: if atrial fibrillation present for >48 hours, anticoagulate for 3-4 weeks prior to cardioversion unless transesophageal echocardiogram (TEE) rules out atrial thrombus.
* Postcardioversion, continue anticoagulation for at least 4 weeks.
* Risk factors for nonvalvular atrial fibrillation thromboembolism:
  • Previous stroke or TIA
  • Hypertension
  • Congestive heart failure
  • Increasing age
  • Diabetes mellitus
  • Coronary artery disease

Recommended antithrombotic therapy
* *Aspirin 325 mg daily*:
  Age <60 years and no heart disease
  Age <60 years and heart disease but no risk factors (risk factors: heart failure, hypertension, left ventricular ejection fraction <35%)
  Age ≥60 years and no risk factors
* *Warfarin (INR 2-3)*:
  Age ≥75 and diabetes or coronary artery disease
  Heart failure
* *Warfarin (INR 2.5-3.5 or higher)*:
  Rheumatic heart disease
  Prosthetic heart valve
  Prior thromboembolism
  Persistent atrial thrombus

Warfarin (Coumadin®)
Dosage forms
• Tablets (Coumadin):
  * 1 mg (pink), 2 mg (lavender), 2.5 mg (green), 3 mg (tan), 4 mg (blue), 5 mg (peach), 6 mg (teal), 7.5 mg (yellow), 10 mg (white)

• Injections (intravenous):
  * 5 mg powder for reconstitution (2 mg/mL)

Mechanism of action
• Inhibits vitamin K epoxide-reductase and vitamin K reductase, preventing the conversion of vitamin K-epoxide to vitamin K. Ultimately inhibits formation of vitamin K-dependent coagulation factors II, VII, IX, and X, as well as proteins C and S.

Pharmacokinetics
Absorption
• Bioavailability 80-100% following oral administration

• Absorbed in upper gastrointestinal tract

• Food/enteral feedings may decrease rate and extent of absorption.

Distribution
• 99.0-99.5% protein bound, primarily to albumin

Metabolism and elimination
• Metabolized in the liver via CYP 2C9 (S-(–)-enantiomer) and mixed function CYP enzymes to inactive metabolites

• Low extraction pharmacokinetic characteristics

• Clearance decreases with increasing age

• Half-life: R-(+)-enantiomer, 45 hours; S-(-)-enantiomer, 33 hours

Pharmacodynamics
• The S-isomer is approximately 2-5 times more potent than the R-isomer in inhibiting vitamin K reductase.

• Pharmacodynamic effect (change in INR) is an indirect effect of the decreased formation of coagulation factors II, VII, IX, and X. The long half-lives of these factors results in delayed onset of action and delayed response to dosage changes.

Adverse effects
• Bleeding, roughly proportional to the degree of anticoagulation

• Skin necrosis; related to depletion of or deficiency of protein C. Usually occurs within 10 days of warfarin initiation; incidence is rare.

• Purple-toe syndrome: usually occurs 3-8 weeks after warfarin initiation; incidence is rare.

Common drug interactions

- Medications decreasing warfarin anticoagulant response:
  * Rifampin
  * Barbiturates
  * Carbamazepine
  * Phenytoin (chronic therapy)
  * Cholestyramine
  * Griseofulvin
  * Nafcillin

- Medications increasing warfarin anticoagulant response:
  * Amiodarone
  * Propafenone
  * Cimetidine
  * Clofibrate
  * Omeprazole (R-enantiomer)
  * Erythromycin
  * Metronidazole
  * Trimethoprim-sulfamethoxazole
  * Phenytoin (acute therapy)
  * Allopurinol
  * Phenylbutazone
  * Azole antifungal agents
  * Ciprofloxacin
  * Sulfinpyrazone

Dosing management

- Once-daily dose of 1-10 mg orally; patient response is highly variable.

- Management of elevated INR (Table 2)

Monitoring

- Standard in the international normalized ratio (INR)

- INR = (observed prothrombin ratio)^{ISI} where ISI is the international standardized index which corrects for variability in thromboplastin sensitivity.

- Initially INR is monitored every 1-2 days until the desired INR is achieved and has stabilized at a given dose. Periodic INR monitoring (ie, monthly) is recommended thereafter unless dosage changes are made.

Paroxysmal supraventricular tachycardia (PSVT)

Diagnostic criteria and characteristics
  * PSVT, rate 160-240, that is abrupt in onset and termination, regular QRS interval; 1:1 AV conduction

Mechanism of arrhythmia
  * Reentry

Clinical etiology (Figure 3)
  * Idiopathic, fever, drug-induced (sympathomimetics, anticholinergics, β-agonists)

Treatment goals
  * Acute: terminate reentry circuit by prolonging refractoriness and slowing conduction
  * Chronic: prevent or minimize the number and severity of episodes

- Acute nonpharmacologic therapy:
  * Vagal maneuvers may terminate PSVT: carotid

Table 2

Management of Elevated International Normalized Ratio

INR	Significant bleeding	Recommendations
<5.0 but above therapeutic range	No	Lower dose or omit single dose and restart at lower dose
>5.0 and <9.0	No	Omit 1-2 doses, resume when INR in therapeutic range; alternatively, omit dose and give 1-2.5 mg vitamin K orally (2-4 mg if urgent surgery is required); restart warfarin when INR therapeutic or clinically appropriate
>9.0	No	Hold warfarin and give 3-5 mg vitamin K orally; resume when INR therapeutic
>20.0	Yes	Hold warfarin; give 10 mg vitamin K IV slow infusion[1]; supplement with fresh frozen plasma or prothrombin complex concentrate if necessary; repeat vitamin K 10 mg IV q12h if necessary
Therapeutic and above	Yes, life-threatening	Hold warfarin. Give prothrombin complex concentrate with vitamin K 10 IV slow infusion[1]; repeat as necessary

[1]Infused over at least 10 minutes.

Figure 3.

Treatment algorithm for paroxysmal supraventricular tachycardia.

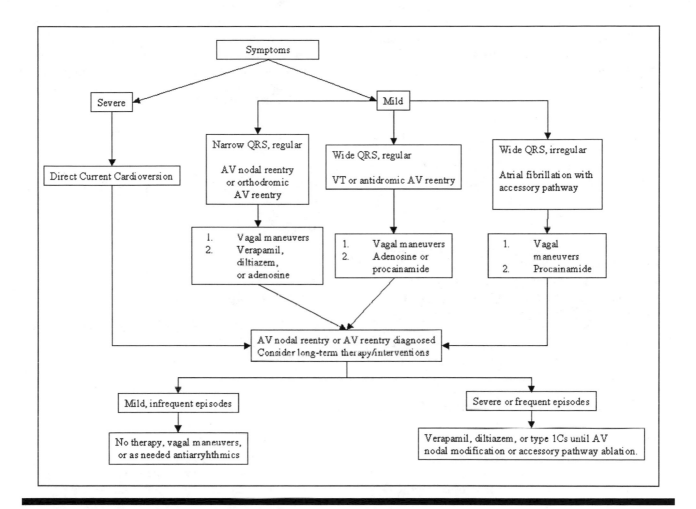

Reproduced with permission from Baurnan et al, 2002.

massage and Valsalva maneuver (most common), squatting, deep breathing, coughing, inducing eyeball pressure, and diving reflex (less common)

Ventricular Arrhythmias

Major classifications and diagnostic criteria and characteristics
Ventricular tachycardia (VT)
- Three or more consecutive premature ventricular contractions (PVCs) at rate >100 bpm; wide QRS interval (>0.12 seconds), usually regular pattern

- Nonsustained VT (NSVT): episode lasting <30 seconds

- Sustained VT: episode lasting >30 seconds

Ventricular fibrillation
- Rapid ventricular rate, irregular pattern, wide QRS interval (>0.12)
  Mechanism of arrhythmia
- Reentry

  Clinical etiology
- Acute myocardial infarction

  Treatment goals
- Restore sinus rhythm

- Minimize recurrences

2. Drug and Nondrug Therapy

Nonsustained ventricular tachycardia
- Patients with heart disease and ejection fraction ≥40%
  * If asymptomatic, no drug therapy is warranted.
  * If symptomatic (palpitations), β-blocker therapy

- Patients with heart disease and ejection fraction <40%, there are three treatment options:
  * Aggressive approach: if rhythm is inducible by electrophysiology studies, treat with intracardiac defibrillator or amiodarone; if rhythm not inducible, treat with β-blockers.
  * Empirically treat with amiodarone
  * Treat with β-blockers

Sustained ventricular tachycardia or ventricular fibrillation (postresuscitation)
- If secondary to myocardial infarction or other reversible causes, no antiarrhythmic drug therapy needed except β-blockers.

- If not secondary to myocardial infarction or other reversible cause, placement of intracardiac defibrillator (ICD) is recommended.

- Antiarrhythmic drugs (ie, amiodarone) may still be required to decrease the number of defibrillator discharges, increase patient comfort, and prolong battery life.

- Amiodarone recommended if patient refuses ICD placement.

- Lidocaine (acute treatment only) or procainamide (acute and chronic treatment) may also be used in place of amiodarone.

Torsades de pointes
- QRS complexes that appear to twist around an axis; associated with prolonged QT interval

Clinical etiology
- Hereditary

- Acquired
  * Hypokalemia, hypomagnesemia
  * Myocardial ischemia or infarction
  * Subarachnoid hemorrhage
  * Hypothyroidism
  * Myocarditis or cardiomyopathy
  * Arsenic poisoning

- Drug-induced (known association with torsades de pointes)
  - Antiarrhythmics: quinidine, procainamide, disopyramide, sotalol, ibutilide, dofetilide, amiodarone
  - Antipsychotics: chlorpromazine, haloperidol, droperidol. mesoridazine, thioridazine, pimozide
  - Antibiotics: erythromycin, clarithromycin, sparfloxacin, pentamidine, trimethoprim-sulfamethoxazole

Treatment
- Stop offending drug, if applicable

- Direct current cardioversion for hemodynamically unstable patient

- Magnesium sulfate 2 g over 1 minute intravenously

- Atrial or ventricular pacing

- Isoproterenol infusion

- Correct hypokalemia or hypomagnesemia

Drug therapy (Tables 3, 4, and 5)

- Antiarrhythmic drugs terminate or minimize dysrhythmia via:
  * Decreasing automaticity of abnormal pacemaker tissues
  * Altering conduction characteristics of reentry
    - Increasing refractory period
  * Eliminating premature impulses that trigger reentry

Table 3

Mechanism of Action of Antiarrhythmic Drugs

Drug class	Ion block	Conduction	Refractory period	Automaticity
Ia	Sodium	↓	↑	↓
Ib	Sodium	0/↓	↓	↓
Ic	Sodium	↓↓	↑	↓
II	Calcium	↓	↑	↓
III	Potassium	0	↑↑	0
IV	Calcium	↓	↑	↓

Sotalol also possesses β-blocking activity

Amiodarone also possesses sodium and calcium channel blockade.

Table 4

Antiarrhythmic Drug Availability and Standard Dosing Regimens

Generic name (trade name)	Dosage forms	Loading dose	Maintenance dose
Class Ia			328-648 mg PO tid
Quinidine gluconate (Quinaglute Dura-Tabs®, Duraquin®, Quinalan®, Quinatime®)	324 mg tablets 80 mg/mL inj	IV: not recommended	
Quinidine sulfate (Quinidex Extentabs®, Cin-Quin®, Quinora®)	200, 300 mg tablets	PO: 200 mg q 2-3 h for 5-8 doses (sulfate salt only)	200-400 mg PO qid
Quinidine polygalacturate (Cardioquin®)	275 mg tablets		275 mg PO bid-tid
Procainamide (Procanbid®, Pronestyl®)	IR: 250, 375, 500 mg capsules/tablets SR: 250, 500, 750 1000 mg tablets 100 and 500 mg/mL inj	IV: 15-18 mg/kg at 20-50 mg/min	IV: 1-6 mg/min PO: up to 50 mg/kg divided q3-6h for immediate release; divided q6h for sustained release
Disopyramide (Norpace®, Norpace CR®)	100, 150 mg capsules 100, 150 mg capsules		150-300 mg q6h 300-600 mg q12h
Moricizine (Ethmozine®)	200, 250, 300 mg tablets		200-300 mg q8h
Class Ib			
Lidocaine	10 mg/mL (5 mL and 10 mL) 20 mg/mL (5 mL) IV infusion: 2 (500 mL), 4 (250, 500, 1000 mL), 8 (250, 500 mL) mg/mL in D5%	IV: 100 mg repeat up to 2 times	IV: 1-4 mg/min
Tocainide (Tonocard®)	400, 600 mg tablets		400-600 mg q8h
Mexiletine (Mexitil®)	150, 200, 250 mg capsules		100-300 mg q8h
Class Ic			
Flecainide (Tambocor®)	50, 100, 150 mg tablets		50-200 mg q12h
Propafenone (Rythmol®)	150, 225, 300 mg tablets		150-300 mg q8h
Class II: β-*blockers*			
Metoprolol (Lopressor®, Toprol XL®)	50, 100 mg tablets 25, 50, 100, 200 mg tablets; 1 mg/mL injection	IV: 2.5-5 mg up to 3 doses	25-450 mg PO daily
Propranolol (Inderal®, Inderal LA®)	10, 20, 40, 60, 80 mg tablets 60, 80, 120, 160 mg capsules 20, 40 mg/mL oral soln 1 mg/mL (5 mL) inj	IV: 0.15 mg/kg IV: 0.5 mg/kg	PO: 80-240 mg daily
Esmolol (Brevibloc®)	10 mg/mL and 250 mg/mL injection		IV: 0.05-0.2 mg/kg/min
Class III			
Bretylium (Bretylol®)	50 mg/mL (10 and 20 mL) for inj In D_5W 2 mg/mL (250 mL), 4 mg/mL (250, 500 mL)		IV: 1-4 mg/min
Amiodarone (Cordarone®)	200, 400 mg tablets 50 mg/mL IV solution	800-1600 mg/d in divided doses x 2-4 weeks IV (VT/VF): 150 mg/10 min or 900 mg in 500 mL D_5W at 1 mg/min x 6 h IV (cardiac arrest): 300 mg	PO: 100-400 mg qd IV: 0.5 mg/min

(continued)

Table 4

Antiarrhythmic Drug Availability and Standard Dosing Regimens (continued)

Generic name (trade name)	Dosage forms	Loading dose	Maintenance dose
Sotolol (Betapace®)	80, 120, 160, 240 mg tablets	0.01 mg/kg IV over 10 min; repeat x 1 if needed	80-320 mg q12h
Ibutilide (Corvert®)	0.1 mg/mL (10 mL) inj		N/A
Dofetilide (Tikosyn®)	125, 250, 500 μg capsules		
			CrCl >60 mL/min = 500 μg bid; 40-60 mL/min = 250 μg bid; 20-39 mL/min = 125 μg bid; <20 mL/min = not recommended
Class IV: calcium channel blockers			
Verapamil (Calan®, Calan SR®, Isoptin SR®, Covera-HS® Verelan®, Verelan-PM®)	40, 80, 120 mg tablets 120, 180, 240 mg tablets 180, 240 mg tablets 120, 180, 240, 360 mg capsules 100, 200, 300 mg capsules	0.25 mg/kg	PO: 120-360 mg/d IV: 5-15 mg/h Calan: tid-qid Calan SR, Isoptin SR, Covera-HS, Verelan: qd
Diltiazem (Cardizem®, Cardizem CD®, Cardizem Monovial Cardizem Lyo-ject Cardizem SR® Cartia XT® Dilacor XR®, Diltiar XT®, Tiazac®)	30, 60, 190, 120 mg tablets; 25 mg/mL injection 120, 180, 240, 300, 360 mg capsules 100 mg/mL injection 25 mg injection 60, 90, 120 mg capsules 120, 180, 240, 300 mg capsules 120, 180, 240 mg tablets 120, 180, 240, 300 mg capsules		IV: 5-15 mg/h; PO: 120-360 mg/d Cardizem: qid Cardizem SR: bid Cardizem CD, Dilacor XR, Tiazac: qd
Miscellaneous			
Atropine	0.1, 0.3, 0.4, 0.5 0.8, 1.0 mg/mL inj	0.5-1.0 mg q 5 min up to 3 mg total	Initial dose: 6 mg IV bolus; if necessary, can be followed by 12 mg q 2 min as IV bolus; flush IV line after each administration
Adenosine (Adenocard®)	3 mg/mL injection	IV and PO: 0.25 mg q 2 h up to 1.5 mg	IV and PO: 0.125-0.375 mg qd
Digoxin (Lanoxin®)	125, 250 500 μg tablets 50 μg/mL elixir 100 μg/mL, 250 μg/mL injection		
Digoxin (Lanoxicaps®)	50, 100, 200 μg capsules		

Patient Counseling

• Take medication as prescribed. If a dose is missed, have the patient take the dose as soon as they remember, unless it is close to next scheduled dose. In this case, the patient should skip the missed dose and continue the regular regimen; do not double doses.

• Many drug interactions are possible; patients should inform health care providers of medications prescribed prior to starting new medications, including over-the-counter medications (Table 6).

Table 5

Pharmacokinetics of Antiarrhythmics Drugs

Drug	Bioavailability (%)	Protein binding (%)	Primary route of elimination	Substrate for	Inhibitor of	Half-life	Therapeutic range (mg/L)
Quinidine	70-80	80-90	Hepatic	CYP 3A4	CYP 2D6, CYP 3A4, P-GP	5-9 h	2-6
Procainamide	75-95	10-20	Hepatic/renal	NAT		2.5-5.0 h	4-15
Disopyramide	70-95	50-80	Hepatic/renal	CYP 3A4		4-8 h	2-6
Moricizine	34-38	92-95	Hepatic			1-6 h	
Lidocaine	20-40	65-75	Hepatic	CYP 3A4, CYP 2B6, CYP 1A2	CYP 1A2	60-180 min	1.5-5.0
Tocainiade	90-95	10-30	Hepatic			12-15 h	4-10
Mexilitine	80-95	60-75	Hepatic	CYP 2D6, CYP 1A2	CYP 1A2	6-12 h	0.8-2.0
Flecainide	90-95	35-45	Hepatic/renal	CYP 2D6	CYP 2D6	13-20 h	0.3-2.5
Propafenone	11-39	85-95	Hepatic	CYP 2D6, CYP 1A2, CYP 3A4	CYP 2D6	12-32 h	
Bretylium	15-20	0	Renal	CYP 3A4		5-10 h	0.5-2.0
Amiodarone	22-88	95-99	Hepatic	CYP 3A4	CYP 1A2, CYP 2C9, CYP 2D6, CYP 3A4, P-GP	15-100 d	1.0-2.5
Sotalol	90-95	30-40	Renal			12-20 h	
Ibutilide		40	Hepatic			6	
Dofetilide	>90	60-70	Renal	CYP 3A4		8-10 h	
Digoxin	60-85 (90-100 for lanicaps)	20-30	Renal	P-GP		34-44	0.5-2.2 ng/mL
Diltiazem	35-50	70-85	Hepatic	CYP 3A4	CYP 3A4, P-GP	4-10 h	>0.05
Verapamill	20-40	95-99	Hepatic	CYP 3A4, CYP 1A2	CYP 3A4, P-GP	4-12 h	>0.05

- Periodic ECG and laboratory assessments may be required to minimize or prevent adverse effects.

- Patients should be educated that complete remission of their arrhythmia is unlikely. However, symptomatic arrhythmias that have increased in frequency or severity should be reported to their physician immediately.

- Patients with atrial fibrillation/flutter should be educated about the importance of antithrombotic therapy as well as the signs and symptoms of stroke. Patients with symptoms including sudden onset of slurred speech, facial drooping, or muscle weakness should seek emergent care.

- Antiarrhythmic drugs that are administered as extended-release formulations should not be crushed, opened, or chewed. Advise patient to swallow dose whole.

Drug-specific information
Amiodarone
- Visual disturbances are rare but should be reported immediately to the physician.

- Difficulty breathing or shortness of breath should be reported immediately to the physician.

- Periodic laboratory tests to evaluate thyroid function, liver function, and pulmonary function, as well as diagnostic tests such as chest x-ray, ECG, and eye exams may be necessary to assess and prevent adverse events (Table 7).

- May cause skin photosensitivity. Patients should be advised to wear protective clothing and sunscreen when exposed to sunlight or ultraviolet light.

- Prolonged use may cause blue-gray skin discoloration.

Table 6

Antiarrhythmic Drug Interactions and Significant Adverse Effects

Drug	Effect of disease/drugs on drug concentration	Effect of antiarrhythmic on other drug concentrations	Common or severe adverse effects
Quinidine	*Elevated:* cimetidine, amiodarone, verapamil, diltiazem, ketoconazole, urine alkalinization; *reduced:* enzyme inducers	*Elevated:* warfarin, digoxin, β-blockers, disopyramide, procainamide, propafenone, mexiletine, flecainide	QTc prolongation, torsades de pointes
Procainamide	*Elevated:* cimetidine, trimethoprim, amiodarone		Lupus-like syndrome, QTc prolongation, torsades de pointes, hypotension, dizziness, blurred vision, GI distress
Disopyramide	*Reduced:* enzyme inducers; *elevated:* erythromycin, protease inhibitors, cimetidine (		Anticholinergic side effects, decreased cardiac contractility, heart failure, QTc prolongation, torsades de pointes, hypoglycemia
Moricizine	*Elevated:* cimetidine	*Elevated:* theophylline	Dizziness, nausea, paresthesias, proarrhythmia
Lidocaine	*Decreased:* with decreased cardiac output		CNS toxicity: paresthesias, dizziness, confusion, nausea and vomiting, seizures
Tocainide	*Decreased:* cimetidine, enzyme inducers		GI distress; CNS: dizziness, paresthesias, confusion, seizures; pulmonary fibrosis/pneumonitis; agranulocytosis
Mexiletine	*Reduced:* enzyme inducers; elevated: quinidine, amiodarone, ritonavir	*Elevated:* theophylline	GI distress; CNS: tremor, dizziness, confusion, vertigo, nystagmus, diplopia; hypotension, sinus bradycardia, AV block
Flecainide	*Elevated:* cimetidine, amiodarone	*Elevated:* digoxin	Proarrhythmia, prolonged PR interval and QRS complex; dizziness, blurred vision, heart failure
Propafenone	*Reduced:* enzyme inducers; elevated: cimetidine, quinidine	*Elevated:* warfarin, digoxin, cyclosporine, theophylline	Metallic/bitter taste; CNS: dizziness, paresthesias, fatigue; GI distress; heart failure, liver injury, agranulocytosis
Bretylium			Adrenergic blocking effects: initial hypertension followed by hypotension; GI distress; hyperthermia
Amiodarone[1]		*Elevated:* quinidine, procainamide, warfarin, digoxin, phenytoin, cyclosporine	IV: phlebitis; general: corneal microdeposits, photophobia, increased liver enzymes, photosensitivity, blue-gray skin discoloration, pulmonary fibrosis, hyper- and hypothyroidism, polyneuropathy
Sotalol			β-blocking effects: bradycardia, fatigue, dyspnea, bronchospasm, heart failure; QTc prolongation, torsades de pointes
Ibutilide			QTc prolongation, torsades de pointes
Dofetilide	*Elevated:* verapamil, cimetidine, ketoconazole, trimethoprim, megestrol, prochlorperazine		QTc prolongation, torsades de pointes
Digoxin	*Elevated:* quinidine, amiodarone, verapamil, diltiazem		
Diltiazem	*Elevated:* cimetidine	*Elevated:* cyclosporine, carbamazepine, digoxin	Hypotension, bradycardia, heart failure
Verapamil	*Reduced:* rifampin, phenobarbital	*Elevated:* theophylline, digoxin, carbamazepine, cyclosporine	Hypotension, bradycardia, heart failure, constipation

[1]See Table 7.

Table 7

Suggested Monitoring Guidelines for Amiodarone

Test	Baseline	3 Months	6 Months	12 Months
Electrocardiogram	•	•	•	•
Pulmonary function tests	•	Routine monitoring controversial; may repeat tests if patient becomes symptomatic		
Ophthalmologic examination	•	Periodic exam recommended		
Chest x-ray	•	•	•	•
Thyroid function tests	•		•	•
Liver enzymes	•		•	•

- Frequent administration with grapefruit juice may increase oral absorption. Encourage patients to drink water with amiodarone or separate grapefruit juice consumption by at least 2 hours.

β-Blockers (including sotalol)
- Patients with asthma and chronic obstructive pulmonary disease should be advised that β-blockers may worsen their symptoms of airway disease. Patients should notify their physician immediately.

- Patients with diabetes should be advised that β-blockers may mask symptoms of hypoglycemia.

- Patients should avoid abrupt withdrawal of β-blocker therapy. If withdrawal of β-blocker therapy is desired, the patient should contact the physician for dosage tapering regimen, if necessary.

Digoxin
- Refer to congestive heart failure chapter.

Quinidine
- Frequent administration with grapefruit juice may increase oral absorption; encourage patients to drink water with amiodarone or separate grapefruit juice consumption by at least 2 hours.

- Take 1 hour before or 2 hours after meals.

Warfarin
- Warfarin should be avoided at any time during pregnancy.

- To determine the correct dosage, your physician may need to check your blood regularly.

- Encourage patients to maintain consistency in their diet. Abrupt changes, particularly in the intake of green leafy vegetables, may alter the effectiveness of warfarin.

- Minor cuts may take longer to stop bleeding. If a cut or injury fails to stop bleeding, contact your health care provider.

- Excessive alcohol intake may alter the effectiveness of this medication.

3. Key Points

- All antiarrhythmic drugs are proarrhythmic.

- Cardiac arrhythmias range from benign to lethal.

- Antiarrhythmic drug therapy should be individualized to patient response while minimizing adverse effects.

- Most antiarrhythmic drugs are hepatically eliminated and are associated with significant drug interactions.

- Nonpharmacologic therapy is an important treatment modality, particularly for life-threatening ventricular tachycardia and ventricular fibrillation.

- Treatment of atrial fibrillation should always include an assessment of antithrombotic therapy.

- Direct current cardioversion is typically the treatment of choice for severely symptomatic arrhythmias.

- Anticoagulant response to warfarin therapy is influenced by numerous factors, including diet, drug interactions, and disease.

- The treatment of excessive anticoagulation secondary to warfarin should be based on the INR, the presence of an active bleed, and the risk of recurrent thromboembolism.

- Patient education and appropriate monitoring are important aspects of successful therapy while minimizing adverse effects.

4. Questions and Answers

1. Which of the following is (are) an adverse effect(s) of orally administered amiodarone?

   I. Gastrointestinal upset
   II. Pulmonary fibrosis
   III. Phlebitis

   A. I only
   B. III only
   C. I and II only
   D. II and III only
   E. I, II, and III

2. Which of the following antiarrhythmic agents' mechanism of action is primarily the result of sodium ion transport blockade?

   A. Quinidine
   B. Ibutilide
   C. Sotalol
   D. Verapamil
   E. Diltiazem

3. First-degree atrioventricular heart block can be categorized as a disorder of

   I. Automaticity
   II. Reentry
   III. Conduction

   A. I only
   B. III only
   C. I and II only
   D. II and III only
   E. I, II, and III

4. Each of the following can be symptoms of atrial fibrillation except

   A. Dizziness
   B. Palpitations
   C. Angina
   D. Hypertension
   E. Sudden-onset slurred speech

5. Each of the following are recommended monitoring tools for patients requiring chronic amiodarone therapy except

   A. Electrocardiogram
   B. Coagulation tests
   C. Thyroid function tests
   D. Liver function tests

E. Chest x-ray

6. For the treatment of persistent atrial fibrillation with chronic warfarin therapy, the target INR should be 2.0-3.0 for each of the following, except patients with:

   A. Heart failure
   B. Age ≥60 years plus hypertension
   C. Prosthetic heart valve
   D. Age ≥75 years plus diabetes
   E. Age ≥75 years plus coronary artery disease

7. Patients with which type of arrhythmia should be educated on performing vagal maneuvers to restore sinus rhythm?

   A. Paroxysmal supraventricular tachycardia
   B. Torsades de pointes
   C. Atrial flutter
   D. Sinus bradycardia
   E. Ventricular fibrillation

8. In the absence of an acute myocardial infarction, what is the treatment of choice for resuscitated patients with sustained ventricular tachycardia?

   A. β-blocker
   B. Amiodarone
   C. No antiarrhythmic therapy
   D. Digoxin
   E. Intracardiac defibrillator

9. Which of the following medications have been associated with torsades de pointes?

   I. Dofetilide
   II. Droperidol
   III. Erythromycin

   A. I only
   B. III only
   C. I and II only
   D. II and III only
   E. I, II, and III

10. Which of the following would result in the greatest risk of lidocaine toxicity?

    A. Rifampin
    B. Cimetidine
    C. Amiodarone
    D. Congestive heart failure
    E. Bradycardia

11. What is the recommended dosage regimen for dofetilide in a patient with a calculated creatinine clearance of 30 mL/min?

    A. Dofetilide therapy not recommended
    B. 125 μg PO bid
    C. 125 mg PO bid
    D. 500 μg PO bid
    E. 500 mg PO bid

12. Quinidine is metabolized by and inhibits the metabolism of which cytochrome P450 enzymes, respectively?

    A. CYP 3A4 and CYP 2D6
    B. CYP 2D6 and CYP 3A4
    C. P-GP and CYP 2D6
    D. P-GP and CYP 3A4
    E. CYP 1A2 and CYP 3A4

13. Which of the following antiarrhythmic agents does not increase digoxin concentrations when used concomitantly?

    A. Quinidine
    B. Procainamide
    C. Amiodarone
    D. Diltiazem
    E. Sotalol

14. J.S. is a 66-year-old male with a past medical history of congestive heart failure and hypertension for which he is receiving lisinopril 10 mg PO qd, digoxin 0.25 mg PO qd, and spironolactone 25 mg PO qd at home. J.S. now presents to the emergency room with a 1-week history of intermittent palpitations and dizziness. A stat EKG reveals atrial fibrillation with a ventricular rate of 130 bpm. The decision is made to attempt to restore normal sinus rhythm. Which of the following represents the best therapeutic approach to cardioverting this patient?

    A. Perform transesophageal echocardiogram; if no thrombus is present, cardiovert. No need for anticoagulation.
    B. Perform transesophageal echocardiogram; if no thrombus present, cardiovert. Anticoagulate for at least 4 weeks postcardioversion.
    C. Anticoagulate for 4 weeks prior to cardioversion. Discontinue anticoagulation postcardioversion.
    D. Anticoagulate for 2 weeks prior to cardioversion. Continue anticoagulation for at least 4 weeks postcardioversion.
    E. Direct current cardiovert immediately.

15. After the initial successful cardioversion, J.S. continues to have recurrent atrial fibrillation episodes. Chronic therapy to maintain sinus rhythm is to be initiated. Which of the following antiarrhythmic drugs would be the best choice to maintain sinus rhythm?

    A. Flecainide
    B. Amiodarone
    C. Sotalol
    D. Ibutilide
    E. Esmolol

16. In a patient with mildly symptomatic paroxysmal supraventricular tachycardia, verapamil should be used for which rhythm(s)?

    I. Narrow QRS complex, regular interval
    II. Wide QRS complex, regular interval
    III. Wide QRS complex, irregular interval

    A. I only
    B. III only
    C. I and II only
    D. II and III only
    E. I, II, and III

17. R.J. is a 53-year-old male with a past medical history of coronary artery disease and hypertension. He presents to his doctor complaining of short (about 10 seconds in duration), intermittent palpitations during the last 2 days. Tests rule out an acute myocardial infarction and an echocardiogram shows a left ventricular ejection fraction of 52%. The patient is sent home with a Holter monitor to identify any arrhythmias. The Holter monitor reveals episodes of ventricular tachycardia. What is the most appropriate intervention for R.J.?

    A. No therapy
    B. Place intracardiac defibrillator
    C. Start amiodarone
    D. Start a β-blocker
    E. Direct current cardioversion

18. Treatment of torsades de pointes may include all of the following except

    A. Discontinue any drugs associated with prolonged QT interval
    B. Isoproterenol infusion
    C. Adenosine
    D. Magnesium sulfate
    E. Atrial/ventricular pacing

19. Which of the following antiarrhythmic agents has anticholinergic properties?

    A. Sotalol
    B. Amiodarone
    C. Lidocaine
    D. Disopyramide
    E. Propafenone

20. Which of the following is not a characteristic of atrial fibrillation?

    A. No discernable p waves
    B. Ventricular rate 100-130 bpm
    C. Regular QRS pattern
    D. Narrow QRS complex
    E. Chaotic atrial contractions

21. Which of the following would be the best choice for ventricular rate control in atrial fibrillation secondary to hyperthyroidism?

    A. Adenosine
    B. Digoxin
    C. Verapamil
    D. Propranolol
    E. Atropine

22. A dose-limiting adverse effect of sotalol is

    A. Bradycardia
    B. Polyneuropathy
    C. Metallic taste
    D. Agranulocytosis
    E. Lupus-like syndrome

23. Which of the following is not available in both intravenous and oral dosage forms?

    A. Procainamide
    B. Amiodarone
    C. Verapamil
    D. Digoxin
    E. Ibutilide

24. Warfarin dosage adjustment should be considered for the following drugs except

    A. Amiodarone
    B. Sotalol
    C. Quinidine
    D. Propafenone
    E. Diltiazem

Answers

1. **C.** Gastrointestinal upset is common, particularly with larger oral doses (ie, during the loading dose phase) and pulmonary fibrosis occurs during prolonged therapy. Phlebitis would only be expected to occur during intravenous amiodarone infusion, particularly through a peripheral intravenous line. To decrease risk of phlebitis, a central line is preferred.

2. **A.** Quinidine blocks sodium entry into the cardiac cell, slowing polarization. Ibutilide and sotolol act primarily by blocking potassium transport, whereas verapamil and diltiazem inhibit the calcium channel.

3. **B.** Atrioventricular heart block is caused by slowed conduction through the atrioventricular node.

4. **D.** Due to loss of functional atrial contraction and rapid ventricular rate (producing palpitations), cardiac output may decrease, resulting in decreased perfusion of major organs, particularly the brain (dizziness, confusion, etc) and heart (angina and heart failure exacerbation). Depending on the vascular tone, blood pressure may remain stable or fall as a direct result of decreased cardiac output; however, hypertension would not be expected. Patients with atrial fibrillation are at increased risk of thrombosis, particularly stroke, secondary to poor blood flow in the left atrium.

5. **B.** See Table 7 for recommended monitoring parameters and schedule. Coagulation tests are not routinely recommended for patients receiving amiodarone therapy. Coagulation tests may be required if a patient develops severe hepatotoxicity secondary to amiodarone or simply requires concomitant warfarin therapy for atrial fibrillation.

6. **C.** Patients with prosthetic heart valves require higher INR to prevent thromboembolism. In general an INR of 2.5-3.5 is appropriate.

7. **A.** Vagal maneuvers are effective nonpharmacologic therapy for PSVT since the reentry impulse circuit exists in the atrioventricular node. Although vagal maneuvers will slow the rate in atrial fibrillation/flutter, it will not terminate the arrhythmia since the reentry circuit is in the atrial tissue. Vagal maneuvers will have no effect on ventricular arrhythmia since the impulse arises from below the AV node.

8. **E.** Based on the results of the AVID trial, intracardiac defibrillator treatment has a significant mortality benefit over antiarrhythmic therapy alone. Antiarrhythmic therapy may be indicated if the patient refuses surgical placement of the defibrillator or to decrease the number of discharges from the defibrillator if recurrences are frequent.

9. **E.**

10. **D.** Lidocaine is nearly 100% metabolized in the liver. Lidocaine metabolism is dependent upon liver blood flow rather than enzymatic activity (ie, high extraction ratio). Therefore, poor cardiac output secondary to congestive heart failure may decrease lidocaine delivery to the liver for metabolism. Bradycardia typically does not decrease cardiac output secondary to a compensatory increase in left ventricular stroke volume.

11. **B.** Dofetilide is renally eliminated and therefore must be adjusted to decrease the significant risk of torsades de pointes.

12. **A.**

13. **E.**

14. **B.** Since the patient appears to have been in atrial fibrillation for 1 week by history, there is a significant risk of thromboembolism during conversion to sinus rhythm. Proper treatment would require at least 3-4 weeks of anticoagulation prior to cardioversion, followed by at least 4 weeks of anticoagulation postcardioversion. Alternatively, a transesophageal echocardiogram can be used to rule out an atrial thrombus, allowing immediate cardioversion. Since the atria will require time to recover normal contractile activity, anticoagulation will be required for at least 4 weeks postconversion.

15. **B.** Since the patient has heart failure, the results of the CAST trials indicate the avoidance of class Ic agents due to increased risk of death. Sotolol may worsen congestive heart failure. Ibutilide is indicated for chemical conversion only, not for maintenance of sinus rhythm. Esmolol will only control the ventricular rate but will have no effect on maintaining sinus rhythm.

16. **A.** A wide QRS complex signifies conduction via an accessory pathway other than the AV node. Since calcium channel blockers prolong

conduction in the AV node and not in the accessory pathways, administration of these agents will block the AV node and force impulses to be conducted via the accessory pathways, which have shorter refractory periods. Consequently, the ventricular response will significantly increase.

17. **D.** According to the patient's presentation, he has nonsustained ventricular tachycardia since the duration of each event is less than 30 seconds. Since he is symptomatic and has no heart failure, the treatment of choice is β-blocker therapy.

18. **C.** Adenosine is typically only used to terminate paroxysmal supraventricular tachycardia. Discontinuation of drugs that prolong the QT interval is essential to terminate torsades de pointes and prevent recurrences. Treatment should consist of intravenous magnesium sulfate and electrical pacing. An isoproterenol infusion can be used while waiting for electrical pacing.

19. **D.**

20. **C.** Atrial fibrillation represents chaotic atrial activity resulting in no identifiable p wave. Since atrial fibrillation originates above the AV node, the QRS complex is narrow and the ventricular rate is typically >100.

21. **D.** β-Blockers are the preferred rate-controlling agent for hyperthyroidism since they inhibit the adrenergic response and decrease thyroid hormone conversion (especially propranolol). Digoxin is not as effective in controlling the ventricular rate related to an hyperadrenergic state (hyperthyroidism).

22. **A.** Sotalol possesses significant β-blocking activity and therefore the patient may experience adverse effects similar to traditional β-blockers.

23. **E.**

24. **B.** Warfarin is metabolized via multiple cytochrome P450 isoenzymes, including CYP 2C9, CYP 1A2, and CYP 3A4. Amiodarone inhibits CYP 2C9, CYP 1A2, and CYP 3A4, quinidine via unknown mechanisms, propafenone via CYP 1A2 and CYP 3A4, and diltiazem via CYP 3A4. Sotalol is primarily renally eliminated and does not result in cytochrome P450–mediated drug interactions.

5. References

ACC/AHA/ESC guidelines for the management of patients with atrial fibrillation: executive summary. *Circulation*. 2001;104:2118-2150.

Ansell J, Hirsh J, Dalen J, et al. Managing oral anticoagulant therapy. *Chest*. 2001;119:22s-38s.

Bauman JL, Schoen MD. Arrhythmias. In: Dipiro JT, Talbert RL, Yee GC, et al, eds. *Pharmacotherapy: A Pathophysiologic Approach*, 5th ed. New York: McGraw-Hill; 2002:273-303.

Echt DS, Liebson PR, Mitchell LB, et al. Mortality and morbidity in patients receiving encainide, flecainide, or placebo. *N Engl J Med*. 1991;324:781-788.

Ganz LI, Friedman PL. Supraventricular tachycardia. *N Engl J Med*. 1995;332:162-173.

Harder S, Thurmann P. Clinically important drug interactions with anticoagulants: an update. *Clin Pharmacokinet*. 1996;30:416-444.

Klein AL, Grimm RA, Murray RD, et al. Use of transesophageal echocardiography to guide cardioversion in patients with atrial fibrillation. *N Engl J Med*. 2001;344:1411-1420.

Ommen SR, Odell JA, Stanton MS. Atrial arrhythmias after cardiothoracic surgery. *N Engl J Med*. 1997;336:1429-1434.

Robinson DC, Gill MA. Cardiac arrhythmias. In: Herfindal ET, Gourley DR, eds. *Textbook of Therapeutics: Drug and Disease Management*, 7th ed. Baltimore: Lippincott Williams & Wilkins; 2000:867-916.

Trujillo TC, Nolan PE. Antiarrhythmic agents: drug interactions of clinical significance. *Drug Safety*. 2000;23:509-512.

The Antiarrhythmics Versus Implantable Defibrillators (AVID) Investigators. A comparison of antiarrhythmic-drug therapy with implantable defibrillators in patients resuscitated from near fatal ventricular arrhythmias. *N Engl J Med*. 1997;337:1576-1583.

The Atrial Fibrillation Follow-up Investigation of Rhythm Management (AFFIRM) Investigators. A comparison of rate control and rhythm control in patients with atrial fibrillation. *N Engl J Med*. 2002;347:1825-1833.

11. Ischemic Heart Disease

Shannon W. Finks, PharmD, BCPS
Assistant Professor, Department of Pharmacy
University of Tennessee College of Pharmacy
Clinical Pharmacy Specialist
Baptist Memorial Hospital, Memphis, Tennessee

Carrie S. Oliphant, PharmD
Assistant Professor, Department of Pharmacy
University of Tennessee College of Pharmacy
Clinical Pharmacy Specialist, Cardiology
Methodist Healthcare–University Hospital

Kelly C. Rogers, PharmD
Assistant Professor, Department of Pharmacy
University of Tennessee College of Pharmacy
Clinical Pharmacy Specialist
Baptist Memorial Hospital, Memphis, Tennessee

Contents

1. Introduction

Definitions

Ischemia
- Lack of oxygen from inadequate perfusion due to an imbalance between oxygen supply and demand.

Ischemic heart disease (IHD)
- Disease caused most frequently by atherosclerosis.

- May present as silent ischemia, chest pain (at rest or on exertion), or myocardial infarction (MI).

Angina
- Syndrome described as discomfort or pain in the chest, arm, shoulder, back, or jaw.

- Frequently worsened by physical exertion or emotional stress and usually relieved by sublingual (SL) nitroglycerin (NTG).

- Patients with angina usually have coronary artery disease (CAD) in at least one large epicardial artery.

Atypical angina
- Transient pain or discomfort lacking one or more of the criteria of classic angina.

- More common presentation for women.

Acute coronary syndrome (ACS)
- ACS encompasses the following:
  * Unstable angina (UA)
  * Non ST-segment myocardial infarction (NSTEMI)
  * ST-segment myocardial infarction (STEMI)

Coronary artery disease (CAD)
- Chronic disorder that typically cycles in and out of the clinically defined phases of ACS and asymptomatic, stable, or progressive angina.

Percutaneous coronary intervention (PCI)
- Procedure to reopen a partially or completely occluded coronary vessel to restore blood flow.

Coronary artery bypass graft (CABG)
- Surgical procedure in which a vein is harvested from the leg and attached to the heart as a new coronary vessel in order to bypass a diseased vessel.

Epidemiology of Ischemic Heart Disease

- Leading cause of death in the U.S.
  * Causes more deaths than the next two leading causes combined (cancer and cerebrovascular disease)

- Approximately 61 million Americans have some type of cardiovascular (CV) disease.

- Approximately 950,000 Americans die of CV disease per year.

- Every 33 seconds an American will die of heart disease or stroke.

- There are ~6 million hospital admissions per year for CV disease.

- Each year in the U.S., the cost of CAD (including MI) totals over a billion dollars in direct and indirect costs.

2. Normal Physiology vs. Pathophysiology

Normal Physiology

- The arterioles change their resistance and dilate as needed to enable the heart to receive a fixed amount of O_2.

- In response to physical exertion, an increase in blood pressure (BP), or increased myocardial oxygen demand (MVO_2), the arterioles dilate to maintain O_2 supply to the heart.

- *Note:* In atherosclerosis, plaque narrows the conductance vessel causing the arterioles to dilate under normal or resting conditions to prevent ischemia. With stress or exercise, the vasodilator response is minimal, which causes ischemia and angina.

Pathophysiology

Determinants of MVO_2
- Heart rate (HR).
    * Tachycardia will increase MVO_2

- Contractility.
    * Increases will increase MVO_2

- Myocardial wall tension.
    * Dependent on ventricular volume and pressure
    * Increased pressure or enlargement of the ventricle will increase systolic wall force and MVO_2

Determinants of Myocardial Oxygen Supply and Flow

- Limits on flow: thrombi, spasm, congenital abnormalities, severe anemia, severe ventricular hypertrophy due to hypertension (HTN) and aortic stenosis (abnormally high oxygen demands).

- Autoregulation of coronary blood flow.
    * Adenosine, a potent vasodilator, is released from myocardial cells in response to decreased O_2 supply (ie, occlusion), increased sympathetic activity (exercise, mental stress, exposure to cold), BP, and HR, which leads to increased MVO_2

- Normal arteries respond to increased demand with increased blood flow and some vasodilation of the large epicardial vessels.

- *Note:* Atherosclerotic vessels lose this vasodilator response and develop constriction.

- Vascular endothelium:
    * Protective surface of the artery wall
    * Promotes smooth muscle relaxation and inhibits thrombogenesis
    * If damaged, the endothelium produces nitric oxide (NO), which produces vasodilation similar to the therapeutic effects of nitroglycerin (NTG)
    * Loss of the vascular endothelium due to primary transluminal coronary angioplasty (PTCA), cigarette smoking, oxidized LDL, HTN, or atherosclerosis results in loss of NO and the defense mechanism

- Diastole:
    * Normally, the distribution of blood flow between the epicardial and endocardial layers is equal during the period when coronary artery filling occurs
    * In atherosclerosis, there is a reduction in subendocardial blood flow

- Coronary vasospasm:
    * Reduces blood flow, thereby causing ischemia in areas of atherosclerotic plaques

- Atherosclerosis is the most common cause of myocardial ischemia.
    * Decrease in the lumen of coronary arteries due to stenosis leads to reduced myocardial perfusion and subsequent ischemia
    * Segmental atherosclerotic narrowing is most commonly caused by a plaque which can fissure, hemorrhage, and cause thrombosis, which then worsens the obstruction, reduces blood flow further, and leads to ACS

3. Diagnostic Procedures

- History and physical examination.

- Laboratory work-up (see Table 1).

- Resting electrocardiogram.

Exercise Tolerance Test (ETT, treadmill)

Drugs can interfere with test

- Digoxin causes abnormal exercise-induced ST depression in ~30% of healthy patients.

- β-Blockers and vasodilators alter hemodynamic response to BP.
    * Hold 4-5 half-lives before ETT
    * Withdraw β-blockers gradually to avoid precipitating an attack

- Nitrates can attenuate angina.

- Flecainide may cause exercise-induced ventricular tachycardia.

Stress Imaging

Thallium treadmill (Exercise thallium test)

Pharmacologic stress imaging
- Drugs "do the exercise" by increasing MVO_2.

Dobutamine
- High doses up to 40 µg/kg/min cause positive inotropic and chronotropic effects which increase myocardial blood flow and lead to ischemia.

- Commonly used with ECHO. Side effects (SE): nausea, anxiety, tremor, arrhythmias, angina, headache.

Dipyridamole and adenosine
- Induce coronary vasodilation; used in conjunction with myocardial perfusion scintigraphy.

- Dipyridamole SEs occur in up to 50% of patients: angina, headache, nausea, dizziness, flushing, severe bronchospasm in patients with COPD or asthma.

- Adenosine SEs occur in up to 80% of patients: chest pain, headache, flushing, shortness of breath (SOB), first-degree AV block, severe bronchospasm in patients with COPD or asthma.

Drug interactions:
- Xanthines (theophylline, caffeine) are adenosine receptor antagonists that attenuate the effects of adenosine and dipyridamole.

- β-Blockers interact with dobutamine, but the interaction can be overcome by increasing the dose of dobutamine.

Cardiac catheterization (cath, angiography)
- A catheter is inserted in the femoral artery and guided to the heart.

- Radiocontrast dye is injected directly into the coronary arteries.

- The dye shows which arteries are involved and the extent of occlusion.

- Complications:
    * Allergic reaction to iodine in the dye
    * Dye is nephrotoxic
    * Arterial bleeding from access site, stroke, MI, death (rare)

Table 1

Pertinent Laboratory Tests in Ischemic Heart Disease

Complete blood cell count (CBC) with platelet count

Serial creatine kinase myocardial bound (CK-MB) and troponin levels
(enzyme markers specific for myocardial necrosis)

Activated partial thromboplastin time (aPTT)

Prothrombin time (PT) and international normalized ratio (INR)

Fasting lipid panel (FLP) within 24 hours of admission

4. Chronic Stable Angina, Prinzmetal's (or Variant) Angina, and Silent Ischemia

Clinical Presentation

Chronic stable angina
- Symptoms are caused by decreased O_2 supply due to reduced flow.

- Considered stable if symptoms have been occurring for several weeks without worsening (Table 2).

Prinzmetal's or variant angina (uncommon)
- Usually due to spasm without increased MVO_2.

- Most patients have severe atherosclerosis.

- Characterized by recurrent, prolonged attacks of severe ischemia.

- Patients are often between 30 and 40 years old.

- Pain usually occurs at rest or awakens patient from sleep.

- Electrocardiogram (ECG) shows ST segment elevation, which returns to baseline when the patient is given NTG.

Silent ischemia (SI)
- SI is ischemia in the absence of symptoms.

- ~75% of ischemic episodes in patients with stable angina are undetected.

- ECG shows ST segment changes, and there is eleva-tion or depression during activity, but patient experiences no symptoms.

- Occurs in ~20-30% of post-MI patients.

- 50% of patients with stable angina have silent ischemia; common in diabetics.

Pharmacologic Management

Chronic stable angina
Goals of therapy
- Prevent MI and death.

- Reduce symptoms of angina and occurrence of ischemia to improve quality of life (QOL).

Agents
Antiplatelet therapy
- Aspirin decreases the incidence of MI, adverse CV events, and sudden death.

- Clopidogrel (Plavix®) has a greater antithrombotic effect than ticlopidine and has fewer SEs.

- *Note:* Ticlopidine (Ticlid®) has not been shown to reduce CV events in stable angina.

- Indications for therapy (see Table 3)

Anti-ischemic therapy
- β-*Blockers (BBs)*
- Effects on MVO_2.
  - * Inhibit catecholamine effects, thereby decreasing MVO_2
  - * Decreases HR (negative chronotrope decreases conduction through the AV node)
  - * Decreases contractility (negative inotrope decreases force of contraction)
  - * Reduces BP

- Effects on oxygen supply (no direct improvement of oxygen supply):

Table 2

Characteristics of Stable Angina

1. Pain located over sternum and may radiate to left shoulder or arm, jaw, back, right arm, or neck
2. Description of symptoms: pressure or heavy weight on chest, burning, tightness, deep, squeezing, aching, vise-like, suffocating, crushing
3. Duration of 0.5-30 minutes
4. Precipitating factors: exercise, cold weather, postprandial, emotional stress, sexual activity
5. Pain relief: sublingual (SL) nitroglycerin or rest

Table 3

Antiplatelet Use in Stable Angina

- Aspirin (75-325 mg qd) in all patients with acute and chronic IHD (with or without symptoms) in the absence of contraindications
- Clopidogrel is chosen when aspirin is absolutely contraindicated
- Ticlopidine is not recommended due to poor side effect profile

* Increases diastolic perfusion time (coronary arteries fill during diastole) due to decreased HR, which may enhance left ventricle (LV) perfusion
* Ventricular relaxation causes increased subendocardial blood flow
* Unopposed α stimulation may lead to coronary vasoconstriction

- Dosing:
    * Start low, go slow
    * Titrate to resting HR of 50-60 bpm, maximal exercise HR $\leq$100
    * Avoid abrupt withdrawal, which can precipitate more severe ischemic episodes and MI. Taper over 2 days

- BB selection:
    * Cardioselectivity to decrease adverse effects; lose cardioselectivity at higher doses
    * The intrinsic sympathomimetic activity (ISA) with acebutolol, carteolol, penbutolol, and pindolol may not be as effective because the reduction in HR would be minimal; therefore, there is a small reduction in MVO_2 BBs are generally reserved for patients with low resting HR who experience angina with exercise
    * Lipophilicity is associated with more central nervous system (CNS) SEs
    * Preferred in young patients who are hypertensive, post-MI, with high resting HR, fixed angina threshold, and mild heart failure (HF)

- Indications for therapy (see Table 4).

Nitrates (endothelium-independent vasodilators)
- Effects on MVO_2.
    * Peripheral vasodilation leads to decreased blood return to the heart (preload) which leads to decreased LV volume, wall stress, and O_2 demand
    * Arterial vasodilation leads to decreased peripheral resistance (afterload), systolic BP (SBP), and O_2 demand
    * Nitrates can cause a reflex increase in sympathetic activity, which may increase HR/contractility and lead to increased O_2 demand in some patients. This can be overcome with the use of a BB

- Effects on O_2 supply.
    * Dilation of large epicardial coronary arteries and collateral vessels in areas with or without stenosis leads to increased O_2 supply

- Indications for therapy (see Table 5).

Calcium channel blockers (CCBs)
- Effects on MVO_2.
    * Primarily by decreasing systemic vascular resistance (SVR) and arterial BP by vasodilation of systemic arteries
    * Decreased contractility and decreased O_2 requirement (all CCBs exert varying degrees of negative inotropic effects: verapamil > diltiazem > nifedipine)
    * Verapamil and diltiazem promote additional decrease in MVO_2 by decreasing conduction through the AV node, thereby decreasing HR

- Effects on O_2 supply.
    * Increased diastolic perfusion time due to

Table 4

β-Blocker Use in Stable Angina

- First-line therapy if not contraindicated in patients with prior MI
- Initial therapy if not contraindicated in patients without prior MI
- More effective than nitrates and calcium channel blockers (CCBs) in silent ischemia
- Effective as monotherapy and in combination with nitrates and/or CCBs
- Avoid in Prinzmetal's angina
- Improves symptoms 80% of the time
- All BBs are effective, but not all are FDA-indicated

Table 5

Nitrate Use in Stable Angina

- Sublingual nitroglycerin or NTG spray for the immediate relief of angina
- Long-acting nitrates as initial therapy to reduce symptoms if BBs are contraindicated
- Long-acting nitrates in combination with BBs when initial treatment with BBs is ineffective
- Long-acting nitrates as a substitute for BBs if BBs cause unacceptable side effects
- In patients with CAD or other vascular disease
- Preferred agents in treatment of Prinzmetal's/vasospastic angina
- Improves exercise tolerance
- In combination with BBs or CCBs, nitrates produce greater effects

decreased HR, which may enhance LV perfusion
* Decreased coronary vascular resistance and increased coronary blood flow by vasodilation of coronary arteries
* Coronary vasodilation at sites of stenosis
* Prevents/relieves vasospastic angina by dilation of the epicardial coronary arteries

• Indications for therapy (see Table 6).

Combination therapy
BBs and nitrates
• BBs can potentially increase LV volume and LVEDP.
* Nitrates attenuate this effect

• Nitrates increase sympathetic tone and may cause a reflex tachycardia.
* BBs attenuate this response

BBs and CCBs
• BBs and long-acting dihydropyridine CCBs are usually efficacious and well-tolerated.

• CCBs, especially the dihydropyridines, increase sympathetic tone and may cause reflex tachycardia.
* BBs attenuate this effect

• BBs and nondihydropyridine CCBs should be used together cautiously as the combination can lead to excessive bradycardia or AV block. The combination can also precipitate symptoms of HF.

Miscellaneous therapy
Angiotensin-converting enzyme inhibitors (ACEIs)
• Potential CV protective effects.
* Reduce the incidence of MI, CV death, and stroke in patients at high risk for vascular disease (Data from the Heart Outcomes Prevention Evaluation [HOPE] trial).
* Controversy exists as to whether all ACEIs are equally effective or if "tissue ACEIs" provide better protection

• Indications for therapy (see Table 7).

Lipid-lowering therapy
• Clinical trials have proved that lipid-lowering therapy should be recommended in patients with established CAD, including chronic stable angina, even if only mild to moderate elevations of LDL cholesterol are present.

• Indications for therapy (see Table 8).

Prinzmetal's or variant angina
• BBs have no role in management and may increase painful episodes.

Table 6

Calcium Channel Blocker Use in Stable Angina

• Initial therapy for reduction of symptoms when BBs are contraindicated
• In combination with BBs when initial treatment with BBs is not successful
• As a substitute for BBs if initial treatment with BBs causes unacceptable side effects
• Slow-release/long-acting dihydropyridines and nondihydropyridines are effective in stable angina
• Avoid short-acting dihydropyridines
• Newer-generation dihydropyridines such as amlodipine or felodipine can be used safely in patients with depressed LV systolic function

Table 7

Angiotensin-Converting Enzyme Inhibitor Use in Stable Angina

• In all patients with CAD (by angiography or previous MI) who also have diabetes mellitus (DM) and/or left ventricular dysfunction
• In patients with CAD or other vascular disease
• In all patients with DM who do not have contraindications due to severe renal disease

Table 8

Low Density Lipoprotein–Lowering Therapy in Stable Angina

• In patients with documented or suspected CAD and LDL cholesterol >130 mg/dL, with a target LDL of <100 mg/dL
• In patients with documented CAD and LDL of 100-129 mg/dL, with a target of <100 mg/dL

- BBs may induce coronary vasoconstriction and prolong ischemia.

- Nitrates are often used for acute attacks.

- CCBs may be more effective, dosed less frequently, and have fewer SEs than nitrates.

- Nifedipine, diltiazem, or verapamil are all equally effective as single agents.

- Nitrates can be added if there is no response to CCBs.

- Combination therapy with nifedipine + diltiazem and nifedipine + verapamil have been reported to be useful.

- Dose titration is recommended to obtain efficacy without unacceptable SEs.

- Treat acute attacks and provide prophylactic treatment for 6-12 months.

Silent ischemia
- Goal is to decrease the number of episodes, both symptomatic and asymptomatic.

- The initial step is to modify risk factors for IHD (ie, smoking, hypercholesterolemia, HTN).

- BBs have shown improvement in patients with ischemic episodes and are preferred in patients post-MI.

- CCBs are somewhat less effective than BBs.

5. Unstable Angina/Non-ST-Segment Elevation Myocardial Infarction

Pathophysiology

- The process of ischemic syndromes involves two essential events:
    * Disruption of an atherosclerotic plaque
    * Formation of a platelet-rich thrombus

- The clinical manifestations depend on the extent and duration of the thrombotic occlusion.

- In unstable angina/non-ST-segment elevation myocardial infarction (UA/NSTEMI) the thrombus does not completely occlude the vessel.

- Pathogenesis and clinical presentations of UA and NSTEMI are similar but differ in severity.

Presentation

- Central/substernal or crushing chest pain that can radiate to the neck, jaw, back, shoulders, and arms.

- Patients may present with diaphoresis, nausea, vomiting, arm tingling, weakness, shortness of breath, or syncope.

- Pain may be similar to typical angina except that the occurrences are more severe, may occur at rest, and may be caused by less exertion.

- May be incorrectly interpreted as dyspepsia or indigestion.

- Pain is not relieved by NTG.

- May evolve into STEMI without treatment.

Diagnosis

- Chest pain persisting longer than 5 minutes that is unrelieved by NTG.

- Cardiac enzymes and ECG changes (Table 9).

Pharmacologic Management of Unstable Angina/Non-ST-Segment Elevation Myocardial Infarction

Goals of therapy
- Complete restoration of blood flow to the myocardium.

Table 9

Cardiac Enzymes and Electrocardiographic Changes: UA vs. NSTEMI

	UA	NSTEMI
Cardiac enzymes	Negative	Positive
ECG changes	If present, are transient	ST-segment, T-wave changes

- Prevent myocardial infarction, arrhythmias, and ischemia.

Agents
Morphine, oxygen, nitrates, aspirin (MONA)
- Indications for therapy (see Table 10).

Anti-ischemic therapy
- β-Adrenergic blockade.
  * Preference is for an agent without ISA

  * Agents with β_1 selectivity are preferred in patients with bronchoconstrictive disease
  * No evidence that one agent is superior to another
  * Initial choices include metoprolol, atenolol, and propranolol
  * Indications for therapy (see Table 11)

- Nitrates (see MONA).

- Calcium channel blockers (CCBs).
  * There is no mortality benefit from the use of CCBs, therefore they are not recommended as first-line therapy
  * Indications for therapy (see Table 12)

- Angiotensin-converting enyzme inhibitors (ACEIs).
  * Indications for therapy (see Table 13)

Antiplatelet therapy
- Aspirin (see MONA).

- Thienopyridines (ie, clopidogrel [Plavix®] and ticlopidine [Ticlid®]).
  * Inhibition of platelet aggregation is irreversible

Table 10

Morphine, Oxygen, Nitrates, and Aspirin (MONA) Therapy

Morphine	**Rationale:** vasodilatory properties on both arterial and venous sides, therefore decreases both preload and afterload. Pain relief decreases tachycardia, along with decrease in preload and afterload; all work to decrease myocardial O_2 demand **Dosing:** increments of 2-4 mg IV every 5-15 minutes until pain relief **Adverse effects:** nausea, vomiting, hypotension, sedation, and respiratory depression **Cautions and contraindications:** produces a vagotonic effect that may be contraindicated in patients with bradycardia. Watch closely for hypotension, respiratory depression, and allergic reactions.
Meperidine	Can be used in patients who are intolerant to morphine. Has vagolytic effects, so it is the analgesic of choice in patients who are bradycardic; 25-75 mg IV
Oxygen	Supplemental O_2 2-4 L/min by nasal cannula is recommended to correct and avoid hypoxia, particularly within the first 2-3 hours. More aggressive ventilatory support should be considered and given as needed.
Nitroglycerin (NTG)	• All patients should receive NTG as an sublingual tablet or spray, followed by IV administration for the relief of ischemia. • Long-acting nitrates (oral, transdermal) should be used as secondary prevention in patients who do not tolerate BBs and CCBs. These nitrates can be used in patients who have continual chest pain despite the use of BBs and CCBs.
Aspirin (ASA)	• Aspirin 160-325 mg should be given at the onset of chest pain unless contraindicated. Chew and swallow the first dose. • Daily dose of 75-325 mg for life. • Other antiplatelet agents such as clopidogrel or ticlopidine may be substituted if true aspirin allergy is present or if the patient is unresponsive to ASA.

Table 11

β-Blocker use in UA/NSTEMI

- All patients without contraindications
- In patients with continued chest pain, the first dose should be given IV

Table 12

Calcium Channel Blocker Use in UA/NSTEMI

- In patients with contraindications to BBs, a nondihydropyridine CCB (verapamil, diltiazem) should be used in the absence of severe LV dysfunction or other contraindication
- Oral long-acting CCBs provide additional control of anginal symptoms in patients who are already receiving BBs and nitrates
- Immediate-release dihydropyridine CCBs should not be used without a BB

Table 13

Angiotensin-Converting Enzyme Inhibitor Use in UA/NSTEMI

- Not indicated for the immediate treatment of UA/NSTEMI
- Based on the results from the HOPE trial, which showed a mortality reduction when ramipril was used in patients with vascular disease and no history of HF, may consider in all patents without contraindications
- Consider in all patients without contraindications

and takes 2-5 days to achieve full effect. Often clopidogrel or ticlopidine is given in a loading dose for a more rapid effect (within 2 hours)
* Clopidogrel is the preferred agent in this class
* Ticlopidine is rarely used as a result of severe toxicities
* The mechanism of platelet aggregation for clopidogrel and ASA differ; therefore their effects are additive
* Indications for therapy (clopidogrel) (see Table 14)

Table 14

Clopidogrel Use in UA/NSTEMI

- Alternative for patients who are allergic to ASA or who have a gastrointestinal intolerance to ASA
- Clopidogrel should be combined with ASA in patients with or without a planned PCI procedure for at least 1 month and up to 1 year

Glycoprotein IIb/IIIa Receptor Inhibitors (GPIs)
- Agents:
    * Abciximab (Reopro®)
    * Eptifibatide (Integrilin®)
    * Tirofiban (Aggrastat®)

- Uses:
    * All of the agents can be used as adjunctive therapy to patients undergoing PCI
    * Eptifibatide and tirofiban can also be used in patients who will be managed medically. Medical management can be used in patients who refuse a PCI procedure or in patients who are at high risk of complications related to a PCI procedure
    * In combination with heparin and ASA, eptifibatide and abciximab have been shown to reduce the incidence of combined death, MI, and recurrent ischemia in patients with UA/NSTEMI who undergo PCI
    * Indications for therapy (see Table 15)

Anticoagulant therapy
- Unfractionated heparin (UFH).
    * Indications for therapy (Table 16)

Table 15

Glycoprotein IIb/IIIa Receptor Inhibitor Use in UA/NSTEMI

- In addition to heparin, ASA and clopidogrel should be given to all patients with a planned PCI procedure. The GPI can be given during the interventional procedure just before stent deployment or angioplasty.
- Eptifibatide or tirofiban should be given in combination with ASA and LMWH/UFH to patients with ACS who will not undergo a PCI procedure.

Table 16

Heparin Use in UA/NSTEMI

- Heparin or LMWH should be given to all patients in combination with ASA and clopidogrel
- Heparin is continued for a total of 24-48 hours or until a PCI procedure is completed
- In patients with a planned CABG within 24 hours, heparin use is preferred to LMWH

- Low molecular weight heparin (LMWH).
  - * Agents
    - Enoxaparin
    - Dalteparin
  - * Differ from UFH in size and affinity for thrombin
  - * Advantages of LMWH over UFH include: better bioavailability, a more predictable response, ease of administration, fewer SEs, and no recommended routine monitoring
  - * A total of four clinical trials have compared UFH to LMWH for the treatment of UA/NSTEMI. Two of the trials showed superiority of enoxaparin (Lovenox) over UFH. The remaining two trials with dalteparin (Fragmin) showed equivalence to UFH
  - * Indications for therapy (see Table 17)

Table 17

Low Molecular Weight Heparin (LMWH) Use in UA/NSTEMI

- LMWH or heparin, in combination with ASA and clopidogrel, should be given to all patients
- Enoxaparin may be superior to heparin in patients with UA/NSTEMI

6. Acute Myocardial Infarction (ST-Segment Elevation MI or STEMI)

Pathophysiology

Acute myocardial infarction
- More than 85% of all MIs occur by thrombus formation precipitated by atherosclerotic plaque rupture.

- Aggregated platelets after plaque rupture can serve as a substrate for thrombus propagation, leading to formation of an occlusive thrombus.

- This complete occlusion results in abrupt and persistent ischemia that clinically manifests as ST-segment elevation MI. Left untreated, occlusion of the coronary arteries can lead to sudden cardiac death.

STEMI vs. UA/NSTEMI (Table 18)

Location
- Patients with RV wall infarction should be managed similarly to LV infarction with the exception that NTG, diuretics, and other preload-reducing agents should be avoided in RV wall MIs because these patients are dependent on preload.

Table 18

STEMI vs. UA/NSTEMI

STEMI	NSTEMI
Totally occlusive thrombus	Platelet-rich thrombi, which do not completely block coronary blood flow
More extensive damage	Smaller, less extensive damage
Results in an injury that affects the entire thickness of the myocardial wall	NSTEMI involves only the subendocardial myocardium
Occlusion persists long enough to compromise myocardial function and leads to myocardial necrosis	Unstable angina is ischemia; NSTEMI may still result in necrosis, but not to the extent of STEMI
ST-segment elevation on ECG	ST depression or no ST elevation on ECG
Lytic therapy or primary reperfusion is a main treatment strategy	Antiplatelet agents such as GPIs are used to target platelet-rich thrombus

- RV MI may require volume loading with IV fluids to maintain preload and cardiac output (CO).

- Symptoms differ from a LV wall MI in that a RV wall MI can cause hypotension, elevated jugular venous pressure, and cardiogenic shock because of inadequate filling of the LV.

Ventricular remodeling
- Can occur as a result of myocardial necrosis and may continue for months following MI.

- Leads to activation of the neurohormonal and renin-angiotensin systems that will ultimately affect ventricular shape, size, and function.

- Precipitates chronic changes in ventricular volume, ventricular dilation, hypertrophy, and eventually heart failure (HF).

- ACEIs and BBs reduce the progression of ventricular remodeling. Carvedilol may reverse ventricular remodeling.

Prognosis

Mortality
- The highest risk of death from MI is generally within the first 48 hours.

- Anterior MIs usually involve a larger area of the myocardium than do inferior MIs, and thereby have a higher mortality.

- An important prognostic factor following MI is LV function, as HF is one of the most serious complications of MI.

- Large anterior wall MIs, LV dysfunction, and complex ventricular ectopy carry the highest mortality rate post-MI.

- Early identification and risk stratification can reduce mortality following MI.

Predictors of death
- High troponin concentration correlates with higher death rates in STEMI and NSTEMI.

- Predictors of death within 30 days post-MI include: age >70 years, HTN, atrial fibrillation (afib), tachycardia, large infarct size, previous MI, and female gender.

- Lower-risk patients include those younger than 71

years of age with an LV ejection fraction (EF) ≥40%.

- Patients who continue to have frequent ventricular arrhythmias following MI are at a high risk of sudden cardiac death.

Presentation

- Symptoms similar to UA/NSTEMI.

- Atypical presentation is common in women and in those with DM.

Diagnosis (see Table 19)

Goals of Therapy in Acute Myocardial Infarction

- Limit infarct size.

- Reverse myocardial ischemia and thereby salvage myocardium.

- Minimize complications.

- Reduce mortality.

MONA therapy (see Table 10)

Nitrate use in AMI (Table 20)

Reperfusion therapy
Primary PTCA
- Intervention designed to re-open a partially or completely occluded coronary artery to re-establish blood flow.

Table 19

Criteria for the Diagnosis of Myocardial Infarction
(Two of these three must be met)

Chest pain	Generally lasting for >30 minutes
ECG changes	ST-segment elevation of 0.1 mV in two limb leads or 0.1-0.2 mV elevation in at least two precordial leads
Cardiac isoenzymes	Troponin T or I elevation
	CK-MB elevations

Table 20

Nitrate Use in STEMI

- Nitrates may be used for the first 24 hours in all patients with MI who do not have hypotension, bradycardia, or tachycardia. Nitrates salvage ischemic myocardium by relaxation of vascular smooth muscle in veins, arteries, and arterioles.
- Insignificant reductions in mortality beyond 48 hours. Use is reserved for those patients with large AMIs, persistent chest discomfort, HF, HTN, or persistent pulmonary congestion.
- Cautions and contraindications: carefully titrate in patients with inferior wall MI because of its frequent association with RV infarction. Such patients are especially dependent on adequate RV preload to maintain CO and can experience profound hypotension during nitrate administration.

- Mechanical reperfusion (PTCA such as balloon angioplasty and coronary stenting) has been shown to be more successful than fibrinolysis, but only 20% of hospitals have 24-hour cath lab capability to perform these procedures.

- PTCA immediately following full-dose fibrinolytic therapy is not beneficial and may actually contribute to morbidity and mortality due to increased bleeding.

Fibrinolytic therapy
(also known as thrombolytic therapy)
- Improves myocardial O_2 supply, limits infarct size, and decreases mortality.

- Controversy exists with regard to one lytic agent's superiority over another.

- A door-to-needle time <30 minutes is an important goal.

- Signs of successful reperfusion include relief of chest pain, resolution of ST-segment changes, and reperfusion arrhythmias, usually ventricular in nature.

- Fibrinolytic therapy is unsuccessful in approximately 22-30% of patients.

- Indications for therapy (see Table 21).

Heparin therapy
- Indications for therapy (see Table 22).

Table 21

Use of Fibrinolytic Therapy in STEMI

- ST-segment elevation >1 mm in two or more contiguous leads or bundle branch block (BBB) (obscuring ST observational changes)
- Presentation within 12 hours or less of symptom onset
- Patient has no contraindications to fibrinolytic therapy and has an indication for therapy
- STEMI in patients age >75 years may be useful and appropriate
- Can be used in STEMI when time to therapy is 12-24 hours if chest pain is ongoing
- Should not be used if the time to therapy >24 hours, and the ischemic pain is resolved
- Should not be used for ST depression

β-Adrenergic blockade (BB)
- Early BB use post-MI decreases infarct size, CV mortality, reinfarction rate, and nonfatal cardiac arrests, and increases the probability of long-term survival.

- Late administration of a BB (at least 24 hours after MI) improves left ventricular diastolic filling and reduces risk of recurrent MI and death.

- Indications for therapy (Table 23).

Table 22

Heparin Use in STEMI

- Adjunct with fibrinolytics for the prevention of recurrent coronary thrombosis.
- Combination of UFH with streptokinase (SK) is less clear because it is a nonspecific fibrinolytic. UFH may increase the risk of bleeding because of SK's long half-life.
- Patients at high risk for systemic emboli (large or anterior MI, afib, previous embolus, or known LV thrombus) should have UFH held for 6 hours (post-thrombolytic) and aPTT monitoring begun at that time. After 48 hours a change to SQ heparin, warfarin, or ASA alone should be considered.
- Can use SQ UFH (7500 U bid x 7 days or until the patient is fully ambulatory) or LMWH (enoxaparin 1 mg/kg SQ bid or dalteparin 120 U/kg bid) in all patients not treated with a thrombolytic (who have no contraindications to UFH). IV UFH preferred in patients at high risk for systemic emboli.

Table 23

β-Blocker Use Post-Myocardial Infarction

Early therapy: BBs should be given to all patients with acute MI who can be treated within 12 hours of MI, regardless of administration of concomitant thrombolytic therapy. IV treatment should be started as soon as possible in all patients within 12-24 hours after onset of symptoms, and oral therapy should be given to patients presenting later.

Late therapy: BBs should be given to all patients without a clear contraindication to BB therapy. Treatment should begin within a few days of event (if not initiated early) and be continued indefinitely.

Glycoprotein IIb/IIIa inhibitors (GPIs)

- The role of platelet GPIs in STEMI is rapidly evolving. Trials to date in combination with full- and half-dose fibrinolytic agents have shown a more complete reperfusion at the price of higher bleeding rates.

- Abciximab reduces the incidence of combined death, MI, and recurrent ischemia in patients with STEMI.

Angiotensin-converting enzyme inhibitors (ACEIs)

- Primary goal is to limit postinfarction LV dilatation and hypertrophy so that pump function is preserved or improved. ACEIs attenuate the remodeling process and thereby slow the progression to HF post-MI.

- Benefits are clearly most pronounced in patients with evidence of ventricular dysfunction (either objective evidence such as LVEF <40% or subjective evidence such as HF symptoms).

- Marked benefit in other high-risk patients (previous MI, HF, and anterior MI without thrombolytic therapy).

Table 24

Angiotensin-Converting Enzyme Inhibitor Use Post-STEMI

- Patients within the first 24 hours of a suspected MI or with clinical HF without contraindications
- All other patients without contraindications within the first 24 hours

- Recent studies suggest acute treatment should be given to patients considered at higher risk due to a history of HTN, DM, or previous MI, and should be continued indefinitely.

- Indications for therapy (see Table 24).

Calcium channel blockers (CCBs)
- Indications for therapy (see Table 25).

Treatment of ventricular fibrillation (VF) post-MI
- The risk of VF is highest during the first 4 hours post-MI and then declines sharply.

- Prophylactic lidocaine use has been shown to increase all-cause mortality when used to prevent VF. The use of lidocaine for VF prophylaxis is not recommended.

- Lidocaine should be utilized if patients experience VF or hemodynamically compromising ventricular tachycardia following MI.

Table 25

Calcium Channel Blockers Post-Myocardial Infarction

- Verapamil or diltiazem only with continuing ischemia when BB use is either contraindicated or used at maximum dose with nitrate.
- Verapamil or diltiazem should not be used in patients with systolic dysfunction, AV block, or bradycardia.

7. Primary Prevention: Risk Factor Modification

Background

- The majority of the causes of cardiovascular disease are known and modifiable.

- Risk factor screening should begin at age 20 with the hope that all adults know the levels and significance of risk factors as routinely assessed by their primary care provider.

Nonmodifiable Risk Factors

Age
- Men >45; women >55 (or those who had an early hysterectomy regardless of age).

Race
- Higher risk in African-American males and females compared to Caucasian males and females.

Family history
- Father or brother with a coronary event before age 55.

- Mother or sister with a coronary event before age 65.

Modifiable Risk Factors

- Smoking.

- Hypertension.

- Hyperlipidemia.

- Hyperhomocysteinemia.

- Diabetes.

- Metabolic syndrome.

- Obesity.

- Physical inactivity.

- Alcohol consumption

Pharmacologic Therapy

Aspirin
- Fifth ACCP Consensus Conference on Antithrombotic Therapy (Chest Guidelines) recommends that ASA (80 to 325 mg/d) be considered for individuals >50 years old who have at least one major risk factor for CAD and who are free of contraindications.

- The ACC/AHA recommends doses of 75-160 mg/d in persons at higher risk of CVD (especially those with a 10-year risk of CHD >10%).

- The American Diabetes Association recommends ASA therapy to prevent CV events in most patients with DM who are >50 years of age and have no contraindications to ASA.

Angiotensin-converting enzyme inhibitors (ACEIs)
- In the HOPE study, ramipril demonstrated effectiveness in reducing the risk of MI, stroke, and death from cardiovascular causes in patents at high risk of a major cardiovascular event. ACEIs may be used as protective agents.

Antioxidants
- Although the results of trials have been conflicting, at this point, there is no consistent evidence with vitamin E or other antioxidant therapy to recommend its use for primary prevention of heart disease.

Nonpharmacologic Therapy for Ischemic Heart Disease

Revascularization
PCI
- Procedure types include balloon angioplasty (PTCA), coronary stenting, and ablative technologies (laser, atherectomy).

- Recommended for patients with multivessel disease with normal LV function (who do not have DM).

- Can be used in patients who are poor surgical candidates and in those who refuse surgery.

Coronary artery bypass graft surgery (CABG)
- Indicated in patients with multivessel disease with LV dysfunction or significant disease of a major coronary vessel.

Diet
- Diets low in saturated fat and high in fruits, vegetables, whole grains, and fiber are associated with a reduced risk of CVD.

- Omega-3 fatty acids: the AHA Dietary Guidelines recommends inclusion of at least two servings of fish per week (particularly fatty fish).

- Food sources high in alpha-linolenic acid (eg, soybean, canola, walnut, and flaxseed oil, and walnuts and flaxseeds) are also recommended.

Exercise

- Regular aerobic physical activity increases a person's capacity for exercise. Exercise plays a role in both primary and secondary prevention of cardiovascular disease.

- Current guidelines from the CDC and NIH recommend that Americans should accumulate at least 30 minutes of moderate-intensity physical activity on most, preferably all, days of the week to prevent risk of chronic disease in the future.

- The Institute of Medicine recommends 60 minutes of physical activity per day.

Weight loss

- Weight loss can reduce blood pressure, lower blood glucose levels, and improve blood lipid abnormalities.

- A goal of 5-10% of body weight loss is associated with a decreased morbidity and mortality.

- Pharmacotherapy used for weight loss should be reserved for those with a BMI >30, or in those with BMI >25 with other risk factors for comorbid diseases.

Alcohol consumption

- Lowest CV mortality occurs in those who consume 1 or 2 drinks per day. People with no alcohol consumption have higher total mortality than those drinking 1 to 2 drinks per day.

- In the absence of alcohol-related illnesses, 1 to 2 drinks per day in males and 1 alcoholic drink per day in females may be considered for high-risk patients.

- A drink equivalent amounts to a 12-ounce bottle of beer, a 4-ounce glass of wine, or a 1.5-ounce shot of 80-proof spirits.

- A general increase in alcohol consumption at the population level is not recommended.

Pharmacology

Anti-ischemic drug therapy

β-Blockers (see hypertension chapter)

Nitrates

Mechanism of action

- Organic nitrates are prodrugs that must be transformed to exert pharmacologic effect.

- NTG leads to denitration of the nitrate, liberation of nitric oxide (NO), guanylyl cyclase stimulation, the conversion of guanosine triphosphate to cGMP, and vasodilation.

- NO also reduces platelet adhesion and aggregation and affects endothelial function and vascular growth.

Properties

- Oral: isosorbide dinitrate (ISDN) and NTG undergo extensive first-pass metabolism when given PO. Mononitrate does not; it is completely bioavailable.

- IV: achieves highest concentrations; usually used for only 24 hours to avoid developing tolerance.

- SL tablet/spray for immediate-release.

- Spray does not degrade when exposed to air like tablets.

- Half-life: 1-5 minutes regardless of route.

Doses

- See Table 26.

Monitoring parameters

- Blood pressure, heart rate

Adverse drug reactions

- See Table 27.

Drug-drug interactions

- See Table 28.

Drug-disease interactions:

- Glaucoma.
  * Intraocular pressure may increase
  * Caution in patients with glaucoma.

- Hypertrophic obstructive cardiomyopathy.

- Severe aortic stenosis.
  * Can cause hypotension and syncope

Contraindications

- Sildenafil (Viagra®): use within 24 hours.

- Hypersensitivity to nitrates.

Table 26

Pharmacologic Properties and Doses of Nitrates

Drug	Route	Onset (min)	Duration of action	Dose
Nitroglycerin sublingual tablet (Nitrostat®, Nitroquick®)	Sublingual	1-3	30-60 min	0.2-0.6 mg every 5 minutes. Maximum of 3 tablets in 15 minutes. Seek emergency treatment if chest pain is unrelieved after 3 doses
Nitroglycerin spray (Nitrolingual®)	Translingual	2	30-60 min	0.4 mg every 5 minutes. Maximum of 3 sprays in 15 minutes. Seek emergency treatment if chest pain unrelieved after 3 sprays
Nitroglycerin transmucosal tablets (Nitroguard®)	Buccal	1-2	3-5 h	Insert 1 tablet into cheek every 3-5 h
Nitroglycerin ointment (Nitrobid®, Nitrol®)	Topical	30-60	2-12 h	1-2 inches every 8 hours up to 4-5 inches every 4 h
Nitroglycerin transdermal patches (Nitro-dur®, Transderm Nitro®, Nitrek®, Nitrodisc®, Deponit®, Minitran®)	Topical	30-60	Up to 24 h	Starting dose: 0.2-0.4 mg/h. Apply and allow patch to stay in place for 12 h. Remove the patch after 12 h to allow for a nitrate-free interval
Nitroglycerin sustained release tablets/capsules (Nitrong®, Nitroglyn®, Nitro-Time®)	Oral	20-45	3-8 h	Starting dose: 2.5 mg tid-qid. Increase the dose by 2.5 mg two to four times daily to reach effective dose
Nitroglycerin intravenous (Tridil®, Nitro-Bid IV®)	IV	1-2	3-5 minutes	Starting dose: 5 µg/min. Titrate to response
Isosorbide mononitrate (Ismo®, Monoket®)	Oral	30-60	No data	20 mg bid (given 7 hours apart). May need to start with 5 mg bid for low-weight patients
Isosorbide mononitrate, extended release (Imdur®, Isotrate ER®)	Oral	30-60	No data	Starting dose: 30-60 mg qd. Maximum dose: 240 mg qd
Isosorbide dinitrate (Isordil Titradose®, Sorbitrate®)	Oral	20-40	4-6 h	Starting dose: 5-20 mg q6h. Maintenance dose: 10-40 mg q6h
Isosorbide dinitrate, sustained release tablets/capsules (Isordil Tembids®, Dilatrate-SR®)	Oral	Up to 4 h	6-8 h	Initial dose: 40 mg q8h. Maintenance dose: 40-80 mg q8-12 h

Table 27

Adverse Reactions of Nitrates

Tolerance	Tolerance to the vasodilatory effects can develop if dosing does not allow for a nitrate-free interval (10-12 h)
CNS	Headache (up to 50%), dizziness, anxiety, nervousness
CV	Hypotension, tachycardia, palpitations, syncope
GI	Nausea, vomiting, dyspepsia
Dermatologic	Rash, dermatitis
Other	Blurred vision, muscle twitching, perspiration, edema, arthralgia

Table 28

Nitrate Drug-Drug Interactions

Interacting medication	Effect
Sildenafil (Viagra®)	Significant reduction of systolic and diastolic blood pressure. Do not give sildenafil within 24 hours of nitrate use
Calcium channel blockers	Marked symptomatic hypotension may occur
Alcohol	Severe hypotension may occur

Patient instructions/counseling

- Avoid alcohol consumption.

- May cause dizziness. Use caution when driving or engaging in hazardous activities until drug effect is known.

- When standing from a sitting position, rise slowly to avoid an abrupt drop in blood pressure.

- Notify physician of acute headache, dizziness, or blurred vision.

- Sublingual tablets.
    * Keep tablets in their original container.
    * Dissolve tablet under the tongue. Lack of tingling does not indicate a lack of potency.
    * Take at the first sign of chest pain. May repeat every 5 minutes for a total of 3 tablets. If chest pain is unrelieved, seek emergency medical attention.

- Translingual spray.
    * Spray under tongue or onto tongue.
    * Hold spray nozzle as close to your mouth as possible and spray medicine onto or under your tongue.
    * Do not inhale the spray or use near heat, open flame, or while smoking.
    * Close mouth immediately after spraying.
    * Avoid eating, drinking, or smoking for 5-10 minutes.
    * Do not use more than 3 sprays in 15 minutes. If your pain does not go away after 3 sprays, seek emergency medical attention.

- Transmucosal tablets.
    * Place between cheek and gum. Do not chew tablet; allow to dissolve over a 3-5-hour period.
    * Release of medication from the tablet may be increased by touching the tablet with the tongue or hot liquids.

- Ointment.
    * Measure the correct amount using the papers provided with the product.
    * Use papers for the application, not fingers.
    * Apply to the chest or back.

- Transdermal patches.
    * Tear the wrapper open carefully. Never cut the wrapper or patch with scissors. Do not use any patch that has been cut by accident.
    * Apply to a hairless area and rotate sites to avoid irritation. Be sure to remove the old patch before applying a new one.
    * Do not put the patch over burns, cuts, or irritated skin.
    * Remove patch approximately 12-14 hours after placing it on every day. This prevents tolerance to the beneficial effects of NTG.
    * Used patches may still contain residual medication; use caution when disposing around children and pets.
    * Store the patches at room temperature in a closed container, away from heat, moisture, and direct light. Do not refrigerate.

- Sustained-release tablets.
    * Take at the same time each day as directed.
    * Do not chew or crush tablets or capsules.

- Others: calcium channel blockers (see hypertension chapter); angiotensin-converting enzyme inhibitors (see heart failure chapter).

Antiplatelet drug therapy
Aspirin

Mechanism of action

- Blocks prostaglandin synthesis, which prevents the formation of thromboxane A_2.

Dose

- At the onset of chest pain: 160-325 mg chewed and swallowed.

- Maintenance dose: 75-325 mg for life.

- Monitoring parameters: signs of bleeding, renal function, tinnitus.

Table 29

Aspirin Adverse Reactions

CV	Hypotension, edema, tachycardia
CNS	Fatigue, nervousness, dizziness
Dermatologic	Rash, urticaria, angioedema
GI	Nausea, vomiting, dyspepsia, gastrointestinal ulceration, gastric erosion, duodenal ulcers
Hematologic	Bleeding, anemia
Otic	Hearing loss, tinnitus
Renal	Renal impairment, increased serum creatinine, proteinuria
Respiratory	Asthma, bronchospasm, dyspnea, tachypnea, respiratory alkalosis

Adverse drug reactions
- See Table 29.

Drug-drug interactions
- Clopidogrel, GPI, UFH, LMWH, NSAIDs, and warfarin may all increase the risk of bleeding if used in combination with ASA.

Drug-disease interactions
- Peptic ulcer disease (PUD).
    * May cause gastric ulceration
    * Recommend the enteric coated tablet

- Other active bleeding.

Patient instructions and counseling
- Avoid over-the-counter (OTC) products containing ASA, NSAIDs, or salicylate ingredients without the direction of a physician.

- Notify physician of dark, tarry stools, persistent stomach pain, difficulty breathing, unusual bruising/bleeding, or skin rash.

- Do not crush an enteric-coated product.

Thienopyridines
Mechanism of action
- Blocks adenosine diphosphate (ADP)-mediated activation of platelets by selectively and irreversibly blocking ADP activation of the glycoprotein IIb/IIIa complex.

Dose
- Clopidogrel.
    * Loading dose: 300-600 mg PO
    * Maintenance dose: 75 mg qd for at least 1 year, possibly life-long

- Ticlopidine.
    * Loading dose: 500 mg PO
    * Maintenance dose: 250 mg bid

Monitoring parameters
- Clopidogrel.
    * Signs of bleeding

- Ticlopidine.
    * CBC with differential every 2 weeks for the first 3 months of therapy; liver function tests periodically; signs of bleeding
    * Discontinue ticlopidine if the absolute neutrophil count <1200 or platelet count <80,000

Adverse drug reactions
- See Table 30.

Table 30

Thienopyridine Adverse Reactions

Clopidogrel	Chest pain, headache, dizziness, abdominal pain, vomiting, diarrhea, arthralgia, back pain, upper respiratory infections, flu-like symptoms; <1% blood dyscrasias, bleeding
Ticlopidine	Rash, nausea, dyspepsia, diarrhea; 2.4% neutropenia; <1% blood dyscrasias, thrombotic thrombocytopenic purpura (TTP), bleeding

Drug-drug interactions
- See Table 31.

Drug-disease interactions
- PUD or other active bleeding.

Contraindications
- Hypersensitivity to an individual product.

- Active bleeding (PUD, intracranial hemorrhage).

- Severe liver disease.

- Ticlopidine—neutropenia, thrombocytopenia.

Patient instructions and counseling
- Avoid OTC ASA, salicylate, and NSAID products unless under the direction of a physician.

- Notify physician for unusual bleeding or bruising; blood in the urine, stool, or emesis; skin rash or yellowing of the skin or eyes.

Table 31

Thienopyridine Drug-Drug Interactions

Interacting medication	Effect
ASA, GPI, UFH, LMWH, NSAIDs, warfarin	Combination may increase the risk of bleeding
CYP2C9 substrates (phenytoin, fluvastatin, NSAIDs, losartan, irbesartan, valsartan)	May have increased serum levels

Glycoprotein IIb/IIIa receptor inhibitors (GPIs)

Mechanism of action
- Blockade of the GP receptor prevents fibrinogen binding, thus inhibiting platelet aggregation; receptor is the final common pathway for platelet aggregation.

Properties of individual agents
- See Table 32.

Indications and dose
- See Table 33.

Monitoring parameters
- Hematocrit/hemoglobin, platelet count, PT/aPTT, activated clotting time (ACT) with PCI.

Adverse drug reactions
- Bleeding, thrombocytopenia, allergic reaction from repeated exposure (abciximab).

Drug-drug interactions
- ASA, clopidogrel, UFH, LMWH, NSAIDs, and warfarin may increase the risk of bleeding if used in combination with GPIs.

Drug-disease interactions
- PUD or other active bleeding.

Contraindications
- Active bleeding.

- Platelet count <100,000.

Table 32

Pharmacologic Properties of the Glycoprotein IIb/IIIa Receptor Inhibitors

Drug	Chemical nature	Duration of effect	Renal elimination
Abciximab (Reopro®)	Antibody	>12 h. Note: action can be reversed by a platelet infusion	No
Eptifibatide (Integrilin®)	Nonpeptide	4-8 h	Yes
Tirofiban (Aggrastat®)	Peptide fragment	4 h	Yes

- History of intracranial hemorrhage, neoplasms, AV malformations, or aneurysm.

- History of stroke within the past 30 days or any history of hemorrhage or stroke.

- Severe HTN (>180/110 mm Hg).

- Major surgery within the past 6 weeks.

Table 33

Indications and Doses of the Glycoprotein IIb/IIIa Receptor Inhibitors

Drug	Indication	Dose
Abciximab (Reopro)	Adjunct to PCI or when PCI is planned w/in 24 hours	0.25 mg/kg IV bolus, 0.125 mg/kg infusion continued for 12 hours post-procedure; Maximum length of infusion: 18-24 h
Eptifibatide (Integrilin)	Adjunct to PCI	180 µg/kg IV bolus x 2, 10 minutes apart; 2 µg/kg/min infusion started after the 1st bolus and continued for 18-24 h postprocedure
	Patients with ACS managed with or without PCI	180 µg/kg IV bolus, 2 µg/kg/min infusion continued for 18-24 h postprocedure; Maximum length of infusion: 96 hours
Tirofiban (Aggrastat)	Adjunct to PCI	0.4 µg/kg IV bolus over 30 minutes, 0.1 µg/kg/min infusion for 72 h; Minimum infusion time: 48 h
		OR
	Patients with ACS managed with or without PCI	10 µg/kg IV bolus over 3 minutes followed by 0.15 µg/kg/min infusion for 36 h 0.4 µg/kg IV bolus over 30 minutes, 0.1 µg/kg/min infusion for 72 h

- SCr >4 mg/dL or dialysis dependent (eptifibatide only).

Anticoagulants
Heparin
Mechanism of action
- Enhances the action of antithrombin III, thereby inactivating thrombin and preventing the conversion of fibrinogen to fibrin.

Dose
- UA/NSTEMI: 60-70 U/kg (maximum 5000 U) IV bolus, 12-15 U/kg/h (maximum 1000 U/h) infusion titrated to an aPTT 1.5-2.5 times control.

- STEMI (in combination with tPA, rPA or tenecteplase):
  * 5000 U bolus IV, 1000 U/h infusion
  * 60 U/kg (maximum 4000 U) IV bolus, 12 U/kg/h (maximum 1000 U/h) infusion
  * Titrate to an aPTT of 1.5-2.5 times control for 48 hours

Monitoring parameters
- aPTT, PT, platelet count, hemoglobin/hematocrit, signs of bleeding, ACT (w/PCI).

Adverse drug reactions
- Bleeding, thrombocytopenia, hemorrhage, epistaxis, allergic reactions, osteoporosis.
  * Protamine can be used to reverse the effects of heparin. Dose: 1 mg of protamine neutralizes 100 U of heparin

Drug-drug interactions
- ASA, clopidogrel, GPI, NSAIDs, and warfarin may increase the risk of bleeding if used in combination with UFH.

- LMWH: combination may increase the risk of bleeding and has been reported to cause death.

Drug-disease interaction
- PUD or other active bleeding.

Contraindications
- History of heparin-induced thrombocytopenia (HIT).

- Severe thrombocytopenia.

- Active bleeding.

- Suspected ICH.

Low molecular weight heparin (LMWH)
Mechanism of action
- Same mechanism as heparin, stronger inhibitor of thrombin (Factor Xa).

Properties
- See Table 34.

Dose
- Enoxaparin (Lovenox): 1 mg/kg SQ q12h.

- Dalteparin (Fragmin): 120 IU/kg q12h (Maximum 10,000 IU q12h).

Monitoring parameters
- Platelet count, hemoglobin/hematocrit, anti-Xa levels, signs of bleeding.

- Note: It is not necessary to monitor aPTT or PT.

Adverse drug reactions
- Bleeding, thrombocytopenia, hemorrhage, epistaxis.

Drug-drug interactions
- ASA, clopidogrel, GPI, NSAIDs and warfarin may increase the risk of bleeding if used in combination with LMWH.

- UFH: combination may increase the risk of bleeding and has been reported to cause death.

Drug-disease interactions
- PUD or any active bleeding.

Warnings
- Patients with recent or anticipated epidural or spinal anesthesia are at risk of hematoma and subsequent paralysis.

Contraindications
- Severe thrombocytopenia.

Table 34

Properties of Low Molecular Weight Heparin vs. Unfractionated Heparin

Drug	Half-life	MW (daltons)	Anti-Xa: Anti-IIa	Renal elimination
Enoxaparin	4.5 h	4500	2.7:1	Yes
Dalteparin	3-5 h	5000	2.0:1	Yes
UFH	1 h	15,000	1:1	No

- Active bleeding.

- Suspected ICH.

Thrombolytic therapy
Thrombolytics
Mechanism of action
- Acts either directly or indirectly to activate or convert plasminogen to plasmin to lyse a formed clot. The conversion of plasminogen to plasmin activates the body's natural thrombolytic/fibrinolytic system, which lyses the clot and releases fibrin degradation products.

Dose
- See Table 35.

Monitoring parameters
- CBC, ECG, aPTT, signs of bleeding, signs of reperfusion.

Adverse drug reactions
- Bleeding, ICH (<1%), stroke (<2%), epistaxis.

Drug-drug interactions
- ASA, clopidogrel, GPI, UFH, LMWH, NSAIDs, and warfarin may increase the risk of bleeding if used in combination with thrombolytics.

Contraindications
- See Table 36

Table 36

Contraindications and Cautions for Fibrinolytic Use

Contraindications:
1. Previous hemorrhagic stroke at any time; other strokes or cerebrovascular events within 1 year
2. Known intracranial neoplasm
3. Active internal bleeding (does not include menses)
4. Suspected aortic dissection

Cautions and relative contraindications:
1. Severe uncontrolled hypertension (BP >180/110)
2. History of prior CVA or known intracerebral pathology not covered in contraindications
3. Current use of anticoagulants in therapeutic doses (INR >2-3)
4. Known bleeding diathesis
5. Recent trauma (within 2-4 weeks), including head trauma or traumatic or prolonged (>10 min) CPR or major surgery (<3 wk)
6. Noncompressible vascular punctures
7. Recent (within 2-4 weeks) internal bleeding
8. For streptokinase: prior exposure (especially within 5 d-2 y) or prior allergic reaction
9. Pregnancy
10. Active peptic ulcer
11. History of chronic severe hypertension

Table 35

Thrombolytic Doses

Drug	Dose
Streptokinase (SK, Streptase®)	1.5 million units in 50 mL of normal saline or D_5W given over 60 minutes
Tissue plasminogen activator (tPA, Alteplase®)	15 mg IV bolus, followed by 0.75 mg/kg IV infusion over 30 minutes (not to exceed 50 mg); then 0.5 mg/kg IV infusion over 1 hour (not to exceed 35 mg)
Reteplase (rPA, Retevase®)	10 U IVP over 2 minutes, followed in 30 minutes by a repeat 10 U IV bolus over 10 minutes
Tenecteplase (TNK, TNKase®)	<60 kg give 30 mg IV bolus; 60-69.9 kg give 35 mg IV bolus; 70-79.9 kg give 40 mg IV bolus; 80-89.9 kg give 45 mg IV bolus; >90 kg give 50 mg IV bolus; Note: each bolus is given over 5 seconds

8. Key Points

- Angina is a syndrome described as discomfort or pain in the chest, arm, shoulder, back, or jaw. Angina is frequently worsened by physical exertion or emotional stress and is usually relieved by sublingual nitroglycerin (NTG). Patients with angina usually have coronary artery disease (CAD).

- Anginal symptoms are caused by a decrease in O_2 supply due to reduced flow.

- The goals for treating stable angina are to prevent death, reduce symptoms, and improve quality of life.

- Aspirin has been shown to decrease the incidence of MI, adverse CV events, and sudden death in patients with coronary artery disease.

- β-Blockers are first-line therapy for treatment of angina in patients with or without a history of MI if there are no contraindications.

- Patients prescribed nitrates for treatment of angina need to be counseled on their appropriate use.

- Upon hospital presentation with UA/NSTEMI/ STEMI, initial therapy for all patients is MONA (morphine, oxygen, nitroglycerin, and aspirin). If there are no contraindications, all patients should be given aspirin therapy for life.

- The first-line anti-ischemic therapy for the treatment of UA/NSTEMI is a β-blocker. If chest pain continues or a β-blocker is contraindicated, a calcium channel blocker or long-acting nitrate should be considered, in that order.

- In addition to aspirin therapy for life, clopidogrel should be combined with aspirin in all patients with or without planned PCI for at least 1 month and up to 1 year.

- Any of the available GP IIb/IIIa agents should be considered in patients undergoing a PCI procedure. In patients without a planned PCI, eptifibatide or tirofiban can be used for medical treatment.

- All patients presenting with UA/NSTEMI should receive anticoagulation with UFH or LMWH.

- STEMI differs from UA/NSTEMI in that there is a totally occlusive clot that causes damage across the entire thickness of the myocardial wall. The damage to the heart is more extensive with STEMI and ECG changes differ.

- Primary reperfusion (either percutaneous coronary intervention or fibrinolytic therapy) is the main treatment strategy for STEMI.

- Ventricular remodeling (post-MI) resulting after myocardial damage can be slowed and possibly reversed by using long-term ACE inhibition and β-blockade.

- Secondary prevention of MI should include aspirin, β-blockers, ACEIs, and statin therapy (to achieve a LDL goal of <100 mg/dL) in all patients without contraindications.

9. Questions and Answers

Mr. Smith is a 66-year-old white male who presented to his local physician with complaints of chest pain. He described the pain as sharp, aching, and nonradiating. The pain, which he has had for the past few weeks, has occurred mainly during his daily walk and is usually relieved when he stops to rest.

PMH: HTN, PUD, asthma, CAD
FH: Father died of a stroke at 86; mother age 82 with DM, HF; sister died of MI at 52
SH: Smokes 1 ppd x 40 years; drinks alcohol socially 1-2 times a week
Meds: Proventil MDI 2 puffs prn
     Flovent 44 µg 2 puffs bid
     Prilosec 20 mg qd
     Aspirin 75 mg qd
     Hydrochlorothiazide 25 mg qd
VS: BP 148/92; HR 82; RR 18; Ht 72"; Wt 200 lb
Labs: (Fasting) total cholesterol 226 mg/dL, TG 110 mg/dL, HDL 38 mg/dL, LDL 166 mg/dL
Chem-12, WNL
ECG: Normal (patient currently pain-free)
Cath 6 years ago: Minimal two-vessel disease

1. How would you classify Mr. Smith's chest pain?

    A. Unstable angina
    B. Stable angina
    C. Variant angina
    D. Silent ischemia
    E. NSTEMI

2. Considering Mr. Smith's situation, which of the following would be the most appropriate therapeutic intervention?

    A. SL NTG prn
    B. Propranolol
    C. Tirofiban
    D. Verapamil and SL NTG prn
    E. Atenolol, amlodipine, and SL NTG

3. What additional medication should be considered for Mr. Smith?

    A. Ticlopidine
    B. Lipitor
    C. Plavix
    D. Eptifibatide
    E. Reteplase

4. Which of the following effects on myocardial oxygen demand do β-blockers NOT cause?

    A. Decrease HR by decreasing conduction through the AV node
    B. Decreases BP
    C. Decreases contractility
    D. Peripheral vasodilation
    E. Decrease conduction through the AV node

5. Which of the following statements is true regarding the use of calcium channel blockers in IHD?

    A. Amlodipine and felodipine reduce MVO_2 by decreasing conduction through the AV node.
    B. They should be used as first-line therapy in patients with stable angina.
    C. Newer-generation dihydropyridines like nifedipine immediate-release are safe in the treatment of IH**D**.
    D. They can be used in combination with β-blockers to attenuate the effect of increased sympathetic tone that some dihydropyridines may cause.
    E. The combination of verapamil and metoprolol in a patient with reduced LV systolic function is safe and well-tolerated by most patients.

6. Which of the following counseling points should be made to a patient being prescribed SL NTG?

    I.   Take at the same time each day as directed.
    II. Keep tablets in their original container.
    III. Take at the first sign of chest pain. May repeat every 5 minutes for a total of 3 tablets. If chest pain is unrelieved, seek emergency medical attention.

    A. III only
    B. I, II, and III
    C. I and III only
    D. I and II only
    E. II and III only

7. Which of the following is not considered a potential cardiovascular benefit of ACEIs in IHD?

    A. Reduce the incidence of MI
    B. Reduce the incidence of CV death and stroke in patients at high risk for vascular disease
    C. Agents with high tissue ACE inhibition have been proven to be superior and provide better protection
    D. ACE-inhibitors should be used in all stable angina patients with known CAD who also have diabetes

E. ACEIs should be used in all patients post-MI, regardless of LV function.

8. Which of the following drugs do not appear to interact with an exercise tolerance test (ETT)?

A. Nitrates
B. Digoxin
C. Atenolol
D. Flecainide
E. Clopidogrel

9. Ideal properties for a β-blocker in the treatment of UA/NSTEMI include all of the following EXCEPT:

A. Available in both IV and PO forms
B. Low lipophilicity
C. Has intrinsic sympathomimetic activity (ISA)
D. Does not have ISA
E. Cardioselectivity

10. Nitrates decrease oxygen demand via the following mechanism(s):

I. Peripheral vasodilation
II. Arterial vasodilation
III. Decreasing contractility

A. I only
B. II only
C. I and II only
D. II and III only
E. I, II, and III

11. The possible benefits of LMWH over UFH include all of the following EXCEPT:

A. Predictable response
B. Ease of administration
C. No recommended routine monitoring
D. Stronger affinity for thrombin
E. No renal adjustment necessary

12. Which of the following β-blocker has ISA activity?

A. Tenormin
B. Sectral
C. Inderal
D. Lopressor
E. Coreg

13. Which of the following medications is contraindicated within 24 hours of a nitrate?

A. Metoprolol
B. Quinapril
C. Verapamil
D. Sildenafil
E. Felodipine

14. The preferred narcotic to relieve chest pain after the use of SL NTG is:

A. Meperidine
B. Oxycodone
C. Morphine
D. Hydromorphone
E. Fentanyl

Use Patient Case #1 to answer Questions 15-16:

Patient Case #1
J.O. is a 54-year-old male who presents to the hospital with crushing substernal chest pain and radiation to his left arm. Past medical history is significant for HTN, COPD, and gout. J.O. has a history of smoking x 30 years and occasionally consumes alcohol. Vital signs on admission include BP 170/85; Pulse 72; RR 18; Temp 97. Before admission the patient was taking enteric coated aspirin 81 mg qd; Combivent inhaler two puffs qid; Tiazac 240 mg qd; Zyloprim 300mg qd.

Allergies: sulfa
Lab/Diagnostic tests:
1. ECG ST-segment depression, T-wave changes
2. Troponin T-positive x 3
3. Ejection fraction <35%
4. LDL 135 mg/dL

Diagnosis:
1. NSTEMI
2. Heart failure

15. What is the preferred β-blocker for this patient?

A. Propranolol
B. Carvedilol
C. Labetalol
D. Atenolol
E. Nadolol

16. All of the following therapies should be considered in this patient, EXCEPT:

A. Reteplase
B. Clopidogrel
C. Enalapril
D. Simvastatin
E. Eptifibatide

Use Patient Case #2 to answer Questions 17-18:

Patient Case #2
S.D. is a 56-year-old female who presents to the local ER complaining of crushing, substernal CP x 3 hours, which has been unrelieved by SL NTG. PMH is pertinent for HTN, T2DM, hypercholesterolemia, and metabolic syndrome. Heart rate and rhythm are regular and no S_3 or S_4 sounds are present. Vital signs include BP 184/119 mm Hg, HR 100 bpm, and RR 32 breaths/min. S.D.'s ECG shows ST-segment elevation >1 mm in leads II, III, and aVF. She is immediately admitted to the chest pain center and started on oxygen.

17. Which of the following criteria for the diagnosis of MI are present in S.D.?

    A. Chest pain symptoms relieved by SL NTG
    B. ST elevation >1 mm in two or more noncontiguous leads
    C. Chest pain symptoms with ECG changes that are consistent with myocardial ischemia or necrosis
    D. S.D. does not meet the criteria for MI based on the above presentation, because myocardial enzymes have not been evaluated.
    E. Since SD has negative enzymes, MI is ruled out

18. Which of the following agents should be administered to S.D.?

    A. tPA 100 mg IV over 90 minutes
    B. IV magnesium
    C. Prophylactic lidocaine
    D. Metoprolol 5 mg IV
    E. Cardizem 240 mg

19. What medications should a patient who is post-MI receive as discharge therapy?

    A. Aspirin, Plavix, Cardizem, and simvastatin
    B. Aspirin, metoprolol, enalapril, atorvastatin, and SL NTG
    C. Plavix, metoprolol, enalapril, and simvastatin
    D. Morphine, aspirin, SL NTG, and Lovenox
    E. Morphine, IV NTG, aspirin, and oxygen

20. The anticoagulant effect of unfractionated heparin requires binding to which plasma co-factor?

    A. Thrombospondin
    B. Antithrombin III
    C. Plasminogen

D. Factor XIIa
E. Factors II, VII, IX, and X

S.P. is a 45-year-old marathon runner. He presents to the emergency department with complaints of chest pain during his morning run. His father died of a myocardial infarction at age 48. His past medical history is positive for angina, hyperlipidemia, and hypertension. His current medications include aspirin, pravastatin, nifedipine, and clonidine. His electrocardiogram is consistent with acute ischemia. His HR is 52, and BP is 170/100. CBC and Chem-7 are within normal limits.

21. All of the following interventions are appropriate EXCEPT:

    A. Enoxaparin 1 mg/kg SC bid
    B. IV metoprolol followed by PO metoprolol
    C. Nitroglycerin SL PRN and IV drip titrated to pain and blood pressure
    D. Continue aspirin
    E. Morphine if NTG does not control the pain

22. Which one of the following agents is not indicated in the setting of STEMI?

    A. Eptifibatide
    B. LMWH
    C. Aspirin
    D. tPA
    E. Metoprolol

23. Which of the following agents would not be administered at the same time as heparin?

    A. tPA
    B. Reteplase
    C. Eptifibatide
    D. TNKase
    E. Streptokinase

24. Which of the following statements about the GPIs is NOT true?

    A. Abciximab, eptifibatide, and tirofiban are all administered as a bolus followed by a continuous infusion.
    B. It is possible to experience an allergic reaction after repeat exposure of abciximab.
    C. Eptifibatide, tirofiban, and abciximab can all be reversed by a platelet infusion.
    D. Tirofiban and eptifibatide are renally eliminated; therefore dosage adjustment is required for patients with renal dysfunction.

E. Abciximab, eptifibatide and tirofiban are all indicated as adjunct to PCI.

Answers

1. **B.** Angina is considered stable if symptoms have been occurring for several weeks without worsening, it lasts <30 minutes, and is relieved by rest or SL NTG.

2. **D.** This regimen will help control the angina without β_1-blocking effects in this asthmatic patient, as well as lowering his BP. SL NTG will be useful for acute attacks. **A** is not the best answer, as this patient also needs a medication to lower his BP. **B** is incorrect as propranolol is not β_1-selective and could worsen his asthma. **C** is incorrect as GP IIb/IIIa inhibitors are not indicated in stable angina. **E** is incorrect; combination therapy is not recommended as first-line therapy and should only be considered when initial treatment with a β-blocker is not successful.

3. **B.** Mr. Smith has an elevated LDL with known heart disease and he needs to be treated to a goal LDL of <100 mg/dL. **A** and **C** are incorrect; these antiplatelet agents are not indicated for treating stable angina unless a patient cannot tolerate aspirin. **D** and **E** are incorrect as glycoprotein IIb/IIIa inhibitors and thrombolytics are not indicated in stable angina.

4. **D.** β-Blockers do not cause peripheral vasodilation like nitrates or calcium channel blockers.

5. **D.** The increased sympathetic tone caused by some dihydropyridines can lead to reflex tachycardia, which would be detrimental in an IHD patient. Therefore, using a β-blocker to block this effect would be desirable. **A** is incorrect; the dihydropyridines do not decrease conduction through the AV node like verapamil or diltiazem. **B** is incorrect; CCBs are not indicated as first-line therapy unless a patient has a contraindication to a β-blocker. **E** is incorrect as both verapamil and metoprolol can lead to worsening systolic function, and used in combination would be unsafe.

6. **E.** SL NTG should be kept in the original amber bottle as exposure to light or extreme temperatures will cause it to lose potency. III. is correct, and patients should be counseled to take no more than three doses of SL NTG in an acute setting. I. is incorrect; SL NTG is used on a prn basis and should not be taken at the same time each day.

7. **C.** It has not been proven that so-called "tissue" ACEIs are better than other ACEIs.

8. **E.** Clopidogrel, or Plavix, does not have any pharmacologic interaction with ETT. Digoxin can cause an abnormal exercise-induced ST depression in ~30% of healthy patients. β-Blockers and vasodilators can alter hemodynamic response to BP and should be withdrawn gradually 4-5 half-lives before ETT. Nitrates can attenuate angina, and flecainide may cause exercise-induced ventricular tachycardia.

9. **C.** It has ISA. β-Blockers with ISA reduce heart rate to a lesser degree than non-ISA β-blockers, thus producing a smaller decrease in oxygen demand. Ideally, a β-blocker used for the treatment of UA/NSTEMI should be available in both IV and PO dosage forms. In addition, it would have β_1-receptor selectivity, no ISA, and low lipophilicity.

10. **C.** Nitrates are vasodilators acting on both arteries and in the periphery, thereby decreasing preload and afterload. As far as anti-ischemic therapy, only β-blockers and nondihydropyridine calcium channel blockers reduce contractility.

11. **E.** Renal adjustment is necessary with LMWH. UFH does not require dosage adjustment in renal patients, and is preferred to LMWH in patients with a CrCl <30 mL/min. LMWH does appear to have advantages over UFH in ease of administration, its affinity to thrombin (stronger than UFH), its more predictable response, and the fact that it does not require monitoring.

12. **B.** β-Blockers with ISA activity include Sectral (acebutolol), Cartrol (carteolol), Levatol (penbutolol), and Visken (pindolol). Tenormin (atenolol), Inderal (propranolol), Lopressor (metoprolol), and Coreg (carvedilol) do not have ISA activity.

13. **D.** Sildenafil. Viagra (sildenafil citrate) use is contraindicated within 24 hours of a nitrate. Likewise, if sildenafil has been used within 24 hours, a nitrate cannot be used. β-Blockers (metoprolol), ACEIs (quinapril), and calcium channel blockers (verapamil, felodipine) can be safely combined with nitrates.

14. **C. Morphine.** Morphine has vasodilator properties, thereby decreasing both preload and afterload, which decrease oxygen demand. In addition, morphine lowers heart rate by relieving pain and anxiety. If a true morphine allergy exists, meperidine may be used as an alternate. Oxycodone, hydromorphone, and fentanyl are not recommended agents for the treatment of anginal pain.

15. **D. Atenolol.** With the patient's history of COPD, a β-blocker with β_1-receptor selectivity is preferred. The only agent with β_1 selectivity in this list is atenolol. All of the remaining agents are nonselective.

16. **A. Reteplase.** Reteplase is a thrombolytic agent, which does not have a role in the treatment of NSTEMI. Thrombolytic therapy is indicated for the treatment of STEMI. Clopidogrel and GPI (eptifibatide) should be considered in all patients with NSTEMI with or without PCI. Eptifibatide and tirofiban can be used in patients who are medically managed; abciximab is reserved for patients with a scheduled PCI procedure. Lipid lowering therapy with an HMG-CoA reductase inhibitor (simvastatin) should be initiated in this patient due to his LDL level >130. This patient has a clear indication for an ACEI (enalapril) due to his EF <40%.

17. **C.** A is incorrect, as chest pain unrelieved by NTG is a diagnostic criterion for MI, but two criteria must be present before the diagnosis can be made. **B** is incorrect because ST-segment elevation >1 mm must be found in two or more contiguous leads. S.D. has both CP symptoms and ECG changes that are consistent with myocardial infarction. **C** is correct because she meets two of the three criteria for diagnosing MI. S.D. does not have positive enzymes, which would meet the third diagnostic criterion. **D** is incorrect because positive enzymes do not have to be present for the diagnosis of MI to be made (as in the case with S.D.).

18. **D.** One of the absolute contraindications to fibrinolytic therapy is severe uncontrolled HTN (BP >180/110 mm Hg). **A** is not appropriate in this patient with BP of 184/119. Routine use of magnesium post-MI is not recommended and should only be reserved for patients with hypomagnesemia. No labs were given for S.D., so answer **B** is not appropriate at this time. Prophylactic lidocaine has been shown to increase all-cause mortality, and is not recommended in the early man-

agement of STEMI for prevention of VF; therefore **C** is incorrect. β-Blockers reduce the incidence of ventricular arrhythmias, recurrent ischemia, re-infarction, infarct size, and mortality in patients with STEMI. Since S.D. does not have any contraindications to β-blockade, **D** is the correct choice. Calcium channel blockers do not have a role in STEMI when a β-blocker can be given.

19. **B.** ACE inhibitors, β-blockers, aspirin, and statin therapy (when LDL >100), and SL NTG should be given to all patients post-MI without contraindications. Plavix can be combined with aspirin, given in the setting of UA/NSTEMI, and can be continued for 1-9 months. All of the answers including Plavix are not correct, however, because **A** omits β-blockade, and **C** omits aspirin therapy. Calcium channel blockers can be given if a patient has contraindications to β-blockade, but it is not recommended as first-line treatment. Answers **D** and **E** are incorrect because ACE inhibition and β-blockade are omitted. Answer **E** would be a correct choice for the immediate treatment of someone who presents with STEMI, but not as discharge medications.

20. **B.** Heparin's anticoagulant effect requires binding to antithrombin (previously antithrombin III), and that binding converts antithrombin from a slow, progressive thrombin inhibitor to a very rapid inhibitor of thrombin and factor Xa.

21. **B.** One of the contraindications to β-blockade is a HR <55 bpm. Since S.P. has a HR of 52 at this time, the only inappropriate therapy out of the above choices would be **B**. Enoxaparin, NTG, morphine, and aspirin are all therapies that should be continued.

22. **A.** GP IIb/IIIa inhibition is still controversial in the setting of STEMI, especially when a fibrinolytic agent is administered. The role of platelet GPI in STEMI is rapidly evolving, and trials to date in combination with full- and half-dose fibrinolytic agents have shown a more complete reperfusion at the price of higher bleeding rates. At this point, there is no formal recommendation on using eptifibatide or other GPI in STEMI.

23. **E.** GPI should be administered with heparin, and therefore **C** is not the correct answer. Combination of UFH with streptokinase (SK) is less clear, because it is a nonspecific fibrinolytic

UFH, and it may increase the risk of bleeding because of streptokinase's long half-life. Therefore, answer **E** is the correct choice. Heparin should be administered for at least 48 hours with the other lytic choices to reduce the risk of reocclusion.

24. **C.** The only GPI that is reversed by a platelet infusion is abciximab. All of the remaining selections are true statements. All of the available GPI agents are administered as a bolus and infusion, so **A** is true. Abciximab is a monoclonal antibody; therefore it is possible to develop an allergic reaction upon rechallenge, so **B** is true. There are only two GPIs that are renally eliminated: eptifibatide and tirofiban, so **D** is true. All of the agents are indicated as adjunct to PCI, so **E** is true.

10. References

Braunwald E, Antman EM, Beasley JW, et al. ACC/AHA 2002 guideline update for the management of patients with unstable angina and non-ST-segment elevation myocardial infarction. A report of the American College of Cardiology/American Heart Association Task Force on Practice Guidelines (Committee on the Management of Patients with Unstable Angina). *Circulation.* 2002;106:1893-1900.

Cardiovascular agents. In: Wickersham RM, Novak KK, Schweain SL, eds. Drug Facts and Comparisons. St. Louis: Facts and Comparisons; 395-571.

Dagenais GR, Yusuf S, Bourassa MG, et al. Effects of ramipril on coronary events in high-risk persons. Results from the Heart Outcomes Prevention Evaluation Study. *Circulation.* 2001;104:522-526.

Ginnons RJ, Abrams J, Chatterjee K, et al. ACC/AHA 2002 guideline update for the management of patients with chronic stable angina: a report of the American College of Cardiology/American Heart Association Task Force on Practice Guidelines (Committee to Update the 1999 Guidelines for the Management of Patients with Chronic Stable Angina). 2002. Available at: http://www.acc.org/clinical/guidelines/stable/stable.pdf.

Guidelines for the management of patients with acute myocardial infarction. A report of the American College of Cardiology/American Heart Association task force on practice guidelines. *J Am Coll Cardiol.* 1996;28:1328-1428.

Hirsh J, Anand S, Halperin JL. Guide to anitcoagulant therapy: heparin. A statement for healthcare professionals from the American Heart Association. *Circulation.* 2001;103:2994-3018.

Malinow MR, Bostom AG, Krauss RM. Homocysteine, diet, and cardiovascular diseases. *Circulation.* 1999;99:178-182.

Mehta SR, Yusuf S, Peter RJ, et al. Effects of pretreatment with clopidogrel and aspirin followed by long-term therapy in patients undergoing percutaneous coronary intervention: the PCI-CURE study. *Lancet.* 2001;358:527-533.

Meister FL, Stringer KA, Spinler SA, et al. Thrombolytic therapy for acute myocardial infarction. *Pharmacotherapy.* 1998;18:686-698.

Phillips BG, Somers VK. Drug information handbook for cardiology, 2000-2001. Hudson: Lexi-Comp, Inc.; 2000.

Ryan TJ, Antman EM, Brooks NH, et al. ACC/AHA guidelines for the management of patients with acute myocardial infarction: 1999 update: a report of the American College of Cardiology/American Heart Association Task Force on Practice Guidelines (Committee on Management of Acute Myocardial Infarction). *J Am Coll Cardiol.* 1999;34:890-911.

Smith SC, Blair SN, Bonow RO, et al. AHA/ACC Guidelines for Preventing Heart Attack and Death in Patients with Atherosclerotic Cardiovascular Disease: 2001 Update. *Circulation.* 2001;104:1577-1579.

Steinhubl SR, Berger PB, Mann JT, et al. Early and sustained dual oral antiplatelet therapy following percutaneous coronary intervention. A randomized controlled trial. *JAMA.* 2002;288:2411-2420.

Stringer KA, Lopez LM. Acute myocardial infarction. In: DiPiro JT, Talbert RL, Hayes PE, et al, eds. *Pharmacotherapy: A Pathophysiologic Approach,* 3rd ed. Norwalk, CT: Appleton & Lange; 1997:295-322.

Summary of the Second Report of the National Cholesterol Education Program (NCEP). Expert Panel on Detection, Evaluation, and Treatment of High Blood Cholesterol in Adults (Adult Treatment Panel III). *JAMA.* 2001;285:2486-2497.

Talbert RL. Ischemic heart disease. In: DiPiro JT, Talbert RL, Yee GC, et al, eds. *Pharmacotherapy: A Pathophysiologic Approach,* 5th ed. New York: McGraw-Hill; 2002:219-250.

The Sixth ACCP Consensus Conference on Antithrombotic Therapy. *Chest.* 2001;119(Suppl 1):1S-370S.

Wong GC, Giugliano RP, Antman EM. Use of low-molecular-weight heparins in the management of acute coronary artery syndromes and percutaneous coronary intervention. *JAMA.* 2003;289:331-342.

12. Hyperlipidemia

J. Chris Bradberry, PharmD
Professor, Department of Pharmacy
University of Tennessee College of Pharmacy

Contents

1. Hyperlipidemia

- *Hyperlipidemia* is an elevation in the blood concentration of a lipid such as cholesterol or triglyceride (in the form of lipoprotein).

- *Dyslipidemia* refers to any lipid disorder.

- *Lipids* include cholesterol, triglycerides (TG), and phospholipids.

- Lipoproteins: apolipoproteins + cholesterol + triglyceride + phospholipids

- Major lipoproteins are chylomicrons, very-low density lipoproteins (VLDL), intermediate-density lipoproteins (IDL), low-density lipoproteins (LDL), high-density lipoproteins (HDL), and lipoprotein (a)

- Apolipoproteins: structural components of lipoproteins

- Friederwald equation: formula used to calculate LDL:

$$LDL = \text{total cholesterol} - (HDL + TG/5)$$

Classification of Lipids

- Total cholesterol, LDL, HDL, and triglycerides measured in mg/dL

- ATP III (Adult Treatment Panel III recommendations from the National Cholesterol Education Program [NCEP]) (Table 1)

Clinical Presentation

- Hyperlipidemia is caused by atherosclerosis, atheroma formation, atherothrombosis, and the subsequent consequences of these disease processes:
  * Coronary artery disease (angina and myocardial infarction)
  * Cerebrovascular disease (TIA and/or stroke)
  * Peripheral arterial disease (intermittent claudication)
  * A state of elevated lipids alone generally promotes no symptoms except in some familial lipid disorders, in which there may be cutaneous manifestations of lipid deposition (eg, tendon xanthomas, planar xanthomas, xanthelasmas, and eye manifestations [corneal arcus]).

Table 1

Classification of Lipids

LDL cholesterol: Primary target of therapy	
<100	Optimal
100-129	Near optimal/above optimal
130-159	Borderline high
160-189	High
≥190	Very high

Total cholesterol	
<200	Desirable
200-239	Borderline high
≥240	High

HDL cholesterol	
<40	Low
≥60	High

Triglycerides: secondary target of therapy after LDL	
<150	Normal
150-199	Borderline high
200-499	High
>500	Very high

Pathophysiology of Atherosclerosis

- Progressive, systemic disease starting early in life
  * Atheroma lesions, called fatty streaks, develop in the arterial vascular walls and result from the accumulation of cholesterol within vessel walls.
  * Atheroma lesions may lead to occlusion by thrombus or embolus formation.
  * LDL cholesterol accumulates below the intimal surface of the artery. General guideline: the higher the cholesterol elevation in the blood, the more LDL migrates into the artery.
  * Endothelial dysfunction occurs, and this increases LDL cholesterol's permeability.
  * LDL becomes oxidized and recruits monocytes.
  * Monocytes are transformed into macrophages and ingest the oxidized LDL.
  * This process results in lipid-filled cells called foam cells.
  * Foam cells are the initial lesion of atherosclerosis. Growth factors are produced by macrophages.
  * Other processes are also occurring, ie, additional endothelial cell injury and inflammatory

responses which can further accelerate the development of plaque.

* Elevated cholesterol and hyperlipidemia enhance this process.
* Plaque may continue to develop, may become stable, or it may rupture.
* Plaque rupture exposes atherogenic materials in the lesion to blood.
* Platelets are activated and a clot may form.
* Partial occlusion or obstruction can result in angina; complete occlusion results in myocardial infarction.
* Other vascular beds promote similar outcomes.

Diagnostic Criteria

- Lipid disorders (dyslipidemias) are classified as familial or secondary.
    * Familial disorders usually are caused by a defect in the way lipid metabolism occurs.
        - Categorized into the hypercholesterolemias and the combined hyperlipidemias
        - Assessment of fasting lipid panels provides diagnostic information and classification of lipid disorders.
        - Familial hypercholesterolemia (FH): LDL = 250-450 mg/dL
        - Familial defective apolipoprotein B-100
        - Polygenic hypercholesterolemia is the most common form (LDL = 160-250 mg/dL).
    * Combined hyperlipidemias:
        - Familial combined hyperlipidemia (FCH): (LDL = 160-250 mg/dL and triglycerides = 200-800 mg/dL)
        - Familial hyperapobetalipoproteinemia
        - Hypoalphalipoproteinemia
        - Dysbetalipoproteinemia
        - Elevated Lp(a)

- These disorders are characterized by variations in the amounts of LDL, HDL, VLDL, and HDL.

- Most common secondary causes of lipid disorders:
    * Diabetes mellitus
    * Hypothyroidism
    * Renal failure
    * Obstructive liver disease
    * Drugs such as β-blockers, thiazide diuretics, oral contraceptives, oral estrogens, glucocorticosteroids, and cyclosporine

- Risk factors are used to assess the potential for an individual to develop coronary heart disease (CHD) or another equivalent atherosclerotic process over the next 10 years. The Framingham Global Risk Score is calculated to provide this information. The major nonlipid risk factors for CHD are counted and used to assess the 10-year risk of developing CHD.

- Major nonlipid risk factors for CHD:
    * Cigarette smoking
    * Hypertension (BP ≥140/90 mm Hg or on antihypertensive medication)
    * Low HDL cholesterol (<40 mg/dL)
    * Family history of premature CHD (CHD in a male first-degree relative <55 years and CHD in female first-degree relative <65 years)
    * Age (men ≥45 years; women ≥55 years)

- HDL ≥60 mg/dL counts as a "negative" risk factor and acts to remove one of the other risk factors from the total count.

Treatment Principles

- Treatment and target lipid goals are based on the estimation of risk for coronary heart disease using the Framingham Global Risk Score.

- If patient has a form of clinical CHD, such as angina, myocardial infarction, stroke, or transient ischemic attack, he or she is considered to be at high risk of another ischemic event within the next 10 years.

- Those at highest risk require the most aggressive therapy, (ie, drug therapy and achieving the lowest target LDL goal). The major nonlipid risk factors above are used in the risk analysis for those individuals who do not have CHD or a CHD risk equivalent. Table 2 identifies risk categories, lipid goals, and risk of event.

Table 2

Risk Categories, Lipid Goals, and Risk of Event

Risk category	LDL goal	Risk of event
CHD and CHD risk equivalent[1]	<100 mg/dL	>20% over 10 years
Multiple risk factors (2+)	<130 mg/dL	10-20% over 10 years
0-1 Risk factor	<160 mg/dL	<10% over 10 years

[1]CHD risk equivalent = clinical CHD, symptomatic carotid artery disease, peripheral arterial disease, abdominal aortic aneurysm and diabetes.

treatment consists of lifestyle changes, ie, therapeutic lifestyle changes (TLC), which are discussed in the nonpharmacologic and pharmacotherapy sections of this chapter.

- Algorithm for drug therapy in primary prevention (<20% risk):
  * Initiate LDL lowering drug therapy (statins, niacin, resin) for 6 weeks. If LDL goal is not met, intensify LDL-lowering therapy (higher dose or combination) for 6 weeks. If LDL goal still not achieved, intensify drug therapy or refer to lipid specialist for 4-6 months. Monitor response and adherence.

- Drug therapy in secondary prevention (>20% risk):
  * The most aggressive treatment is required.
  * A large LDL reduction requires a statin and possibly a statin in combination with another agent. Follow the same algorithm as outlined in primary prevention above.

Monitoring (Clinical Evaluation)

- Screening: The National Cholesterol Education Program (NCEP) Adult Treatment Panel III (ATP III) recommends that starting at age 20, adults receive a fasting lipid profile (FLP). If this is normal, then repeat in 5 years.

- Children do not need to be screened unless there is significant family history or other reasons to test the lipids.

Monitoring
- The main tool is fasting lipid profile (FLP).
  * Baseline FLP is done before drug or dietary intervention.
  * After therapeutic lifestyle changes and/or drug therapy is started, monitor every 6 weeks times two initially, again in 4-6 months, and then periodically thereafter (usually annually). Results of FLP will show the effects of lifestyle and drug therapy interventions and help direct changes in therapy.

2. Drug Therapy

- See Tables 3, 4, and 5 for details on dosing, efficacy, and drug combinations.

Statins
- Conduct baseline liver function tests (LFTs) and creatine kinase (CK) before therapy is initiated. LFTs should be repeated again in 4-6 weeks, at 3 months, and then periodically (usually annually).

- Creatine kinase needs to be monitored only if the patient has suspected muscle damage. Assess effectiveness at 6 weeks.

Resins
- Determine baseline FLP to screen for hypertriglyceridemia.
  * If TG >200 mg/dL, use with caution.
  * Contraindicated if TG >400 mg/dL. Assess effectiveness at 6 weeks.

Nicotinic acid
- Determine baseline fasting glucose, LFTs, and serum uric acid levels before initiating therapy.

- Repeat these tests 4-6 weeks after each dose level is reached.

- Sustained-release niacin requires monthly LFT readings while dosage is titrated; subsequent LFT readings should occur every 12 weeks for the first year and then periodically.

- Diabetics require routine fasting glucose tests.

- Monitor serum uric acid after the highest dose level is achieved in those with a history of hyperuricemia or gout. Assess effectiveness at 6 weeks.

Fibric acids
- Determine baseline fasting lipid panel (TC, HDL, LDL, TG) before therapy and again at 3 and 6 months.

- Monitor changes in triglycerides at 3 months and assess effectiveness.

Cholesterol inhibitors
- Determine baseline lipid panel. Assess effectiveness at 6 weeks.

Table 3

Drug Products and Dosage

Generic name (trade name)	Dosage range and schedule	Dosage form and strength
Statins		
Atorvastatin (Lipitor®)	10-80 mg/d hs	10-, 20-, 40-, 80-mg tablet
Fluvastatin (Lescol®)	20-80 mg/d hs	20- and 40-mg capsule; 80-mg XL tablet
Lovastatin (Mevacor®)	20-80 mg/d hs	10-, 20-, 40-mg tablet
Lovastatin (Altocor®)	20-80 mg/d hs	10-, 20-, 40-, 60-g tablet
Pravastatin (Pravachol®)	20-80 mg/d hs	10-, 20-, 40-, 80-mg tablet
Simvastatin (Zocor®)	20-80 mg/d hs	5-, 10-, 20-, 40-, 80-mg tablet
Bile acid sequestrants		
Cholestyramine (Questran®)	4-16 g/d divided	Powder
Colestipol (Colestid®)	5-20 g/d divided	Powder/tablet
Colesevelam (Welchol®)	2.6-3.8 g/d (once or bid)	625-mg tablet
Nicotinic acid		
Immediate release (Niacor®)	1.5-3 g/d (divided tid)	500-mg tablet
Sustained release (Slo-Niacin®)	1-2 g/d hs	250-, 500-, 750-mg tablet
Extended release (Niaspan®)	1-2 g/d hs	500-, 750-, 1000-mg tablet
Fibric acids		
Gemfibrozil (Lopid®)	600 mg before meals bid	600-mg tablet
Fenofibrate (Tricor®)	200 mg/d with food	200-mg capsule
	160 mg/d with food	160-mg tablet
Cholesterol inhibitors		
Ezetimibe (Zetia®)	10 mg/d	10-mg tablet
Combinations		
Lovastatin + Niaspan (Advicor®)	20/1000-40/2000 daily	20/500-mg tablets
		20/750-mg tablets
		20/1000-mg tablets

Mechanism of action

HMG-CoA reductase inhibitors (statins)
- Competitively inhibit HMG-CoA reductase, which is the enzyme responsible for conversion of HMG-CoA to mevalonate.

- Mevalonate is an early precursor and a rate-limiting step in cholesterol synthesis. This reduction in liver cholesterol synthesis results in upregulation of liver LDL receptors and increased clearance of LDL and VLDL particles in the blood. These actions induce a decrease in total cholesterol and LDL cholesterol, promote a slight increase in HDL cholesterol, and affect a modest decrease in triglycerides.

Bile acid sequestrants (BAS or resins)
- Nonabsorbable anion exchange resins exchange chloride ions for bile acids and other anions in the intestine.

- This inhibits enterohepatic recycling, which results in bile excretion and a decrease in the cholesterol pool in the liver.

- LDL receptors are upregulated, increased LDL is cleared, and LDL is lowered.

Niacin
- Reduces LDL cholesterol and triglycerides, increases HDL.

Table 4

Efficacy of Drugs Used to Treat Hyperlipidemia

Drug class	Lipid/lipoprotein effect
Statins	LDL ↓18-55%
	HDL ↑5-15%
	TG ↓7-30%
Resins	LDL ↓15-30%
	HDL ↑3-5%
	TG (no change)
Nicotinic acid	LDL ↓5-25%
	HDL ↑15-35%
	TG ↓20-50%
Fibric acids	LDL ↓5-20%
	HDL ↑10-20%
	TG ↓20-50%
Cholesterol inhibitors	LDL ↓17%
	HDL (1.3%
	TG ↓6%

- May decrease VLDL synthesis, thereby leading to decreased LDL cholesterol and triglycerides.

- Niacin may inhibit metabolism of apolipoprotein A-I, which increases HDL cholesterol.

Fibric acids (fibrates)
- Reduce triglycerides by reduction of apolipoproteins B, C-III, and E.

Table 5

Pharmacotherapeutic Options for Treatment of Hyperlipidemia

Lipid target	Pharmacotherapy
LDL	Statin most potent and effective for large LDL reductions
	Niacin and resins effective for moderate LDL reductions
	Combination of statin + niacin; statin + ezetimibe; statin + resin
LDL + TG	Statin + niacin or statin + fibric acid
TG	Fibric acid or niacin

- Increase HDL by increasing apolipoproteins A-I and A-II.

Cholesterol inhibitors (ezetimibe)
- Selectively inhibit intestinal absorption of dietary and biliary cholesterol at the brush border of the small intestine, which results in a decrease in the absorption of cholesterol and a decrease in cholesterol in the blood.

Patient Instructions and Counseling

Statins
- Usually administered in the evening because most hepatic cholesterol production occurs during the night.

- Lovastatin should be given with the evening meal since absorption is better with food.

- Non–extended release statins can be dosed once daily.

- Other regular dosage forms should be divided as the doses are raised above 40 mg/d.

- Atorvastatin may be given any time of the day because of its longer half-life.

- Monitor LFTs and muscle toxicity as described in this chapter

Bile acid sequestrants (resins)
- Cholestyramine and colestipol: start with 1 dose daily with the largest meal. May be increased (after the patient adjusts to the resin) to 2 doses daily with the largest meal or divided between breakfast and dinner.

- Titrate doses slowly to avoid gastrointestinal side effects.

- Powered doses can be mixed with food or liquid such as soup, oatmeal, nonfat yogurt, applesauce, etc. The mixture can also be chilled overnight to improve palatability.

- Do not use carbonated beverages to mix as this promotes increased air swallowing.

- Drinking through a straw may also help.

- Patients who suffer constipation with the resins may mix with psyllium; however, this mixture should be ingested immediately after mixing in order to prevent a gel from forming.

- Counsel the patient to rinse the glass to ensure ingestion of all resin.

- Colesevelam is a tablet formulation, which may be easier for some patients to self-administer. However, the tablets are large, and some patients may not be able to swallow them.

- Monitor for adherence and gastrointestinal side effects for all resins.

Fibric acids (fibrates)
- Gemfibrozil should be taken twice daily 30 minutes before meals.

- Fenofibrate (200 mg is micronized) can be taken with food once daily.

- Reduce dose in renal insufficiency and monitor for muscle toxicity, especially when used in combination with statins and niacin.

Nicotinic acid (niacin)
- Immediate-release (IR) niacin should be started at a low dose and slowly titrated upward:
  * Start with 100 mg tid and adjust upward the second week to 200 mg tid; the next week increase to 350 mg tid; the following week raise to 500 mg tid. When 1500 mg/d is reached and maintained for 4 weeks, assess effectiveness at 4 weeks before increasing dose.
  * If further titration is needed, go to 750 mg tid and assess effectiveness after 4 weeks before increasing. Maximum dose is 1000 mg tid.
  * Aspirin 325 mg or ibuprofen 200 mg must be given 30 minutes before the morning dose to minimize flushing and itching.
  * Caution patient to avoid hot beverages and hot showers so as not to exacerbate the flushing effect.

- Extended-release formulation (ER) should be taken at bedtime (500 mg) and titrated weekly to a maximum of 1500 mg/d. Aspirin should be taken 30 minutes before the dose.

- Sustained-release formulations are started at 250 mg bid and increased at weekly intervals to a maximum of 2000 mg/d. Aspirin should be given 30 minutes before the dose.

- Monitor for adherence and side effects. The titration schedule for some patients may have to be done more gradually due to flushing and itching.

Cholesterol inhibitors
- Dosed once daily without regard to food.

- Can be taken simultaneously in combination with statins.

Adverse Drug Events

HMG-CoA reductase inhibitors (statins)
- Myopathy due to muscle damage

- Myalgia from muscle soreness or tenderness

- Myositis occurs in 0.2% of patients.

myalgia + ↑creatine kinase
(3-10 times upper limit of normal)

- Rhabdomyolosis occurs rarely, but can cause acute renal failure. Stop drug immediately.

severe myositis + creatine kinase
10 x upper limit of normal, ↑serum
creatinine and urine myoglobin

- Elevated liver enzymes occurs 0.1-2.3%. Obtain baseline liver function test (LFT), repeat at 4-6 weeks, again at 6 months, and yearly thereafter.

- Flu-like symptoms and headache

- Mild GI complaints

- Absolute contraindication in active or chronic liver disease

- Relative contraindication in combination with certain drugs (see drug interactions)

Bile acid sequestrants (resins)
- Gastrointestinal distress

- Palatability problems with the resin slurry.

- Constipation that increases with dose and in elderly

- Decreased absorption of other drugs:
  * Dose other drugs 1 hour before or 4 hours after resin

- Absolute contraindication is dysbetalipoproteinemia (higly elevated VLDL) and TG >400 mg/dL.

- Relative contraindication when TG >200 mg/dL.

Nicotinic acid (niacin)

- Flushing is common. Pretreat with aspirin (325 mg) 30 minutes before first niacin dose of the day

- Hyperglycemia risk; use with caution in diabetics.

- Hyperuricemia (or gout)
  * Upper GI distress
  * Hepatotoxicity
  * Absolute contraindication in chronic liver disease and severe gout
  * Relative contraindication in diabetes, hyperuricemia or severe gout

Fibric acids (fibrates)

- Dyspepsia

- Gallstones

- Myopathy increases when combined with statins.

- Absolutely contraindicated in severe renal or severe hepatic disease

Cholesterol inhibitors

- Elevated liver enzymes (same as placebo)

- GI distress (less than with resins)

- Absolutely contraindicated in moderate to severe hepatic disease

Drug-Drug and Drug-Disease Interactions

HMG-CoA reductase inhibitors (statins)

- CYP450 mixed function oxidase enzymes metabolize statins, and drugs that inhibit this process can cause increases in statin concentrations, thus predisposing to myopathy and liver toxicity.
  * Common CYP450 3A4 inhibitors include amiodarone, clarithromycin, cyclosporine, Danazol, dedlavirdine, diltiazem, erythromycin, fluoxetine, fluvoxamine, grapefruit juice, indinivir, itraconazole, ketoconazole, miconazole, nefazadone, nelfinavir, nicardipine, nifedipine, pimozide, propoxyphene, quinidine, ritonavir, saquinavir, sildenafil, tacrolimus, tamoxifen, testosterone, troleandomycin, verapamil, and zafirlukast.
  * Pravastatin is not metabolized by the CYP450 system; therefore, these drug-drug interactions are avoided.

- Absolute contraindication in active or chronic liver disease.

Bile acid sequestrants (resins)

- Avoid concomitant use with all other drugs, especially warfarin, digoxin, levothyroxine, tetracycline, fat-soluble vitamins, and minerals.

- Always separate other drugs by 1 hour before use and 4 hours after.

- Colesevelam does not appear to have these drug and nutrient interactions.

- Absolute contraindication in dysbetalipoproteinemia.

Nicotinic acid (niacin)

- Use caution in combination with resins.

- Combination therapy with statins and gemfibrozil may cause an increased risk of myopathy.

- Absolute contraindications in chronic liver disease and severe gout.

Fibric acids (fibrates)

- Highly protein-bound and metabolized by the CYP450 3A4 enzyme system.

- Increased warfarin effect

- Cyclosporine may increase gemfibrozil concentrations.

- Fenofibrate may have less interaction potential with warfarin and cyclosporine.

- BAS (resins) decrease fibrate absorption.
  * Combinations with statins and niacin may increase the risk of myopathy.
  * Absolute contraindications are severe renal disease and severe liver disease.

Cholesterol inhibitors

- Cyclosporine may increase ezetimibe concentrations.

- Combination with a resin may decrease absorption.

- Combination with a fibric acid may predispose to gallbladder disease.

- Absolute contraindication in moderate to severe hepatic disease.

Landmark Clinical Trials with Statins

Primary prevention trials
West of Scotland Study (WOSCOPS)
- This trial with pravastatin showed decreased coro-

nary morbidity and mortality in hypercholes-terolemic men with no clinical evidence of coronary heart disease (CHD).

Air Force/Texas Coronary Atherosclerosis Prevention Study (AFCAPS/TexCAPS)

- This trial with lovastatin showed reduced incidence of first acute major coronary events in patients who did not have CHD but did have normal to mildly elevated total cholesterol and LDL with low HDL.

Secondary prevention trials

Scandinavian Simvastatin Survival Study (4S)

- This trial with simvastatin showed decreased cardiac morbidity and mortality in patients with CHD and elevated cholesterol.

Cholesterol and Current Events Study (CARE)

- This trial with pravastatin showed reduced incidence of myocardial infarction (MI), death from CHD, stroke, and need for revascularization procedures in patients with recent MI and normal cholesterol levels.

Long-term Intervention with Pravastatin in Ischemic Disease Study (LIPID)

- This trial with pravastatin showed reduced mortality and incidence of MI and stroke in patients with CHD and a broad range of cholesterol.

Heart Protection Study (HPS)

- This trial with simvastatin is the largest single cholesterol trial (as of 2002) in patients at high-risk of CHD (prior MI, diabetes, or hypertension) and LDL >135 mg/dL. Antioxidants studied included vitamins E and C and beta-carotene. Simvastatin therapy showed a reduced incidence of CHD regardless of age (also elderly) or pre-existing condition. There was not a threshold for LDL at 100 mg/dL (ie, benefits extended below this level). In addition, there was no cardiovascular protective effect from vitamins E and C and beta-carotene.

3. Nondrug Therapy

- Nonpharmacologic therapy focuses on therapeutic lifestyle changes (TLC), which incorporate dietary changes, physical activity, and weight reduction.
    * "Heart healthy" nutrition is the foundation for any therapeutic interventions.

General Therapeutic Lifestyle Change Recommendations

- Decrease the amount of high-fat foods consumed (especially foods high in saturated fat).

- Decrease intake of high-cholesterol foods.

- Replace saturated fats with monounsaturated fats and fish oils.

- Use foods high in complex carbohydrates (fiber, starch, fruits, vegetables).

- Strive for and maintain an acceptable weight.

- Patients should be instructed in how to read a nutrition label.

- Recommended nutrient makeup of the TLC diet shown in Table 6.

Table 6

Nutrient Makeup of the TLC Diet

Nutrient	Recommended Intake
Saturated fat	<7% of total calories
Polyunsaturated fat	Up to 10% of total calories
Monounsaturated fat	Up to 20% of total calories
Total fat	25-35% of total calories
Carbohydrate	50-60% of total calories
Fiber	20-30 g/d
Protein	About 15% of total calories
Cholesterol	<200 mg/d
Total calories	Individualize to balance energy intake and expenditure to maintain desirable weight and/or prevent weight gain

Algorithm for Therapeutic Lifestyle Changes

- Begin lifestyle therapies and continue for 6 weeks. Evaluate LDL response, and if the LDL goal is not achieved, intensify LDL-lowering therapy (diet + weight management + physical activity) for 6 more weeks. Evaluate LDL response, and if LDL goal is not achieved, consider adding drug therapy (if not already added). Monitor adherence to TLC every 4-6 months.

Other Nonpharmacologic Therapies

- Soluble fiber and plant sterols/stanols can help lower LDL.

- Viscous or soluble fiber such as psyllium or pectin in the amount of 5-10 g/d, or other sources of fiber such as vegetables, fruits, and whole grains can reduce LDL by up to 8%.

- Fish oils
  - * Active ingredient is omega-3-fatty acid.
  - * Can reduce triglycerides as much as 30-60%
  - * Can be added when niacin or fibrates do not control triglycerides.

- Antioxidant and vitamin therapy
  - * Recent clinical trials have shown that the antioxidants, vitamins A, C, E, and beta-carotene are not protective for cardiovascular disease.

- Alcohol
  - * Light to moderate alcohol use (1 drink per day for women, 2 drinks per day for men) has been associated with reductions in coronary heart disease rates. The benefit may be potentially due to a rise in HDL.
  - * Use of alcohol should not be encouraged as a means of lowering cholesterol.
  - * Excessive alcohol can cause elevations of triglycerides.

- Alternative therapies
  - * Herbal therapies have not been systematically studied in hyperlipidemia and should not be recommended for treatment of hyperlipidemia or other lipid disorders.

4. Key Points

- Hyperlipidemia is the elevation of the blood concentration of a lipid such as cholesterol or triglyceride (in the form of lipoprotein).

- There are four major classifications of lipids: total cholesterol, low-density lipoproteins (LDL), high-density lipoproteins (HDL), and triglycerides.

- The process of atherosclerosis begins with atheroma lesions in the arterial vascular walls resulting from the accumulation of cholesterol within vessel walls.

- Polygenic hypercholesterolemia (LDL = 160-250 mg/dL) is the most common form of familial dyslipidemia.

- Major nonlipid risk factors for coronary heart disease (CHD) are cigarette smoking, hypertension, family history of premature CHD, and age (men over 45 years, women over 55 years).

- Persons with a history of CHD such as angina, MI, stroke, or transient ischemic attack are considered at highest risk of having another ischemic event in the next 10 years and require the most aggressive therapy and the lowest target LDL goal (less than 100 mg/dL).

- Monitoring for drug therapy of hyperlipidemia includes laboratory monitoring for adverse effects (eg, liver function tests, uric acid, and creatine kinase) and fasting lipid profiles (FLPs) for effectiveness.

- The mechanism of action of statin agents to treat hyperlipidemia is to competitively inhibit HMG-CoA reductase, which is the enzyme responsible for conversion of HMG-CoA to mevalonate, which is an early precursor and a rate-limiting step in cholesterol synthesis.

- The statins are usually administered in the evening because most hepatic cholesterol production occurs during the night, except for atorvastatin, which has a longer half-life than the other agents in this class.

- The only class of agents to control hyperlipidemias that is not contraindicated in patients with active or chronic liver disease is the bile acid sequestrant (resin) type.

- Pravastatin is not metabolized by the CYP450 enzyme system and thus avoids most of the drug interactions with the other statin agents.

- The bile acid sequestrants (resins) may decrease the absorption of warfarin, digoxin, levothyroxine, tetracycline, fat-soluble vitamins, and minerals.

- Therapeutic lifestyle changes (TLC) which incorporate dietary changes, increased physical activity, and weight reduction are the first recommended therapy for hyperlipidemia for 6-12 weeks prior to addition of drug therapy.

5. Questions and Answers

Case Presentation: Medication Profile—Community

H.L. is a 50-year-old man who comes to your pharmacy for cholesterol and medication monitoring. His medical history is positive for stage 1 hypertension, recent-onset type 2 diabetes, and hypercholesterolemia. Family history is noncontributory. Social history indicates he neither smokes nor uses alcohol. He has no known allergies. His medication history reveals that he occasionally takes acetaminophen for headaches and no other OTC medications or herbal products. Current medications include hydrochlorothiazide 25 mg/d (for 4 years) and a new prescription today for atorvastatin 10 mg/d. Your physical assessment reveals the following:

BP 144/90 mm Hg, pulse 70 and regular, weight 185 lb, height 5'9"
FLP today reveals total cholesterol = 250 mg/dL, HDL = 40 mg/dL, triglycerides = 145 mg/dL.

Answer Questions 1-5 using the above case.

1. What is H.L.'s LDL cholesterol?

   A. 130 mg/dL
   B. 153 mg/dL
   C. 162 mg/dL
   D. 178 mg/dL
   E. 181 mg/dL

2. What is H.L.'s LDL goal?

   A. <100 mg/dL
   B. 130-160 mg/dL
   C. 160-189 mg/dL
   D. <200 mg/dL
   E. >40 mg/dL

3. H.L. is started on TLC and atorvastatin because of his high LDL. When should you assess the effectiveness of therapy?

   A. 12 weeks
   B. 6 months
   C. 3 weeks
   D. 6 weeks
   E. Annually

4. H.L. is most likely to have which of the following?

A. Familial hypercholesterolemia
B. Polygenic hypercholesterolemia
C. Familial combined hyperlipidemia
D. Elevated triglycerides
E. Isolated low HDL

5. H.L. returns for reassessment at the appropriate time. His FLP shows that his LDL is now 100 mg/dL. What is your recommendation?

A. Stop the statin since you have achieved optimal LDL
B. Increase statin dose
C. Intensify TLC
D. Add gemfibrozil
E. Add cholestyramine

6. The National Cholesterol Education Program (NCEP) Expert Panel identifies which of the following as a positive risk factor for coronary heart disease (CHD)?

A. Hypertension
B. Low HDL (<40 mg/dL)
C. Family history of premature CHD
D. Current cigarette smoking
E. All are correct

7. Which of the following is NOT a secondary cause of hyperlipidemia?

A. High LDL
B. Hypothyroidism
C. Diabetes
D. Renal disease
E. β-Blockers

8. Cholesterol biosynthesis can be decreased by which of the following?

A. Statins
B. Oat bran
C. Bile acid sequestrants (resins)
D. Ezetimibe
E. Aspirin

9. Choose the medication with the greatest effect in raising HDL.

A. Lovastatin
B. Pravastatin
C. Gemfibrozil
D. Niaspan
E. Colesevalam

10. Choose the drug class with the most potent lowering effect on LDL.

A. Nicotinic acid
B. Fibric acids
C. Bile acid sequestrants (resins)
D. Cholesterol inhibitors
E. HMG-CoA reductase inhibitors

11. The initial lesion in the development of atherosclerosis is

A. Development of foam cells
B. Increase in HDL reverse transport
C. Rupture of a vulnerable plaque
D. Clot formation in the artery lumen
E. Development of a thin cap over the lipid pool

12. Choose the correct statement.

A. Diabetes is an absolute contraindication to use of nicotinic acid.
B. Aspirin is dosed three times per day in order to prevent flushing from niacin.
C. Gemfibrozil may reduce triglycerides by as much as 50%.
D. Colesevelam has similar patient tolerability problems as cholestyramine.
E. Ezetimibe frequently causes muscle toxicity.

13. Hyperlipidemia refers to

A. Elevation of apolipoproteins
B. Hypercholesterolemia
C. High levels of white blood cells
D. Increased ingestion of protein
E. Endothelial dysfunction

14. Which of the following indicates an optimal LDL?

A. >190 mg/dL
B. <40 mg/dL
C. >60 mg/dL
D. <100 mg/dL
E. <150 mg/dL

15. Polygenic hypercholesterolemia is characterized by which of the following?

A. LDL = 150-450 mg/dL
B. LDL = 160-250 mg/dL
C. Triglycerides >400 mg/dL
D. HDL = 50 mg/dL
E. LDL = 160-250 mg/dL + triglycerides >400 mg/dL

16. Identify a baseline laboratory test required before statin treatment.

    A. White blood cell count
    B. Complete blood count
    C. Liver function test
    D. Serum creatinine
    E. Creatinine clearance

17. The major troublesome side effect in nicotinic acid therapy is:

    A. Diarrhea
    B. Vomiting
    C. Hair growth
    D. Flushing
    E. Dizziness

18. A patient has elevated cholesterol and requires drug therapy. The most potent drug therapy for LDL reduction is:

    A. Gemfibrozil
    B. Niaspan
    C. Colestipol
    D. Atorvastatin
    E. Ezetimibe

19. Identify the drug interaction that involves the CYP450 system.

    A. Ezetimibe + niacin
    B. Colestipol + simvastatin
    C. Gemfibrozil + cholestyramine
    D. Fenofibrate + ezetimibe
    E. Lovastatin + itraconazole

20. A TLC diet could include

    A. Antioxidant therapy such as vitamin E
    B. <7% of total calories from saturated fat
    C. 150-250 g/d of fiber
    D. 2-4 drinks of alcohol per day
    E. Assessing the effectiveness of TLC at 12-week intervals

Answers

1. **E.** Use the Friederwald equation to calculate LDL.

$$LDL = TC - (HDL + TG/5)$$

2. **A.** H.L. has type 2 diabetes that is a CHD risk equivalent, therefore he is at highest risk for an event in the future and his LDL goal should be optimal or <100 mg/dL.

3. **D.** Both TLC and drug therapy measures should be assessed at 6-week intervals.

4. **B.** H.L.'s LDL is 181 mg/dL, which falls into the range for polygenic hypercholesterolemia (160-250 mg/dL) and he does not have elevated triglycerides or low HDL.

5. **C.** Since H.L.'s LDL is still slightly above optimal; intensify TLC. That is, continue to decrease saturated fat in the diet and to intensify weight reduction and physical activity. If after the next assessment in 6 weeks the LDL is still above 100 mg/dL, options would be to increase the statin dose (double it), or add another agent such as niacin or ezetimibe.

6. **E.** All of the answers are positive risk factors for CHD as defined by the NCEP ATP III. The remaining positive risk factors are gender and age (ie, males 45 and over and females 55 and over).

7. **A.** Causes of hyperlipidemia must be ruled out. The common secondary causes are renal failure, hypothyroidism, obstructive liver disease, and diabetes, and drugs such as β-blockers, thiazide diuretics, oral contraceptives, oral estrogens, glucocorticoids and cyclosporine.

8. **A.** Statins competitively inhibit HMG-CoA reductase, which is the enzyme responsible for converting HMG-CoA to mevalonate. Inhibition of mevalonate reduces cholesterol synthesis.

9. **D.** Nicotinic acid (Niaspan) has the most efficacy in raising HDL compared to other therapies. HDL may be raised 15-35%.

10. **E.** Statins (HMG-CoA reductase inhibitors) have the most efficacy in lowering LDL. LDL may be lowered 18-55%.

11. **A.** Foam cells represent the initial lesion of atherosclerosis and develop as a result of the ingestion of oxidized LDL by macrophages in the subintimal space of the artery.

12. **C.** Diabetes is a relative contraindication to the use of nicotinic acid. Aspirin is dosed once daily, before the first nicotinic acid dose of the day. Gemfibrozil can reduce TGs 20-50%. Colesevelam is a tablet and avoids most of the

palatability problems of other resins. Ezetimibe does not cause muscle toxicity.

13. **B.** Hyperlipidemia is defined as an elevation of a lipid in the blood. The lipid can be cholesterol or triglyceride in the form of a lipoprotein.

14. **D.** Level <100 = optimal; 100-129 = near optimal/above optimal; 130-159 = borderline high; 160-189 = high; ≥190 = very high.

15. **B.** Polygenic hypercholesterolemia is the most common cause of mild to moderately elevated LDL (LDL = 160-250 mg/dL).

16. **C.** Baseline tests before statin use include liver function tests (LFTs) and creatine kinase (CK).

17. **D.** The most common side effect is flushing, which may occur in many patients. To decrease flushing intensity, aspirin 325 mg should be taken 30 minutes prior to the first dose of nicotinic acid. Itching may also occur with flushing.

18. **D.** Statins (atorvastatin) have the most potent LDL-reducing properties. LDL reductions of 18-55% are possible.

19. **E.** Lovastatin is metabolized by CYP450 3A4 enzymes, and itraconazole will inhibit this enzyme system. Inhibition causes lovastatin blood and tissue concentrations to rise thus predisposing to potential muscle or liver toxicity.

20. **B.** TLC diet includes <7% saturated fat, 20-30 g/d fiber, avoidance of alcohol, and assessment at 6 weeks. Vitamin E is not recommended for cardiovascular risk reduction.

6. References

ACC/AHA/NHLBI Clinical Advisory on the Use and Safety of Statins. *J Am Coll Cardiol*. 2002;40:568-573.

Beaird SL. HMG-CoA reductase inhibitors: assessing differences in drug interactions and safety profiles. *J Am Pharm Assoc*. 2000;40:6337-6344.

Downs JR, Clearfield M, Weis S, et al. Primary prevention of acute coronary events with lovastatin in men and women with average cholesterol levels: results of AFCAPS/TexCAPS. Air Force/Texas Coronary Atherosclerosis Prevention Study. *JAMA*. 1998;279:1615-1622.

Executive Summary of the Third Report of the National Cholesterol Education Program (NCEP) Expert Panel on Detection, Evaluation, and Treatment of High Blood Cholesterol in Adults (Adult Treatment Panel III). *JAMA*. 2001;285:2486-2497.

Heart Protection Study Collaborative Group. *Lancet*. 2002;360:7-22.

Knopp RH. Drug treatment of lipid disorders. *N Engl J Med*. 1999;341:498-511.

McKenney JM, Hawkins DW, eds. *Handbook on the Management of Lipid Disorders*. Springfield, New Jersey: Scientific Therapeutics Information/National Pharmacy Cardiovascular Council; 2001.

Scandinavian Simvastatin Survival Study Group. Randomized trial of cholesterol lowering in 4444 patients with coronary heart disease: The Scandinavian Simvastatin Survival Study (4S). *Lancet*. 1994;344:1383-1389.

Sudhop T, Lutjohann D, Kodal A, et al. Inhibition of intestinal cholesterol absorption by ezetimibe in humans. *Circulation*. 2002;106:1943-1948.

The Long-Term Intervention with Pravastatin in Ischaemic Disease (LIPID) Study Group. *N Engl J Med*. 1998;338:1349-1357.

Talbert RL. Hyperlipidemia. In: DiPiro JT, Talbert RL, Yee GC, et al, eds. *Pharmacotherapy: A Pathophysiologic Approach,* 5th ed. New York: McGraw-Hill; 2002.

West of Scotland Coronary Prevention Study Group. Influence of pravastatin and plasma levels on clinical events in the West of Scotland coronary Prevention Study (WOSCOPS). *Circulation.* 1998;97:1440-1445.

Wolf MI, Vartnian SF, Ross JL, et al. Safety and effectiveness of Niaspan when added sequentially to a statin for treatment of dyslipidemia. *Am J Cardiol.* 2001;87:476-479.

13. Diabetes Mellitus

Greta K. Gourley, MSN, PharmD, PhD
Associate Professor, Department of Pharmaceutical Sciences
University of Tennessee College of Pharmacy

Kent B. Stoneking, PharmD, CDE
University of Tennessee College of Pharmacy

Contents

1. **Diabetes**

2. **Drug Therapy**

3. **Nondrug Therapy**

4. **Key Points**

5. **Questions and Answers**

6. **References**

1. Diabetes

Definition and Epidemiology

- Diabetes mellitus is a group of chronic metabolic diseases due to defects in insulin secretion and/or action, which result in hyperglycemia; abnormal metabolism of carbohydrates, fats and proteins; and long-term macrovascular and microvascular complications.

Prevalence

- It affects 17 million people, 6.2% of the population (type 1: 1.7 million people; type 2 :15.3 million people).

- Diagnosed: 11.1 million people; undiagnosed: 5.9 million people

Age range
- <20 years of age: 0.19%; approximately 1 in every 400-500 has type 1 diabetes mellitus (DM)

- 20 years or older: 16.9 million have DM

- 65 years or older: 7 million have DM

Gender
- Males: 7.8 million have DM

- Females: 9.1 million have DM

Race and ethnicity
- 20 years of age or older: non-Hispanic whites: 11.4 million have DM; non-Hispanic blacks: 2.8 million; they have a two times greater chance of having DM than do non-Hispanic whites of comparable age

- Hispanic/Latino Americans: 2 million have DM; they also have a two times greater chance of having DM than do non-Hispanic whites of comparable age

- American Indians and Alaska Natives: 105,000; they have a 2.6 times greater chance of having DM than non-Hispanic whites of comparable age

Incidence
- 1 million people age 20 years or older are affected

Mortality
- Sixth leading cause of death
  - * Risk of death two times that of people without diabetes; greatest risk for people aged 25-44

years vs. those 65-74 years (3.6 times vs. 1.5 times)
  - * Risk of death for females with DM 2.7 times that of nondiabetics for those aged 45-64 years vs. 2 times higher risk for similar males in that age group

Types of Diabetes Mellitus

Type 1 diabetes
- Originally called insulin-dependent diabetes mellitus (IDDM) or juvenile onset diabetes

- Generally occurs in children and young adults who require exogenous insulin for survival

- 5-10% of all diagnosed cases

Type 2 diabetes
- Originally called non–insulin dependent diabetes mellitus (NIDDM) or adult onset diabetes

- Generally occurs in adults

- 90-95% of all diagnosed cases

- Increasingly being diagnosed in children and adolescents

Gestational diabetes mellitus (GDM)
- Glucose intolerance with onset or first recognition during pregnancy (second and third trimesters)

- Approximately 7% of all pregnancies; >200,000 annually

- More common in the following groups: African-Americans, Hispanic/Latino Americans, American Indians; obese females and females with a family history of diabetes

- Postpregnancy 5-10% have type 2 diabetes; the remainder have a 20-50% chance of developing DM in the 5-10 years postpregnancy

- Primary fetal complication of concern: macrosomia (abnormally large fetal body size)

Other types (secondary DM)
- 1-5% of all diagnosed cases

- Due to genetic conditions (eg, maturity onset diabetes of youth [MODY]), surgery, drugs, malnutrition, infections, and other illnesses (eg, pancreatitis)

Clinical Presentation
(Onset, Signs, and Symptoms [S&S])

- Findings that distinguish type 1 from type 2 DM:
  * Type 1: rapid, abrupt onset; moderate to severe classic S&S; unexplained weight loss; potentially in ketoacidosis
  * Type 2: gradual onset; asymptomatic or mild classic S&S to progressive changes of advanced DM; obesity

- Classic S&S include polydipsia (excessive thirst), polyuria (excessive urination), and polyphagia (excessive hunger)

- Other common findings include fatigue, blurred vision, frequent infections

- Persons with type 1 DM may experience a "honeymoon" period, a phase of erratic insulin secretion during destruction of beta cells by islet cell antibodies; an apparent short-lived remission, lasting months to a year

Pathophysiology

- Pathophysiology associated with abnormalities of glucose metabolism and regulation involving insulin and counterregulatory hormones (glucagon, epinephrine, norepinephrine, growth hormone, cortisol)

- Glucose metabolism dysfunction leads to life-threatening diabetic ketoacidosis (DKA) or hyperglycemic hyperosmolar nonketotic syndrome (HHNS)

- Mild, moderate, and severe DKA are differentiated by level of acidosis and mental status (ie, alert, alert/drowsy, stupor/coma)

Type 1 (ketosis-prone; DKA)
- Type 1 due to β-cell destruction causing absolute insulin deficiency and increased counterregulatory hormones; progressive hyperglycemia
  * Renal threshold for glucose exceeded (180 mg/dL)
    • Glucose excreted in urine
    • Osmotic diuresis leading to dehydration and electrolyte imbalances
  * Impaired glucose uptake in peripheral tissues (primarily muscles)
  * Protein metabolized for glucose (energy) source
  * Triglycerides metabolized to free fatty acids and glycerol (lipolysis)
  * Increased glycerol results in increased hepatic

production of glucose and greater hyperglycemia
  * Decreased conversion of glucose to glycogen (primarily in the liver); decreased insulin-induced suppression of hepatic glucose production
  * Ketone bodies formed in excess due to fatty acid metabolism in the liver leading to ketonuria and ketonemia and ultimately diabetic ketoacidosis
  * Kussmaul's respirations (deep and rapid); attempt to compensate for metabolic acidosis
  * Requires prompt intervention with insulin, fluids and electrolytes to prevent coma and death
  * Complications associated with treatment: hypokalemia, cerebral edema, and hypoglycemia

Type 2 (ketosis-resistant; HHNS)
- Type 2 diabetes is due to relative insulin deficiency, often accompanied by insulin resistance, and increased counterregulatory hormones; progressive hyperglycemia
  * Renal threshold for glucose exceeded
    • Glucose excreted in urine
    • Osmotic diuresis leading to dehydration and electrolyte imbalances
  * Impaired glucose uptake in peripheral tissues (primarily muscles)
  * Protein metabolized for glucose (energy) source
  * Minimal blood levels of endogenous insulin prevent ketoacidosis
  * Requires intervention with insulin, fluids, and electrolytes to prevent severe dehydration
  * Coma and death may occur without timely treatment
  * Complications associated with treatment: hypokalemia, cerebral edema, and hypoglycemia

Etiology

Type 1 DM
- β-Cell destruction, usually leading to absolute insulin deficiency; manifested by low or undetectable levels of plasma C-peptides

- Immune mediated
  * Strong HLA (human leukocyte antigen) associations
  * Genetic predisposition; higher risk in children of persons diagnosed with diabetes
  * Related to environmental factors; stimulus (eg, virus) required for expression of genetic propensity

* Common in childhood and adolescence; can occur at any age

- Idiopathic diabetes: no known etiology

Type 2 DM
- Ranges from primarily insulin resistance with some insulin deficiency to predominantly a secretory defect with insulin resistance

- Specific etiologies unknown

- Though genetic links are not clearly defined, type 2 is associated with stronger genetic predisposition than type 1 diabetes

- Obesity observed with this disease causes some degree of insulin resistance

- Risk increases on either end of the age continuum with obesity and physical inactivity; common in adulthood; can occur at any age

- Autoimmune destruction of β-cells does not occur

Sequelae (Acute/Short- and Long-Term Complications)

Acute/Short-term complications
Hyperglycemia
- Rapid onset; causative or associated factors:
    * Stress related (eg, illness, infection, or trauma)
    * Somogyi effect: rebound hyperglycemia; early morning hyperglycemia secondary to nocturnal hypoglycemia
    * Dawn phenomenon: fasting hyperglycemia (pre-breakfast) due to plasma insulin decrease during the night or the anti-insulin effect of nocturnal growth hormone
    * Excessive chronic alcohol (ETOH) intake
    * Inadequate or inappropriate insulin or oral anti-diabetic therapy
    * Excessive caloric intake
    * Inadequate physical activity/exercise
    * Use of glucogenic drugs; dose dependent, direct effect (eg, corticosteroids, thiazide diuretics, nicotinic acid, phenytoin, furosemide, isoniazid, protease inhibitors, sympathomimetics)

- DKA

- HHNS

Hypoglycemia
- Rapid onset, causative or associated factors:
    * Excessive or inappropriate use of drug(s) to treat DM, either insulin or oral antidiabetic agent
    * Acute ETOH intake
    * Inadequate caloric intake
    * Excessive physical activity/exercise therapy
    * Rotation to a new insulin injection site (due to increase in absorption; eg, buttock to abdomen)
    * Gastroparesis (delayed emptying of stomach after a meal)
    * Drug interactions leading to decreased blood glucose (BG) (hypoglycemia); altered protein binding or other drug interactions with sulfony-lureas: ETOH, salicylates, NSAIDs, methyl-dopa, MAO inhibitors, antifungals (azoles), fluoxetine
    * Use of β blockers (prolonged decreased BG and masked symptoms)

- Patient may be unaware of hypoglycemia

- Acute treatment for mild to moderate and severe presentations of hypoglycemia
    * Treatment for mild to moderate presentation in conscious patient: 10-15 g of fast-acting oral carbohydrate (eg, $\frac{1}{2}$ cup of regular soda, 3 glucose tablets, $\frac{1}{2}$ cup of orange juice, 5 small sugar cubes, or 6-7 hard candies containing sugar); repeat in 10-15 minutes as needed after rechecking BG
    * Treatment for severe presentation in unconscious patient: glucagon 0.5-1 mg injection SC or IM (glucagon is a pancreatic hormone from alpha cells; antagonistic effect on hypoglycemia) or 50% dextrose solution IV

Long-term complications
Macrovascular disease
- Peripheral vascular disease: pain due to intermittent claudication; insufficient circulation impairing healing, increased risk of gangrene and amputation (DM accounts for >60% of nontraumatic lower limb amputations in the U.S.)

- Cerebrovascular disease: increased incidence of stroke

- Coronary artery disease (CAD) major cause of mortality and major contributor to morbidity; hypertension (HTN) is a major risk factor for cardiovascular disease (CVD); increased prevalence of lipid abnormalities contribute to higher rates of CVD

Microvascular disease

- Retinopathy: leading cause of new cases of blindness among adults 20-74 years of age; duration of diabetes strongest predictor for development and progression; nearly all persons with type 1 diabetes and >60% of persons with type 2 have retinopathy during the first 20 years of disease; hypertension is a risk factor for macular edema and is associated with proliferative diabetic retinopathy (PDR)

- Nephropathy
  - * DM is the predominant cause of end-stage renal disease (ESRD) in the U.S. and Europe; in the U.S., diabetic nephropathy accounts for about 40% of new cases of ESRD; ESRD develops in 50% of type 1 diabetic individuals with overt nephropathy within 10 years and in >75% by 20 years; after onset of overt nephropathy, only ~20% of persons with type 2 DM will progress to ESRD
  - * Hypertension, usually caused by underlying DM nephropathy, markedly accelerates progression

Neuropathy

- Peripheral: sensorimotor nervous system dysfunction; pain and diminished sensation with "stocking glove" pattern (progression from lower to upper extremities); poor detection of trauma which increases risk for ulcers and infection, particularly in lower extremities and feet

- Autonomic: several systems affected adversely
  - * Genitourinary: neurogenic bladder and sexual dysfunction
  - * Gastrointestinal: gastroparesis
  - * Cardiovascular: orthostatic hypotension

Increased risk for infectious disease (especialy in integumentary system and mucous membranes; approximately one-third of patients have periodontal disease)

- Etiologic organisms: staphylococci, beta-hemolytic streptococci, and fungi

- Causative or associated factors: neuropathy; poor peripheral circulation; hyperglycemia resulting in decreased immunity and slower healing

Diagnostic Criteria

Diagnostic criteria for type 1 and type 2 DM (Table 1)
- Plasma values are used because they are unaffected by hematocrit changes

Table 1

Criteria for the Diagnosis of Diabetes Mellitus[1]

- Symptoms of DM plus casual plasma glucose concentration ≥200 mg/dL ("casual" means level taken any time of day regardless of time of last meal)
- Classic symptoms include polyuria, polydipsia, polyphagia, and unexplained weight loss

OR

- Fasting plasma glucose (FPG) ≥126 mg/dL (level taken after no caloric intake for 8 hours)

OR

- 2-Hour plasma glucose ≥200 mg/dL during an oral glucose tolerance test (OGTT) using 75 g anhydrous glucose dissolved in water (not recommended for routine clinical use)

[1]In the absence of unequivocal hyperglycemia with acute metabolic decompensation, criteria should be confirmed by repeat testing on a different day.
Report of the Expert Committee on the Diagnosis and Classification of Diabetes Mellitus. "Copyright ©1997 American Diabetes Association from Diabetes Care, Vol. 20, 1997;1183-1197. Reprinted with permission from *The American Diabetes Association*."

- Normal fasting plasma glucose (FPG): 70-110 mg/dL
- Abnormal results not meeting above criteria outlined in Table 1 are classified as: impaired fasting glucose (IFG), or impaired glucose tolerance (IGT), or prediabetic
  - * IFG: FPG ≥110 mg/dL and <126 mg/dL
  - * IGT: 2-hour OGTT plasma glucose ≥140 mg/dL and <200 mg/dL

- Serum C peptide level: diagnostic for functioning of β cells (rarely done to reduce cost; may be used for classification)

Diagnostic criteria for gestational diabetes mellitus
- OGTT preferred screening test in pregnancy

- For high-risk patients (marked obesity, history of GDM, glycosuria, or strong family history of DM): Perform first prenatal visit risk assessment and test as soon as possible; if negative at initial screenings, retest between 24 and 28 weeks of gestation

- For average-risk patients: test at 24-28 weeks of gestation
- If FPG >126 mg/dL or casual PG >200 mg/dL (if not confirmed on subsequent day, in average- or high-risk patients use one of two approaches):
  * One-step approach (diagnostic 75-g or 100-g OGTT) or
  * Two-step approach (1-hour 50-mg glucose challenge test followed by diagnostic OGTT if 1-hour level ≥140 mg/dL)

- Test criteria with 100-g glucose load—fasting: 95 mg/dL; 1-hour: 180 mg/dL; 2-hour: 155 mg/dL; 3-hour: 140 mg/dL

- Test criteria with 75-g glucose load—fasting: 95 mg/dL; 1-hour: 180 mg/dL; 2-hour: 155 mg/dL

- Diagnosis positive if two glucose values meet or exceed those listed for 100-mg or 75-g load

- At least 6 weeks postpartum re-evaluation and reclassification should be conducted using the criteria for the diagnosis of DM per the Report of the Expert Committee on the Diagnosis and Classification of Diabetes

Diagnostic criteria for sequelae (acute/short- and long-term)

Ketoacidosis (DKA of one to several days' duration)
- Laboratory findings: increased PG (>250 mg/dL); ketosis (serum and urine ketones positive); low arterial pH (<7.20); low arterial PCO_2 (<35 mm Hg); low serum bicarbonate (<15 mEq/L); abnormal serum electrolyte values; and leukocytosis

- Clinical findings: history of classic DM S&S, Kussmaul respirations, acetone (fruity) breath odor, dehydration, abdominal pain, nausea and vomiting, weakness, lethargy, headache, decreased consciousness level (confusion to coma)

Hyperglycemic hyperosmolar nonketotic syndrome (HHNS of days' to weeks' duration)
- Laboratory findings: greatly increased BG (>600 mg/dL); absence of ketosis; serum osmolarity ≥320 mOsm/kg; abnormal serum electrolyte values

- Clinical findings: history of classic DM S&S, dehydration, rapid respirations, decreased level of consciousness (confusion to coma), seizures

Hypoglycemia
- Laboratory findings: BG eliciting S&S and magnitude varies per individual (eg, mild: 60-70 mg/dL;

moderate: 50-60 mg/dL; severe: <50 mg/dL [biochemical hypoglycemia])

- Clinical findings: Mild—alert (may not exhibit S&S), tachycardia, pallor, palpitations, shakiness (tremor), paresthesia, diaphoresis, inability to concentrate, dizziness, hunger, blurred vision; moderate—confused, inappropriate behavior, impairment of motor functions, appears inebriated; severe—unconscious, coma, seizures, and/or impairment of motor function (life-threatening)

Hypoglycemic unawareness
- Laboratory findings: vary per individual

- Clinical findings: no or few S&S noted by the person with DM

Nephropathy
- Laboratory findings: Microalbuminuria elevated (>30 mg albumin/24 h); clinical microalbuminuria (dipstick) screening of urinary albumin excretion positive if ≥300 mg/24 h; decrease in glomerular filtration with increasing serum creatinine until ESRD occurs

- Clinical findings: Peripheral edema, fatigue, uremia with GI disturbances, anemia, and renal osteodystrophy

Treatment Principles and Goals

- Achieve and maintain glycemic control

- Prevent or slow progression of long-term complications

- Prevent or resolve acute and short-term complications

- Help the patient with DM to achieve an acceptable quality of life and satisfaction with care

- Blood pressure, lipid, and weight normalization and control in adults with DM

Monitoring glycemic control
- This is best evaluated by self-monitored blood glucose (SMBG) and hemoglobin A_{1c} (A_{1c}) results in combination

Hemoglobin A_{1c}
- With good control, A_{1c} level should be <6.5% (normal range: 4-6%), using a Diabetes Control and Complications Trial (DCCT)–recommended assay

* Hemoglobin A_{1c} test (previously abbreviated HbA_{1c}, recently changed to A_{1c}): glycosylated hemoglobin test reflects average blood glucose level over previous 2-3 months; assesses glycemic control and compliance with therapy
  * For type 1 DM: insulin therapy in combination with medical nutritional therapy (MNT) and physical activity/exercise essential for glycemic control; may use oral antidiabetic agents as adjunct to insulin
  * For type 2 DM: monotherapy with MNT and physical activity/exercise may be sufficient for glycemic control; graduated therapy recommended, beginning with MNT and exercise therapy alone, then in combination with oral antidiabetic agents, and finally all three with insulin as needed
* Use individualized goals (eg, less intensive goals in certain populations, such as children, the elderly, and pregnant women; and in certain situations, such as those with severe or frequent hypoglycemia, hypoglycemic unawareness, or advanced severe complications)
* Factors that may affect A_{1c} results: decreased levels—hemoglobinopathies, anemias (eg, hemolytic or untreated iron deficiency), blood loss, antioxidants; increased levels—uremia

Preprandial plasma glucose (PPG): <110 mg/dL

Peak postprandial plasma glucose: <140 mg/dL

Prevention, recognition, and treatment of acute hypoglycemic and hyperglycemic episodes:
* Periodic testing of A_{1C}
  * Twice per year if stable glycemic control is achieved
  * Test quarterly (or every 2-3 months) if therapy changed or glycemic control is inadequate

BP normalization and control: <130/80 mm Hg
* BP 130-139/80-89 mm Hg: give lifestyle and behavioral therapy for maximum of 3 months; if goal is not achieved, add drug therapy

* BP ≥140/≥90 mm Hg: give pharmacologic therapy and lifestyle and behavioral therapy

* Initial drug therapy: any drug class presently used for treatment of hypertension
  * Drug classes shown to be beneficial in reducing CVD events are: ACE inhibitors (angiotensin-converting enzyme inhibitors), β blockers, and diuretics
  * Monitor renal function and serum potassium level if using ACE inhibitors or ARBs

(angiotensin II-receptor blockers)
* ACE inhibitors delay the progression of nephropathy (ie, renal protective effect) in type 1 and type 2 DM

Lipid and weight normalization and control
* LDL: <100 mg/dL

* Triglycerides: <150 mg/dL

* HDL: >40 mg/dL (increase goal by 10 mg/dL for women)

* Medical nutritional therapy (MNT) and physical activity/exercise therapy variably effective alone; emphasis should be on reduction of saturated fat and cholesterol intake, weight loss, and increased physical activity/exercise to improve lipid profile

* Non-achievement of lipid goals with lifestyle modifications requires drug therapy

* Statins are first-line drug therapy for LDL reduction

* Therapy with fibrates in patients with low HDL has been shown to reduce CVD rates

* Fibrates or niacin in combination with a statin require care to minimize the risk of adverse effects

* Initial therapy for increased triglycerides is increased glycemic control

Smoking cessation (discontinue nicotine use), nephropathy, and retinopathy
* Smoking cessation: counseling and other forms of treatment as a routine component of care

* Nephropathy
  * Optimize glucose and BP control to reduce risk and slow progression
  * Use either ACE inhibitors or ARBs for both micro- and macroalbuminuria
  * If ACE inhibitors or ARBs are used, monitor serum potassium levels for hyperkalemia
  * If unable to tolerate ACE inhibitors and/or ARBs consider use of non-DCCBs (dihydropyridine calcium channel blockers) or β-blockers
  * Protein restriction to ~10% of daily calories (current adult recommended allowance)

* Retinopathy
  * Optimize glucose and BP control to reduce risk and slow progression
  * Promptly refer to specialty ophthalmologist in

DM when any level of the following is present: macular edema, severe nonproliferative diabetic retinopathy, or any proliferative diabetic retinopathy (PDR)

Prevention

- Smoking: advise all patients not to smoke (avoid nicotine use)

- Antiplatelet therapy: to prevent CV events
  * Enteric-coated aspirin (ASA) 81-325 mg/d in adults with DM, no contraindications to ASA, and macrovascular disease

- Immunization
  * Annual influenza vaccine if 6 months of age or older and no contraindications
  * At least one lifetime pneumonia vaccine for adults with no contraindications (one-time revaccination >64 years of age, no contraindications, previously immunized at <65 years of age, vaccine administered >5 years ago)

- Foot inspection and care daily; prompt medical attention for any problems noted (eg, wounds, blisters, signs of infection); annual comprehensive and visual inspection at each visit

- Skin inspection and care daily; prompt medical attention if problems observed

- Dental care: annual examination recommended

- Eye care: routine ophthalmologic screening and an annual dilated eye examination

- Reduce modifiable risk factors: hyperglycemia; hypertension; dyslipidemia; nicotine use; obesity; physical inactivity; alcohol use; excessive protein, carbohydrate, and fat intake

Self-monitoring in special situations

- Intercurrent illness or other conditions
  * Reduced glycemic control (due to illness [sick day], infection or trauma) necessitates more frequent blood glucose and blood ketone monitoring (ie, q4h)
  * Ketone monitoring on early morning voiding in persons with GDM or pregnant women with DM to assess adequate caloric intake

Routine self-monitoring of blood glucose (SMBG)

- Individualized and indicated for most persons with DM; urine glucose monitoring (does not reflect current BG) ONLY for those persons unable or unwilling to do SMBG

- Engages the patient in treatment regimen

- Provides short-term immediate evaluation of glycemic control

- Provides data to use for decision making about diet, exercise, insulin and/or oral agent dosing adjustment

- Factors that may alter results of SMBG:
  * Inadequate sample (lower)
  * Decreased Hct (lower)
  * Increased Hct (higher)
  * Dehydrated (lower)
  * HHNS (lower)

Patient education and self-care

- Provides means for person with DM to become empowered and assist with self-care

- Education content includes the disease process; acute/short- and long-term complications; drug and nondrug treatment; monitoring; preventive measures; decision-making skills; specific self-care measures relative to foot, skin, dental and eye care; goal setting; and psychosocial adjustment

- National Standards for Diabetes Self-Management education published by the American Diabetes Association, 2003 (see ADA, 2003).

2. Drug Therapy

Insulin and Insulin Analogues

- Drug class, mechanism of action, types, generic and trade name, and administration route (Table 2).

Source
- Pork pancreas or chemical modification of pork insulin to human insulin: Pork semisynthetic human (being replaced by biosynthetic human)

- Recombinant DNA technology: biosynthetic

- Chemical alteration of human insulin: human insulin analogue

Indications
- Type 1 DM

Table 2

Insulin and Insulin Analogues

Pharmacologic class: Pancreatic hormone   Therapeutic class: Injectable antidiabetic

Type and generic name[1]	Trade name	Onset (h)[1]	Peak (h)[1]	Duration (h)[1]	Administration route[1]
Rapid-acting:					
Lispro (analogue)	Humalog®	<0.25	0.5-1.5	3-4	SC (injection/CSII)
Aspart (analogue)	Novolog®	<0.25	0.7-1	3-5	SC (injection/CSII)
Short-acting:					
Regular (human)	Humulin R®; Novolin®; Velosulin BR®	0.5-1	2-3	3-6	SC (injection/CSII) for daily maintenance therapy; continuous intravenous (IV; insulin drip) for DKA, HHNS, surgery, delivery
Regular (purified)	Regular Iletin II (pork)®				
Intermediate-acting:					
NPH (isophane insulin susp.; purified)	NPH Iletin II (pork)®	2-4	6-10	10-16	SC
Human	Humulin N®; Novolin N®				
Lente (insulin zinc susp.; purified)	Lente Iletin II (pork)®	3-4	6-12	12-18	SC
Human	Humulin L®; Novolin L®				
Long-acting:					
Ultralente (extended insulin zinc suspension; human)	Humulin U®; Ultralente®	6-10	10-16	18-20	SC
Insulin glargine (analogue; human)	Lantus®	5	N/A	20-24	SC

Mechanism of action:

Decreases blood glucose and assists with glucose control by:
- Increasing glucose uptake and utilization by peripheral tissues (primarily in muscle)
- Increasing glycogenesis (glucose → glycogen; primarily in liver)
- Decreasing glycogenolysis (glycogen → glucose)
- Decreasing gluconeogenesis (amino acids → glucose)
- Decreasing lipolysis and ketogenesis (fats → ketone bodies)
- Converting amino acids to increase protein
- Converting triglycerides and fatty acids to increase adipose tissue

[1]Parenteral administration of insulin is required because it is destroyed in the GI tract. Insulin is metabolized primarily in the liver and kidneys; ~30-80% is cleared by the kidneys.

CSII, continuous subcutaneous insulin infusion (insulin pump); DKA, diabetic ketoacidosis; HHNS, hyperglycemic hyperosmolar nonketotic syndrome; SC, subcutaneous (factors limiting the rate of absorption include the type of insulin and other factors (eg, site of injection).

[1]Campbell RK, White JR. "Copyright ©2000 American Diabetes Association. From Medications for the Treatment of Diabetes. Reprinted with permission from *The American Diabetes Association.*"

- Type 2 DM as monotherapy or combination therapy when MNT and physical activity/exercise and/or oral antidiabetes medications are ineffective in controlling DM (eg, advancing disease process, periods of stress, acute illness)

- GDM not controlled by diet

- DKA and HHNS

- Secondary DM (eg, pancreatitis)

- Parenteral nutrition or high caloric therapy

Concentrations and other product considerations
- Concentrations available in the United States
    * U-100: 100 U/mL
    * U-500: 500 U/mL used in insulin resistance

- Premixed products
    * 50/50: 50% regular insulin with 50% NPH insulin (rapid acting for premeal bolus and intermediate-acting to control later hyperglycemia)
    * 70/30: 30% regular insulin with 70% NPH insulin
    * 70/30 analogue: 30% aspart insulin analogue with 70% neutral protamine aspart insulin analogue
    * 75/25: 25% lispro insulin analogue with 75% neutral protamine lispro insulin analogue

- Individualized mixtures
    * Based on SMBG results, periodic A_{1c} results, dietary intake, physical activity/exercise, and other influencing factors (eg, stress, illness, infection, other drug therapy and/or diseases)

- Human insulin or insulin analogue preferred over animal source insulins due to reduced antigenicity

- Lispro and aspart: increase lifestyle flexibility, decrease 2-hour PPG levels, and decrease risk for high PPG and nocturnal hypoglycemia

- Glargine (long-acting); once-daily administration; mimics basal insulin secretion (like CSII); acidic pH (4.0); should not be mixed with other insulins or given IV; has same advantages as lispro and aspart

Physical appearance
    * Clear (solution): aspart, lispro, glargine, regular
    * Milky (suspension): NPH, lente, ultralente, all premixed insulin products

- Route of administration: onset more rapid and duration shorter; IV more so than IM, which is more so than SC (Table 2)

Insulin Dosing and Administration Considerations

- No universal formula for the appropriate dose and no typical maintenance dose

- Therapy individualized based on target BG range, SMBG results, periodic A_{1c} results, daily diet, physical activity/exercise, and other influencing factors (eg, stress, other drug therapy and/or diseases)

- Conventional therapy changing to intensive as appropriate (considerations are frequency of hypoglycemic events and the patient's willingness and ability to comply)

Conventional (split-mixed dosing)
- Assumptions: lifestyle includes waking time in the morning, meals routinely spaced during the day and waking hours, and a late evening bedtime

- Two injections per day of intermediate-acting insulin or mixed doses of rapid-acting or short-acting insulin with intermediate-acting insulin

- Two-thirds of total daily dose (TDD) prebreakfast (using a ratio of 1:2, 1 part rapid- or short-acting insulin to 2 parts intermediate-acting insulin) and $^1/_3$ of TDD pre-supper (using a ratio of 1:1 or 1:2, rapid- or short-acting to intermediate-acting insulin)

Intensive therapy (individualized dosing)
- Multiple injections (3 or more) of short- or rapid-acting insulin as required throughout the day
- Adjustments based on SMBG results, physical activity/exercise, and food intake; attempt to mimic normal insulin secretion

Recommended initial starting doses
- Type 1 DM: TDD if within 20% of IBW = 0.5-1.0 U/kg per day in divided doses

- Type 2 DM: TDD varies with the degree of insulin resistance; 0.15-0.3 U/kg per day in divided doses

- Numerous types of individualized regimens; see Koda-Kimble et al, 2001 and Setter et al, 2000 for more information.; sliding dosage scale primarily used in the acute care setting

Continuous subcutaneous insulin infusion (CSII; insulin pump)

- Short- or rapid-acting insulin in continuous low doses to mimic basal insulin (0.5-1.0 U/h)

- Premeal bolus dose delivered as needed, per sliding scale or carbohydrate counting regimens

- Assists with tighter glycemic control

- Frequent SMBG required

Patient instructions or counseling

- Review mechanism of action of insulin and peak action (time most vulnerable to low BG) of each insulin taken

- Review drug-drug and drug-disease interactions and reporting (Table 3)

- Regular meal times are necessary and meals must not be omitted; discuss use of ETOH

- Spread carbohydrates throughout day and eat regularly so intake is matched to dose and action of insulin

- Lispro and aspart (rapid-acting insulins) should be given within 15 minutes before a meal; do not delay eating

- Regular (short-acting insulin) should be given within 30 minutes before a meal

- Insulin glargine is given once daily, and NEVER mixed with other insulins

- Insulin should be injected SC (demonstrate SC injection initially and then periodically verify that the patient is using proper technique)

- Injection sites should be rotated within an anatomical area to aid in consistent absorption and to prevent lipohypertrophy
    * Sites: abdomen > arm > hip > thigh > buttock (in order of greater and more rapid absorption to lesser and slower absorption)
    * Exercise of injection area increases absorption
    * Heat applied to injection area increases absorption; cold applied decreases absorption
    * Local massage of injection area increases absorption
    * Use of an area with lipohypertrophy decreases absorption

Table 3

Drug Interactions for Injectable Antidiabetic Agents: Insulins

Drugs that decrease insulin effect (cause an increase in blood glucose levels; hyperglycemia)

Acetazolamide	Estrogens
AIDS antivirals	Ethacrynic acid
Albuterol	Isoniazid
Asparaginase	Lithium carbonate
Calcitonin	Morphine sulfate
Corticosteroids	Niacin
Cyclophosphamide	Nicotine
Danazol	Oral contraceptives
Dextrothyroxine	Phenothiazines
Diazoxide	Phenytoin
Diltiazem	Somatropin
Diuretics	Terbutaline
Dobutamine	Thiazide diuretics
Epinephrine	Thyroid products

Drugs that increase insulin effect (cause a decrease in blood glucose levels; hypoglycemia)

ACE inhibitors	MAO inhibitors
Alcohol	Mebendazole
Anabolic steroids	Oral antidiabetic products
β-Blockers[1]	Pentamidine
Calcium	Phenylbutazone
Chloroquine	Propoxyphene
Clofibrate	Pyridoxine
Clonidine	Salicylates
Disopyramide	Somatostatin analog
Fluoxetine	(eg, octreotide)
Guanethidine	Sulfinpyrazone
Lithium carbonate	Sulfonamides
	Tetracyclines

[1]Nonselective β-blockers may mask the signs and symptoms of hypoglycemia; cardioselective agents may be better alternatives (eg, atenolol).

Adapted from Drug Facts and Comparisons, copyright 2003 by Wolters Kluwer Health, Inc.

- Carry fast-acting oral carbohydrate for emergency use

- Review signs and symptoms of hypoglycemia and how to treat

- Review signs and symptoms of hyperglycemia and need to report to health care provider

- Monitoring of blood glucose or urine glucose (if patient not able or unwilling to test BG) is an essential guide to accurate dosage and therapeutic success; avoid extremes of temperature for storage of test strips (demonstrate use of meter initially and periodically verify patient is using proper technique)

- Storage requirements: open insulin vials may be kept at room temperature (68-75°F) for 10-28 days, depending on the type (refer to package insert); after 1 month, discard unopened vial if kept at room temperature or opened vial if kept refrigerated; if unopened insulin is refrigerated, use by expiration date on vial (do not freeze); excessive agitation should be avoided to prevent loss of potency; gentle rolling of vial in palms of hands to warm it is allowed to decrease painful injections due to cold insulin

- When mixing two insulins, draw regular, lispro, or aspart (these clear insulins ONLY) into the syringe first; NEVER MIX GLARGINE (another clear insulin) WITH OTHER INSULINS; mixing of short-acting and lente insulins is not recommended; NPH (phosphate buffered insulin) should not be mixed with lente insulins; review mixing and measuring techniques periodically

- Inspect vial for change in appearance, including cloudiness or discoloration of clear insulin, clumping or frosting of insulin suspensions. *Note:* regular, lispro, aspart, and glargine are clear solutions and all other insulins are milky suspensions

- Wear medical identification

- Carry insulin and supplies on your person rather than leaving them in a checked bag or car when traveling

- Review use of insulin on sick days

Adverse drug events
- Hypoglycemia

- Weight gain

- Local and systemic allergic reactions

- Lipodystrophies
  * Atrophy: concavity or pitting of adipose tissue due to immune response
  * Hypertrophy: bulging of adipose tissue due to nonrotation of injection sites

Drug-drug and drug-disease interactions (Table 3)

Parameters to monitor
- Blood or urine glucose (if patient unable or unwilling to perform BG monitoring)

Glycosylated hemoglobin (A_{1c}) periodically (every 3 months if BG is not well controlled; every 6 months if BG is well controlled)

Pharmacokinetics: see Table 2

Storage requirements; other administration information (see section on patient instructions or counseling above)

Oral Antidiabetic Agents

Insulin secretagogues (Table 4)
- First-generation sulfonylureas
  * Acetohexamide
  * Chlorpropamide
  * Tolazamide
  * Tolbutamide

- Second-generation sulfonylureas
  * Glimepiride
  * Glipizide
  * Glyburide, glyburide micronized

- Meglitinides (nonsulfonylurea secretagogues)
  * Repaglinide
  * Nateglinide

Indications
- Type 2 DM (failed MNT and physical activity/exercise; sufficient functioning of β cells)
  * Monotherapy; combination therapy with other oral antidiabetic agents
  * Combination therapy with insulin

- Not recommended for children, pregnant and lactating women, or in type 1 DM

- Not used for control of type 2 DM during stressful situations (eg, surgery, infection); insulin should be used during these situations

Drug class, mechanism of action, generic and trade names, dosing, administration, and adverse drug effects (Table 4)
- Primary difference with sulfonylureas: duration of action

- All sulfonylureas highly protein bound (90-100%) to albumin; metabolized extensively in liver

Table 4

Oral Antidiabetic Agents

Trade name (generic name)	Mechanism of action	Dosage range: initial/d (maximum/d)	Dosage forms	Administration schedule; $t_{1/2}$; DA; PA	Adverse drug effects
INSULIN SECRETAGOGUES					
First-generation sulfonylureas					
Dymelor® (acetohexamide)	Stimulates pancreatic β cells to secrete insulin	250 mg (1.5 g)	Tablets 250 mg, 500 mg	qd-bid (when dosed @ 1.5 g/d); $t_{1/2}$ = 5 h; DA = 12-24 h; PA = unknown	GI, hematologic, disulfiram-like reaction, SIADH, wt. gain, hypoglycemia
Diabinese® (chlorpropamide)	Stimulates pancreatic β cells to secrete insulin	250 mg (500 mg); older adults 100 mg (125 mg)	Tablets 100 mg, 250 mg	qd; $t_{1/2}$ = 35 h; DA 60 h; PA = 3-6 h	GI, hematologic, disulfiram-like reaction, dilutional hyponatremia, SIADH, wt. gain, prolonged hypoglycemia
Tolinase® (tolazamide)	Stimulates pancreatic β cells to secrete insulin	100 mg (1000 mg); older adults 100 mg	Tablets 100 mg, 250 mg, 500 mg	qd-bid (when dosed @ >500 mg/d); older adults qd; $t_{1/2}$ = 7 h; DA = 12-24 h; PA = 3-4 h	GI, hematologic, disulfiram-like reaction, wt. gain, hypoglycemia
Orinase® (tolbutamide)	Stimulates pancreatic β cells to secrete insulin	1-3 g; older adults 500-1000 mg	Tablets 500 mg	qd-bid (when dosed @ 3 g/d); $t_{1/2}$ = 4.5-6.5 h; DA = 6-12 h; PA = 3-5 h	GI, hematologic, disulfiram-like reaction, dilutional hyponatremia, SIADH, wt. gain, hypoglycemia
Second-generation sulfonylureas					
Amaryl® (glimepiride)	Stimulates pancreatic β cells to secrete insulin	1 mg (8 mg)	Tablets 1 mg, 2 mg, 4 mg	qd $t_{1/2}$ = 9 h; DA = 8-12 h; PA = 2-3 h	GI, hematologic, cholestatic jaundice, wt. gain, hypoglycemia
Glucotrol®, Glucotrol XL® (glipizide)	Stimulates pancreatic β cells to secrete insulin	5 mg (40 mg); older adults 2.5 mg (5 mg)	Tablets 5 mg, 10 mg	qd-bid/tid (when dosed @ >15 mg/d) $t_{1/2}$ = 2-4 h; DA = 10-24 h; PA = 1-3 h XL $t_{1/2}$ = 4-13 h; DA = 24 h; PA = 6-12 h	GI, hematologic, cholestatic jaundice, wt. gain, hypoglycemia
Diabeta®, Micronase® (glyburide)	Stimulates pancreatic β cells to secrete insulin	2.5 mg (20 mg); older adults 1.25 mg (2.5 mg)	Tablets 1.25 mg, 2.5 mg, 5 mg	qd-bid (when dosed @ 20 mg/d); $t_{1/2}$ = 10 h; DA = 16-24 h; PA = 4 h	GI, blurred vision, hematologic, cholestatic jaundice, hepatitis, increased LFTs, wt. gain, hypoglycemia
Glynase® (glyburide micronized[1])	Stimulates pancreatic β cells to secrete insulin	1.5 mg (12 mg) micronized	Tablets 1.5 mg, 3 mg, 6 mg (micronized)	qd-bid (when dosed @ >6 mg/d; micronized) $t_{1/2}$ = 4 h; DA = 24 h; PA = 2-4 h	GI, blurred vision, hematologic, cholestatic jaundice, hepatitis, increased LFTs, wt. gain, hypoglycemia

[1]Micronized formulation is significantly absorbed; a 3-mg tablet has similar blood levels to a 5-mg conventional tablet.

GI (gastrointestinal): first-generation sulfonlyureas—nausea, epigastric distress, heartburn; second-generation sulfonylureas—dyspepsia, nausea, vomiting, constipation, diarrhea, flatulence; DA, duration of action; hematologic: leukopenia, thrombocytopenia, aplastic anemia, agranulocytosis; LFTs, liver function tests; PA, peak of action; SIADH, syndrome of inappropriate secretion of antidiuretic hormone; $t_{1/2}$, half-life.

Table 4

Oral Antidiabetic Agents (continued)

Trade name (generic name)	Mechanism of action	Dosage range: initial/d (maximum/d)	Dosage forms	Administration schedule; $t_{1/2}$; DA; PA	Adverse drug effects
ENZYME INHIBITORS					
Alpha-glucosidase inhibitors (AGIs)					
Precose® (acarbose)	Delays carbohydrate metabolism and absorption (due to competitive and reversible inhibition of intestinal alpha-glucoside hydrolase and pancreatic alpha-amylase)	25 mg (300 mg); ≤60 kg: 150 mg; >60 kg: 300 mg	Tablets 50 mg, 100 mg	tid (with first bite of each meal; titrate q 4-8 wk to a maximum dose of 50-100 mg tid); $t_{1/2}$ = 2 h; DA = 2-4 h; PA = 1 h	GI and increased LFTs
Glyset® (miglitol)	Delays carbohydrate metabolism and absorption (due to competitive and reversible inhibition of intestinal alpha-glucoside hydrolase and pancreatic alpha-amylase)	25 mg (300 mg)	Tablets 25 mg, 50 mg; 100 mg	tid (with first bite of each meal; titrate q 4-8 wk to a maximum dose of 100 mg tid); $t_{1/2}$ = 2 h; DA = unknown; PA = 2-3 h	GI, decreased serum iron
INSULIN SENSITIZERS					
Biguanide					
Glucophage® (metformin)	Increases hepatic and peripheral insulin sensitivity and decreases hepatic glucose production	1000 mg (2550 mg)	Tablets 500 mg, 850 mg, 1000 mg	bid-tid (titrate 500 mg/wk or 850 mg q2wk; when dosed @ 2550 mg/d); $t_{1/2}$ = 6.25 h; DA = 6-12 h; PA = 4-8 h	GI, megaloblastic anemia, lactic acidosis
Thiazoladinediones ("glitazones"/TZDs)[1]					
Actos® (pioglitazone)	Increases skeletal muscle, adipose tissue, and liver insulin sensitivity and decreases hepatic glucose production	15 g (45 mg)	Tablets 15 mg, 30 mg, 45 mg	qd; $t_{1/2}$ = 3-7 h; DA = unknown; PA = 2 h	Edema, anemia, wt. gain, exacerbation of CHF, URIs, resumption of ovulation
Avandia® (rosiglitazone)	Increases skeletal muscle, adipose tissue, and liver insulin sensitivity and decreases hepatic glucose production	4 mg (8 mg)	Tablets 2 mg, 4 mg, 8 mg	qd-bid; $t_{1/2}$ = 3-4 h; DA = unknown; PA = 1 h	Edema, anemia, wt. gain, exacerbation of CHF, URIs, resumption of ovulation
Rezulin® (troglitazone)	Increases skeletal muscle, adipose tissue, and liver insulin sensitivity and decreases hepatic glucose production	Withdrawn from market on 3/21/2000 due to severe liver toxicity			

[1]Based on the history of Rezulin®, Actos®, and Avandia® should be monitored for the adverse drug effect of potential liver toxicity.

CHF, congestive heart failure; DA, duration of action; GI (gastrointestinal): AGIs—flatulence, diarrhea, abdominal pain; biguanide—unpleasant or metallic taste, diarrhea, nausea, vomiting, abdominal bloating, flatulence, anorexia; LFTs, liver function tests; PA, peak of action; $t_{1/2}$, half-life; URI, upper respiratory infection.

Table 4

Oral Antidiabetic Agents (continued)

Trade name (generic name)	Mechanism of action	Dosage range: initial/d (maximum/d)	Dosage forms	Administration schedule; $t_{1/2}$; DA; PA	Adverse drug effects
INSULIN SENSITIZERS					
Meglitinides/nonsulfonylurea secretagogues					
Prandin® (repaglinide)	Stimulates pancreatic β cells to secrete insulin	0.5 mg (16 mg)	Tablets 0.5 mg, 1 mg	bid-qid (varies with meal patterns); $t_{1/2}$ = 1 h; DA = 2-4 h; PA = 1 h	Hypoglycemia, wt. gain, URIs, GI, arthropathy, back pain, dizziness, flu symptoms
Starlix® (nateglinide)	Stimulates pancreatic β cells to secrete insulin	180 mg (360 mg)	Tablets 60 mg, 120 mg	tid before meals; $t_{1/2}$ = 1.5 h; DA = 2-4; PA = unknown	Hypoglycemia, wt. gain, URIs, GI, arthropathy, back pain, dizziness, flu symptoms
Combination therapy (second-generation sulfonylureas or TZD and biguanide)					
Glucovance® (glyburide & metformin)	See mechanism of action for these two drugs	1.25 mg/250 mg (20 mg/ 2000 mg)	Tablets 1.25 mg/ 250 mg, 2.5 mg/ 500 mg, 5 mg/ 500 mg	qd with a meal; bid with meals as dose increases	See adverse effects for these two drugs
Metaglip® (glipizide & metformin)	See mechanism of action for these two drugs	2.5 mg/250 mg (20 mg/ 2000 mg)	Tablets 2.5 mg/ 250 mg, 2.5 mg/ 500 mg, 5 mg/ 500 mg	qd with a meal; bid with meals as dose increases	See adverse effects for these two drugs
Avandamet® (rosiglitazone & metformin)	See mechanism of action for these two drugs	4 mg/1000 mg (8 mg/ 2000 mg)	Tablets 1 mg/ 500 mg, 2 mg/ 500 mg, 4 mg/ 500 mg	bid with meals	See adverse effects for these two drugs

DA, duration of action; GI (gastrointestinal): meglitinides—nausea, diarrhea, constipation, vomiting, dyspepsia; PA, peak of action; $t_{1/2}$, half-life; URI, upper respiratory infection.

Adapted from Setter SM, White JR, Campbell RK. Diabetes (Table 19.19). Copyright 2000 by Lippincott, Williams & Wilkins. From Herfindahl ET, Gourley DR, eds. Textbook of Therapeutics, 7th ed., 2000:402-403. With permission from Lippincott, Williams & Wilkins.

- Treatment failure rate high; secondary failure due mainly to disease progression (ie, decreasing number of functioning β cells
  * Primary failure: failure within first 4 weeks; did not respond to drug
  * Secondary failure: failure to maintain control >5 years

Patient instructions or counseling
Drug class–specific points
Sulfonylureas and meglitinides
- Review MOA of insulin secretagogues and peak action (time most vulnerable to low BG) of drug taken

Table 5

Drug Interactions for Oral Antidiabetic Agents

Interacting drug/agent	Antidiabetic drug or class	Effect and explanation
Androgens, anticoagulants, antifungals (azoles; eg, itraconazole, fluconazole), chloramphenicol, clofibrate, fenfluramine, gemfibrozil, magnesium salts, methyldopa, histamine antagonists (eg, cimetidine), MAO inhibitors, probenecid, salicylates, sulfinpyrazone, sulfonamides, tricyclic antidepressants, urinary acidifiers	Sulfonylureas	Decreased BG (hypoglycemia): Hypoglycemic effect of sulfonylureas may be increased by various MOA: decreasing hepatic metabolism; inhibition of renal excretion; displacement from protein-binding sites; alteration of carbohydrate metabolism
β-Blockers, calcium channel blockers, cholestyramine, corticosteroids (eg, prednisone), diazoxide, estrogens, hydantoins (eg, phenytoin), isoniazid, nicotinic acid (niacin), oral contraceptives, phenothiazines, rifampin, sympathomimetics, thiazide diuretics, thyroid products, urinary alkalinizers	Sulfonylureas	Potential increase in BG (hyperglycemia): Hypoglycemic effect of sulfonylureas may be decreased by various MOA: increased hepatic metabolism; decreased insulin release; increased renal excretion
Alcohol (ethanol)	Glipizide	Prolong but not augment glipizide-induced decrease in blood glucose
Alcohol (ethanol)	Tolbutamide	Chronic ETOH use may decrease $t_{1/2}$
Alcohol (ethanol)	Chlorpropamide	ETOH ingestion may cause disulfiram-like reaction
Anticoagulants	Glyburide	Potentiates or weakens effects of coumarin derivatives
Barbiturates	Chlorpropamide	Disulfiram-like reaction; prolong action of barbiturates
Charcoal	Sulfonylureas	Decrease absorption and decrease efficacy and toxicity of sulfonylureas
Ciprofloxacin	Glyburide	Potentiation of hypoglycemic action
Digitalis glycosides	Sulfonylureas	Increase digitalis serum levels
Digestive enzymes	Acarbose	Decrease effect of acarbose
Digoxin	Acarbose	Decreases digoxin serum concentrations
Charcoal	Acarbose	Decreases effect of acarbose
Digestive enzymes	Miglitol	Decrease effect of miglitol
Charcoal	Miglitol	Decreases effect of miglitol
Digoxin	Miglitol	Decreases digoxin plasma concentrations
Glyburide	Miglitol	Decreases AUC and C_{max} values for glyburide (not statistically significant)
Metformin	Miglitol	Decreases mean AUC and C_{max} values for metformin (not statistically significant)
Propranolol	Miglitol	Bioavailability of propranolol decreased by 40%
Ranitidine	Miglitol	Bioavailability of ranitidine decreased by 60%
Alcohol (ethanol)	Metformin	Potentiates metformin's effect on lactate metabolism
Cationic drugs: amiloride, digoxin, morphine, procainamide, quinine, ranitidine, triamterene, trimethoprim, vancomycin	Metformin	Competition for common renal tubular transport systems and increased metformin effect
Cimetidine	Metformin	81% increase in peak metformin plasma concentrations; 50% increase in AUC and 27% decrease in average renal clearance of metformin
Furosemide	Metformin	Increases metformin plasma and blood C_{max} and AUC without significant change in renal clearance; decreases furosemide C_{max}, AUC, and $t_{1/2}$ without significant change in renal clearance

Table 5

Drug Interactions for Oral Antidiabetic Agents (continued)

Interacting drug/agent	Antidiabetic drug or class	Effect and explanation
Iodinated contrast medium	Metformin	Acute renal failure associated with lactic acidosis
Nifedipine	Metformin	Increases metformin plasma C_{max} and AUC and increases amount excreted in the urine; absorption of metformin enhanced
Ketoconazole	Pioglitazone	Inhibits metabolism of pioglitazone
Barbiturates, carbamazepine, rifampin	Repaglinide	Increase metabolism of repaglinide
β-Blockers, chloramphenicol, MAO inhibitors, NSAIDs, probenecid, salicylates, sulfonamides	Repaglinide	Potentiate hypoglycemic action of repaglinide
Calcium channel blockers, corticosteroids, estrogens, isoniazid, nicotinic acid (niacin), oral contraceptives, phenothiazines, phenytoin, sympathomimetics, thiazide diuretics, thyroid products	Repaglinide	Reduce hypoglycemic action of repaglinide; produce hyperglycemia
Erythromycin, ketoconazole	Repaglinide	Inhibit metabolism of repaglinide
Corticosteroids, sympathomimetics, thiazide diuretics, thyroid products	Nateglinide	Reduce hypoglycemic action of repaglinides; produce hyperglycemia
β-Blockers, MAO inhibitors, NSAIDs, salicylates	Nateglinide	Potentiate hypoglycemic action of nateglinide

AUC, area under the curve; BG, blood glucose, C_{max}, maximum concentration; MAO, monoamine oxidase; NSAIDs, nonsteroidal anti-inflammatory drugs; $t_{1/2}$, half-life.
Adapted from Drug Facts and Comparisons, copyright 2003 by Wolters Kluwer Health, Inc.

- Review drug-drug and drug-disease interactions and reporting for insulin secretagogues (Table 5)

- Regular meal times are necessary and meals must not be omitted; discuss use of ETOH

- Spread carbohydrates throughout the day and eat regularly so intake is matched to dose and action of drug

- Carry fast-acting oral carbohydrate for emergency use

- Review signs and symptoms of hypoglycemia and how to treat

- Review signs and symptoms of hyperglycemia and need to report to health care provider

- Monitoring of blood glucose or urine glucose (if patient is unable or unwilling to test BG) is an essential guide to accurate dosage and therapeutic success; avoid extremes of temperature for storage of test strips (demonstration of meter use initially and then periodically verify proper technique)

- Wear medical identification

- Store in a cool dry place (not bathroom)

- Review use of oral antidiabetic agents on sick day

- Weight gain possible

Drug class–specific points
Meglitinides
- Must be taken 30 minutes before main meals

- If meal is omitted, do not take

- Enhances postprandial glucose utilization

Drug class–specific points
Sulfonylureas
- Report signs and symptoms of hematologic adverse events: fever, sore throat, rash, unusual bruising or bleeding

- Tolbutamide, glyburide, and glipizide are more effective if taken 30 minutes before a meal

Adverse drug events and significant precautions
Drug class–specific points:
Sulfonylureas and meglitinides
- Hypoglycemia

- Weight gain

Drug class or individualized drugs:
Sulfonylureas
- Sulfonylureas are contraindicated in persons with a sulfa allergy

- Sulfonylureas are associated with increased risk of cardiovascular mortality and morbidity (see University Group Diabetes Program, 1970)

- Chlorpropamide and tolbutamide more likely to produce disulfiram-like reaction when ingested with ETOH than other sulfonylureas

- Avoid certain sulfonylureas in persons with decreased renal or hepatic function (ie, acetohexamide, chlorpropamide, and glyburide)

- Chlorpropamide use can result in dilutional hyponatremia and syndrome of inappropriate antidiuretic hormone secretion (SIADH)

- Chlorpropamide should be avoided in the elderly due to long duration of activity and greater risk for prolonged hypoglycemia; glyburide also associated with hypoglycemia in the elderly but not to same extent

- Acetohexamide-active metabolite primarily responsible for hypoglycemia; avoid in the elderly and those with renal dysfunction (like chlorpropamide, it is no longer widely used); second-generation agents have higher potency, fewer reported significant adverse drug events (eg, disulfiram-like reaction with ETOH) and drug interactions

Other adverse drug events (see Table 4)

Drug-drug and drug-disease interactions (Table 5)

Parameters to monitor
- Routine blood or urine glucose monitoring (if patient is unable to unwilling to test BG)

- Glycosylated hemoglobin (A_{1c}) periodically (every 3 months if BG not well controlled; every 6 months if BG is well controlled)

- CBC

Pharmacokinetics (see Table 4)

Storage requirements; other administration information (see section on patient instructions or counseling, above)

Enzyme inhibitors:
Alpha-glucosidase inhibitors (AGIs) (Table 4)
- Acarbose

- Miglitol

Indications
- Type 2 DM: failed MNT and physical activity/exercise; patient with adequate endogenous or exogenous insulin; monotherapy

- Type 2 DM: combination with other oral antidiabetic agents

- Persons with significant postprandial hyperglycemia

- During periods of stress, insulin therapy may be required

- Type 1 DM as adjunct to insulin; not as monotherapy

- Not indicated in children and pregnant or breastfeeding women

Drug class, mechanism of action, generic and trade name, dosing, administration, and adverse drug effects (see Table 4)

Patient instructions or counseling
Drug class–specific points
AGIs
- Review MOA of AGIs and peak action (time most vulnerable to low BG) of drug taken

- Review drug-drug and drug-disease interactions and reporting for AGIs (see Table 5)

- Take with first bite of each meal

- Initially gas and diarrhea will occur but will decrease with time; increase dose gradually to minimize these effects

Note: Does not cause hypoglycemia, but it may occur if used with other antidiabetic drugs; no weight gain

- Treat hypoglycemia due to combination therapy with other oral antidiabetic agents or insulin with oral glucose (dextrose or glucose tablets) instead of carbohydrate sources with sucrose (cane sugar) or fructose because absorption of these is inhibited

- Review signs and symptoms of hypoglycemia

- Review signs and symptoms of hyperglycemia and need to report to health care provider

- Monitoring of blood or urine glucose (if patient unable or unwilling to perform BG testing) is an essential guide to accurate dosing and therapeutic success; avoid extremes of temperature for storage of test strips (demonstrate meter use and then periodically check to verify that patient is using proper technique)

- Wear medical identification

- Store in a cool dry place (not bathroom)

- Review use of oral antidiabetic agents on sick day

Adverse drug effects or significant precautions (see Table 4)
- Initially gas and diarrhea will occur but will decrease with time

- Titrate dose slowly to minimize GI effects of flatulence, diarrhea, and abdominal pain

- Contraindicated in inflammatory bowel disease, colonic ulceration, or obstructive bowel disease

- Contraindicated in cirrhosis of the liver

- Avoid use if serum Cr levels >2 mg/dL

Drug-drug and drug-disease interactions (see Table 5)

Parameters to monitor
- LFTs every 3 months during first year of therapy and periodically thereafter with acarbose dose >50 mg tid

- Routinely monitor blood or urine glucose (if patient unable or unwilling to perform routine BG monitoring)

- Glycosylated hemoglobin (A_{1c}) periodically (every 3 months if BG not well controlled; every 6 months if BG well controlled)

Pharmacokinetics (see Table 4)

Storage requirements; other administration infor-

mation (see patient instructions or counseling section, above)

Insulin sensitizers (antihyperglycemic agents)
Biguanide
- Metformin

Thiazolidinediones (TZDs)
- Pioglitazone

- Rosiglitazone

- Troglitazone (withdrawn from U.S. market on 3/21/00 due to severe liver toxicity)

Indications
- Type 2 DM: failed MNT and physical activity/exercise; monotherapy

- Combination with other oral antidiabetic agents

- Combination therapy with insulin

- Type 1 DM adjunct to insulin

- Patient with adequate endogenous or exogenous insulin

- Not indicated in children or pregnant or breastfeeding women

Drug class, mechanism of action, generic and trade names, dosing, administration, and adverse drug effects (see Table 4)

Patient instructions or counseling
Drug class–specific points
Insulin sensitizers
- Review MOA of each insulin sensitizer taken

- Review drug-drug and drug-disease interactions and reporting for insulin sensitizers (see Table 5)

- GI discomfort or diarrhea occur initially; this will decrease over time and lessen if taken with meals and dose is increased gradually

Note: Does not cause hypoglycemia, but it may occur if used with other antidiabetic drugs; no weight gain.

- Review signs and symptoms of hypoglycemia and how to treat

- Review signs and symptoms of hyperglycemia and need to report to health care provider

- Monitoring blood or urine glucose (if patient is unable or unwilling to perform BG testing) is an essential guide to accurate dosage and therapeutic success; avoid extremes of temperature for storage of test strips (demonstrate use of meter and periodically verify that the patient is using proper technique)

- Wear medical identification

- Store in a cool dry place (not bathroom)

- Review use of oral antidiabetic agents on sick day

Individual drug-specific points
Metformin
- No hypoglycemia or weight gain; may experience modest weight loss

- GI discomfort or diarrhea occur initially; this will decrease over time and lessen if drug is taken with meals and dose is increased gradually

- Must be discontinued 48 hours before radiologic procedures requiring parenteral iodinated contrast media and resumed 48 hours after the procedure if kidney function is normal; remind the health care provider and radiologist that metformin (also called Glucophage; give both names) is being taken

- Immediately report the following symptoms of lactic acidosis (a potentially fatal problem) to the health care provider: weakness, malaise, heavy labored breathing

- Avoid excessive ethanol intake

- Avoid use in patients with renal dysfunction (contraindicated in female DM patients having serum creatinine ≥1.4 mg/dL; also contraindicated in male DM patients having serum creatinine ≥1.5 mg/dL), or those predisposed to potentially fatal lactic acidosis.

Thiazolidinediones
- Take once or twice daily with or without food

- Persons with polycystic ovarian syndrome may have resumption of menstrual periods and pregnancy may occur

- If taking low-dose birth control pills, consult physician about taking one with greater amounts of estrogen

- If taking estrogen replacement therapy, report to physician any reappearance of menopausal signs and symptoms

- Report the following symptoms to the health care provider: fatigue, GI distress, increased abdominal girth, swollen ankles/feet, shortness of breath, jaundice

Adverse drug effects or significant precautions (see Table 4)

Individual drug-specific points
Metformin
- Avoid use in persons with renal dysfunction or those predisposed to potentially fatal lactic acidosis (eg, alcoholics or those with CHF, severe respiratory disorders, or liver disease)

- Must be discontinued 48 hours before radiologic procedures requiring parenteral iodinated contrast media and resumed 48 hours after the procedure if kidney function is normal; remind the health care provider and radiologist that metformin (also called Glucophage; give both names) is being taken

- Immediately report the following symptoms of lactic acidosis (a potentially fatal problem) to the health care provider: weakness, malaise, heavy labored breathing

- Avoid excessive ethanol intake

- Titrate dose slowly to minimize GI discomfort and diarrhea

Thizolidinediones
- Should not be used in persons with ALT >2.5 normal

- Discontinue if ALT >3 times normal, serum bilirubin levels increase, or symptoms of hepatitis (ie, jaundice) occur

- Contraindicated in severe CHF (NYHA class III or IV cardiac status) and hepatic disease

- Persons with polycystic ovarian syndrome may have resumption of menstrual periods and pregnancy may occur

- If taking low-dose birth control pills, consult physician about taking one with greater amounts of estrogen

- If taking estrogen replacement therapy, report to physician any reappearance of menopausal signs and symptoms

- Report the following symptoms to the health care provider: fatigue, GI distress, increased abdominal girth, swollen ankles/feet, shortness of breath, jaundice

Drug-drug and drug-disease interactions: see Table 5

Parameters to monitor
- Metformin: renal and liver function tests; serum B_{12}, folic acid, Hgb, Hct, and CBC at baseline and then annually

- TZDs: LFTs at baseline, every 2 months during first year of therapy, and then periodically

- Routinely monitor blood or urine glucose (if patient is unable or unwilling to perform BG monitoring)

- Glycosylated hemoglobin (A_{1c}) periodically (every 3 months if BG not well controlled; every 6 months if BG is well controlled)

Pharmacokinetics (see Table 4)

Storage requirements; other administration information (see patient instructions or counseling section, above)

3. Nondrug Therapy

- Medical nutrition therapy and physical activity/exercise (may be sufficient treatment for type 2; however, the progressive nature of DM may ultimately require the use of drug therapy)

Medical nutrition therapy (MNT)
- Individualized with consideration of usual dietary habits, metabolic profile, lifestyle, and treatment goals
  - Adequate carbohydrates to cover peak action of insulin and oral hypoglycemic agents; regularly scheduled snacks and meals to prevent hypoglycemia
  - Normalization and control of BG, weight, lipid levels, and BP
  - Prevent or assist with treatment of complications
  - Meet increased metabolic needs during stressful periods

- Carbohydrate (CHO) 45-60% of total daily caloric intake; if intensive insulin therapy used with premeal bolus dose of short- or rapid-acting insulin, then insulin should be adjusted to cover the daily CHO intake; with conventional insulin therapy (when the premeal bolus is not used) or oral antidiabetic drug therapy, then CHO intake must be adjusted so it is consistent with the effects of therapy

- Protein 15-20% of total daily caloric intake; should be modified if renal function is reduced

- Fat <30% of total daily caloric intake; cholesterol <300 mg/d

- Fiber intake should be encouraged, but there is no reason to recommend a greater amount than in persons without DM

- Sodium intake: <3000 mg/d

- Daily ETOH intake
  - Adult females: one drink
  - Adult males: two drinks
  - One drink = 12 oz. beer, 5 oz. wine or 1.5 oz. distilled spirits
  - Consume with food to decrease hypoglycemia

- Dietary algorithms: assist patient when changes arise with regard to food intake, physical activity/exercise, medication regimen, and increased stress or other factors that affect glycemic control

Physical activity/exercise

- Individualized; pre-exercise program history and detailed medical examination essential

- Program adjusted in the presence of macro- and microvascular complications that may be worsened (eg, those with retinopathy in the presence of PDR should avoid anaerobic exercise or exercise that involves straining, jarring, or Valsalva-like maneuvers, and in the presence of cardiovascular disease a stress test may be necessary)

- Consistent frequency (daily, or at least 3-4 days/week), intensity, and duration; proper warm-up and cool-down essential

- SMBG necessary before and after exercise

- Types of exercise
    * Aerobic (eg, swimming, walking, or running)
    * Anaerobic (eg, weightlifting): generally avoided in persons with DM unless specifically approved by appropriate medical specialist

- Side effects: hypoglycemia, hyperglycemia, and increased ketosis (if insulin used and BG >240 mg/dL)

- Fast-acting oral carbohydrates should be available during and post exercise

4. Key Points

- Diabetes mellitus (DM) is a group of chronic metabolic diseases exhibiting hyperglycemia resulting from defects in insulin secretion and/or action.

- The principal treatment goals include maintaining blood glucose levels in the normal or near normal range and preventing acute/short- and long-term complications.

- The specific etiology for type 1 DM is immune mediated β-cell destruction, which usually leads to absolute insulin deficiency (Table 6). The immune-mediated destruction of β-cells may be related to a stimulus such as a virus. The specific etiologies for type 2 DM are unknown. However, type 2 DM is associated with a stronger genetic predisposition than type 1, and it is characterized by relative insulin deficiency and/or insulin resistance.

- Type 1 DM generally occurs in children and young adults who require insulin for survival, and it represents 5-10% of all diagnosed cases. Type 2 DM most commonly affects adults, but is increasingly being diagnosed in children and adolescents. Type 2 represents 90-95% of all diagnosed cases.

- Diabetic ketoacidosis (DKA) predominates in type 1 DM (ketosis-prone DM), and hyperglycemic hyperosmolar nonketotic syndrome (HHNS) predominates in type 2 DM (ketosis-resistant DM). Both conditions are life threatening.

- Standards of medical care for monitoring patients with DM include measurement of glycosylated hemoglobin (A_{1c}), which reflects the average blood glucose level over the previous 2-3 months (or lifespan of the red blood cell (RBC), which is approximately 120 days). This test should be done on all patients periodically (ie, quarterly if BG is poorly controlled; at least semiannually if BG is well controlled).

- Most patients should do self-monitoring of blood glucose (SMBG) and the results of the monitoring should be reviewed routinely by their health care provider. Periodic SMBG review with the health care provider is a good opportuinty for decision making about diet, exercise, and insulin and/or oral agent dosing adjustments.

- Outcomes of uncontrolled BG include cardiovascular, kidney, eye, and nerve disease, all of which decrease the quality of life in the patient with DM.

Table 6

Comparison of Type 1 and Type 2 Diabetes Mellitus

	Type 1	Type 2
Previous names	Insulin-dependent diabetes mellitus (IDDM); juvenile onset; type I	Non-insulin dependent diabetes mellitus (NIDDM); type II
Current names	Type 1	Type 2
Percentage of all DM cases	5-10%	90-95%
Age of occurrence	<30 years of age (usually childhood or adolescence); at any age following autoimmune stimulus (eg, virus)	>30 years of age (usually older); increase in childhood/adolescence in association with obesity and inactivity
Onset	Rapid, abrupt	Gradual
Family history	Negative/weak	Positive/strong
Primary etiology	Autoimmune mediated mechanism with genetic predisposition	Genetic and environmental (eg, family history, ethnicity, obesity, inactivity)
Pathogenesis	Destruction of β cells resulting in absolute insulin deficiency and abnormal glucose control	Increasing resistance of tissue (liver and skeletal muscle) to insulin; impaired insulin secretion resulting in relative deficiency of insulin; increased hepatic glucose production
Signs and symptoms	Polyuria, polydipsia, polyphagia, and unexplained weight loss, fatigue, blurred vision; possibly ketoacidosis	Polyuria, polydipsia, polyphagia, obesity, fatigue, blurred vision; possibly asymptomatic
Diagnostic criteria	See Table 1	See Table 1
Ketoacidosis	Ketosis prone (diabetic ketoacidosis; DKA)	Not ketosis prone due to residual insulin (hyperglycemic hyperosmolar nonketotic syndrome [HHNS])
Treatment:		
Nondrug therapy	Essential adjunct to insulin therapy: • Medical nutrition therapy (MNT) • Physical activity/exercise therapy approved by physician; type based on presence of factors such as retinopathy, neuropathy, and cardiovascular status	Essential adjunct to oral antidiabetic therapy **OR** may be sufficient as monotherapy to control blood glucose
Drug therapy	• Insulin monotherapy **OR** oral antidiabetic drugs as adjuct to insulin therapy (rarely)	• Oral antidiabetic drugs **OR** • MNT monotherapy **OR** • Oral antidiabetic drugs in combination therapy **OR** • Insulin monotherapy **OR** • Insulin and oral antidiabetic drugs

Adapted from Setter SM, White JR, Campbell RK. Diabetes (Table 19.3). Copyright 2000 by Lippincott, Williams & Wilkins. From Herfindahl ET, Gourley DR, eds. Textbook of Therapeutics, 7th ed., 2000:379. With permission from Lippincott, Williams & Wilkins.

• The drug treatment options to control DM include subcutaneous insulin therapy, oral antidiabetic agents, or a combination of both.
  * Insulin therapy is essential for type 1 DM. Intensive insulin therapy (>3 doses/day or use of CSII) is replacing conventional insulin therapy (split-mix dosing: two-thirds of total daily dose [TDD] is taken before breakfast and one-third of the TDD is taken before the evening meal; two injections per day of intermediate-acting insulin or mixed doses of rapid- or short-acting insulin with intermediate-acting insulin). Oral antidiabetic agents as monotherapy or in combination with insulin are used for type 2 DM.
  * Insulins vary principally by their source, appearance, time-activity profiles (onset, peak, and duration), dosing, and route of administration. Main adverse events are hypoglycemia, weight gain, and lipodystrophies. Mechanism of action is the same for all types (Table 2).
  * Oral antidiabetic agents vary in their time activity profiles, dosing and administration, site and mechanism of action, and adverse events. Hypoglycemia is an adverse drug event for all these agents EXCEPT alpha-glucosidase

inhibitors, biguanides, and thiazolidinediones. Main adverse events for other oral agents are as follows: chlorpropamide (Diabinese®)—prolonged hypoglycemia (especially in the elderly), dilutional hyponatremia, SIADH, disulfiram-like reaction when ETOH is ingested; acarbose (Precose®) and miglitol (Glyset®)—flatulence, diarrhea, abdominal pain, increased LFTs (acarbose only); metformin (Glucophage®)—diarrhea, lactic acidosis (ie, associated with use of parenteral iodinated contrast media; potentially fatal), and megaloblastic anemia; thiazolidinediones—edema, exacerbation of CHF, URI, resumption of ovulation, and potential liver toxicity; meglitinides—hypoglycemia, weight gain, URI, and arthropathy (see Table 4). Added beneficial effects with metformin are lack of weight gain and potential modest weight loss.

* See Tables 3 and 5 for drug interactions for insulin and oral antidiabetic agents.

- Nondrug treatment includes medical nutrition therapy (MNT) and physical activity/exercise. These therapies are essential adjuncts to drug treatment. In the case of type 2 DM, nondrug therapy may be sufficient as monotherapy to control blood glucose.

- The Diabetes Control and Complications Trial (DCCT) demonstrated that tight control of blood glucose in persons with type 1 DM could delay the onset and slow the progression of long-term microvascular complications (ie, retinopathy, nephropathy, and neuropathy). The United Kingdom Prospective Diabetes Study (UKPDS) demonstrated that increased control of blood glucose in persons with type 2 DM could reduce the incidence of microvascular complications as it does in type 1 diabetes. It also showed that lowering blood pressure reduces the incidence of cardiovascular and microvascular long-term complications.

- Patient education is essential for the management of DM as it provides a means for persons with this chronic disease to become empowered, cope effectively, and engage in appropriate self-care.

5. Questions and Answers

Use Patient Profile #1 to answer Questions 1-5.

1. Chlorpropamide would be problematic in this case for which of the following reasons?

   I. Alcohol intake
   II. Sulfa allergy
   III. Asthma
   IV. Hypertension
   V. Drug-drug interaction

   A. I only
   B. III only
   C. I and II only
   D. II, III, and IV
   E. I, II, and V

2. Due to a renal protection mechanism, the drug class of choice for B.E.'s hypertension is

   A. β-Blocker
   B. Loop diuretic
   C. Thiazide diuretic
   D. Alpha adrenergic blocker
   E. Angiotensin-converting enzyme inhibitor

3. One of the most common adverse drug events caused by B.E.'s oral antidiabetic agent is

   A. Flatulence
   B. Hypoglycemia
   C. Renal failure
   D. Hyperglycemia
   E. Weight gain

4. Which of the following medications on the medication list in this case can mask the symptoms of hypoglycemia?

   A. Propranolol
   B. Albuterol
   C. Acarbose
   D. Prednisone
   E. Aspirin

5. What change in the following laboratory tests might be observed with the addition of prednisone to B.E.'s drug regimen?

   A. Increase in liver function tests (LFTs)
   B. Decrease in BUN
   C. Decrease in serum creatinine
   D. Increase in serum creatinine

E. Increase in blood glucose

Use Patient Profile #2 to answer Questions 6-10.

6. What is the principal drug-related problem in this patient's medication record?

   A. Insulin therapy is not indicated for persons with type 2 DM
   B. Therapeutic duplication of sulfonylurea therapy
   C. Potential decrease of BG due to drug-drug interaction between phenytoin and tolazamide
   D. Potential increase of BG due to drug-drug interaction between glimepiride and itraconazole

E. Use of an ACE inhibtor for hypertension in type 2 DM

7. All of the following monitoring parameters are necessary for T.R. EXCEPT

   A. Periodic glycosylated hemoglobin A_{1c}
   B. SMBG levels
   C. Phenytoin levels
   D. Blood pressure readings
   E. Quarterly serum C-peptide level

8. Which of the following is inappropriate treatment for a mild hypoglycemic episode?

   A. $^1/_2$ cup of diet soda
   B. 6-7 hard candies containing sugar

Patient Profile #1—Institution or Nursing Home Care

Patient Name: Barbara Evens
Address: 413 Summit Street
Age: 68
Height: 5' 5"
Weight: 190 lb
Sex: Female
Race: African-American
Allergies: Penicillin, sulfa drugs

Diagnosis:

	Primary	1) Type 2 DM
	Secondary	1) Hypertension
		2) Asthma

Lab/Diagnostic Tests:

	Date	Test
1)	2/1	LFTs
2)	2/1	Serum K
3)	5/1	LFTs
4)	5/1	Serum K
5)	6/1	A_{1c}

	Date	Test
6)	6/1	Serum creatinine
7)	6/1	BUN
8)	6/1	Serum K

Additional Orders:
1) Referral to dietitian for weight reduction diet
2) Low impact exercise 30 mins 3 days per week

Dietary Consideration:
1) Dietary changes per dietitian conslut.
2) Enteral and parenteral

Pharmacist Notes and Other Patient Information:

	Date	Comment
1)	2/1	Advise patient to continue SMBG and to report any hypoglycemic episodes. Instruct patient to treat hypoglycemia with glucose or lactose products. Instruct patient to take acarbose with first bite of meal. Foot exam negative. Patient reports having 1-2 drinks of bourbon per day.
2)		Inform patient to report any changes in BG.

Medication Orders:

Date	RX No	Physician	Drug & strength	Qty	Sig	Refills
2/1	834924	Jones	Propranolol 20 mg	30	1 PO bid	3
2/1	834925	Jones	Albuterol inhaler	1	1-2 inhalations q4-6h	3
2/1	834926	Jones	Acarbose 25 mg	90	1 tab PO w/meals	2
5/1	834927	Jones	Acarbose 50 mg	90	1 tab PO w/meals	2
6/1	834928	Jones	Prednisone 10 mg	30	1 tab PO daily	0
6/1	834929	Jones	Propranolol 20 mg	30	1 tab PO bid	3
6/1	834930	Jones	Albuertol inhaler	1	1-2 inhalations q4-6h	3
6/1	834931	Jones	ASA 81 mg	30	1 tab PO daily	3

Patient Profile #2—Community

Patient Name: Tom Right

Address:	20 Blue Ridge Drive
Age:	48
Height:	5' 6"
Weight:	135 lb
Sex:	Male
Race:	Caucasian
Allergies:	NKDA

Diagnosis:

Primary	1) Type 2 DM
	2) Epilepsy
Secondary	1) Hypertension
	2) Fungal infection under toenails

Pharmacist Notes and Other Patient Information:

	Date	Comment
1)	4/8	Patient should be monitored closely for hypoglycemia. Teach patient signs and symptoms of hypoglycemia and treatment measures.

Medication Orders:

Date	RX No	Physician	Drug & strength	Qty	Sig	Refills
1/6	765321	Smith	Tolazamide 250 mg	90	1 tab PO daily	0
4/8	765323	Smith	Glimepiride 2 mg	90	1 tab PO daily	0
8/6	765324	Smith	Lisinopril 5 mg	90	1 tab PO daily	0
8/6	765325	Thomas	Phenytoin extended	60	300 mg PO daily	0
8/6	765366	Smith	Itraconazole	14	50 mg PO daily	0
8/6	765367	Smith	Regular insulin	Trial	5 units SC before meals	0

C. 3 glucose tablets

D. $1/_2$ cup of regular soda

E. 5 small sugar cubes

9. Persons on insulin therapy should be advised to rotate their injection sites for the following reason

   A. Reduces the risk of infection
   B. Reduces the risk of lipoatrophy
   C. Reduces the risk of lipohypertrophy
   D. Reduces the risk of generalized myalgia
   E. This advice is outdated due to the use of human insulin

10. Which of the following is the most appropriate treatment for a severe hypoglycemic episode?

    A. $1/_2$ cup of diet soda
    B. 3 hard candies containing sugar
    C. 1 glucose tablet
    D. Glucagon injection
    E. 2-3 small sugar cubes

11. Commercially available insulin may be administered by which of the following routes?

    I   Intravenously
    II. Subcutaneously
    III. Via inhalation

    IV. Transdermally
    V. Sublingually

    A. I only
    B. II only
    C. I and II only
    D. II, III, and IV
    E. I, II, and V

12. Insulin therapy is indicated in all of the following except

    A. Newly diagnosed type 1 DM
    B. Gestational diabetes mellitus (GDM) not controlled by diet
    C. Hyperglycemic hyperosmolar nonketotic syndrome (HHNS)
    D. Newly diagnosed type 2 DM
    E. Diabetic ketoacidosis (DKA)

13. Insulin dosing is adjusted based on the following parameters

    I.   Liver function test results
    II. Dietary intake
    III. Physical activity/exercise
    IV. Blood glucose levels
    V.   Ophthalmic examinations

    A. I only

B. II only
C. I and II only
D. II, III, and IV
E. I, II, and V

14. Which of the following oral antidiabetic agents is a micronized formulation?

    A. Micronase®
    B. Glynase®
    C. Glucotrol XL®
    D. Amaryl®
    E. Orinase®

15. Insulin that has been stored in a refrigerator should be allowed to reach room temperature prior to administration in order to

    A. Allow for proper mixing
    B. Minimize painful injections
    C. Prevent frosting or clumping
    D. Delay systemic absorption
    E. Prevent change in clarity

16. When mixing rapid- or short-acting insulin with intermediate- or long-acting insulin, which insulin in the list below should be drawn up first?

    A. Regular
    B. NPH
    C. Lente
    D. Ultralente
    E. Glargine

17. Uniform dispersion of insulin suspensions can be obtained by

    A. Vigorously shaking the vial
    B. Rolling the vial gently between the hands
    C. Warming the vial in a microwave
    D. Packing the vial in dry ice
    E. Keeping the vial at room temperature (68-75°F)

18. Of the following types of insulin, which can be administered intravenously?

    A. Glargine
    B. Lente
    C. Regular
    D. Ultralente
    E. NPH

19. Diabetes mellitus is the leading cause of which of the following complications?

    A. Pancreatitis
    B. Fatty liver
    C. Blindness
    D. Stroke
    E. Deafness

20. Which of the following is an indication that a patient is developing a long-term complication from diabetes mellitus?

    A. Tachycardia
    B. Glucosuria
    C. Leukocytosis
    D. Proteinuria
    E. Tinnitus

21. What sulfonylurea has been associated with the greatest incidence of prolonged hypoglycemia in the elderly?

    A. Tolazamide
    B. Tolbutamide
    C. Chlorpropamide
    D. Glimepiride
    E. Glipizide

22. Which of the following drugs taken with alcohol can cause a disulfiram-like reaction?

    A. Chlorpropamide
    B. Acarbose
    C. NPH insulin
    D. Glucagon
    E. Pioglitazone

23. Metformin should be withheld for 48 hours prior to and for 48 hours after any procedure requiring the use of parenteral iodinated contrast media due to the potential for this adverse drug event

    A. Optic neuritis
    B. Metabolic alkalosis
    C. Lactic acidosis
    D. Purple toe syndrome
    E. Tinnitus

24. The use of insulin in a woman with GDM helps reduce the incidence of the which complication in the fetus?

    A. Macrosomia
    B. Cystic fibrosis
    C. Deafness
    D. "Soft bones"
    E. Eczema

25. Metformin would not be an option for the patient with the following diagnosis

    A. Iron deficiency anemia
    B. Impaired renal function
    C. Hypertension
    D. Type 2 diabetes
    E. Frequent hypoglycemic episodes

26. Nocturnal hypoglycemia resulting in rebound hyperglycemia in type 1 DM is termed

    A. Honeymoon period
    B. Somogyi effect
    C. Dawn phenomenon
    D. Hyperglycemic phase
    E. Insulin resistance syndrome

27. Which of the following is a potentially fatal adverse drug event of Glucophage®?

    A. Weight gain
    B. Frequent urination
    C. Diarrhea
    D. Lactic acidosis
    E. Angioedema

28. All of the following are true of acarbose therapy EXCEPT

    A. Contraindicated in inflammatory bowel disease
    B. Should be taken with first bite of each meal
    C. Does not cause hypoglycemia or weight gain
    D. Hypoglycemia due to combination therapy should be treated with sucrose
    E. LFTs are monitored every 3 months during the first year and periodically thereafter (if the dose is >50 mg tid)

29. Prandin® is a nonsulfonylurea secretagogue. Adverse drug events include all of the following EXCEPT

    A. Upper respiratory infection (URI)
    B. Arthropathy
    C. Hypoglycemia
    D. Back pain
    E. Hyperglycemia

30. Patient counseling relative to meglitinides should include the following points

    I. Must be taken 30 minutes before main meals
    II. If a meal is omitted, do not take
    III. Enhances preprandial glucose utilization

IV. Hyperglycemia is a potential adverse drug event
V. Disulfiram-like reaction possible when ingested with ETOH

    A. I only
    B. III only
    C. I and II only
    D. II, III, and IV
    E. I, II, and V

31. Which one of the following anti-diabetic agents does not require liver function tests for monitoring?
    A. Glargine
    B. Miglitol
    C. Rosiglitazone
    D. Acarbose
    E. Metformin

32. Adverse drug events reported for pioglitazone (Actos), a thiazolidinedione, include all of the following EXCEPT

    A. Exacerbation of CHF
    B. Resumption of ovulation
    C. Edema
    D. Upper respiratory infection (URI)
    E. Megaloblastic anemia

33. All of the following drugs have a direct glucogenic effect EXCEPT

    A. Thiazide diuretics
    B. Corticosteroids
    C. Nicotinic acid
    D. Sympathomimetics
    E. Acetohexamide

34. Which of the following is the mechanism of action (MOA) for the sulfonylureas?

    A. Stimulates pancreatic β-cells to secrete insulin
    B. Delays carbohydrate metabolism and absorption (due to inhibition of intestinal and pancreatic enzymes)
    C. Increases hepatic insulin sensitivity and decreases hepatic glucose production
    D. Increases skeletal muscle and adipose tissue insulin sensitivity and decreases hepatic glucose production
    E. Decreases blood glucose and assists with blood glucose control by increasing glucose uptake and utilization by peripheral tissues

35. All of the following are signs or symptoms of hypoglycemia EXCEPT

    A. tachycardia
    B. diaphoresis
    C. shakiness
    D. polyuria
    E. pallor

Answers

1. **E.** Chlorpropamide is contraindicated in persons with a sulfa allergy. Alcohol (ETOH) ingestion with chlorpropamide could lead to a disulfiram-like reaction. Also, acute ingestion of ETOH (especially in the fasting state) includes the risk of severe hypoglycemia. Chlorpropamide and prednisone may produce a drug-drug interaction resulting in hyperglycemia. Items 3 and 4 are non-problematic in this case in relation to chlorpropamide.

2. **E.** Angiotensin-converting enzyme inhibitors (ACEIs) exhibit a renal protective mechanism in persons with DM. None of the remaining drugs exhibit such an effect.

3. **A.** The most common adverse drug events for acarbose are flatulence, abdominal pain, and diarrhea. These adverse effects may be decreased by titrating the dose gradually and taking the drug with the first bite of each meal. There may also be an increase in LFTs.

4. **A.** Propranolol (a nonselective beta-blocker) can mask the symptoms of hypoglycemia (ie, tachycardia [palpitations], pallor, shakiness [tremor], paresthesia, hunger, diaphoresis [sweating], dizziness and blurred vision). None of the remaining drugs listed have this effect.

5. **E.** The increase in LFTs may be due to acarbose, and the increase in serum creatinine may represent the development or progression of nephropathy, a long-term complication of DM. The decrease in the serum creatinine and BUN are incorrect answers. Prednisone, a corticosteroid, has a dose-dependent, direct glucogenic and glycosuric effect, and therefore an increase in BG might be observed.

6. **B.** Though tolazamide and glimepiride are first- and second-generation sulfonylureas, duplication of drug class is inappropriate. These agents are both intermediate-acting and therefore might potentiate the adverse drug event of hypoglycemia. Insulin may be indicated in the person with type 2 DM as the disease progresses. The potential drug-drug interaction between phenytoin and tolazamide could result in an increased BG and the potential drug-drug interaction between glimepiride and itraconazole could result in a decreased BG. An ACEI for hypertension in type 2 DM is appropriate as this drug is renal protective.

7. **E.** The A_{1c} and SMBG tests are essential for monitoring the success of glucose control therapy. The SMBG gives an immediate determination of BG level and the A_{1c} gives an average reading over the previous 2-3 months (or 120 days, the life span of a RBC). Phenytoin levels are necessary for monitoring therapeutically appropriate levels, and BP readings are for monitoring success of antihypertensive therapy. A serum C-peptide might be diagnostic for the determination of functioning β-cells; however, if performed, it is done very infrequently to reduce cost.

8. **A.** One-half cup of diet soda would be inappropriate, because a mild hypoglycemic episode requires a fast-acting oral carbohydrate for resolution and diet soda has none. The other options would all be appropriate for resolution of the event.

9. **C.** Lipohypertrophy (a bulging of the injection site) is due to nonrotation of injection sites. Risk of infection may be reduced by using aseptic injecting technique. Lipoatrophy (a pitting of the injection site) may be due to an antigenic response to insulin. The advice regarding rotation of injection site is not outdated.

10. **D.** Glucagon, a pancreatic hormone which is given parenterally, is the most appropriate treatment for a severe hypoglycemic episode (life-threatening) as the patient may be unconscious and not able to take a fast-acting carbohydrate by mouth. The other items represent inappropriate treatment for mild to moderate hypoglycemia (the amounts of items B, C, and E are inadequate, and the soda in item A should be regular soda).

11. **C.** Pharmaceutical research has developed an inhaled insulin product which is still being tested. Presently, the commercially available insulins may only be administered intravenously or subcutaneously.

12. **D.** Newly diagnosed type 2 DM should first have a trial with MNT and exercise, and if this nondrug therapy fails, then oral antidiabetic monotherapy should be added. Combination oral therapy would be indicated next with failure of monotherapy, and then following its failure, insulin monotherapy or in combination with oral agents is indicated. Insulin is indicated in all the other situations.

13. **D.** Dietary intake, physical activity/exercise, and blood glucose levels are the parameters used in adjusting insulin dosing (eg, if the parameters of dietary intake and blood glucose levels are decreased and physical activity/exercise is increased, then the insulin dosing would require reduction to avoid hypoglycemia). Monitoring of these parameters is critical to adjusting the insulin regimen. Items 1 and 5 are incorrect.

14. **B.** Glynase® is a micronized formulation of glyburide that is significantly absorbed (eg, a 3-mg tablet provides blood levels similar to a 5-mg conventional tablet). Micronase® is a trade name for nonmicronized glyburide. Glucotrol XL® is the name of an extended formulation of glipizide. Orinase® is the trade name for tol-butamide (the only first-generation sulfonylurea listed here) and Amaryl is the trade name for glimepiride.

15. **B.** Refrigerated insulin is allowed to reach room temperature prior to administration to minimize painful injections. Proper mixing, prevention of frosting or clumping, or maintenance of clarity have nothing to do with reaching room temperature. Systemic absorption would actually be enhanced by increasing to room temperature, not delayed.

16. **A.** Regular or clear insulin is always drawn up first (to assure that all persons mixing insulins will use the same procedure and no intermediate- or long-acting insulin will be placed in the regular insulin vial and potentially cause contamination and dose variance). Glargine is also a clear insulin; however, it is NEVER to be mixed with other insulins due to the low pH (4.0) of its diluents.

17. **B.** Uniform dispersion of insulin suspensions can be obtained by gently rolling the vial between the hands. Insulin is a fragile molecule and all the other means listed could cause molecular degradation.

18. **C.** Of these insulins, regular is the only one that can be administered intravenously. Though glargine is clear like regular insulin, its pH is 4.0 and it should NEVER be given intravenously. The remaining insulins are suspensions and also should NEVER be given intravenously.

19. **C.** DM is the leading cause of new cases of blindness among adults 20-74 years of age in the U.S. There is also an increased incidence of stroke with DM, but DM is not the leading cause of this problem. The other items are incorrect.

20. **D.** Proteinuria is an indication that a patient is developing the long-term complication of nephropathy. Items A, B, and C could be related to acute complications such as DKA (glucosuria and leukocytosis) and hypoglycemia (tachycardia). Item E is incorrect.

21. **C.** Chlorpropamide has a $t_{1/2}$ of 35 hours and a duration of action of 60 hours, therefore it has been associated with prolonged hypoglycemia in the elderly (perhaps due to their declining renal function). The other sulfonylureas have reported less hypoglycemia.

22. **A.** Chlorpropamide has had the greatest reporting of this drug interaction relative to the first-generation sulfonylureas. The remaining drugs listed have not had reports of this adverse drug event.

23. **C.** Lactic acidosis can result if metformin (Glucophage®) is given in this situation and it can be potentially fatal. Renal function must be evaluated following such a procedure, and it must be normal before metformin may be resumed. The other items are incorrect.

24. **A.** Macrosomia (abnormally large fetal body size) is one of the fetal complications of concern in GDM. The primary benefit of insulin therapy is reduction in the incidence of macrosomia. The other items are incorrect.

25. **B.** Contraindications for metformin are renal dysfunction for those predisposed to lactic acidosis. Metformin does not cause hypoglycemia and it is indicated in type 2 DM. Hypertension and iron deficiency anemia are incorrect answers. Metformin may cause megaloblastic anemia.

26. **B.** The Somogyi effect is rebound hyperglycemia or early morning hyperglycemia secondary to nocturnal hypoglycemia. The person with type 1 DM may experience a honeymoon period—a phase of erratic insulin secretion during destruction of β cells by islet cell antibodies. This apparent short-lived remission, lasts months to a year. The dawn phenomenon is fasting hyperglycemia (pre-breakfast) due to decreased plasma insulin during the night or the anti-insulin effect of nocturnal growth hormone. Items D and E are incorrect.

27. **D.** Lactic acidosis is a potentially fatal adverse drug event of Glucophage® (metformin). It does not cause weight gain. Modest weight loss is possible and no hypoglycemia is reported when metformin is used as monotherapy. Diarrhea is an adverse drug event, but with gradual dose titration and administration with food, it decreases over time. Items B and E are incorrect.

28. **D.** Oral glucose instead of carbohydrate sources with sucrose (cane sugar) or fructose is used because absorption of these is inhibited. The remaining items are true of acarbose therapy.

29. **E.** Prandin® may cause hypoglycemia like the sulfonylureas. Hyperglycemia is not one of the adverse drug events (ADEs) reported. All the other ADEs may be caused by Prandin®.

30. **C.** Meglitinides should be taken 30 minutes before main meals and if a meal is omitted, the drug should not be taken. It enhances postprandial glucose utilization, hypoglycemia and not hyperglycemia may occur, and disulfiram-like reactions are not reported.

31. **A.** The alpha-glucosidase inhibitors (eg, acarbose), biguanides (eg, metformin), and thiazolidinediones (eg, rosiglitazone) all require LFTs for monitoring. Glargine, a long-acting insulin, dose not require LFTs for monitoring; rather it requires blood glucose monitoring.

32. **E.** Megaloblastic anemia is a reported adverse drug effect for metformin but not for Actos®. All the other items listed are reported ADEs. Since troglitazone (Resulin®), a thiazolidinedione, was withdrawn from the market in 2000 due to severe liver toxicity, this ADE could potentially occur with Actos®; therefore LFTs should be done.

33. **E.** Acetohexamide has a hypoglycemic effect. All the other drugs listed have a direct glucogenic effect.

34. **A.** The sulfonylureas stimulate pancreatic β cells to secrete insulin. Item B is the MOA for alpha-glucosidase inhibitors, item C is the MOA for the biguanide metformin, item D is the MOA for the glitizones, and item E is the MOA for insulin.

35. **D.** Polyuria (excessive urination) is one of the classic signs and symptoms of DM. All of the other answers listed are some of the signs and symptoms of hypoglycemia, which can be life threatening.

6. References

American Hospital Formulary Service Drug Information, 2003 Edition. Bethesda, MD: American Society of Health-System Pharmacists, Inc.

America Diabetes Association (ADA). Clinical practice recommendations 2003. *Diabetes Care.* 2003;26(suppl 1):S3-S156.

Atkinson MA, Maclaren NK. The pathogenesis of insulin-dependent diabetes mellitus. *N Engl J Med.* 1994;331:1428-1436.

Campbell RK, White JR. *Medications for the Treatment of Diabetes.* Alexandria, VA: American Diabetes Association; 2000.

Cox DJ, Gonder-Frederick L, Antoun B, Cryer PE, Clarke WL. Perceived symptoms in the recognition of hypoglycemia. *Diabetes Care.* 1993;6:519-527.

Diabetes Control and Complications Trial Research Group. The effect of intensive treatment on the development and the progress of long-term complications in insulin-dependent diabetes mellitus. *N Engl J Med.* 1993;329:977-986.

DeFronzo RA, Bonadonna RC, Ferrannini E. Pathogenesis of NIDDM. A balanced overview. *Diabetes Care.* 1992;15:318-368.

Funnell MM, Hunt C, Kulkarni K, et al. *A Core Curriculum for Diabetes Education,* 3rd ed. Chicago: American Association of Diabetes Educators; 1998.

Facts and Comparisons, drug information monthly update service. St. Louis, MO: Wolters Kluwer Health, Inc.; 2000-2003 editions.

Koda-Kimble, MA, Carlisle, BA. Diabetes mellitus. In: Koda-Kimble, MA, Young LY, eds. *Applied Therapeutics: The Clinical Use of Drugs,* 7th ed. Philadelphia: Lippincott, Williams & Wilkins; 2001:48-1 to 49-92.

McEvoy GK, Litvak K, Welsh OH, et al. *Pharmacist's Drug Handbook.* Bethesda, MD: American Society of Health-System Pharmacists and Springhouse; Springhouse Corp., 2001.

National Institute of Diabetes and Digestive and Kidney Diseases. National diabetes statistics fact sheet: general information and national estimates on diabetes in the United States, 2000. Bethesda, MD: U.S. Department of Health and Human Services, National Institutes of Health; 2002.

Physician's Desk Reference (PDR), 56th ed. Montvale, NJ: Medical Economics Co.; 2002.

Report of the Expert Committee on the Diagnosis and Classification of Diabetes Mellitus. *Diabetes Care.* 1997;20:1183-1197.

Setter SM, White Jr JR, Campbell RK. Diabetes. In: Herfindal ET, Gourley DR, eds. *Textbook of Therapeutics,* 7th ed. Philadelphia: Lippincott, Williams & Wilkins; 2000:377-406.

The University Group Diabetes Program. A study of the effects of hypoglycemic agents on vascular complications in patients with adult onset diabetes. *Diabetes.* 1970;19(Suppl 2):1-26.

UK Prospective Diabetes Study (UKPDS) Group. Effect of intensive blood-glucose control with metformin on complications in overweight patients with type 2 diabetes (UKPDS 34). *Lancet.* 1998;352:854-865.

UK Prospective Diabetes Study (UKPDS) Group. Efficacy of atenolol and captopril in reducing risk of macrovascular and microvascular complications in type 2 diabetes (UKPDS 39). *BMJ.* 1998;317:13-20.

UK Prospective Diabetes Study (UKPDS) Group. Intensive blood-glucose control with sulphonylureas or insulin compared with conventional treatment and risks of complications in patients with type 2 diabetes (UKPDS 33). *Lancet.* 1998;352:837-853.

UK Prospective Diabetes Study (UKPDS) Group. Tight blood pressure control and risk of macrovascular and microvascular complications in type 2 diabetes (UKPDS 38). *BMJ.* 1998;317:703-713.

United States Pharmacopeia Dispensing Information. Drug Information for the Health Care Professional, Vol. 1, 22nd ed. Greenwood Village, CO: Micromedex; 2002.

White JR, Campbell RK. Drug/drug and drug/disease interactions and diabetes. *Diabetes Educator.* 1995;21:283-289.

Yarborough PC, Rodgers ST. Diabetes mellitus. In: Shargel L, Mutrick AH, Souney PF, Swanson LN, eds. *Comprehensive Pharmacy Review,* 4th ed. Philadelphia: Lippincott, Williams & Wilkins; 2001:970-992.

14. Thyroid, Adrenal, and Miscellaneous Endocrine Drugs

Bob L. Lobo, PharmD, BCPS
Associate Professor, Department of Pharmacy
University of Tennessee College of Pharmacy
Clinical Specialist, Medicine and Neurosciences
Methodist Healthcare-University Hospital

Contents

1. Thyroid

Hypothyroidism

Disease overview
Definition and epidemiology
- Hypothyroidism is a syndrome resulting from deficient thyroid hormone production that results in a slowing down of all bodily functions
- Retardation of growth occurs in infants and children
- Prevalence greater in women and increases with age; affects 1.5-2% of women and 0.2% of men

Types
- Most cases are caused by thyroid gland failure (primary hypothyroidism)
- Hashimoto's disease (chronic lymphocytic thyroiditis) is the cause of 90% of primary hypothyroidism
- Pituitary failure causes secondary hypothyroidism
- Hypothalamic failure causes tertiary hypothyroidism
- Iatrogenic hypothyroidism follows exposure to radiation with radioiodine or external radiation
- Other causes may include thyroidectomy, iodine deficiency, enzymatic defects, iodine, lithium, and interferon-alpha

Clinical presentation
- Symptoms include cold intolerance, fatigue, somnolence, constipation, menorrhagia, myalgias, and hoarseness
- Signs include thyroid gland enlargement or atrophy, bradycardia, edema, dry skin, and weight gain
- Myxedema coma is an end stage of hypothyroidism characterized by weakness, confusion, hypothermia, hypoventilation, hypoglycemia, hyponatremia, coma, and shock

Pathophysiology
- Thyroxine (T_4) is the major hormone secreted by the thyroid, which is converted to the more potent triiodothyronine (T_3) in tissues
- Thyroxine secretion is stimulated by thyroid-stimulating hormone (TSH)
- TSH secretion is inhibited by T_4, forming a negative feedback loop
- Hashimoto's disease is an autoimmune-mediated disease resulting from cell- and antibody-mediated thyroid injury
- Antimicrosomal antibodies are directed against thyroidal antigens

Diagnosis
- Plasma TSH assay is the initial test of choice if hypothyroidism is suspected clinically

- TSH levels are elevated in primary hypothyroidism
- Low plasma free T_4 (or T_4 index) confirms the diagnosis of hypothyroidism

Treatment principles
- Synthetic thyroxine (levothyroxine) is the drug of choice for hypothyroidism because it is chemically stable, inexpensive, free of antigenicity, and has uniform potency
- Typical dose is 100-125 µg PO once daily; reduce dose to 50 µg in elderly and 25 µg in patients with coronary artery disease to reduce risk of precipitating angina
- The goal of therapy is to maintain plasma TSH in the normal range
- Dose changes are made at 6- to 8-week intervals until the TSH is normal
- Overtreatment is detected by subnormal TSH and is associated with osteoporosis and atrial fibrillation
- Failure to respond to appropriate doses is most often due to poor compliance
- Do not use thyroid hormones to facilitate weight loss in euthyroid patients

Drug therapy of hypothyroidism (Table 1)
Mechanism of action
- Thyroid hormones enhance oxygen consumption by most tissues and increase basal metabolic rate and metabolism of carbohydrates, lipids, and proteins

Patient counseling
- Take once daily, 30 minutes before breakfast since food may decrease absorption
- Replacement therapy is usually to be taken for life; don't discontinue without advice of prescriber
- Notify prescriber if you experience rapid or irregular heartbeat, chest pain, shortness of breath, nervousness, irritability, tremors, heat intolerance, or weight loss
- Don't take antacids, calcium, or iron supplements within 4 hours of levothyroxine

Adverse effects
- Cardiovascular: tachycardia, arrhythmia, angina, MI
- CNS: tremor, headache, nervousness, insomnia, irritability, hyperactivity
- GI: diarrhea, vomiting, cramps
- Miscellaneous: weight loss, fatigue, menstrual irregularities, excessive sweating, heat intolerance, fever, muscle weakness, hair loss, decreased bone mineral density, hypersensitivity

Drug interactions
- Amiodarone may cause hypothyroidism or hyperthyroidism

Table 1

Thyroid Preparations for the Treatment of Hypothyroidism

Trade name	Generic name	Dosage forms	Usual dosage range
Synthroid® Levothroid® Levoxyl® Unithroid® Thyro-Tabs®	Levothyroxine sodium (T$_4$)	Tablets: 0.025, 0.05, 0.075, 0.088, 0.1, 0.112, 0.125, 0.137, 0.15, 0.175, 0.2 and 0.3 mg Injection: 200 and 500 µg	0.1-0.15 mg PO qd for hypothyroidism (dosage is individualized); higher doses are used in treating thyroid cancer
Armour Thyroid® Nature-Throid® Westhroid®	Desiccated thyroid USP	Tablets: 15, 30, 32.4, 60, 64.8, 65, 90, 120, 129.6, 130, 180, 194.4, 195, 240 and 300 mg	60-120 mg PO qd for hypothyroidism; (dosage is individualized); higher doses used in treating thyroid cancer
Cytomel® Triostat®	Liothyronine (T$_3$)	Tablets: 5, 25, 50 µg Injection: 10 µg	25 µg PO qd for hypothyroidism
Thyrolar®	Liotrix (T$_4$ and T$_3$ in a 4:1 ratio)	Tablets: 15, 30, 60, 120, 180 mg	60-120 mg PO qd for hypothyroidism

- Antacids decrease absorption of levothyroxine; separate administration by at least 4 hours
- Antidiabetic agents may be less effective with levothyroxine; increase in insulin or oral hypoglycemic dose may be needed
- Bile acid sequestrants reduce absorption of levothyroxine; separate by at least 4 hours
- Enzyme-inducing antiepileptic agents increase hepatic degradation of levothyroxine; may need to increase thyroxine dosage
- Estrogens may decrease response to levothyroxine; may need to increase levothyroxine dosage
- Lithium commonly causes hypothyroidism
- Warfarin effect may be enhanced by levothyroxine; may need to decrease warfarin dosage
- Digoxin levels may be reduced by levothyroxine supplementation
- Sucralfate may decrease levothyroxine absorption; separate by at least 4 hours
- Soybean formula decreases levothyroxine absorption
- Sympathomimetic drugs may potentiate the effects of levothyroxine
- Theophylline clearance may be enhanced by levothyroxine

Monitoring parameters
- Plasma TSH every 6-8 weeks until normalization
- Signs and symptoms of hypothyroidism should improve within a few weeks
- Once optimum replacement dose attained, physical examination and TSH every 6-12 months
- Patients at risk for coronary artery disease should be monitored for angina

Pharmacokinetics
- Oral absorption is improved by fasting but decreased by dietary fiber, drugs, and foods
- Half-life of 7 days allows once-daily dosing
- Average bioavailability of levothyroxine products is 80%; a variety of AB rated generic products are available

Other
- Use of natural thyroid hormones such as desiccated thyroid USP is discouraged due to less predictable potency and stability compared to synthetic levothyroxine
- Synthetic T$_3$ (liothyronine) has a shorter half-life than levothyroxine, a higher incidence of cardiac side effects and is more difficult to monitor

Hyperthyroidism

Disease overview
Definition and epidemiology
- Hyperthyroidism (thyrotoxicosis) is the clinical syndrome that results when tissues are exposed to high levels of thyroid hormone

- Thyrotoxicosis is more common in women than men, occurring in 3 per 1000 women

Types

- Graves' disease is the most common cause of hyperthyroidism
- Toxic multinodular goiter (MNG), toxic adenoma, and exogenous thyroid hormone ingestion may also cause hyperthyroidism
- Thyroid storm is a life-threatening, sudden exacerbation of all of the symptoms of thyrotoxicosis characterized by fever, tachycardia, delirium, and coma
- Hyperthyroidism may be caused by drugs such as amiodarone and iodine

Clinical presentation

- Symptoms include heat intolerance, weight loss, weakness, palpitations, and anxiety
- Signs include tremor, tachycardia, weakness and eyelid lag, and warm, moist skin
- Other manifestations include atrial fibrillation and congestive heart failure

Pathophysiology

- Graves' disease is an autoimmune disease in which thyroid-stimulating antibodies are produced; these antibodies mimic the action of TSH on thyroid tissue
- Toxic adenomas and MNGs are masses of thyroid tissue that secrete thyroid hormones independent of pituitary control

Diagnosis

- Elevated T_4 or T_3 in the presence of a decreased TSH confirms diagnosis of hyperthyroidism

Treatment principles

- There are three primary methods for controlling hyperthyroidism: surgery, radioactive iodine (RAI), and antithyroid (thionamide) drugs
- The goal is to minimize symptoms and eliminate excess thyroid hormone
- RAI is often considered the treatment of choice in Graves' disease, toxic adenomas, and MNGs
- Drug therapy is preferred in pregnancy since RAI is contraindicated
- Thionamide drugs (propylthiouracil and methimazole) have no permanent effect on thyroid function
- Adjunctive treatments for hyperthyroidism include beta-adrenergic receptor blockers or calcium channel blockers in order to control tachycardia associated with hyperthyroidism

Drug therapy of hyperthyroidism (Table 2)
Thionamides
Mechanism of action

- Propylthiouracil (PTU) and methimazole inhibit the synthesis of thyroid hormones by preventing the incorporation of iodine into iodotyrosines and by inhibiting the coupling of monoiodotyrosine and diiodotyrosine to form T_4 and T_3
- Propylthiouracil inhibits the peripheral conversion of T_4 to T_3

Patient counseling

- This medication prevents excessive thyroid hormone production
- It must be taken regularly in order to be effective
- Do not discontinue use without first consulting your physician

Table 2

Antithyroid Medications

Drug name	Drug contains	Dosage forms	Usual dosage range
PTU	Propylthiouracil	Tablets: 50 mg	150-300 mg PO daily at 8-hour intervals
Tapazole®	Methimazole	Tablets: 5, 10 mg	5-40 mg PO daily in singe daily dose or divided
Lugol's solution	Strong iodine solution	Solution: 5% iodine and 10% potassium iodide; delivers 6.3 mg iodine per drop	0.1-0.3 mL (3-5 drops) PO tid
SSKI	Saturated solution of potassium iodide	Solution: 1 g/mL; delivers 38 mg iodine per drop of saturated solution	1-5 drops PO tid in water or juice

- Notify physician if fever, sore throat, unusual bleeding, rash, abdominal pain, or yellowing of the skin occurs

Adverse effects
- CNS: fever, headache, paresthesia
- General: rash, arthralgia, urticaria
- GI: jaundice, hepatitis
- Hematologic: agranulocytosis, leukopenia, bleeding

Drug interactions
- Potentiation of warfarin effect

Monitoring parameters
- Monitor for improvement in signs and symptoms of hyperthyroidism
- Thyroid function tests, signs and symptoms of agranulocytosis (fever, malaise, sore throat)

Pharmacokinetics
- Propylthiouracil has a short half-life requiring more frequent dosing than methimazole

Iodides
Mechanism of action
- Blocks hormone release, inhibits thyroid hormone synthesis
- May be used when rapid reduction in thyroid hormone secretion is desired such as in thyroid storm or to decrease glandular vascularity prior to thyroidectomy

Patient instructions
- Dilute with water or fruit juice to improve taste
- Notify physician if fever, skin rash, metallic taste, swelling of the throat, or burning of the mouth occurs

Adverse effects
- Rash, swelling of salivary glands, metallic taste, burning of the mouth, GI distress, hypersensitivity, goiter

Drug Interactions
- Lithium potentiates antithyroid effect of iodides

Monitoring parameters
- Monitor for improvement in signs and symptoms of hyperthyroidism and adverse effects

2. Adrenal

Cushing's Syndrome

Disease overview

Definition and epidemiology
- Syndrome resulting from chronic glucocorticoid excess
- Incidence of 2-4 per million cases each year

Types
- Usually iatrogenic due to therapy with glucocorticoid drugs
- Endogenous Cushing's syndrome is usually caused by overproduction of adrenocorticotropic hormone (ACTH) by pituitary gland adenomas (Cushing's disease)

Clinical presentation
- Obesity involving face, neck, trunk, and abdomen, hypertension, hirsutism, acne, amenorrhea, depression, thin skin, easy bruising, diabetes, osteopenia, and depression

Pathophysiology
- The hypothalamus produces corticotropin-releasing hormone (CRH) which stimulates the anterior pituitary gland to release ACTH. Circulating ACTH stimulates the adrenal cortex to produce cortisol

Diagnosis
- Based on signs and symptoms of hypercortisolism
- Dexamethasone suppression test or 24-hour urine cortisol measurement may be used

Treatment principles
- If syndrome is iatrogenic, minimization of corticosteroid exposure is essential
- Pharmacotherapy of Cushing's disease is aimed at reducing cortisol production or activity with drugs, radiation, or surgery

Drug therapy of Cushing's disease (Table 3)
Mechanism of action
- Drugs that are used to treat Cushing's disease suppress synthesis of cortisol
- Ketoconazole inhibits cytochrome P-450–dependent enzymes and cortisol synthesis
- Aminoglutethimide inhibits conversion of cholesterol to pregnenolone
- Mitotane is a cytotoxic drug that suppresses ACTH secretion and reduces synthesis of cortisol
- Metyrapone decreases cortisol synthesis by inhibition of 11-hydroxylase activity

Table 3

Drugs for Cushing's Syndrome

Trade name	Generic name	Dosage forms	Usual dosage range
Nizoral®	Ketoconazole	Tablets: 250 mg	800-1200 mg PO qd
Cytadren®	Aminoglutethimide	Tablets: 200 mg	250 mg PO q6h
Lysodren®	Mitotane	Tablets: 500 mg	9-10 g/d PO in divided doses
Metopirone®	Metyrapone	Capsules: 250 mg	1-6 g/d PO in 4-6 divided doses

Patient counseling
- Ketoconazole should be taken with food; separate from antacids by at least 2 hours; notify physician if abdominal pain, yellow skin, or pale stool occurs
- Aminoglutethimide may cause drowsiness, rash, weakness, nausea, and loss of appetite
- Metyrapone may cause nausea, vomiting, dizziness, and sedation
- Mitotane may cause nausea, vomiting, diarrhea, and tiredness

Adverse effects
- Ketoconazole causes nausea, vomiting, headache, impotence and hepatotoxicity
- Aminoglutethimide causes drowsiness, rash, weakness, hypotension, nausea, loss of appetite, hypothyroidism, and blood dyscrasias
- Metyrapone causes nausea, vomiting, dizziness, and sedation
- Mitotane may cause nausea, vomiting, diarrhea, and tiredness

Drug interactions
- Ketoconazole is a CYP-P450 3A4 enzyme inhibitor and may increase serum concentrations of cyclosporine, warfarin, cisapride, and triazolam; drugs that lower gastric acidity will decrease ketoconazole absorption; rifampin decreases ketoconazole levels
- Aminoglutethimide may induce metabolism of warfarin

Monitoring parameters
- Cortisol monitoring is required with mitotane

Adrenal Insufficiency

Disease overview
Definition and epidemiology
- Primary adrenocortical deficiency (Addison's disease) is caused by autoimmune-mediated destruction of the adrenal cortex, and results in glucocorticoid and mineralocorticoid deficiency
- Addison's disease occurs in 5-6 people per million per year

Types
- Primary adrenal insufficiency (Addison's disease) involves autoimmune destruction of the adrenal cortex
- Secondary insufficiency occurs after cessation of chronic exogenous corticosteroid use
- Acute adrenal insufficiency, or Addisonian crisis, is an endocrine emergency precipitated by severe stress

Clinical presentation
- Glucocorticoid deficiency (weight loss, malaise, abdominal pain, and depression)
- Mineralocorticoid deficiency (dehydration, hypotension, hyperkalemia, and salt craving)

Pathophysiology
- Cortisol is synthesized in the adrenal cortex when cholesterol is converted to pregnenolone by ACTH
- The adrenal cortex secretes aldosterone, cortisol, and androgenic hormones
- Mineralocorticoids (eg, aldosterone) enhance reabsorption of sodium and water from the distal tubule of the kidney and increase urinary potassium excretion

- Glucocorticoids affect glucose, carbohydrate and fat metabolism, produce anti-inflammatory and immunosuppressive effects, and affect other physiologic processes
- Chronic administration of corticosteroids produces inhibition of pituitary ACTH secretion and reduced cortisol production (hypothalamic-pituitary-adrenocoritical [HPA] axis suppression)
- Abrupt cessation of steroids may precipitate adrenal insufficiency

Diagnosis
- Cosyntropin (ACTH) stimulation test may be used to assess hypocortisolism

Treatment principles
- Addison's disease requires lifelong glucocorticoid and mineralocorticoid replacement
- Hydrocortisone 100 mg IV q8h is the drug of choice for acute adrenal crisis
- "Stress doses" of corticosteroids are given for minor illness, injury, or surgery; if stress is severe, hydrocortisone 100 mg IV q8h is used
- Gradual tapering of corticosteroids reduces the risk

of adrenal insufficiency in patients with HPA axis suppression
- Non-adrenal uses for corticosteroids are numerous, including allergic reactions; inflammatory conditions; hematologic disorders; rheumatic disorders; neurologic diseases; cancer; immunosuppression; pulmonary, renal, skin and thyroid diseases; hypercalcemia; and others
- Fludrocortisone has minimal anti-inflammatory activity and is used only when mineralocorticoid activity is needed, such as when increased blood pressure is desired

Drug therapy of adrenal insufficiency (Table 4)
Mechanism of action
- Glucocorticoids increase blood glucose by stimulating gluconeogenesis and glycogenolysis; increased fat deposition
- Catabolic effects in lymphoid, connective tissue, bone, muscle, fat, and skin
- Inhibition of inflammation and immunosuppression, vasoconstriction, reduction in prostaglandin and leukotriene synthesis, decreased neutrophils at site of inflammation and inhibition of macrophage function

Table 4

Corticosteroids and Dose Equivalents

Trade name	Generic name	Anti-inflammatory potency	Sodium retaining potency	Equivalent dose (mg)	Half-life
Cortone®	Cortisone	0.8	2	25	Short
Cortef®, Hydrocortone®, Solu-Cortef®	Hydrocortisone	1	2	20	Short
Deltasone®, Liquid Pred®	Prednisone	4	1	5	Medium
Prelone®, Pediapred®, Delta-Cortef®	Prednisolone	4	1	5	Medium
Medrol®, Solu-Medrol®, Depo-Medrol®, A-Methapred®	Methylprednisolone	5	0	4	Medium
Aristocort®, Kenacort®, Kenalog®	Triamcinolone	5	0	4	Medium
Decadron®, Dexameth®, Dexone®, Hexadrol®	Dexamethasone	30	0	0.75	Long
Celestone®	Betamethasone	25	0	0.75	Long
Florinef®	Fludrocortisone	15	150	2	Medium

Patient counseling
- May cause stomach upset, so take with food
- It is preferable to take dose prior to 9 AM
- Wear or carry identification if on chronic steroid therapy
- May mask signs of infection
- May increase insulin or oral hypoglycemic requirements if diabetic
- Notify physician if weight gain, muscle weakness, sore throat, or infection occurs
- Report tiredness, stomach pain, weakness, and high or low blood sugar to your physician
- Do not discontinue abruptly if taking long-term

Adverse effects
- Cardiac: hypertension, sodium and fluid retention, atherosclerosis
- CNS: insomnia, anxiety, depression, psychosis
- Metabolic: obesity, hyperglycemia, hypokalemia, amenorrhea, impotence
- Ophthalmic: cataracts, glaucoma
- Immune: Infections, impaired wound healing, leukocytosis
- Musculoskeletal: myopathy, osteoporosis

Drug interactions
- Rifampin and other enzyme-inducing drugs increases metabolism of corticosteroids and decreases their effectiveness
- Concomitant use of NSAIDs and corticosteroids increases risk of peptic ulcer disease
- Immunologic response to vaccines may be impaired by corticosteroids
- Estrogens may increase corticosteroid clearance
- Ketoconazole, macrolides, and other CYP-P450 3A4 enzyme-inhibiting drugs may decrease clearance of corticosteroids
- Corticosteroids increase insulin and oral hypoglycemic drug requirements

Monitoring parameters
- Weight gain, edema, increased blood pressure, electrolytes, blood glucose, infection

Pharmacokinetics
- Many dosage forms, doses, and schedules are used, including tablets, topicals, enemas, oral liquids, injections, and depot injection forms for intra-articular or intramuscular use

3. Miscellaneous Endocrine Drugs

ACTH and Cosyntropin (Table 5)

Therapeutic uses
- For diagnosis of adrenal insufficiency and occasionally as an alternative to corticosteroids

Mechanism of action
- ACTH stimulates the adrenal cortex to secrete adrenal hormones
- If ACTH fails to elicit an appropriate cortisol response, adrenal insufficiency is present
- Cosyntropin is a synthetic peptide which is similar to human ACTH, but less allergenic

Patient counseling
- Same as for corticosteroids

Adverse effects
- Same as for corticosteroids

Drug interactions
- Enzyme-inducing drugs will decrease effects

Monitoring parameters
- Same as for corticosteroids

Vasopressin and Desmopressin (Table 6)

Therapeutic uses
- Vasopressin: diabetes insipidus, variceal hemorrhage, shock, ventricular fibrillation
- Desmopressin: nocturnal enuresis, diabetes insipidus, hemophilia A, von Willebrand's disease

Mechanism of action
- Vasopressin is also known as antidiuretic hormone (ADH); it increases water resorption
- Vasopressin causes vasoconstriction in portal and splanchnic vessels (GI tract)
- Desmopressin is a synthetic derivative of vasopressin with ADH activity and only minimal vasoconstrictive properties; increases clotting factor VII levels

Patient counseling
- Intranasal desmopressin: Bottle should be discarded after 25 or 50 doses; don't transfer solution to another bottle; may cause nasal irritation; notify physician if bleeding is not controlled or if headache, shortness of breath or severe abdominal cramps occur; instruct on proper intranasal use

Table 5

ACTH and Cosyntropin

Trade name	Generic name	Dosage forms	Usual dosage range
Cortrosyn®	Cosyntropin	Injection: 0.25 mg	0.25-0.75 mg for testing
Acthar® (ACTH)	Corticotropin	Injection: 25, 40 units	10-25 units for testing
H.P. Acthar Gel®		Repository injection: 40, 80 units/mL	40-80 units of repository injection every 1-3 days

Adverse effects
- Vasopressin: angina, MI, vasoconstriction, hyponatremia, gangrene, abdominal cramps, tissue necrosis if extravasation occurs, hypersensitivity
- Desmopressin: Abdominal pain, headache, flushing, nausea, nasal irritation, vulvar pain, nosebleed, rhinitis, hypersensitivity

Drug interactions
- May enhance effects of other pressors
- Carbamazepine and chlorpropamide potentiate effect of desmopressin on ADH

Monitoring parameters
- Diabetes insipidus: urine volume, plasma osmolality
- von Willebrand's disease: factor VIII levels, bleeding time
- When intravenous vasopressin is used, monitor blood pressure and pulses

Androgens and Anabolic Steroids (Table 7)

Therapeutic uses
- Hypogonadism, delayed puberty, metastatic breast cancer, anemia

- C-III controlled substances since they are intentionally misused for performance enhancing effects and enhanced muscular development and endurance

Mechanism of action
- Androgens promote growth and development of male sex organs and maintenance of secondary sex characteristics
- Androgens also cause retention of nitrogen, sodium, potassium, and phosphorus; increase protein anabolism and decrease protein catabolism
- Androgens are responsible for growth spurt of adolescence and termination of linear growth by fusion of epiphyseal growth centers
- Exogenous androgens stimulate production of red blood cells and suppress endogenous testosterone release through feedback inhibition of LH and spermatogenesis through feedback inhibition of FSH

Patient counseling
- May cause stomach upset, notify physician if swelling of ankles or persistent erections of the penis occur
- Controlled substance; do not misuse or abuse this product

Table 6

Vasopressin and Desmopressin

Trade Name	Generic name	Dosage forms	Usual dosage range
Pitressin®	Vasopressin	Injection: 20 units/mL	10-20 units IM, SC or IV daily at 3- to 4-hour intervals or as continuous infusion
Stimate® (DDAVP)	Desmopressin	Tablets: 0.1, 0.2 mg Nasal solution: 0.1 mg/mL, 1.5 mg/mL Injection: 4 µg/mL	Nocturnal enuresis: 20 -40 µg intranasally qhs Diabetes insipidus: 0.1-0.2 mg PO bid, 0.1-0.4 mL intranasally in single or divided doses

Table 7

Androgens and Anabolic Steroids

Trade name	Generic name	Dosage forms	Usual dosage range
Testoderm® Androderm®	Testosterone transdermal system	Patch: 2.5, 4, 5, 6 mg/24 h	Patch: 2.5-6 mg for 24 h
AndroGel® 1% Testim®	Testosterone	1% Gel	5 grams applied once daily
Depo-Testosterone®	Testosterone cypionate (in oil)	Injection in oil: 100 mg/mL & 200 mg/mL	50-400 mg every 2-4 weeks
Android® Testred®	Methyltestosterone	Tablets: 10, 25 mg Capsules: 10 mg	10-50 mg once daily
Halotestin®	Fluoxymesterone	Tablets: 2, 5, 10 mg	5-10 mg once daily
Anadrol-50®	Oxymetholone	Tablets: 50 mg	50-100 mg once daily
Winstrol®	Stanozolol	Tablets: 2 mg	2 mg qd-tid
Oxandrin®	Oxandrolone	Tablets: 2.5, 10 mg	2.5-10 mg qd
Deca-Durabolin®	Nandrolone decanoate	Injection: 100, 200 mg/mL (in oil)	100-200 mg once weekly

- For females, notify physician if deepening of the voice, increased facial hair, or menstrual irregularities occur

Adverse effects
- General: jaundice, hepatitis, edema, abuse potential in an effort to enhance athletic performance, hypercholesterolemia and atherosclerosis, increased aggression and libido
- Women: hirsutism, voice deepening, acne, decreased menses, clitoral enlargement
- Men: acne, sleep apnea, gynecomastia, azoospermia, prostate enlargement, decreased testicular size

4. Key Points

- Levothyroxine is the drug of choice for hypothyroidism
- Lower doses of levothyroxine are used in the elderly and cardiac patients
- Overtreatment with thyroid hormones causes osteoporosis and atrial fibrillation
- Antacids, bile acid sequestrants, sucralfate, calcium, and iron supplements decrease absorption of levothyroxine and must be separated by at least 4 hours
- Propylthiouracil (PTU) and methimazole (Tapazole) are thionamide derivatives that are used to treat hyperthyroidism
- Thionamides may cause life-threatening agranulocytosis or hepatitis, so patients must report to their physician if they experience fever, sore throat, abdominal pain, or jaundice
- Drugs used to treat Cushing's disease inhibit synthesis of cortisol
- Corticosteroid should be used at the lowest dose for the shortest time in order to reduce the risk of HPA axis suppression and adrenal insufficiency

- Patients with adrenal insufficiency must receive supplemental corticosteroids in times of physiologic stress
- Vasopressin and desmopressin are antidiuretic hormones
- Androgens and anabolic steroids are abused by athletes seeking to enhance performance

5. Questions and Answers

Use Patient Profile #1 to answer Questions 1 and 2.

1. The Synthroid prescription dispensed to Mrs. Ricardo on 3/21 requires advising her to:

   A. take 4 hours before or 4 hours after Questran
   B. take with food
   C. watch for signs of infection
   D. take as needed to keep desired level of energy
   E. discontinue if you experience nausea

2. Which of the following of Mrs. Ricardo's conditions could the Synthroid exacerbate?

   A. hypercholesterolemia
   B. anemia
   C. coronary artery disease
   D. hypertension
   E. constipation

Patient Profile #1—Corn State Community Pharmacy

Patient Name	Jasmine Ricardo				
Address	189 Jonesbourough Road				
Age	78		Height	48 in	
Sex	Female	Race Hispanic	Weight	103 lbs	
Allergies	Cats				

DIAGNOSIS	Primary	1.	Hypercholesterolemia
		2.	Anemia
		3.	Coronary artery disease
	Secondary	1.	Hypertension
		2.	

MEDICATION RECORD

Date	Rx #	Physician	Drug/Strength	Quantity	Sig	Refills
3/21	89995	Stubie	Synthroid 0.025 mg	30	1 PO qd	0
2/23	88768	Hooper	Zocor 40 mg	30	1 PO qhs	5
2/23	88769	Hooper	Questran 4 g	60	1 packet bid mix with juice	5
2/23	88770	Hooper	Tenormin 50 mg	30	1 PO qd	5
2/23	88771	Hooper	Enalapril 5 mg	60	1 PO bid	5

PHARMACIST NOTES

Date	Note
2/23	Patient reminded to continue taking aspirin 325 mg for CAD
2/23	Patient to take OTC ferrous sulfate 325 mg daily for 3 months for anemia, advised patient to begin docusate 100 mg QD if constipation occurs

3. Excessive doses of levothyroxine may cause

   A. weight gain
   B. osteoporosis
   C. cold intolerance
   D. bradycardia
   E. sedation

4. Which of the following drugs may produce hypothyroidism?

   1. amitriptyline
   2. lithium
   3. amiodarone
   A. 1 only
   B. 3 only
   C. 1 and 2 only
   D. 2 and 3 only
   E. 1, 2 and 3

5. All of the following may decrease the effect of thyroid hormone supplementation EXCEPT:

   A. antacids
   B. bile acid sequestrants
   C. estrogens
   D. sucralfate
   E. theophylline

6. A patient who is suffering from heat intolerance, weight loss, tachycardia, tremor, and anxiety may be treated with

   A. acetaminophen
   B. mitotane
   C. cyproheptadine
   D. propylthiouracil
   E. diazepam

7. The patient with atrial fibrillation may require a decreased Coumadin dosage when the following drug is initiated

   A. liothyronine
   B. rifampin
   C. methimazole
   D. phenytoin
   E. diphenhydramine

8. Which of the following drugs is used to treat Cushing's disease?

   I.   ketoconazole
   II. aminoglutethimide
   III. mitotane

A. I only
B. III only
C. I and II only
D. II and III only
E. I, II, and III

9. Which of the following drugs works by decreasing cortisol synthesis?

   A. Cortrosyn
   B. ACTH
   C. oxandrolone
   D. prednisone
   E. metyrapone

10. Decreased ketoconazole absorption may occur if it is administered concomitantly with

   A. antacids
   B. food
   C. warfarin
   D. cyclosporine
   E. CYP-P450 3A4 inhibitors

11. Close monitoring of adrenal hormone secretion may be required when administering

   A. methyltestosterone
   B. mitotane
   C. desmopressin
   D. iodides
   E. propylthiouracil

12. Which of the following is used to treat adrenal crisis?
   A. cosyntropin
   B. aminoglutethimide
   C. fluoxymesterone
   D. vasopressin
   E. hydrocortisone

13. Which of the following is NOT an effect of glucocorticoids?

   A. immunosuppression
   B. decreased prostaglandin synthesis
   C. inhibit glycogenolysis
   D. decreased neutrophils at site of infection
   E. inhibition of macrophages

Use Patient Profile #2 to answer Questions 14 and 15.

14. Which of the following is LEAST likely to contribute to the increased blood glucose seen in this patient?

Patient Profile #2—Big Sky Hospital

Patient Name	Stuart Big		Date of Admission 4/21 @ 1526
Address	440 Mountain Lane		
Age	28	Height	5' 8"
Sex	Male	Race	White
Allergies	Aspirin	Weight	178 lbs

DIAGNOSIS

Admit Diagnosis	1.	anaphylactic reaction to aspirin	
	2.		
Secondary	1.	Type 2 diabetes mellitus	
	2.	Hypertension	

LABORATORY

Date	Time	Lab	Result	(Normal Range)
4/23	1232	Glucose	443	(60-110 mg/dL)
4/23	0620	Glucose	391	(60-110 mg/dL)
4/22	1915	Glucose	352	(60-110 mg/dL)
4/22	1221	Glucose	289	(60-110 mg/dL)
4/22	0600	Glucose	240	(60-110 mg/dL)
4/21	1920	Glucose	181	(60-110 mg/dL)
4/21	1529	Glucose	144	(60-110 mg/dL)

ACTIVE MEDICATION ORDERS

Date	Time	Name & Strength	Route	Frequency/Schedule
4/21	1530	Solu-Medrol 125 mg	IV	q6h
4/21	1530	Dextrose 5%/NaCl 0.9%	IV	200 mL/h
4/21	1530	Diphenhydramine 50 mg	IV	q6h
4/21	1703	Glipizide 5 mg	PO	bid
4/21	1703	Glucophage 850 mg	PO	bid
4/21	1703	Captopril 50 mg	PO	tid

DISCONTINUED MEDICATION ORDERS

Date	Time	Name & Strength	Route	Frequency/Schedule
4/21	1530	Epinephrine 0.1 mg	SQ	Stat
4/21	1530	Diphenhydramine 50 mg	IV	Stat

DIETARY

Date	
4/21	1800 Kcal American Diabetes Association Diet

A. dextrose 5%/NaCl 0.9% solution
B. captopril
C. epinephrine
D. methylprednisolone
E. anaphylaxis

15. The patient in Profile #2 is discharged on a new prescription for Deltasone 40 mg qd for 7 days. He should be instructed to

A. check feet closely for wounds
B. take ibuprofen for musculoskeletal pain
C. take on an empty stomach
D. take at bedtime
E. wear identification for steroid therapy

16. Chronic administration of glucocorticoids predisposes patients to

A. arthritis
B. obesity
C. Alzheimer's disease
D. osteoporosis
E. hepatitis

17. A patient is taking prednisone 40 mg daily for 6 months. Upon abrupt cessation, the following may occur:

A. myopathy

B. diabetes
C. infection
D. adrenal crisis
E. psychosis

18. An increased risk of peptic ulcer disease occurs when NSAIDs are combined with

A. ranitidine
B. ferrous sulfate
C. dexamethasone
D. carbamazepine
E. acetaminophen

19. Which of the following drugs may be used to diagnose adrenal insufficiency?

A. desmopressin
B. clemestine
C. captopril
D. cosyntropin
E. aminoglutethimide

20. Decreased urine production is an effect of

A. BCNU
B. PTU
C. ACTH
D. DDAVP
E. SSKI

21. Which of the following hormones is secreted by the pituitary gland?

    A. adrenocorticotropic hormone
    B. testosterone
    C. cortisol
    D. thyroxine
    E. corticotropin-releasing hormone

22. Chronic administration of Winstrol may produce all of the following complications EXCEPT:

    A. prostate enlargement
    B. increased testicular size
    C. gynecomastia in men
    D. accelerated atherosclerosis
    E. decreased menses in women

23. Androderm is administered

    A. once daily
    B. three times per week
    C. once weekly
    D. every 2 weeks
    E. monthly

24. Which of the following is NOT an acceptable indication for testosterone?

    A. anemia
    B. hypogonadism
    C. delayed puberty
    D. body building
    E. metastatic breast cancer

Answers

1. **A.** Bile acid sequestrants reduce levothyroxine absorption and must be separated from levothyroxine administration by at least 4 hours. Levothyroxine should be administered before a meal on an empty stomach in order to maximize absorption.

2. **C.** Thyroid hormones enhance oxygen consumption and increase the oxygen demand. Mrs. Ricardo has a past medical history of coronary artery disease (CAD), and is elderly. Thyroid supplementation would actually lower her cholesterol in the long run, but may precipitate angina acutely.

3. **B.** Levothyroxine decreases bone mineral density and when given in supratherapeutic doses may cause osteoporosis. For this reason,

the lowest possible replacement dose should be administered.

4. **D.** Lithium and amiodarone have both been associated with hypothyroidism. Amiodarone contains iodine, and may cause hypo- or hyperthyroidism.

5. **E.** Numerous drugs are known to decrease thyroid hormone absorption, including antacids that contain divalent and trivalent cations, calcium salts, magnesium, sucralfate, and bile-acid sequestrants. Estrogens and enzyme-inducing drugs may decrease circulating thyroid hormone levels and necessitate a dose increase of thyroxine.

6. **D.** Heat intolerance, weight loss, tachycardia, tremor and anxiety are cardinal features of hyperthyroidism. Propylthiouracil is effective at reducing the excessive thyroxine level.

7. **A.** Liothyronine (Cytomel) is T_3, a potent thyroid hormone. In states of hypothyroidism, metabolism is decreased. However, if thyroid hormone is supplemented, blood clotting factors will be metabolized more quickly, leading to decreased warfarin requirements.

8. **E.** Ketoconazole, aminoglutethimide, and mitotane are all used to treat Cushing's disease. Ketoconazole is most commonly known as an antifungal agent, but it inhibits cortisol synthesis at high doses (800-1200 mg daily).

9. **E.** Metyrapone (Metopirone) inhibits 11-hydroxylase activity, and thus decreases cortisol synthesis.

10. **A.** Ketoconazole requires the presence of stomach acid in order to be absorbed. Any drug that decreases gastric acidity will decrease the extent of ketoconazole absorption. Food increases ketoconazole absorption since food stimulates release of gastric acid.

11. **B.** Mitotane is cytotoxic to adrenal cells and thus reduces cortisol synthesis and release. ACTH increases cortisol release. Close monitoring of cortisol levels is important when this drug is used.

12. **E.** Hydrocortisone is the drug of choice for adrenal crisis since it possesses both mineralocorticoid and glucocorticoid properties. Although cosyntropin increases cortisol release,

patients with adrenal crisis may not have enough adrenal reserve to meet their increased demand.

13. **C.** Glucocorticoids have potent effects on glucose and carbohydrate metabolism. They promote glycogen breakdown, rather than inhibit it.

14. **B.** Captopril increases insulin sensitivity and would not be expected to contribute to increased blood glucose. This patient's blood glucose began rising shortly after admission. Her IV fluids contain glucose, epinephrine increases blood glucose by increasing glycogen breakdown, methylprednisolone (Solu-Medrol) promotes glycogenolysis, and anaphylaxis would be expected to increase stress response leading to increased epinephrine release and increased blood glucose.

15. **A.** The patient has a history of diabetes and will be given prednisone, which would be expected to increase blood glucose. When diabetes is poorly controlled, infections are more likely to occur. For this reason, he should monitor more closely for wounds that may become infected. He will not be taking prednisone long enough to develop adrenal insufficiency, so there is no need for him to wear identification for steroid therapy.

16. **D.** Glucocorticoids have catabolic effects on a number of tissues, including muscle, fat, skin, and bone. Chronic administration leads to osteopenia and osteoporosis.

17. **D.** Chronic administration of glucocorticoids such as prednisone (Deltasone) will lead to feedback inhibition of pituitary ACTH release, and atrophy of the adrenal cortex. When prednisone is abruptly stopped, the adrenals will not be able to meet the body's demand for cortisol during severe stress and adrenal crisis may occur.

18. **C.** Corticosteroids such as dexamethasone (Decadron) are known to increase the risk of peptic ulcers when used in combination with NSAIDs.

19. **D.** Cosyntropin (Cortrosyn) is a synthetic analog of ACTH that is used to diagnose adrenal insufficiency. It works by stimulating the adrenal cortex to secrete cortisol. If cosyntropin administration does not result in an appropriate increase in cortisol release, adrenal insufficiency is present.

20. **D.** Desmopressin (DDAVP) is a synthetic analog of vasopressin, or antidiuretic hormone. Thus it decreases urine production by increasing water resorption.

21. **A.** Adrenocorticotropic hormone, or ACTH, is released by the pituitary and acts on the adrenal glands to increase cortisol release. Corticotropin-releasing hormone is released by the hypothalamus and acts on the pituitary to stimulate ACTH release.

22. **B.** Stanozolol (Winstrol) is an androgen that would be expected to promote growth and development of male sex organs. However, chronic administration leads to feedback inhibition of testosterone secretion which leads to testicular atrophy.

23. **A.** Testosterone transdermal systems (Androderm, Testoderm) are both applied once a day and remain in place for 24 hours. Longer acting androgens are available, such as nandrolone decanoate (Deca-Durabolin), for once-weekly administration.

24. **D.** Anabolic steroids may be abused by those who are seeking enhanced muscular development and endurance, such as athletes. For this reason, all of these agents are subject to the Controlled Substances Act (C-III).

6. References

American Association of Clinical Endocrinologists Medical Guidelines for Clinical Practice for the evaluation and treatment of hyperthyroidism and hypothyroidism (AACE Thyroid Task Force). *Endocr Pract.* 2002;8:457-469.

Chrousos GP, Margioris AN. Adrenocorticosteroids & adrenocortical antagonists. In: Katzung BG, ed. *Basic & Clinical Pharmacology*, 8th ed. Stamford, CT: Appleton & Lange; 2000:660-678.

Chrousos GP, Zoumakis EN, Gravanis A. The gonadal hormones & inhibitors. In: Katzung BG, ed. *Basic & Clinical Pharmacology*, 8th ed. Stamford, CT: Appleton & Lange; 2000:679-710.

Dayan CM, Daniels GH. Chronic autoimmune thyroiditis. *N Engl J Med.* 1996;335:99-106.

Dong, BJ, Hauck WW, Gambertoglio JG, et al. Bioequivalence of generic and brand name levothyroxine products in the treatment of hypothyroidism. *JAMA.* 1997;277:1205-1213.

Dong BJ. Thyroid disorders. In: Herfindal ET, Gourley DR, eds. *Textbook of Therapeutics: Drug and Disease Management*. Baltimore, MD: Lippincott Williams & Wilkins; 2000:325-358.

Fitzgerald PA. Hypothalamic & pituitary hormones. In: Katzung BG, ed. *Basic & Clinical Pharmacology*, 8th ed. Stamford, CT: Appleton & Lange; 2000:625-643.

Greenspan FG, Dong BJ. Thyroid & antithyroid drugs. In: Katzung BG, ed. *Basic & Clinical Pharmacology*, 8th ed. Stamford, Ct: Appleton & Lange; 2000:644-659.

Hoffmeister AM, Tietze KJ. Adrenocortical dysfunction and clinical use of steroids. In: Herfindal ET, Gourley DR, eds. *Textbook of Therapeutics: Drug and Disease Management*. Baltimore, MD: Lippincott Williams & Wilkins; 2000:305-324.

McEvoy GK, ed. AHFS Drug Information 2003. Bethesda, MD: American Society of Health-System Pharmacists, Inc.; 2003.

15. Women's Health

Samantha Eichner, PharmD
Assistant Professor, Department of Pharmacy
University of Tennessee College of Pharmacy

Contents

1. Postmenopausal Hormone Replacement Therapy

- Menopause is permanent cessation of menses resulting from diminishing ovarian follicular function.
    * Defined as 12 consecutive months of amenorrhea
    * Median age of onset in U.S. is 51 years of age
    * Physiologic changes and symptoms of menopause may present up to 4 years prior to the menopause

- Perimenopause, also called the climacteric, is the time just before the menopause and the first year following menopause. Ovarian function and production of estrogen decline during this time.

Clinical Presentation

- Cessation of menses for at least 12 consecutive months

- Symptoms of perimenopause related to declining estrogen:
    * Anovulation
    * Dysfunctional uterine bleeding
    * Extended menstrual cycle intervals
    * Oligomenorrhea

- Symptoms of menopause directly related to lack of estrogen:
    * Vaginal dryness, vulvar or vaginal atrophy
    * Hot flashes
    * Night sweats

- Symptoms associated with menopause, but without a proven link to estrogen deficiency:
    * Arthralgia
    * Depression
    * Insomnia
    * Migraines
    * Mood swings
    * Myalgia
    * Urinary frequency

Pathophysiology

- Loss of ovarian follicular activity results in endocrine, biologic, and clinical changes.

- Ovarian production of estradiol and progesterone diminishes.

- FSH and LH concentrations increase.

- Primary estrogen available is now estrone (which is converted peripherally from androstenedione and is less potent), not estradiol.

Treatment Principles

- Women with an intact uterus must be treated with estrogen plus progestin to reduce the risk of endometrial hyperplasia and endometrial cancer.

- Women who have had a hysterectomy are treated with unopposed estrogen.

- Hormone replacement therapy should be initiated on an individual basis with careful consideration of the risks and benefits.

- Contraindications to use:
    * Abnormal, undiagnosed genital bleeding
    * Breast cancer
    * Deep vein thrombosis or pulmonary embolism
    * Estrogen-dependent neoplasia
    * Pregnancy
    * Stroke or myocardial infarction in the last year
    * Thromboembolic disorder
    * Thrombophlebitis

Drug Therapy (Table 1)

Estrogen and progestin
Mechanism of action
Estrogen
- Acts as a replacement for diminished estrogen levels and restores estrogenic activity

Progestin
- Acts as a replacement for diminished progesterone

- Protects the uterus by:
    * Decreasing nuclear estradiol receptor concentrations
    * Suppressing DNA synthesis
    * Decreasing estrogen bioavailability

Patient instructions and counseling
- Side effects due to estrogen may be diminished by starting with a low dose and may be alleviated by changing products. Fewer side effects are associated with the transdermal preparation.

- Side effects due to progestin may be alleviated or diminished by changing products or changing from a continuous to cyclic regimen.

- Immediately report any unusual vaginal bleeding.

Table 1

Hormone Replacement Therapy Products

Medication	Available strengths and dosing
Oral formulations	
Conjugated equine estrogens (CEE) (Premarin®)	0.625, 0.9, 1.25, 2.5 mg qd
Micronized estradiol (Estradiol®, Estrace®, Gynodiol®)	0.5, 1, 1.5, 2 mg qd
Estrone sulfate (Estropipate®, Ortho-Est®, Ogen®)	0.625, 1.25, 2.5, 5 mg qd
Esterified estrogens (Estratab®, Menest®)	0.3, 0.625, 1.25, 2.5 mg qd
17-β-Estradiol	2 mg qd
Synthetic conjugated estrogen	0.3, 0.625, 0.9, 1.25 mg qd
Estradiol transdermal formulations	
Estradiol transdermal system (Estraderm®)	0.05, 0.1 mg/24 h
Alora®, Climara®	0.025, 0.5, 0.075, 0.1 mg/24 h
Esclim®, Vivelle®, Vivelle-Dot®	0.025, 0.0375, 0.5, 0.075, 0.1 mg/24 h
	Apply to skin once weekly (Climara) or twice weekly
Injectable formulations	
Estradiol valerate in oil (Delestrogen®)	10, 20, 40 mg/mL in 5 mL multidose vials; dose: 10-20 mg q 4 weeks
Estradiol cypionate in oil	5 mg/mL in 5-mL vials; dose: 1-5 mg q 3-4 weeks
Vaginal estrogen formulations	
Estrace® vaginal cream	0.1 mg estradiol/g; dose: 2-4 g qd for 1-2 weeks; maintenance dose: 1 g 1-3 times/week
Ogen® vaginal cream	1.5 mg estropipate/g; dose: 2-4 g qd
Premarin® vaginal cream	0.625 mg conjugated estrogen/g; dose: 0.5-2 g qd for 3 weeks, then 1 week off
Estring® vaginal ring	2 mg estradiol ring releases 7.5 µg/24 h; ring remains in vagina for 3 months
Vagifem® vaginal tablet	25 µg estradiol/tablet; dose: 1 tablet once daily for 2 weeks; maintenance dose: 1 tablet twice/week
Combination estrogen-progestin products	
Activella®	1 mg estradiol, 0.5 mg norethindrone acetate
femhrt®	5 µg ethinyl estradiol, 1 mg norethindrone acetate
Prempro®	0.625 mg conjugated estrogen, 2.5 or 5 mg medroxyprogesterone
Premphase®	0.625 mg conjugated estrogen; 0.625 mg conjugated estrogen, 5 mg medroxyprogesterone (2 weeks of estrogen alone, 2 weeks of combination)
Combipatch® (transdermal patch)	0.05 mg estradiol, 0.14 or 0.25 mg norethindrone acetate
Combination estrogen-androgen products	
Estratest H.S.®, Syntest H.S.®	0.625 mg esterified estrogens, 1.25 mg methyltestosterone
Estratest®, Syntest D.S.®	0.625 mg esterified estrogens, 2.5 mg methyltestosterone

Adapted from Burnham et al, 2003 and Kalantaridou et al, 2002.

- Contact your physician promptly if any of the following events occur:
    * Abdominal tenderness, pain, or swelling
    * Coughing up blood
    * Disturbances of vision or speech
    * Dizziness or fainting
    * Lumps in the breast
    * Numbness or weakness in an arm or leg
    * Severe vomiting or headache
    * Sharp chest pain or shortness of breath
    * Sharp pain in the calves

Adverse drug events
Estrogen
- Most common:
    * Breast tenderness
    * Heavy bleeding
    * Headache
    * Nausea

Progestin
- Most common:
    * Depression

* Headache
* Irritability

Drug-drug and drug-disease interactions

* Estrogen may exacerbate illness in the following disease states:
  * Depression
  * Diabetes (glucose intolerance has been observed with estrogen)
  * Hypertriglyceridemia
  * Hepatic adenoma
  * Thyroid disorder (patients may require an increased dose of thyroid supplement)
  * Impaired hepatic function (poor metabolism of estrogens)
  * Cardiovascular disorders (coronary heart disease and venous thromboembolism risk may be increased with estrogens)

* Interaction may result in decreased pharmacologic effect of estrogens:
  * CYP 3A4 inducers: barbiturates, carbamazepine, rifampin, St. John's wort
  * Hydantoins
  * Topiramate

* Interaction with estrogen may result in decreased pharmacologic effect of interacting drug:
  * Hydantoins
  * Thyroid hormones
  * Oral anticoagulants

* Interaction with estrogen may result in increased pharmacologic effect of interacting drug:
  * Corticosteroids
  * Tricyclic antidepressants (interaction may alter the effects and may increase toxicity of antidepressant)

* Interaction may result in increased pharmacologic effect of estrogens:
  * CYP 3A4 inhibitors: itraconazole, ketoconazole, macrolide antibiotics, ritonavir
  * Food interaction: grapefruit juice

* Drug-drug interactions with progestins:
  * Concomitant administration with aminoglutethimide may increase the metabolism of medroxyprogesterone
  * Concomitant administration with rifampin may increase the metabolism of norethindrone

Parameters to monitor

* Laboratory monitoring not recommended

Androgens (testosterone)

Mechanism of action

* Androgens are the precursor hormones to estrogen production by the ovaries and peripheral sites. Ovarian testosterone production declines with menopause.

* Act at androgen receptor sites or exhibit action following conversion to estrogen

* Replaces androgen to improve deficiency-related symptoms (ie, decreased sexual desire, decreased energy, diminished well-being)

Patient instructions and counseling

* Testosterone therapy should only be administered to postmenopausal women who are receiving concurrent estrogen therapy.

* Relative contraindications to testosterone therapy
  * Androgenic alopecia
  * Clinical hirsutism
  * Moderate to severe acne

Adverse drug events

* Fluid retention

* Possible undesirable changes in lipid profile

* Virilization (lower HDL)

Parameters to monitor

* Laboratory monitoring not recommended

Nondrug Therapy

Phytoestrogens

* Plant compounds (isoflavones, lignans, coumestans)

* Food sources of phytoestrogens: soybeans, flaxseed, alfalfa sprouts

* Some studies have shown improvement in vaginal symptoms

* No evidence supporting improvement in other symptoms of menopause (ie, hot flashes, depression, anxiety, headache, myalgia)

* May have beneficial effects on lipids

2. Birth Control: Contraceptive Options

- Contraception is the prevention of pregnancy by one of two methods:
  * Preventing implantation of the fertilized ovum in the endometrium
  * Inhibiting contact of sperm with mature ovum

Prescription Contraceptive Options

Oral contraceptives
- Estrogen plus progestin (combined oral contraceptives [COC])

- Progestin-only (minipill)
  * Appropriate for use in breastfeeding women
  * Efficacy is less than COCs
  * Free of cardiovascular risks associated with estrogen-containing products

- Long-term injectables or implantation products
  * Progestin only

- Estrogens and progestins used in prescription contraceptives (Table 2)
  * Estrogens
    • Ethinyl estradiol
    • Mestranol
  * Progestins
    • Desogestrel
    • Norgestrel; levonorgestrel
    • Ethynodiol diacetate
    • Norethindrone, norethindrone acetate, norethynodrel

Drug Therapy

Mechanism of action
Estrogens
- Prevent development of a dominant follicle by suppression of follicle-stimulating hormone (FSH). Does not block ovulation

Progestin
- Blocks ovulation. Contributes to production of thick and impermeable cervical mucus. Contributes to involution and atrophy of the endometrium

Patient instructions and counseling
- Efficacy is high but dependent on proper scheduled use
- Oral contraceptives do not prevent the transmission of sexually transmitted diseases.

- Warning signs of important complications:
  * Severe abdominal pain
  * Severe chest pain, shortness of breath, coughing up blood
  * Severe headache
  * Eye problems (ie, blurred vision, flashing lights, or blindness)
  * Severe leg pain in the calf or thigh

- Expect changes in characteristics of menstrual cycle

- Use of a back-up contraceptive method is advised if more than one dose is missed per cycle.

Adverse drug events
- The World Health Organization suggests refraining from prescribing combined oral contraceptives to women with certain diagnoses (Table 3).

- Most common:
  * Nausea and vomiting (usually resolves within 3 months)
  * Breakthrough bleeding, spotting, amenorrhea, altered menstrual flow
  * Melasma
  * Headache, migraine
  * Weight change, edema

- Serious and less common:
  * Venous thrombosis, pulmonary embolism, MI, coronary thrombosis, arterial thromboembolism, cerebral thrombosis

- Potential hormonal effects associated with an imbalance in estrogen and progestin (Table 4)

Drug-drug and drug-disease interactions
- Interaction may result in decreased pharmacologic effect of oral contraceptives:
  * Ampicillin, griseofulvin, sulfonamides, tetracycline
  * Anticonvulsants (barbiturates, carbamazepine, felbamate, phenytoin, topiramate)
  * Non-nucleoside reverse transcriptase inhibitors, protease inhibitors
  * Pioglitazone
  * Phenytoin
  * Protease inhibitors
  * Rifampin
  * Theophylline

- Interaction may result in increased plasma levels of oral contraceptives:
  * Atorvastatin
  * Vitamin C
  * CYP 3A4 inhibitors

Table 2

Prescription Contraceptive Products

Product	Estrogen (μg)	Progestin (mg)
Progestin-only oral contraceptives		
Ortho Micronor®, Errin®, Nor-QD®, Nora-BE®, Camila®	—	Norethindrone (0.35)
Ovrette®	—	Norgestrel (0.075)
Monophasic low-dose estrogen oral contraceptives		
Alesse®, Aviane®, Lessina®, Levlite®	Ethinyl estradiol (20)	Levonorgestrel (0.1)
Loestrin 21 1/20®, Loestrin Fe 1/20®, Microgestin Fe 1/20®	Ethinyl estradiol (20)	Norethindrone acetate (1)
Yasmin®	Ethinyl estradiol (30)	Drospirenone (3)
Levlen®, Levora®, Nordette®, Portia®	Ethinyl estradiol (30)	Levonorgestrel (0.15)
Cryselle®, Lo/Ovral®, Low-Ogestrel®	Ethinyl estradiol (30)	Norgestrel (0.3)
Apri®, Desogen®, Ortho-Cept®	Ethinyl estradiol (30)	Desogestrel (0.15)
Ovcon-35®	Ethinyl estradiol (35)	Norethindrone (0.4)
Brevicon®, Modicon®, Necon 0.5/35®, Nortrel 0.5/35®	Ethinyl estradiol (35)	Norethindrone (0.5)
Necon 1/35®, Norinyl 1+35®, Nortrel 1/35®, Ortho-Novum 1/35®	Ethinyl estradiol (35)	Norethindrone (1)
Kariva®	Ethinyl estradiol (20)/ Ethinyl estradiol (10)	Desogestrel (0.15)
Mircette®	Ethinyl estradiol (20)/ Ethinyl estradiol (10)	Desogestrel (0.15)
Monophasic high-dose estrogen oral contraceptives		
Ovral®, Ogestrel 0.5/50®	Ethinyl estradiol (50)	Norgestrel (0.5)
Demulen 1/50®, Zovia 1/50E®	Ethinyl estradiol (50)	Ethynodiol diacetate (1)
Ovcon-50®	Ethinyl estradiol (50)	Norethindrone (1)
Necon 1/50®, Norinyl 1+50®, Ortho-Novum 1/50®	Mestranol (50)	Norethindrone (1)
Biphasic oral contraceptives		
Ortho-Novum 10/11®, Necon 10/11®	Ethinyl estradiol (35)	Norethindrone (0.5 x 10 d); (1 x 11 d)
Triphasic oral contraceptives		
Enpresse®, Tri-Levlen®, Triphasil®, Trivora®	Ethinyl estradiol (30) x 6 d; (40) x 5 d; (30) x 10 d	Levonorgestrel (0.05) x 6 d; (0.075) x 5 d; (0.125) x 10 d
Tri-Norinyl®	Ethinyl estradiol (35) x 21 days	Norethindrone (0.5) x 7 d; (1) x 9 d; (0.5) x 5 d
Necon 7/7/7®, Ortho-Novum 7/7/7®	Ethinyl estradiol (35) x 21 days	Norethindrone (0.5) x 7 d; (0.75) x 9 d; (1) x 5 d
Cyclessa®	Ethinyl estradiol (25) x 21 days	Desogestrel (0.1) x 7 d; (0.125) x 7 d; (0.15) x 7 d
Ortho Tri-Cyclen Lo®	Ethinyl estradiol (25) x 21 days	Norgestimate (0.18) x 7 d; (0.215) x 7 d; (0.25) x 7 d
Ortho Tri-Cyclen®	Ethinyl estradiol (35) x 21 days	Norgestimate (0.18) x 7 d; (0.215) x 7 d; (0.25) x 7 d
Estrostep 21®, Estrostep Fe®	Ethinyl estradiol (20) x 5 d; (30) x 7 d; (35) x 9 d	Norethindrone (1) x 21 days
Transdermal contraceptive system		
Ortho Evra®	Ethinyl estradiol (20 released per 24 hours)	Norelgestromin (0.15 released per 24 h)
Vaginal ring contraceptive system		
NuvaRing®	Ethinyl estradiol (0.015 mg released per 24 hours)	Etonogestrel (0.12 released per 24 h)
Contraceptive implants		
Norplant® system	—	Levonorgestrel (set of 6 capsules, each containing 36 mg)
Contraceptive injection		
Depo-Provera®	—	Medroxyprogesterone (150 mg/mL injection)
Lunelle®	Estradiol cypionate 5 mg/mL	Medroxyprogesterone acetate 25 mg/mL
Intrauterine contraceptive systems		
Progestasert®	—	Progesterone (unit reservoir contains 38 mg)
Mirena®	—	Levonorgestrel (unit reservoir contains 52 mg)

Adapted from Burnham et al, 2003 and Dickerson et al, 2002.

Table 3

World Health Organization Contraindications for Combined Oral Contraceptive Use

- Breast cancer
- Current history of deep vein thrombosis or pulmonary embolism
- Current history of cerebrovascular accident or coronary artery or ischemic heart disease
- Diabetes with nephropathy, neuropathy, retinopathy, or other vascular disease
- Headaches
- Hypertension (≥160/100 mm Hg) or hypertension with vascular disease
- Lactation (<6 weeks postpartum)
- Liver disease
- Pregnancy
- Surgery with prolonged immobilization or any surgery on the legs
- Smoker (20 or more cigarettes a day) ≥35 years of age
- Structural heart disease complicated by pulmonary hypertension, atrial fibrillation, or history of acute bacterial endocarditis

Adapted from Dickerson et al, 2002 and Ruggiero et al, 2001.

- Interaction may result in decreased pharmacologic effect of interacting drug:
  - Anticoagulants
  - Benzodiazepine tranquilizers
  - β-Blockers
  - Hypoglycemics (tolbutamide, Diabinese®, Orinase®, Tolinase®)
  - Methyldopa
  - Phenytoin

- Interaction may result in increased pharmacologic effect of interacting drug:
  - Tricyclic antidepressants
  - Benzodiazepine tranquilizers
  - β-Blockers
  - Theophylline

- Interaction may result in increased toxicity of interacting drug:
  - Cortisone

Parameters to monitor
- Patients must monitor themselves for warning signs of serious complications as listed above.

- Laboratory monitoring is not recommended with use of oral contraceptives.

Table 4

Potential Hormonal Effects Associated with an Imbalance in Estrogen or Progestin

Estrogen excess	• Breast tenderness, fullness
	• Cervical mucorrhea
	• Edema
	• Hypertension
	• Melasma
	• Migraine
	• Nausea, bloating
Progestin excess	• Acne or oily scalp
	• Breast regression
	• Depression
	• Hypomenorrhea
	• Increased appetite
	• Monilial vaginitis
	• Tiredness, fatigue
	• Weight gain
Estrogen deficiency	• Breakthrough bleeding (early or mid-cycle)
	• Hypomenorrhea
	• Spotting
Progestin deficiency	• Amenorrhea
	• Breakthrough bleeding (late)
	• Hypermenorrhea

Adapted from Burnham et al, 2003.

Nondrug Therapy

- Condoms

- Diaphragms

- Intrauterine devices

- Spermicides

3. Osteoporosis

- Osteoporosis is characterized by low bone mineral density and deterioration of bone tissue, increasing fragility of bone and subsequent risk of fracture.

Types of Osteoporosis

- Postmenopausal (most common and the focus of this chapter)

- Age related

- Osteoporosis in men

- Drug-induced

Diagnostic Criteria

- T scores are used in the diagnosis and decision to treat osteoporosis.
  * The National Osteoporosis Foundation (NOF) and the American Association of Clinical Endocrinologists (AACE) recommend initiation of therapy in the following situations:
    - T score < –2 and no risk factors
    - T score < –1.5 with risk factors
  * The National Institutes of Health (NIH) recommends choice of when to initiate therapy on an individual basis.

- The World Health Organization (WHO) classification of bone mass based on T scores:
  * Osteopenia: T score –1 to –2.5 SD below the young adult mean
  * Osteoporosis: T score ≤ –2.5 SD below the young adult mean

- Risk factors for osteoporosis:
  * Advanced age
  * Amenorrhea
  * Anorexia
  * Cigarette smoking
  * Current low bone mass
  * Estrogen deficiency as a result of menopause
  * Ethnicity (Caucasian or Asian)
  * Excessive alcohol use
  * Family history of osteoporosis or history of fracture in a primary relative
  * Female gender
  * History of fracture over the age of 50
  * Inactive lifestyle
  * Long-term use of corticosteroids or anticonvulsants
  * Low lifetime calcium intake
  * Low testosterone levels in men
  * Thin or small frame

- Recommendations for the initial evaluation of patients for osteoporosis are as follows:
  * AACE and NOF: screen all women 65 years of age and older; postmenopausal women less than 65 years of age with family history or clinical risk factors; and women with a fracture history unrelated to trauma
  * NIH: decision to screen is individualized

Clinical Presentation

- Shortened stature

- Vertebra, hip, or forearm fracture

- Kyphosis

- Lordosis

- Bone pain

Pathophysiology

- Two types of bone: trabecular (ie, vertebrae, wrist and ankle, and ends of long bones, which are the most susceptible to fracture) and cortical

- Osteoblasts (formation) and osteoclasts (destruction) create a constant state of bone remodeling.

- Bone formation exceeds destruction during childhood

- Peak bone mass is reached around age 25-35, then bone density begins to decline
  * 3-4% decline per decade in men
  * 8-12% decline per decade in women 10 years after menopause

- Following menopause (postmenopausal osteoporosis), estrogen production declines and osteoclastic activity increases.

Treatment Principles

- Adequate calcium and vitamin D intake, through diet or supplementation is recommended for everyone (calcium 100-1500 mg daily plus 400-800 IU vitamin D daily) (Table 5).

- Lifestyle modifications are recommended: weight-

Table 5

Select Calcium Supplement Products

Product	Calcium (mg)
Calcium citrate	
(24% calcium content)	
Citracal®	Tablet: 200; liquitab: 500
Citracal® + vitamin D	316 plus 200 IU
Calcium carbonate	
(40% calcium content)	
Caltrate 600®	600
Titralac®	Chewable: 168, 300;
	liquid: 400/5 mL
Tums®	Chewable: 200, 300, 500
Viactiv Chews®	500
Mylanta® lozenges	240
Calcium carbonate + vitamin D	
Caltrate 600 + D®	600 plus 200 IU
Calcilyte® + vitamin D	500 plus 200 IU
Oscal® + vitamin D	500 plus 125 IU
Calcium phosphate tribasic	
(39% calcium content)	
Posture®	600
Posture-D®	600 plus 125 IU

Adapted from Dickerson et al, 2002 and Burnham et al, 2003.

bearing exercise, smoking cessation, limited alcohol intake

- Prescription drug therapy should be initiated on an individual basis, considering risk factors, bone mineral density, fracture history, and concomitant diseases and medications.

Drug Therapy

Calcium and vitamin D
Mechanism of action
  Calcium
- Necessary to improve bone mass; calcium is absorbed through the GI tract, stored in the skeleton, and made available when calcium levels become low.

  Vitamin D
- Facilitates absorption and regulation of calcium levels

Patient instructions and counseling
- Approximately 500 mg of calcium can be absorbed

from the GI tract at a time; separate doses appropriately to achieve dose of 1000-1500 mg per day.

- Calcium carbonate contains the highest level of elemental calcium; take with food to facilitate absorption.

- Calcium citrate products may be administered without regard to meals.

Adverse drug events
- Most common:
  * GI upset (nausea, vomiting, cramping, flatulence)
  * Headache
  * Hypophosphatemia, hypercalcemia

Drug-drug and drug-disease interactions
- Concomitant administration may decrease the bioavailability of fluoroquinolones or tetracyclines.

Parameters to monitor
- Laboratory monitoring is not recommended.

Bisphosphonates: alendronate (Fosamax), risedronate (Actonel) (Table 6)
Mechanism of action
- Binds to bone (hydroxyapatite) and incorporates into bone to increase and stabilize bone mass

Patient instructions and counseling
- Bisphosphonates must be taken with a full glass of water (8 ounces) 30 minutes prior to the first meal of the day.

- Remain in an upright position for at least 30 minutes following ingestion.

- Take medication on a regularly scheduled basis.

- Compliance may be increased by once-weekly dosing.

Adverse drug events
- Most common:
  * GI: abdominal pain, dyspepsia, constipation, diarrhea, flatulence, nausea, acid regurgitation, gastritis
  * CNS: headache

Drug-drug and drug-disease interactions
- Interaction may result in decreased pharmacologic effect of bisphosphonates:
  * Calcium supplements, antacids (separate administration by 1 hour)

- Interaction may result in increased pharmacologic effect of bisphosphonates:
  - * Ranitidine (IV ranitidine may double bioavailability of alendronate)

- Interaction may result in increased toxicity of interacting drug:
  - * Aspirin (alendronate >10 mg/d may increase risk of upper GI side effects of aspirin)

Parameters to monitor
- Laboratory monitoring is not recommended.

Estrogen replacement therapy
Mechanism of action
- Replaces the natural estrogen in postmenopausal women to restore protective skeletal benefits provided by the hormone (see Table 6).

Patient instructions and counseling
- Patient must discuss and weigh benefits and risks of

Table 6

Antiresorptive Agents

Medication	Dosing	FDA Indication
Bisphosphonates		
Alendronate (Fosamax®)	Prevention: 5 mg qd or 35 mg weekly; treatment: 10 mg qd or 70 mg weekly	Prevention and treatment of postmenopausal osteoporosis.
Risedronate (Actonel®)	Prevention: 5 mg qd; treatment: 5 mg qd or 30 mg weekly	Prevention and treatment of osteoporosis in men.
Estrogen replacement therapy		
Conjugated equine estrogens (CEE) (Premarin®)	0.625 mg qd	Prevention of osteoporosis
Ethinyl estradiol (Estinyl®)	0.02 mg qd	
Estropipate (Ortho-Est®, Ogen®)	0.625 mg qd	
Esterified estrogens (Estratab®, Menest®)	0.625 mg qd	
Micronized estradiol (Estrace®)	1 mg qd	
17-β-Estradiol	2 mg qd	
Estrone sulfate	1.5 mg qd	
Transdermal estradiol (Estraderm®, Alora®, Climara®, Esclim®, Vivelle/Vivelle-Dot®)	0.05 mg qd	
Combination estrogen/progestin products:		
Prempro® (conjugated estrogens/ medroxyprogesterone acetate)	0.45 mg/1.5 mg, 0.625/1.5 mg qd	
Premphase® (conjugated estrogens/ medroxyprogesterone acetate)	0.625 mg/5 mg qd	
femhrt 1/5® (norethindrone acetate/ ethinyl estradiol)	1 mg/ 5 µg qd	
Activella® (estradiol/norethindrone acetate)	1 mg/0.5 mg qd	
Selective estrogen receptor modulator		
Raloxifene (Evista®)	60 mg qd	Prevention and treatment of postmenopausal osteoporosis
Other agents		
Calcitonin (Miacalcin®)	Intranasal: 200 IU qd; IM or SC: 100 IU qd	Treatment of postmenopausal osteoporosis
Teriparatide (Forteo®)	Injection: 20 µg qd	Treatment of postmenopausal women with osteoporosis who are high risk for fractures or who have failed or are intolerant to other therapies; treatment of men with primary or hypogonadal osteoporosis who are at high risk for fractures

Adapted from Dickerson et al, 2002 and Burnham et al, 2003.

estrogen or combined hormone replacement therapy with her physician.

Contraindications to use of these medications
- History of thromboembolism

- History of breast or endometrial cancer

- Undiagnosed abnormal genital bleeding

- Pregnancy

Adverse drug events
- Most common:
  * Genitourinary: vaginal bleeding or spotting
  * Other: breast enlargement and tenderness, increased weight
  * Cardiovascular: increased triglycerides

Drug-drug and drug-disease Interactions
- Interaction may result in decreased serum concentrations of estrogen:
  * Rifampin

- Interaction may result in increased toxicity of interacting drug:
  * Hydrocortisone
  * Anticoagulants: increased potential for thromboembolic events

Parameters to monitor
- Laboratory monitoring is not recommended.

Selective estrogen receptor modulator: raloxifene (Evista)
Mechanism of action
- Estrogen receptor agonist at the skeleton; decreases resorption of bone and overall bone turnover

Patient instructions and counseling
- This medication may be taken without regard to food.

- Concomitant use with estrogen therapy is not recommended.

- This medication will not treat symptoms of menopause such as hot flashes.

- In the event of prolonged immobilization, discontinue raloxifene 3 days prior to and during the immobile period when possible.

Adverse drug events
- Most common:
  * Cardiovascular: hot flashes, chest pain, syncope

  * GI: nausea, diarrhea, vomiting
  * Musculoskeletal: arthralgia, myalgia
  * CNS: insomnia, neuralgia
  * Skin: rash, sweating

Drug-drug and drug-disease interactions
- Interaction may result in decreased pharmacologic effect of raloxifene:
  * Ampicillin (peak levels reduced by 28%; overall absorption reduced by 14%). Coadministration is not contraindicated due to maintained systemic exposure and elimination.
  * Cholestyramine (absorption and enterohepatic cycling reduced). Do not administer together.

- Interaction may result in decreased pharmacologic effect of interacting drug:
  * Warfarin (prothrombin time may decrease up to 10%)

Parameters to monitor
- Laboratory monitoring is not recommended.

Calcitonin (Miacalcin)
Mechanism of action
- Participates in the regulation of calcium and bone metabolism. Inhibits bone resorption by binding to osteoclast receptors.

Patient instructions and counseling
- If this medication is administered as an injection, it should be given in the upper arm, thigh, or buttocks.

- Proper education regarding administration of the injection and the nasal spray preparation is necessary.

- If you miss a shot, administer it as soon as possible. Do not administer the shot if it is almost time for your next dose.

- Store the nasal spray in the refrigerator until time for use. Warm the spray to room temperature prior to first use and then store at room temperature.

Adverse drug events
- Most common:
  * Skin: facial flushing and hand flushing (most common overall)
  * GI: nausea, diarrhea, vomiting, abdominal pain
  * Taste disorder: salty taste
  * Genitourinary: nocturia, urinary frequency
  * Nasal (with nasal spray): rhinitis, nasal dryness, irritation, itching, congestion
  * Ophthalmic: blurred vision, abnormal lacrimation

Drug-drug and drug-disease interactions
- Interaction may result in decreased pharmacologic effect of interacting drug:
  * Lithium: concomitant administration may decrease lithium levels

Parameters to monitor
- Laboratory monitoring is not recommended.

Teriparatide (Forteo)
Mechanism of action
- Increases the rate of bone formation by increasing the birth rate of osteoclasts and preventing apoptosis, resulting in improved bone mineral density.

Patient instructions and counseling
- Patients must read the user guide and pen manual prior to use.

Adverse drug events
- Most common:
  * Musculoskeletal: pain, arthralgia
  * CNS: paresthesias
  * GI: nausea, diarrhea, abdominal cramps
  * Taste disorder: metallic taste
  * Skin: injection pain, urticaria

Drug-drug and drug-disease interactions
- None known

Parameters to monitor
- Laboratory monitoring is not recommended.

Nondrug Therapy

- Weight-bearing exercise

- Smoking cessation

- Limited alcohol consumption

- Calcium-rich diet

4. Key Points

Postmenopausal hormone replacement therapy
- Therapy must be selected on an individual basis while considering risks and benefits, concomitant diseases, and medications. Important patient parameters to consider include menopause symptoms, risk of coronary artery disease, risk of osteoporosis, risk of breast cancer, and risk of thromboembolism.

- Primary indication for initiating hormone replacement therapy is to relieve vasomotor and other menopause symptoms to improve quality of life.

- Another indication is to continue estrogen's protective benefits, ie, the preservation of bone mass and prevention of osteoporosis.

- Hormone replacement therapy is not recommended for use in the primary prevention of any other disease states at this time.

- Estrogen plus progestin therapy is indicated in patients with a uterus.

- Estrogen alone is indicated in women who no longer have a uterus.

Contraceptives
- Oral contraceptives are highly effective and safe when used properly according to manufacture recommended dose and administration.

- Selection of prescription contraceptives requires careful consideration of patient medical history, lifestyle, compliance, and preference.

- In addition to the contraceptive benefit of these products, other menstrual-related health problems may be resolved or lessened (eg, menstrual pain, irregular menses, headache, and spotting).

- Changes in dose or product are often necessary to achieve an appropriate balance of estrogen and progestin that minimizes undesirable adverse effects associated with deficiencies or excess amounts of the hormones.

- Patients must be educated to immediately report the onset of severe abdominal pain, severe chest pain, shortness of breath, apoptosis, severe headache, visual disturbances, or severe pain in the leg or calf.

Osteoporosis

- Therapy must be selected on an individual basis considering risks and benefits, concomitant diseases, and medications.

- Appropriate calcium and vitamin D intake is an important component of prevention and treatment. If this is not obtained in the diet, supplementation is recommended for all individuals, even in patients receiving prescription therapy for osteoporosis.

- Bisphosphonates must be taken with a full glass of water 30 minutes prior to the first meal of the day. The patient must remain upright for at least 30 minutes.

- Estrogen replacement therapy is not approved for the treatment of osteoporosis and should not be initiated for this reason. It is approved for prevention of osteoporosis.

5. Questions and Answers

1. A.J. is a 35-year-old, premenopausal woman who is concerned about her family history of osteoporosis. She states that she does not eat dairy products due to lactose intolerance. Her recent bone mineral density screening revealed a T score of 1.0. Select the appropriate therapy recommendation from the choices below.

    A. Daily estrogen replacement therapy
    B. Daily calcium and vitamin D supplementation
    C. Daily combined estrogen/progestin replacement therapy
    D. Daily teriparatide (Forteo) injections
    E. Daily calcitonin nasal spray

2. The pharmacist receives a prescription for Fosamax 70 mg qd for prevention of osteoporosis with instructions to take with food and remain upright for at least 30 minutes following ingestion. From the choices below, identify the errors in this prescription.

    A. The dose of Fosamax should be 35 mg weekly for prevention.
    B. Fosamax should be taken at least 30 minutes prior to a meal; it should not be taken with food.
    C. Patients should lie down for 1 hour following administration of Fosamax.
    D. Choices B and C are correct.
    E. Choices A and B are correct.

3. What is the recommended dosage range of daily calcium intake for an adult?

    A. 200-400 mg
    B. 250-500 mg
    C. 300-600 mg
    D. 500-1000 mg
    E. 1000-1500 mg

4. Which of the following dose and schedule is correct for prevention of osteoporosis?

    A. Alendronate 35 mg weekly
    B. Risedronate 5 mg weekly
    C. Alendronate 70 mg weekly
    D. Risedronate 30 mg weekly
    E. Alendronate 10 mg daily

5. Which of the following products is available in an injectable and nasal spray dosage form?

A. Raloxifene
B. Alendronate
C. Teriparatide
D. Calcitonin
E. Prempro

6. Which agents are FDA approved for treatment of osteoporosis in men?

    A. Prempro and Premphase
    B. Alendronate and teriparatide
    C. Alendronate and raloxifene
    D. Raloxifene and calcitonin
    E. Risedronate and calcitonin

7. What is the recommended dose of raloxifene (Evista) in the prevention and treatment of post-menopausal osteoporosis?

    A. 10 mg daily
    B. 15 mg daily
    C. 40 mg daily
    D. 60 mg daily
    E. 120 mg daily

8. S.T. is a 32-year-old woman who wants to begin use of a prescription contraceptive product. S.T. is a new mother and would like to know if any products are safe for use during breastfeeding. S.T. states that she is not interested in using a device intravaginally, and experiences irritation and inflammation with condom use. Which of the following product(s) would be an appropriate choice for S.T.?

    A. Ortho Tri-Cyclen
    B. Micronor
    C. Depo-Provera
    D. A or B
    E. B or C
    F. A, B, or C

9. T.H. is a 27-year-old woman currently taking Nordette oral contraceptive. She presents to your pharmacy with a prescription of ampicillin 500 mg qid for 1 week. Which of the following choices describes appropriate action taken by the pharmacist?

    A. Call the physician and request a change to amoxicillin to avoid a drug interaction with Nordette and ampicillin.
    B. Dispense the ampicillin and counsel T.H. on the appropriate administration and duration of therapy for the antibiotic.
    C. Dispense the ampicillin and counsel T.H.

regarding the potential for ampicillin to interfere with the efficacy of Nordette, and instruct T.H. to use a back-up method of contraception until her next menstrual period begins.
    D. Refuse to fill the ampicillin prescription, and counsel T.H. that she should never take antibiotics while she is on birth control.

10. Which of the following oral contraceptives is a biphasic product?

    A. Ortho Tri-Cyclen
    B. Ortho-Novum 10/11
    C. Ortho-Novum 1/35
    D. Mircette
    E. Alesse

11. Which of the following products is a progestin-only oral contraceptive?

    A. Nordette
    B. Ortho Tri-Cyclen
    C. Ovrette
    D. Demulen 1/50
    E. Necon 1/35

12. Which of the following triphasic oral contraceptives varies the dose of both the estrogen and progestin component?

    A. Triphasil
    B. Ortho-Novum 7/7/7
    C. Ortho Tri-Cyclen
    D. Cyclessa
    E. Tri-Norinyl

13. What is highest dose of estrogen (ethinyl estradiol) offered in an oral contraceptive?

    A. 25 µg
    B. 30 µg
    C. 35 µg
    D. 40 µg
    E. 50 µg

14. Which triphasic oral contraceptive provides constant progestin dose and varies the estrogen?

    A. Necon 7/7/7
    B. Tri-Norinyl
    C. Ortho Tri-Cyclen
    D. Estrostep 21
    E. Tri-Levlin

15. A.J. is a 55-year-old woman who presents to

your pharmacy with a prescription for Premarin 0.625 mg daily. She has an intact uterus and has been recently diagnosed with menopause. Which of the following statements describes the appropriate action to be taken by the pharmacist?

A. Refuse to fill the prescription and recommend a phytoestrogen supplement
B. Call the physician and confirm that the patient has an intact uterus and recommend a product containing estrogen plus progestin
C. Fill the prescription and counsel the patient regarding administration instructions and potential adverse effects
D. None of the above

16. Which of the following factors is a contraindication to the use of hormone replacement therapy in postmenopausal women?

A. Diabetes
B. Basal cell skin cancer
C. Thromboembolic disease
D. Depression
E. Obesity

17. From the choices below, please select the most common side effects associated with estrogen replacement.

A. Breast tenderness
B. Depression
C. Nausea
D. Brittle fingernails
E. A and C

18. Which of the following products is available in a vaginal cream dosage form?

A. Estrace
B. Vagifem
C. Vivelle
D. Estratest
E. Premphase

19. Which of the following product dosing regimens is correct?

A. Climara Transdermal: apply to skin once daily
B. Vagifem: one tablet vaginally once daily for 2 weeks, then one tablet vaginally twice weekly
C. Delestrogen: 10-20 mg injections once weekly
D. Premarin caplets: 0.625-2.5 mg tid

E. Ogen vaginal cream: 20-40 g vaginally once daily

20. Which of the following drug interactions may result in increased pharmacologic effect of estrogen?

A. Macrolide antibiotics
B. Itraconazole
C. Ketoconazole
D. A and C
E. A, B, and C

Answers

1. **B.** A.J. has neither osteopenia nor osteoporosis with a T score of 1.0. At this point, preventive therapy is appropriate with adequate calcium and vitamin D intake. Prescription therapy is not indicated at this point in time.

2. **E.** The appropriate use of Fosamax for prevention of osteoporosis includes a 35-mg weekly or 5-mg daily dose. The 70-mg weekly dose is for treatment of osteoporosis. The medication should be taken with a full glass of water at least 30 minutes prior to ingesting food or beverage. Patients should remain in the upright position for at least 30 minutes following ingestion of Fosamax.

3. **E.** 1000-1500 mg is the recommended dosage range of daily calcium intake for an adult.

4. **A.** Choices C, D, an E are treatment doses. Choice B is not an accurate dose or frequency for treatment or prevention.

5. **D.** Injectable and nasal spray dosage forms of calcitonin are available. Teriparatide is available as an injection only. Prempro, raloxifene, and alendronate are only available in oral dosage forms.

6. **B.** Alendronate and teriparatide are FDA approved for treatment of osteoporosis in men.

7. **D.** 60 mg once daily is the approved and recommended dose of raloxifene.

8. **E.** Micronor is a progestin only (minipill) oral contraceptive and is considered compatible with breastfeeding. Depo-Provera is an injectable progestin-only contraceptive option that is considered safe and appropriate for women who desire to breastfeed. Ortho Tri-Cyclen is a combined oral contraceptive known to decrease the

quantity of breast milk available and may adversely affect the infant.

9. **C.** Ampicillin is known to interact with combined oral contraceptives. Although clinical studies have not consistently demonstrated an interaction, more than 25 case reports of unintended pregnancies have been attributed to concomitant use of ampicillin and oral contraceptives. Concomitant administration of ampicillin, as well as other antibiotics, may decrease the effectiveness of combined oral contraceptives, resulting in pregnancy. Patients must be counseled to use a back-up method of contraception until menses occurs.

10. **B.** Ortho-Novum 10/11 and Necon 10/11 are the two biphasic oral contraceptives available.

11. **C.** Ovrette is a progestin-only oral contraceptive.

12. **A.** Triphasil is a triphasic oral contraceptive which varies the dose of **both** the estrogen and progestin component.

13. **E.** 50 μg is the highest dose of estrogen (ethinyl estradiol) offered in an oral contraceptive.

14. **D.** Estrostep 21 is a triphasic oral contraceptive that provides a constant progestin dose and varies the estrogen.

15. **B.** Unopposed estrogen is not recommended in women with an intact uterus due to increased risk of endometrial hyperplasia and endometrial cancer. Women with an intact uterus should receive a product containing estrogen plus progestin.

16. **C.** Thromboembolic disease is a definite contraindication to use of hormone replacement therapy in postmenopausal women.

17. **E.** Breast tenderness and nausea are the most common side effects associated with estrogen replacement.

18. **A.** Estrace is available in a vaginal cream dosage form.

19. **B.** Vagifem dosage is one tablet vaginally once daily for 2 weeks, then one tablet vaginally twice weekly.

20. **E.** Macrolide antibiotics, itraconazole, and ketoconazole may result in increased pharmacologic effect of estrogen.

6. References

Postmenopausal hormone replacement therapy
Burnham TH, Wichersham RN, Novak KK, eds. Drug Facts and Comparisons Updated Monthly. St Louis: Facts and Comparisons; 2003.

Hutchison TA, Shahan DR, eds. DRUGDEX® System. MICROMEDEX, Greenwood Village, CO. (Edition expired 6-2003.)

Kalantaridou SN, Davis SR, Calis KA. Hormone replacement therapy. In: Dipiro JT, Talbert RL, Yee GC, eds. *Pharmacotherapy: A Pathophysiologic Approach*, 5th ed. New York: McGraw-Hill; 2002:1491-1504.

Loose-Mitchell DS, Stancel GM. Estrogens and progestins. In: Hardman JG, Limbird LE, Goodman Gilman A, eds. *Goodman and Gilman's The Pharmacological Basis of Therapeutics,* 10th ed. New York: McGraw-Hill; 2001:1597-1622.

Sagraves R, Parent-Stevens L, Hardman J. Gynecologic disorders. In: Koda-Kimble MA, Young LY, eds. *Applied Therapeutics: The Clinical Use of Drugs,* 7th ed. Philadelphia: Lippincott Williams & Wilkins; 2001:46-32.

Contraceptives
Burnham TH, Wichersham RN, Novak KK, eds. Drug Facts and Comparisons Updated Monthly. St Louis: Facts and Comparisons; 2003.

Dickerson LM, Bucci KK. Contraception. In: Dipiro JT, Talbert RL, Yee GC, eds. *Pharmacotherapy: A Pathophysiologic Approach*, 5th ed. New York: McGraw-Hill; 2002:1445-1462.

Hutchison TA, Shahan DR, eds. DRUGDEX® System. MICROMEDEX, Greenwood Village, CO. (Edition expired 6-2003.)

Loose-Mitchell DS, Stancel GM. Estrogens and progestins. In: Goodman LS, Hardman JG, Limbird LE, et al, eds. *Goodman and Gilman's The Pharmacological Basis of Therapeutics,* 10th ed. New York: McGraw-Hill; 2001:1597-1629.

Ruggiero R. Contraception. In: Koda-Kimble MA, Young LY, eds. *Applied Therapeutics: The Clinical Use of Drugs,* 7th ed. Philadelphia: Lippincott Williams & Wilkins; 2001:41-43.

Osteoporosis

American Association of Clinical Endocrinologists 2001 Medical Guidelines for Clinical Practice for the Prevention and Management of Postmenopausal Osteoporosis. *Endocr Pract.* 2001;7:294-312.

Burnham TH, Wickersham RN, Novak KK, eds. Drug Facts and Comparisons Updated Monthly. St Louis: Facts and Comparisons; 2003.

Consensus Development Panel. Osteoporosis prevention, diagnosis, and therapy consensus conference. National Institutes of Health. *JAMA.* 2001;285:785-795.

Dickerson LM, Bucci KK. Contraception. In: Dipiro JT, Talbert RL, Yee GC, eds. *Pharmacotherapy: A Pathophysiologic Approach,* 5th ed. New York: McGraw-Hill; 2002:1445-1462.

Hutchison TA, Shahan DR, eds. DRUGDEX® System. MICROMEDEX, Greenwood Village, CO. (Edition expired 6-2003.)

Marcus R. Agents affecting calcification and bone turnover. In: Hardman JG, Limbird LE, Goodman Gilman A, eds. *Goodman and Gilman's The Pharmacological Basis of Therapeutics,* 10th ed. New York: McGraw-Hill; 2001:1715-1743.

National Osteoporosis Foundation. Physician's Guide to Prevention and Treatment of Osteoporosis, 2000. Available at: http://www.nof.org/physguide. Accessed April 1, 2003.

Sagraves R, Parent-Stevens L, Hardman J. Gynecologic disorders. In: Koda-Kimble MA, Young LY, eds. *Applied Therapeutics: The Clinical Use of Drugs,* 7th ed. Philadelphia: Lippincott Williams & Wilkins; 2001:46-49.

16. Kidney Disease

Joanna Q. Hudson, PharmD, BCPS
Assistant Professor, Department of Pharmacy
University of Tennessee College of Pharmacy

Contents

1. Acute Renal Failure

- Acute renal failure (ARF) is defined as rapid (hours to days) deterioration of kidney function resulting in *azotemia* (retention of nitrogenous waste products such as urea) and failure of the kidney to maintain fluid, electrolyte, and acid-base homeostasis.

- A reduced urine output is frequently seen: *oliguria* (urine output <400 mL/d), *anuria* (urine output <50 mL/d), *nonoliguria* indicates urine output >400 mL/d.

- Objective definition: Increase in serum creatinine of 0.5 mg/dL over a 24-hour period when baseline creatinine is less than 3.0 mg/dL, or an increase of 1.0 mg/dL when baseline creatinine is greater than 3.0 mg/dL.

Epidemiology

Incidence and prevalence
- Community-acquired ARF accounts for 1% of hospital admissions.

- Hospital-acquired ARF occurs in 2-5% of hospitalized patients.

Mortality
- Best prognosis when renal replacement therapy not required.

- 10-25% mortality rate in patients who require renal replacement therapy

- >50% mortality rate in patients with multiple organ failure

Types and Classifications

- ARF is classified according to precipitating factors.

Prerenal
- Characterized by a decrease in renal perfusion with or without systemic arterial hypotension; most common type; usually reversible. *Functional ARF* describes conditions that decrease glomerular ultrafiltrate production without damage to the kidney (similar to prerenal).

Intrinsic (intrarenal)
- Results from structural damage to the parenchymal tissue of the kidney. Divided into vascular, glomerular, interstitial, and tubular disorders (most common).

Postrenal
- Obstruction of urine flow occurring at any level of the urinary outflow tracts

Clinical Presentation

- Decreased urine output

- Signs of hypovolemia (prerenal causes): tachycardia, decreased venous and arterial pressure, orthostasis

- Unique color and composition of urine: cola-colored urine suggests bleeding; foaming is indicative of proteinuria.

- Symptoms of *uremia* (the clinical syndrome resulting from azotemia):
  * Weakness, shortness of breath, fatigue, mental confusion, nausea and vomiting, bleeding, loss of appetite, edema

- Flank pain (suggestive of swelling of the kidneys)

- Increased weight (suggesting fluid accumulation)

- Increased blood pressure (suggesting fluid accumulation)

- Signs and symptoms of electrolyte abnormalities (hyperkalemia, hypocalcemia), metabolic acidosis (see section on fluids and electrolytes)

- Bladder distention or prostate enlargement (postrenal causes)

- Other findings specific to the cause of ARF (see section on pathophysiology)

Pathophysiology

Prerenal/functional ARF
- Caused by conditions that decrease glomerular hydrostatic pressure leading to a decrease in glomerular filtration rate (GFR) (see section on etiologies)

- Hypoperfusion leads to increased sodium and water reabsorption by the kidney and stimulates compensatory mechanisms.

- Compensatory mechanisms to increase hydrostatic pressure and GFR:
  * Vasodilation of the afferent arteriole (mediated by prostaglandins)
  * Vasoconstriction of the efferent arteriole (mediated by angiotensin II)

- Alterations in afferent and efferent arteriolar tone can affect compensatory mechanisms.

- Nonsteroidal anti-inflammatory drugs (NSAIDs) and cyclooxygenase II (COX II) inhibitors can prevent compensatory vasodilation of the afferent arteriole.

- Angiotensin-converting enzyme inhibitors (ACEIs) and angiotensin receptor blockers (ARBs) can prevent compensatory vasoconstriction of the efferent arteriole

Etiologies
- Intravascular volume depletion: excessive diuresis, vomiting, excessive GI fluid loss, bleeding

- Severe hypotension

- Hypocalcemia

- Decreased effective blood volume (volume perceived by arterial baroreceptors): congestive heart failure, cirrhosis, nephrotic syndrome, hepatorenal syndrome

- Systemic vasodilatation: sepsis, liver failure, anaphylaxis

- Large-vessel renal vascular disease: renal artery thrombosis or embolism, renal artery stenosis

- Medications: see Table 1

Intrinsic acute renal failure
- The primary anatomic sites of the kidney are prone to structural damage from prolonged ischemia and/or direct toxicity due to the high metabolic activity and concentrating ability of the kidney.

Etiologies by anatomic site
- Vascular: inflammation, emboli

- Glomerular (glomerulonephritis): systemic lupus erythematosus, medications (see Table 1)

- Interstitial: ischemia, allergic interstitial nephritis, infections, medications (see Table 1)

- Tubular: accounts for 90% of cases of intrinsic cases
  * Intrarenal vasoconstriction, direct tubular toxicity, intratubular obstruction
  * Prolonged ischemia from prerenal causes
  * Toxins
    • Endogenous: myoglobin, hemoglobin, uric acid

Table 1

Drug-Induced Causes of Kidney Disease

Clinical syndrome	Causative drugs[1]
Prerenal	ACEIs, ARBs, COX-2 inhibitors, cyclosporine, diuretics, NSAIDs, radiocontrast dye, tacrolimus
Intrinsic	
Vascular	Amphetamines, cisplatin, cyclosporine, mitomycin C
Glomerular	Gold, heroin, lithium, NSAIDs, phenytoin
Interstitial nephritis	Analgesic combinations, aristolochic acid (Chinese herbs), cyclosporine, lithium, NSAIDs, penicillins, sulfonamides, tacrolimus
Acute tubular necrosis	Aminoglycosides, amphotericin B, chemotherapeutic agents, cidofovir, cocaine, foscarnet, ifosfamide, radiocontrast dye, tacrolimus
Postrenal	
Obstructive	Acyclovir, methotrexate, oxalate, sulfonamides, uric acid
Nephrolithiasis	Allopurinol, indinavir, sulfadiazine, triamterene

[1]Not inclusive of all potential nephrotoxins.

- Exogenous:
  * Medications (see Table 1): aminoglycosides common nephrotoxins leading to nonoliguric ARF after 5-7 days of therapy
  * Other: ethylene glycol, pesticides

Postrenal acute renal failure
- Obstruction of urinary flow at any level from the urinary collecting system to the urethra

- Must involve both kidneys, or one kidney in a patient with a single functioning kidney

Etiologies by anatomic site
- Renal pelves or tubules: crystal deposition

- Ureteral: tumor, stricture, stones

- Bladder neck obstruction: prostatic hypertrophy, bladder carcinoma

- Medications: see Table 1

Diagnostic Criteria (see Table 2)

- Physical findings: assess for signs and symptoms listed in clinical presentation

- Medication history: identify potentially nephrotoxic agents (see Table 1)

- Estimate GFR: normal 100-125 mL/min

Creatinine clearance (CrCl)
- Measured using urine collection methods:

$$CrCl = \frac{Ucr \times V}{SCr \times t}$$

where Ucr = urinary creatinine concentration (mg/dL)
V = volume of urine (mL)
SCr = serum creatinine concentration (mg/dL)
t = time period of urine collection (min)

- Estimated using the Cockcroft-Gault equation (assumes stable kidney function):

$$CrCl = \frac{(140 - age)(IBW \text{ in kg})}{72 \times SCr \text{ (mg/dL)}}$$

(multiply result by 0.85 for females)
where IBW = ideal body weight in kg

Modification of diet in renal disease (MDRD) equation
GFR = 170 $\times$ (serum creatinine)$^{-0.999}$ $\times$ (age)$^{-0.176}$ $\times$ (BUN)$^{-0.170}$ $\times$ (serum albumin)$^{0.318}$ $\times$ (0.762 if female) $\times$ (1.18 if black)
(Other assessments are available to assess GFR in patients with acute changes in kidney function)

Blood tests
- Elevated: blood urea nitrogen, serum creatinine, electrolytes (potassium, phosphorus)

- Decreased: calcium (consider albumin concentration), bicarbonate

Urinalysis (consider whether fluids and/or diuretics were previously administered)
- Specific gravity, osmolality: high values indicate prerenal causes and stimulation of sodium and water retention

- Proteinuria (indicates loss of filtering ability by glomeruli): microalbuminuria (>30 mg/d), overt proteinuria (>300 mg/d)

- Hematuria: red blood cells

- Glucose, ketones

- Urine sediment: hyaline casts normal, granular casts and cellular debris suggests structural damage

- White blood cells: suggest inflammation

Urine chemistries: sodium, potassium, chloride, creatinine, urinary anion gap
- Fractional excretion of sodium [FE$_{Na}$]: useful to differentiate prerenal from acute intrinsic renal failure. Low value (<1%) suggests retention of sodium and water (prerenal etiology) versus intrinsic cause.

$$FE_{Na} = \frac{U_{Na} \times P_{Cr}}{U_{Cr} \times P_{Na}}$$

where U$_{Na}$ = urine sodium
U$_{Cr}$ = urine creatinine
P$_{Cr}$ = plasma creatinine
P$_{Na}$ = plasma sodium

- Radiographic procedures: ultrasound, plain film radiograph, radioisotope scan, computed tomography

Table 2

Laboratory Findings to Differentiate Prerenal and Intrinsic Renal Failure

Diagnostic test	Prerenal	Intrinsic
BUN:Cr ratio	>20:1	<10-15:1
Urinalysis	Normal with few cells or casts (hyaline casts normal)	Granular casts present with tubular epithelial cells
Urine osmolality	>500 mOsm/kg	300-350 mOsm/kg
Urinary Cr:Plasma Cr	>40:1	<20:1
Specific gravity	>1.020	<1.015
Urine sodium	<25 mEq/L	>40 mEq/L
FE$_{Na}$	<1%	>2%

- Renal biopsy: indicated for patients without cause of ARF identified by other diagnostic tests

Treatment Principles and Goals

Prevention
- Identify high risk patients
  * Volume depleted
  * Undergoing surgical procedures: consider current renal function, age, cardiovascular status, volume status
  * Receiving potentially nephrotoxic medications
  * Preexisting renal or hepatic disease
  * Diabetes mellitus
  * Undergoing diagnostic tests (radiocontrast media exposure)

- Strategies for prevention: hydration, sodium loading

Treatment
- Correct underlying causes of ARF (eg, discontinue nephrotoxic agents, correct fluid status, treat underlying infection, remove urinary tract obstructions)

- Return to baseline kidney function or highest kidney function possible

- Prevent development of chronic kidney disease and the need for chronic renal replacement therapies (dialysis or transplantation)

- Avoid nephrotoxic agents or take measures to reduce exposure if possible (eg, select liposomal amphotericin B over conventional amphotericin)

- Adjust doses of medications based on kidney function

- Avoid agents contraindicated in patients with kidney disease (eg, metformin, Glucophage®)

- Address complications of ARF: eg, electrolyte abnormalities (hyperkalemia), fluid overload, metabolic acidosis (see sections on fluids and electrolytes and acid-base disorders), hyperphosphatemia (see section on chronic kidney disease)

Strategies for treatment
- Diuretic therapy (loop diuretics) are first-line agents to improve fluid status and urine output

Experimental therapies
- Fenoldopam (Corlopam®), a dopamine agonist, is used in ARF patients to increase renal blood flow and promote diuresis

- Calcium channel blockers

- Acetylcysteine (Mucomyst®) to prevent radiocontrast-induced renal failure

Drug therapy (Table 3)
Diuretics
Mechanism of action
- *Loop diuretics:* delivered to the tubular lumen of the kidney by proximal tubular cells. Cause inhibition of sodium and chloride reabsorption in the thick ascending limb of the loop of Henle to promote water excretion.

- *Osmotic diuretics:* freely filtered into the tubular lumen in the proximal tubule. Increases the osmolarity of the glomerular filtrate, which inhibits tubular reabsorption of water and electrolytes and increases urinary output.

- *Thiazide and thiazide-like diuretics:* inhibit the Na^+-Cl^- cotransport in the early distal convoluted tubules. Generally used in combination with loop diuretics for resistant edema and fluid overload, particularly metolazone, which is effective at GFRs <30 mL/min. Other thiazide diuretics generally not effective when GFR is <30 mL/min.

Patient instructions and counseling
- Take the last dose of the day early in the evening if possible to minimize nocturia (excessive urination at night).

- Follow all dietary instructions (generally low sodium, fluid restricted diet).

- Move slowly from sitting to standing position (potential for orthostatic hypotension).

- Make note of any changes in urine output.

- Contact your health care provider if you experience hearing loss or ringing in the ears.

- This medicine may make your skin more sensitive to sunlight. Use a sunscreen when you are outdoors.

- Tell your health care provider if you have any known drug allergies, particularly to sulfa.

Adverse drug events
Loop diuretics
- Hypokalemia, hypomagnesemia, hyponatremia, hypovolemia, hyperuricemia, hyperglycemia

Table 3

Drug Therapy for Acute Renal Failure by Drug Classification

Classification	Generic name (trade name)	Dosage range	Dosage forms	Frequency of administration
Diuretics[1]				
Loop	Furosemide (Lasix®)	20-400 mg	PO	q 6-12 h
		20-200 mg	IV	
	Bumetanide (Bumex®)	0.5-10 mg	PO, IV	q 12-24 h
	Torsemide (Demadex®)	10-100 mg	PO, IV	q 24 h
	Ethacrynic acid (Edecrin®)	50-400 mg	PO	q 8-12 h
		50-100 mg	IV	
Osmotic	Mannitol (Osmitrol®, Resectisol®)	Initial "test" dose: 12.5-25 g over 3-5 min; maintenance dose: 0.25-0.5 g/kg	IV	q 4-6 h
Thiazide	Hydrochlorothiazide (Hydrodiuril®, Dyazide®, Maxzide®)	25-200 mg/d	PO	qd, bid
	Chlorothiazide (Diuril®)	500 mg-2 g/d	PO	qd, bid
		100-500 mg/d	IV	
Thiazide-like	Metolazone (Zaroxolyn®, Mykrox®)	5-10 mg	PO	qd
Sympathomimetic	Dopamine (Intropin®)	0.5-2.0 µg/kg per min	IV	Continuous

[1]Loop diuretics also administered as a continuous infusion. Higher dose ranges for intermittent dosing are reserved for patients unresponsive to initial smaller doses.

- Hypercalciuria

- Orthostatic hypotension, dehydration

- Metabolic alkalosis (partly due to extracellular fluid volume contraction)

- Ototoxicity

- Diarrhea, nausea

- Furosemide, bumetanide, and torsemide have a sulfonamide substituent (potential for hypersensitivity reactions). Ethacrynic acid generally reserved for patients allergic to sulfa compounds.

Osmotic diuretics
- Acute expansion of extracellular fluid volume and increased risk of pulmonary edema, acute rise in serum K^+, nausea and vomiting, headache, blurred vision, rash

Thiazide and thiazide-like diuretics (used in combination with loop diuretics)
- Hypokalemia, hyponatremia, hypercalcemia

- Hypovolemia, orthostatic hypotension

- Hyperglycemia, hypochloremic alkalosis, hyperlipidemia

- Hypersensitivity reactions from sulfonamide substituents

- Chest pain (metolazone, more common with the brand Mykrox, which is more rapidly and extensively absorbed than Zaroxolyn)

Drug-drug and drug-disease interactions
- Loop diuretics and aminoglycosides: increased potential for ototoxicity

- Diuretics and other nephrotoxins: increased risk of nephrotoxicity if hypovolemia occurs

- Diuretics and lithium: decreased renal clearance of lithium, monitor lithium concentrations more closely

- Diuretics and digoxin: hypokalemia from diuretic use may increase risk of toxicity with digoxin (monitor potassium and digoxin)

- Loop and thiazide diuretics and gout: potential for increased gouty attacks from hyperuricemia

- Thiazide diuretics and diabetes: hyperglycemia from thiazides; increase monitoring

- Conditions that decrease secretion of diuretic to its site of action in the renal tubule:
  * proteinuria (diuretic binds to protein and not available at site of action);
  * decreased renal blood flow;
  * competitive inhibition of transport system (NSAIDs, probenecid, cephalosporins)

Parameters to monitor
- Blood pressure (sitting and standing), pulse, urine output, fluid intake, kidney function, serum electrolytes, blood urea nitrogen, bicarbonate, calcium, glucose, uric acid

- Osmotic diuretics: serum osmolality (310-320 mOsm/kg); assess urine output after initial test dose (goal urine flow at least 30-50 mL/h)

Kinetics if appropriate
Loop diuretics
- Oral bioavailability: furosemide (60%), bumetanide (85%), torsemide (85%)

- PO:IV dose ratios: furosemide (1.5), bumetanide (1), torsemide (1)

- Equivalent doses: 1 mg bumetanide = 20 mg torsemide = 40 mg furosemide

- Elimination route: furosemide (primarily renal), bumetanide (hepatic and renal), torsemide (primarily hepatic), ethacrynic acid (hepatic and renal)

Thiazide and thiazide-like diuretics
- Metolazone absorption differs between brands. Mykrox is more rapidly and extensively absorbed than Zaroxolyn

Other (eg, unusual storage requirements, administration, etc.)
- Patients with kidney disease generally require larger doses of diuretics to achieve adequate concentrations of the drug at the site of action in the kidney.

- The brands of metolazone (Zaroxolyn and Mykrox) are not bioequivalent and should not be interchanged.

Dopamine
Mechanism of action
- At low doses (0.5-2 µg/kg per min) selectively dilates the renal vasculature and may cause an increase in renal blood flow and GFR. Dose is titrated to desired response.

Patient instructions and counseling
- Administered to hospitalized patients (see parameters to monitor)

Adverse drug events
- Hypotension, tachycardia, arrhythmias, dyspnea

- Headache, nausea, vomiting

- At higher doses (>10 µg/kg per min) stimulates α- and β_1-adrenergic receptors, causing peripheral vasoconstriction and hypertension.

Drug-drug and drug-disease interactions
- Prolonged and intensified effect when given with MAO inhibitors, α- and β-adrenergic blockers, general anesthetics, and phenytoin

- Use with caution in patients with cardiovascular disease or cardiac arrhythmias and patients with occlusive vascular disease.

Parameters to monitor
- Blood pressure, pulse, urine output, ECG, heart rate

- Monitor for extravasation

Kinetics if appropriate
- Onset of action: 5 minutes

- Duration: <10 minutes (continuous infusion necessary)

- Half-life: 2 minutes

- Metabolized to inactive metabolites (75%) and active metabolite norepinephrine (25%). Metabolites excreted in urine.

Other (eg, unusual storage requirements, administration, etc.)
- Administer in large vein to prevent extravasation and tissue necrosis; phentolamine (Regitine®) used as antidote

Nondrug Therapy

Fluid management
- Fluid intake and output should be equal (consider sensible and insensible losses)

- Fluid selection and rate of correction dependent on clinical condition of the patient (eg, crystalloids, colloids, normal saline)

Nutritional
- High calorie, low protein diet
- Consider restriction of sodium, potassium, phosphorus

Renal replacement therapies
- Procedures by which the blood is artificially cleared of waste and some essential metabolic products to augment the function of a failed or failing kidney. Includes *hemodialysis* and *hemofiltration*, in which the semipermeable membrane is a dialyzer, and *peritoneal dialysis*, in which the peritoneal cavity serves as this membrane. Procedures may be intermittent or continuous. Kidney transplantation is also considered a form of renal replacement therapy.

- Consider the potential for drug removal by dialysis.

Indications for renal replacement therapy
- Any of the following refractory to more conservative measures:
    * Acidosis
    * Electrolyte abnormalities (hyperkalemia)
    * Drug-induced renal failure (if drug removed by dialysis)
    * Volume overload
    * Uremia or uremic symptoms

2. Chronic Kidney Disease

- *Chronic kidney disease* (CKD) is kidney damage with or without a decrease in GFR or a GFR <60 mL/min per 1.73 m^2 for ≥3 months. *Kidney damage* is defined as pathologic abnormalities or markers of damage, including abnormalities in blood or urine tests or imaging studies.

- CKD refers to five stages (1-5) classified based on GFR (see section on classifications). *End-stage renal disease* (ESRD) occurs when patients require renal replacement therapy (either dialysis or transplantation) to sustain life and is classified as stage 5 CKD.

Epidemiology of CKD

Incidence
- ESRD continues to increase by 3-5% each year, with approximately 96,000 new patients per year.

- Incidence is approximately four times higher in the black population.

- Median age of patients is 64 years.

Prevalence
- Estimated prevalence of CKD based on stage (see classifications)
    * Stage 1 (5.9 million), stage 2 (5.3 million), stage 3 (7.6 million), stage 4 (400,000), stage 5 (300,000) (Table 4)

- Approximately 370,000 patients treated for ESRD (including hemodialysis, peritoneal dialysis, and transplant patients)

Mortality
- Life expectancy is four to five times less in dialysis patients than in the general population.

- The primary causes of death in the ESRD population are cardiac diseases and infection.

- Comorbidities, estimated GFR, and albumin at initiation of dialysis are strong predictors of mortality in the dialysis population.

Classifications of Chronic Kidney Disease (Table 4)

Clinical presentation
- Changes in urine output (may not occur in earlier stages of CKD)

Table 4

Stages of Chronic Kidney Disease

Stage	Description	GFR (mL/min per 1.73 m²)	Action
	Increased risk	≥90 (with CKD risk factors)	Screening, CKD risk reduction
1	Kidney damage with normal or increased GFR	≥90	Diagnosis and treatment, treatment of comorbid conditions, slowing progression, CVD risk reduction
2	Kidney damage with mildly decreased GFR	60-89	Estimating progression
3	Moderately decreased GFR	30-59	Evaluating and treating complications
4	Severely decreased GFR	15-29	Preparation for kidney replacement therapy
5	Kidney failure (defined as ESRD if renal replacement therapy needed)	<15 (or need for renal replacement therapy)	Renal replacement therapy (if uremia present)

- "Foaming" of urine: indicates proteinuria (or albuminuria)
    * *Microalbuminuria:* the presence of albumin in the urine in amounts of 30-300 mg/d
    * *Albuminuria:* the presence of albumin in the urine in amounts greater than 300 mg/d
    * *Clinical proteinuria:* total protein in the urine in amounts greater than 300 mg/d (Table 5)

- Increased blood pressure (hypertension is a common etiology and result of CKD)

- Signs and symptoms of hyperglycemia, glucosuria (diabetes is a common etiology)

- Signs and symptoms associated with fluid and electrolyte abnormalities (eg, hyperkalemia, fluid overload; see section on fluids and electrolytes)

Secondary complications of CKD
    * Anemia: decreased hemoglobin and hematocrit; may also present with iron deficiency
    * Hyperphosphatemia: increased phosphorus; decreased calcium
    * Secondary hyperparathyroidism: increased parathyroid hormone
    * Metabolic acidosis: decreased serum bicarbonate, increased anion gap
    * Malnutrition: decreased albumin and prealbumin (See section on nutrition)

- Signs of uremia (see section on acute renal failure) in later stages of CKD, stage 4-5 CKD

Table 5

Definitions of Proteinuria and Albuminuria

	Total protein			Albumin		
	24-hour collection (mg/d)	Spot urine dipstick (mg/dL)	Spot urine protein:SCr ratio (mg/g)	24-hour collection (mg/d)	Spot urine dipstick (mg/dL)	Spot urine albumin:SCr ratio (mg/g)
Normal	<300	<30	<200	<30	<3	<17 (men); <25 (women)
Microalbuminuria	NA	NA	NA	30-300	>3	17-250 (men); 25-355 (women)
Albuminuria or clinical proteinuria	>300	>30	>200	>300	NA	>250 (men); >355 (women)

Pathophysiology of Progressive Kidney Disease and Selected Secondary Complications

Progressive kidney disease
- Progressive loss of nephron function results in adaptive changes in remaining nephrons to increase single nephron glomerular filtration pressure.

- Over time the compensatory increase in single nephron GFR leads to hypertrophy from sustained increases in pressure and loss of individual nephron function.

- Proteinuria, one of the initial diagnostic signs, may also contribute to the progressive decline in kidney function.

- Loss of kidney function progresses slowly and is usually irreversible.

Etiology of progressive kidney disease
- Each of the following may result in damage to the kidney that over time leads to a decrease in functioning nephrons and decreased total GFR:
  * Diabetes (accounts for primary cause in 44% of patients with ESRD)
  * Hypertension (accounts for primary cause in 26% of patients with ESRD)
  * Glomerulonephritis
  * Cystic kidney disease
  * HIV nephropathy
  * Other factors (hyperlipidemia, genetic factors, gender differences)

Anemia of CKD
- Primary etiology is a decrease in production of the hormone erythropoietin by the kidney as kidney disease progresses (>90% of erythropoietin production occurs in the kidney, approximately 10% by the liver)

- Results in a normochromic, normocytic anemia

- Red blood cell lifespan is also decreased from 120 days to approximately 64 days in patients with kidney failure.

- Other contributors include iron deficiency and blood loss (eg, from uremic bleeding, dialysis, etc.)

Hyperphosphatemia and hypocalcemia
- Decrease in phosphorus elimination as kidney function declines

- Results in accumulation of phosphorus (hyperphosphatemia) and a reciprocal decrease in serum calcium concentrations (hypocalcemia)

- Active vitamin D (1,25-dihydroxyvitamin D_3) promotes increased intestinal absorption of calcium. This process is impaired as kidney disease progresses due to decreased conversion of vitamin D to its active form in the kidney. (As kidney disease progresses the final hydroxylation step that normally occurs in the kidney is altered and patients become deficient in active vitamin D.)

Secondary hyperparathyroidism
- Hypocalcemia stimulates the release of parathyroid hormone (PTH) by the parathyroid glands.

- Hyperphosphatemia and vitamin D deficiency also contribute to development of hyperparathyroidism.

- To normalize ionized calcium PTH causes:
  * Decreased phosphorus reabsorption within the kidney
  * Increased calcium reabsorption by the kidney
  * Increased calcium mobilization from bone

- As kidney disease progresses:
  * Hyperphosphatemia and subsequent hypocalcemia progressively worsen and hyperparathyroidism results.
  * The renal effects of PTH are no longer maintained and PTH predominantly stimulates calcium resorption from bone.
  * Decreased production of active vitamin D worsens hypocalcemia and stimulus for release of PTH.

- Secondary hyperparathyroidism leads to hyperplasia of the parathyroid gland

Metabolic acidosis
- Decreased excretion of acid by the kidney

- Accumulation of endogenous acids due to impaired kidney function (eg, phosphates, sulfates)

Diagnostic Criteria

Progressive kidney disease
- Progressive increase in serum creatinine: >1.1-1.2 mg/dL for females, >1.2-1.3 mg/dL for males (consider factors that may alter serum creatinine such as decreased muscle mass and nutritional status)

- Decreased creatinine clearance (see sections on classifications of CKD and diagnostic criteria for acute renal failure)

- Microalbuminuria, albuminuria, or clinical proteinuria

- Abnormal serum chemistries
  * Increase in serum creatinine, BUN
  * Increased potassium, decreased serum bicarbonate, increased phosphorus, decreased calcium (indicative of secondary complications)

- Development of secondary complications

Anemia of CKD
- Hemoglobin <12 g/dL (premenopausal females), <13.5 g/dL (males and postmenopausal females)

- Hematocrit <36% (premenopausal females), <41% (males and postmenopausal females)

- Guidelines for anemia management in patients with CKD: recommend a work-up for anemia when hemoglobin is <11 g/dL in premenopausal females and <12 g/dL in males and postmenopausal females

- Iron deficiency: evaluate red blood cell indices and iron indices to identify deficiency as a contributing factor; iron deficiency manifests as a microcytic anemia
  * Red blood cell count <4.2 x 10^6 cells/mm^2
  * Mean corpuscular volume (MCV): <80 fl
  * Serum iron: <50 mg/dL
  * Total iron binding capacity (TIBC): <250 mg/dL
  * Transferrin saturation (TSat): <16%
  * Serum ferritin: <12 ng/mL
    • Transferrin saturation and serum ferritin should be maintained at higher values for patients receiving erythropoietin therapy (TSat ≥20%, serum ferritin ≥100 ng/mL).

- Evaluate for folate and B_{12} deficiencies (manifests as a macrocytic anemia), sources of blood loss (eg, GI bleeding), and confounding disease states (eg, cancer, HIV)

Hyperphosphatemia and hypocalcemia
- Serum phosphorus >4.6 mg/dL (>5.5 mg/dL in stage 5 CKD)

- Also evaluate serum calcium and the calcium times phosphorus product in conditions of hyperphosphatemia

- Hypocalcemia: corrected serum calcium <8.5 mg/dL
  * Corrected calcium = measured serum calcium + 0.8 (normal albumin – measured albumin concentration); normal serum albumin = 4.0 g/dL

- Elevated calcium times phosphorus product: >55 mg^2/dL^2 (elevated product increases risk for metastatic calcifications)

Secondary hyperparathyroidism
- Intact parathyroid hormone (iPTH) >200 pg/mL (normal iPTH ~5-65 pg/mL)

- Radiographic evidence of bone abnormalities (eg, osteitis fibrosa cystica)

Metabolic acidosis
- Serum bicarbonate (HCO$_3$) <20-22 mEq/L

- Typically have an increased anion gap: anion gap = $[Na^+] – ([Cl^-] + [HCO_3^-])$

- Signs and symptoms of chronic metabolic acidosis that develops as CKD progresses are generally not of the same magnitude as with acute metabolic acidosis (eg, hyperventilation, cardiovascular and CNS manifestations)

Treatment Principles and Goals

Progressive kidney disease
- Control underlying cause of progressive CKD (eg, diabetes, hypertension; see corresponding chapters on hypertension and diabetes)
  * Blood glucose: 80-120 mg/dL fasting, 100-140 mg/dL nonfasting
  * Target hemoglobin A$_{1c}$ ≤7.0%
  * BP goals
    • BP <130/80 mm Hg for patients with evidence of kidney disease and/or diabetes

- Prevent or minimize microalbuminuria/proteinuria.

- Slow the rate of progression of CKD (by achieving diabetes and hypertension goals and minimizing proteinuria).

- Prevent drug-induced causes of kidney disease.
  * Avoid chronic use of combinations of analgesics.
  * Minimize use of agents known to cause ARF (can develop an acute or chronic kidney disease).

- Manage secondary complications of CKD (anemia, secondary hyperparathyroidism, electrolyte abnormalities).

- Control hyperlipidemia.

- Address cardiovascular risk factors (cardiovascular disease leading cause of death in stage 5 CKD or ESRD population).

- Adjust drug doses based on kidney function.

- Avoid medications contraindicated in patients with reduced kidney function.
  * *Example:* Metformin (Glucophage®) is contraindicated in patients with elevated serum creatinine (>1.5 mg/dL for men, >1.4 mg/dL for women); increased risk of lactic acidosis.

- Preparation for kidney failure and kidney replacement therapy (ie, dialysis, transplantation) as needed

- Replacement of kidney function by dialysis and transplantation, if signs and symptoms of uremia are present

- Smoking cessation

Treatment strategies
- Diuretics for fluid balance and management of hypertension (diuretic selection based on kidney function)

- Antihypertensives with diet and lifestyle modifications for control of blood pressure (see chapter on hypertension)

- Antidiabetic agents with diet and lifestyle modifications for control of blood glucose (see chapter on diabetes)

- Angiotensin-converting enzyme inhibitors (ACEIs) and angiotensin receptor blockers to delay progression of kidney disease

- Protein restriction to 0.6-0.8 g/kg per day
  * Recommended for patients with >1 g/d proteinuria despite optimal blood pressure control with a regimen that includes an ACEI
  * Must be cautious to maintain adequate caloric intake and avoid malnutrition
  * Not to be implemented for patients <80% of their ideal body weight or with >10 g/d proteinuria

- Chronic dialysis therapy
  * Plans for dialysis therapy (hemodialysis or peritoneal dialysis) should be considered during stage 4 CKD (when GFR <25 mL/min) (see section on acute renal failure for description of dialysis)

Anemia of CKD
- Target hemoglobin 11-12 g/dL, target hematocrit 33-36%

- Iron indices: transferrin saturation ≥ 20% (range 20-50%), serum ferritin ≥100 ng/mL (range 100-800 ng/mL)

- Other goals: improve symptoms of anemia (eg, fatigue, shortness of breath), improve quality of life, improve other conditions affected by decreased oxygenation (eg, heart failure)

Treatment strategies
- Erythropoietic growth factors to stimulate red blood cell production
  * Epoetin alfa (Epogen, Procrit): subcutaneous (SC) administration preferred to intravenous (IV) administration; lower doses may be adequate with SC to achieve target hemoglobin and hematocrit (approximately $^2/_3$ the dose required for IV administration)
  * Initial doses: SC: 80-120 U/kg per week divided into 2-3 doses per week; IV administration: 120-180 U/kg per week in 3 divided doses
  * Darbepoetin alfa (Aranesp): initial dose 0.45 µg/kg IV or SC administered once weekly
  * Dose conversion required from epoetin alfa (U/wk) to darbepoetin alfa (µg/week) (Table 6)

Table 6

Dose Conversion from Epoetin Alfa to Darbepoetin Alfa

Weekly epoetin alfa dose (U/wk)	Weekly darbepoetin alfa dose (µg/wk)
<2500	6.25
2500-4999	12.5
5000-10,999	25
11,000-17,999	40
18,000-33,999	60
34,000-89,999	100
≥90,000	200

- Darbepoetin (Aranesp) package insert:
  * For patients receiving epoetin alfa 2-3 times per week, darbepoetin alfa should be administered weekly. For patients receiving epoetin alfa once per week, darbepoetin alfa should be administered every other week. To determine the darbepoetin alfa dose for every-other-week administration, multiply the weekly epoetin alfa dose by 2.

- Dose titration: allow at least 2-4 weeks before change in dose of epoetin alfa or darbepoetin alfa is made based on change in hemoglobin or hematocrit
  * If change in hemoglobin <1 g/dL (hematocrit <2-3%), increase dose by 50% (epoetin alfa) or 25% (darbepoetin alfa)
  * If change in hematocrit >6-8% (hemoglobin >2-3 g/dL), reduce dose by 25% (epoetin alfa and darbepoetin alfa)

- Iron supplementation to prevent iron deficiency as a cause of resistance to therapy with erythropoietic growth factors
  * Oral iron supplementation limited by poor absorption and often inadequate to achieve goal iron indices. May be reasonable for stage 3-4 CKD and peritoneal dialysis population. Recommended dose is 200 mg elemental iron per day.
  * Intravenous iron supplementation preferred to treat true iron deficiency and in hemodialysis patients with regular intravenous access. May administer a full course of iron, typically a 1-g total dose divided over 8-10 hemodialysis sessions (100 mg per dose for iron sucrose [Venofer] and iron dextran [InFeD, Dexferrum] or 125 mg per dose for Ferrlecit) or a larger dose administered over several hours to minimize adverse reactions. Weekly doses of of 25-125 mg may be administered to provide a maintenance dose of iron.

- Blood transfusions may be required for more severe anemia or when blood loss is a major contributing factor.

Hyperphosphatemia and hypocalcemia
- Serum phosphorus <4.6 mg/dL (stages 1-4 CKD), <5.5 mg/dL (stage 5 CKD)

- Serum calcium 8.5-10 mg/dL (recommend upper range of approximately 9.5 mg/dL in stage 5 CKD due to risk of hypercalcemia and calcifications)

- Calcium times phosphorus product <55 mg^2/dL^2

Treatment strategies
- Dietary phosphorus restriction: 800-1000 mg/d phosphorus (consult with dietitian)

- Phosphate binding agents: elemental (calcium, aluminum, magnesium) and nonelemental (sevelemer)
  * Titrate doses based on phosphorus and calcium times phosphorus product

- Removal by dialysis for stage 5 CKD patients (continue phosphorus restriction and use of phosphate binding agents with dialysis)

Hyperparathyroidism
- Intact PTH (iPTH)
  * Stage 1-3 CKD: iPTH within normal range (5-65 pg/mL)
  * Stage 4 CKD: iPTH 1-2 times normal
  * Stage 5 CKD: iPTH 2-3 times normal

- Maintain goal calcium and phosphorus concentrations

Treatment strategies
- Implement strategies to control calcium and phosphorus.

- Provide vitamin D supplementation based on stage of CKD; supplementation with the active form (calcitriol) or a vitamin D analog necessary in more severe stages of CKD (stages 4-5), supplementation with precursors (eg, ergocalciferol) may be sufficient in earlier stages.

- Control metabolic acidosis (causes bone demineralization if not controlled)

Metabolic acidosis
- Serum bicarbonate: 22-26 mEq/L

- pH: 7.35-7.45

Treatment strategies
- Administration of sodium bicarbonate or other alkali preparation
  * Gradual correction (over days to weeks) is usually appropriate for asymptomatic patients with mild to moderate acidosis (serum bicarbonate 12-20 mEq/L, pH 7.2-7.4).

- Dialysis: bicarbonate or lactate solution contained within the dialysate solution diffuses from dialysate to plasma and effectively treats metabolic acidosis.

Monitoring

Progressive kidney disease
- Patients at high risk for progressive CKD (eg, patients with diabetes and/or hypertension) should have the following monitored regularly:
  * Serum creatinine (consider limitations)
  * Creatinine clearance: assess rate of progression (mL/min per year)
  * Proteinuria: monitor at least every 5 years in patients with type 1 diabetes and at diagnosis for patients with type 2 diabetes
  * Assessment of control of hypertension and diabetes

Other monitoring
- Serum electrolytes

- Serum lipoprotein

- Drug doses based on kidney function

Anemia of CKD
- Hemoglobin, hematocrit: every 1-2 weeks after initiation of erythropoietic therapy or following a dose change and every 2-4 weeks once stable target hemoglobin and hematocrit are achieved

- Iron indices (transferrin saturation, serum ferritin), signs and symptoms of anemia

Hyperphosphatemia
- Phosphorus, calcium

Secondary hyperparathyroidism
- Parathyroid hormone, phosphorus, calcium

Metabolic acidosis
- Serum bicarbonate

- Potassium

Drug Therapy

Progressive kidney disease
- ACEIs, ARBs (see chapter on hypertension)

- Antihypertensive agents (see chapter on hypertension)

- Antidiabetic agents (see chapter on diabetes)

Anemia
- Erythropoietic agents (Table 7)

Mechanism of action
- Stimulates the division and differentiation of erythroid progenitor cells and induces the release of reticulocytes from the bone marrow into the bloodstream where they mature into erythrocytes

Patient instruction and counseling
- For self-administration (subcutaneous injections)
  * Patients may experience pain at site of injection with subcutaneous administration.
  * Always wipe the top of the vial with an alcohol pad before each use.
  * Do not shake the bottle and do not inject if you see solid material in the solution.
  * Use a new syringe with each injection.
  * Stick the need into the rubber stopper at the top of the bottle then turn the bottle upside down and hold at eye level.
  * Pull the plunger until it lines up with the appropriate number for your dose.
  * Gently tap the syringe with your finger to make any air bubbles float to the top of the syringe.
  * Inject the medication into a different place on you body each time.
  * Store vials in the refrigerator, do not freeze.

Adverse drug events
- Hypertension

- Red blood cell aplasia

Table 7

Erythropoietic Growth Factors

Generic name (trade name)	Dosage range	Dosage forms	Frequency of administration
Epoetin alfa (Epogen®, Procrit®)	80-180 U/kg	IV, SC	Divided in 1-3 doses per week
Darbepoetin alfa (Aranesp®)	0.45 µg/kg	IV, SC	Once weekly or once every other week

- Seizures (low incidence)

- Polycythemia

- Thrombocytosis

Drug-drug and drug-disease interactions
- ACEIs and ARBs may decrease the effectiveness of erythropoietic therapy.

- Causes of resistance to erythropoietic therapy:
  * Iron deficiency
  * Secondary hyperparathyroidism
  * Inflammatory conditions
  * Aluminum accumulation
  * Other disease states causing anemia (eg, cancer, HIV)

Parameters to monitor
- Hemoglobin and hematocrit

- Iron indices

- Blood pressure

Kinetics if appropriate
- Half-life:
  * Epoetin alfa: approximately 8.5 h IV, 24 h SC
  * Darbepoetin alfa: approximately 25 h IV, 48 h SC

- Effect on hematologic parameters observed over approximately 7 days to 6 weeks

- Steady-state dependent on lifespan of red blood cells and rate of red blood cell production stimulated by erythropoietin.

Other
- Epoetin alfa is supplied as single-dose, preservative-free solution (2000-, 3000-, 4000-, 10,000-, and 40,000-U/mL vials) and as a multidose, preserved solution (10,000- and 20,000-U/mL vials)

- Darbepoetin alfa is available in two solutions: a polysorbate solution and an albumin solution, supplied as single-dose vials (25-, 40-, 60-, 100-, and 200-mg/mL vials containing polysorbate) and (25-, 40-, 60-, 100-, 150-, 200-, 300-, and 500-mg/mL vials containing albumin); contains no preservative.

Iron supplementation (Table 8)
Mechanism of action
- Repletes iron stores and iron available for red blood cell production in the bone marrow. Incorporated

into hemoglobin within the red cells and facilitates transport of oxygen

Patient instructions and counseling
- Oral iron
  * May color stool black
  * Take between meals to increase absorption
  * May take with food if GI upset occurs
  * Do not take with dairy products or antacids

Adverse drug events
- Oral iron: stomach cramping, constipation, nausea, vomiting, dark stools

- Intravenous iron:
  * Anaphylactic reactions have occurred with iron dextran (InFed, Dexferrum); administer a 25-mg test dose prior to administration of the full dose. Reduced incidence of hypersensitivity reactions with sodium ferric gluconate (Ferrlecit) and iron sucrose (Venofer).
  * All preparations: observe patients for diaphoresis, nausea, vomiting, lower back pain, dyspnea, hypotension

- Iron overload: may be treated with deferoxamine (Desferal)

Drug-drug and drug-disease interactions
- Oral iron: decreased GI absorption when given with antacids, quinolones, and tetracycline; increased absorption when administered with vitamin C

- Intravenous iron: potential for increased risk of infection (administration to patients with severe systemic infections controversial)

Parameters to monitor
- Iron indices: ferritin, transferrin saturation

- Hemoglobin and hematocrit

- Monitor for anaphylactic or hypersensitivity reactions after IV administration.

Other
- Sodium ferric gluconate (Ferrlecit): supplied as colorless glass ampules containing 62.5 mg elemental iron in 5 mL (12.5 mg/mL). The 125-mg dose may be diluted in 100 mL of 0.9% sodium chloride administered IV over 1 hour or administered undiluted as an IV injection at a rate of up to 12.5 mg/min.

- Iron sucrose (Venofer): supplied in 5-mL single-dose vials containing 100 mg elemental iron (20 mg/mL).

Table 8

Iron Supplements

Generic name (trade name)	Dose	Dosage forms	Frequency of administration[1]
Ferrous sulfate (Fer-In-Sol®, Feosol®, Slow FE®)	200 mg elemental iron per day	PO	bid-tid
Ferrous fumarate (Femiron®, Vitron-C®)	200 mg elemental iron per day	PO	bid-tid
Ferrous gluconate (Fergon®)	200 mg elemental iron per day	PO	bid-tid
Polysaccharide iron (Hytinic®, Niferec®)	200 mg elemental iron per day	PO	qd-bid
Heme iron polypeptide (Proferrin-ES®)	200 mg elemental iron per day	PO	tid-qid
Sodium ferric gluconate (Ferrlecit®)	62.5-125 mg	IV	Weekly or three times per week
Iron sucrose (Venofer®)	20-100 mg	IV	Weekly or three times per week
Iron dextran (InFeD®, Dexferrum®)	25-100 mg	IV	Weekly or three times per week

[1]For oral formulations, frequency of administration dependent on amount of elemental iron per unit; must give 200 mg elemental iron per day.

The 100-mg dose may be diluted in 100 mL of 0.9% sodium chloride administered IV over at least 15 minutes or administered undiluted by slow IV injection at a rate of 20 mg/min.

- Iron dextran (InFeD, Dexferrum): supplied in 2-mL single-dose vials containing 50 mg of elemental iron per mL.

Hyperphosphatemia
- Phosphate binding agents (Table 9)

Mechanism of action
- Combines with dietary phosphate in the GI tract to form insoluble calcium phosphate that is excreted in the feces.

Patient instructions and counseling
- Take with meals and snacks.

- Do not take with oral iron salts or certain antibiotics (quinolones, tetracyclines).

- Aluminum and magnesium products are generally for short-term use (concern of accumulation in patients with kidney disease).

- Use in conjunction with dietary phosphorus restriction.

Adverse drug events
- Calcium products: hypercalcemia, nausea, vomiting, abdominal pain, constipation

Table 9

Phosphate Binding Agents

Classification	Generic name (trade names)	Dosage range
Calcium-containing	Calcium carbonate [40% elemental calcium] (Tums®, Os-Cal-500®, Nephro-Calci®, Caltrate 600®, CalCarb HD®, CaCO₃ [multiple preparations])	0.8-2 g elemental Ca
	Calcium acetate [25% elemental calcium] (Phos-Lo®)	1334-2001 mg
Nonelemental (polymer based)	Sevelamer (Renagel®)	800-1600 mg
Aluminum-containing	Aluminum hydroxide (AlternaGel®, Amphojel®, Alu-Cap®, Alu-tab®, Basaljel®)	300-600 mg
Magnesium-containing	Magnesium carbonate (Mag-Carb®)	70 mg
	Magnesium hydroxide (milk of magnesia)	300-400 mg

All these agents are taken orally and all should be taken with meals.

- Sevelamer (Renagel): decreased LDL cholesterol, increased HDL cholesterol (may be a beneficial effect)

- Aluminum: constipation, aluminum toxicity, chalky taste, cramps, nausea, vomiting

- Magnesium products: diarrhea, hypermagnesemia, cramps, muscle weakness

- All products: hypophosphatemia

Drug-drug and drug-disease interactions
- Calcium, aluminum, and magnesium products may bind with antibiotics (quinolones, tetracyclines) in the GI tract, thus decreasing their absorption.

- Sevelamer (Renagel): may contribute to metabolic acidosis and decreased lipid LDL cholesterol

Parameters to monitor
- Phosphorus, calcium, PTH

- Aluminum, magnesium (if receiving aluminum- or magnesium-containing products)

- Sevelamer (Renagel): serum bicarbonate, LDL cholesterol

Other
- Calcium carbonate: 40% elemental calcium

- Calcium acetate: 25% elemental calcium

- Aluminum and magnesium not recommended for long-term use due to potential for accumulation in patients with kidney disease

Secondary hyperparathyroidism
- Vitamin D therapy (Table 10)

Mechanism of action (active vitamin D)
- Increases intestinal absorption of calcium, tubular reabsorption of calcium by the kidney (in patients with sufficient kidney function) and suppresses release of parathyroid hormone. May also increase phosphorus via similar intestinal and renal effects

Patient instructions and counseling
- Use in conjunction with dietary recommendations for phosphorus restriction and phosphate binding agents. Therapy may need to be temporarily discontinued if calcium and phosphorus are elevated.

- Notify health care provider of any of the following (signs of hypercalcemia): weakness, headache, decreased appetite, lethargy

Adverse drug events
- Hypercalcemia: decreased potential with vitamin D analogs

- Hyperphosphatemia: decreased potential with vitamin D analogs

- Adynamic bone disease: caused by oversuppression of PTH

Drug-drug and drug-disease interactions
- Cholestyramine may decrease intestinal absorption of oral products.

- Magnesium absorption may be increased with concomitant administration.

Table 10

Vitamin D Therapy

Classification	Generic name (trade name)	Dosage range	Dosage forms	Frequency of administration
Vitamin D precursor	Ergocalciferol (Drisdol®)	400-50,000 IU	PO	qd; once per month
	Ergocalciferol (Calciferol®)	400-50,000 IU	PO, IV	qd; once per month
Active vitamin D	Calcitriol (Calcijex®)	0.5-5 µg	IV	Three times per week
	Calcitriol (Rocaltrol®)	0.25-5 µg	PO	qd; every other day, three times per week
Vitamin D analogs	Paricalcitol (Zemplar®)	2.5-15 µg	IV	Three times per week
	Doxercalciferol (Hectorol®)	5-20 µg	PO	Three times per week
		2-8 µg	IV	Three times per week

Parameters to monitor
- Parathyroid hormone

- Calcium

- Phosphorus

- Calcium times phosphorus product: vitamin D therapy may need to be temporarily discontinued if product is elevated.

- Alkaline phosphatase

- Signs of vitamin D intoxication and hypercalcemia (eg, weakness, headache, somnolence, nausea, vomiting, bone pain, polyuria)

Kinetics if appropriate
- Ergocalciferol: requires hydroxylation within the liver to calcifediol and a second hydroxylation within the kidney to the active form, calcitriol. Do not give to patients with severe kidney and/or liver disease.

- Doxercalciferol: requires conversion to its active form 1α,25-dihydroxyvitamin D_2 in the liver

Other
- Calcitriol (Calcijex): 1-mg/mL, 2-mg/mL ampules

- Calcitriol (Rocaltrol): 0.25-mg, 0.5-mg capsules

- Paricalcitol (Zemplar): 5-mg/mL vials

- Doxercalciferol: IV: 2-mg/mL ampules; PO: 2.5-mg capsules

Metabolic acidosis
- Drug therapy: see chapter on critical care

Table 11

Water-Soluble Vitamin Supplements

Generic name (trade names)

Vitamin B complex, vitamin C, folic acid (Nephrocaps®, Nephrovite®, Nephrovite Rx®, Renavite®, Biotin Forte®)

Vitamin B complex, vitamin C, folic acid, and iron (Neprhvite Rx + Iron®, NephrPlex Rx®)

Vitamin B complex (Allbee with C®)

All these are taken orally, one capsule or tablet once a day.

Nutrition
- Vitamin supplements (Table 11)

Mechanism of action
- Replace water-soluble vitamins lost during dialysis without providing supratherapeutic amounts of fat-soluble vitamins.

Patient instructions and counseling
- Take daily to replace water-soluble vitamins.

- Hemodialysis patients should take after dialysis.

Adverse drug events
- General: nausea, headache, pruritus, flushing (dependent on specific vitamin)

- Vitamin B_6 (pyridoxine): neuropathy, increased aspartate transaminase

- Vitamin C (ascorbic acid): hyperoxaluria, dizziness, diarrhea, fatigue, nausea

- Folic acid: headache, rash, pruritus

Drug-drug and drug-disease interactions
- Folic acid may decrease phenytoin concentrations by increasing metabolism.

Parameters to monitor
- Periodic folate levels

Nondrug therapy
- Preparation for renal replacement therapy when patients reach stage 4 CKD
  * Includes choice of chronic dialysis (hemodialysis or peritoneal dialysis) if patient is candidate for both modalities
  * Placement of dialysis access (graft or fistula for hemodialysis, catheter for peritoneal dialysis)

- Patient education

Diet
- Consider risk/benefit of protein restriction (0.6-0.8 g/kg per day) if patient has >1 g/d proteinuria

- Increased protein requirements for patients on dialysis (approximately 1.2 g/kg per day)

- Nutritional supplementation as needed

- Counseling by a renal dietitian beneficial to tailor diet based on stage of CKD

Renal replacement therapies
Hemodialysis
- Generally performed three times per week for 3-5 hours for patients with stage 5 kidney disease (end-stage renal disease)

- Requires a viable permanent access site (graft or fistula) or a temporary site for patients requiring immediate dialysis or with failed permanent access sites

- Complications (infection, hypotension during dialysis, clotting, dialyzer reactions)

- Drug removal: drug removal by hemodialysis most likely to occur for drugs with low molecular weight, low protein binding, and small volume of distribution.

Peritoneal dialysis
- Requires insertion of a catheter into the peritoneum

- CAPD: continuous ambulatory peritoneal dialysis

- CCPD: continuous cyclic peritoneal dialysis

- IPD: intermittent peritoneal dialysis

- Complications
  * Peritonitis
    - Most common gram-positive organisms are *Staphylococcus epidermidis, Staphylococcus aureus*
    - Most common gram-negative organisms are *Escherichia coli, Pseudomonas aeruginosa*
    - Empiric therapy should include gram-positive coverage (first-generation cephalosporin) and gram-negative coverage (ceftazidime).
    - *Note:* An aminoglycoside may be used in patients with residual urine output <100 mL/d; if used in patients with greater residual urine output, the risk of further loss of renal function increases.
    - Intraperitoneal administration of antibiotics is common.
  * Hyperglycemia from glucose content of dialysate solution.
  * Malnutrition from increased protein loss

Transplantation
- See chapter on transplantation

3. Key Points

Acute renal failure
- Prevention of kidney dysfunction in high-risk patients is the most effective strategy to address ARF.

- Conditions that put patients at increased risk of ARF include decreased perfusion to the kidney (dehydration, poor effective circulating volume such as with CHF) and administration of potential nephrotoxic agents, particularly under conditions of decreased perfusion.

- Nephrotoxic agents should be avoided when possible in patients at risk for ARF.

- Immediate recognition and treatment of ARF may prevent irreversible kidney damage.

- Goals of treatment for patients with ARF are achievement of baseline kidney function and prevention of chronic kidney disease and the need for chronic renal replacement therapy.

- Diuretics are first-line therapy in patients with ARF to maintain fluid balance and hemodynamic stability.

- A review of medications is frequently necessary to ensure appropriate dose adjustments based on kidney function (see appendix: drugs in renal failure).

Chronic kidney disease
- Chronic kidney disease is classified into stages 1-5 based on estimated glomerular filtration rate and evidence of pathological abnormalities or markers of kidney damage, including abnormalities in blood or urine tests or imaging studies.

- Screening for microalbuminuria and proteinuria is important for identifying patients with kidney disease and monitoring progression of the disease.

- Therapy to delay progression of kidney disease includes control of diabetes and hypertension, initiation of therapy with angiotensin-converting enzyme inhibitors or angiotensin receptor blockers, and protein restriction if indicated.

- Common secondary complications of CKD include anemia, fluid and electrolyte abnormalities, hyperphosphatemia, secondary hyperparathyroidism, and malnutrition.

- Management of anemia includes administration of erythropoietic agents [epoetin alfa (Epogen, Procrit) and darbepoetin alfa (Aranesp)] and iron supplementation with oral (multiple preparations) or intravenous iron [sodium ferric gluconate (Ferrlecit), iron sucrose (Venofer), iron dextran (InFeD, Dexferrum)] to achieve target hemoglobin (11-12 g/dL) and hematocrit (33-36%), while preventing iron deficiency.

- Hyperphosphatemia is managed by dietary phosphorus restriction, use of phosphate binding agents [calcium-containing products, sevelamer (Renagel), and short-term use of aluminum-containing products], and dialysis.

- Management of secondary hyperparathyroidism includes control of serum calcium and phosphorus and administration of vitamin D therapy including vitamin D precursors in early CKD based on kidney function [ergocalciferol (Drisdol, Calciferol)] and active vitamin D therapy for more severe kidney disease [calcitriol (Calcijex, Rocaltrol), paricalcitol (Zemplar), doxercalciferol (Hectorol)].

- Nutritional requirements must be re-evaluated based on severity of kidney disease (eg, protein restriction to delay progression of CKD versus increased protein requirements for patients on dialysis]

4. Questions and Answers

1. R.T. is a 45-year-old female admitted to the hospital after fainting while at work. Her past medical history includes type 1 diabetes and rheumatoid arthritis. Her only complaint is that she has had difficulty over the last 5 days keeping down anything she eats or drinks. She has also noticed a decrease in urination over the last 24 hours. Regular medications include aspirin 325 mg qd, celecoxib 200 mg qd for arthritis, metformin 500 mg qd, Triphasil 1 qd, and Tylenol prn headache. Laboratory values in the emergency department showed a serum creatinine of 2.0 mg/dL and BUN 56 mg/dL, consistent with acute renal failure. Her labs from one month ago at a regular check up had been normal. The most likely etiology of RT's acute renal failure is:

    A. Dehydration from poor oral intake
    B. Trauma from fainting
    C. Age-related decreases in kidney function
    D. Kidney failure caused by diabetes
    E. Obstruction of urine outflow

2. Which of the following medications may have contributed to R.T.'s acute renal failure?

    A. Aspirin
    B. Celecoxib
    C. Metformin
    D. Triphasil
    E. Tylenol

3. Which of the following diuretics may retain its effectiveness at glomerular filtration rates less than 30 mL/min?

    A. Hydrochlorothiazide
    B. Chlorothiazide
    C. Metolazone
    D. Spironolactone
    E. Aldactone

4. Which of the following fluid and electrolyte abnormalities typically occur in patients with severe kidney dysfunction (ie, creatinine clearance <15 mL/min)?

    I. Metabolic alkalosis
    II. Hyperkalemia
    III. Hyperphosphatemia

    A. I only

B. III only
C. I and II only
D. II and III only
E. I, II, and III

5. Which set of laboratory values is most consistent with a patient in acute intrinsic renal failure?

A. Urinary granular casts absent, FE_{Na} <1, urinary osmolality 600 mOsm/kg
B. Urinary granular casts absent, FE_{Na} >1, urinary osmolality 600 mOsm/kg
C. Urinary granular casts present, FE_{Na} <1, urinary osmolality 300 mOsm/kg
D. Urinary granular casts present, FE_{Na} >1, urinary osmolality 300 mOsm/kg
E. Acute intrinsic kidney failure can only be diagnosed by biopsy

6. Which of the following diuretics would be most appropriate for the initial treatment of a patient with acute renal failure?

I. Metolazone
II. Spironolactone
III. Furosemide

A. I only
B. III only
C. I and II only
D. II and III only
E. I, II, and III

7. A patient with nephrotoxicity caused by genta-micin would likely present with an increase in serum creatinine

A. Immediately after starting therapy and nonoliguria
B. Immediately after starting therapy and oliguria
C. 5-7 days after starting therapy and oliguria
D. 5-7 days after starting therapy and nonoliguria
E. Within 24 hours with excessive diuresis

8. Lisinopril may cause hemodynamically-mediated renal failure by preventing which of the following compensatory mechanisms by the kidney?

A. Vasodilation of the afferent arteriole
B. Vasoconstriction of the afferent arteriole
C. Vasodilation of the efferent arteriole
D. Vasoconstriction of the efferent arteriole

E. Vasodilation of both the afferent and efferent arterioles

9. The estimated creatinine clearance for a 47-year-old male patient with an ideal body weight of 176 lbs (less than actual body weight) and a serum creatinine of 2.2 mg/dL is

A. 32 mL/min
B. 40 mL/min
C. 47 mL/min
D. 93 mL/min
E. 120 mL/min

10. D.K. is a 53-year-old female (ideal body weight = 65 kg) with hypertension and hypercho-lesterolemia who is seen in the outpatient nephrology clinic for evaluation of kidney disease progression. Her current BP is 156/82, SCr 2.6 mg/dL, BUN 44 mg/dL, and urinary protein 800 mg/d. Her medications are enalapril 20 mg/d x 1 year and simvastatin 20 mg qd x 2 years. Based on D.K.'s estimated creatinine clearance, she would be classified in which of the following stages of chronic kidney disease (CKD)?

A. Stage 1
B. Stage 2
C. Stage 3
D. Stage 4
E. Stage 5

11. The recommended target blood pressure for D.K. is

A. <110/70 mm Hg
B. <130/85 mm Hg
C. <130/80 mm Hg
D. <140/95 mm Hg
E. <140/90 mm Hg

12. Which of the following would be most beneficial in a patient with type I diabetes and microalbuminuria to delay progression of CKD?

I. Angiotensin-converting enzyme inhibitor
II. Angiotensin receptor blocker
III. Loop diuretic

A. I only
B. III only
C. I and II only
D. II and III only
E. I, II, and III

13. Epoetin alfa and darbepoetin alfa stimulate erythropoiesis by which of the following?

    A. Preventing excessive red blood cell destruction
    B. Preventing degradation of bone marrow stem cells
    C. Differentiation of peritubular interstitial cells of the kidney
    D. Increasing the size of red blood cells produced in the bone marrow
    E. Differentiation of erythroid progenitor stem cells in the bone marrow

14. When administered intravenously, darbepoetin alfa has a terminal half-life approximately ___ that of epoetin alfa.

    A. equal to
    B. twofold longer than
    C. twofold shorter than
    D. threefold longer than
    E. threefold shorter than

15. One of the most commonly reported adverse reactions with epoetin alfa and darbepoetin alfa is

    A. Nausea
    B. Hypertension
    C. Constipation
    D. Anemia
    E. Anaphylaxis

16. At least _____ should be allowed to lapse before a change in dose of epoetin alfa or darbepoetin alfa is made based on change in hemoglobin and hematocrit.

    A. 1 week
    B. 2-4 weeks
    C. 6-8 weeks
    D. 2 months
    E. 4 months

17. R.A. is a 42-year-old 70-kg male on hemodialysis three times per week (TIW) who receives epoetin alfa for treatment of anemia. He has been stable on an epoetin dose of 4000 U intravenously TIW with an average hemoglobin of 11 g/dL (hematocrit of 33%). Over the last 3 months, his hematocrit has dropped to 28%. Iron indices reveal the following: ferritin 78 ng/mL, transferrin saturation 12%. The best initial treatment for RA is to

    A. Increase the dose of epoetin alfa to maintain a hemoglobin of 11-12 g/dL (hematocrit of 33-36%)
    B. Withhold epoetin alfa therapy until hemoglobin increases to 12g/dL
    C. Administer intravenous iron (sodium ferric gluconate) at a maintenance dose of 125 mg per week
    D. Administer a 1-gram total dose of intravenous iron (sodium ferric gluconate) divided over eight hemodialysis sessions
    E. Begin oral ferrous sulfate 325 mg three times per day

18. In the gastrointestinal tract, calcitriol promotes

    A. Absorption of calcium and inhibits absorption of phosphorus
    B. Absorption of phosphorus and inhibits absorption of calcium
    C. Absorption of both calcium and phosphorus
    D. Decreased binding of calcium and phosphorus
    E. Increased elimination of calcium and phosphorus

19. J.T. is a 63-year-old female with stage 5 CKD (end-stage renal disease) receiving peritoneal dialysis. Her most recent laboratory analysis reveals the following: BUN 58 mg/dL, SCr 5.2 mg/dL, phosphorus 7.4 mg/dL, calcium 9.0 mg/dL, albumin 2.5 g/dL, and iPTH 542 pg/mL (normal 10-65 pg/mL). In addition to dietary restriction, which one of the following agents is best for initial management of R.J.'s hyperphosphatemia?

    A. Sevelamer
    B. Aluminum hydroxide
    C. Calcium carbonate
    D. Calcium acetate
    E. Ferrous sulfate

20. J.T. should be instructed to take her phosphate binder

    A. With meals to enhance phosphorus absorption
    B. With meals to minimize phosphorus absorption
    C. Between meals to avoid food-drug interactions
    D. Between meals to minimize GI side effects
    E. There are no specific instructions to follow with regard to meals

21. Which of the following agents is appropriate for a patient with stage 5 CKD and secondary hyperparathyroidism requiring treatment to reduce iPTH?

    I. Calcitriol
    II. Paricalcitol
    III. Ergocalciferol

    A. I only
    B. III only
    C. I and II only
    D. II and III only
    E. I, II, and III

22. A drug with which of the following characteristics is most likely to be removed by hemodialysis (fu = fraction unbound, Vd = volume of distribution, MW = molecular weight)?

    A. fu 0.05, Vd 0.2 L/kg, MW 800
    B. fu 0.05, Vd 0.2 L/kg, MW 400
    C. fu 0.30, Vd 0.6 L/kg, MW 1500
    D. fu 0.95, Vd 0.2 L/kg, MW 800
    E. fu 0.95, Vd 6 L/kg, MW 400

23. The best antibiotic selection for empiric treatment of peritonitis in a patient with urine output >100 mL/d is

    A. Cefazolin + gentamicin
    B. Cefazolin + ceftazidime
    C. Vancomycin alone
    D. Cefazolin alone
    E. Gentamicin alone

24. Which of the following supplements should be recommended daily in a patient with stage 5 CKD requiring chronic hemodialysis?

    A. Multivitamin
    B. Nephrocaps
    C. Vitamin A
    D. Nephrocaps + Vitamin A
    E. Folic acid only

Answers

1. **A.** Dehydration is the most likely cause of ARF in R.T. since she has had a decrease in oral intake over the last 5 days. This would be classified as a prerenal cause of ARF. Fainting was likely a result of dehydration and not the cause of her decline in kidney function. A serum creatinine of 2.0 mg/dL would not be considered normal in a 45-year-old, eliminating age as a rationale for kidney disease. Diabetes would be more likely to cause a chronic decrease in her kidney function as opposed to an acute change (labs from 1 month ago were normal, ruling out evidence of chronic kidney disease). She has had some urine output in the last 24 hours, which rules out obstruction.

2. **B.** COX-II inhibitors are associated with hemodynamic changes (in particular they prevent the compensatory vasodilation of the afferent arteriole that occurs in conditions of prerenal acute renal failure). Metformin is not a cause of ARF in this case, but would need to be discontinued at this time because of the risk of lactic acidosis in a patient with decreased renal function (serum creatinine >1.4 in females, >1.5 in males).

3. **C.** There is some evidence that metolazone is beneficial in patients with kidney disease and a GFR <30 mL/min. This is not the case with other thiazide or thiazide-like diuretics or with potassium-sparing diuretics. Metolazone is frequently used in combination with loop diuretics for this reason.

4. **D.** Hyperkalemia and hyperphosphatemia are common electrolyte abnormalities observed as kidney function decreases. Metabolic acidosis is also common, not metabolic alkalosis.

5. **D.** Acute intrinsic renal failure is generally characterized by the presence of granular casts (indicating structural damage), a fractional excretion of sodium greater than 1, and a urine osmolality similar to that of plasma osmolality (indicating changes in concentrating ability of the kidney).

6. **B.** A patient with acute renal failure generally requires aggressive diuresis (while avoiding dehydration). Furosemide is a loop diuretic that is more potent than a thiazide-like diuretic (metolazone) or a potassium-sparing diuretic (spironolactone) and would be a rational choice for initial therapy of ARF.

7. **D.** Aminoglycoside-induced nephrotoxicity is characterized by a delay in changes in serum creatinine (approximately 5-7 days) and relatively normal urine output (nonoliguria).

8. **D.** Angiotensin-converting enzyme inhibitors may contribute to development of acute renal

failure in patients with conditions resulting in prerenal kidney disease (eg, conditions resulting in decreased perfusion of the kidney such as hypovolemia, heart failure, liver disease, etc). ACEIs (and angiotensin receptor blockers) prevent the compensatory vasoconstriction of the efferent arteriole mediated by angiotensin II that occurs in an attempt to increase GFR.

9. **C.** Using the Cockcroft-Gault equation to estimate creatinine clearance, this patient has an estimated creatinine clearance of 47 mL/min.

$$CrCl = \frac{(140 - age) \ (IBW \ in \ kg)}{72 \times SCr \ (mg/dL)}$$

IBW (kg) = 176 lbs/2.2 = 80 kg
SCr = 2.2 mg/dL

10. **D.** D.K.'s estimated creatinine clearance determined using the Cockcroft-Gault equation is 26 mL/min, classified as stage 4 CKD (GFR 15-29 mL/min).

$$CrCl = \frac{(140 - age) \ (IBW \ in \ kg)}{72 \times SCr \ (mg/dL)}$$

with the result multiplied by .85 for a female.

11. **C.** The recommended BP for D.K. is <130/80 mm Hg since she has kidney disease.

12. **C.** ACEIs and angiotensin receptor blockers (ARBs) are advocated for patients with diabetes and microalbuminuria. The decreases in glomerular pressure caused by these agents that are detrimental in patients with acute renal failure are beneficial in a chronic condition such as diabetes, in which sustained elevations in glomerular pressure result in worsening kidney disease over time.

13. **E.** Erythropoietic agents including epoetin alfa and darbepoetin alfa work in the bone marrow to stimulate differentiation of erythroid progenitor stem cells and result in an increase in red blood cell production (increase erythrocytes).

14. **D.** The half-life of darbepoetin alfa is three times longer than epoetin alfa, giving this agent the added benefit of reduced frequency of administration.

15. **B.** Hypertension is the most common adverse effect in patients receiving erythropoietic agents.

16. **B.** Stimulation of erythropoiesis by epoetin alfa and darbepoetin alfa occurs immediately;

however, it will take at least 2-4 weeks before substantial changes in hemoglobin and hematocrit are observed as a result of any change in dose of erythropoietic therapy.

17. **D.** R.A. is iron deficient as indicated by his low serum ferritin (<100 ng/mL) and transferrin saturation (<20%). No change in epoetin alfa should be made until iron deficiency is corrected (this is the leading cause of resistance to epoetin alfa/darbepoetin alfa therapy). R.A. will require a full course of iron (1 gram administered intravenously in divided doses with each dialysis session) as opposed to a maintenance dose, which should be administered once R.A. is iron replete. Sodium ferric gluconate may be administered in doses of 125 mg per dialysis session for 8 dialysis sessions to give the total 1-gram dose (iron sucrose and iron dextran would be administered in 100-mg increments over 10 hemodialysis sessions). Absorption of oral iron is poor, making intravenous iron preferred in this hemodialysis patient.

18. **C.** Active vitamin D (calcitriol) promotes absorption of both calcium and phosphorus in the GI tract. This is one reason that therapy with calcitriol or a vitamin D analog may need to be withheld if the calcium times phosphorus product is elevated.

19. **A.** Sevelamer (Renagel) is best for initial management since J.T. has a corrected calcium of 10.2 mg/dL [corrected calcium = measured calcium + (0.8 x (4 − measured serum albumin))] and a calcium times phosphorus product of 75 mg^2/dL^2. This elevated product increases the risk of metastatic calcifications. She requires a phosphorus binding agent without calcium to minimize calcium absorbed in the GI tract.

20. **B.** Phosphate binders must be taken with meals to allow binding with dietary phosphorus.

21. **C.** Calcitriol and paricalcitol are active forms of vitamin D that do not require conversion in the liver or kidney. Ergocalciferol is a vitamin D precursor that does require activation and would not be beneficial for a patient with stage 5 CKD without the necessary activity of the enzyme in the kidney (α-1-hydroxylase) responsible for final conversion to the active form.

22. **D.** Drug characteristics that make an agent more

likely to be removed by dialysis include low protein binding, small volume of distribution, and small molecular weight. Among the choices the agent that best meets these criteria is choice D, which has a high fraction unbound in the plasma, a low volume of distribution, and a relatively small molecular weight.

23. **B.** Empiric therapy should include antibiotics with gram-positive and gram-negative coverage (choices A and B). Choice B is most appropriate since this patient has some residual renal function (urine output >100 mL/d) and use of gentamicin for a patient with this degree of urine output is not preferred over other agents such as ceftazidime.

24. **B.** Nephrocaps include water soluble vitamins (vitamin B complex + vitamin C + folic acid) recommended for a patient with kidney failure. Supplementation with fat-soluble vitamins is not recommended in patients with kidney failure due to toxicities associated with accumulation.

5. References

**Acute renal failure and
drug-induced kidney disease**
DuBose TD, Warnock DG, Mehta RL, et al. Acute renal failure in the 21st century: recommendations for management and outcomes assessment. *Am J Kidney Dis.* 1997;29:793-799.

Hock R, Anderson RJ. Prevention of drug-induced nephrotoxicity in the intensive care unit. *J Crit Care.* 1995;10:33-43.

Nolin TD, Abraham PA, Matzke GR. Drug-induced renal disease. In: DiPiro J, et al. eds. *Pharmacotherapy: A Pathophysiologic Approach*, 5th ed. New York: McGraw-Hill; 2002:889-905.

Wood AJJ. Diuretic therapy. *N Engl J Med.* 1998; 339:387-395.

Chronic kidney disease and progression
Chobanian AV, et al and the National High Blood Pressure Education Program Coordinating committee. The Seventh Report of the Joint National Committee on Prevention, Detection, Evaluation, and Treatment of High Blood Pressure: the JNC 7 report. *JAMA.* 2003;289:2560-2572.

National Kidney Foundation. NKF-K/DOQI Clinical Practice Guidelines for Chronic Kidney Disease: Evaluation, Classification, and Stratification. *Am J Kidney Dis.* 2002;39:S1-S266.

U.S. Renal Data System, USRDS 2002 Annual Data Report: Atlas of End-Stage Renal Disease in the United States. National Institutes of Health, National Institute of Diabetes and Digestive and Kidney Diseases, Bethesda, MD: 2002.

National Kidney Foundation Task Force on CVD Report. *Am J Kidney Dis.* 1998;32:853-906.

Anemia
American Reagent Laboratories, Inc. Venofer® (iron sucrose injection) package insert. Shirley, NY: American Reagent Laboratories, Inc., 2000.

Amgen Inc. Aranesp® (darbepoetin alfa) package insert. Thousand Oaks, CA: Amgen Inc, 2001.

Macdougall IC, Gray SJ, Elston O, et al. Pharmacokinetics of novel erythropoiesis stimulating protein compared with epoetin alfa in dialysis patients. *J Am Soc Nephrol.* 1999;10:2392-2395.

National Kidney Foundation. K/DOQI Clinical Practice Guidelines for Anemia of Chronic Kidney Disease. Update 2000 . *Am J Kidney Dis.* 2001; 37(suppl 1):S182-238 [erratum in *Am J Kidney Dis.* 2001;38:442].

Watson Pharmaceuticals, Inc. Ferrlecit® (sodium ferric gluconate complex in sucrose injection) package insert. Corona, CA: Watson Pharmaceuticals, Inc., 2001.

Hyperphosphatemia and secondary hyperparathyroidism
Chertow GM, Dillon M, Burke SK, et al. A randomized trial of sevelamer hydrochloride (RenaGel) with and without supplemental calcium. Strategies for the control of hyperphosphatemia and hyperparathyroidism in hemodialysis patients. *Clin Nephrol.* 1999;51:18-26.

Hruska KA, Teitelbaum SL. Renal osteodystrophy. *N Engl J Med.* 1995;333:166-174.

Yudd M, Llach F. Current medical management of secondary hyperparathyroidism. *Am J Med Sci.* 2000; 320:100-106.

Nutrition
National Kidney Foundation. K/DOQI Clinical Practice Guidelines for Nutrition in Chronic Renal Failure. *Am J Kidney Dis.* 2000;35(suppl 2):S1-S140.

Other
Aronoff GR, Bennett WM, Berns JS, et al. *Drug Prescribing in Renal Failure: Dosing Guidelines for Adults,* 4th ed. American College of Physicians: 1999.

Ifudu O. Care of patients undergoing hemodialysis. *N Engl J Med.* 1998;339:1054-1062.

National Kidney Foundation. Kidney Disease Outcomes Quality Initiative. Clinical practice guidelines for peritoneal dialysis adequacy: update 2000. Available at http://www.kidney.org/professionals/doqi/guidelines/doqi_uptoc.html#pd

17. Critical Care, Fluids, and Electrolytes

G. Christopher Wood, PharmD, BCPS
Assistant Professor, Department of Pharmacy
University of Tennessee College of Pharmacy
Clinical Pharmacist
Regional Medical Center, Memphis, Tennessee

1. Sedation, Analgesia, and Neuromuscular Blockade

Overview

Definition and classifications
- Pain: critically ill patients may experience both acute and chronic pain
- Anxiety/agitation: psychophysiologic response to real or imagined danger ("agitation" for rest of chapter)
- ICU delirium ("delirium" for rest of chapter): see clinical presentation

Clinical presentation
- Pain/agitation: examples in patients with impaired consciousness:
  * Pulling tubes/lines, writhing, kicking, restlessness, hypertension, tachycardia, tachypnea, diaphoresis, moaning
- Delirium: fluctuating, disorganized thinking or inattentiveness not due to an obviously reversible cause; with or without agitation

Pathophysiology
- Injuries
- Medical procedures/equipment (eg, mechanical ventilation, catheters)
- Mental status changes (eg, fear, infection, hypoxia, sleep deprivation, adverse drug effects/withdrawal)
- Preexisting medical conditions (eg, chronic pain)

Diagnostic Criteria
- Pain: use a verbal or visual scale to assess severity
  * For unconscious patients, use physical signs/symptoms
- Agitation: use a validated scale to assess (eg, Riker sedation-agitation scale)
- Delirium: use Confusion Assessment Method for the ICU (CAM-ICU scale)

Treatment goals
- Find and remove the cause of pain/agitation/delirium
- Achieve a balance between patient comfort, adverse effects, and ability to provide care
- Reserve neuromuscular blocking agents (NMBs) for patients who are not controlled with maximum doses of sedation and analgesia

Mechanism of action (Table 1)
- Opiates, NSAIDs: see chapter on pain management
- Benzodiazepines, haloperidol: see chapter on psychiatric disease

- Propofol: unknown, possible GABA-related activity
- NMBs: postsynaptic cholinergic receptor antagonists; do not provide analgesia or sedation

Patient instructions
- Patient-controlled analgesia (PCA) pumps; make sure patient understands how to activate a dose

Adverse drug events
- Opiates, NSAIDs: see chapter on pain management
- Benzodiazepines, haloperidol: see chapter on psychiatric disease
- Propofol: respiratory depression, hypotension, hypertriglyceridemia
- Neuromuscular blockers: respiratory depression, prolonged weakness/paralysis after discontinuation, tachycardia with pancuronium (this is the reason for using vecuronium if hemodynamically unstable or history of cardiac disease)

Drug interactions
- Opiates, NSAIDs: see chapter on pain management
- Benzodiazepines, haloperidol: see chapter on psychiatric disease
- Propofol: actions potentiated by other sedatives
- Neuromuscular blockers:
  * Action potentiated by corticosteroids, aminoglycosides, clindamycin, calcium channel blockers, anesthetics
  * Action inhibited by anticholinesterase inhibitors (eg, neostigmine)

Parameters to monitor
- Opiates, NSAIDs: use visual or verbal scale to assess efficacy, monitor HR, BP, RR (see also chapter on pain management)
- Benzodiazepines, haloperidol: use validated scale, monitor HR, BP, RR (see also chapter on psychiatric disease)
- Propofol:
  * Level of sedation (use validated scale)
  * BP, HR, RR, ICP
  * Serum triglycerides at baseline and 1-2 times a week if long term use
- Neuromuscular blockers:
  * Peripheral nerve stimulation ("train of four") highly recommended
  * Movement/spontaneous breathing
  * BP, HR, ICP (acute increases may indicate suboptimal sedation/analgesia)
- In patients with continuous sedation, a daily wakening and assessment period results in decreased sedative use and ICU length of stay

Table 1

Select Drug Therapy Based on Guidelines for Use in ICU Patients

Generic (trade) name	Dosage range	Forms[1]	Schedule[2]	Notes on usage
Morphine sulfate (generic)	0.5-10 mg	IV, IM, PO	Continuous; q6h	General opiate of choice
Hydromorphone (Dilaudid®)	0.3-1.5 mg	IV	Continuous; q6h	Use in morphine intolerance, hemodynamic instability, or renal dysfunction
Fentanyl (Sublimaze®)	50-200 µg/h	IV	Continuous	Same as hydromorphone
Acetaminophen (Tylenol®)	Up to 4 g/d	PO, PR	q4-6h	NSAIDs may be added to opiates
Ketorolac (Toradol®)	10-30 mg	IV, IM, PO	q6h	Maximum use 5 days
Lorazepam (Ativan®)	0.5-4 mg	IV, PO	Continuous; q6h	Long-term sedation (>24-72 h)
Midazolam (Versed®)	1-5 mg	IV	Continuous; q2h	Acute and short term (<24-72 h)
Propofol (Diprivan®)	0.5-5 mg/kg/h	IV	Continuous	Use when rapid awakening needed
Haloperidol (Haldol®)	2-5 mg	IV, PO	q1-4h	Drug of choice for delirium
Pancuronium (Pavulon®)	0.05-0.1 mg/kg	IV	Continuous; q2h	General NMB of choice (low cost)
Vecuronium (Norcuron®)	0.05-0.1 mg/kg	IV	Continuous; q1h	Use in hemodynamic instability, renal dysfunction, cardiac disease
Cisatracurium (Nimbex®)	0.05-0.1 mg/kg	IV	Continuous; q1h	Use in renal and hepatic dysfunction

[1]Long-acting drugs and dosage forms generally not used in ICU (eg, fentanyl patch, CR morphine, doxacurium).

[2]Continuous analgesia and sedation with frequent titration (PCA pump, IV infusion, or scheduled) preferred to prn therapy alone. NMBs used prn are preferred.

Kinetics

- Opiates, NSAIDs: see chapter on pain management
- Benzodiazepines, haloperidol: see chapter on psychiatric disease
- Propofol: highly lipophilic (may accumulate long term), rapid onset (1 min), short duration (~10 min)
- Neuromuscular blockers:
  * Onset for all <5 min
  * Duration: pancuronium, 60-90 min; vecuronium, cisatracurium; 30-60 min
  * Excretion: pancuronium, mostly renal; vecuronium, ~50:50 hepatic:renal; cisatracurium, not organ dependent

Other

- Propofol is in a lipid vehicle
  * Provides 1 kcal/mL
  * Potential growth medium for bacteria; 12-hour maximum hang time for a bottle
  * Use with caution in egg allergy; uses egg-based emulsifier

2. Traumatic Brain Injury

Overview

Definition
• Neurologic deficit secondary to brain trauma

Classifications
• Severe
• Mild/moderate

Clinical Presentation
• Use Glasgow Coma Scale (GCS) for assessment; sum of eye, motor, and verbal scores (range 3-15)
• Wide range of presentation from mild confusion to totally nonresponsive coma

Pathophysiology
• Motor vehicle accidents (most common), falls/accidents, assaults, gunshot wounds
• Most common in 15-24 year age group; 375,000 cases and 75,000 deaths per year
• Consists of: direct neuronal damage ± edema ± secondary ischemia-related neuronal death

Diagnostic criteria
• CT scan
• GCS
• Intracranial pressure (ICP) monitoring in severe patients (GCS 3-8)

Treatment goals
• Improved outcomes with cerebral perfusion pressure (CPP) kept >60 mm Hg and intracranial pressure (ICP) <20 mm Hg (CPP = mean arterial pressure – ICP)
• Seizure prevention

Strategies to decrease ICP
• Osmotic agents/diuretics
    * Mannitol 0.25-1 g/kg IV q4h
    * Loop diuretics IV (eg, furosemide)
    * Hypertonic NaCl IV (eg, 3%, 7.5%)
• Sedation: short-acting agent preferred to allow frequent patient assessment (propofol, morphine, fentanyl, midazolam)
    * Pentobarbital 1-3 mg/kg/h IV: long-acting agent for refractory intracranial hypertension
• NMBs: short-acting agent preferred (vecuronium); used for refractory intracranial hypertension

Nondrug interventions
• Raise head of the bed 30°
• Ventricular drainage of CSF via ventriculostomy

• Mild/moderate hyperventilation (PCO_2 30-35 mm Hg)
• Surgery

Strategies to increase MAP
• Maximize fluid status; overall goal is euvolemia
• Vasopressors/inotropes may be used in shock after fluid status is optimized

Seizure prevention (may be started based on severity and type of injury)
• Phenytoin (Dilantin®, generic) 20 mg/kg IV loading dose + 4-8 mg/kg/d x 7 days
    * Continue beyond 7 days if patient has a seizure
    * Alternative agent: carbamazepine
• See chapter on epilepsy for mechanism of action, adverse drug events, drug interactions, and kinetics

Parameters to Monitor
• Overall goal of CPP >60 mm Hg and ICP <20 mm Hg; drug classes covered elsewhere

3. Acute Spinal Cord Injury

Overview

Definition
- Traumatic spinal cord injury with neurologic impairment

Classifications
- Complete: total loss of motor and sensory function in affected areas
- Incomplete: some motor and/or sensory function retained in affected areas
- Paraplegia: neurologic deficit in the lower extremities
- Quadriplegia: neurologic deficit in the upper and lower extremities
- Central cord syndrome: atypical presentation of symptoms

Clinical presentation
- Loss of motor and/or sensory function from nerves distal to level of vertebral injury
- Symptoms usually bilaterally symmetrical

Pathophysiology
- See traumatic brain injury

Diagnostic criteria
- Physical examination consistent with SCI plus CT and/or radiographic evidence of injury

Treatment goals
- Preservation/restoration of motor and sensory function

Drug Therapy

- Methylprednisolone: 30 mg/kg IV loading dose, then 5.4 mg/kg/h IV infusion:
    * Continued for a total of 24 hours if loading dose given within 3 hours of injury
    * Continued for a total of 48 hours if loading dose given 3-8 hours from injury
- No methylprednisolone if >8 hours from injury or for penetrating injuries

Mechanism of action
- Protects neurons by inhibiting lipid peroxidation

Adverse drug effects
- Increased infections (48 h worse than 24 h)
- Hyperglycemia

Parameters to monitor
- Neurologic status
- Serum glucose

4. Venous Thromboembolism Prophylaxis

Overview

Definition
• Venous thromboembolism (VTE): pathogenic blood clot formation

Classifications
• Deep venous thrombosis (DVT): VTE in a large vein, generally in lower extremity
• Proximal (iliac) more likely to embolize; distal (popliteal) 4-5 times more common
• Pulmonary embolism (PE): DVT that has embolized to the pulmonary vasculature
  * 10-100 times less common than DVT

Clinical presentations
• DVT: often asymptomatic
  * Unilateral leg symptoms: swelling, pain, tenderness, erythema, warmth, ± palpable cord
  * Pain behind the knee upon dorsiflexion (Homan's sign)
• PE: often asymptomatic
  * Pulmonary symptoms: chest pain, cough, dyspnea, tachypnea, hemoptysis
  * May proceed rapidly to life-threatening shock and hypoxia

Pathophysiology
Three general risk factors
• Hypercoagulable states
  * Clotting factor deficiencies/abnormalities (eg, protein C or S deficiency)
  * Malignancy, pregnancy, estrogen use
• Direct vessel trauma
• Venous stasis: poor blood flow allows clot formation

Specific risk factors
• Age: risk increases with age; >40 and >60 years of age are important cutoffs
• Immobility, previous VTE, obesity, CHF
• Major surgery or trauma: worse in lower extremity, pelvis; GU, neurologic injury

Epidemiology
• ~600,000 hospitalizations in U.S. yearly with ~60,000 deaths (10% mortality)
• Incidence of distal DVT ranges from 2-80% based on risk factors

Diagnostic criteria
• Radiocontrast dye studies (venography for DVT, pulmonary angiography for PE)
  * Considered the gold standard
  * Invasive, expensive, require expertise, significant adverse events (eg, nephropathy)
• Ultrasonography (for DVT)
  * Noninvasive, inexpensive, performed at bedside, but less sensitive for diagnosis
• Ventilation/perfusion scan (for PE)
  * Less invasive, but inconclusive results are common and require further testing
• Serum D-dimer concentrations: normal levels may rule out VTE

Treatment goals
• Decrease the significant morbidity (VTE recurrence), mortality, and costs of VTE
• VTE prophylaxis is underused: only 35-50% of at-risk patients receive it

Drug Therapy to Treat Venous Thromboembolism

• Full-dose IV heparin (80 units/kg load + 18 units/kg/h) or high-dose low molecular weight heparin (LMWH) SC (enoxaparin 1 mg/kg q12h or 1.5 mg/kg qd)
  * LMWH may be used outpatient in stable DVT patients
  * May give full-dose heparin SC bid (rarely done)
• Warfarin: begin concurrently, discontinue heparin/LMWH when INR therapeutic (usually 2-3) and stable
  * Duration: 3-6 months in most patients, 12 months or longer in recurrence or high risk
• Direct thrombin inhibitors: use in place of heparin for heparin-induced thrombocytopenia
• Thrombolytic therapy: (eg, alteplase [tPA, tissue plasminogen activator]); reserve for very severe cases; highly individualized
• Inferior vena cava filter: reserve for select patients with contraindication to anticoagulation

Drug Therapy to Prevent Venous Thromboembolism (Table 2)

Mechanism of action
• Heparin: binds to antithrombin and potentiates its anticoagulation (anti IIa activity > anti Xa)
• LMWHs – same as heparin but anti Xa activity > anti IIa
  * There is some controversy over the interchangeability of these drugs because different LMWHs have different Xa:IIa activity ratios
• Fondaparinux: factor Xa inhibitor
• Warfarin: see chapter on arrhythmias

Table 2

Drug and Nondrug Therapy for Prevention of Venous Thromboembolism

Patient group	Recommended therapy
Medical conditions	
General medical patient with risk factor	LDUH, LMWH
Acute MI	LDUH, full dose IV heparin
Ischemic stroke	LDUH, LMWH; alternatives: IPC, ES
General surgery: begin preoperatively, generally continue until ambulatory or discharged	
Low risk	
Minor procedure without risk factors	Early ambulation
Moderate to high risk	
Minor procedure + risk factor or major procedure ± risk factor	LDUH, LMWH, IPC, or ES
Highest risk	
Major procedure + multiple risk factors	LDUH, LMWH + IPC and/or ES (combine drug + mechanical)
Orthopedic surgery or trauma	
Hip replacement	LMWH, warfarin (INR 2-3) ± IPC or ES; alternatives: full dose IV heparin ± IPC or ES, fondaparinux
Knee replacement	LMWH, warfarin (INR 2-3); alternatives: fondaparinux
Hip fracture	LMWH, warfarin (INR 2-3); alternatives: LDUH, fondaparinux
Neurosurgery	IPC ± ES; may add LDUH, LMWH when bleeding stopped
Major trauma	LMWH, use IPC ± ES if actively bleeding
Acute spinal cord injury	LMWH ± IPC, ES; convert to warfarin (INR 2-3) in rehabilitation

LDUH = low-dose unfractionated heparin (generic) 5000 units SC q8-12h.

LMWH = low molecular weight heparin:

    Dalteparin (Fragmin®): 2500-5000 units SC qd; enoxaparin (Lovenox): 20-40 mg SC qd or 30 mg SC q12h; tinzaparin (Innohep®): 3500 units to 75 units/kg SC qd.

Fondaparinux (Arixtra®): 2.5 mg SC qd.

IPC = intermittent pneumatic compression; may add to efficacy of drugs; noncompliance is high.

ES = elastic compression stockings; may add to efficacy of drugs.

Hip replacement, knee replacement, or hip fracture: optimal duration unknown, treat at least 7-10 days.

Major trauma: start within 36 h of injury; routine vena cava filter placement not recommended.

- Direct thrombin inhibitors (lepirudin [Refludan®], argatroban): directly inhibit thrombin

Patient instructions and counseling

- Heparin, fondaparinux, thrombin inhibitors, thrombolytics: not applicable
- LMWHs: patients can be taught to self-inject after hospital discharge
    * Monitor for signs and symptoms of bleeding or VTE recurrence
    * Avoid NSAIDs
- Warfarin: see chapter on arrhythmias

Adverse drug events
- Bleeding: all agents
    * LDUH and low-dose LMWH have similar bleeding risks
    * Protamine sulfate reverses heparin, LMWH
- Thrombocytopenia: heparin, LMWH
    * Early: occurs about in first week; transient; no therapy needed
    * Late: immune mediated; if severe must discontinue heparin/LMWH; less frequent with LMWH
      - If full anticoagulation, switch to thrombin

inhibitor; if VTE prophylaxis, use thrombin inhibitor and/or IPC/ES
- • May result in severe thrombosis/limb amputation
- • May happen immediately upon rechallenge with heparin or LMWH
- Spinal hematoma with epidural: LMWH or full anticoagulation worse than LDUH; do not use LMWHs
- Osteoporosis: heparin worse than LMWH; occurs with long-term therapy

Drug interactions
- NSAIDs may increase bleeding risk with all agents
- Warfarin: see chapter on arrhythmias

Parameters to monitor
- Heparin (full-dose IV) and thrombin inhibitors:
  - * PTT is goal 1.5-2.5 times control, monitor q6h until therapeutic; then monitor qd-bid
  - * LDUH doesn't affect PTT
- LMWHs: anti Xa levels (goal 0.5-1 units/mL [treatment]; 0.3-0.7 units/mL [prophylaxis]
  - * No routine monitoring; may monitor in renal impairment, obesity, prolonged use, pregnancy
- Fondaparinux: no monitoring; affects anti Xa levels
- Warfarin: see chapter on arrhythmias

Kinetics
- Heparin: cleared by endothelial cell enzymes ($t_{1/2}$ ~90 min); higher doses also renally cleared
- LMWHs: renally cleared; $t_{1/2}$ 2-4 times longer than heparin
- Fondaparinux: renally cleared; longer $t_{1/2}$ (~24 h)
- Thrombin inhibitors: $t_{1/2}$ 30-90 min; lepirudin renally cleared; others hepatically cleared

5. Stress Ulcer Prophylaxis

Overview

Definition and classifications
- GI mucosal damage related to metabolic stress in the ICU

Clinical presentation
- Similar to peptic ulcer disease (see chapter on gastrointestinal disorders)

Pathophysiology
- Shunting of blood from the GI tract to vital organs during critical illness results in breakdown of gastric mucosal defenses (eg, bicarbonate production, epithelial cell turnover)

Risk factors
- Mechanical ventilation >48 h
- Coagulopathy
- Other disease states/organ dysfunction where GI perfusion may be compromised (eg, sepsis, burns, traumatic brain injury)

Diagnostic criteria
- Based on signs/symptoms; diagnosis can be confirmed with endoscopy.

Treatment goals
- Prevent stress ulcers

Drug Therapy

- See chapter on gastrointestinal disorders for full drug information
- Histamine$_2$ (H$_2$) antagonists or sucralfate are standard of therapy; both are equally effective
  - * Cimetidine continuous infusion is only agent with this indication
  - * Intermittent IV bolus therapy of H$_2$ antagonists common; PO efficacy unknown
  - * H$_2$ antagonists may be associated with a higher incidence of nosocomial pneumonia than sucralfate
  - * Sucralfate must be used PO/per gastric tube; can be difficult in ICU patients
- Proton pump inhibitors: likely effective, but few data

- Antacids: less effective; not recommended; higher aspiration risk; require frequent dosing

6. Severe Sepsis and Septic Shock

Overview

Definition
- Severe sepsis is sepsis (see chapter on infectious diseases) plus dysfunction of one or more major organs (eg, hypotension responsive to fluids, oliguria, acute mental status change, lactic acidosis, respiratory insufficiency, coagulopathy)
- Septic shock is severe sepsis plus hypotension that is not fully responsive to fluids (ie, requires vasopressor therapy)

Classifications
- Severe sepsis
- Septic shock

Clinical presentation
- See sepsis criteria (see chapter on infectious diseases) and definitions above

Pathophysiology
- Progression of the systemic manifestations of sepsis; imbalances in the inflammatory, immune, and coagulation systems lead to organ hypoperfusion and organ dysfunction with or without refractory hypotension
- Causative organisms vary by institution, but broad patterns are known:
  * Common community-acquired organisms include *Streptococcus pneumoniae*, *Staphylococcus aureus*, *Haemophilus influenzae*, *Escherichia coli*, and "atypicals" (*Mycoplasma pneumoniae*, *Chlamydia pneumoniae*, *Legionella* spp.)
  * Common nosocomial organisms include *Pseudomonas aeruginosa*, *S aureus* (methicillin-resistance more common), *Enterobacter* spp., *Klebsiella* spp., *Proteus* spp., *Citrobacter* spp., *Serratia* spp., *Candida* spp.

Diagnostic criteria
- See sepsis criteria (see chapter on infectious diseases) and definitions above

Treatment goals
- Rapid stabilization of hemodynamic parameters and organ dysfunction
- Identification of causative organism(s), starting appropriate antimicrobial therapy, and elimination of the source of infection if applicable (eg, vascular or urinary catheter, abscess); duration of antimicrobial therapy is typically 7-14 days

- Modulation of inflammatory, coagulation, and hormonal derangements if applicable

Drug and Nondrug Therapy

- See chapter on infectious diseases for antimicrobial information (mechanism of action, dosing, adverse effects, etc)
- Empiric antimicrobial selection is also covered in the chapter on infectious diseases; definitive therapy should be streamlined to a narrower-spectrum agent if possible based on the final culture and sensitivity reports
- See section on fluid and electrolytes for details on fluid therapy; fluid therapy for severe sepsis and septic shock can be colloids and/or isotonic crystalloids; vasopressors should only be used after appropriate fluid therapy fails to adequately normalize BP (Table 3)

Mechanism of action
- Vasopressors/inotropes: adrenergic receptor agonists
- Drotrecogin alfa: the drug is recombinant human activated protein C (an endogenous anticoagulant), and the exact MOA is unknown; it modulates coagulation and inflammatory cascades

Adverse drug events
- Vasopressors/inotropes: tachycardia, arrhythmias, organ and extremity ischemia, hypertension
- Drotrecogin alfa: bleeding
  * Contraindicated in active internal bleeding, recent trauma, stroke, or other clinical condition at high bleeding risk, presence of epidural catheter

Drug-drug interactions
- Vasopressors/inotropes: none
- Drotrecogin alfa: increased bleeding risk with concomitant anticoagulation or antiplatelet therapy

Parameters to monitor
- Vasopressors/inotropes: BP, HR, cardiac output, urine output, extremity perfusion on physical exam
- Drotrecogin alfa:
  * Signs and symptoms of bleeding on physical exam, BP, HR
  * Improvement in signs and symptoms of infection; temperature, WBC, organ dysfunction
  * May prolong aPTT

Kinetics
- Drotrecogin alfa: dose adjustment is not required in renal or hepatic dysfunction

Table 3

Vasopressors and Inotropes Used in Severe Sepsis and Septic Shock

Name	Dosage range	Adrenergic receptor activity	Comments
Dopamine	<5 µg/kg/min	Increased renal perfusion (dopaminergic receptors)	Use of low-dose "renal tonic" dopamine
	5-10 µg/kg/min	Increased CO/HR (β_1) > increased BP (α_1)	is not supported by clinical data
	10-20 µg/kg/min	Increased CO/HR and BP	
Epinephrine	0.01-0.5 µg/kg/min	Increased CO/HR and BP (all receptors)	
Norepinephrine	0.01-3 µg/kg/min	Increased BP (α_1) > increased CO/HR (β_1)	
Phenylephrine	0.01-5 µg/kg/min	Increased BP only (α_1)	
Dobutamine	5-20 µg/kg/min	Increased CO/HR (β_1)	

Immunomodulator used in severe sepsis and septic shock

Drotrecogin alfa (Xigris®)	24 µg/kg/h x 96 h IV infusion		Add to antimicrobial therapy within 48 h of onset of severe sepsis; significantly decreases mortality, more effective in higher illness severity; monitor for bleeding; very expensive but likely cost effective

Note: All vasoactive agents are given as continuous IV infusions and are titrated to effect.

Other

- Patients with severe sepsis or septic shock may have cortisol and/or vasopressin deficiency; limited data suggest that such patients may benefit from low-dose hydrocortisone therapy or vasopressin therapy; however, current guidelines do not address such use of these agents

7. Fluids and Electrolyte Abnormalities in Critically Ill Patients

(See chapter on nutrition, chapter on renal disorders for hyperphosphatemia, and chapter on oncology for hypercalcemia)

Overview

Definition
- Pathologic alterations in fluid and electrolyte homeostasis

Classifications
- Classified by electrolyte (see below)

Clinical presentation
- *FOR ALL:* Mild to moderate abnormalities are usually asymptomatic

Sodium (normal range: 135-145 mEq/L)
- Hyponatremia or hypernatremia: lethargy, nausea, headache, dry mucous membranes, poor skin turgor (depends on hydration status), confusion
- Coma, seizures, or central pontine myelinolysis may occur in severe hyponatremia or if Na increases or decreases rapidly (>12 mEq/L/d)

Chloride (normal range: 96-106 mEq/L)
- Symptoms are related to acid/base or fluid abnormalities, not Cl itself

Water (moves osmotically with sodium)
- Dehydration: dry mucous membranes, poor skin turgor, lethargy, nausea, headache, hypotension, tachycardia, seizures/coma/death if severe, decreased urine output, metabolic acidosis, hypotension, tachycardia
- Edema/fluid overload: see chapter on heart failure

Potassium (normal range: 3.5-5.0 mEq/L)
- Hypokalemia: confusion, muscle cramps, weakness, cardiac arrhythmias
- Hyperkalemia: muscle cramps, weakness, cardiac arrhythmias

Magnesium (normal range: 1.5-2.2 mEq/L)
- Hypomagnesemia: similar to hypocalcemia
- Hypermagnesemia: lethargy, weakness, cardiac arrhythmias, coma if severe

Phosphorus (normal range: 2.6-4.5 mg/dL)
- Hypophosphatemia: confusion, anxiety, weakness, respiratory depression, paresthesias, lethargy; seizures and coma if severe
- Hyperphosphatemia: see chapter on kidney disorders

Calcium (normal range: 8.5-10.5 mg/dL)
- Hypocalcemia: confusion, anxiety, paresthesias, muscle cramps, tetany; coma and cardiac arrhythmias if severe
- Hypercalcemia: see chapter on oncology

Pathophysiology
Normal distribution of fluids and electrolytes:
- Electrolytes with high serum concentrations are primarily extracellular (Na, Cl); those with low serum concentrations are mostly intracellular or in bone (K, P, Mg, Ca)
- Total body water is ~60-70% of total body weight (differs by age, gender, disease states)
  * Of all water: intracellular ~2/3, extracellular ~1/3
  * Of extracellular: ~3/4 is interstitial and ~1/4 is intravascular (plasma)
- Fluid requirements: typical requirements for adults ~35 mL/kg/d, can be much higher in critical illness due to extrarenal losses (GI tract, wounds) and fluid shifts (trauma, sepsis)
- Primary hormonal controls: aldosterone (Na retention), antidiuretic hormone (water retention)

Hyponatremia (the first three below are hypotonic):
- Hypovolemic (high urine osmolality): Na and water loss
  * Extrarenal fluid losses (GI, wounds), diuretics, adrenal insufficiency
- Euvolemic: moderate water retention
  * SIADH, renal failure, carbamazepine, NSAIDs, chlorpropamide
- Hypervolemic: Na and water retention
  * CHF, cirrhosis, nephrotic syndrome, glucocorticoids
- Hypertonic: dilutional effect of abnormal osmotic agents in the vasculature (severe hyperglycemia)

Hypernatremia: water loss or excessive Na intake (eg, from IV fluids)
- Extrarenal fluid losses (GI, wounds), diabetes insipidus

Hypochloremia:
- GI losses

Hypokalemia:
- Diuretics, beta$_2$ agonists, amphotericin B, glucocorticoids, cisplatin, GI losses

Hyperkalemia:
- Renal dysfunction, acidosis, ACE inhibitors, K-sparing diuretics, trimethoprim, PO salt substitutes, adrenal insufficiency

Hypomagnesemia:
- GI losses, diuretics, amphotericin B, alcohol, cisplatin
  * Treat prior to treating hypokalemia; Na/K-ATPase pumps require Mg to work

Hypermagnesemia:
- Renal dysfunction, Mg-containing antacids, adrenal insufficiency, hyperparathyroidism

Hypophosphatemia:
- Refeeding syndrome, phosphate binders, diuretics, hypercalcemia, vitamin D deficiency, glucocorticoids

Hypocalcemia:
- Hypoparathyroidism, hypomagnesemia, vitamin D deficiency, loop diuretics
  * Total Ca artificially low in hypoalbuminemia (Ca is highly albumin bound)

Diagnostic criteria
- Serum concentration, signs, and symptoms
- Sodium analysis may use urine Na, urine osmolality

Treatment goals
- Find and treat underlying cause of abnormality
- Treat abnormality to avoid sequelae

Drug and Nondrug Therapy

Fluid replacement
- Crystalloids: salt solutions—1/2 or 1/4 NS ± dextrose 5% ± KCl 20 mEq/L (approximates urine electrolytes), NS (154 mEq/L of Na), lactated Ringer's, 1/4 NS, or D_5W chosen based on Na and fluid needs; NS or LR typically used for fluid resuscitation (Na is the major osmotic cation in plasma)
- Colloids: osmotic agents—albumin 5-25%, hetastarch, used for fluid resuscitation or to raise oncotic pressure (eg, cirrhosis)
- Vasopressors ± isotropic activity may be used after fluids are optimized (see chapter on heart failure)

Edema
- Fluid restriction ± diuretics (see chapters on heart failure and kidney disorders)

Hyponatremia
- If severe, titrate 3% NaCl to maximum serum Na increase of 12 mEq/d
    * Hypovolemic: replace fluid losses with IV NS (0.9% NaCl, 154 mEq/L)
    * Euvolemic (SIADH): fluid restriction ± demeclocycline
    * Hypervolemic: fluid restriction ± diuretics
    * Hypertonic: correct hyperglycemia

Hypernatremia
- Titrate low Na fluids (eg, D_5W, 1/4 NS) to a normal serum Na
    * Diabetes insipidus: use DDAVP

Hyperchloremia
- Give Na acetate or LR instead of NS, especially if acidemic (acetate is converted to bicarbonate by the liver)

Hypokalemia
- IV (KCl) or PO (KCl, K phosphate, or K acetate); each 10-mEq dose increases serum K ~0.1 mEq/L
    * IV administration faster than 10 mEq/h requires ECG monitoring for arrhythmias

Hyperkalemia
- K removal (slower onset of action): Na polystyrene sulfonate (kayexalate) PO or PR, loop diuretics, hemodialysis (if severe)
- Intracellular K shifting (rapid onset of action): Regular insulin + dextrose IV, albuterol, Na bicarbonate

- K antagonism of cardiac effects (rapid onset of action): IV calcium

Hypomagnesemia
- Large percentage of dose is renally wasted, repletion requires 3-5 days treatment
    * IV: 0.5-1 mEq/kg/d (8 mEq = 1 gram), administration rate = 8 mEq/h
    * Can give IM but painful
    * PO: Mg-containing antacid or laxative tid-qid as tolerated or Mg oxide 300-600 mg bid-qid

Hypermagnesemia
- Diuretics, IV Ca, hemodialysis (similar to hyperkalemia)

Hypophosphatemia
- If severe, IV Na or K phosphate 0.16-0.64 mmol/kg at 7.5 mmol/h to avoid K overdose (if K phosphate is used) and/or Ca precipitation
    * PO: 1-2 g/d (5-60 mmol/d) eg, Neutra-Phos®, Neutra-Phos-K®, Fleet Phospho-soda®

Hyperphosphatemia
- See chapter on kidney disorders

Hypocalcemia
- If symptomatic, IV Ca gluconate (2-3 g) or IV Ca chloride (1 g) over 10 min
    * ± IV infusion of 0.5-2.0 mg/kg/h of elemental Ca
    * PO: calcium salts (eg, calcium carbonate) 1-3 g elemental Ca/d ± vitamin D

Patient counseling
- PO administration: advise patient about potential adverse events (see below)

Adverse drug events
- Sodium: edema, central pontine myelinolysis if serum Na changes rapidly (>12 mEq/d)
- Crystalloids: vein irritation with hypotonic (1/4 NS, 1/2 NS) or hypertonic fluids (3% NaCl)
    * D_5W is approximately isotonic; often added to low-Na fluids
- Potassium: cardiac arrhythmias (>10 mEq/h), vein irritation (IV), GI upset (PO; worse with wax matrix CR tablets), bad taste (PO liquid)
    * Na polystyrene sulfonate: constipation (usually mixed with sorbitol)
- Magnesium: diarrhea (PO), flushing, sweating (IV), vein irritation (IV)
- Phosphorus: diarrhea (oral), Ca phosphate precipitation (IV)
- Calcium: IV Ca gluconate less irritating than Ca chloride, cardiac dysfunction if administered >60

mg/min (elemental Ca), Ca phosphate precipitation (IV), constipation (oral)

Drug interactions
- Hypokalemia and/or hypomagnesemia predisposes to digoxin toxicity
- Binding of drugs in the GI tract by Ca, Mg (see nutrition chapter)

Parameters to monitor
- Serum concentrations
- Resolution of signs and symptoms
- Fluid replacement (normalization of the following): BP, HR, urine output (goal >0.5 mL/kg/h), skin turgor, mucous membrane hydration, edema, cardiac output, pulmonary artery wedge pressure (see chapter on heart failure), serum lactate/base deficit

Other/Miscellaneous
- Glucose control in critically ill patients (hyperglycemia increases infection risk)
  * Tight glucose control (80-110 mg/dL) with insulin infusion has been shown to reduce mortality in one large trial; however, it is not practical in many centers to use insulin infusions routinely, because they are labor intensive, plus the higher risk of hypoglycemic events versus insulin given as needed on a sliding scale
- Pharmacotherapy of anemia with recombinant erythropoietin
  * Anemia is very common in critically ill patients; causes include blood loss, low production of RBCs, and dilution from large volume intake
  * RBC transfusion is common but associated with adverse reactions, infection risk, high cost, and possibly increased mortality
  * Recombinant erythropoietin therapy (40,000 units SC per week) has been shown to decrease the need for RBC transfusions by ~20%
  * Pending issues include: clinical outcome studies; pharmacoeconomic analysis; optimal hemoglobin levels (thresholds for therapy) in critically ill patients remain controversial

8. Key Points

- Appropriate sedation and analgesia are essential because pain and agitation are common in critically ill patients. Drug selection should be based on clinical guidelines and patient parameters.
- Sedation and analgesia should be monitored using a validated assessment tool.
- Neuromuscular blockers should only be used after sedation and analgesia have been maximized.
- Drug selection should be based on clinical guidelines and patient parameters.
- Neuromuscular blockade should be monitored using peripheral nerve stimulation in addition to clinical signs and symptoms.
- Appropriate stress ulcer prophylaxis (H_2 antagonists or sucralfate) is recommended in patients at risk.
- Appropriate VTE prophylaxis is recommended for patients at risk. Optimal therapy is determined by clinical guidelines and patient risk factors.
- High-dose methylprednisolone therapy within 8 hours of injury can improve outcomes after acute spinal cord injury.
- ICP and CPP should be optimized after severe traumatic brain injury using drug and nondrug therapies. Phenytoin is effective at preventing early posttraumatic seizures.
- Severe sepsis and septic shock are progressions of sepsis. Therapy includes hemodynamic stabilization, appropriate antimicrobial agents, and removal of infectious foci if possible.
- Drotrecogin alfa is the first modulator of the sepsis cascade approved for use. It decreases mortality in severe sepsis if given within 48 hours of the onset of symptoms. Bleeding is the most common adverse event.
- Maintaining adequate fluid status is vital to maintaining tissue perfusion and organ function. However, many clinical factors can affect fluid and electrolyte status in critically ill patients. Finding and treating underlying causes of fluid and electrolyte abnormalities is essential.
- Fluid and electrolyte abnormalities are generally asymptomatic unless severe.
- Fluid and electrolyte therapy should be monitored closely because of patient instability and the risk of iatrogenic abnormalities (eg, cardiac arrhythmias, fluid overload).

9. Questions and Answers

1. In most critically ill patients, the opiate of choice for analgesia is:

   A. Morphine
   B. Hydromorphone
   C. Fentanyl
   D. Acetaminophen
   E. Ketorolac

2. In which situations should hydromorphone or fentanyl be used for analgesia in critically ill patients?

   I. Morphine allergy
   II. Renal dysfunction
   III. Hemodynamic instability

   A. I only
   B. III only
   C. I and II only
   D. II and III only
   E. I, II, and III

3. What is the maximum duration of therapy for ketorolac?

   A. 5 days
   B. 7 days
   C. 14 days
   D. 30 days
   E. There are no restrictions on length of use

4. Which agent is recommended for general long-term sedation in the ICU (>24-72 hours)?

   A. Diazepam
   B. Propofol
   C. Midazolam
   D. Pentobarbital
   E. Lorazepam

5. In most critically ill patients, the NMB agent of choice is:

   A. Propofol
   B. Vecuronium
   C. Cisatracurium
   D. Pancuronium
   E. Any agent may be used first line

6. The primary advantage of cisatracurium over pancuronium and vecuronium is:

   A. Elimination is not organ dependent
   B. Shorter duration of action
   C. Longer duration of action
   D. More effective
   E. Doesn't require monitoring

7. Which of the following is preferred as a first-line sedative agent for ICP control in patients with traumatic brain injury?

   A. Pentobarbital
   B. Lorazepam
   C. Propofol
   D. Vecuronium
   E. Sedation is not recommended

8. The regimen of choice for posttraumatic seizure prophylaxis is:

   A. Phenytoin indefinitely
   B. Phenytoin x 7 days
   C. Carbamazepine x 7 days
   D. Benzodiazepines prn if seizures occur
   E. Propofol x 7 days

9. Which of the following best describes the use of high-dose methylprednisolone in acute spinal cord injury?

   A. Duration of therapy is 24 hours if started within 12 hours of injury
   B. Duration of therapy is 48 hours if started within 8 hours of injury
   C. Duration of therapy is 24 hours if started 0-3 hours from injury; 48 hours if started 3-8 hours from injury
   D. High-dose methylprednisolone may be started at any time after injury
   E. Both blunt and penetrating spinal cord injuries should be treated with high-dose methylprednisolone

Use this case to answer Questions 10 and 11:

Patient name:	DG
Address:	N/A
Age:	24 years
Race:	Caucasian
Sex:	M
Height:	5'10"
Allergies:	NKDA
Weight:	70 kg
Diagnosis:	Motor vehicle accident
	Multiple rib fractures
	Moderate liver contusion

Lab/diagnostic tests:	CT scan of liver shows no active bleeding	
Medication orders:	Cimetidine 300 mg IV q8h	
	Morphine 1-4 mg IV q1h prn pain	
Additional orders:	Pharmacy consult for VTE prophylaxis	
Dietary:	N/A	
Pharmacist notes:	N/A	

10. Which of the following is the most appropriate VTE prophylaxis regimen for DG?

A. Low-dose LMWH
B. Heparin 5000 units SC q12h
C. Full-dose IV heparin infusion
D. Warfarin to INR 2-3
E. IPC and ES

11. The following day DG requires placement of an epidural catheter for pain control for his rib fractures. Which of the following is true regarding VTE prophylaxis in DG?

A. LMWH should be started and monitored closely with anti Xa levels
B. LMWH should be avoided because of the risk of perispinal hematoma
C. Full-dose IV heparin should be used for VTE prophylaxis
D. Warfarin should be started
E. A full-dose direct thrombin inhibitor should be started

Use this case to answer Questions 12 and 13:

Patient name:	AC
Address:	N/A
Age:	65 years
Race:	Caucasian
Sex:	F
Height:	5'4"
Allergies:	Penicillin (rash)
Weight:	60 kg
Diagnosis:	Severe community-acquired pneumonia
	Acute pain and swelling in left leg 7 days after admission
Lab/diagnostic tests:	Bedside ultrasound shows acute DVT in left leg

Below is a comparison of AC's CBC on admission and day 7:

	Admission	Day 7
WBC	18.0	4.0
% neutrophils/% bands	80/10	60/0
Hematocrit %	42	48
Platelets	175,000	8000

Medication orders:	Ranitidine 50 mg IV q8h
	Heparin 5000 units SC q12h changed to IV heparin infusion 1100 units/h after DVT is diagnosed
	Gatifloxacin 400 mg IV qd
Additional orders:	N/A
Dietary:	N/A
Pharmacist notes:	N/A

12. Which of AC's hematologic changes over time is most likely due to heparin?

A. Leukopenia
B. Leukocytosis
C. Increased hematocrit
D. Bandemia (left shift)
E. Thrombocytopenia

13. What should be done regarding heparin therapy in AC?

A. Switch to a direct thrombin inhibitor
B. Continue heparin; monitor CBC closely
C. Switch to high-dose LMWH
D. Switch to aspirin
E. Discontinue heparin; do not anticoagulate

14. In most patients with an acute DVT who are hemodynamically stable, what is the initial treatment of choice?

A. Heparin 5000 units SC q12h
B. Full-dose IV heparin or full-dose LMWH
C. Thrombolytic therapy (eg, rt-PA)
D. Aspirin
E. Low-dose LMWH

15. All of the following are risk factors for the development of stress ulcers EXCEPT:

A. Sepsis
B. Coagulopathy
C. Mechanical ventilation
D. Age >40 years
E. Burns

16. Which of the following is correct regarding stress ulcer prophylaxis?

A. H$_2$ antagonists or sucralfate are equally effective; considered drugs of choice

B. Proton pump inhibitors are more effective than H$_2$ antagonists or sucralfate

C. Antacids have the most direct effect on gastric pH; are considered drugs of choice

D. Sucralfate is more effective; causes less pneumonia than H$_2$ antagonists

E. All agents (H$_2$ antagonists, sucralfate, PPIs, antacids) are equally effective

17. Which of the following is the most likely adverse event associated with drotrecogin alfa use in severe sepsis?

   A. Renal dysfunction
   B. Allergy/anaphylactic shock
   C. Tachycardia
   D. Bleeding
   E. Rash

18. Which of the following will NOT increase blood pressure via α_1 adrenergic activation?

   A. Phenylephrine
   B. Dopamine
   C. Epinephrine
   D. Norepinephrine
   E. Dobutamine

19. MW is a 25-year-old pregnant female who is admitted to the medical ICU following several days of severe nausea and vomiting. She is hypotensive, tachycardic, and confused, and her urine output is very low. Her serum sodium is 128. Which of the following should be given to treat her fluid and sodium abnormalities?

   A. IV NS or LR
   B. IV D$_5$W
   C. PO water
   D. IV furosemide
   E. DDAVP

20. Common fluid and electrolyte abnormalities associated with loop diuretics include all of the following EXCEPT:

   A. Hypokalemia
   B. Hyperkalemia
   C. Hypomagnesemia
   D. Dehydration
   E. Hypocalcemia

21. RT is a 40-year-old male admitted to the medical ICU following a severe asthma exacerbation. RT's serum phosphorus is 0.9 and his body weight is 70 kg (100% of ideal). Which of the following acute phosphorus supplementation regimens is most appropriate?

   A. 45 mmol of sodium phosphate IV over 6 hours
   B. 45 mmol of sodium phosphate IV over 10 minutes
   C. 15 mmol of PO phosphorus (eg, Neutra-phos) over the next 24 hours
   D. 15 mmol of IV sodium phosphate over 2 hours
   E. No acute phosphorus therapy is required

22. The most common electrolyte abnormality associated with ACE inhibitors is:

   A. Hypomagnesemia
   B. Hypokalemia
   C. Hyperkalemia
   D. Hyperphosphatemia
   E. Hypernatremia

23. All of the following are useful in the rapid treatment of severe hyperkalemia EXCEPT:

   A. Potassium restriction
   B. IV calcium
   C. IV regular insulin and dextrose
   D. IV sodium bicarbonate
   E. PO Kayexalate

24. The most common electrolyte abnormalities associated with amphotericin B are:

   I.   Hypokalemia
   II. Hypomagnesemia
   III. Hypocalcemia

   A. I only
   B. III only
   C. I and II only
   D. II and III only
   E. I, II, and III

25. All of the following are side effects of K replacement therapy EXCEPT:

   A. Constipation (PO)
   B. GI upset (PO)
   C. Cardiac arrhythmias (IV)
   D. Vein irritation (IV)
   E. Poor taste (PO liquid)

26. Which of the following best describes GI side effects of antacids containing Mg and Ca salts?

    A. Mg causes constipation; Ca causes diarrhea
    B. Mg causes diarrhea; Ca causes constipation
    C. Both cause diarrhea
    D. Both cause constipation
    E. Neither has GI side effects

Answers

1. **A.** Morphine is recommended by the current Society of Critical Care Medicine (SCCM) guidelines on sedation and analgesia as the opiate of choice for most critically ill patients. Morphine is inexpensive, relatively short acting, and well tolerated by many patients.

2. **C.** Based on SCCM guidelines, hydromorphone or fentanyl is recommended for critically ill patients with any of the three conditions mentioned. Morphine may cause more hemodynamic instability than hydromorphone or fentanyl because of more histamine release. In addition, morphine has a renally-excreted, partially active metabolite that may accumulate in renal dysfunction. Hydromorphone and fentanyl do not have such a metabolite. The reason for using these agents in morphine allergy is self-explanatory.

3. **A.** Per the manufacturer, ketorolac should not be used longer than 5 days due to the high risk of GI bleeding with this drug.

4. **E.** Based on SCCM guidelines, lorazepam is the sedative of choice in most critically ill patients requiring long-term sedation. Lorazepam is less expensive than propofol and has a longer duration of action than propofol or midazolam.

5. **D.** Based on SCCM guidelines, pancuronium is the NMB of choice for most critically ill patients. Pancuronium is less expensive than other agents.

6. **A.** Cisatracurium is metabolized by nonspecific plasma esterases while pancuronium and vecuronium have varying degrees of hepatic and renal elimination. Thus cisatracurium is recommended by SCCM guidelines for use in patients with renal and hepatic dysfunction.

7. **C.** Based on SCCM guidelines, propofol is the sedative of choice for patients that require neurologic assessment often. Traumatic brain injury patients may require multiple neurologic assessments daily. The short duration of action of propofol allows rapid wakening.

8. **B.** Based on the Brain Trauma Foundation guidelines, phenytoin for 7 days postinjury is the regimen of choice for posttraumatic seizure prophylaxis in patients requiring such therapy.

9. **C.** This regimen is based on the results of the NASCIS III trial. There is some controversy regarding the study design of this trial and the actual efficacy of the drug for this indication; however, most clinicians treat acute SCI with high-dose methylprednisolone.

10. **A.** Based on American College of Chest Physicians (ACCP) guidelines, low-dose LMWH is the drug of choice for VTE prophylaxis in a patient with multiple trauma. LMWH is acceptable in this patient because the organ injury is not actively bleeding. If the patient had active bleeding, then mechanical methods (IPC, ES) would be indicated instead of LMWH.

11. **B.** Manufacturers of LMWHs do not recommend using these agents in patients with epidural catheters because of case reports of clinically significant spinal hematomas. Full anticoagulation should also be avoided.

12. **E.** Thrombocytopenia is a common hematologic side effect of heparin. A severe drop in platelets during the first 7-14 days is a typical presentation.

13. **A.** Based on ACCP guidelines, all forms of heparin must be discontinued. However, this patient requires acute, full anticoagulation for treatment of an active DVT. A direct thrombin inhibitor should be started. These agents do not cross react with heparin and potentiate thrombocytopenia.

14. **B.** Based on ACCP guidelines, rapid, full anticoagulation with IV heparin or SC LMWH is recommended in most patients with uncomplicated DVT. Thrombolytic therapy is only recommended in selected patients with hemodynamic instability or a massive VTE.

15. **D.** Increased age is not an independent risk factor for stress ulcers.

16 **A.** Based on ASHP guidelines, H_2 antagonists and sucralfate are generally considered to be equally effective and the drugs of choice. However, there is some controversy over the effect of H_2 antagonists on pneumonia development. Because of this, some clinicians prefer sucralfate.

17. **D.** Drotrecogin alfa is a recombinant form of the endogenous anticoagulant activated protein C. The anticoagulant activity increases the risk of bleeding.

18. **E.** Dobutamine has no α_1 adrenergic (vasoconstriction) activity.

19. **A.** MW is hyponatremic and her clinical signs and symptoms indicate severe dehydration from GI losses of water and sodium. She requires rapid fluid resuscitation with a fluid that has an approximately physiologic amount of sodium (either NS 154 mEq/L or LR 130 mEq/L). This amount of sodium will increase her serum sodium into the normal range over time and the osmotic effect will hold water in the extracellular compartment (the vasculature and interstitium) to help restore organ perfusion.

20. **B.** Loop diuretics enhance renal excretion of water, K, Mg, and Ca.

21. **A.** RT is severely hypophosphatemic and requires high-dose IV therapy (0.64 mmol/kg x 70 kg = 44.8 mmol). The dose should be infused at 7.5 mmol/h (total time ~6 h) to avoid precipitation with Ca.

22. **C.** ACE inhibitors cause hyperkalemia because of aldosterone inhibition.

23. **E.** Oral Kayexalate does not act very quickly. It requires transit time through the intestines to bind potassium and create a gradient that pulls more potassium into the lumen of the GI tract.

24. **C.** Amphotericin B causes renal wasting of potassium and magnesium.

25. **A.** Oral potassium replacement therapy does not normally cause constipation. Cardiac arrhythmias are a concern if IV potassium is given faster than 10 mEq/h.

26. **B.** Magnesium salts (eg, milk of magnesia) are often used as osmotic laxatives and may cause diarrhea. Calcium salts may cause constipation.

10. References

ASHP Commission on Therapeutics. ASHP therapeutic guidelines on stress ulcer prophylaxis. *Am J Health Syst Pharm.* 1999;56:347-379.

Ateshkadi A, Pelter MA. Electrolytes, other minerals, and trace elements. In: Traub SL, ed. *Basic Skills in Interpreting Laboratory Data,* 2nd ed. Bethesda, MD: ASHP; 1996:93-130.

Bernard GR, Vincent JL, Laterre PF, et al. Efficacy and safety of recombinant human activated protein C for severe sepsis. *N Engl J Med.* 2001;344:699-709.

Boucher BA, Clifton GD, Hanes SD. Critical care therapy. In: Herfindal ET, Gourley DR, eds. *Textbook of Therapeutics: Drug and Disease Management,* 7th ed. Philadelphia, PA: Lippincott Williams & Wilkins; 2000:2077-2094.

Boucher BA, Phelps SJ. Acute management of the head injury patient. In: DiPiro JT, Talbert RL, Yee GC, et al, eds. *Pharmacotherapy: A Pathophysiologic Approach,* 5th ed. New York, NY: McGraw-Hill; 2002:1077-1088.

Bracken ME, Shepard MJ, Holford TR, et al. Administration of methylprednisolone for 24 or 48 hours or tirilazad mesylate for 48 hours in the treatment of acute spinal cord injury. Results of the third national acute spinal cord injury randomized controlled trial. National Acute Spinal Cord Injury Study. *JAMA.* 1997;277:1597-1604.

Brophy DF, Gehr TWB. Disorders of potassium and magnesium homeostasis. In: DiPiro JT, Talbert RL, Yee GC, et al, eds. *Pharmacotherapy: A Pathophysiologic Approach,* 5th ed. New York, NY: McGraw-Hill; 2002:981-994.

Corwin HL, Gettinger A, Pearl RG, et al. Efficacy of recombinant human erythropoietin in critically ill patients: a randomized trial. *JAMA.* 2002;288:2827-2835.

Geerts WH, Heit JA, Clagett GP, et al. Prevention of venous thromboembolism. *Chest.* 2001;119:132S-175S.

Jacobi J, Fraser GL, Coursin DB, et al. Clinical practice guidelines for the sustained use of sedatives and analgesics in the critically ill adult. *Crit Care Med.* 2002;30:119-141.

Joy MS, Hladik GA. Disorders of sodium, water, calcium, and phosphorus homeostasis. In: DiPiro JT, Talbert RL, Yee GC, et al, eds. *Pharmacotherapy: A Pathophysiologic Approach,* 5th ed. New York, NY: McGraw-Hill; 2002:953-980.

Kang-Birken SL, DiPiro JT. Sepsis and septic shock. In: DiPiro JT, Talbert RL, Yee GC, et al, eds. *Pharmacotherapy: A Pathophysiologic Approach,* 5th ed. New York, NY: McGraw-Hill; 2002:2029-2041.

Murray MJ, Cowen J, DeBlock H, et al. Clinical practice guidelines for sustained neuromuscular blockade in the critically ill patient. *Crit Care Med.* 2002;30:142-156.

The Brain Trauma Foundation. The American Association of Neurologic Surgeons. The Joint Section on Neurotrauma and Critical Care. Management and prognosis of severe traumatic brain injury. *J Neurotrauma.* 2000;17:451-627.

18. Nutrition

Rex O. Brown, PharmD
Professor and Executive Vice Chair, Department of Pharmacy
University of Tennessee College of Pharmacy

1. Overview

General Nutrition

U.S. dietary guidelines (food pyramid)
- Maintain healthy weight
- Low-fat diet (<30% of total calories)
- Plenty of fruits, vegetables, and grain products
- Salt, sugar, and alcohol in moderation

Malnutrition
- Causes of undernutrition (protein-calorie malnutrition)
    * Depressed intake of nutrients (starvation, semi-starvation)
    * Alteration in nutrient metabolism (trauma, major infection)
- Obesity and its causes
    * Excessive caloric intake (especially carbohydrate and fat)
    * Alteration in nutrient metabolism (genetic predisposition)
    * Sedentary lifestyle

Dietary reference intakes (DRIs) of selected nutrients
- Fiber: 20-35 g per day (many people find this goal unpalatable)
- Calcium: 1200-1500 mg/d in adolescents and young adults; 1000 mg/d in men until age 65 and women until age 50; 1200-1500 mg/d for life (usually requires supplements)
- Multivitamins help to meet daily requirements of pregnant and lactating women, elderly persons, and those who eat vegetarian or low-calorie diets

Nutritional assessment components
History and physical examination
- Dietary intake (anorexia, hyperphagia, taste alterations)
- Underlying pathology affecting nutrition (cancer, burns)
- End-organ effects (diarrhea, constipation)
- General appearance (edema, cachexia)
- Skin appearance (scaling skin, decubitus ulcers)
- Musculoskeletal (depressed muscle mass, growth retardation)
- Neurologic (depressed sensorium, encephalopathy)
- Hepatic (jaundice, hepatomegaly)

Anthropometrics
- Skinfold measurements for assessment of fat (triceps, calf)
- Arm muscle circumference for assessment of skeletal muscle
- Weight for height to determine undernutrition or obesity
- Head circumference in infants to document appropriate growth
- Percent of ideal body weight (IBW) after calculation of IBW for patient
    * IBW of males (kg) = 50 + (2.3 x height in inches over 5 feet)
    * IBW of females (kg) = 45.5 + (2.3 x height in inches over 5 feet)
- Body mass index (BMI) for assessment of undernutrition or obesity calculated from body weight (kg) and height (meters): BMI = wt (kg)/ht (m)^2

Biochemical assessment
Serum albumin concentration
- Good prognostic indicator and good for assessment of long-term nutritional status
- Poor for repletion marker because of long half-life (21 days) and large body pool
Serum prealbumin concentration
- Good for short-term assessment of nutrition support because of short half-life (2 days) and small body pool
- Serum transferrin concentration is also good for short-term assessment because of short half-life (7 days) and small body pool
    * Elevated in iron deficiency anemia
Creatinine height index
- Requires 24-hour urine collection to determine levels of creatinine

Immune assessment
- Total lymphocyte count from complete blood count with differential (insensitive)
- Cell-mediated immunity
- Skin test with common antigens, eg, *Candida*, mumps (usually takes 48-72 hours for skin induration to occur to give positive response)
Other methods of nutritional assessment
- Muscle strength testing
- Bioelectrical impedance (ie, a low-grade electrical current runs through the body to identify body protein stores and fat stores)

Types of malnutrition
Marasmus
- Features depleted fat and muscle stores, normal biochemical measurements, and intact immune status

Kwashiorkor
- Features normal or elevated fat and body weight with abnormally low biochemical measurements and depressed immune function

Kwashiorkor-marasmus mix
• All measurements are depressed

Obesity
• Demonstrated as elevated body weight to at least 120% of IBW or BMI >27.8 (male) and >27.3 (female)

Selected definitions
• Hypermetabolism: An increase in energy expenditure above normal (usually >10% above normal)
• Hypercatabolism: An increase in protein losses above normal (usually via urinary excretion of nitrogen)
• Specialized nutrition support: Parenteral nutrition (PN) or enteral nutrition (EN)
• Basal energy expenditure (BEE): A calculation of normal energy needs of healthy adult men or women using gender, age, height, and weight (Harris-Benedict equations)
    * Male (kcal/d) = 66 + 13.7 (wt in kg) + 5 (ht in cm) – 6.8 (age in years)
    * Female (kcal/d) = 655 + 9.6 (wt in kg) + 1.8 (ht in cm) – 4.7 (age in years)
• Resting energy expenditure (REE): A measured value of energy expenditure (generally ~10% above BEE in health, can be 100% above BEE in severe burns)
• Respiratory quotient (RQ): The value that results when carbon dioxide production (VCO_2) is divided by oxygen consumption (VO_2)
    * RQ for carbohydrate oxidation = 1
    * RQ for fat oxidation = 0.7
    * RQ for protein oxidation = 0.8
    * RQ for fat synthesis = 8
• Body cell mass: Lean, metabolically active tissue (skeletal muscle, body organs)
• Lean body mass: body cell mass, extracelluar fluid, and extracellular solids (bone, serum proteins)

2. Nutritional Requirements

Calorie requirements
• Most clinicians dose specialized nutrition support in total calories (ie, using carbohydrate, fat, and protein calorie contributions to obtain the desired dose)
    * 25 kcal/kg/d for adults with little stress (eg, elective surgery)
    * 30 kcal/kg/d for patients with infections, skeletal trauma
    * 35 kcal/kg/d for patients with major trauma (head injury, long-bone fractures)
    * 40 kcal/kg/d for patients with major thermal injury (>50% body surface area burn)
• Basal energy expenditure (BEE) times the stress factor to determine calorie requirements
    * 1 x BEE for patient with little stress
    * 1.3 x BEE for minor trauma, infections
    * 1.5 x BEE for major trauma
    * 2 x BEE for severe thermal injury
• Measurement of the resting energy expenditure (REE) via indirect calorimetry for calorie requirements

Caloric contribution of the major macronutrients
• Glucose: 3.4 kcal/g because hydrated glucose is used in PN (glucose powder would be 4 kcal/g)
• Fat: 9 kcal/g
• Protein: 4 kcal/g
    * Protein requirements are usually dosed in g/kg/d
    * 0.8 g/kg/d is the adult recommended daily allowance (RDA) for protein in the U.S.
    * 1 g/kg/d for patients with minor stress (elective operations)
    * 1.5 g/kg/d for patients with major trauma, infection
    * 2 g/kg/d for patients with severe head injury, sepsis, severe thermal injury

Measurement of nutritional efficacy using nitrogen balance (NB)
NB = nitrogen in, nitrogen out
• Nitrogen in (g) is determined by dividing the grams of protein taken in on the day of balance divided by 6.25
• Nitrogen out (g) is determined by measuring the grams of urea nitrogen excreted during a 24-hour urine collection and then adding a factor of 2 or 4 g for insensible nitrogen loss/stool loss
• Positive nitrogen balance can be used to document adequacy of nutritional support
    * +4 to 6 g/d is desired in undernourished patients
    * Nitrogen equilibrium (–2 to +2 g/d) is usually adequate in critically ill patients

Water requirements during nutrition support
- Up to 35 mL/kg/d for average size adults
- 40 mL/kg/d for smaller adults and adolescents
- >40 mL/kg/d for patients with extra-renal losses (eg, gastrointestinal drains)

Electrolytes
- Sodium requirements
  - * 60-100 mEq/d in adults
  - * 2-6 mEq/kg/d in children
- Chloride requirements
  - * 60-100 mEq/d in adults
  - * 2-6 mEq/kg/d in children
- Potassium requirements
  - * 60-100 mEq/d in adults
  - * 2-5 mEq/kg/d in children
- Calcium requirements
  - * 5-15 mEq/d in adults
  - * 2-3 mEq/kg/d in children
- Phosphorus requirements
  - * 20-45 mmol/d in adults
  - * 1-2 mmol/kg/d in children
- Magnesium requirements
  - * 10-20 mEq/d in adults
  - * 0.25-1 mEq/kg/d in children

Vitamins
- Vitamins are provided daily in both PN (added) and EN (endogenous)
  - * Most enteral formulations provide the RDI for vitamins in a volume of 1000-1500 mL
- Parenteral vitamin products
  - * Adult products contain 12 (MVI-12) or 13 vitamins (Infuvite Adult®); vitamin K is added when the product with 12 vitamins is used
  - * Pediatric products (MVI-Pediatric®, Infuvite Pediatric®) contain all 13 vitamins

Trace elements
- Zinc: 3-5 mg/day in adults with PN; 50-250 µg/kg/d in children in PN
- Copper: 0.5-1.2 mg/d in adults with PN; 20 µg/kg/d in children in PN (maximum of 300 µg/d)
- Chromium: 10-15 µg/d in adults with PN; 0.14-0.2 µg/kg/d in children in PN (maximum of 5 µg/d)
- Manganese: 50-100 µg/d in adults with PN; 1 µg/kg/d in children in PN (maximum of 50 µg/d)
- Selenium: 40-80 µg/d in adults with PN; 1.5-3 µg/kg/d in children in PN

3. Specialized Nutrition Support

Parenteral Nutrition

Indications: PN is generally used for patients who cannot be fed via the gastrointestinal tract

Severe acute pancreatitis
- Oral food or tube feeding will usually exacerbate condition

Short bowel syndrome
- PN from a few weeks to lifelong as needed

Ileus
- Secondary to lack of bowel function (eg, acute renal failure secondary to sepsis)

- Crohn's disease exacerbation with fistula or obstruction
- Neonates who cannot eat in the first day of life
- Preoperatively for undernourished patients who are undergoing an elective operation and there is no direct access to the gastrointestinal tract (eg, partial small bowel obstruction from cancer)
- Pregnancy with severe hyperemesis gravidarum (ie, there is an inability to tolerate PO or EN)
- Gastrointestinal fistulae where EN/PO should be restricted

Components of parenteral nutrition
Protein
- Protein should be included in all PN formulations
- Standard amino acids from 10 or 15% stock solutions can be used for most patients
- Final concentrations in the PN formulation vary from 2-7%
- Rarely need doses >2 g/kg/d

Fat
- Fat provided as intravenous fat emulsion either as a separate infusion or admixed with the rest of the PN formulation, making a total nutrient admixture (TNA)
- Products are manufactured as 10%, 20%, and 30% fat emulsions (30% can be used only for TNAs, not for direct infusion)
- Provides essential fatty acids to the patient who is most likely not eating PO
- Provides nonprotein calories other than glucose
- Common doses used in adults are ~1 g/kg/d (9-10 kcal/kg/d)
- Intravenous fat emulsions contain phospholipid to emulsify the product and glycerol to make the emul-

sion isotonic (both of these components provide modest calories)

Dextrose
- Common doses of dextrose in critically ill patients: 3-4 mg/kg/min (~15-20 kcal/kg/d)
- In all PN formulations for obligate needs (CNS, renal medulla, WBCs, RBCs, and wound healing)
- PN formulations are usually made from 70% dextrose in water
- Final concentrations in the PN formulation vary from $D_{10}W$ to $D_{35}W$
- Should never exceed a dose of 5 mg/kg/min (~25 kcal/kg/d)

Sodium
- Can be provided as chloride, acetate, or phosphate salts in PN
- After phosphate addition, the remaining anions are added based on acid/base status (eg, acetate with metabolic acidosis, chloride with metabolic alkalosis)
- Requirements can be increased when the patient has extra-renal losses from nasogastric suction, abdominal drains, or ostomy losses

Potassium
- Can be provided as chloride, acetate, or phosphate salts in PN
- Requirements can be increased with administration of potassium-wasting drugs (diuretics, steroids) or in severe undernutrition
- Like sodium, the remaining potassium can be added as acetate or chloride after the proper dose of phosphate is determined

Calcium
- Most practitioners add calcium as the gluconate salt
- Higher doses of calcium (~20-25 mEq/d) in patients receiving long-term PN to help prevent metabolic bone disease
- Addition of calcium is limited in PN formulations because of the potential to precipitate with phosphate salts, which ultimately results in insoluble calcium phosphate

Phosphate
- Added as the sodium or potassium salt
- Higher doses of phosphorus (eg, 30 mmol/L) are needed to prevent refeeding syndrome in severely undernourished patients
- Phosphorus should be decreased or removed in patients with renal failure
- Addition of phosphorus is limited in PN formulation because of the potential to precipitate with calcium or magnesium salts to form an insoluble compound

Magnesium
- Most practitioners add magnesium as the sulfate salt
- Higher doses should be used in patients with alcoholism or large bowel losses, or in patients receiving drugs causing renal wasting of magnesium (cisplatin, amphotericin B, aminoglycosides, loop diuretics)
- Magnesium should be restricted or deleted in patients with renal failure

Multivitamins
- Given daily as part of PN
- A multivitamin preparation contains 12 or 13 vitamins (vitamin K should be administered separately if the 12-vitamin preparation is used)
- Additional thiamine and folic acid are often given to patients with alcoholism who are receiving PN
- Additional folic acid (at least 600 μg/d) should be given to pregnant patients receiving PN

Trace elements
- Given daily as a cocktail of 4 or 5 trace metals
- Extra zinc should be given in patients with ostomy or diarrhea losses
- Copper and manganese should be reduced or eliminated in patients with cholestasis
- Extra selenium is usually needed in home PN patients

Total nutrient admixtures (TNAs) versus 2-in-1 admixtures
Advantages of TNAs
- Decreased nursing time for administration
- Potentially decreased touch contamination
- Decreased pharmacy preparation time (assuming a 24-hour hang-time)
- Financial savings (only 1 pump, 1 tube)
Disavantages of TNAs
- Better media for bacterial growth than 2-in-1
- Impossible to visualize particulate matter
- Cannot filter formulation with a 0.22 micron filter
- Some additives like calcium and phosphorus are less compatible in TNAs

Central vein PN versus peripheral vein PN
Advantages of central vein PN
- Can maximize caloric intake
- Can volume-restrict patients
- Long-term catheter can be maintained
Disadvantages of central vein PN
- Mechanical complications during catheter placement (eg, pneumothorax)
- Potential hyperosmolar complications (eg, from using hypertonic dextrose)
- Potential septic catheter complications

Advantages of peripheral vein PN
- Easier to place the catheter (ie, peripheral vein stick)
- Avoid hyperosmolar complications because dilute formulations must be used

Disadvantages of peripheral vein PN
- High incidence of thrombophlebitis
- Requires frequent vein rotation
- Energy intake is limited
- Volume restriction is not possible (using dilute formulations)
- Higher cost because more lipid calories are generally used (lipids are isotonic)

Parenteral nutrition calculations

$D_{20}W$ (final concentration of PN formulation)
- $D_{20}W$ = 20% dextrose = 20 g/100 mL = 200 g/L x 3.4 kcal/g = 680 kcal/L
- 2 L/d of $D_{20}W$ (final concentration of PN) = 1360 kcal/d

Amino acids 5% (final concentration of PN formulation)
- 5% amino acids = 5 g/100 mL = 50 g/L x 4 kcal/g = 200 kcal/L
- 2 L/d of 5% amino acids = 100 g/d = 400 kcal/d

Lipid 2% (final concentration of TNA formulation)
- 2% lipid will deliver 200 kcal/L (includes calories from glycerol/phospholipid)
- 2 L/d of lipid 2% = 400 kcal/d

Lipid 20% infused at 20 mL/h x 24 h (separate infusion given with 2-in-1 PN)
- 20% lipid = 2 kcal/mL
- 20 mL/h x 24 h = 480 mL/d
- 480 mL/day x 2 kcal/mL = 960 kcal/d

Example: $D_{30}W$; amino acids 4%; lipid 3%, at 60 mL/h
- 60 mL/h x 24 h/d = 1440 mL/day (1.44 L/d)
- $D_{30}W$ = 30% dextrose = 300 g/L = 1020 kcal/L x 1.44 L = 1469 kcal
- 4% amino acids = 40 g/L = 160 kcal/L x 1.44 L = 230 kcal
- 3% lipid = 300 kcal/L x 1.44 L = 432 kcal
- 1469 kcal + 230 kcal + 432 kcal = 2131 total kcal/d

Example: dextrose 400 g; amino acids 100 g; lipids 40 g; 85 mL/h
- Dextrose 400 g x 3.4 kcal/g = 1360 kcal/d
- Amino Acids 100 g x 4 kcal/g = 400 kcal/d
- Lipids 40 g x 10 kcal/g (includes phospholipid/glycerol) = 400 kcal/d

General principles of compounding parenteral nutrition
- Each component of the PN prescription should be reviewed to ensure a balanced PN formulation is provided
- Each component should be assessed for dose and potential compatibility programs
- All compounded PN formulations should be visually inspected to ensure no gross contamination or precipitation is present
- Manufacturers of automated compounders should provide the additive sequence to ensure safety in PN preparation

General principles of stability and compatibility of parenteral nutrition
- Parenteral multivitamins should be added shortly before dispensing and administering the PN formulation because vitamins A and C degrade fairly quickly
- Preparation of TNAs using dual-chambered bags (lipid is in separate compartment until administration) can enhance the shelf life of a PN formulation
- Dibasic calcium phosphate ($CaHPO_4$) can precipitate in PN formulations if the additives of calcium gluconate and sodium or potassium phosphate are excessive
- Generally, phosphate should be added first to the PN formulation
- Generally, calcium should be added last to the PN formulation
- Calcium chloride should not be used in PN because it is highly reactive with phosphate
- Iron dextran can be added to 2-in-1 PN formulation, but should not be added to TNAs

Parenteral nutrition filtration
- Filters are used to prevent administration of particulate matter, microorganisms, and air
- Use a new 0.22-micron filter each day with 2-in-1 PN formulations (0.22-micron filters with positive charged nylon can be used up to 96 hours in 2-in-1 PN formulations)
- Use a 1.2-micron filter each day with TNAs

Complications of parenteral nutrition
Metabolic
Hyperglycemia
- Patients with stress of trauma or infection or those with diabetes often need regular human insulin added to the PN to control hyperglycemia

Electrolyte disorders
Hypokalemia
- Patients often require extra potassium in PN (eg, 60 mEq/L)

Hypophosphatemia
- Patients often require extra phosphorus in PN (eg, 30 mmol/L)

Hypomagnesemia
- Patients often require extra magnesium in PN (eg, 16 mEq/L)

Hyponatremia
- Electrolyte disorder must be interpreted with an assessment of extracellular fluid status (ie, volume status)
  * Volume depleted: add sodium and water to PN or increase intravenous fluid administration
  * Volume overloaded: remove sodium from PN and concentrate the formulation
  * Euvolemic: generally, water restriction is first-line therapy (PN concentration)

Acid-base disorders
- Increase acetate anions if patient has metabolic acidosis
- Increase chloride anions if patient has metabolic alkalosis

Essential fatty acid deficiency
- During PN, at least 4% of total calories need to be provided as intravenous lipid (easily attained when lipid is used daily as a calorie source)

Trace element disorders
- Patients with increased ostomy output or chronic diarrhea need extra zinc
- Hold copper and manganese in patients with cholestasis

Hepatic steatosis
- Fatty infiltration of the liver has been reported with long-term PN
- Thought to be primarily caused by administration of excessive dextrose calories
- Prevention is the key via administration of an appropriate dose of dextrose (eg, <5 mg/kg/min)

Mechanical complications
- Pneumothorax (punctured lung) can occur during central vein access
- Subclavian artery injury can occur when artery is cannulated instead of vein
- Subclavian vein thrombosis can occur with long-term central vein access (heparin is used in some PN patients to prevent this)

Infectious complications
- Usually catheter-related breakdown in sterile technique
- Rarely solution-related

Monitoring of parenteral nutrition
- Frequency/intensity of monitoring is based on patient acuity
  * Electrolytes and glucose
  * Acid-base status via arterial blood gases
  * Intake and output for assessment of fluid balance
  * Serum prealbumin concentrations and/or nitrogen balance to document efficacy

Enteral Nutrition

Indications
- Generally used in patients who cannot or will not eat, but have a functional and accessible gastrointestinal tract
- Neonates should begin EN as early as possible, even if receiving PN
- Elderly patients without the ability to take in PO food

Cardiac
- May need fluid-restricted EN with fluid overload

Pulmonary failure
- Used frequently in patients receiving mechanical ventilation

Hepatic failure
- Used frequently in this population
- In severe hepatic encephalopathy, use formulation with high branched-chain amino acids and low aromatic amino acids
- In the absence of encephalopathy or mild encephalopathy, use EN with standard protein.

- In short-bowel syndrome, EN is used to enhance small bowel hypertrophy after major resection
- Inflammatory bowel syndrome: preferred method of nutrition support in these patients

Neurologic impairment
- EN is preferred because patient may not be able to eat, but the gastrointestinal tract is functional and accessible

Cancer/HIV infection
- Use EN (if possible) in these patients to prevent or treat undernutrition

Types of enteral access
Feeding enterostomy
- Usually placed for long-term EN
- Gastrostomy: G-tube or PEG (percutaneous endoscopic gastrostomy)

- Jejunostomy: requires an exploratory laparotomy to place

Oral route (by drinking supplements)

Nasal tube feeding
- Usually placed for short-term EN
- Nasogastric tube
- Nasoduodenal tube
- Nasojejunal tube

Products for enteral nutrition
- Polymeric, nutritionally-complete tube feeding for patients with normal digestive processes (eg, 1 kcal/mL)
- Concentrated, nutritionally-complete tube feeding for patients who need severe fluid restriction (eg, 2 kcal/mL)
- Polymeric, nutritionally-complete, oral supplements to supplement a PO diet (eg, 1 or 1.5 kcal/mL)
- Chemically-defined, nutritionally complete tube feeding for patients with impaired digestive processes like short bowel syndrome or pancreatic insufficiency (eg, 1 kcal/mL)
- Fiber-containing, nutritionally-complete tube feeding is beneficial in patients who receive long-term tube feeding (can prevent diarrhea and constipation; eg, 1 or 1.2 kcal/mL)
- Concentrated, low-protein, low-electrolyte tube feeding is generally used for patients with renal failure
- High branched-chain amino acid, low aromatic amino acid EN formula is used for patients with liver failure and severe hepatic encephalopathy (eg, 1 or 1.5 kcal/mL)
- High-fat, low-carbohydrate, nutritionally-complete tube feeding is helpful in management of diabetic or other glucose-intolerant patients (eg, 1 kcal/mL)
- Immune-enhancing formulas that contain arginine, glutamine, and omega-3 fatty acids are marketed and used in patients with high metabolic stress (eg, severe trauma or infection; 1 or 1.3 kcal/mL)

Complications of enteral nutrition
Pulmonary aspiration pneumonia
- The most severe complication of EN
- Caused by regurgitation of gastric contents into the lung (with or without tube feeding)
- Prevention is important
  * Elevate the head of the bed to 30° if possible
  * Frequently assess the patient's abdomen to ensure tolerance
  * Frequently assess the placement of the feeding tube (especially nasally placed tubes)

Gastrointestinal
- Diarrhea is often associated with the administration of EN, and is not necessarily the reason for using EN
  Increased frequency or volume of stools
- Pharmacotherapy is often the cause due to sorbitol in liquid vehicles; lack of fiber and excessive infusion rate advancements can also be causes
- Decreasing or at least not advancing the infusion rate is appropriate
- Change to a fiber-containing formulation if the patient is not receiving one
- Pseudomembranous enterocolitis from antibiotic therapy
- Use pharmacotherapeutic treatment if the above factors are ruled out (kaolin-pectin, loperamide)
  Constipation (decrease in stool frequency)
- Lack of fiber can be a cause
- Lack of water can be a cause
- Poor mobility and drugs with anticholinergic activity can contribute
- Keep patient well hydrated and use a fiber-containing EN formulation
- Elevated gastric residuals is suggestive of poor gastric emptying of EN formulation

Mechanical complications of EN
- In the event of nasal necrosis, use a small-bore feeding tube and do not tape it too firmly to the nose
- In the event of esophageal injury, use small-bore feeding tube
- In the event of tube clogging, frequently flush the feeding tube with water
- In the event of tube displacement, discourage removing the tube; the tube may have to be anchored with a bridle

Metabolic complications of EN
  Hyperglycemia
- Use regular human insulin
- Consider a high-fat, low-carbohydrate EN formulation
  Hypokalemia
- Provide additional potassium as an IV or per tube supplement
- Some institutions allow the addition of potassium salts to the EN formulation
  Hypophosphatemia
- Provide additional phosphorus as an IV supplement (eg, potassium phosphate)
- Some institutions allow the addition of phosphorus salts to the EN formulations (eg, Fleet Phosphosoda 5 or 10 mL/L)

Monitoring of enteral nutrition

- The intensity of monitoring will be dictated by the condition of the patient
    * Electrolytes and glucose
    * Acid-base status via arterial blood gases (critical care only)
    * Intake and output for assessment of fluid balance

Assessment of the patient's abdomen

- Positive bowel sounds usually should be present
- Abdomen should be soft, nontender, nondistended in most cases
- A profoundly distended abdomen usually requires the EN to be decreased or discontinued temporarily
- Serum prealbumin concentrations and/or nitrogen balance to document efficacy

Home Nutrition Support

Parenteral nutrition

- Can be given from weeks to lifetime (eg, severe short bowel syndrome)
- Usually cycled at night over 10-16 hours
- Must be monitored closely for iron deficiency because it is not routinely added to PN
- Regular assessment of hemoglobin, hematocrit, and MCV
- Serum iron, TIBC, and ferritin are commonly used in the diagnosis of iron deficiency
- Metabolic bone disease is another long-term complication of home PN
    * Supplemental calcium in the PN formulation is usually required (15-25 mEq/d)
    * Adequate vitamin K for osteocalcin is important on a long-term basis

Enteral nutrition

- Can be given indefinitely as full nutrition support or as supplement to PO diet
- Permanent feeding ostomies are used almost exclusively in home EN
- Patients in nursing homes and extended-care facilities usually receive EN as a continuous infusion over 12-24 hours
- Patients who receive home EN via gastrostomy usually receive bolus feeding (eg, two 240-mL cans tid via PEG)
- Patients who receive home EN as a supplement to PO intake are often cycled at night (eg, 1000 mL at 85 mL/h from 7 PM to 7 AM each night)

4. Major Drug-Nutrient Interactions

Phenytoin and enteral tube feeding

- It has been demonstrated that enteral feeding will bind to phenytoin, thus impairing the absorption dramatically (possibly the protein component of EN [caseinates])

Management of phenytoin/enteral nutrition interaction

- Hold the EN 2 hours before and after the daily dose of phenytoin capsules
- Hold the EN 1 hour before and after each dose of phenytoin suspension (usually given bid or tid)
- Increase the EN infusion rate to allow the desired nutritional dose of EN to be given (ie, to make up the lost time while the EN is being held for drug administration)

Fluoroquinolones and enteral tube feeding/oral food

- It has been demonstrated that enteral feedings will decrease the absorption of many of the fluoroquinolones during concurrent administration (eg, >80% decrease with ciprofloxacin)

Management of ciprofloxacin/enteral nutrition interaction

- Hold the EN 1 hour before and after each dose of ciprofloxacin (usually given qd or bid)
- Increase the EN infusion rate to allow the desired dose of EN to be given

Warfarin and enteral tube feeding

- It has been reported that adequate anticoagulation with warfarin is very difficult to achieve with concurrent EN (low INRs)

Management of warfarin/enteral nutrition interaction

- Some practitioners hold EN 1 hour before and after the daily warfarin dose. If this is done, the EN rate should be increased to attain the desired nutritional dose

Grapefruit juice interacts with many drugs (eg, amlodipine, carbamazepine, cyclosporine)

- Grapefruit juice from frozen concentrate has been reported to inhibit gastrointestinal cytochrome P450-3A4 resulting in enhancement of oral absorption of some drugs (toxicity)

Management of grapefruit juice/drug interaction

- When taking drugs that are known to interact with grapefruit juice, patients should be advised to avoid these products (ie, substitute another fruit juice such as apple or orange juice)

5. Key Points

- Malnutrition can present as either undernutrition or obesity
- The components of a nutritional assessment include a history and physical exam, anthropometric measurements, biochemical tests, and immune competence assessment
- An increase in energy expenditure (energy needs) is defined as hypermetabolism and an increase in nitrogen excretion (protein needs) is defined as hypercatabolism
- Most patients receiving specialized nutrition support (parenteral or enteral nutrition) require from 25-30 kcal/kg/d and 1-2 g protein/kg/d
- Water requirements for most adult patients without substantial extra-renal losses is from 30-40 mL/kg/d
- Parenteral nutrition (PN) should be reserved for patients whose gastrointestinal tract is not functional or accessible (eg, severe acute pancreatitis, severe short bowel syndrome)
- Total nutrient admixtures (TNAs) contain dextrose, amino acids, lipid emulsion, electrolytes, vitamins, and trace elements in one container
- The advantages of TNAs include decreased nursing administration time, decreased potential for touch contamination, and reduced expense (use of only 1 pump and 1 intravenous administration set)
- The advantages of central vein PN over peripheral vein PN include ability to concentrate the formulation, administer adequate calories and protein, and use the catheter for long-term administration
- For PN calculations: 1 g hydrated dextrose = 3.4 kcal, 1 g amino acids = 4 kcal, and 1 g lipid = 9 kcal (intravenous fat emulsion actually provides 10 kcal/g because it includes calories provided as glycerol and phospholipid)
- All PN formulations should be filtered during administration (0.22-micron filter for 2-in-1 PN formulations and 1.2-micron filter for TNAs)
- Enteral nutrition support is generally used in patients who cannot or will not eat, but have a functional and accessible gastrointestinal tract
- Enteral tube feeding can be provided by one of the following methods: nasogastric, nasoduodenal, nasojejunal, gastrostomy, or jejunostomy
- Diarrhea associated with enteral tube feeding is often caused by pharmacotherapy (eg, sorbitol in liquid drug preparations as a vehicle)
- Patients receiving phenytoin, ciprofloxacin, or warfarin concurrently with enteral tube feeding should have the tube feeding held at least 1 hour before and after each dose.

6. Questions and Answers

1. What is the most appropriate calcium intake (mg/d) for adults >65 years of age?

   A. 600-800 mg
   B. 800-1000 mg
   C. 1000-1200 mg
   D. 1200-1500 mg
   E. 1500-1800 mg

Use this case for Questions 2 and 3:

A patient presents for a comprehensive nutritional assessment. She is 35 years old, 5'8" in height, and weighs 52 kg. She has a history of Crohn's disease involving both the small bowel and colon. She has had no surgeries, but has intermittent diarrhea.

Medications:
Prednisone 5 mg qod
Mesalamine 1 g tid
Kaolin-pectin 30 mL q6h prn diarrhea

Measurements:
Triceps skinfold = 3 mm (normal, 10-14 mm)
Calf skinfold = 4 mm (normal, 10-15 mm)
Serum albumin concentration = 2.5 g/dL
Serum prealbumin concentration = 13 mg/dL
  (normal, 15-45 mg/dL)

2. The triceps skinfold measurement for this patient is an anthropometric measurement for assessment of:

   A. Somatic protein stores
   B. Fat stores
   C. Visceral protein stores
   D. Immune competence
   E. Body cell mass

3. What type of malnutrition does this patient have?

   A. Kwashiorkor
   B. Marasmus
   C. Obesity
   D. Kwashiorkor-marasmus mix
   E. Fat overload syndrome

4. A patient with a bone fracture and gram-negative pneumonia excretes 15 g (normal, 6-8 g/d) of urea nitrogen during a 24-hour urine collection. Based on these data, the patient is:

A. Hypercatabolic
B. Hypermetabolic
C. Hypocatabolic
D. Hypometabolic
E. Euvolemic

5. During nutritional assessment, the measurement of body cell mass includes:

    A. Bone
    B. Interstitial fluid
    C. Skeletal muscle
    D. Intravascular fluid
    E. Extracellular fluid solids

Use this case for Questions 6-9

Following major gastrointestinal resection, a patient with severe short bowel syndrome is started on parenteral nutrition (PN). It is anticipated that this patient may need this therapy for 6 months to 1 year. The PN prescription for this patient includes:

* $D_{20}W$ amino acids 5% (final concentrations) at 105 mL/h (2500 mL/d)
*   Intravenous fat emulsion 20% at 10 mL/h x 24 hours (240 mL/d)
*   0.45% sodium chloride injection at 50 mL/h x 24 hours (1200 mL/d)

6. How many calories from dextrose will this patient receive each day?

    A. 1100
    B. 1300
    C. 1500
    D. 1700
    E. 1900

7. How many grams of protein will this patient receive each day?

    A. 25
    B. 50
    C. 75
    D. 100
    E. 125

8. How many calories from intravenous lipid will this patient receive each day?

    A. 240
    B. 360
    C. 480
    D. 600
    E. 720

9. Calculate the daily nitrogen balance (g/d) in this patient if she excretes 12 g of urea nitrogen during the urine collection and 4 g is used as insensible and stool loss each day.
    A. –4
    B. –2
    C. 0
    D. 2
    E. 4

10. What would be an appropriate water/fluid requirement (mL) for a 60-kg patient with no extra-renal fluid losses?

    A. 800 mL
    B. 1200 mL
    C. 2400 mL
    D. 3600 mL
    E. 4800 mL

11. Which of the following disease states or clinical conditions would usually require the administration of parenteral nutrition?

    A. Severe acute pancreatitis
    B. Motor vehicle crash resulting in femur fracture and head injury
    C. 20% body surface area burn from a house fire
    D. Laparoscopic cholecystectomy
    E. Acute exacerbation of hepatic encephalopathy

12. What is the maximum dose (kcal/kg/d) of dextrose in parenteral nutrition for adult patients?

    A. 5
    B. 10
    C. 15
    D. 20
    E. 25

13. In a patient with metabolic acidosis, what anion salt would you use to add the majority of sodium and potassium to a PN formulation?

    A. Chloride
    B. Gluconate
    C. Phosphate
    D. Acetate
    E. Sulfate

14. If excessive amounts of calcium are added to a standard parenteral nutrition formulation, it will likely precipitate with:

A. Phosphate
B. Gluconate
C. Magnesium
D. Chloride
E. Sodium

15. Which vitamin should be supplemented during nutrition support of a pregnant patient?

   A. Cyanocobalamin
   B. Folic acid
   C. Biotin
   D. Chromium
   E. Pantothenic acid

16. Which of the following is an advantage of central vein parenteral nutrition over peripheral vein parenteral nutrition?

   A. Easier catheter placement
   B. Does not require a pump for administration
   C. Allows for fluid restriction
   D. Does not have to be filtered
   E. Dilute formulations are used in most cases

17. Which component of a total nutrient admixture should be added last before storing it in a refrigerator?

   A. Phosphorus
   B. Magnesium
   C. Trace elements
   D. Calcium
   E. Intravenous fat emulsion

18. The advantages of using a 0.22-micron filter when administering a 2-in-1 parenteral nutrition formulation include:

   I. Traps particulate matter
   II. Prevents precipitations from entering the patient
   III. 389Filters most bacteria

   A. I only
   B. III only
   C. I and II only
   D. II and III only
   E. I, II, and III

19. Which trace element should be reduced or removed in patients with cholestasis who are receiving parenteral nutrition?

   A. Zinc
   B. Chromium

C. Selenium
D. Copper
E. Iodine

20. A 70-year-old female who has mild congestive heart failure, GERD, type II diabetes mellitus, and rheumatoid arthritis had a recent CVA. She will not regain her premorbid degree of mental status, so it is decided to give her long-term nutritional support. Which method would be most appropriate for this patient?

   A. central parenteral nutrition
   B. nasogastric tube feeding
   C. peripheral parenteral nutrition
   D. jejunostomy tube feeding
   E. nasoduodenal tube feeding

21. A common cause of diarrhea in patients receiving enteral nutrition is from the:

   A. osmotic load of the enteral nutrition formulation
   B. sorbitol in drug vehicles
   C. addition of fiber to the enteral nutrition formulation
   D. solute load from the protein component of the enteral nutrition formulation
   E. improper placement of a nasogastric feeding tube

22. What is the drug of choice for enhancing gastric emptying in a patient receiving enteral nutrition support?

   A. kaolin-pectin
   B. azithromycin
   C. metoclopramide
   D. loperamide
   E. acyclovir

23. A patient is receiving phenytoin capsules 300 mg each day for seizure control. She requires tube feeding with a 1 kcal/mL formulation at 85 mL/h (2000 mL/d). What would be the most appropriate intervention to maintain a therapeutic drug concentration and maintain the required nutrition support?

   I. increase the dose of phenytoin to 600 mg/d
   II. hold the enteral nutrition 2 hours before and after the dose
   III. increase the enteral nutrition to 100 mL/hr x 20 hrs

   A. I only

B. III only
C. I and II only
D. II and III only
E. I, II, and III

24. What is the mechanism for grapefruit juice to inhibit the metabolism of some drugs that can result in drug toxicity?

A. decreased renal excretion of drug
B. inhibition of gastrointestinal cytochrome P450-3A4
C. decreased systemic clearance of drug
D. inhibition of hepatic cytochrome P450-3A4
E. expanded apparent volume of distribution

Answers

1. **D.** Calcium requirements are 1000 mg/d for male adults until age 65, when they increase to 1200-1500 mg/d. Calcium requirements are 1000 mg/d for female adults until age 50, when they increase to 1200-1500 mg/d.

2. **B.** Skinfold measurements measure body fat stores, which assess the lipid component of the body. Visceral protein stores are serum proteins. Body cell mass and somatic protein stores assess skeletal muscle and visceral organs. Immune competence assessment requires a skin test with a common antigen.

3. **D.** All measurements of nutritional assessment are depressed (ie, weight for height, anthropometric measurements, and biochemical serum markers of protein status).

4. **A.** Catabolism is related to loss of body protein. Since it is increased, the patient would be considered hypermetabolic in this case.

5. **C.** Lean body mass includes bone, skeletal muscle, visceral organs, and extracellular solids. Body cell mass includes only the lean, metabolically active tissue like skeletal muscle and visceral organs (eg, liver).

6. **D.** $D_{20}W = 20$ g/100 mL = 200 g/L x 2.5 L/d = 500 g/d x 3.4 kcal/g = 1700 kcal/d

7. **E.** 5% amino acids = 5 g/100 mL = 50 g/L x 2.5 L/d = 125 g/d

8. **C.** Intravenous lipid emulsion 20% = 2 kcal/mL x 240 mL/d = 480 kcal/d.

9. **E.** The nitrogen intake is calculated by dividing the protein intake (125 g) by 6.25 which results in 20 g. The nitrogen output would be the sum of the urinary urea nitrogen and insensible losses (12 g + 4 g = 16 g/d). Therefore, the nitrogen balance would be 20 g – 16 g = 4 g. A nitrogen balance of +4 would be suggestive of nutritional adequacy with this PN formulation.

10. **C.** Water requirements are 30-40 mL/kg/d for patients without extra-renal fluid losses: 60 kg x 40 mL/kg/d = 2400 mL/d.

11. **A.** It is difficult to feed patients with severe pancreatitis enterally unless there is access to the small bowel (eg, jejunostomy). The other clinical conditions like trauma and burns would occur in patients in whom the gastrointestinal tract could and should be used for nutrition support. A patient receiving laparoscopic cholecystectomy would not need nutrition support. Most patients with hepatic encephalopathy can be fed enterally if they require nutrition support.

12. **E.** The dose of dextrose in PN should never exceed 5 mg/kg/min in adult patients. This can be converted to 25 kcal/kg/d.

13. **D.** Acetate is converted to bicarbonate in the liver and would thus help or at least not exacerbate the metabolic acidosis.

14. **A.** Calcium phosphate is a relatively insoluble compound so manufacturer guidelines for the concentrations of these two elements must be followed closely to prevent precipitation. The order of mixing these components in the PN formulation is also important.

15. **B.** Folic acid should be given at a dose of at least 600 µg/d during pregnancy. Many practitioners administer 1 mg/d above what the patient is eating or receiving via nutrition support. This has been shown to prevent neural tube defects in the newborn.

16. **C.** Hyperosmolar nutrients (dextrose, amino acids) can be used to concentrate the PN formulation, but it would have to be administered via a central vein.

17. **D.** If calcium is added last, the PN formulation will contain the final volume including all other nutrients. The chance of calcium causing a precipitate will be decreased since all other

components (eg, phosphorus) are diluted in the entire volume of the PN.

18. **E.** A 0.22-micron filter will do all three. In contrast, a 1.2-micron filter (used with TNAs) will not filter most bacteria.

19. **D.** Copper is excreted via the biliary tract. Patients with severe cholestasis should have copper removed during short-term parenteral nutrition. In long-term PN, copper may be required in reduced doses to prevent anemia. Serum copper concentrations should be monitored regularly in long-term patients who have cholestasis.

20. **D.** She is not a candidate for long-term PN because her gastrointestinal tract would be accessible and functional. Nasogastric and nasoduodenal methods are only used for short-term use of enteral nutrition. A jejunostomy would be ideal because she also has GERD and perhaps gastroparesis from her diabetes.

21. **B.** Several liquid preparations for drugs contain sorbitol as a pharmaceutical vehicle. These liquid preparations are commonly used in patients with tubes because the drugs can be given easily this way, especially if the patient cannot swallow. Most enteral nutrition formulations are close to being isotonic, ie, the osmotic load or solute load are not big factors in causing diarrhea. Fiber will prevent or improve diarrhea in most cases.

22. **C.** Metoclopramide enhances gastric emptying and is used commonly in patients with gastrointestinal intolerance. This is true in both diabetics and nondiabetics.

23. **D.** Phenytoin absorption is markedly impaired when it is given concurrently with enteral tube feeding. The enteral tube feeding should be held 2 hours before and after the daily dose of phenytoin capsules. To maintain the current dose of enteral nutrition, the rate of feeding should be increased to 100 mL/h x 20 h (2000 mL/d).

24. **B.** Drugs such as amlodipine, carbamazepine, and cyclosporine are profoundly metabolized in the gastrointestinal tract before absorption. Grapefruit juice from frozen concentrate has been shown to inhibit gastrointestinal CYP 3A4 and thus allows more of the drug to be absorbed. This has caused drug toxicity for drugs with a narrow therapeutic index.

7. References

Brown RO, Dickerson RN. Drug-nutrient interactions. *Am J Managed Care.* 1999;5:345-351.

Brown RO. Parenteral and enteral nutrition in adult patients. In: Herfindal ET, Gourley DR, eds. *Textbook of Therapeutics: Drug and Disease Management,* 7th ed. Philadelphia: Lippincott, Williams, & Wilkins; 2001:193-211.

Chessman KH, Teasley-Strausburg KM. Assessment of nutrition status and nutrition requirements. In: Dipiro JT, Talbert RL, eds. *Pharmacotherapy: A Pathophysiologic Approach*, 5th ed. New York: McGraw-Hill; 2002:2445-2463.

DeHart RM, Worthington MA. Nutritional considerations in major organ failure. In: Dipiro JT, Talbert RL, eds. *Pharmacotherapy: A Pathophysiologic Approach*, 5th ed. New York: McGraw-Hill; 2002:2519-2542.

Guidelines for the use of parenteral and enteral nutrition in adult and pediatric patients. *J Parenter Enteral Nutr.* 2002;26(1 Suppl):1SA-138SA.

Janson DD, Chessman KH. Enteral nutrition. In: Dipiro JT, Talbert RL, eds. *Pharmacotherapy: A Pathophysiologic Approach*, 5th ed. New York: McGraw-Hill; 2002:2495-2517.

Malone M. General nutrition. In: Herfindal ET, Gourley DR, eds. *Textbook of Therapeutics: Drug and Disease Management,* 7th ed. Philadelphia: Lippincott, Williams, & Wilkins; 2001:163-174.

Mattox TW. Parenteral nutrition. In: Dipiro JT, Talbert RL, eds. *Pharmacotherapy: A Pathophysiologic Approach*, 5th ed. New York McGraw-Hill; 2002:2475-2494.

National Advisory Group on Standards and Practice Guidelines for Parenteral Nutrition. Safe practices for parenteral nutrition formulations. *J Parenter Enteral Nutr.* 1998;22:49-66.

Reiter PD, Sacks G. Prevalence and significance of malnutrition. In: Dipiro JT, Talbert RL, eds. *Pharmacotherapy: A Pathophysiologic Approach*, 5th ed. New York: McGraw-Hill; 2002:2465-2474.

Van Den Berghe G, Wouters P, Weekers F, et al. Intensive insulin therapy in critically ill patients. *N Engl J Med.* 2001;345:1359-1367.

19. Oncology

Susannah Motl, PharmD
Assistant Professor, Department of Pharmacy
University of Tennessee College of Pharmacy

Contents

1. **Overview**

2. **Drug Therapy**

3. **Nondrug Therapy**

4. **Key Points**

5. **Questions and Answers**

6. **References**

1. Overview

Definition

- Oncology can be defined as the science dealing with the etiology, pathogenesis, and treatment of cancers (synonymous with malignant neoplasms).

- It encompasses more than 100 different diseases that share characteristics of uncontrollable cell growth, invasion of local tissues, and metastases (eg, spread from original site).

- In the United States, men have roughly a 1 in 2 lifetime risk of developing cancer and women have a 1 in 3 risk.

Classifications

- Malignancies arise from four tissue types (epithelial, connective, lymphoid, and nerve) and are classified based on this origin. Table 1 shows the tissue origin of each type of malignancy.

Table 1

Tissue Origin of Malignant Tumor Types

Origin	Tissue type	Malignant tumor
Epithelial	Surface epithelium	Carcinoma
	Glandular tissue	Adenocarcinoma
Connective	Fibrous	Fibrosarcoma
	Bone	Osteosarcoma
	Smooth/striated muscle	Leiomyosarcoma/ rhabdomyosarcoma
	Fat	Liposarcoma
Lymphoid	Bone marrow	Leukemia
	Lymphoid	Hodgkin's, non-Hodgkin's lymphoma
	Plasma	Multiple myeloma
Neural	Glial	Glioblastoma, astrocytoma
	Nerve sheath	Neurofibrosarcoma
	Melanocytes	Malignant melanoma
Mixed	Gonadal tissue	Teratocarcinoma

Adapted from Balmer et al, 2002.

Table 2

Warning Signs of Cancer in Adults

*C*hange in bowel or bladder habits
A sore that does not heal
*U*nusual bleeding or discharge
*T*hickening of lump in breast or elsewhere
*I*ndigestion or difficulty swallowing
*O*bvious change in wart or mole
*N*agging cough or hoarseness

Clinical Presentation

- The first signs and symptoms of cancer develop when the tumor has grown to approximately 10^9 cells (1 cm in diameter or 1 g mass).

- The type of cancer determines the presentation of signs and symptoms, which vary widely across tumor types.

- Positive screening tests (see section on nondrug therapy) or generalized signs of anorexia, fatigue, fever, weight loss, and anemia must also be evaluated.

- Tables 2 and 3 show the American Cancer Society's seven warning signs of cancer for adults and the warning signs for children.

Pathophysiology and Etiology

- Cancer promoting factors include:
  - * External factors: tobacco, chemicals, radiation, infectious organisms, diet

Table 3

Warning Signs of Cancer in Children

*C*ontinued, unexplained weight loss
*H*eadaches with vomiting in the morning
*I*ncreased swelling or persistent pain in bones or joints
*L*ump or mass in abdomen, neck, or elsewhere
*D*evelopment of a whitish appearance in the pupil of the eye
*R*ecurrent fevers not caused by infection
*E*xcessive bruising or bleeding
*N*oticeable paleness or prolonged tiredness

* Internal factors: genetics, hormones, immune conditions

- Development of cancer is genetically regulated and is a multistage process:
    * Initiation: normal cells are exposed to chemical, physical, or biological carcinogens. This results in irreversible damage, genetic mutations, and selective growth advantages.
    * Promotion: reversible environmental changes favor the growth of the mutated cells.
    * Transformation: the cells becomes cancerous.
    * Progression: additional genetic changes occur resulting in increased cancerous proliferation. Tumors invade local tissues and metastases occur.

- Oncogene activation and tumor suppressor gene (TSG) inhibition are necessary for the development and growth of cancer.
    * Oncogenes promote growth advantages in mutated cells and cause excessive proliferation.
    * Inactivation of TSGs results in inappropriate cell growth, as TSGs normally regulate the cell cycle (eg, halt growth for repairs and corrections in normal cell development).

- Malignant tumor cells do not resemble their tissue of origin (in contrast to benign tumors). They are unstable and are incapable of performing normal cell functions.

Diagnostic Criteria

- A sample of suspected malignant tissues or cells is needed for a definitive diagnosis. Radiation or chemotherapy should not begin without pathological staging.

- This can be done with a biopsy, fine-needle aspiration, or exfoliative cytology.

- Further imaging may include:
    * Chest x-ray: evaluates spread to bones or lungs
    * Computed tomography (CT): assesses the size, shape, and position of tumor; detects masses in lymph nodes, brain, or adrenal glands via a three-dimensional view
    * Magnetic resonance imaging (MRI): evaluates spread to the brain or spinal cord
    * Positron emission tomography (PET) scanning: evaluates lymph and other metastatic involvement
    * Bone scanning: assesses bone metastasis

- Laboratory work may include: complete blood counts (CBCs), blood chemistries, and tumor markers (see section on nondrug therapy).

- If a diagnosis of cancer is made, the malignancy will need to be staged or categorized based on severity. Staging guides the oncology practitioner in determining the prognosis and the treatment regimen for the patient.
    * The TNM staging system is the most commonly used tool for solid tumors. Tumors are scored numerically based on the size of the tumor (T), the extent of lymph node involvement (N), and presence or absence of metastases (M). This allows classification of tumors by stage, from stage 0 to stage IV, with stage IV denoting the presence of metastasis (eg, most severe disease). A stage 0 tumor is called a *carcinoma in situ,* in which case the malignancy has not yet invaded the basement membrane of the epithelial surface.
    * Lymphoid tumors are staged differently and beyond the scope of this review. Refer to Balmer et al, 2002, Chaps. 129, 131, and 132, for more information.

Treatment Principles and Goals

- Treatment regimens are based on the type of cancer, stage, the age of the patient, and other prognostic factors (eg, presence of a tumor marker, poor performance status, and ethnicity, among others).

- *Neoadjuvant therapy* is therapy given prior to the main treatment regimen. The goal is to shrink the tumor and to increase the efficacy of the primary treatment.

- *Adjuvant therapy* is additional therapy given after the main treatment. The goal is to make sure that all residual disease has been eradicated.

- The four main cancer treatments include: surgery, radiation, chemotherapy, and biologic therapy. Most regimens are a combination of modalities.
    * Surgery alone is reserved for solid localized tumors, where the entire cancer can be resected. It may also be combined with other modalities in later stages of disease. This is not an option for patients with lymphoid-based disease (eg, Hodgkin's disease).
    * Radiation alone is also reserved for curing localized tumors, as it treats a very focused area. It also can be combined with other treatments as neoadjuvant or adjuvant therapy to reduce disease-related symptoms.
        · Patients need to be aware that the affected area may become irritated, dry, or appear sunburned after radiation therapy.

* Chemotherapy is a means of systemic treatment, in contrast to the two types of local treatment just described. It can be used to treat the primary tumor as well as metastases. This is generally not administered to patients with local disease that can be fully resected.
* Biologic therapy is another systemic treatment and includes agents such as monoclonal antibodies, interferons, interleukins, and tumor vaccines. It is a new type of treatment and acts by stimulating the host immune system.

• The goals of cancer chemotherapy are based on the type and stage of cancer, as well patient characteristics (eg, an older patient with a short life expectancy may not be offered intense treatment that may impair their quality of life).
* *Localized or regional disease* (ie, stages 0, I, II, and early III): curative intent, inhibit recurrence of disease.
  • Stage 0 diseases are often not treated, but monitored until clinically apparent.
* *Advanced or metastasized disease* (ie, advanced stage III and all stage IV): palliation of symptoms, reduce tumor load, prolongation of survival time, and increase quality of life.

Survival and response to treatment
• In 2002, it was predicted that 1500 people a day would die of a cancer-related process.

• Survival depends on patient characteristics, type of disease, stage of disease, and treatment regimen. Older patients with more severe disease and faster-growing tumors have a poor prognosis.

• Response to treatment modalities for solid tumors are classified as:
* *Cure*: 5 years of cancer-free survival for most tumor types
* *Complete response (CR)*: absence of all neoplastic disease for a minimum of 1 month after cessation of treatment
* *Partial response (PR)*: ≥50% decrease in tumor size or other disease markers for a minimum of 1 month
* *Stable disease*: ≤25% decrease in tumor size or no change
* *Progression*: ≥25% increase in tumor size or new lesion

• Response to treatment for hematologic cancers are measured by the elimination of abnormal cells, a decrease in tumor markers to normal, and the improved function of affected cells.

2. Drug Therapy

Chemotherapy

• Chemotherapeutic agents have a very narrow therapeutic index and toxic side effects.

• They are generally more effective in combination due to synergism through biochemical interactions.
  * It is important to choose drugs with different mechanisms of action, resistance, and toxicity profiles to get the full benefit of combination therapy.

• Chemotherapy has the greatest effect on rapidly-dividing cells, as most of the potent chemotherapy drugs act by damaging DNA.
  * These agents are more active in different phases of the cell cycle. A therapeutic effect is seen on cancer cells, but adverse effects are also seen on human cells that rapidly divide (eg, hair follicles, gastrointestinal tract, blood cells).
  * Agents can be phase-specific or phase-nonspecific. Nonspecific agents are effective in all phases.

Cell Cycle Phase

• G_0 = resting phase: no cell division occurs and cancer cells are generally not susceptible to chemotherapy. This is problematic for slow-growing tumors that exist primarily in this phase.

• G_1 = postmitotic phase: enzymes for DNA synthesis are manufactured.

• S = DNA synthesis phase: DNA separation and replication occurs.

• G_2 = premitotic phase: specialized proteins and RNA are made.

• M = mitosis: actual cell division occurs.

Drug Classes

There are numerous chemotherapy agents. Drugs will be grouped by class. Please refer to the corresponding table for each class of drugs.

Alkylating agents (Table 4)
Mechanism of action
• Covalent bond formation of drugs to nucleic acids and proteins. Results in the cross-linking of two

Table 4

Alkylating Agents

Generic name (trade name)	Dosage range	Dosage forms	Frequency	Diseases
Nitrogen mustard				
Mechlorethamine (Mustargen®)	6-10 mg/m²	IV	q 28 days	HL, NHL
Cyclophosphamide (Cytoxan®, Neosar®)	40-50 mg/kg, 1-5 mg/kg	IV, PO	qd 2-5 days, qd	ALL, CLL, HL, NHL, myeloma, testis, neuroblastoma, breast ovary, lung, cervix
Ifosfamide (Ifex®)	1.2 g/m², 4 g/m²	IV	qd x 5 days q 3 wk, qd x 6 d	Testis, BMT
Melphalan (Alkeran®)	16 mg/m², 6 mg	IV, PO	q 2 wk x 4, 2-3 wk	Myeloma, breast, ovarian
Chlorambucil (Leukeran®)	0.1-0.2 mg/kg	PO	qd x 3-6 wk	CLL, HL, NHL
Ethylenimines and methylmelamines				
Altretamine (Hexalen®)	260 mg/m²	PO	qd x 14-21 d	Ovarian
Thiotepa (Thioplex®)	0.3-0.8 mg/kg	IV	q 1-4 wk	Bladder, breast, ovarian
Alkyl sulfonates				
Busulfan (Myleran®, Busulfex®)	0.8 mg/kg (pre-BMT), 1-8 mg/kg	IV, PO	q6h, qd	CML, BMT
Nitrosureas				
Carmustine (BICNU®)	150-200 mg/m²	IV, implant	q 6 wk	HL, NHL, brain, myeloma
Streptozocin (Zanosar®)	500 mg/m²	IV	qd 5 d	Islet cell carcinoma

ALL, acute lymphocytic leukemia; BMT, bone marrow transplant; CLL, chronic lymphocytic leukemia; CML, chronic myelogenous leukemia; HL, Hodgkin's lymphoma; NHL, non-Hodgkin's lymphoma.

DNA strands and inhibition of DNA replication. These are non–phase specific agents. Most commonly used agents include: cyclophosphamide (C), ifosfamide (I), carmustine, dacarbazine, and temozolomide.

Patient instructions and counseling
• All drugs are carcinogenic, teratogenic, and mutagenic. Male and female patients should not try to conceive a baby while on these drugs. Medications may cause sterility. Let your dentist know you are on chemotherapy, due to an increased risk of bleeding and infections. Hydration therapy is recommended for C and I. Let your MD know if you have burning upon urination.

Adverse drug events
• Myelosuppression, primarily leukopenia; mucosal ulceration; pulmonary fibrosis and interstitial pneumonitis; alopecia; nausea and vomiting; amenorrhea and azoospermia; hemorrhagic cystitis with C and I.

Drug interactions
• Drugs with specific interactions of moderate to major severity include:
  * Altretamine: tricyclic antidepressants, monoamine oxidase inhibitors
  * Busulfan: itraconazole, pheytoin
  * Carmustine: cimetidine, ethyl alcohol, pheytoin
  * Cyclophosphamide: allopurinol, barbiturates, digoxin, phenytoin, hydrochlorothiazide, tamoxifen, steroids, trastuzumab
  * Ifosfamide: allopurinol, phenytoin, warfarin

Monitoring parameters
• Pulmonary function tests; renal and hepatic tests; chest x-ray; CBC with differential (baseline and expected nadir prior to next cycle) and electrolytes; urinalysis for RBC detection; signs of bleeding (bruising, melena); infection (sore throat, fever); nausea or vomiting.

Antimetabolites (Table 5)
Mechanism of action
• Structural analogues of natural metabolites. Act by falsely inserting themselves in place of a pyrimidine

Table 5

Antimetabolites

Generic name (trade name)	Dosage range	Dosage forms	Frequency	Disease
Folic acid antagonists				
Methotrexate (Rheumatrex®)	12-15 g/m², 30-50 mg/kg	IV, PO, IM, SC, intrathecal, intra-arterial	qd	Pancreatic, NSCLC, ovarian
Pyrimidine analogs				
Fluorouracil, 5-FU (Adrucil®)	12 mg/kg (max 800 mg/d)	IV	qd x 4 d	ALL, NHL, breast, head, neck, lung, bone
Cytarabine (Cytosar-U®, DepoCyt®)	100-300 mg/m², 50 mg	IV, intrathecal	qd x 7 d, q14d	Colorectal, breast, gastric, pancreatic, bladder, stomach
Capecitabine (Xeloda®)	2500 mg/m²	PO	qd x 14 d q 3 wk	ALL, CML, ANLL, leukemia, NHL
Gemcitabine (Gemzar®)	100-1250 mg/m²	IV	q wk	Breast, colorectal
Purine analogs				
Mercaptopurine (Purinethol®)	1.5-2.5 mg/kg	PO	qd	ALL
Thioguanine (Tabloid®)	2-3 mg/kg	PO	qd	ALL, ANLL
Pentostatin (Nipent®)	4 mg/m²	IV	q 2 wk	CLL, hairy cell leukemia
Cladribine (Leustatin®)	0.09-0.1 mg/kg	IV	qd x 7 d	NHL, hairy cell leukemia
Fludarabine (Fludara®)	25 mg/m²	IV	qd x 5 d	CLL, NHL

ALL, acute lymphocytic leukemia; ANLL, acute nonlymphocytic leukemia; CLL, chronic lymphocytic leukemia; CML, chronic myelogenous leukemia; NHL, non-Hodgkin's lymphoma; NSCLC, non–small cell lung cancer.

or purine ring, causing an interference in nucleic acid synthesis. Phase-specific agents that are most active in the S phase and in tumors with a high growth fraction. Subdivided into three groups: folate, purine, and pyrimidine antagonists.

Patient instructions and counseling
• Avoid crowds and sick people. You may be asked to chew ice if receiving 5-FU or capecitabine. This is to reduce damage to the mucosal lining in your mouth. Contact your MD if you have uncontrollable nausea or vomiting, excessive diarrhea, or pain, swelling, or tingling in palms and soles of feet (hand-foot syndrome).

Adverse drug events
• Hand-foot syndrome, stomatitis (5-FU, capecitabine), severe diarrhea, GI mucosal damage, myelosuppression, alopecia, neurotoxicity (cytarabine and fludarabine), rash and fever, flu-like symptoms (gemcitabine), renal toxicity and mucositis (methotrexate)

Interactions
• Specific interactions include:
  * Capecitabine: warfarin, phenytoin
  * Cytarabine: digoxin
  * Fluorouracil: hydrochlorothiazide, metronidazole, warfarin
  * Gemcitabine: warfarin
  * Mercaptopurine: warfarin, allopurinol
  * Methotrexate: NSAIDs, amiodarone, amoxicillin, sulfasalazine, doxycycline, erythromycin, hydrochlorothiazide, leucovorin, mercaptopurine, omeprazole, phenytoin, procarbazine, rotavirus, tamoxifen
  * Pentostatin: cyclophosphamide, fludarabine
  * Thioguanine: busulfan, mesalamine, sulfasalazine

Monitoring parameters
• Note any complaints of mucositis or mouth soreness, monitor for neurotoxicity, CBC with differential prior to each dose of drug, hepatic and renal function, monitor for tingling or swelling of palms and soles of hands and feet, bruising or bleeding, INR (capecitabine), monitor weight and question patient about diarrhea, jaundice, and hepatomegaly (mercaptopurine).

Antitumor antibiotics (Table 6)

Mechanism of action

- Bleomycin is the only cell cycle–specific agent. Anthracyclines: block DNA and RNA transcription through the intercalation (insertion) of adjoining nucleic acid pairs in DNA, which results in DNA strand breakage. Mitomycin: alklyating-like agent that cross-links DNA. Dactinomycin: blocks RNA synthesis. Bleomycin: inhibits DNA synthesis in mitosis and G_2 stages of growth. All agents are too toxic to treat bacterial infections.

Patient instructions and counseling

- Contact MD with fast, slow, or irregular heartbeats and/or breathing difficulties; anthracyclines may cause a change of urine color or whites of eyes to a bluish-green or orangish-red. Bleomycin may cause a change in skin color or nail growth.

Adverse drug events

- Severe nausea and vomiting, alopecia, and stomatitis. Anthracyclines: cardiac toxicity, acute or chronic (doxorubicin = daunorubicin > idarubicin > epirubicin > mitoxantrone). All drugs have limits on cumulative lifetime dosing. Avoid in patients with a cardiac history. Myelosuppression with all agents, although mitomycin demonstrates a delayed effect. Dactinomycin: renal toxicity, leukopenia, increased pigmentation of previously radiated skin. Bleomycin: pulmonary fibrosis and interstitial pneumonitis.

Interactions

- Specific interactions include:
  * Bleomycin: phenytoin, digoxin
  * Doxorubicin: cisplatin, digoxin, paclitaxel, phenyoin, phenobarbital, trastuzumab, zidovudine
  * Epirubicin: cimetidine, paclitaxel, trastuzumab
  * Idarubicin: trastuzumab

Monitoring parameters

- Hepatic, renal, CBC with differential monitoring. Pulmonary function tests pre- and post-treatment with bleomycin, cardiac monitoring via left ventricular ejection fraction (LVEF) measurements for anthracyclines, extravasation and necrosis with anthracyclines. Local bladder symptoms after instillation (frequency, pain, hematuria, bladder spasms) with valrubicin.

Table 6

Antitumor Antibiotics

Generic name (trade name)	Dosage range	Dosage forms	Frequency	Disease
Anthracyclines				
Doxorubicin (Adriamycin®, Doxil® [liposomal])	60-75 mg/m², 20-50 mg/m² (lipo)	IV	q 3 wk	ALL, ANLL, NHL, HL, solid tumors of every major organ
Daunorubicin (Cerubidine®, Daunoxome® [liposomal])	45 mg/m², 40-100 mg/m² (lipo)	IV	qd x 3 d, q 2-3 wk	ANLL, ALL
Epirubicin (Ellence®, Pharmarubicin®)	100-120 mg/m²	IV	q 3 wk	Breast, bladder, lung, ovarian
Idarubicin (Idamycin®)	12 mg/m²	IV	qd x 3 d	ANLL
Mitoxantrone (Novantrone®)	12-14 mg/m²	IV	qd x 3 d	ANLL, prostate, NHL
Valrubicin (Valstar®)	800 mg	Intravesically	q wk x 6 wk	Bladder
Alkylating like				
Mitomycin (Mutamycin®)	10-20 mg/m²	IV	q 6-8 wk	Bladder, breast, NSCLC, cervix pancreatic, colon
Chromomycin				
Dactinomycin (Cosmegen®)	12-15 µg/kg	IV	qd x 5 d	Wilms', testis, sarcoma
Miscellaneous				
Bleomycin (Blenoxane®)	10-20 USP U/m²/wk	IV, IM, SC	q wk	HL, NHL, testis, head, neck, lung, skin

ALL, acute lymphocytic leukemia; ANLL, acute nonlymphocytic leukemia; CLL, chronic lymphocytic leukemia; CML, chronic myelogenous leukemia; NHL, non-Hodgkin's lymphoma; NSCLC, non–small cell lung cancer.

Pharmacokinetics
- Anthracyclines are extensively bound in the tissue, have large volumes of distribution, long half-lives, and are excreted in the bile. They need dosing adjustments in hepatic impairment. Bleomycin is renally excreted and needs dosing adjustments in impaired patients.

Other
- Lifetime doses of doxorubicin should not exceed 450-550 mg/m^2, taking into account other anthracycline agents received; lifetime maximum of epirubicin is 900 mg/m^2, idarubicin <150 mg/m^2.

Hormones and antagonists (Table 7)
Mechanism of action
- A diverse group of compounds that act on hormone-dependent tumors by inhibiting or decreasing the production of the disease-causing hormone.

Patient instructions and counseling
- Avoid use in pregnant women; several agents may cause weight gain and menstrual irregularities in women. Be aware of leg swelling or tenderness, breathing problems, and sweating. Transient muscle or bone pain or problems urinating may occur initially in patients receiving LHRH agonists.

Adverse drug events
- Edema, menstrual disorders, hot flashes, transient urinary or bone pain, gynecomastia, elevated liver enzymes, nausea and vomiting, diarrhea, body pain, erectile impotence, decreased libido, endometrial cancers with tamoxifen

Interactions
- Specific interactions include:
  * Aminoglutethimide: dexamethasone, warfarin, tamoxifen, theophylline
  * Megestrol: dofetilide contraindication
  * Diethylstilbestrol: warfarin
  * Medroxyprogesterone acetate: aminoglutethimide, rifampin
  * Tamoxifen: contraceptives, anticoagulants, cyclophosphamide, chemotherapy agents
  * Fluoxymesterone: cyclosporine, anticoagulants, valerian

Monitoring parameters
- Check WBCs with differential, platelets, liver function tests, thyroid function, and serum creatinine regularly. Note any weight changes, abnormal vaginal bleeding, body or bone pain, galactorrhea, or decreased libido. Monitor for embolic disorders and uterine cancer (in females).

Pharmacokinetics
- The majority of agents are available orally with longer half-lives, allowing once-daily dosing.

Other
- Agents are often contraindicated if patient has more than one hormone-dependent tumor. With the exception of tamoxifen and LHRH agonists, the majority of agents are not indicated for first-line therapy.

Plant alkaloids (Table 8)
Mechanism of action
- Inhibit the replication of cancerous cells. Taxanes and vincas interfere with microtubule assembly; camptothecins and epipodophyllotoxins inhibit topoisomerase I and II enzymes, respectively.

Patient instructions and counseling
- Contact MD with uncontrollable diarrhea (irinotecan), nausea or vomiting, signs and symptoms of an infection; should receive prophylaxis for emesis, pretreatment for anaphylaxis (taxanes).

Adverse drug events
- Myelosuppression (dose-limiting toxicity for all except vincristine), mucositis, nausea and vomiting, alopecia, edema (docetaxel), hypotension upon administration (taxanes), neurotoxicity (vincristine).

Interactions
- Specific interactions include:
  * Docetaxel: itraconazole
  * Etoposide: cyclosporine, St. John's wort
  * Irinotecan: St. John's wort
  * Paclitaxel: phenytoin
  * Teniposide: Phenobarbital, phenytoin
  * Topotecan: granulocyte colony-stimulating factor (G-CSF)
  * Vincas: CYP 3A4 inhibitors; itraconazole, voriconazole
  * Vincristine: phenytoin, l-asparaginase, carbemazepine, digoxin, filgrastim, nifedipine, pheytoin, zidovudine
  * Vinblastine: phenytoin, erythromycin, mitomycin, zidovudine

Monitoring parameters
- Monitor WBCs with differential for all agents, peripheral neuropathy, liver and renal function, constipation, painful mouth sores, blood pressure (taxanes and epipodophyllotoxins), acute and late-onset diarrhea or dyspnea on exertion (irinotecan), bilirubin elevations (taxanes and camptothecins), fluid retention (docetaxel); neuropathy, shortness of breath and bronchospasm (vincas).

Table 7

Hormones and Antagonists

Generic name (trade name)	Dosage range	Dosage forms	Frequency	Disease
Adrenocorticoids				
Aminoglutethimide (Cytadren®)	250 mg	PO	bid x 2 wk	Adrenal, breast, prostate
Progestins				
Hydroxyprogesterone caproate (Duralutin®)	1000 mg	IM	q wk	Endometrial cancer
Megestrol acetate (Megace®)	40 mg, 40-320 mg	PO	qid, qd divided	Breast, endometrial
Medroxyprogesterone acetate (Provera®, Depo-Provera®)	400-1000 mg			
Estrogens				
Diethylstilbestrol (Diastyl®)	150 mg to 1 g, 15 mg	IM	q wk	Endometrial, renal cell
Ethinyl estradiol (Estinyl®)	150 µg-3 mg, 100 µg to 1 mg	PO	qd	Prostate, breast
Antiestrogen				
Tamoxifen (Nolvadex®)	20-40 mg	PO	qd, tid	Prostate, breast
Fulvestrant (Faslodex®)	250 mg	IM	qd	Breast, DCIS, breast cancer prophylaxis
Aromatase inhibitors				
Anastrozole (Arimidex®)	1 mg	PO	q month	Metastatic breast
Letrozole (Femara®)	2.5 mg	PO	qd	Breast
Androgens				
Testosterone propionate (Delatestryl®)	200-400 mg	IM	qd	Breast
Fluoxymesterone (Halotestin®)	10-40 mg	PO	q 2-4 wk	Mammary
Antiandrogens				
Flutamide (Eulexin®)	750 mg	PO	qd	Breast
Bicalutamide (Casodex®)	50 mg	PO	qd	Prostate
Nilutamide (Nilandron®)	300 mg	PO	qd	Prostate
LHRH agonists				
Leuprolide (Lupron®)	7.5 mg, 1 implant	IM, SC	q month, q year	Prostate, breast
Goserelin (Zoladex®)	3.6 mg	SC	q month	Prostate, breast

DCIS, ductal carcinoma in situ.

Pharmacokinetics
- Taxanes and epipodophyllotoxins are extensively bound to plasma and tissues.

Other
- Drug resistance may occur via p-glycoprotein pumps for all agents; topotecan needs dose adjustments for patients with a CrCl <40 mL/min; vincas are vesicants and need close monitoring for extravasation; vincas are contraindicated in the diagnosis of granulocytopenia.

Biologic response modifiers (Table 9)
Mechanism of action
- Activate the body's immune-mediated host defense mechanisms to malignant cells. In contrast to immunotherapy, these agents have direct biological effects on malignancies.

Patient instructions and counseling
- Let your MD know if you have severe fatigue, trouble breathing, or irregular heart rhythms. Chills, fever, and flu-like symptoms are common. Taste and smell alterations occur with levamisole.

Table 8

Plant Alkaloids

Generic name (trade name)	Dosage range	Dosage forms	Frequency	Disease
Taxanes				
Docetaxel (Taxotere®)	60-100 mg/m²	IV	q 3 wk	NSCLC, breast, ovarian, head, neck
Paclitaxel (Taxol®)	135-175 mg/m²	IV	q 3 wk	NSCLC, breast, ovarian, head
Epipodophyllotoxins				
Etoposide (Vepesid®)	35-100 mg/m², 50 mg/m²	IV, PO	qd x 4-5 d, qd x 21 d	SCLC, testis
Teniposide (Vumon®)	165 mg/m²	IV	q wk x 4 doses	ALL, SCLC
Camptothecins				
Irinotecan (Camptosar®)	100-125 mg/m²	IV	3 x wk x 8 doses	Colorectal
Topotecan (Hycamtin®)	1.5 mg/m²	IV	qd x 5 d q 21 d	Ovarian
Vinca alkaloids				
Vincristine (Oncovin®)	1.4 mg/m²	IV	q wk	ALL, HL, NHL, Wilms
Vinblastine (Velban®)	3.7-18.5 mg/m²	IV	q wk	HL, NHL, testis
Vinorelbine (Navelbine®)	25-30 mg/mm²	IV	q wk	NSCLC

ALL, acute lymphocytic leukemia; HL, Hodgkin's lymphoma; NHL, non-Hodgkin's lymphoma; NSCLC, non–small cell lung cancer; SCLC, small cell lung cancer.

Adverse drug events

- Hypotension and hypersensitivity upon infusion, cardiac, pulmonary, and renal impairment. Avoid in patients with autoimmune disorders. Mental status changes, fever, chills, nausea, and musculoskeletal pain with all agents. Tumor lysis syndrome with rituximab.

Interactions

- Specific drug interactions include:
  * Aldesleukin: glucocorticoids
  * Interferon-alpha 2b: zidovudine, theophylline
  * Levamisole: warfarin, alcohol
  * Rituximab: cisplatin

Table 9

Biologic Response Modifiers

Generic name (trade name)	Dosage range	Dosage forms	Frequency	Disease
Immune therapies				
Aldesleukin (Proleukin®)	0.037 mg/kg	IV	q8h x 14 doses	Metastatic renal cell, metastatic melanoma
Interferon-alpha 2b (Intron A®)	10-20 x 10⁶ U, 2 x 10⁶ U (hairy)	IV and SC	qd x 5 d per wk,[1] 3 x wk x 6 mo	Malignant melanoma, hairy cell leukemia
Levamisole (Ergamisol®)	50 mg	PO	q8h x 3 d	Adjuvant colon with 5-FU
Monoclonal antibodies				
Rituximab (Rituxan®)	375 mg/m²	IV	q wk x 4-8 doses	NHL, CLL
Trastuzumab (Herceptin®)	2-4 mg/kg	IV and SC	q wk	Metastatic breast
Gemtuzumab (Mylotarg®)	9 mg/m²	IV	q 2 wk	AML
Alemtuzumab (Campath®)	3-10 mg	IV	qd, then 30 mg/d 3 x wk	B-cell CLL

[1]Induction dose.

AML, acute myelogenous leukemia; CLL, chronic lymphocytic leukemia; NHL, non-Hodgkin's lymphoma.

* Trastuzumab: anthracyclines, cyclophosphamide, warfarin

Monitoring parameters
• Baseline and follow-up pulmonary, cardiac, and renal function tests. Check CBCs with differential, LFTs, TSH, electrolytes, and glucose regularly. Premedicate with acetaminophen and diphenhydramine for monoclonal antibodies. Observe blood pressure during infusion for all agents.

Other
• Make sure correct form of interferon alpha is being used (four forms). Do not administer gemtuzumab and alemtuzumab as an IV push or bolus.

Miscellaneous
Platinum compounds
• Alkylating-like agents causing the inhibition of DNA synthesis. Adverse effects include: nephrotoxicity, peripheral neurotoxicity, myelosuppression, ototoxicity, nausea and vomiting.
    * Cisplatin: hydration therapy and premedications are needed. Interactions: doxorubicin, rituximab, tacrolimus, topotecan

Asparaginase
• Removes exogenous asparagines from leukemic cells, which are required for their survival. Intradermal skin testing is needed due to severe anaphylactic reactions. Myelosuppression, hyperuricemia, hyperglycemia, and renal problems. Interactions: methotrexate, prednisolone, prednisone, vincristine

Hydroxyurea
• Inhibits DNA synthesis without interfering with RNA and protein synthesis. Myelosuppression (leukopenia), development of secondary leukemias, nausea, vomiting, diarrhea, constipation, mucositis, and rare fatal hepatotoxicity and pancreatitis. Interactions: didanosine, stavudine.

Imatinib
• Selective inhibitor of the Philadelphia chromosome (biomarker in CML). Causes hepatotoxicity, fluid retention (pleural effusions, weight gain), neutropenia, GI effects, muscle cramps, nausea and vomiting. Interactions: CYP 3A4 substrates (cyclosporine, simvastatin, erythromycin, itraconazole), CYP 2C9 substrates (warfarin).

Common Toxicities and Treatments

• Rapidly dividing cells, including mucous membranes, hair, skin, GI tract, and bone marrow are the most adversely affected.

Common toxicities of chemotherapeutic agents (Table 11)
The prevention and treatment of chemotherapy-induced nausea and vomiting (CINV) is an important area in which pharmacists may play a role in drug selection in oncology patients. The selection of anti-emetic agents should be based primarily on the emetogenic potential of the drug regimen. Other factors that increase the risk of CINV include: female gender, young age, prior chemotherapy exposure, lack of chronic alcohol use, combination chemotherapy, high dosage and numerous cycles, and short infusion times.

Table 10

Miscellaneous Agents

Generic name (trade name)	Dosage range	Dosage forms	Frequency	Disease
Platinum compounds				
Cisplatin (Platinol-AQ®)	50-100 mg/m²	IV	q 3-4 wk	NSCLC, ovarian, testis, bladder
Carboplatin (Paraplatin®)	300-400 mg/m²	IV	q 3-4 wk	Ovarian, testis, NSCLC, head and neck
Oxaliplatin (Eloxatin®)	85-200 mg/m²	IV	qd x 2 d q 2 wk	Colorectal
Enzymes				
Asparaginase (Elspar®)	200 IU/kg	IV	q 28 d	ALL
Cell-specific				
Hydroxyurea (Hydrea®)	20-30 mg/kg	PO	qd	CML, myeloma, head, neck
Tyrosine kinase inhibitor				
Imatinib mesylate (Gleevec®)	400-600 mg	PO	qd	CML, gastrointestinal stromal tumors

AML, acute myelogenous leukemia; CML, chronic myelogenous leukemia; NSLC, non–small cell lung cancer.

Table 11

Common Toxicities of Chemotherapeutic Agents

Toxicity	Causative drugs[1]	Recommended therapy
Alopecia	Cyclophosphamide, doxorubicin, paclitaxel, mechlorethamine	N/A
Cardiac toxicity	Anthracyclines	Limit cumulative doses
Diarrhea	Irinotecan, fluorouracil	Premedicate with atropine (irinotecan); treat with loperamide
Extravasation	Anthracyclines, mitomycin, vinka alkaloids, paclitaxel, mechlorethamine	Treat with heat packs for vincas, cold compresses for all other causes or instill normal saline to dilute drug
Hemorrhagic cystitis	Cyclophosphamide, ifosfamide	Premedicate: hydration therapy, mesna
Hepatotoxicity	Asparaginase, cytarabine, mercaptopurine, methotrexate	N/A
Hypersensitivity	Paclitaxel, asparaginase, cisplatin, carboplatin, etoposide, teniposide	Premedicate with ranitidine or cimetidine, diphenhydramine, dexamethasone or test dose; treat with emergency resuscitation
Infertility	Cyclophosphamide, chlorambucil, melphalan, mechlorethamine	N/A
Myelosuppression	Alklyating agents, fluorouracil, methotrexate, lomustine, cyclophosphamide, methotrexate	Treat with G-CSF, platelet transfusions
Nausea and vomiting	Cisplatin, cyclophosphamide, cytarabine, dacarbazine, ifosfamide, melphalan, mitomycin, mechlorethamine	Premedicate with phenothiazines (eg, compazine) and 5-HT3-receptor antagonists (eg, granisetron)
Neurotoxicity	Paclitaxel, cisplatin, cytarabine, methotrexate, vincristine, asparaginase	N/A
Pulmonary toxicity	Bleomycin, busulfan, carmustine, mitomycin	Treat with corticosteroids
Renal toxicity	Cisplatin, ifosfamide, methotrexate, streptozocin	Premedicate with hydration therapy, mannitol
Stomatitis	Fluorouracil, methotrexate	Hold ice chips in mouth
Edema	Docetaxel	Prophylactic dexamethasone

[1]Adverse effects are not limited to the listed drugs.

Table 12 summarizes the pertinent antiemetic drugs used in the prophylactic setting. Please note that treatment regimens are different, although the drugs are the same.

- For highly to moderately emetogenic drug regimens, dexamethasone and a 5-HT3 receptor antagonist are recommended for the prevention of CINV.

- For low to unlikely emetogenic drug regimens, dexamethasone and a phenothiazine are recommended.

- For delayed CINV (>24 hours after administration of chemotherapy), metoclopramide and dexamethasone are recommended.

- All patients receiving agents with emetogenic potential should receive prophylactic therapy for CINV with rescue medication readily available.

Miscellaneous Commonalities across Chemotherapy Agents

- All patients should not receive live and rotavirus vaccines during chemotherapy due to suppressed immune systems.

- The majority of agents are teratogenic and mutagenic.

- Patients should avoid becoming pregnant or breastfeeding during and immediately after chemotherapy.

- Patients should receive lab work on a regular basis to check for common toxicities, such as myelosuppression, renal and hepatic impairment, and electrolyte disturbances.

Table 12

Pharmacologic Management for the Prevention of Chemotherapy-Induced Nausea and Vomiting

Generic name (trade name)	Dosage range	Dosage forms	Frequency	Side effects
5-HT3 receptor antagonists				
Dolasetron (Anzemet®)	100-200 mg	PO	30 min before treatment	Headache, dizziness, constipation, blurred
Granisetron (Kytril®)	5-20 mg	PO	30 min before treatment	vision, elevated liver enzymes
Ondansetron (Zofran®)	10-25 mg	PO	30 min before treatment	
Phenothiazines				
Prochlorperazine (Compazine®)	10-25 mg	PO	q4h prn	Sedation, hypotension, extrapyramidal effects,
Chlorpromazine (Thorazine®)	1.25-5 mg	PO	q4-6h prn	lethargy
Promethazine (Phenergan®)	1-4 mg	PO	q4-6h prn	
Butyrophenones				
Droperidol (Inapsine®)	10-20 mg	IV	q4h prn	Sedation, tachycardia, hypotension
Haloperidol (Haldol®)	5-15 mg/m²	IV, IM, PO	q4-6h prn	
Corticosteroids				
Dexamethasone (Decadron®)	0.5-2 mg	PO	Varies	Anxiety, insomnia, GI upset, psychosis
Cannabinoids				
Dronabinol (Marinol®)	10-20 mg	PO	q3-6h	Drowsiness, euphoria, dry mouth
Benzodiazepines				
Lorazepam (Ativan®)	2 mg	PO	q6h	Sedation, amnesia
Benzamides				
Metoclopramide (Reglan®)	24 mg	PO	tid-qid	Diarrhea, sedation, agitation

[1]**Note:** Most agents are available in more than one dosage form. Due to space limitations, oral dosing has been given preference.

3. Nondrug Therapy

• As mentioned, cancer treatment is generally a combination of modalities. Chemotherapy is the mainstay, as most patients present with advanced disease upon diagnosis.

• Surgery plays a role in resecting primary tumors or metastases and can be part of neoadjuvant therapy to debulk large tumors. It can also be used diagnostically to biopsy tumors or conduct explorative laparotomies.

• Radiation is used to shrink primary tumors in local disease or metastases. It can be used in both neoadjuvant therapy to downsize tumors and in adjuvant therapy to eradicate residual disease.
    * Adverse effects include: skin irritation, nausea and vomiting, fatigue, and myelosuppression.

• Screening is also an important part of cancer therapy, as it can allow the detection of disease in very early stages, when the survival rates are much more acceptable. Table 13 refers to American Cancer Society (ACS) screening recommendations for patients at average risk of developing cancer.

• Tumor markers make possible additional screening tests, and are found in the plasma, serum, or other body fluids, and may be used to identify neoplastic growth.
    * These markers are often not sensitive to diagnose cancer and may produce false-positive results (ie, falsely identify people with a disease that do not have the disease).
    * They are helpful in identifying the recurrence of advanced disease in patients that had elevated levels upon diagnosis. Table 14 lists some commonly used tumor markers.

Table 13

American Cancer Society Screening Recommendations

Disease[1]	Sex	Age (y)	Procedure	Frequency
Colorectal	M and F	50+	Fecal occult blood test (FOBT)	q year
	M and F	50+	Flexible sigmoidoscopy OR colonoscopy OR double contrast barium enema	q 5 years OR q 10 years OR q 5 years
Breast	F	20+	Breast self-exam	q month
	F	20-39 OR 40+	Clinical breast exam	q 3 years OR q year
	F	40+	Mammography	q year
Cervical	F	21+[2]	Pap smear and pelvic exam	q 3 years
Prostate	M	50+	Digital rectal exam (DRE)	q year
	M	50+	Prostate-specific antigen (PSA) test	q year

[1]No specific screening recommendations have been made for lung, skin, and testicular cancer in patients with average risk. However, after the age of 40, it is recommended that all men and women receive health counseling and a physical exam every year.
[2]Earlier if sexually active.
Adapted from the American Cancer Society.

4. Key Points

- Oncology includes over 100 diverse diseases that share properties of abnormal and detrimental cell growth.

- Diseases are classified based on the tissue they originate in (eg, breast cancer metastasized to the brain is classified as breast cancer).

- Signs and symptoms of cancer do not follow a specific pattern. Any unusual or persistent change in body appearance or function should be evaluated by a health care provider.

Table 14

Common Tumor Markers and Associated Cancers

Tumor marker	Abnormal level	Cancer
Alpha-fetoprotein (AFP)	>20 ng/mL	Hepatocellular, ovarian
β-2 Microglobulin (β2M)	>3 ng/mL	Multiple myeloma, lymphoma
CA 15-3	>25 U/mL	Breast
CA 125	>30 U/mL	Ovarian
CA 19-9	>37 U/mL	Pancreatic, colorectal
Calcitonin[1]	>70 pg/mL	Thyroid
Carcinoembryonic antigen (CEA)	>5 U/mL	Colorectal, breast, non–small cell lung
Chromogranin A	>76 ng/mL (men); >51 (women)	Neuroendocrine, lung, prostate
Gamma globulin	>2-3 g/100 mL	Multiple myeloma
Her-2/neu	>450 fmol/mL	Breast
Human chorionic gonadotropin (HCG)	>5 mIU/mL	Testicular
Prostate-specific antigen (PSA)[1]	>4-10 ng/mL	Prostate
Thyroglobulin	>10 ng/mL	Thyroid

[1]Can be used to diagnose early disease.

- Before a diagnosis of cancer can be made and systemic treatment can begin, a positive biopsy or blood examination must confirm the presence of the disease.

- Further imaging and lab work-up should be done to evaluate the extent of the disease (ie, determine the stage of disease).

- Cancer therapy must be individualized to each patient based on the type and severity of disease, patient characteristics, and patient and family preferences.

- Surgery, radiation, chemotherapy, and biologic therapy are all cancer treatment modalities that are often used in combination.

- Pharmacists can impact patients' chemotherapy and biologic therapy by counseling the patients and educating health care providers on details of the individual drug regimens.

- Chemotherapy is often employed in combinations to take advantage of different mechanisms of action, avoid resistance, and minimize toxicities.

- Most chemotherapy is aimed at rapidly proliferating cancerous cells. However, many chemotherapy-related side effects occur in normal highly proliferative cells of the body, such as hair follicles, the GI tract lining, and blood cells.

- Patient counseling should include a discussion of the teratogenic effects of chemotherapy and taking measures to avoid the conception of a child. Additionally, all patients should not receive live vaccines or the rotavirus vaccine during treatment.

- Patients should be aware of expected toxicities of chemotherapy, which are not limited to alopecia, diarrhea, nausea and vomiting, infertility, myelosuppression, neurotoxicity, nephrotoxicity, hepatotoxicity, stomatitis, and pulmonary toxicity.

- Lab work and the importance of follow-up appointments to treatment should be stressed to the patient.

- All prophylactic and post-treatment medications for chemotherapy-related complications should be made available to the patient. Counsel the patient to keep a diary of events that occur prior to and after treatments. Use this record to make interventions and increase the patient's quality of life.

- All pharmacists should be aware of the accepted cancer screening recommendations and discuss these with all pertinent patients. Many diseases can be cured if they are caught early enough.

- It is the pharmacist's responsibility to make sure that the patient and family are educated enough to participate in making decisions about their care.

5. Questions and Answers

Use Patient Profile #1 to answer Questions 1-5

1. Which of the following agents that Ms. Tiny is taking can be used to treat breast and prostate cancer?

    I. Arimidex
    II. Zoladex
    III. Megace

    A. I only
    B. III only
    C. I and II only
    D. II and III only
    E. I, II, and III

2. When the patient presents with the Megace prescription, you notice that the Sig. is missing. You call the doctor to clarify what the instructions are. Which of the following is a correct Sig.?

    A. 20 mL PO tid
    B. 10 mL PO qid
    C. 10 mL PO tid
    D. 5 mL PO qid
    E. 5 mL PO tid

3. You notice that Ms. Tiny did not pick up her Lo-Estrin prescription last month. Which of her medications are contraindicated in pregnant women and/or breastfeeding mothers?

    I. Megace
    II. Goserelin
    III. Arimidex

    A. I only
    B. III only
    C. I and II only
    D. II and III only
    E. I, II, and III

4. Ms. Tiny calls you 2 days after her 03/01 visit to your pharmacy. She has been feeling a lot of bone pain and describes an "achy, creaky feeling all over." She is worried that her cancer has

Patient Profile #1—Medication Profile: Community

Patient Name	Tina Tiny		
Address	234 Small St.		
Age	33	Height	5'8"
Sex	Female	Weight	150 lb
Allergies	Sulfa, penicllin		

DIAGNOSIS	1. Diagnosed on 12/00 with metastatic breast cancer
	2. Mastectomy to right breast on 12/15/00
	3. Weight loss of 20 lb
	4. Allergies

MEDICATION RECORD

Date	Rx #	Physician	Drug/Strength	Quantity	Sig	Refills
12/00	12345	Buford	Percocet 325/5	30	1-2 q4h prn	0
1/01	12346	Charles	Lo-Estrln FE 1.5/30	28	1 PO qd	prn
3/01	12347	Buford	Armidex 1 mg	30	1 PO qd	2
3/01	12349	Buford	Megace 40 mg/mL	80 mg/d	—	2
3/01	12350	Charles	Zyrtec 10 mg	30	1 PO qd	2

PHARMACIST NOTES

Date	Note
1/01	Patient complained of soreness after mastectomy and swelling of right arm
3/01	Patient did not pick up birth control last month (2/01)
3/01	Patient is receiving Zoladex 3/6 mg SC q28d at oncology clinic. Received dose today.

spread to her bones. What advice can you give her?

I. She should call her oncology caretaker and be formally evaluated.
II. This could be a side effect of her Zoladex therapy and the pain should subside.
III. This could be a side effect of her Megace therapy and the pain should subside.

A. I only
B. III only
C. I and II only
D. II and III only
E. I, II, and III

5. Ms. Tiny's mother (age 59) is worried that she will develop breast cancer like her daughter. Which of the following is *not* an appropriate initial screening test for breast cancer?

A. Monthly breast self-examination
B. Clinical breast examination
C. Mammography
D. Biopsy
E. Mammography and clinical breast examination

6. Which of the following is (are) an absolute contraindication(s) for patients receiving chemotherapy?

I. Rotavirus vaccines
II. Flu vaccines
III. Tobacco

A. I only
B. III only
C. I and II only
D. II and III only
E. I, II, and III

7. Your patient has just received 5-FU and irinotecan for the treatment of colorectal cancer. Before he leaves the clinic, you make sure that he has a prescription to prevent and/or treat which of the following side effects from irinotecan?

A. Nausea
B. Diarrhea
C. Headache
D. Delayed allergic reaction
E. Change in urine color

8. Which of the following drugs is an oral prodrug of 5-FU?

A. Fluorouracil
B. Xeloda
C. Fludara
D. Cytoxan
E. Alkeran

9. An elderly male patient comes to your pharmacy and is worried that he might have prostate cancer. He just had some lab work done and his doctor told him that some level was abnormal, indicating potential prostate cancer. Which lab test might he be talking about?

I. PSA
II. Cortisol
III. ESR

A. I only
B. III only
C. I and II only
D. II and III only
E. I, II, and III

10. Stomatitis is the clinical term for which of the following chemotherapy-related adverse effects?

I. Nausea and projectile vomiting
II. Inflammation of the epithelial lining of the stomach
III. Inflammation of the mucosal lining of the mouth

A. I only
B. III only
C. I and II only
D. II and III only
E. I, II, and III

11. Which of the following does *not* describe characteristics of most chemotherapy agents?

A. A wide therapeutic index
B. Interfere with DNA synthesis and replication
C. More effective in combination
D. Adverse effects occur primarily in rapidly dividing normal cells
E. Phase-specific and non–phase specific actions

Use Patient Profile #2 to answer Questions 12-17.

12. A nurse would like to know if she can administer the diphenhydramine and the cimetidine in the same IV line simultaneously. Which of the following resources will provide you with this information?

I. *Facts and Comparisons*
II. *Trissel's*
III. Micromedex

A. I only
B. III only
C. I and II only
D. II and III only
E. I, II, and III

13. Which of the following agents that Mr. Migash is taking requires the premedication regimen of dexamethasone, diphenhydramine, and raniti-

dine or cimetidine to prevent an anaphylactic reaction?

I. Taxotere
II. Paraplatin
III. Taxol

A. I only
B. III only
C. I and II only
D. II and III only
E. I, II, and III

14. Based on the patient's weight and height, you calculate Mr. Migash's body surface area to be 2.1 m². Paclitaxel is supplied as 6 mg/mL in 5-mL, 16.7-mL, and 50-mL vials. Your pharmacy has all quantities available. What is the best way to correctly dose this patient?

A. One 50-mL vial

Patient Profile #2—Medication Profile: Institution

Patient Name	Cassimer Migash		
Address	579 Hunter's Ridge		
Age	60	Height	180 cm
Sex	Male	Weight	200 lb
Allergies	NKDA		

DIAGNOSIS	1. Diagnosed on 2/03 with metastatic non–small cell lung cancer
	2. Chronic obstructive pulmonary disease
	3. Asthma

LABS AND DIAGNOSTIC TESTS

Date	Test
5/03	WBC: 2500/μL
5/03	RBC: $2.8 \times 10^6/mm^3$
5/03	PLT: $100 \times 10^3/μL$
5/03	Theophylline: 10 μg/mL

MEDICATION RECORD

Date	Route	Drug	Sig.
4/03	IV	Paclitaxel 135 mg/m²	135 mg/m³ over 3 h q 3 wk
4/03	IV	Carboplatin AUC 6	AUC 6 over 2 h q 3 wk
4/03	PO	Theophylline SR 400 mg	1 tab PO bid
4/03	INH	Albuterol inhaler	2 puffs prn
4/03	INH	Cromolyn inhaler	1 puff qid
4/03	INH	Beclomethasone inhaler	2 puffs qid
4/03	PO	Dexamethasone 20 mg	1 tab 12 h and 6 h prior to chemo
4/03	IV	Diphenhydramine 50 mg	Infuse 30 min and 60 min prior to chemo
4/03	IV	Cimetidine 300 mg	Infuse 30 min and 60 min prior to chemo

B. One 50-mL vial and one 5-mL vial
C. Two 16.7-mL vials
D. Two 16.7-mL vials and one 5-mL vial
E. Three 16.7-mL vials

15. If Mr. Migash were to have an anaphylactic reaction, which of the following orders would *not* be helpful to treat this?

   A. Administer epinephrine STAT
   B. Administer diphenhydramine STAT
   C. Administer IV fluids STAT
   D. Administer cimetidine STAT
   E. Discontinue the infusion STAT

16. Based on the patient's lab values, which of the following adverse reactions appear to have occurred as a likely result of the chemotherapy?

   I. Thrombocytopenia
   II. Leukopenia
   III. Anemia

   A. I only
   B. III only
   C. I and II only
   D. II and III only
   E. I, II, and III

17. The goal of Mr. Migash's treatment regimen is:

   I. To cure his disease
   II. To palliate his disease-related symptoms
   III. To increase his quality of life

   A. I only
   B. III only
   C. I and II only
   D. II and III only
   E. I, II, and III

18. Doxorubicin is an antineoplastic agent that

   A. Is *not* related to epirubicin and daunorubicin
   B. Interacts with the microtubules of cells during mitosis
   C. Has an oral dosage form commercially available
   D. Causes cumulative cardiac toxicity
   E. Can also be used to treat tuberculosis

19. Which of the following agents is used to treat cancer, but is not considered an antineoplastic agent?

   A. Methotrexate

B. Levamisole
C. Doxorubicin
D. Cyclophosphamide
E. Gemcitabine

20. Methotrexate (Rheumatrex®) is not available as which of the following dosage forms?

   A. An intravenous injection
   B. An oral tablet or capsule
   C. An intrathecal injection
   D. An ointment
   E. An intramuscular injection

Answers

1. **E.** All three agents can be used to treat breast cancer. However, the Megace used in this patient is more likely to treat the cachexia or weight loss that this patient appears to be experiencing.

2. **D.** 5 mL PO qid equates to 20 mL of Megace a day. The strength of the Megace is stated in the patient profile (40 mg/mL). 20 mL times 40 mg/mL equals 800 mg/d.

3. **E.** All three agents are contraindicated in pregnant women *and* breastfeeding mothers. This is an important point. No patient, male or female, should be receiving chemotherapy treatment and trying to conceive a child.

4. **C.** While the bone pain is most likely a side effect of her Zoladex therapy, she should notify her oncology practitioner so they can document this side effect. If other factors point to metastatic disease, this patient may need additional evaluation.)

5. **D.** Biopsies should never be performed as initial screening tests. However, if results from the mammography and other tests point to disease, a biopsy is needed to make a diagnosis. However, there is some debate about the usefulness of clinical breast examinations (CBEs) for women that are reluctant to perform breast self-examinations; CBEs should be offered.

6. **A.** Rotavirus and live vaccines should not be given to any patient that has a suppressed immune system. The flu vaccine is an inactivated product and should be administered to chemotherapy patients.

7. **B.** Diarrhea is a dose-limiting toxicity of irinotecan. Late diarrhea can be life threatening.

All patients should receive a prescription for loperamide to treat delayed-onset diarrhea. Patients should be instructed to take 2 mg PO q2h while awake and 4 mg PO q4h during the night until the diarrhea has stopped for at least 12 hours. Acute-onset diarrhea can be treated with atropine.

8. **B.** Xeloda, generic name capecitabine, is an oral prodrug of 5-FU. Fluorouracil is another name for 5-FU. Fludara is the brand name for fludarabine and is used to treat CLL and NHL intravenously. Cytoxan is the brand name for cyclophosphamide and is available in IV and PO dosage forms. Alkeran is the brand name for melphalan and is also available in IV and PO dosage forms.

9. **A.** PSA is a lab test that is commonly done in men over the age of 40. It should be tested annually in men over the age of 50 to check for prostate cancer. PSA stands for prostate-specific antigen.

10. **B.** Stomatitis is used to describe an irritation or ulceration of the mucosal lining. This side effect is common with fluorouracil and methotrexate. It can be prevented by having the patient hold ice chips in their mouth during treatment. The cold is thought to cause vasoconstriction of the lining and prevent damage.

11. **A.** Chemotherapy agents have a very narrow therapeutic index. This is one of the main reasons why there are so many toxic effects with these drugs. They can be phase-specific or non–phase specific drugs and cause many adverse reactions to normal cells that undergo rapid proliferation.

12. **D.** Both *Trissel's Handbook of Injectable Drugs* and the Micromedex IV compatibility tool can be used to assess whether the diphenhydramine and cimetidine are compatible.

13. **B.** Taxol is the brand name of paclitaxel. This agent has been shown to cause hypersensitivity reactions in patients. It is unclear if these reactions are due to the drug itself or the drug's vehicle (Cremophor®). All patients receiving paclitaxel should receive a premedication regimen of dexamethasone, diphenhydramine, and ranitidine or cimetidine.

14. **A.** The patient requires 283.5 mg of drug, which can be rounded up to 300 mg. Both choices A

and E will provide 300 mg of drug; however, using one large vial is more economical than using three smaller vials.

15. **D.** The patient needs to undergo emergency resuscitation treatment. Standard of care would include discontinuing the causative infusion, and administering IV fluids, diphenhydramine, and epinephrine to begin with.

16. **E.** Myelosuppression is a common adverse reaction to most chemotherapy agents. Both paclitaxel and carboplatin can cause anemia, thrombocytopenia, and leukopenia. It is very important to monitor blood levels in these patients. If myelosuppression is too severe, the length of time between chemotherapy cycles may be increased so all or some of the blood cells can return to normal levels.

17. **D.** Mr. Migash has metastatic disease. Anytime a solid tumor is diagnosed as stage IV, this is representative of the fact that their disease is incurable. The treatment goals for these patients include relieving any disease-related symptoms, minimizing toxicity from treatments, and increasing the patient's quality of life through treatment or supportive care measures.

18. **D.** Doxorubicin is an antitumor antibiotic related to epirubicin and daunorubicin. These agents act by binding tightly to DNA via intercalation. Doxorubicin does have a liposomal IV product, but it is not available orally. All anthracyclines are associated with cardiac toxicity and have cumulative dosing limits to prevent this.

19. **B.** Levamisole is an anthelmintic agent that is approved for combination therapy with 5-FU in the treatment of colorectal cancer.

20. **D.** Methotrexate is not commercially available for topical use.

6. References

ASHP Therapeutic Guidelines on the Pharmacologic Management of Nausea and Vomiting in Adult and Pediatric Patients Receiving Chemotherapy or Radiation Therapy or Undergoing Surgery. *Am J Health Syst Pharm.* 1999;56:729-764.

Balmer CM, Valley AW. Cancer treatment and chemotherapy. In: Dipiro JT, Talbert RL, Yee GC, et al, eds. *Pharmacotherapy: A Pathophysiologic Approach,* 5th ed. New York: McGraw-Hill; 2002:2175-2222.

Calabresi P, Chabner BA. Chemotherapy of neoplastic diseases. In: Hardman JG, Limbird LE, eds. *Goodman & Gilman's: The Pharmacological Basis of Therapeutics,* 10th ed. New York; McGraw-Hill: 2001:1381-1388.

Chabner BA, Ryan DP, Paz-Ares L, Garcia-Carbonero R, Calabresi P. Antineoplastic agents. In: Hardman JG, Limbird LE, eds. *Goodman & Gilman's: The Pharmacological Basis of Therapeutics,* 10th ed. New York: McGraw-Hill; 2001:1389-1459.

DeVita VT, Hellman S, Rosenberg SA, eds. *Cancer: Principles & Practices of Oncology,* 6th ed. Philadelphia: Lippincott Williams & Wilkins; 2001.

Dorr RT, Fritz WL. *Cancer Chemotherapy Handbook.* New York: Elsevier North Holland; 1980.

Mueller BA, Schumock GT, Bertch KE, et al, eds. *Pharmacotherapy Self-Assessment Program*, 4th ed. Book 10, Hematology Oncology. Kansas City; ACCP: 2002.

National Comprehensive Cancer Network (NCCN) Antiemesis Practice Guidelines [on CD-ROM]. Rockledge, PA: NCCN; 2003.

20. Solid Organ Transplantation

Marsha R. Honaker, PharmD
Assistant Professor, Department of Pharmacy
University of Tennessee College of Pharmacy
Director, Pharmacy Division of Transplantation
Director, Solid Organ Transplantation/
Immunology Pharmacy Residency
University of Tennessee Health Sciences Center

Contents

1. **Organ Transplantation**

2. **Immunosuppressants**

3. **Key Points**

4. **Questions and Answers**

5. **References**

1. Organ Transplantation

Principles of Transplantation

Types of allografts
- Heart: first successfully transplanted in 1968. In 2002, 3196 heart transplants were performed in U.S.

- Intestinal: first successfully transplanted in 1987. In 2002, 108 intestinal transplants were performed in U.S.

- Kidney: first successful cadaveric transplant in 1954. In 2002, 15,641 kidney transplants were performed in U.S.

- Liver: first successful cadaveric transplant in 1967. In 2002, 5329 liver transplants were performed in U.S.

- Lung: first successful cadaveric single-lung transplant in 1983. In 2002, 2084 lung transplants were performed in U.S.

- Pancreas: first successful solitary pancreas transplant in 1968. In 2002, 1457 pancreas transplants were performed in U.S.

Goal
- Improve patients' quality of life and survival by stabilizing and/or improving end-organ failure–related complications

Outcome
- See Table 1.

Definitions
- *acute rejection:* a systemic immunologic response to donor antigens primarily mediated by T lymphocytes

- *adaptive immunity:* involves stimulation of cells and soluble mediators in response to specific antigens with a markedly enhanced response on repeat exposure

- *complement:* an enzyme system that is a crucial part of the basic immune response on primary exposure to an antigen, and also provides augmented signaling during memory immunity

- *human leukocyte antigen (HLA):* antigen binding proteins that rescue protein fragments from intracellular catabolism (class I or II) or select antigens from the extracellular milieu that are then presented to lymphocytes (class II)

- *innate immunity:* involves stimulation of cells and soluble mediators that nonspecifically recognize antigens and have no ability to alter response with repeat exposure

- *major histocompatibility complex (MHC):* group of genes that encode for human leukocyte antigens class I and II

- *opsonization:* occurs when antigens or immune complexes become coated with a molecule that facilitates binding with a phagocyte

- *panel reactive antibody (PRA):* a test which quanti-

Table 1

Kaplan-Meier Patient and Graft Survival Rates for Transplants Performed: 1996-2001

Organ	Patient survival (%)	Graft survival (%)
Heart		
1 year	85.3	84.9
3 years	78.1	77.4
Intestinal		
1 year	71.3	66.7
3 years	53.8	46.9
Kidney: cadaveric		
1 year	94.4	88.3
3 years	89.3	77.8
Kidney: living		
1 year	97.7	94.4
3 years	94.9	87.7
Liver: cadaveric		
1 year	85.3	80.0
3 years	77.7	70.6
Liver: living		
1 year	87.9	77.7
3 years	80.1	71.6
Lung: cadaveric		
1 year	76.6	76.1
3 years	57.7	56.6
Lung: living		
1 year	73.4	72.2
3 years	50.7	49.2
Pancreas		
1 year	95.0	78.5
3 years	86.9	60.5

Based on the Organ Procurement and Transplantation Network data as of February 7, 2003.

tates a patient's immunologic reactivity to a given pool of antigens

- *phagocytosis:* process by which recognized antigens are engulfed and subsequently undergo intracellular catabolism

Basic Immunology and Acute Rejection

Fundamental types of immunity
Innate immunity
Cellular components
- Macrophages: phagocytic cells found throughout the body, which may function as antigen presenting cells

- Neutrophils: highly motile cells whose major physiologic role is the destruction of invading microorganisms via phagocytosis/opsonization

- Natural killer cells: a subset of non-B, non-T lymphocytes that survey for the normal biosynthesis and expression of HLA class I, making them important in immunity against viral infection and malignancy

Humoral component
- Complement: activation leads to formation of lipophilic complexes, called membrane-attack complexes, in the cell membrane of the target cell and results in osmotic leakage
    * Physiologic function: defense against pyogenic bacterial infections
    * Bridges innate and adaptive immunity
    * Mediates disposal of immune complexes
Acute phase proteins

Adaptive immunity
Cellular components
- Thymus-derived lymphocytes (T cells): mature T cells become activated when they encounter an antigen presenting cell presenting an antigen; T-cells *do not* recognize antigens directly:
    * CD4$^+$ T cells ("T helper cells") recognize antigen presented via HLA class II
    * CD8$^+$ T cells ("cytotoxic T cells") recognize antigen presented via HLA class I

- Bone marrow-derived lymphocytes (B cells): B cells encounter the antigen to which their surface immunoglobulin has specificity, through either its APC function or via interaction with an activated CD4$^+$ T cell. B-cell/CD4$^+$ T-cell interaction is required for translocation into a follicle within secondary lymphoid tissue, where a germinal center forms and where high-affinity memory B cells and plasma cells are produced/selected (somatic hypermutation).

Humoral components
- Complement: as above

- Immunoglobulins (Ig): complex proteins of various isotypes formed as a consequence of B-cell activation for the purpose of binding and elimination of the activating antigen

Acute rejection
Pathophysiology
- During transplantation, the recipient is exposed to donor antigens to which he or she has no previous exposure. While undesirable, acute rejection is the normal physiologic response of the immune system to these donor antigens. This response can be divided into 5 basic phases:
    1. Recognition: recognition of foreign antigen via self/nonself recognition mediated via MHC
    2. Presentation: upon recognition, antigen presenting cells present antigens in association with native HLA class II to inactive CD4+ T cells
    3. Activation/proliferation: activation is dependent on antigen/HLA binding to the T-cell receptor (TCR) complex and the subsequent binding of a second signal or "co-stimulatory pathway." Subsequently, the active CD4+ T cell produces and releases various lymphokines, particularly interleukin-2 (IL-2), important for activation and proliferation of numerous lymphocyte lineages.
    4. Recruitment: recruitment is mediated via several lymphokines produced as a consequence of lymphocyte activation.
    5. Antigen/tissue destruction: tissue injury is mediated via induction of polyclonal immune response.

Incidence
- The incidence is organ specific and dependent on many pre- and post-transplant factors. There are several known factors that increase risk:
    * Increasing HLA mismatch
    * Factors affecting previous sensitization: history of pregnancy, previous transplantation, previous rejection, or panel reactive antibody >20%
    * Ethnicity: African-American recipients
    * Age: pediatric recipients
    * Donor source: cadaveric donor
    * Prolonged preservation time
    * Noncompliance

Immunosuppressive Strategies

Balance of immunosuppression
- Selection of an immunosuppression regimen for the prevention of acute rejection should be individual-

ized based on known risk and potential for toxicity. Subsequent adjustment must focus on the balance of the triad: rejection, infection, and toxicity.

Phases of preventive immunosuppression
Induction
- Early phase intended to provide highly potent, multi-focal suppression of the immune system for several days to a few weeks. Ccommonly used agents include:
  * Corticosteroids
  * Monoclonal antibody: muromonab, basilix-amab, daclizumab
  * Polyclonal antibody: antithymocyte globulin (equine or rabbit)

Maintenance
- Immunosuppression regimen designed to provide chronic, balanced immunodeficiency. Some commonly used regimens:
  * Double therapy:
    • Calcineurin inhibitor + steroids
    • Calcineurin inhibitor + antimetabolite
    • Calcineurin inhibitor + mTOR inhibitor
    • mTOR inhibitor + steroids
    • mTOR inhibitor + antimetabolite
    • Antimetabolite + steroids
  * Triple therapy:
    • Calcineurin inhibitor + antimetabolite + steroids
    • mTOR inhibitor + calcineurin inhibitor + steroids
    • mTOR inhibitor + antimetabolite + steroids

Phases of immunosuppression during treatment
Treatment
- Selection of agent is organ specific and dependent on severity of acute rejection. Commonly used agents include:
  * Corticosteroids
  * Calcineurin inhibitor: tacrolimus may be used as the primary treatment of acute rejection in liver recipients; may also have a role as adjuvant therapy in refractory acute rejection in various other solid organ recipients
  * Monoclonal antibody: muromonab
  * Polyclonal antibody: antithymocyte globulin (horse or rabbit)

Maintenance re-evaluation
- Decision to heighten maintenance immunosuppression is dependent on cause for rejection (ie, failure of regimen versus noncompliance)

Immunosuppressive Complications

Infectious
- Infectious complications are an important cause of early morbidity and mortality. The incidence is organ specific and closely linked to the net degree of immunodeficiency. Prevention is a key management strategy post-transplant.

Bacterial
- Tuberculosis: *Mycobacterium tuberculosis*
- Nocardiasis: various species of *Nocardia*

Fungal
- Aspergillosis: various species of *Aspergillus*
- Blastomycosis: *Blastomyces dermatitidis*
- Candidiasis: various species of *Candida*
- Coccidioidomycosis: *Coccidioides immitis*
- Cryptococcosis: *Cryptococcus neoformans*
- Histoplasmosis: *Histoplasma capsulatum*
- Mucormycosis: various species of *Mucor*
- *Pneumocystis carinii*

Parasitic
- Toxoplasmosis: *Toxoplasma gondii*

Viral
- Cytomegalovirus
- Epstein-Barr virus: including post-transplant lymphoproliferative disease (PTLD)
- Herpes simplex virus
- Varicella-zoster virus
- Human herpes viruses (ie, HHV-6, HHV-8)
- Parvovirus
- Polyomavirus

Noninfectious
- The noninfectious complications are specific to the agents included in the immunosuppressive regimen.

2. Immunosuppressants

• See Table 2.

Calcineurin Inhibitors

Cyclosporine
Mechanism of action
• Inhibits calcineurin-dependent translocation of the cytosolic subunit of NFAT, the promoter gene for IL-2, into the nucleus, thereby inhibiting transcription and synthesis of IL-2. Thus it inhibits IL-2–mediated monoclonal T-cell proliferation and polyclonal T-cell activation.

Administration
• Intravenous
  * 5-6 mg/kg per day divided every 12 h or as a continuous infusion. Each milliliter of IV concentrate should be diluted in 20-100 mL of NS or D_5 in a glass container. For bolus dosing, dose should be infused over 2-6 h.

• Oral
  * Capsules: administer daily dose as two equally divided doses every 12 h with meals
  * Oral solution: administer daily dose as two equally divided doses every 12 h with meals. Solution may be diluted with chocolate milk or orange juice in a glass container. Additional diluent should be used to rinse the container to assure administration of total dose.

Drug-drug interactions
• Metabolized primarily via cytochrome P450 3A isoenzymes. Substances known to alter functionality of these enzymes will alter bioavailability and elimination of this drug (Table 3).

• Drug-interactions leading to altered exposure of other drugs by cyclosporine: see Table 4

Drug-disease interactions
• Altered biliary flow: diversion of biliary flow can significantly reduce adsorption. This more profoundly affects cyclosporine USP compared to cyclosporine USP, (modified).

• Diabetes mellitus: administration worsens glycemic control in patients with pre-existing diabetes.

• Vaccination: in general, immunosuppressants may affect efficacy of vaccination. The use of live vaccines should be avoided.

Adverse drug reactions
• CNS: seizure, hallucination, insomnia, tremor, paresthesia

• HEENT: gingival hyperplasia

• CV: hypertension

• GI: hepatotoxicity

• Renal: nephrotoxicity

• Endocrine and metabolic: diabetes mellitus, hyperlipidemia, hyperuricemia, hyperkalemia, hypomagnesemia

• Dermatologic: hirsutism, hypertrichosis, acne

Patient instructions
• Keep cyclosporine stored in its original container. Take the prescribed dose twice daily with meals. Keep timing of dosing consistent. Make sure you take or do not take your medication at the appropriate time prior to therapeutic drug monitoring. Many medications interact with this medication. Do not take anything prescribed by another physician until you verify that there are no drug interactions.

Monitoring
• C_0 (trough): goals dependent on multifactorial risk assessment and assay type

• C_2: concentration 2 hours after dose; goals dependent on multifactorial risk assessment and assay type

Pharmacokinetics
• Cyclosporine USP: highly lipoprotein bound
  * Bioavailability: significant intra- and interpatient variability
  * Mean F = 30%, range 5-92%
  * Elimination: $t_{1/2}$ = 19 h, range 10-28 h (increased with hepatic dysfunction)

• Cyclosporine USP, (modified): highly lipoprotein bound
  * Bioavailability: improved and more consistent absorption (60-70% increased C_{max})
  * Elimination: $t_{1/2}$ = 8 h, range 5-18 h (increased with hepatic dysfunction)

Tacrolimus
Mechanism of action
• Inhibits translocation of the cytosolic subunit of NFAT, the promoter gene for IL-2, into the nucleus via its binding with FKBP-12 and a calcium-calmodulin-calcineurin complex, thereby inhibiting

Table 2

Immunosuppressant Drugs

Trade name	Generic name	Dosage forms	Dose	Generic products
Calcineurin inhibitors				
Sandimmune®	Cyclosporine USP	Injection: 50 mg/mL; oral solution: 100 mg/mL; capsules: 25, 50, 100 mg	**Intravenous:** 5-6 mg/kg/d; **oral:** 8-14 mg/kg/d divided q12h; **adjusted to desired trough concentration**	Injection 50 mg/mL; capsules 25 and 100 mg
Neoral®	Cyclosporine USP (modified)	Oral solution 100 mg/mL; capsules 25 and 100 mg	**Oral:** 5-10 mg/kg/d divided q12h; **adjusted to desired trough concentration**	Oral solution: 100 mg/mL; capsules: 25 and 100 mg
Prograf®	Tacrolimus	Injection: 5 mg ampules; capsules: 0.5, 1, and 5 mg	**Intravenous:** 0.03-0.05 mg/kg/d as continuous infusion; **oral:** 0.1-0.2 mg/kg/d divided q12h; **adjusted to desired trough concentration**	Not available
mTOR inhibitors				
Rapamune®	Sirolimus	Oral solution: 1 mg/mL; tablets: 1 mg	**Initial:** 6-15 mg PO; **maintenance:** 2-5 mg PO qd; **adjusted to desired trough concentration**	Not available
Antiproliferative agents				
Imuran®	Azathioprine	Injection: 100 mg vial; tablets: 50 mg	**Initial:** 3-5 mg/kg IV or PO; **maintenance:** 1-2 mg/kg IV or PO qd	Injection: 100 mg vial; tablets: 50 mg
CellCept®	Mycophenolate mofetil	Injection: 500 mg vial; oral suspension: 200 mg/mL; capsules: 250 mg; tablets: 500 mg	**Maintenance:** Adults: 2-3 g/d divided q8-12h IV or PO; pediatrics: 1200 mg/m^2 divided q8-12h IV or PO	Not available
Arava®	Leflunomide	Tablets: 10, 20, and 100 mg	**Initial:** 100 mg PO qd x 3; **maintenance:** 10-20 mg PO qd	Not available
Monoclonal antibodies				
Orthoclone OKT 3®	Muromonab-CD3	Injection: 5 mg ampules	**Induction:** 2-5 mg IV qd x 7-10 d; **acute rejection:** 5-10 mg IV qd x 10-14 d	Not available
Simulect®	Basiliximab	Injection: 10 and 20 mg vials	**Induction:** adults and pediatrics >35 kg: 20 mg IV on day 0 and day 4; pediatrics <35 kg: 10 mg IV on day 0 and day 4	Not available
Zenapax®	Daclizumab	Injection: 25 mg vials	**Induction:** 1 mg/kg IV q 2 wk x 5	Not available
Polyclonal antibodies				
Atgam®	Anti-thymocyte globulin (equine)	Injection: 50 mg vials	**Induction:** 15 mg/kg IV qd x 7-10 d; **acute rejection:** 10-15 mg/kg IV qd x 14 d	Not available
Thymoglobulin®	Anti-thymocyte globulin (rabbit)	Injection: 25 mg vials	**Induction:** 1.5 mg/kg IV qd x 3-7 d; **acute rejection:** 1.5 mg/kg IV qd x 7-10 d	Not available

Table 3

Drug Interactions Leading to Altered Exposure of Cytochrome P450 3A Isoenzyme Substrates[1]

Cytochrome P450 3A4 enzyme inducers: *Inducers result in increased metabolism and decreased bioavailability of substrates of the same system*	Cytochrome P450 3A4 enzyme inhibitors: *Inhibitors result in decreased metabolism and increased bioavailability of substrates of the same system*
Anticonvulsants: phenytoin, phenobarbital, carbamazepine	Antidepressants: nefazodone
Antimicrobial agents: rifampin, rifabutin	Antiviral agents: delavirdine, indinavir, nelfinavir, ritonavir, saquinavir
Antiviral agents: nevirapine, efavirenz	Azole antifungal agents: ketoconazole, fluconazole, itraconazole, clotrimazole
Herbal products: St. John's wort	Calcium channel blockers: diltiazem, nicardipine, verapamil
	Macrolide antimicrobial agents: erythromycin, clarithromycin, troleandomycin
	Food-drug interaction: grapefruit juice

[1]These are examples only. Numerous other interactions are associated with CYP 3A4 substrates. See current journals or drug interaction texts for a more detailed list.

transcription and synthesis of IL-2. Thus it inhibits IL-2–mediated monoclonal T-cell proliferation and polyclonal T-cell activation.

Administration
- Intravenous
  * Dilute in NS or D_5 to a concentration between 0.004 and 0.02 mg/mL and administer as a continuous infusion via PVC-free container and tubing.

- Oral
  * Two equally divided doses PO every 12 h consistently with or without food

Drug-drug interactions
- Metabolized primarily via cytochrome P450 3A isoenzymes. Substances known to alter functionality of these enzymes will alter bioavailability and elimination of this drug (Table 3).

Drug-disease interactions
- Diabetes mellitus: administration worsens glycemic control in patients with pre-existing diabetes.

- Vaccinations: in general, immunosuppressants may affect efficacy of vaccination. The use of live vaccines should be avoided.

Adverse drug reactions
- CNS: seizure, hallucinations, insomnia, tremor, depression, psychosis, anorexia

- HEENT: alopecia

Table 4

Drug Interactions Leading to Altered Exposure of Other Drugs by Cyclosporine[1]

Mechanism	Drug	Comment
Cytochrome P450 3A4 enzyme substrates	HMG-CoA reductase inhibitors: lovastatin, simvastatin, atorvastatin	Co-administration of these agents with CsA results in significant increases in HMG-CoA reductase inhibitor exposure and may place patient at increased risk of rhabdomyolysis
Cytochrome P450 3A4 enzyme substrates	Sirolimus	Simultaneous administration increased C_{max} and AUC of sirolimus by 120-500% and 140-230%, respectively; administration 4 hours apart increased C_{max} and AUC of sirolimus by 30-40% and 35-80%, respectively
Alteration in enterohepatic recycling	Mycophenolate mofetil	CsA co-administration inhibits MPAG excretion via hepatocytes, thus interfering with MPA enterohepatic recycling, leading to reduced exposure of the active metabolite, MPA

CsA, cyclosporine A; HMG-CoA, 3-hydroxy-3-methyglutaryl coenzyme A; MPA, mycophenolic acid; MPAG, phenolic glucuronide of MPA.
[1]These are examples only. See current journals or drug interaction texts for detailed list.

- CV: hypertension

- GI: hepatotoxicity

- Renal: nephrotoxicity

- Endocrine and metabolic: diabetes mellitus, hyperlipidemia, hyperkalemia, hypercalcemia, hypomagnesemia, hypophosphatemia

- Hematologic: anemia

Patient instructions
- Take the prescribed dose at a consistent time twice daily. It may be taken with or without food, but should be taken the same way to maintain consistency. Make sure you do not take your medication prior to therapeutic drug monitoring. Many medications interact with this medication. Do not take anything prescribed by another physician until you verify that there are no drug interactions.

Monitoring
- C_0 (trough): goals dependent on multifactorial risk assessment; in general, 5-20 ng/mL

Pharmacokinetics
- Highly protein bound

- Bioavailability: F = 14-32%

- Elimination: $t_{1/2}$ = 8 h, range 6-11 h (increased with hepatic dysfunction)

mTOR Inhibitor

Sirolimus
Mechanism of action
- Binds to FKBP-12 to form a complex that binds and inhibits activation of its target protein, mTOR, a kinase that is critical in IL-2–mediated cell cycle progression.

Administration
- To limit variability, administer consistently with or without food.

- Tablets: administer daily dose PO once a day.

- Oral solution: dilute dose in 2 ounces of water or orange juice, stir vigorously, and drink at once. Then refill container with 4 ounces of the chosen fluid, stir vigorously, and drink.

Drug-drug interactions
- Metabolized primarily via cytochrome P450 3A isoenzymes. Substances known to alter functionality of these enzymes will alter bioavailability and elimination of this drug (Table 3).

- Additionally, the pharmacokinetic profile of sirolimus is significantly altered by concomitant cyclosporine (Table 4)

Drug-disease interactions
- Liver transplantation: associated with increased incidence of mortality, graft loss, and hepatic artery thrombosis in de novo liver transplant recipients.

- Lung transplantation: there have been cases of fatal bronchial anastomotic dehiscence in de novo lung transplant recipients.

- Vaccinations: in general, immunosuppressants may affect efficacy of vaccination. The use of live vaccines should be avoided.

Adverse drug reactions
- CNS: anorexia

- HEENT: oral ulcers

- GI: diarrhea, esophagitis, gastritis, gastroenteritis, hepatotoxicity, hepatic artery thrombosis in de novo liver transplant recipients

- Renal: synergistic nephrotoxicity with calcineurin inhibitors

- Endocrine and metabolic: hyperlipidemia, hypertension, hyperkalemia

- Dermatologic: rash, acne

- Hematologic: pancytopenia, thrombosis

- Other: lymphocele, pneumonitis, bronchial anastomotic dehiscence in de novo lung transplant recipients

Patient instructions
- Take the prescribed dose at a consistent time once daily. It may be taken with or without food, but should be taken the same way to maintain consistency. Make sure you do not take your medication prior to therapeutic drug monitoring. Many medications interact with this medication. Do not take anything prescribed by another physician until you verify that there are no drug interactions.

Monitoring
- C_0 (trough): goal dependent on multifactorial risk assessment and assay type; in general, 5-20 ng/mL

Pharmacokinetics
- Bioavailability: tablet: F = 27%; oral solution: F = 15%

- Elimination: $t_{1/2}$ = 57-63 h (increased with hepatic dysfunction)

Antiproliferative Agents

Azathioprine
Mechanism of action
- Azathioprine is a purine analogue prodrug which is cleaved to 6-mercaptopurine. 6-Mercaptopurine is activated intracellularly to several active metabolites, which can be incorporated directly into DNA as thiopurine as well as interfere with the RNA and DNA biosynthesis directly and via feedback inhibition.

Administration
- Intravenous: dilute dose in NS or D_5 and administer IV infusion over 5-60 minutes.

- Oral: administer daily dose PO once a day

Drug-drug interactions
- Allopurinol: xanthine oxidase is responsible for the elimination of the active metabolites of azathioprine. Concomitant use of allopurinol with azathioprine results in significantly increased azathioprine-induced toxicity. Reduce dose of azathioprine by 65-75%.

Drug-disease interactions
- Renal insufficiency: bioavailability significantly reduced in uremic patients.

- Vaccinations: in general, immunosuppressants may affect efficacy of vaccination. The use of live vaccines should be avoided.

Adverse drug reactions
- HEENT: retinopathy

- GI: nausea, vomiting, diarrhea, anorexia, pancreatitis, hepatotoxicity

- Dermatologic: rash, skin cancer

- Hematologic: pancytopenia

Patient instructions
- Take the prescribed dose at a consistent time once daily. It may be taken with or without food, but should be taken the same way to maintain consistency. Do not take anything prescribed by another physician until you verify that there are no drug interactions.

Monitoring
- No clinically important pharmacokinetic or pharmacodynamic monitoring is needed.

Pharmacokinetics
- Bioavailability: F = 41-47%; F_{uremia} = 17%

Mycophenolate mofetil
Mechanism of action
- Metabolized to mycophenolic acid (MPA), which causes noncompetitive, reversible inhibition of inosine monophosphate dehydrogenase (IMPDH), a critical enzyme in the de novo pathway of purine synthesis, which is crucial during lymphocyte activation and proliferation.

Administration
- Intravenous: dilute in D_5 to a concentration of 6 mg/mL and infuse over at least 2 h.

- Oral: administer as equally divided doses PO every 8-12 h consistently with or without food

Drug-drug interactions
- Cyclosporine: see Table 4

Drug-disease interactions
- Severe renal impairment: reduces protein binding of MPA

- Vaccinations: in general, immunosuppressants may affect efficacy of vaccination. The use of live vaccines should be avoided.

Adverse drug reactions
- GI: nausea, vomiting, diarrhea, abdominal pain

- Hematologic: pancytopenia

Patient instructions
- Take the prescribed dose at consistent times during the day. It may be taken with or without food, but should be taken the same way to maintain consistency. Make sure you do not take your medication prior to therapeutic drug monitoring.

Monitoring
- No clinically important pharmacokinetic or pharmacodynamic monitoring is needed.

Pharmacokinetics
- MPA is highly protein bound

- Bioavailability: F = 94%

- Elimination: $t_{1/2}$ = 17 h

Leflunomide
Mechanism of action
- Metabolized to an active metabolite, A77 1726, which inhibits de novo pyrimidine synthesis by selective inhibition of dihydro-orotate dehydrogenase (DHODH). Thus it inhibits proliferation of stimulated lymphocytes.

Administration
- Administer daily dose PO once a day.

Drug-drug interactions
- Cholestyramine: reduces biliary recycling, which significantly shortens $t_{1/2}$. Should not be used during leflunomide therapy.

Drug-disease interactions
- Renal insufficiency: bioavailability significantly reduced in uremic patients.

- Vaccinations: in general, immunosuppressants may affect efficacy of vaccination. The use of live vaccines should be avoided.

Adverse drug reactions
- CNS: headache, dizziness, neuralgia, neuritis

- HEENT: alopecia

- GI: nausea, vomiting, diarrhea, anorexia, gastroenteritis, esophagitis, colitis

- Endocrine and metabolic: diabetes mellitus, hyperlipidemia, hyperthyroidism

- Patient instructions: take the prescribed dose at a consistent time once daily. It may be taken with or without food.

Monitoring
- No clinically important pharmacokinetic or pharmacodynamic monitoring is needed.

Pharmcokinetics
- A77 1726 is highly protein bound.

- Bioavailability: F = 80%

- Elimination: $t_{1/2}$ = 11-14 d

Corticosteroids

Selection of agent
- Selection of the corticosteroid used is based on the ratio of glucocorticoid to mineralocorticoid potency.

Intravenous
- Methylprednisolone, dexamethasone

Oral
- Prednisone, prednisolone, dexamethasone

Mechanism of action
- Corticosteroids bind to cytosolic glucocorticoid receptors, which translocate to the nucleus where the complexes bind to regulatory DNA sequences, glucocorticoid-responsive elements (GREs), within the promoter section of various genes. Activation of these GREs modifies activities of promoter genes such as NFAT, AP-1, and NFκβ. This results in downregulation of expression of HLA and numerous cell adhesion molecules, as well as decreased synthesis of numerous lymphokines responsible for activation, proliferation, and migration (ie, IL-1, IL-2, IL-6, IL-8, IFN-γ, TNF-α).

Administration
- Dependent on individual agent

Drug-drug interactions
- Metabolized primarily via cytochrome P450 3A isoenzymes. Substances known to alter functionality of these enzymes will alter bioavailability and elimination of this drug (Table 3).

Drug-disease interactions
- Diabetes mellitus: administration worsens glycemic control in patients with pre-existing diabetes.

- Osteopenia/osteoporosis: administration alters calcium and phosphate absorption and excretion, as well as osteoblast activity, resulting in progression of bone loss that is common in metabolic diseases such as end-stage renal disease and liver failure.

- Vaccinations: in general, immunosuppressants may affect efficacy of vaccination. The use of live vaccines should be avoided.

Adverse drug reactions
- The incidence and extent of most adverse drug reactions with corticosteroids depend on the ratio of glucocorticoid to mineralocorticoid potency.

- CNS: seizure, psychosis, delirium, hallucinations, mood swings, insomnia, pseudotumor cerebri

- HEENT: cataracts, glaucoma

- CV: hypertension, cardiomyopathy

- GI: increased appetite, GERD, PUD, pancreatitis

- Renal: edema, alkalosis, hyperkalemia

- Endocrine and metabolic: diabetes mellitus, hyperlipidemia, hypothalamic-pituitary-adrenal axis suppression, growth suppression

- Dermatologic: hirsutism, acne, skin atrophy, impaired wound healing

- Hematologic: transient leukocytosis

- Musculoskeletal: arthralgia, myopathy, osteoporosis, avascular necrosis

Patient instructions
- When taking orally, take daily dose in the morning with food. Many drugs interact with these agents. Do not take anything prescribed by another physician until you verify that there are no drug interactions.

Monitoring
- No clinically important pharmacokinetic or pharmacodynamic monitoring is needed.

Pharmacokinetics
- Dependent on individual agent

Monoclonal Antibodies

Orthoclone OKT3
Mechanism of action
- Murine, monoclonal IgG that binds to and facilitates removal of cell lines expressing CD3. CD3, part of the TCR complex, is an important molecule that distinguishes T cells. CD3 is important in antigen recognition and antigen-specific signal transduction.

Administration
- Premedication:
  * Dose 1: intravenous steroids, acetaminophen, and antihistamines taken 1 h prior are strongly recommended to modify first-dose reactions.
  * Subsequent doses: acetaminophen and antihistamines taken 1 h prior with steroids as needed for infusion-related reactions

- Dosing: prior to administration, volume status must be carefully assessed. Patients with evidence of volume overload or uncompensated CHF on chest x-ray should not receive this drug. Dose should be administered via IV bolus over less than a minute.

Drug-drug interactions
- No clinically significant interactions occur.

Drug-disease interactions
- Uncompensated CHF/volume overload: risk of fatal pulmonary edema

- Vaccinations: in general, immunosuppressants may affect efficacy of vaccination. The use of live vaccines should be avoided.

Adverse drug reactions
- CNS: dizziness, headache

- HEENT: photophobia

- CV: tachycardia

- Hematologic: transient lymphopenia, pancytopenia

- Musculoskeletal: rigor, tremor

- Other: fever, chills, dyspnea, pulmonary edema

Patient instructions
- Repeat any shortness of breath, palpitations, lightheadedness, tremor, fever, or itching to your nurse immediately.

Monitoring
- CD3: suppression of CD3 lineage <25 cells/mm^3

Pharmacokinetics
- Elimination: $t_{1/2}$ = 18 h

Basiliximab
Mechanism of action
- Chimeric (murine/human), monoclonal IgG that specifically binds to the α subunit, CD25, of the human high-affinity IL-2 receptor, which is only expressed on activated lymphocytes. In this way

basiliximab competitively inhibits IL-2 and facilitates preferential elimination of activated lymphocytes.

Administration
• Dilute to a concentration of 0.4 mg/mL in NS or D_5. Administer peripherally or centrally as a bolus or continuous infusion over 20-30 minutes.

Drug-drug interactions
• No clinically significant drug interactions occur.

Drug-disease interactions
• Vaccinations: in general, immunosuppressants may affect efficacy of vaccination. The use of live vaccines should be avoided.

Adverse drug reactions
• Severe acute hypersensitivity reactions including anaphylaxis may occur within the 24 hours following administration of the initial dose or on repeat exposure.

Patient instructions
• Repeat any shortness of breath, palpitations, light-headedness, or itching to your nurse immediately.

Monitoring
• No clinically important pharmacokinetic or pharmacodynamic monitoring is needed.

Pharmacokinetics
• Adults: following a 20-mg IV infusion over 20 minutes:
  * Mean C_{max} = 7.1 ± 5.1 mg/L
  * Mean $t_{1/2}$ = 7.2 ± 3.2 days
  * Pediatrics: mean $t_{1/2}$ = 11.5 ± 6.3 days

Pharmacodynamics
• Adults: CD25 saturation at or above serum concentration of 0.2 µg/mL
  * Mean duration of saturation dependent on concomitant immunosuppressive regimen.
• Pediatrics: CD25 saturation similar to adults

Daclizumab
Mechanism of action
• Humanized monoclonal IgG that specifically binds to the α subunit, CD25, of the human high-affinity IL-2 receptor, which is only expressed on activated lymphocytes. In this way daclizumab competitively inhibits IL-2 and facilitates preferential elimination of activated lymphocytes.

Administration
• Dilute in 50 mL of NS and administer peripherally or centrally as a continuous infusion over 15 minutes

Drug-drug interactions
• No clinically significant drug interactions occur.

Drug-disease interactions
• Vaccinations: in general, immunosuppressants may affect efficacy of vaccination. The use of live vaccines should be avoided.

Adverse drug reactions
• Severe acute hypersensitivity reactions including anaphylaxis have rarely occurred within the 24 hours following administration of the initial dose or on repeat exposure.

Patient instructions
• Repeat any shortness of breath, palpitations, light-headedness, or itching to your nurse immediately.

Monitoring
• No clinically important pharmacokinetic or pharmacodynamic monitoring is needed.

Pharmacokinetics
• Adults: at recommended dosing:
  * Mean C_{max}: dose 1 = 21 ± 14 mg/mL; dose 5 = 32 ± 22 mg/mL
  * Mean C_{min}: dose 5 = 7.6 ± 4.0 mg/mL
  * $t_{1/2}$ = 20 days
  * Pediatrics: at recommended dosing:
  * Mean C_{max}: dose 1 = 16 ± 12 mg/mL; dose 5 = 21 ± 14 mg/mL
  * Mean C_{min}: dose 5 = 5.0 ± 2.7 mg/mL
  * $t_{1/2}$ = 13 days

Pharmacodynamics
• Adults: CD25 saturation at serum concentrations of 5-10 mg/mL
  * At recommended dosing, saturation occurs for approximately 120 days

• Pediatrics: CD25 saturation at serum concentrations of 5-10 mg/mL
  * At recommended dosing, saturation occurs for approximately 90 days

Polyclonal Antibodies

Anti-thymocyte globulin (equine)
Mechanism of action
• Purified, sterile, polyclonal IgG harvested from horses immunized with human thymocytes. This preparation includes IgG directed against cell sur-

face markers such as CD2, CD3, CD4, CD8, CD11a, and CD18. In this way horse anti-thymocyte globulin targets multiple phases of immunity, including T-cell activation, homing, and cytotoxic activities.

Administration
- Premedication
    * Dose 1: intravenous steroids, acetaminophen, and antihistamines 1 h prior are strongly recommended to modify first-dose reactions.
    * Subsequent doses: acetaminophen and antihistamines 1 h prior with steroids as needed for infusion reactions

- Dose: Dilute dose to a concentration not to exceed 4 mg/mL in $^1/_2$NS or D_5 and administer centrally over 4-6 h.

Drug-drug interactions
- No clinically significant drug interactions occur.

Drug-disease interactions
- Vaccinations: in general, immunosuppressants may affect efficacy of vaccination. The use of live vaccines should be avoided.

Adverse drug reactions
- Most adverse drug reactions with anti-thymocyte globulin (equine) are related to infusion-related reactions (ie, fever, chills, dyspnea), leukopenia, thrombocytopenia, and/or rash.

Patient instructions
- Report any shortness of breath, palpitations, light-headedness, tremor, fever, or itching to your nurse immediately.

Monitoring
- CD2: goal for treatment of acute rejection is suppression of CD2 lineage to <50 cells/mm^3

Pharmacokinetics
- Elimination: $t_{1/2}$ = 36 h-12 d

Anti-thymocyte globulin (rabbit)
Mechanism of action
- Purified, pasteurized, polyclonal IgG harvested from pathogen-free rabbits immunized with human thymocytes. This preparation includes IgG directed against cell surface markers such as TCRab, CD2, CD3, CD4, CD5, CD6, CD7, CD8, CD11a, CD18, CD28, CD45, CD49, CD54, CD58, CD80, CD86, HLA class I, and β2 microglobulin. In this way, rabbit anti-thymocyte globulin targets multiple phases of immunity, including T-cell activation, homing, and cytotoxic activities.

Administration
- Premedication
    * Dose 1: intravenous steroids, acetaminophen, and antihistamines 1 h prior are strongly recommended to modify first-dose reactions.
    * Subsequent doses: acetaminophen and antihistamines 1 h prior with steroids as needed for infusion reactions

- Dose: dilute dose to a concentration of 0.5 mg/mL in NS or D_5 and administer centrally over 4-6 h.

Drug-drug interactions
- No clinically significant drug interactions occur.

Drug-disease interactions
- Vaccinations: in general, immunosuppressants may affect efficacy of vaccination. The use of live vaccines should be avoided.

Adverse drug reactions
- Most adverse drug reactions with anti-thymocyte globulin (rabbit) are related to infusion-related reactions (ie, fever, chills, dyspnea), leukopenia, thrombocytopenia, and/or rash.

Patient instructions
- Repeat any shortness of breath, palpitations, light-headedness, tremor, fever, or itching to your nurse immediately.

Monitoring
- CD2: Goal for treatment of acute rejection is suppression of CD2 lineage to <50 cells/mm^3

Pharmacokinetics
- Two-compartment model; terminal elimination: $t_{1/2}$ = 2-3 d

3. Key Points

- The goal of solid organ transplantation is to improve patients' quality of life and survival by stabilizing and/or improving end-organ failure related complications.

- The immune system is a highly intricate system with mechanisms for antigen recognition in a highly specific manner, as well as a nonspecific manner.

- Acute rejection is a normal physiologic immune response to transplantation of donor antigens.

- The incidence of acute rejection is organ specific and dependent on multiple pre- and post-transplant factors.

- Selection of the post-transplant immunosuppression regimen for prevention of acute rejection should be individualized based on known risk and potential toxicity.

- Adjustment in the post-transplant immunosuppression regimen should focus on the balance between acute rejection, infection, and toxicity.

- Selection of the agent to be used to treat acute rejection is organ dependent and dependent on the severity of acute rejection.

- Immunosuppressive complications, both infectious and noninfectious, are an important cause of early morbidity and mortality and require close management post-transplant.

- Many agents commonly included in immunosuppression regimens require a clinician with expertise in immunosuppressive therapeutic drug monitoring to optimize efficacy and/or reduce toxicity.

- Many agents commonly included in immunosuppression regimens have the potential for numerous pharmacokinetic and pharmacodynamic drug interactions.

4. Questions and Answers

Use the patient profile provided below to answer Questions 1-4.

Patient name: Doe, John   Age: 52
Address: 101 South First Street
Gender: Male   Ethnicity: African-American
Height: 5'11"   Weight: 240 lbs
Allergies: Sulfa
Diagnoses: h/o ESRD s/p cadaveric renal transplant 3 mo ago
DM x 20 yrs
HTN x 30 yrs
Drug-induced hyperkalemia 1/2003
Laboratory: 3/20/03 Scr = 1.2, K = 4.8, WBC 3.8, Plt 120
Medications:

1/20/03	Prograf 4 mg PO bid
	Amaryl 4 mg PO bid
	Cellcept 750 mg PO bid
	Metoprolol 100 mg PO bid
	Diflucan 200 mg PO qd
	Dapsone 100 mg PO qd
	Valcyte 450 mg PO qd
	EC ASA 81 mg PO qd
	Prednisone 5 mg PO qd
2/1/03	Lasix 40 mg PO bid
	Imuran 100 mg PO qd

1. Which medication(s) should be given with caution due to the patient's sulfonamide allergy?

   I. Lasix
  II. Dapsone
 III. Amaryl

    A. I only
    B. II only
    C. I and III only
    D. II and III only
    E. I, II, and III

2. Which of the following combinations of drugs represent therapeutic duplication?
    A. Prograf and Imuran
    B. Azathioprine and Cellcept
    C. Dapsone and Valcyte
    D. Amaryl and Tacrolimus
    E. Prednisone and Cellcept

3. Which of the following combinations of drugs interact?

   I. Diflucan and tacrolimus
  II. Diflucan and Valcyte
 III. Dapsone and Lasix

A. I only
B. II only
C. I and II only
D. II and III only
E. I, II, and III

4. In the above case, the patient was diagnosed with drug-induced hyperkalemia in 1/2003. Which medication on his profile could be responsible for this?

A. Cellcept
B. Lasix
C. Prednisone
D. Prograf
E. EC ASA

5. Which medication(s) is/are classified as a calcineurin inhibitor?

A. Rapamune
B. Cyclosporine
C. Tacrolimus
D. B and C
E. A and C

6. Which medication(s) cause myelosuppression?

A. Sirolimus
B. Mycophenolate mofetil
C. Valcyte
D. All of the above
E. B and C

7. Which medication(s) require bile for emulsification and absorption?

A. Imuran
B. Cyclosporine
C. Prograf
D. Prednisone
E. All of the above

8. All of the following are known adverse effects of cyclosporine EXCEPT:

A. Hirsutism
B. Nephrotoxicity
C. Oral ulceration
D. Gingival hyperplasia
E. Hyperlipidemia

9. All of the following are contraindications or precautions associated with Rapamune EXCEPT:

A. De novo lung transplant recipient
B. Hyperlipidemia
C. Diabetes mellitus
D. De novo liver transplant recipient
E. Allergy to sirolimus

10. What is the generic name for Arava?

A. Leflunomide
B. Azathioprine
C. Daclizumab
D. Tacrolimus
E. Alemtuzumab

11. Which of the immunosuppressive medication(s) listed may cause diabetes mellitus?

A. Prednisone
B. Azathioprine
C. Tacrolimus
D. A and C
E. All of the above

12. Which medication(s) requires therapeutic drug monitoring via trough concentrations?

A. Mycophenolate mofetil
B. Prograf
C. Daclizumab
D. Leflunomide
E. A and B

13. Which medication(s) selects for destruction of activated lymphocytes by binding to the CD25 subunit of the high affinity IL-2 receptor?

A. Anti-thymocyte globulin (rabbit)
B. Anti-thymocyte globulin (equine)
C. Zenapax
D. A and B
E. All of the above

14. All of the following increase the risk of acute rejection EXCEPT:

A. Pediatric recipient
B. HLA mismatch
C. Living donor
D. Noncompliance
E. History of previous transplantation

15. Which of the following produces a significant pharmacokinetic interaction when administered with azathioprine?

A. Allopurinol
B. Diflucan
C. Sirolimus
D. Probenecid
E. A and D

16. Which of these conditions alter the pharmacokinetic profile of cyclosporine?

   A. Biliary obstruction
   B. Malnutrition
   C. Hyperglycemia
   D. A and B
   E. All of the above

17. Which of the following medication(s) interacts with leflunomide?

   A. Erythromycin
   B. Prevalite
   C. Diltiazem
   D. A and C
   E. B and C

18. Which of the following immunosuppressants should not be administered at the same time secondary to an interaction related to timing of doses?

   A. Prograf and mycophenolate mofetil
   B. Rapamune and cyclosporine
   C. Neoral and leflunomide
   D. None of these interact
   E. B and C

19. Which type of immunity involves stimulation of cells and soluble mediators that nonspecifically recognize alloantigens with no altered response on repeat exposure?

   A. Autoimmunity
   B. Innate immunity
   C. Adaptive immunity
   D. Acute rejection
   E. Hyperacute rejection

20. Which group of genes encode for antigens that are responsible for self/nonself recognition?

   A. Class I human leukocyte antigen (HLA)
   B. Class II human leukocyte antigen (HLA)
   C. Major histocompatibility complex (MHC)
   D. A and B
   E. All of the above

21. Upon binding of antigen displayed by the APC to the T-cell receptor complex, what additional step is required for T-helper cell activation?

   A. Binding of the costimulator pathway (ie, CD58/CD2)
   B. Activation of the promoter gene NFAT
   C. Transcription of the IL-2 gene
   D. No additional step is required
   E. Both B and C

22. Which cytokine released by activated $CD4^+$ lymphocytes plays a major role in the subsequent activation of numerous lymphocyte lineages?

   A. Interleukin-1 (IL-1)
   B. Tumor necrosis factor-α (TNF-α)
   C. Interleukin-2 (IL-2)
   D. Interferon-γ (IFN-γ)
   E. Complement

23. Which solid organ was the first to be successfully transplanted?

   A. Heart
   B. Liver
   C. Kidney
   D. Lung
   E. Pancreas

24. What is the 1-year patient survival rate for renal transplant recipients?

   A. >90%
   B. 60-70%
   C. 25-50%
   D. <25%
   E. Limited data available; currently an experimental procedure

Answers

1. **C.** Lasix and Amaryl are structurally similar to sulfonamides and would be expected to elicit a similar allergic response. Dapsone is a sulfone and would not be expected to elicit an allergic response.

2. **B.** Both azathioprine and Cellcept are classified as antiproliferative agents. Both agents inhibit purine biosynthesis and would not offer a synergy.

3. **A.** Diflucan is an inhibitor of cytochrome P450 3A isoenzymes, which is the enzyme system that is responsible for metabolism of tacrolimus.

4. **D.** Hyperkalemia (incidence 20-40%) is a well documented adverse drug reaction with Prograf.

5. **D.** Both cyclosporine and tacrolimus are calcineurin inhibitors.

6. **D.** All of the above-listed agents have myelosuppressive properties when administered individually. When administered concurrently the myelosuppression is synergistic.

7. **B.** Cyclosporine is highly lipophilic and requires bile for emulsification and absorption.

8. **C.** Hirsutism, nephrotoxicity, gingival hyperplasia, and hyperlipidemia are known adverse effects of cyclosporine. Oral ulceration is not an adverse effect of cyclosporine.

9. **C.** The use of Rapamune in de novo lung and liver transplant recipients is contraindicated due to an increased incidence of fatal adverse drug reactions. Additionally, use of Rapamune in patients with uncontrolled hyperlipidemia is strongly discouraged due to its profound effects on lipid biosynthesis and catabolism.

10. **A.** Leflunomide is the generic name for Arava.

11. **D.** Prednisone and tacrolimus may cause diabetes mellitus. Azathioprine does not produce a diabetogenic effect.

12. **B.** Prograf requires therapeutic drug monitoring via trough concentrations in order to obtain desired therapeutic effects.

13. **C.** Zenepax selects for destruction of activated lymphocytes by binding to the CD25 subunit of the high-affinity IL-2 receptor.

14. **C.** Of the above parameters, all are considered to increase the risk of acute rejection except living donor as donor source.

15. **A.** Xanthine oxidase is responsible for the elimination of the active metabolites of azathioprine. Concomitant use of allopurinol with azathioprine results in significantly increased azathioprine-induced toxicity. Reduce the dose of azathioprine by 65-75%.

16. **D.** Both biliary obstruction and severe malnutrition would change the pharmacokinetic profile of cyclosporine. Cyclosporine requires bile for emulsification and absorption. If bile flow is obstructed, then the bioavailability is significantly decreased. Additionally, cyclosporine is a highly lipoprotein bound drug. In severe malnutrition, total protein stores are depleted, thereby increasing the total free drug.

17. **B.** Cholestyramine reduces biliary recycling which significantly shortens $t_{1/2}$.

18. **B.** Simultaneous administration increased C_{max} and AUC of sirolimus by 120-500% and 140-230%, respectively. Administration 4 hours apart increased C_{max} and AUC of sirolimus by 30-40% and 35-80%, respectively.

19. **B.** Innate immunity is the fundamental type of immunity in which antigens are recognized in a nonspecific manner. This type of immunity is not augmented on repeat exposure.

20. **C.** Class I and II HLA are the actual antigens important for self/nonself recognition. The group of genes that encode for these antigens is the major histocompatibility complex (MHC).

21. **A.** Activation is dependent on antigen/HLA binding to the T-cell receptor complex and the subsequent binding of a second signal or "co-stimulator pathway."

22. **C.** Active $CD4^+$ T cells produce and release various lymphokines, particularly IL-2, important for activation and proliferation of numerous lymphocyte lineages.

23. **C.** The kidney was the first organ to be successfully transplanted, in 1954.

24. **A.** Currently, the 1-year patient survival rate after renal transplantation is 94.4%, based on Organ Procurement and Transplantation Network data.

5. References

Christians U, Jacobsen W, Benet LZ, Lampen A. Mechanisms of clinically relevant drug interactions associated with tacrolimus. *Clin Pharmacokinet.* 2002;41:813-851

Cotts WG, Johnson MR. The challenge of rejection and cardiac allograft vasculopathy. *Heart Fail Rev.* 2001;6:227-240.

Delves PJ, Roitt IM. The immune system—first of two parts. *N Engl J Med.* 2000;343:37-49.

Delves PJ, Roitt IM. The immune system—second of two parts. *N Engl J Med.* 2000;343:108-117.

Dunn CJ, Wagstaff AJ, Perry CM, Plosker GL, Goa KL. Cyclosporin: an updated review of the pharmacokinetic properties, clinical efficacy and tolerability of a microemulsion-based formulation (neoral)1 in organ transplantation. *Drugs.* 2001;61:1957-2016.

Kelly P, Kahan BD. Review: metabolism of immunosuppressant drugs. *Curr Drug Metab.* 2002;3:275-287.

Klupp J, Holt DW, van Gelder T. How pharmacokinetic and pharmacodynamic drug monitoring can improve outcome in solid organ transplant recipients. *Transpl Immunol.* 2002;9:211-214.

Neuberger J. Incidence, timing, and risk factors for acute and chronic rejection. *Liver Transpl Surg.* 1999Jul;5(Suppl 1):S30-S36.

Tejani A, Emmett L. Acute and chronic rejection. *Semin Nephrol.* 2001;21:498-507.

Williams JW, Mital D, Chong A, et al. Experience with leflunomide in solid organ transplantation. *Transplantation.* 2002;15:358-366.

21. Gastrointestinal Diseases

Christa M. George, PharmD, BCPS
Assistant Professor, Department of Pharmacy
University of Tennessee College of Pharmacy

Contents

1. Peptic Ulcer Disease

Definition and Incidence

- Peptic ulcer disease (PUD) is a group of disorders of the upper gastrointestinal tract characterized by ulcerative lesions dependent on acid and pepsin for their formation.

- Approximately 1.5-2 million Americans have an active ulcer at any given time.

- 500,000 new cases are diagnosed in the U.S. annually.

- U.S. lifetime prevalence of PUD ranges from 11-20% for men and 8-11% for women.

- The cost of PUD in the U.S. is $20 billion per year.

Classification

- Ulcers are either duodenal or gastric in nature (duodenal ulcers are more common).

- Duodenal and gastric ulcers are classified as *Helicobacter pylori*–related, nonsteroidal anti-inflammatory drug (NSAID)–related, non–*H pylori*-related, non–NSAID related, or stress related.

Clinical Presentation

- Epigastric pain occurring 1-3 hours after meals that is relieved by ingestion of food or antacids is the classic presentation of PUD.

- Pain typically occurs in episodes lasting weeks to months, and may be followed by variable periods of spontaneous remission and recurrence.

- Ten percent of patients with PUD present with complications and have no prior history of pain.

Pathophysiology

- Duodenal ulcers result from the imbalance between duodenal acid load and the acid-buffering capacity of duodenum.

- Duodenal ulcers are more frequently associated with an antrum-predominant gastritis.

- *H pylori* is a gram-negative microaerophilic bacterium that inhabits the area between the mucosal layer and epithelial cells in the stomach. It can be found anywhere gastric epithelium is present.
  - * Over 50% of the world's population is colonized by *H pylori*, but only 15% of colonized individuals develop clinical symptoms of PUD. The prevalence of *H pylori* is decreasing in developed countries.
  - * *H pylori* causes duodenal inflammation, increases duodenal acid load, and impairs duodenal bicarbonate secretion, which leads to duodenal ulcers.
  - * *H pylori* causes inflammation of gastric epithelium, particularly in the antrum-corpus area. This disrupts mucosal defense, which also leads to gastric ulcers.

- NSAIDs are the leading cause of PUD in patients negative for *H pylori* infection.
  - * NSAIDs are directly toxic to gastric epithelium and inhibit the synthesis of prostaglandins.
  - * Inhibition of prostaglandin synthesis leads to decreased bicarbonate secretion, the presence of epithelial mucus, mucosal perfusion, epithelial proliferation, and mucosal resistance to injury.
  - * NSAIDs may cause gastric or duodenal ulcers (more frequently gastric).

- Gastric ulcers are associated with a corpus-predominant (ie, diffuse-predominant) gastritis.

- This pattern of gastritis is associated with low acid output, gastric atrophy, and adenocarcinoma.

Diagnostic Criteria

- Upper gastrointestinal endoscopy is used to diagnose PUD. The procedure is usually reserved for patients with clinical features that suggest PUD complications (eg, gastric cancer, bleeding).

- Patients who initially present with clinical symptoms of PUD may be treated for *H pylori* if a test is positive for *H pylori* infection.
  - * *H pylori* may be detected noninvasively by serology, urea breath test (UBT), a fecal antigen test, and/or a urine antibody test. The UBT is the test of choice and is commercially available for use in medical offices.
  - * Gastric mucosal biopsies may be obtained during endoscopy for culture, rapid urease tests, and histology.

Treatment Principles and Goals

- The goals of PUD therapy include healing the ulcer and eliminating the cause of the ulcer.

- Additional considerations include preventing complications and relieving symptoms.

- Use of proton pump inhibitors (PPIs) is associated with faster healing rates and symptom relief than treatment with histamine$_2$ receptor antagonists (H$_2$RAs). (*Note:* H$_2$RAs are less expensive.)

- Choice of PUD therapy is based on the etiology of the case. For *H pylori*–related PUD, antibacterial therapy is used with antisecretory therapy.
  * Eradication of *H pylori* reduces the recurrence of PUD and is of prime importance.
  * The ideal treatment regimen for *H pylori* has not been identified.
  * Treatment regimens consist of triple or quadruple drug therapy, eg, with a PPI or an H$_2$RA, bismuth, and one or two antibiotics for 10-14 days. Average cure rates range from 86-94%, depending on the regimen used.
  * The eradication of *H pylori* should be confirmed with UBT or fecal antigen testing 2-4 weeks after completing therapy.
  * If resistance to clarithromycin is suspected, replace it with metronidazole and vice versa. Often metronidazole resistance can be overcome by increasing the dose.
  * If both clarithromycin and metronidazole resistance is suspected, furazolidone may be substituted (as part of a quadruple drug regimen).

- For NSAID-related PUD, discontinuation of the offending agent is imperative.
  * Antisecretory therapy should be instituted to promote healing and to relieve symptoms.
  * If *H pylori* is also present, antibacterial therapy should be initiated. Eradication of *H pylori* does not prevent NSAID-related complications or recurrence.
  * PPIs, H$_2$RAs, or misoprostol should be used to prevent PUD in patients who require chronic NSAIDs and who are at risk of developing PUD (eg, patients who are elderly and/or have concomitant cardiovascular disease, patients with a history of PUD, patients using high-dose NSAID therapy, and/or patients who concomitantly use corticosteroids or anticoagulants).
  * If chronic anti-inflammatory therapy is required, replacing the NSAID with a COX-2 inhibitor should be considered since it may reduce the risk of PUD.

- Sucralfate may also be used to aid in ulcer healing, but it requires multiple daily dosing and is associated with many significant drug interactions.

- Non–*H pylori*, non-NSAID–related PUD should be treated with antisecretory therapy.

Drug Therapy

Mechanism of action
- PPIs suppress gastric acid secretion specifically by inhibiting the H$^+$-K$^+$ ATPase enzyme system of the secretory surface of the gastric parietal cell (Table 1).

- H$_2$RAs suppress gastric acid secretion by reversibly blocking histamine$_2$ receptors on the surface of the gastric parietal cell.

- Clarithromycin, amoxicillin, metronidazole, tetracycline, bismuth subsalicylate, and furazolidone exhibit antibacterial effects against *H pylori*.

- When exposed to gastric acid, sucralfate forms a viscous adhesive that binds positively-charged protein molecules in the ulcer crater. This forms a protective barrier, which protects against back-diffusion of hydrogen ions.

Patient counseling
- Educate patients about the importance of completing the entire course of therapy to ensure the eradication of *H pylori* and to avoid bacterial resistance.

- PPIs are best taken before eating. Lansoprazole granules may be sprinkled onto applesauce for patients who have trouble swallowing pills. Omeprazole capsules should be swallowed whole.

- If antacids are being used to control breakthrough symptoms, the dose should be taken no less than 1-2 hours before or after taking an H$_2$RA. H$_2$RAs may be taken without regard to meals.

- Amoxicillin, clarithromycin, and metronidazole may be taken without regard to meals; however, taking clarithromycin and metronidazole with meals often reduces the incidence of stomach upset.

- Tetracycline is best taken on an empty stomach. Antacids, dairy products, or iron-containing products should be taken 2 hours before or after taking tetracycline.

- Sucralfate should be taken 1 hour before meals and at bedtime.

Table 1

Selected Medications Used in Peptic Ulcer Disease

Generic name (trade name)	Classification	Dosage range and frequency	Dosage forms
Omeprazole (Prilosec®)	Proton pump inhibitor	20-40 mg qd	C
Esomeprazole (Nexium®)	Proton pump inhibitor	20-40 mg qd	C
Lansoprazole (Prevacid®)	Proton pump inhibitor	15 mg qd-30 mg bid	C, DT, L
Rabeprazole (Aciphex®)	Proton pump inhibitor	10-20 mg qd	T
Pantoprazole (Protonix®)	Proton pump inhibitor	40-80 mg qd	T, IV
Cimetidine (Tagamet®)	H_2-receptor blocker	300 mg qid-800 mg hs	T, L, IV
Ranitidine (Zantac®)	H_2-receptor blocker	150 mg bid-300 mg hs	T, L, IV, G, EfT
Nizatidine (Axid®)	H_2-receptor blocker	150 mg bid-300 mg hs	C
Famotidine (Pepcid®)	H_2-receptor blocker	20 mg bid-40 mg hs	T, L, DT, IV
Ranitidine bismuth citrate (Tritec®)	H_2-receptor blocker + bismuth	400 mg bid x 10-14 d	T
Clarithromycin (Biaxin®)	Antibacterial	500 mg bid x 10-14 d	T
Amoxicillin (Amoxil®)	Antibacterial	1 g bid x 10-14 d	C, L
Metronidazole (Flagyl®)	Antibacterial	250-500 mg tid x 10-14 d	T, IV
Tetracycline (various)	Antibacterial	500 mg qid x 10-14 d	C
Furazolidone (Furoxone®)	Antibacterial	100 mg tid x 10-14 d	T
Sucralfate (Carafate®)	Cytoprotective	1 g qid	T, L

T, tablet; C, capsule; L, liquid; EfT, effervescent tablet; DT, delayed-release tablet; IV, intravenous.

Adverse drug effects
- Side effects occur in 15-20% of patients, but they are usually minor.

- PPIs and H_2RAs are generally well-tolerated, but headache, diarrhea, and nausea have been reported.

- Antibiotics may cause diarrhea, nausea, dysgeusia, rash, and monilial vaginitis.

- Bismuth subsalicylate may cause black, tarry stools.

- Constipation is the most common side effect of sucralfate.

- Furazolidone may cause nausea, vomiting, headache, tachycardia, and hypertension.

- PPIs may alter the bioavailability of drugs that require an acidic environment for absorption (eg, ketoconazole, digoxin, and iron).

Drug interactions
- Omeprazole inhibits the cytochrome P450 enzyme system, which decreases the elimination of warfarin, phenytoin, diazepam, and cyclosporine. Lansoprazole has been reported to increase theophylline clearance by approximately 10%.

- Cimetidine is a potent inhibitor of the cytochrome P450 enzyme system, which decreases the elimination of numerous drugs (eg, warfarin, theophylline, and phenytoin).

- Amoxicillin and tetracycline may decrease the effectiveness of oral contraceptives.

- Clarithromycin is a potent inhibitor of the cytochrome P450 enzyme system, which decreases the elimination of warfarin, digoxin, cyclosporine, carbamazepine, theophylline, and cisapride (no longer on the market).

- Tetracycline may decrease the effectiveness of oral contraceptives. Antacids, iron products, and dairy products bind to tetracycline, decreasing its effectiveness. Tetracycline can also increase the therapeutic effect of warfarin. Tetracycline can increase or decrease lithium levels.

- Metronidazole produces a disulfiram-like reaction when ingested with alcohol, and increases the therapeutic effect of warfarin and lithium.

- Sucralfate leads to the absorption of small amounts of aluminum, which may accumulate if given to patients with renal insufficiency (especially when combined with aluminum-containing antacids).

- Sucralfate alters the absorption of numerous drugs, including warfarin, digoxin, phenytoin, ketoconazole, quinidine, and quinolones.

- Furazolidone is a monoamine oxidase inhibitor (MAOI). In order to avoid hypertensive crisis, furazolidone should not be administered with selective serotonin-reuptake inhibitors (SSRIs), tricyclic antidepressants (TCAs), or tyramine-containing foods.

- Disulfiram-like reactions have been reported with the concurrent ingestion of alcohol and furazolidone.

Monitoring parameters
- Patients should monitor for the return of PUD symptoms and for the side effects of medications as discussed in the earlier sections.

Pharmacokinetics
- Several medications are substrates for or have effects on the cytochrome P450 enzyme system in the liver. Please see discussion in drug interactions section.

Nondrug Therapy and Complications

- Patients should be counseled to decrease psychological stress and to discontinue smoking, taking NSAIDs, and ingesting food or beverages that may exacerbate PUD symptoms.

- Major complications occur in approximately 25% of patients with PUD (hemorrhage, perforation, penetration, and obstruction).
  * Patients with active bleeding should initially undergo endoscopic hemostasis, as the procedure is associated with a lower mortality rate than emergency surgery.
  * Due to its safety, laparoscopic repair is beginning to replace laparotomy in the treatment of perforated ulcers.
  * Surgery is reserved for those patients who have refractory ulcers (or hemorrhage or perforation) that cannot be managed with endoscopy or laparoscopic repair.

2. Gastroesophageal Reflux Disease

Definition and Incidence

- Gastroesophageal reflux disease (GERD) is defined as chronic symptoms or mucosal damage produced by the abnormal reflux of gastric contents into the esophagus.

- The prevalence of GERD is highest in Western countries. It occurs equally in men and women, except during pregnancy, when its incidence is higher in women. It may also occur in children.

- Approximately 20% of the population experiences heartburn or regurgitation of gastric acid weekly.

- Approximately 30-50% of pregnant women have symptomatic esophageal reflux; 50% experience heartburn daily.

Classification

- Nonerosive reflux disease (NERD), erosive esophagitis (EE), and Barrett's esophagus (BE) are types of GERD. Esophageal adenocarcinoma rarely develops (2-4 cases per 100,000 persons per year). Patients with BE have an increased risk of developing esophageal adenocarcinoma.

Clinical Presentation

- Symptoms of GERD may be classified as typical, atypical, or complicated.

- The hallmark symptom of GERD is heartburn (pyrosis), which is described as substernal burning or pain that may radiate to the neck, back, or throat.

- Symptoms usually occur shortly after meals or when reclining after meals, or upon lying down at bedtime. Patients are often awakened from sleep by symptoms.

- Symptoms are exacerbated by eating a large meal (especially a high-fat meal), bending over, and occasionally by exercising.

- Additional typical symptoms include hypersalivation, belching, and regurgitation.
  * Typical symptoms are usually relieved with antacids.

- Atypical symptoms (or extraesophageal symptoms) include chronic cough, hoarseness, nonallergic asthma, pharyngitis, and chest pain that resembles angina.

- Symptoms suggestive of complications from GERD include continuous pain, dysphagia, odynophagia, bleeding, unexplained weight loss, and choking.
    * Complications include esophageal ulcers, strictures, and adenocarcinoma.

- Symptom severity does not correlate with the degree of esophagitis present on endoscopy, but severity usually does correlate with the duration of reflux.

Pathophysiology

- The effortless movement of gastric contents into the esophagus is a physiologic process that occurs numerous times daily throughout life and does not produce symptoms. This occurs more frequently in patients with GERD.

- The pathophysiology of GERD involves the prolonged contact of esophageal epithelium with refluxed gastric contents containing acid and pepsin.

- Prolonged contact between esophageal epithelium and gastric contents can overwhelm esophageal defense mechanisms and produce symptoms.

- Higher-potency gastric refluxate may produce symptoms during times of esophageal contact of normal duration.

- The presence of refluxate in an esophagus with impaired defense mechanisms may also produce symptoms.

- Esophageal defenses consist of the antireflux barrier, luminal clearance mechanisms, and tissue resistance.
    * Components of the antireflux barrier are the lower esophageal sphincter (LES) and the diaphragm. The LES is a thickened ring of circular smooth muscle localized to the distal 2-3 centimeters of the esophagus. It is contracted at rest, thereby serving as a barrier to refluxate. The diaphragm encircles the LES and acts as a mechanical support, especially during physical exertion.
    * Luminal clearance factors include gravity, esophageal peristalsis, and salivary and esophageal gland secretions (which contain acid-neutralizing bicarbonate).
    * The three areas of tissue resistance are pre-epithelial, epithelial, and postepithelial defense. Pre-epithelial and epithelial tissues limit the rate of diffusion of H^+ between cell mem-

branes. Postepithelial defense is provided by the blood supply, which removes HCl and supplies oxygen, nutrients, and bicarbonate.

Diagnostic Criteria

- For patients who present with typical symptoms of GERD, a trial of empiric therapy is appropriate. A diagnosis of GERD may be assumed for patients who respond to empiric treatment.

- Further diagnostic testing should be considered for patients who do not respond to empiric therapy, patients who present with atypical symptoms or symptoms suggestive of complications, patients with chronic symptoms at increased risk for developing BE, and patients with the need for continuous chronic therapy.
    * Endoscopy is the preferred method for evaluating the esophageal mucosa for esophagitis and for evaluating for the presence of complications (eg, ulcers, strictures, BE).
    * Endoscopy is a highly specific test, but it is not extremely sensitive. Patients with symptoms may have normal esophageal mucosa (NERD).
    * Ambulatory pH monitoring may be used to confirm the diagnosis of GERD in patients with persistent symptoms (and no esophagitis present on endoscopy [NERD]), patients with noncardiac chest pain (or pulmonary symptoms), and in patients with refractory symptoms.
    * Ambulatory pH monitoring is performed by passing a small electrode to measure pH intranasally to the level of 5 cm above the LES. This allows patient symptoms to be correlated with the timing of episodes of decreased pH levels in the esophagus. This test may not be available at all institutions.
    * The Bernstein test of mucosal sensitivity to acid is highly specific for GERD and is the most commonly used provocative test of the esophagus.
    * An empirical trial of therapy with full- or double-dose omeprazole is similar (in specificity and sensitivity) to ambulatory pH monitoring and may be equally useful for confirming the diagnosis of GERD.
    * Esophageal manometry consists of passing a multilumen tube into the stomach and subsequently measuring pressures as the tube is pulled back across the LES, esophagus, and pharynx.
    * Esophageal manometry should be performed to facilitate placement of ambulatory pH probes

and to aid in determining the best procedure in antireflux surgery candidates.

Treatment Principles and Goals

- Goals of therapy are to alleviate or eliminate symptoms, decrease frequency and duration of reflux, promote healing of the injured mucosa, and prevent the development of complications.

- Therapy is directed at increasing lower esophageal pressure, improving esophageal acid clearance and gastric emptying, protecting esophageal mucosa, decreasing the acidity of refluxate, and decreasing the amount of gastric contents being refluxed.

- Antisecretory therapy with H$_2$RAs and PPIs are the mainstays of therapy for GERD.

- Therapy for patients with GERD may be divided into three phases. Phase I consists of lifestyle modifications and patient-directed therapy with OTC H$_2$RAs and/or antacids. Phase II consists of continuation of lifestyle modifications and therapy with standard or high-dose antisecretory agents. Phase III consists of surgical intervention.

- Phase I therapy is appropriate for patients with mild typical symptoms of GERD. If symptoms persist after 2 weeks of therapy, Phase II therapy is appropriate.

- For patients who present with mild to moderate typical symptoms, phase II therapy is appropriate. If atypical symptoms or symptoms suggestive of complications develop, patients should undergo endoscopic evaluation.

- H$_2$RAs are effective for patients with mild GERD. Patients with more severe symptoms (or patients with documented esophagitis) should receive PPI therapy. PPIs provide faster symptomatic relief and heal esophagitis much more effectively than H$_2$RAs.

- The addition of prokinetic agents to antisecretory drugs may offer modest improvements in symptoms compared to standard doses of H$_2$RAs. This addition is not routinely recommended, however, due to the increased incidence of side effects, higher cost, and only modest improvement of symptoms.

- The decision to progress to phase III (surgery) should be individualized. There is no medical evidence to support medical or surgical therapy as the best treatment for GERD. Surgery should be considered in patients who are intolerant of medical therapy due to side effects, in patients who respond poorly to medical therapy, and in patients who desire a permanent solution to free them from chronic medication regimens.

- GERD is considered a chronic condition, and most patients will require chronic therapy with antisecretory agents. For patients with more severe symptoms (with or without esophagitis) or for patients with complications, maintenance therapy with PPIs is preferred.

- GERD in patients with BE should be managed no differently than GERD in patients without BE. Aggressive GERD therapy for patients with BE is controversial. Patients with BE, no GERD symptoms, and no esophagitis do not require antisecretory therapy.

Drug Therapy

Mechanism of action
- For information on H$_2$RAs and PPIs, see Table 1 in the section on PUD.

- Antacids neutralize gastric acid (which increases LES tone) and inhibit the conversion of pepsinogen to pepsin, thus raising the pH of gastric contents.

- Alginic acid reacts with sodium bicarbonate in saliva to form sodium alginate viscous solution, which floats on the surface of gastric contents. The solution acts as a barrier to protect the esophagus from the corrosive effects of gastric reflux (Table 2).

Patient counseling
- Antacids and alginic acid are appropriate for the management of mild symptoms of GERD (phase I therapy). Symptoms persisting longer than 2 weeks require further evaluation and treatment with prescription medications.

- Refrigeration of liquid antacids may aid in palatability. Chewable tablets may be more effective than liquids due to increased adherence of antacid and saliva to the distal esophagus. Antacids must be taken at least 2 hours apart from tetracyclines, iron, and digoxin. Antacids and quinolones should be taken 4-6 hours apart.

- Alginic acid is effective for the relief of GERD symptoms, but there are no data to indicate esophageal healing on endoscopy. Alginic acid is ineffective if the patient is in the supine position, and must not be taken at bedtime

Table 2

Selected Antacids and Absorbents

Generic name (trade name)	Classification	Dosage range and frequency	Dosage forms
Magnesium hydroxide (milk of magnesia)	Antacid	15-30 mL prn	T, L
Aluminum hydroxide (Amphojel®, Alternagel®)	Antacid	15-30 mL prn	T, L
Aluminum carbonate (Basaljel®)	Antacid	15-30 mL prn	T, L
Magnesium hydroxide + aluminum hydroxide (Maalox®)	Antacid	15-30 mL prn	T, L
Magaldrate (Riopan®)	Antacid	15-30 mL prn	T, L
Calcium carbonate (Tums®, Titralac®)	Antacid	15-30 mL prn	T, L
Sodium bicarbonate (various)	Antacid	15-30 mL prn	T, L
Alginic acid + aluminum hydroxide + magnesium hydroxide (Gaviscon®)	Absorbent + antacid	15-30 mL prn; 2 after meals	T, L

T, tablet; L, liquid.

Adverse drug effects

- Magnesium-containing antacids frequently cause diarrhea. Aluminum-containing antacids frequently cause constipation and bind to phosphate in the gut. This can lead to bone demineralization. Antacids may also cause acid-base disturbances.

- Magnesium and aluminum toxicity may occur when used chronically in patients with renal insufficiency. Sodium bicarbonate may cause sodium overload, particularly in patients with hypertension, congestive heart failure, and chronic renal failure. It may also lead to systemic alkalosis. It should be used on a short-term basis, if at all.

Drug interactions

- When taken with antacids, the absorption and effectiveness of tetracycline, ferrous sulfate, and quinolones is reduced, as the antacids form chelates with them. Antacids decrease the absorption of azoles and sucralfate by increasing gastric pH. Antacids increase urine pH, which decreases the renal clearance of quinidine. Antacids decrease the systemic absorption of digoxin and H$_2$RAs when taken concomitantly with them. Large doses of antacid may decrease the absorption of phenytoin.

- Digoxin and phenytoin levels should be monitored frequently when antacids are used concomitantly. Suspected adverse effects of antacids should be reported to a health care provider.

Monitoring parameters

- Patients should monitor for the return of GERD symptoms and for the side effects of medications as discussed in the earlier section.

Pharmacokinetics

- Several medications are substrates for or have effects on the cytochrome P450 enzyme system in the liver. Please see discussion under drug interactions in the PUD section.

Nondrug Therapy

- Lifestyle modifications should be initiated and maintained throughout the course of GERD therapy.

- Lifestyle modifications include elevating the head of the bed, decreasing fat intake, quitting smoking, avoiding lying down within 3 hours of eating, losing weight, avoiding foods or medications that can exacerbate GERD, avoiding alcohol, and eating smaller meals.

- Fats, chocolate, alcohol, peppermint, and spearmint reduce LES pressure and may exacerbate GERD symptoms. Spicy foods, orange juice, tomato juice, and coffee have direct irritant effects on the esophageal mucosa.

- Calcium channel blockers, β-blockers, nitrates, barbiturates, anticholinergics, and theophylline decrease LES pressure. Tetracyclines, NSAIDs, aspirin, bisphosphonates, iron, quinidine, and potassium chloride have direct irritant effects on the esophageal mucosa.

3. Inflammatory Bowel Disease

Definition and Incidence

- Idiopathic inflammatory bowel disease (IBD) is divided into two major types: (1) ulcerative colitis (UC) and (2) Crohn's disease (CD).

- UC is defined as a mucosal inflammatory condition confined to the rectum and colon.

- CD is defined as a transmural inflammation of the gastrointestinal (GI) tract that can affect any part of the GI tract from mouth to anus.

- The prevalence of UC is approximately 37.5-229 cases per 100,000 persons; the prevalence of CD is approximately 26-198.5 cases per 100,000 persons.

- There are approximately 1.3 million people with UC in North America, and each year 7000-43,000 new cases of UC are diagnosed in this region.

- Approximately 9000-44,000 new cases of CD are diagnosed each year; UC is slightly more predominant in men; CD is more predominant in women.

- North America, Scandinavia, and Great Britain have the highest incidence rates for IBD.

- UC typically occurs between age 30 and 40. CD typically occurs between age 20 and 30. Both may be diagnosed at any stage in life, but of all cases of IBD, 10-15% are diagnosed before adulthood.

- The incidence of IBD is low for Hispanic and Asian-Americans. Its incidence in African-Americans has increased and is equal to that of Caucasians. In addition, its incidence rate is high among the Jewish population in North America, Europe, and Israel.

Classification

- There are two major types of idiopathic inflammatory bowel disease (IBD): ulcerative colitis (UC) and Crohn's disease (CD).

- Clinical presentation and diagnostic tests help to distinguish one form from the other.

Clinical Presentation

- IBD is characterized by acute exacerbations of symptoms followed by periods of remission that are spontaneous or secondary to changes in medical therapy.

- The hallmark clinical symptom of UC is bloody diarrhea that is often accompanied by rectal urgency and tenesmus.

- The extent and severity of UC is characterized by clinical and endoscopic findings. Clinical symptoms are categorized as mild, moderate, or severe. Endoscopic findings are categorized as distal (limited to below the splenic flexure) or extensive (extending proximal to the splenic flexure).

Mild
- Mild UC is characterized by less than four stools per day with or without blood, without systemic disturbance, and with a normal erythrocyte sedimentation rate (ESR).

Moderate
- Moderate UC is characterized by more than four stools per day with little systemic disturbance.

Severe
- Severe UC is characterized by more than six stools per day with blood, systemic disturbance (eg, fever, tachycardia, anemia), and ESR greater than 30.

- The presentation of CD is variable and its onset is often insidious. Typical symptoms include chronic or nocturnal diarrhea and abdominal pain. Additional typical symptoms include weight loss, fever, and rectal bleeding.

- Symptoms differ depending on the site and severity of inflammation.
    * Mild to moderate: patients tolerate oral alimentation without dehydration, toxicity (fever, rigors, prostration), abdominal tenderness, painful mass, and/or obstruction; weight loss >10%.
    * Moderate to severe: patients fail to respond to treatment for mild to moderate disease or have fever, weight loss, abdominal pain, nausea, vomiting (without obstruction), or anemia.
    * Severe to fulminant: patients have persistent symptoms despite the use of steroids (as outpatients), high fever, persistent vomiting, evidence of obstruction, rebound tenderness, cachexia, or abscess.
    * The ileum and colon are the most commonly affected sites. Ileitis may mimic appendicitis. Intestinal obstruction and inflammatory masses or abscesses may also develop. Patients with colonic CD commonly have rectal bleeding, perianal lesions, and extraintestinal manifesta-

tions (eg, spondylarthritis, peripheral arthritis, erythema nodosum, pyoderma gangrenosum, uveitis, fatty liver, chronic active hepatitis, cirrhosis, primary sclerosing cholangitis, gallstones, cholangiocarcinoma, and hypercoagulability).
  * Oral CD is characterized by lesions ranging from a few aphthous ulcers to deep linear ulcers with edema and induration. Gastroduodenal involvement may mimic PUD.

Pathophysiology

* The etiology of UC and CD is unclear, but similar factors may contribute to both diseases. These include infectious agents, genetics, environmental factors, immune deficits, and psychologic factors. Major etiologic theories involve a combination of infectious and immunologic factors.

* UC is confined to the rectum and colon and only affects the mucosa and submucosa. The primary lesion of UC is a crypt abscess, which forms in the crypts of the mucosa. CD most commonly affects the terminal ileum and involves extensive damage to the bowel wall.

* UC and CD complications can be local or systemic. Local complications of UC include hemorrhoids, anal fissures, and perirectal abscesses. Toxic megacolon can lead to perforation and is a major complication that affects 1-3% of patients with UC or CD. Colonic strictures and hemorrhage may also occur. Small bowel strictures, obstruction, and fistulae are common in CD. Systemic complications (extraintestinal) can occur with UC and CD.

Diagnostic Criteria

* The diagnosis of IBD is based on negative stool evaluation for infectious causes. Abdominal ultrasonography, computed tomography, and magnetic resonance imaging aid in the identification of masses, abscesses, and perianal complications.

Treatment Principles and Goals

* Treatment of IBD involves medications that target inflammatory mediators and alter immuno-inflammatory processes. These medications include anti-inflammatory agents and immunosuppressive agents.

* Nutritional considerations are also important since many patients with IBD may be malnourished.

* Goals of therapy for UC and CD include the induction and maintenance of remission of symptoms, resolution of complications and systemic symptoms, and/or surgical palliation or cure.

* In UC patients, remission is likely to last at least 1 year with medical therapy. Without medical therapy, up to two thirds of patients will relapse within 9 months. For mild CD, up to 40% of patients improve in 3-4 months with observation alone. Most will remain in remission for prolonged periods without medical therapy.

* The treatment of choice for distal UC that only involves the rectum (proctitis) is topical therapy with aminosalicylates.
  * Treatment is initiated with a nightly suppository or enema. Improvement usually occurs within 2-3 weeks. Most patients will require maintenance therapy in order remain in remission.
  * Rectally administered steroids may be used in combination with aminosalicylates when patients do not respond to aminosalicylates alone.
  * For patients who do not respond to or cannot tolerate topical therapy, oral therapy with steroids and/or aminosalicylates is necessary.

* Initial therapy for mild to moderate distal or left-sided colitis includes nightly aminosalicylates or corticosteroid enemas.
  * Once remission is achieved, dosing may be tapered to every second or third night.

* For moderate to severe distal or left-sided colitis, twice-daily enemas are required.

* For severe distal or left-sided colitis, combining oral and topical aminosalicylates is required.
  * Oral corticosteroids are reserved for patients who fail initial aminosalicylate therapy.
  * Corticosteroids are tapered once remission is achieved, and topical and oral aminosalicylates are continued as maintenance therapy.

* Extensive UC (pancolitis) requires oral therapy; however, topical therapy is still a useful adjunct in controlling rectal disease. For mild to moderate extensive UC, oral aminosalicylates are first-line therapy.
  * Patients who fail to respond require the addition of high-dose oral corticosteroid therapy.
  * Corticosteroid tapering should begin only when complete remission is achieved.
  * Corticosteroids do not have a role in mainte-

nance therapy, as aminosalicylates are effective at maintaining remission.

* For patients who fail oral therapy, hospitalization and intravenous steroid therapy is necessary

• Hospitalization and complete bowel rest are required for severe or fulminant colitis.
* Intravenous steroids are the mainstays of therapy.
* Topical therapy may be added for patients with significant rectal symptoms.
* Patients who do not respond to 7 days of IV steroids, surgery or intravenous cyclosporine should be considered. Patients who respond to IV cyclosporine are converted to oral cyclosporine and a steroid taper.
* Azathioprine is often added to maintain remission.

• Abdominal x-ray should be performed to exclude toxic megacolon. Surgery is often required for patients with toxic megacolon, and preoperative antibiotics are recommended to reduce the chance of septic complications.

• For mild to moderate CD, oral aminosalicylates are appropriate initial therapy.
* Rectal aminosalicylates are often used treat distal colonic CD; however, controlled studies showing efficacy are lacking
* Alternatively, metronidazole or ciprofloxacin may be used as first-line therapy.
* Both aminosalicylates and antibiotics are more effective for colonic CD than ileal CD.
* In studies, controlled-release budesonide produces a higher remission rate than mesalamine in treating mild to moderate ileal CD. Results of studies comparing budesonide with oral steroids are conflicting.
* No controlled data exist regarding the treatment of mild to moderate oral CD. Lidocaine lozenges may provide symptomatic relief. Lesions will respond to systemic steroids or azathioprine in 50% of patients.
* For mild to moderate cases of gastroduodenal CD, acid suppression therapy with H_2RAs or PPIs is recommended.
* Once remission is achieved, maintenance therapy should be initiated. For patients who do not respond, progression to therapy for moderate-to-severe disease should be considered.

• For patients with moderate to severe disease, oral corticosteroids are the mainstay of therapy.
* Prednisone or budesonide may be used as first-

line agents. Steroids are not appropriate maintenance therapy.
* For steroid-refractory patients, azathioprine or 6-mercaptopurine should be added.
* Alternatively, methotrexate may be added for maintenance therapy. Infliximab is also effective therapy, but requires IV infusion at least every 8 weeks.
* Total parenteral nutrition and enteral nutrition with elemental nutrient formulas are also effective in inducing remission.

• For severe to fulminant CD, hospitalization for intravenous steroids and hydration is required.
* Anemic patients may require blood transfusions.
* Intestinal obstructions related to adhesions should be managed with bowel rest and nasogastric tube suctioning. Obstructions related to inflammatory strictures require antibiotic therapy and IV steroids. Surgery should be considered if obstructive symptoms do not respond to therapy.
* Abscesses should be drained and appropriate antibiotic therapy instituted.
* High-dose metronidazole or ciprofloxacin may be used in the management of fistulas.
* Azathioprine, 6-mercaptopurine, infliximab, and PPIs in combination with octreotide may also be used in the management of fistulas.
* If patients do not respond to IV steroids after 5-7 days of therapy, cyclosporine or tacrolimus therapy may be instituted.
* Maintenance therapy with azathioprine is usually required.
* Patients who do not respond to therapy require surgical intervention.

• 6-Mercaptopurine is the best agent for preventing relapse of CD after surgical intervention.

Drug Therapy (Table 3)

Mechanism of action
• Sulfasalazine is cleaved to sulfapyridine (excreted in the urine) by bacteria in the gut and mesalamine (the active component). The sulfapyridine molecule is responsible for many side effects associated with sulfasalazine.

• Mesalamine's mechanism of action is poorly understood. Mesalamine inhibits cyclooxygenase and may also inhibit production of cyclooxygenase, thromboxane synthetase, platelet-activating factor synthetase, and interleukin-1 in macrophages. It may also act as a superoxide free-radical scavenger.

Table 3

Selected Medications Used in Inflammatory Bowel Disease

Generic name (trade name)	Classification	Dosage range and frequency	Dosage forms
Sulfasalazine (Azulfidine®)	Aminosalicylate	4-6 g/d	T
Mesalamine (Asacol®	Aminosalicylate	2.4-4.8 g/d	DT
Pentasa®		2-4 g/d	DC
Rowasa®, Salofalk® Claversal®, Pentasa®)		1-4 g/d	EN, SU
Metronidazole (Flagyl®)	Antibacterial	10-20 mg/kg/d (Crohn's)	T, IV
Ciprofloxacin (Cipro®)	Antibacterial	500 mg bid (Crohn's)	T, IV
Prednisone (various)	Corticosteroid	40-60 mg/d	T
Methylprednisolone (Solu-Medrol®)	Corticosteroid	16 mg q8h	IV
Budesonide (Entocort EC®)	Corticosteroid	9 mg qd	C
Azathioprine (Imuran®)	Immunosuppressive	1-2.5 mg/kg/d	T, IV
6-Mercaptopurine (Purinethol®)	Immunosuppressive	1.5 mg/kg/d	T
Methotrexate (Abitrexate®)	Antimetabolite	25 mg/wk	IM, SQ
Infliximab (Remicade®)	Immunomodulator	5 mg/kg q 8 weeks	IV
Cyclosporine (Neoral®, Sandimmune®)	Immunosuppressive	4 mg/kg/d	IV, C, L

T, tablet; C, capsule; L, liquid; DT, delayed-release tablet; DC, delayed-release capsule; IV, intravenous; IM, intramuscular; SQ, subcutaneous; EN, enema; SU, suppository.

- Corticosteroids have immunomodulatory effects and inhibit the production of cytokines and other inflammatory mediators.

- Corticosteroids, azathioprine, 6-mercaptopurine, cyclosporine, and tacrolimus are immunosuppressive agents. For full discussion of mechanism of action, patient counseling, side effects, drug interactions, and pharmacokinetics, the reader is referred to the chapter on transplantation.

- The exact mechanism of action of metronidazole and ciprofloxacin in IBD is not known. One theory suggests that antibacterials interrupt the role of bacteria in the inflammatory process.

- Methotrexate inhibits dihydrofolate reductase and purine synthesis, reduces the production of leukotriene B_4 and interleukins 1 and 2, and may induce T-cell apoptosis.

- Infliximab is a chimeric monoclonal antibody that inhibits tumor necrosis factor.

Patient counseling
- Sulfasalazine should be taken after meals. Patients should avoid sun exposure while taking sulfasalazine. Folic acid supplementation should be given during sulfasalazine treatment to avoid ane-

mia. Sulfasalazine may cause orange discoloration of urine and skin. Mesalamine tablets should be swallowed whole. Suppositories should not be handled excessively and foil wrappers should be removed before insertion. Suspension enemas should be shaken well before use.

- Antacids and ciprofloxacin should be taken 4-6 hours apart. Iron- or zinc-containing products should be taken 4 hours before or 2 hours after taking ciprofloxacin. Patients should avoid excessive exposure to sunlight.

- Patients taking methotrexate should avoid alcohol, salicylates, and prolonged exposure to sunlight. Female patients of childbearing age should be counseled on appropriate contraceptive measures during methotrexate therapy.

- Patients receiving therapy with infliximab should be counseled on the possibility of infusion reactions. Live vaccines should not be administered to patients taking infliximab.

Adverse drug effects
- Sulfasalazine may cause nausea, vomiting, anorexia, and headaches. The sulfapyridine moiety leads to hypersensitivity reactions (eg, rash, fever, agranulo-

cytosis, pancreatitis, nephritis, and hepatitis) and altered spermatogenesis in males.

- Mesalamine is better tolerated than sulfasalazine. Olsalazine may cause self-limited watery diarrhea. Balsalazide may cause abdominal pain in 10% of patients.

- Ciprofloxacin may cause nausea, diarrhea, headache, and vaginal candidiasis.

- Methotrexate frequently causes nausea and leukopenia. Asymptomatic elevations in liver function tests may occur.

- Infliximab may cause acute and delayed infusion reactions, autoantibody development, and lupus.

Drug interactions
- Sulfasalazine may decrease the bioavailability of digoxin.

- Allopurinol enhances the effect of azathioprine. The azathioprine dose should be lowered by 50% when the agents are used concurrently.

- Ciprofloxacin binds with antacids, zinc, and iron products. It also increases the therapeutic effects of warfarin, cyclosporine, and theophylline.

- The use of methotrexate and concurrent NSAIDs has caused fatal interactions. Methotrexate may increase levels of 6-mercaptopurine.

Monitoring parameters
- Serum creatinine, complete blood counts, liver function tests, blood glucose concentrations, ESR, response to therapy, and the presence of adverse effects should be monitored.

Pharmacokinetics
- Several medications are substrates for or have effects on the cytochrome P450 enzyme system in the liver. Please see discussion in drug interactions section.

Nondrug Therapy

- Patients with UC and CD are often malnourished due to malabsorption or maldigestion caused by chronic bowel inflammation, "short gut" syndrome from multiple bowel surgeries, or bile salt deficiency in the gut. The catabolic effects of the disease process can also lead to malnutrition.

- Individuals should eliminate foods that exacerbate symptoms. Patients with lactase deficiency should avoid dairy products or take lactase supplements to avoid symptoms.

- Fish oil supplementation may improve weight gain and reduce the rate of relapse in CD.

- Enteral or parenteral supplementation may also be used in patients with severe UC or CD.

- Surgery may be necessary for patients with severe UC or CD. Surgery (proctocolectomy) is curative for UC, but not for CD.
    * Surgery involves removing diseased segments of bowel, repairing fistulas, and draining abscesses.
    * In UC, surgery is indicated for patients who fail maximum medical therapy to correct complications (perforation, strictures, obstruction, hemorrhage, toxic megacolon). It is also used and as prophylaxis against the development of cancer (in patients with long-standing UC) and in patients with premalignant changes found on bowel biopsies.
    * In CD, surgery is reserved for patients with complications from the disease. There is a high recurrence rate after surgery for CD. Other indications for surgery are colon cancer, inflammatory mass, or perforations.

4. Irritable Bowel Syndrome

Definition and Incidence

- Irritable bowel syndrome (IBS) is a functional bowel disorder associated with disturbed defecation. It is characterized by symptoms of abdominal pain or discomfort.

- IBS is classified according to the Rome II diagnostic criteria.

- IBS is the most prevalent digestive disease; it constitutes 12% of visits to primary care physicians and 28% of referrals to gastroenterologists.

- The medical expenses of patients with IBS is 1.6-fold higher than the expenses of an asymptomatic individual. They miss three times as many days of work per annum as persons without IBS.

- Most cases of IBS are diagnosed before age 45. Women develop IBS 2-3 times more often than men. IBS is less common in Asians and Hispanics than in other ethnic groups.

Classifications

- IBS is classified according to the Rome II diagnostic criteria.

- Patients may be categorized as having mild, moderate, or severe disease.

- IBS is also classified as either diarrhea- or constipation-predominant, depending upon the patient's clinical presentation.

Clinical Presentation

- IBS is a heterogeneous disorder with various clinical presentations.
    * Abdominal pain is generally described as crampy or achy, and the intensity and location is highly variable. It may be exacerbated by meals and may last from 1-3 hours. Stress and emotional turmoil can also exacerbate pain.
    * Patients typically present with diarrhea, constipation, or alternating periods of both. Half of patients have a mucoid discharge.
    * Upper gastrointestinal symptoms occur more frequently in patients with constipation (heartburn, dyspepsia, early satiety, and nausea). Women experience abdominal distention, bloating, and nausea more often than men.
    * Extraintestinal symptoms are common.
        • They include genitourinary symptoms (eg, pelvic pain, dysmenorrhea, dyspareunia, urinary frequency, nocturia, and sensation of incomplete bladder evacuation), impaired sexual function (eg, decreased libido), and musculoskeletal complaints (eg, lower back pain, headaches, and chronic fatigue).
        • IBS is strongly associated with fibromyalgia.
        • The triad of IBS, asthma, and GERD occurs three times more often than the expected prevalence.

Pathophysiology

- The pathogenesis is multifactorial and includes abnormal gut sensorimotor activity, central nervous system (CNS) dysfunction, psychologic disturbances, genetic predisposition, enteric infection, and other luminal factors.
    * Colonic motor abnormalities commonly occur in IBS. Patients with IBS may exhibit an exaggerated gastrocolonic response lasting up to 3 hours.
    * Small intestinal motor patterns are frequently disturbed in patients with IBS. Small intestinal transit is delayed in constipation-predominant IBS and is accelerated in diarrhea-predominant IBS.
    * Bloating may be the result of abnormal retrograde reflux of intestinal gas, enhanced perception of the presence of intestinal gas, or obstructive intestinal motor patterns.
    * Motor dysfunction of other smooth muscles may occur in IBS. The following abnormalities may also be found: lowered LES sphincter pressures, abnormal esophageal body peristalsis, gastric slow-wave dysrhythmias, delayed gastric and gallbladder emptying, and dysfunction of the sphincter of Oddi.
    * It is theorized that IBS results from sensitization of visceral afferent fibers, which causes normal physiologic events to be perceived as painful. It is unknown if sensorineural dysfunction is generalized or localized to the gut afferent fibers.
    * It is unknown whether IBS is primarily a CNS disorder with centrally directed changes in gut sensorimotor function, or primarily a gut disorder with inappropriate CNS input. Further investigation is needed in this area.
    * Eighty percent of patients with IBS exhibit psychiatric disturbances. The onset of psychiatric disturbances usually predates or occurs concurrently with the onset of IBS. Psychologic stress

triggers symptoms in many patients. IBS is also associated with a history of sexual abuse.
  * Other factors that may contribute to IBS are alterations in gut flora (controversial), antecedent gastrointestinal infection, carbohydrate malabsorption, food allergies, neurohumoral disturbances, genetic factors, and abnormal stool characteristics (low concentrations of bile or short-chain fatty acids).

- IBS is categorized using the Rome II diagnostic criteria.
  * Abdominal discomfort or pain present for at least 12 weeks (not necessarily consecutive weeks) in the preceding 12 months that has two of three features:
    - Relieved with defecation; and/or
    - Its onset is associated with a change in frequency of stool; and/or
    - Its onset is associated with a change in the form (appearance) of the stool
  * Symptoms that cumulatively support the diagnosis of IBS include the following:
    - Abnormal stool frequency (ie, greater than three bowel movements per day and less than three bowel movements per week)
    - Abnormal stool form (lumpy/hard or loose/watery stool)
    - Abnormal stool passage (straining, urgency, or feeling of incomplete evacuation)
    - Passage of mucus
    - Bloating or feeling of abdominal distention

- Weight loss, bleeding, fever, or palpable masses are warning signs of organic disease and are not common in IBS.

- Relief of pain with defecation, looser stool with pain onset, more frequent stools with pain onset, and abdominal distention are significantly more common in IBS than in organic disease.

Diagnostic Criteria

- Physical examination is usually normal. A complete blood count, serum electrolytes, erythrocyte sedimentation rate (ESR), and thyroid hormone levels should be performed.

- For patients with pain, abdominal x-ray should be used to exclude obstruction.

- In patients with diarrhea, hydrogen breath testing may be used to exclude lactase deficiency (an empiric trial of lactose restriction may also be used).

- Sigmoidoscopy should be performed for patients under age 50 to exclude obstruction in patients with constipation and to exclude IBD in patients with diarrhea.

- In patients over age 50, colonoscopy should be performed to exclude colonic neoplasm.

Treatment Principles and Goals

- Treatment strategy is based on the nature and severity of symptoms, correlation of symptoms with food intake and/or defecation, degree of functional impairment, and the presence of psychosocial/psychiatric comorbidities.

- Generally, mild disease is related to visceral hyperactivity and may be managed with medications aimed at the gut.

- Severe disease is associated with greater psychosocial difficulties and often requires psychological/behavioral therapy with antidepressant medications.

- The most frequently encountered group is patients with mild disease. They are usually managed in primary care settings, maintain normal daily activities, have little or no psychosocial difficulties, and do not frequently use the health care system. Treatment includes dietary modifications, education, and reassurance. Drug therapy with gut-acting agents is appropriate when needed.

- Patients with moderate disease have intermittent symptoms that are disabling at times and are associated with increased gut reactivity. Drug therapy with gut-acting agents, low-dose tricyclic antidepressants (TCA), and psychological treatment is appropriate.

- A small proportion of patients with severe disease have more severe or constant pain symptoms, psychiatric comorbidity, and psychosocial difficulties. They are frequent users of the health care system. They require antidepressant medication and referral to mental health and pain management centers. A long-term relationship with a primary care physician is important to provide support during regular, brief visits.

Drug Therapy (Table 4)

Mechanism of action
- The antispasmodic agent dicyclomine decreases GI motility by relaxing smooth muscle in the gut.

Table 4

Selected Medications Used in Irritable Bowel Syndrome

Generic name (trade name)	Classification	Dosage range and frequency	Dosage forms
Dicyclomine (Bentyl®)	Antispasmodic	10-20 mg qid prn	T, C, L
Hyoscyamine (various)	Anticholinergic	0.25 mg-0.5 mg bid-qid	T, L
Amitriptyline (Elavil®)	Tricyclic antidepressant	10-50 mg qhs	T
Citalopram (Celexa®)	Selective serotonin-reuptake inhibitor	20-40 mg/d	T, L
Paroxetine (Paxil®)	Selective serotonin-reuptake inhibitor	10-60 mg/d	T, L, DT
Tegaserod (Zelnorm®)	Osmotic laxative	6 mg bid	T
Lactulose (various)	Laxative	30-45 mL bid-qid prn	L
Polycarbophil (Fibercon®)	Laxative	1g qd-qid prn	T
Polyethylene glycol (various)	5HT-3 antagonist	250 mL q 10 min up to 4 L	L
Alosetron (Lotronex®)	Antidiarrheal	1 mg qd-bid	T
Loperamide (Imodium®)	Antidiarrheal	2 mg after each loose stool; max 16 mg/d	T, C, L
Diphenoxylate/Atropine (Lomotil®)	5HT-4 agonist	2 tabs qid	T, L

T, tablet; C, capsule; L, liquid; DT, delayed release tablet.

- Hyoscyamine is an anticholinergic agent that decreases GI motility by decreasing smooth muscle tone through antimuscarinic activity in the gut.

- TCAs (eg, amitriptyline) delay intestinal transit and may blunt perception of visceral distention. The effect of TCAs on the cerebral processing of visceral pain is unknown.

- Tegaserod maleate, a partial 5-HT4 agonist that stimulates the peristaltic reflex and intestinal secretion, inhibits visceral sensitivity by binding to 5-HT4 receptors in the gut.

- Lactulose, milk of magnesia, and polyethylene glycol solutions are osmotic laxatives that aid in the treatment of IBS patients with constipation.

- Fiber supplements (bulk laxatives) increase stool bulk and water content.

- Loperamide inhibits peristalsis by directly affecting the circular and longitudinal muscles of the intestinal wall. Diphenoxylate is a meperidine congener that has a direct effect on the circular smooth muscle in the gut, which slows GI transit time.

- Alosetron is a selective 5HT-3–receptor antagonist that inhibits activation of nonselective cation channels in the gut, thereby modulating the enteric nervous system.

- Selective serotonin-reuptake inhibitors (SSRIs) inhibit the neuronal uptake of serotonin in the CNS. Citalopram has peripheral effects on colonic tone and sensitivity. Paroxetine has potent anticholinergic effects.

Patient counseling

- Antispasmodics and anticholinergic agents are best used on an as-needed basis up to three times per day during acute attacks or before meals when postprandial symptoms are present.

- Patients taking a TCA should avoid prolonged exposure to sunlight and avoid concurrent use of CNS depressants.

- Tegaserod should be taken before meals and should not be initiated during an acute exacerbation of IBS.

- Osmotic laxatives should be used on an as-needed basis. Lactulose may be mixed with water or juice to increase palatability. Patients should drink plenty of water.

- Patients must be enrolled in the manufacturer prescribing program in order to receive alosetron. Patients should not initiate therapy with alosetron if they are currently constipated. Alosetron should be discontinued if no improvement in symptoms is seen after 4 weeks of therapy.

- See the chapter on psychiatric disease for a full discussion of SSRIs.

Adverse drug effects
- Dicyclomine, hyoscyamine, and TCAs may cause anticholinergic side effects (CNS depression, dry mouth, urinary retention, constipation, and decreased sweating).

- Tegaserod may cause diarrhea, nausea, headache, and abdominal pain.

- Osmotic laxatives may cause abdominal pain and cramping.

- Alosetron may cause constipation, abdominal pain, and nausea. Intestinal obstruction, perforation, toxic megacolon, ischemic colitis, and death have occurred.

Drug interactions
- Anticholinergics and antispasmodics may decrease the effectiveness of antipsychotic medications. Anticholinergic side effects are increased when given concurrently with a TCA.

- TCA concentrations may be increased or decreased by medications that induce or inhibit the activity of the cytochrome P450 enzyme system in the liver. TCAs should not be given concurrently with monoamine oxidase inhibitors or sympathomimetic agents.

- No significant drug interactions with tegaserod have been reported.

- Other medications should not be taken within 1 hour of the start of therapy with osmotic laxatives.

- Drugs that induce or inhibit the cytochrome P450 enzyme system may affect serum concentrations of alosetron. The clinical significance of this is unknown.

Monitoring parameters
- Patients should monitor for the presence of IBS symptoms and for the side effects of medications as discussed in the earlier section.

Pharmacokinetics
- Several medications are substrates for or have effects on the cytochrome P450 enzyme system in the liver.

Nondrug Therapy

- An effective physician-patient relationship is necessary for successful treatment.

- Education regarding disease pathophysiology and treatment and reassurance that the symptoms are real should be provided.

- Patients should be counseled to avoid foods that exacerbate symptoms. Foods commonly implicated are fatty foods, beans, gas-producing foods, alcohol, caffeine, and lactose (in lactase-deficient individuals), and occasionally excess fiber. Fiber has an established role in managing constipation; however, its value in the management of diarrhea in IBS is controversial.

5. Key Points

Peptic ulcer disease

- Peptic ulcer disease (PUD) is a group of disorders of the upper gastrointestinal tract characterized by ulcerative lesions that require acid and pepsin for their formation.

- Duodenal and gastric ulcers are classified as *Helicobacter pylori*–related, NSAID-related, non-*H pylori*–related, non-NSAID–related, or stress-related.

- Epigastric pain occurring 1-3 hours after meals that is relieved by ingestion of food or antacids is the classic symptom of PUD.

- *H pylori* is a gram-negative microaerophilic bacterium inhabiting the area between the mucous layer and epithelial cells in the stomach. It can be found anywhere gastric epithelium is present.

- NSAIDs are the leading cause of PUD in patients who are negative for *H pylori* infection. NSAIDs are directly toxic to gastric epithelium and inhibit the synthesis of prostaglandins.

- PUD is diagnosed with upper gastrointestinal endoscopy. This is usually reserved for patients with clinical features suggestive of complications from PUD (eg, gastric cancer, bleeding).

- *H pylori* may be detected noninvasively by serology, urea breath test (UBT), fecal antigen testing, and urine antibody testing. UBT is the test of choice and is commercially available for use in medical offices.

- The goals of PUD therapy are ulcer healing and eliminating the cause. Additional considerations are prevention of complications and relief of symptoms.

- For patients with *H pylori*-related PUD, a triple or quadruple drug regimen consisting of a PPI or an H_2RA, bismuth, and antibiotics should be used for 7-14 days. *H pylori* eradication reduces the risk of recurrence of PUD. The ideal treatment regimen for *H pylori* has not been identified.

- For NSAID-related PUD, treatment consists of discontinuing the offending agent and issuing antisecretory therapy for symptom relief. If *H pylori* is present, eradication therapy should be used. A PPI, an H_2RA, or misoprostol should be used for prevention of PUD in patients requiring chronic NSAIDs who are at risk for developing PUD

- Patients with active bleeding should initially undergo endoscopic hemostasis. Laparoscopic repair or surgery may be used to repair perforations. Open surgery is reserved for those patients with refractory ulcers or for hemorrhage/perforations that cannot be managed endoscopically or with laparoscopy.

- Patients should be counseled on the importance of adherence to treatment regimens, proper dosing, and side effects of medications.

- Patients should counseled to decrease psychological stress, discontinue smoking and use of NSAIDs, and avoid food or beverages that exacerbate PUD symptoms.

Gastroesophageal reflux disease

- Gastroesophageal reflux disease (GERD) is defined as chronic symptoms or mucosal damage produced by the abnormal reflux of gastric contents into the esophagus.

- Approximately 20% of the population experience heartburn or regurgitation of gastric acid weekly.

- Patients with GERD may be classified as having nonerosive reflux disease (NERD), erosive esophagitis (EE), or Barrett's esophagus (BE). Adenocarcinoma is rare.

- Symptoms of GERD may be classified as typical, atypical, or complicated. The hallmark symptom of GERD is heartburn (pyrosis), which is described as substernal burning or pain that may radiate to the neck, back, or throat.

- Atypical symptoms (or extraesophageal symptoms) include chronic cough, hoarseness, nonallergic asthma, pharyngitis, and chest pain that resembles angina. Symptoms that are suggestive of complications of GERD include continuous pain, dysphagia, odynophagia, bleeding, unexplained weight loss, and choking. Complications include ulcers, strictures, and adenocarcinoma.

- The pathophysiology of GERD involves the prolonged contact of esophageal epithelium with refluxed gastric contents that contain acid and pepsin.

- Esophageal defenses consist of the antireflux barrier, luminal clearance mechanisms, and tissue resistance. Increased contact time of refluxate and esophageal mucosa or impaired defense mechanisms can lead to the symptoms of GERD.

- For patients who present with typical symptoms of GERD, a trial of empiric therapy is appropriate. A diagnosis of GERD may be assumed for patients who respond to empiric treatment.

- Further diagnostic testing should be considered for patients who do not respond to empiric therapy, patients who present with atypical symptoms or symptoms suggestive of complications, patients with chronic symptoms at increased risk for developing BE, and patients with the need for continuous chronic therapy.

- Goals of therapy are to alleviate or eliminate symptoms, decrease frequency and duration of reflux, promote healing of the injured mucosa, and prevent the development of complications.

- Antisecretory therapy with H_2RAs and PPIs are the mainstay of therapy for GERD. Therapy for patients with GERD may be divided into three phases. Phase I consists of lifestyle modifications and patient-directed therapy with OTC H_2RAs and/or antacids. Phase II consists of continuation of lifestyle modifications and therapy with standard or high-dose antisecretory agents. Phase III consists of surgical intervention.

- Patients should be counseled on medication dosing and administration, side effects, drug interactions, monitoring of GERD symptoms, and lifestyle modifications.

- Lifestyle modifications should be initiated and maintained throughout the course of GERD therapy. These include elevating the head of the bed, decreasing fat intake, smoking cessation, avoiding lying down within 3 hours of eating, losing weight, avoiding foods or medications that can exacerbate GERD, avoiding alcohol, and eating smaller meals.

- GERD is considered a chronic condition, and most patients will require chronic therapy with antisecretory agents.

Inflammatory bowel disease
- Idiopathic inflammatory bowel disease (IBD) is divided into two major types: (1) ulcerative colitis (UC) and (2) Crohn's disease (CD).

- UC is defined as a mucosal inflammatory condition confined to the rectum and colon.

- CD is defined as a transmural inflammation of the gastrointestinal (GI) tract that can affect any part (mouth to anus).

- The hallmark clinical symptom of UC is bloody diarrhea, often with rectal urgency and tenesmus.

- Clinical symptoms are categorized as mild, moderate, or severe. Endoscopic findings are categorized as distal (limited to below the splenic flexure) or extensive (extending proximal to the splenic flexure).

- Typical symptoms of CD include chronic or nocturnal diarrhea and abdominal pain. Additional typical symptoms include weight loss, fever, and rectal bleeding.

- Symptoms differ depending on the site of inflammation, and are categorized as mild, moderate, or severe.

- The etiology of IBD is unclear, but similar factors may contribute to both UC and CD. The diagnosis of IBD is made based on negative stool evaluation for infectious causes.

- Treatment of IBD involves medications that target inflammatory mediators and alter immunoinflammatory processes. These medications include anti-inflammatory agents and immunosuppressive agents.

- Goals of therapy for UC and CD include the induction and maintenance of remission of symptoms, resolution of complications and systemic symptoms, or surgical palliation or cure.

- Patients should be counseled on medication dosing and administration, side effects, drug interactions, monitoring of IBD symptoms, and proper nutrition.

- Patients with IBD are often malnourished due to malabsorption or maldigestion caused by chronic bowel inflammation, "short gut" syndrome from multiple bowel surgeries, or bile salt deficiency in the gut.

- Surgery may be necessary for patients with severe UC or CD. Surgery (proctocolectomy) is curative for UC, but not for CD.

Irritable bowel syndrome
- Irritable bowel syndrome (IBS) is a functional bowel disorder characterized by symptoms of abdominal pain or discomfort associated with disturbed defecation.

- IBS is the most prevalent digestive disease, representing 12% of visits to primary care physicians and 28% of referrals to gastroenterologists.

- IBS is a heterogeneous disorder with various clinical presentations.

- The pathogenesis is multifactorial, including abnormal gut sensorimotor activity, central nervous system (CNS) dysfunction, psychologic disturbances, genetic predisposition, enteric infection, and other luminal factors.

- IBS is categorized using the Rome II diagnostic criteria. Weight loss, bleeding, fever, or palpable masses are warning signs of organic disease, and are not common in IBS.

- Treatment strategy is based on the nature and severity of symptoms, correlation of symptoms with food intake and/or defecation, degree of functional impairment, and the presence of psychosocial/psychiatric comorbidities.

- Patients may be categorized as having mild, moderate, or severe disease. Generally, mild disease may be managed with medications aimed at the gut, education, and reassurance. Patients with moderate disease have increased symptoms. Drug therapy with gut-acting agents, low-dose tricyclic antidepressants (TCAs), and psychological treatments are appropriate. Patients with severe disease have more severe, often constant pain symptoms, psychiatric comorbidity, and psychosocial difficulties. They require antidepressant medication and referral to mental health and pain management centers in addition to gut-directed drug therapy.

- Patients should be counseled on medication dosing and administration, side effects, drug interactions, and monitoring of IBS symptoms.

- An effective physician-patient relationship is necessary for successful treatment.

- Education regarding disease pathophysiology and treatment, and reassurance that the symptoms are real should be provided.

- Patients should be counseled to avoid foods that exacerbate symptoms.

6. Questions and Answers

1. H.B. is a 59-year-old black male recently diagnosed with PUD on endoscopy. Tissue biopsy is positive for *H pylori*. Which of the following is the ideal therapeutic regimen for *H pylori*-related PUD in H.B.?

    A. Omeprazole, bismuth, tetracycline, furazolidone
    B. Omeprazole, amoxicillin, clarithromycin
    C. Omeprazole, amoxicillin
    D. Omeprazole, bismuth, clarithromycin, furazolidone
    E. Omeprazole, sucralfate, clarithromycin, furazolidone

2. H.B. does not respond to omeprazole, clarithromycin, and amoxicillin. Which of the following is the best choice?

    A. Clarithromycin should be replaced by tetracycline
    B. Clarithromycin should be replaced by metronidazole
    C. Clarithromycin dosage should be increased
    D. Clarithromycin should be replaced by furazolidone
    E. Clarithromycin should be replaced by amoxicillin

3. Which one of the following is the leading cause of PUD in *H pylori*–negative patients?

    A. Mineralocorticoids
    B. NSAIDs
    C. DMARDs
    D. Antibiotics
    E. Corticosteroids

4. Which of the following is true of NSAIDs?

    I.   They inhibit production of prostaglandins.
    II. They are directly toxic to gastroduodenal epithelium.
    III. They require dose adjustments in renal insufficiency.
    IV. They only cause gastric ulcers.
    V.   They allow healing of PUD during continued therapy.

    A. I only
    B. III only
    C. I and II only
    D. II and III only

E. I, II, and III

5. Which of the following are goals of therapy for PUD?

I. Reduce episodes of diarrhea
II. Elimination of symptoms
III. Healing of ulcerations
IV. Reduce risk of gastric cancer
V. Avoiding spreading *H pylori*

    A. I only
    B. III only
    C. I and II only
    D. II and III only
    E. I, II, and III

6. The test of choice for identifying *H pylori* infection is:

    A. Serology
    B. Urine antigen test
    C. Urea breath test
    D. Endoscopic biopsy
    E. Blood culture

7. A.B. is a 45-year-old white female with PMH significant only for seizure disorder. She has experienced heartburn soon after meals for 2 weeks. It becomes worse upon reclining at bedtime. Medications: phenytoin 300 mg hs. A.B. wishes to self-treat with an OTC H$_2$RA. Which one of the following should NOT be recommended to AB?

    A. Alginic acid
    B. Cimetidine
    C. Famotidine
    D. Ranitidine
    E. Magnesium hydroxide

8. A.B.'s symptoms are not relieved after 2 weeks of OTC treatment with famotidine and lifestyle modifications. Which one of the following is the best choice?

    A. Add the prokinetic agent metoclopramide to famotidine.
    B. Endoscopy should be performed since A.B. is at high risk for complications
    C. Add alginic acid 2 tablets qhs to famotidine.
    D. Switch to high-dose omeprazole 60 mg qd.
    E. Continue lifestyle modifications and switch to famotidine 20 mg bid.

9. Which of the following is an atypical symptom of GERD?

I. Hoarseness
II. Regurgitation
III. Belching
IV. Hypersalivation
V. Heartburn

    A. I only
    B. III only
    C. I and II only
    D. II and III only
    E. I, II, and III

10. Which of the following diagnoses carries an increased risk for developing esophageal adenocarcinoma?

I. Barrett's esophagus
II. Mild noncrosive reflux disease
III. Mild erosive esophagitis
IV. Moderate nonerosive reflux disease
V. Moderate erosive esophagitis

    A. I only
    B. III only
    C. I and II only
    D. II and III only
    E. I, II, and III

11. Which one of the following may exacerbate GERD symptoms by lowering the LES pressure?

    A. Quinidine
    B. Iron
    C. Potassium chloride
    D. Diltiazem
    E. Tetracycline

12. Which of the following is the best choice for the initial (phase I) treatment of a patient with mild GERD?

    A. Nizatidine 75 mg qid
    B. Pantoprazole 40 mg bid
    C. Metoclopramide 10 mg qid
    D. 3-month trial of lifestyle modifications
    E. Lansoprazole 30 mg bid

13. A.Y. is a 32-year-old white male who presents with bloody diarrhea (less than four stools per day) x 2 days. Complete blood counts and ESR are normal. Physical exam is normal. Colonoscopy reveals distal colitis. Which of the fol-

lowing is the best choice for initial therapy for
A.Y.?

A. Prednisone 40 mg PO qd
B. Sulfasalazine 4-6 g PO qd
C. Mesalamine 1-4 g PR qhs
D. Mesalamine 2-4 g PO qd
E. Methylprednisolone 16 mg IV q8h

14. A.Y. continues to have bloody diarrhea (without
systemic disturbances). Which one of the following is the best choice?

A. Add prednisone 40 mg PO qd and discontinue enema.
B. Add mesalamine 2-4 g PO qd and continue
enema.
C. Add methylprednisolone 16 mg IV q8h until
remission is achieved.
D. Add mesalamine 2-4 g PO qd and discontinue enema.
E. Add azathioprine 1-2.5 mg/kg/d and discontinue enema.

15. Which of the following is true for UC?

I. Aminosalicylates are the drugs of choice for
maintenance therapy.
II. Azathioprine often allows reduction in corticosteroid dose.
III. Oral corticosteroids are the drugs of choice for
maintenance therapy.
IV. Topical aminosalicylates are the drugs of choice
for severe or fulminant disease.
V. Ciprofloxacin is alternative first-line therapy for
mild to moderate disease.

A. I only
B. III only
C. I and II only
D. II and III only
E. I, II, and III

16. Which of the following is true for CD?

I. Ciprofloxacin is an alternative drug of choice
for mild to moderate disease.
II. Infliximab is the drug of choice for mild to
moderate disease.
III. Oral corticosteroids are the drugs of choice for
maintenance therapy.
IV. Topical aminosalicylates are the drugs of choice
for mild to moderate disease.
V. Oral cyclosporine is the drug of choice for
maintenance therapy.

A. I only
B. III only
C. I and II only
D. II and III only
E. I, II, and III

17. Which of the following is true for moderate to
severe CD?

A. Azathioprine is the drug of choice for initial
therapy.
B. Budesonide is appropriate maintenance
therapy.
C. Oral corticosteroids are the drugs of choice
for initial therapy.
D. Methotrexate has no role in CD therapy.
E. Topical aminosalicylates are appropriate
maintenance therapy.

18. Which one of the following may be used in the
management of fistulas?

A. Prednisone
B. Sulfasalazine
C. Mesalamine
D. Methotrexate
E. Infliximab

19. J.J. is a 39-year-old female who presents with
intermittent abdominal pain x 14 weeks and four
episodes of diarrhea per day (worsened after
meals). J.J. has no significant PMH and occasionally misses days from her full-time job.
Which one of the following is the best choice
for initial therapy?

I. Dicyclomine 10 mg qid after meals
II. Amitriptyline 10 mg hs
III. Tegaserod 6 mg bid
IV. Alosetron 1 mg qd
V. Paroxetine 10 mg qd

A. I only
B. III only
C. I and II only
D. II and III only
E. I, II, and III

20. J.J.'s symptoms are controlled for several months
until she loses her job. Her abdominal pain has
returned, she has five episodes of diarrhea per
day, and complains of fatigue and insomnia.
Which of the following is the most appropriate
for J.J.?

I. Psychological counseling should be initiated

II. Amitriptyline 10-50 mg hs
III. Add loperamide 2 mg after each loose stool (16 mg/d)
IV. Add alosetron 1 mg qd
V. Start paroxetine 10-40 mg qd

A. I only
B. III only
C. I and II only
D. II and III only
E. I, II, and III

21. Which of the following is indicated for constipation-predominant IBS?

A. Tegaserod 6 mg bid
B. Alosetron 1 mg bid
C. Loperamide 2-16 mg/d
D. Paroxetine 10-40 mg qd
E. Diphenoxylate + atropine 2 tabs qid

22. Which of the following is affected by medications that induce or inhibit the cytochrome P450 enzyme system?

A. Tegaserod
B. Alosetron
C. Fibercon
D. Hyoscyamine
E. Amitriptyline

23. Which life-threatening complication caused the restriction of alosetron?

A. Stevens-Johnson syndrome
B. Toxic epidermal necrolysis
C. Aplastic anemia
D. Ischemic colitis
E. Chronic diarrhea

24. Alosetron is indicated for which group of IBS patients?

A. Women with diarrhea-predominant IBS
B. Men with diarrhea-predominant IBS
C. Women with constipation-predominant IBS
D. Men with constipation-predominant IBS
E. Children with diarrhea-predominant IBS

Answers

1. **B.** Furazolidone should only be used when resistance to clarithromycin or metronidazole is suspected. Sucralfate is not a part of triple or quadruple drug therapy. Triple and quadruple drug regimens are more effective than two-drug regimens.

2. **B.** Furazolidone should only be used when resistance to clarithromycin or metronidazole is suspected. Increasing dose does not overcome resistance of clarithromycin.

3. **B.** NSAIDs are the leading cause of PUD in patients who are negative for *H pylori* infection.

4. **E.** NSAIDs inhibit production of prostaglandins and are directly toxic to gastroduodenal epithelium. NSAIDs require dose adjustments in renal insufficiency. NSAIDs may cause gastric or duodenal ulcers, and must be discontinued to allow for ulcer healing.

5. **D.** Elimination of symptoms and healing of ulcerations are goals of therapy for PUD.

6. **C.** The urea breath test is commercially available for in-office use and is the test of choice for identifying *H pylori*.

7. **B.** Cimetidine is a potent inhibitor of the cytochrome P450 enzyme system and will increase serum concentrations of phenytoin in A.B.

8. **E.** Prokinetic agents are useful mainly in patients with concurrent gastric motility disorders and are not routinely recommended. Alginic acid is ineffective when lying in the supine position. High-dose omeprazole is used to confirm the diagnosis of GERD in patients not responding to initial therapy with prescription medications.

9. **A.** Hoarseness, chronic cough, nonallergic asthma, pharyngitis, and chest pain that resembles angina are atypical symptoms of GERD.

10. **A.** Patients with Barrett's esophagus have an increased risk of developing esophageal adenocarcinoma

11. **D.** Calcium channel blockers decrease LES pressure. Quinidine, iron, potassium chloride, and tetracycline have direct irritant effects on the esophageal mucosa.

12. **A.** GERD therapy may be divided into three phases. Phase I therapy consists of lifestyle modifications and patient-directed therapy with OTC histamine-receptor antagonists and/or

antacids. Nizatidine 75 mg qid is appropriate for patients with mild typical GERD symptoms. If symptoms persist after 2 weeks, phase II therapy is appropriate. Phase II therapy is for patients with mild to moderate typical GERD symptoms and consists of continuous lifestyle modifications and standard or high-dose antisecretory medications. Phase III therapy consists of surgical intervention and is reserved for patients with severe symptoms.

13. **C.** A.Y. has mild (fewer than four stools per day, no systemic disturbances) distal (below the splenic flexure) ulcerative colitis. Mesalamine or corticosteroid enemas are appropriate first-line therapy.

14. **B.** Oral aminosalicylates should be added if no response is achieved with topical therapy. Oral and IV steroids are reserved for moderate to severe UC or for patients with systemic disturbances. Azathioprine may be added if UC is refractory to aminosalicylates and to allow corticosteroid dose reduction.

15. **C.** Aminosalicylates are the drugs of choice for maintenance therapy of UC, not corticosteroids. Azathioprine often allows a reduction in dose of corticosteroids in the management of active UC. Severe or fulminant UC requires oral therapy, not topical. Ciprofloxacin may be used as an alternative first-line therapy in the treatment of mild to moderate CD, not UC.

16. **A.** Ciprofloxacin or metronidazole is an alternative first-line agent for mild to moderate disease. Infliximab is reserved for moderate to severe disease or patients who do not respond to initial therapy. Oral cyclosporine is not effective maintenance therapy. Topical aminosalicylates may be used as an adjunct to oral therapy.

17. **C.** Moderate to severe disease requires oral corticosteroid therapy initially. Corticosteroids have no role in maintenance therapy. Topical aminosalicylates may be used as adjuncts in colonic CD. Methotrexate is used as maintenance therapy for moderate to severe CD.

18. **E.** Infliximab, high-dose metronidazole, ciprofloxacin, or azathioprine may be used in the management of fistulas.

19. **A.** J.J. has mild, diarrhea-predominant IBS. Symptomatic treatment with dicyclomine is appropriate initial therapy. A TCA may be added

to dicyclomine if needed. Tegaserod is indicated for constipation-predominant IBS. Alosetron is reserved for severe, diarrhea-predominant disease

20. **E.** Alosetron is reserved for patients with severe, diarrhea-predominant IBS (FDA-restricted use). SSRIs have less benefit than TCAs, but may be used for significant depression. Loperamide may be used on an as-needed basis for diarrhea.

21. **A.** Alosetron is approved for restricted use in diarrhea-predominant IBS. Loperamide and diphenoxylate + atropine are antidiarrheal medications which will exacerbate constipation. Paroxetine is an SSRI with potent anticholinergic effects, which could worsen diarrhea. If an SSRI is needed for depression, another should be chosen.

22. **E.** TCA serum concentrations are affected by drugs that alter cytochrome P450 activity.

23. **D.** Severe constipation, ischemic colitis, and death have been reported with alosetron.

24. **A.** Alosetron is approved for women with diarrhea-predominant IBS. It was not found to be effective in men, and is not approved for use in children

7. References

Peptic ulcer disease

Berardi R. Peptic ulcer disease. In: Dipiro JT, Talbert RL, Yee GC, et al, eds. *Pharmacotherapy: A Pathophysiologic Approach,* 5th ed. Stamford, CT: McGraw-Hill/Appleton & Lange; 2002:603-624.

Chan FKL, Leung WK. Peptic ulcer disease. *Lancet.* 2002;360:933-941.

Current European concepts in the management of *Helicobacter pylori* infection. The Maastricht Consensus Report. European Helicobacter Pylori Study Group. *Gut.* 1997;41:8-13.

Del Valle J. Peptic ulcer disease and related disorders. In: Braunwald E, Fauci AS, Casper DL, et al, eds. *Harrison's Principles of Internal Medicine,* 15th ed. New York: McGraw-Hill; 2001:1649-1661.

Henderson RP. Acid-peptic disorders and intestinal gas. In: Berardi RR, DiSimone EM, Newton GD, eds. *Handbook of Nonprescription Drugs,* 13th ed. Washington: American Pharmaceutical Association; 2002:243-272.

Henderson RP, Lander RD. Peptic ulcer disease. In: Herfindal ET, Gourley DR, eds. *Textbook of Therapeutics: Drug and Disease Management,* 7th ed. Philadelphia: Lippincott Williams & Wilkins; 2000:515-531.

NIH Consensus Conference. *Helicobacter pylori* in peptic ulcer diseases. NIH Consensus Development Panel on Helicobacter Pylori in Peptic Ulcer Disease. *JAMA.* 1994;272:65-69.

Shiotani A, Graham DY. Pathogenesis and therapy of gastric and duodenal ulcer disease. *Med Clin North Am.* 2002;86:1447-1466.

Singh G, Triadafilopoulos G. Epidemiology of NSAID-induced GI complications. *J Rheumatol.* 1999;26(Suppl 26);18-24.

Wolfe MM, Lichtenstein DR, Singh G. Gastrointestinal toxicity of nonsteroidal anti-inflammatory drugs. *N Engl J Med.* 1999;340:1888-1889.

Gastroesophageal reflux disease

DeVault KR, Castell DO, et al. Updated guidelines for the diagnosis and treatment of gastroesophageal reflux disease. *Am J Gastroenterology.* 1999;94:1434-1442.

DeVault KR. Overview of medical therapy for gastroesophageal reflux disease. *Gastroenterol Clin North Am.* 1999;28:831-845.

Fass R. Gastroesophageal reflux disease revisited. *Gastroenterol Clin North Am.* 2002;31(Suppl 4):S1-S10.

Goyal RK. Diseases of the esophagus. In: Fauci AS, Braunwald KJ, Wilson JD, et al, eds. *Harrison's Principles of Internal Medicine,* 15th ed. New York: McGraw-Hill; 2001:1642-1649.

Henderson RP. Acid-peptic disorders and intestinal gas. In: Berardi RR, DeSimone EM, Newton GD, et al. *Handbook of Nonprescription Drugs: An Interactive Approach to Self-Care,* 13th ed. Washington: American Pharmaceutical Association; 2002:243-272.

Henderson RP, Lander RD. Peptic ulcer disease. In: Herfindal ET, Gourley DR, eds. *Textbook of Therapeutics: Drug and Disease Management*, 7th ed. Baltimore: Lippincott Williams & Wilkins; 2000:515-531.

Locke GR. Natural history of nonerosive reflux disease: Is all gastroesophageal reflux the same? What is the evidence? *Gastroenterol Clin North Am.* 2002;31(Suppl 4):S59-S66.

Locke GR, Talley NH, Fett SL, et al. Prevalence and clinical spectrum of gastroesophageal reflux: a population-based study in Olmstead county. *Gastroenterology.* 1997;112:1448-1456.

Orlando RC. Pathogenesis of gastroesophageal reflux disease. *Gastroenterol Clin North Am.* 2002;31(Suppl 4):S35-S44.

Spechler SJ. Barrett's esophagus and esophageal adenocarcinoma: pathogenesis, diagnosis, and therapy. *Med Clin North Am.* 2002;86:1423-1445.

Waring JP. Surgical and endoscopic treatment of gastroesophageal reflux disease. *Gastroenterol Clin North Am.* 2002;31(Suppl 4):S89-S109.

Williams DB. Gastroesophageal reflux disease. In: Dipiro JT, Talbert RL, Yee GC, et al, eds. *Pharmacotherapy: A Pathophysiologic Approach,* 5th ed. Stamford, CT: McGraw-Hill/Appleton & Lange; 2002:585-601.

Inflammatory bowel disease
Ardizzone S, Porro GB. Inflammatory bowel disease: new insights into pathogenesis and treatment. *J Intern Med.* 2002;252:475-496.

Banerjee S, Peppercorn MA. Inflammatory bowel disease: Medical therapy for specific clinical presentations. *Gastroenterol Clin North Am.* 2002;31:185-202.

Berardi RR. Inflammatory bowel disease. In: Herfindal ET, Gourley DR, eds. *Textbook of Therapeutics: Drug and Disease Management,* 7th ed. Philadelphia: Lippincott Williams and Wilkins; 2000:533-551.

DiPiro JT, Schade RR. Inflammatory bowel disease. In: Dipiro JT, Talbert RL, Yee GC, et al, eds. *Pharmacotherapy: A Pathophysiologic Approach,* 5th ed. Stamford, CT: McGraw-Hill/Appleton & Lange; 2002:625-639.

Friedman S, Blumberg. Inflammatory bowel disease. In: Braunwald E, et al, eds. *Harrison's Principles of Internal Medicine,* 15th ed. New York: McGraw-Hill; 2001:1679-1692.
Hanauer SB, Sandborn W, et al. Practice guidelines: Management of Crohn's disease in adults. *Am J Gastroenterol.* 2001;96:635-643.

Harrison J, Hanauer SB. Medical treatment of Crohn's disease. *Gastroenterol Clin North Am.* 2002;31:167-184.

Jani N, Regueiro MD. Medical therapy for ulcerative colitis. *Gastroenterol Clin North Am.* 2002;31:147-166.

Kornbluth A, Sachar DB. Ulcerative colitis: Practice guidelines in adults. *Am J Gastroenterol.* 1997;92:204-211.

Irritable bowel syndrome
Brandt LJ, Bjorkman D, Fennerty MB, et al. Systematic review on the management of irritable bowel syndrome in North America. *Am J Gastroenterol.* 2002;97(Suppl 11):S7-S26.

Drossman DA, Camilleri M, Mayer EA, Whitehead WE. AGA technical review on irritable bowel syndrome. *Gastroenterology.* 2002;123:2108-2131.

Hasler WL. The irritable bowel syndrome. *Med Clin North Am.* 2002;86:1525-1551.

Owyang C. Irritable bowel syndrome. In: Braunwald E, et al, eds. *Harrison's Principles of Internal Medicine,* 15th ed. New York: McGraw-Hill; 2001:1692-1695.

Spruill WJ, Wade WE. Diarrhea, constipation, and irritable bowel syndrome. In: Dipiro JT, et al, eds. *Pharmacotherapy: A Pathophysiologic Approach,* 5th ed. New York: McGraw-Hill; 2002:655-669.

Talley NJ, Spiller R. Irritable bowel syndrome: a little understood organic bowel disease? *Lancet.* 2002;360:555-564.

Viera AJ, Hoag S, Shaughnessy J. Management of irritable bowel syndrome. *Am Fam Physician.* 2002;66:1867-1874.

22. Rheumatoid Arthritis, Osteoarthritis, Gout, and Lupus

Kevin L. Freeman, PharmD
Assistant Professor, Department of Pharmacy
University of Tennessee College of Pharmacy
Clinical Pharmacy Specialist
Veterans Affairs Medical Center, Memphis, Tennessee

Contents

1. Rheumatoid Arthritis

- Rheumatoid arthritis (RA) is a highly variable, chronic autoimmune disorder of unknown etiology depicted by symmetric, erosive synovitis. Manifestations may extend to extra-articular sites.

Incidence

- RA affects 1% of the population and is two to three times more common in women than in men. RA has a peak incidence in women between 30 and 60 years of age. There is a greater incidence of RA in certain families, monozygotic twins, and people with specific HLA genetic markers, which suggests a genetic predisposition.

Clinical Presentation

- The onset of RA is unpredictable and varies from rapid to insidious progression.

- The course of the disease is likewise variable. Ten to twenty percent of patients have a short course with remission, 70-80% have mild to moderate disease with cyclic exacerbation, and 10-20% develop progressively destructive disease.

- RA usually affects diarthrodial joints such as the proximal interphalangeal (PIP) joints, metacarpophalangeal (MCP) joints, metatarsophalangeal (MTP) joints, wrists, and ankles. Also commonly involved are the elbows, shoulders, sternoclavicular joints, temporomandibular joints, hips, and knees.

- The initial complaints may include generalized fatigue and multiple joint pain.

- Morning stiffness is a hallmark of RA. Patients describe it as a gel-like sensation in the joints that occurs after attempting to move upon awakening.

- Ulnar deviation, swan-neck deformities, boutonnière deformities, hammertoe formation, and ankylosis are common irreversible joint abnormalities that occur in RA.

- The extra-articular features that occur in RA include rheumatoid nodules, vasculitis, anemia, thrombocytopenia, Felty's syndrome, and Sjögren's syndrome.

Etiology

- The cause of RA remains a mystery. Factors that may be responsible are of environmental, genetic, endocrinologic, gastrointestinal, atmospheric, and infectious origin.

- It is widely held that RA has a strong genetic component. This assertion is supported by the fact that a greater prevalence of RA is found in patients with the major histocompatibility complex (MHC) antigen HLA-DR4. This is a class II antigen expressed on the surface of helper T lymphocytes and macrophages. In combination with environmental factors, an inappropriate immune response may occur, resulting in chronic inflammation.

- It has been demonstrated that patients with RA have increased antibody titers to *Mycobacterium tuberculosis*, *Proteus mirabilis*, *Escherichia coli*, *Klebsiella pneumoniae*, normal human gut flora antigen, Epstein-Barr virus, and the superantigen staphylococcal enterotoxin B.

- There is a greater risk of RA in female patients after breastfeeding, which supports that there are endocrinologic risk factors.

- Gastrointestinal factors may be responsible for hyperactivity of the immune system, ie, antibodies to enteric organisms and gluten develop in the GI tract.

- Atmospheric changes are associated with symptomatic changes in the disease course.

Pathophysiology

- Due to causes still unknown, the body's immune system (starting with macrophages) attacks the cells within the joint capsule, thereby causing synovitis (as indicated by the warmth, swelling, redness, and pain associated with RA). Specifically, helper T lymphocytes stimulate B cells to attack antigen (in this case, the body's own collagen). In addition, helper T lymphocytes release cytokines (interleukins and tumor necrosis factor) which cause further inflammation and injury in the joints. During the inflammatory process, the cells of the synovium grow and divide abnormally, causing a normally thin synovium to become thick (pannus).

- These abnormal synovial cells begin to invade and destroy the cartilage and bone within the joint.

- The above effects are responsible for the pain and deformities seen in patients with RA.

Diagnostic Criteria

- Patients meeting four of the following criteria are classified as having rheumatoid arthritis:
    * Morning stiffness of or near joints lasting 1 hour before maximum improvement. This must be present for 6 weeks.
    * Three or more joint areas, including the right or left proximal interphalangeal (PIP) joint, metacarpophalangeal (MCP) joint, wrist, elbow, metatarsophalangeal (MTP) joint, ankle, or knee joint; must have arthritis as demonstrated by soft tissue swelling or fluid. This must be present for at least 6 weeks and observed by a physician.
    * Arthritis as demonstrated by soft tissue swelling or fluid in the hand joints (MCP, PIP, or wrist). This must be present for at least 6 weeks and observed by a physician.
    * Symmetric arthritis must occur in the areas noted in the second criterion. This must be present for at least 6 weeks and observed by a physician.
    * Subcutaneous nodules (rheumatoid nodules) over bony prominences, extensor surfaces, or in juxta-articular regions.
    * Positive rheumatoid factor (antibodies that collect in the synovium of the joint) as demonstrated by a positive test in less than 5% of normal subjects.
    * Radiologic changes of the hands or wrists, eg, erosions or bone decalcification in or next to involved joints.

Treatment Goals

- According to the American College of Rheumatology, the goals in managing RA are to prevent or control joint damage, prevent loss of function, and decrease pain (Figure 1).

Monitoring

- At each visit, the patient should be evaluated for subjective evidence of active disease based on the following criteria:
    * Degree of joint pain
    * Duration of morning stiffness
    * Duration of fatigue
    * Presence of actively inflamed joints on examination
    * Limitation of function

- Periodically, the patient should be evaluated for disease activity or progression:
    * Evidence of disease progression on physical exam (loss of motion, instability, malalignment, and/or deformity)
    * Erythrocyte sedimentation rate or C-reactive protein elevation
    * Progression of radiographic damage of involved joints

- Other parameters for assessing response to treatment (outcomes):
    * Physician's global assessment of disease activity
    * Patient's global assessment of disease activity
    * Functional status or quality of life assessment using standardized questionnaires

Drug Therapy

- Currently the most popular approach to the pharmacological treatment of RA is the "inverted pyramid," which refers to utilizing aggressive therapy with disease-modifying antirheumatic drugs (DMARDs) (Table 1). Some patients start out immediately with DMARDs with or without nonsteroidal anti-inflammatory drugs (NSAIDs). Others start DMARDs after 3 months if NSAIDs have not relieved symptoms (Table 2).

Nonsteroidal anti-inflammatory drugs (NSAIDs)
- Salicylates, NSAIDs, and selective cyclooxygenase-2 (COX-2) inhibitors are agents with analgesic and anti-inflammatory properties useful in the management of RA. These agents reduce joint pain and swelling; however, they do not inhibit joint destruction or otherwise alter the course of the disease. For this reason, they should not be considered as a sole treatment option. These agents act by inhibiting prostaglandin synthesis and release. Cyclooxygenase is present in many cells, including platelets, endothelial cells, and cells of the gastric and intestinal mucosa. The initial choice of agent is based on the efficacy, safety, cost, and convenience for any given patient. There is a high amount of interpatient variability with regard to clinical effect; several NSAIDs may need to be tried before achieving patient satisfaction.

Aspirin
Mechanism of action
- Aspirin prevents prostaglandin formation by inhibiting the action of the enzyme cyclooxygenase. The antithrombotic effect of aspirin occurs by an irreversible inhibition of platelet cyclooxygenase. This irreversible inhibition is unique to aspirin as the remaining NSAIDs do so in a reversible manner.

Figure 1.

Outline of the management of rheumatoid arthritis.

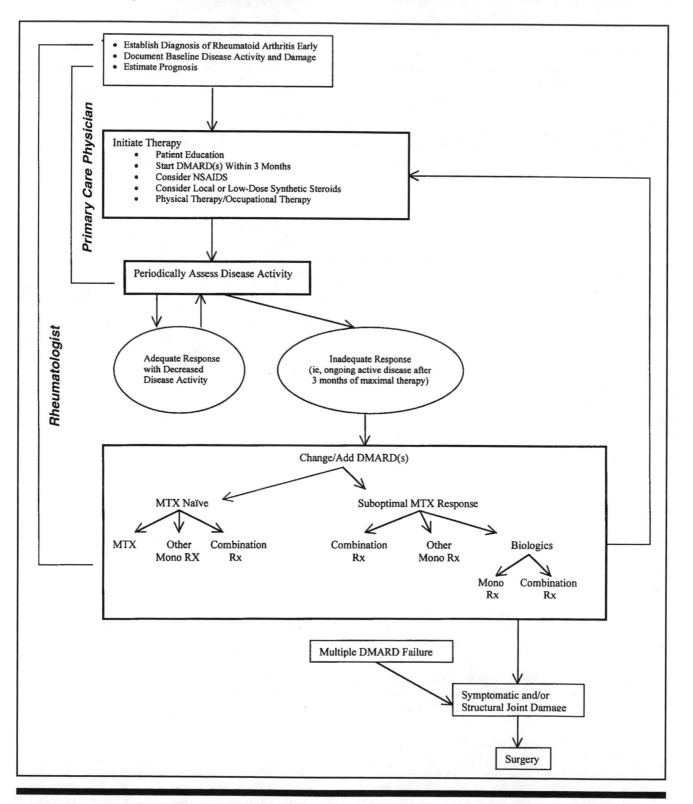

Boxes with heavy borders represent major decision points in management. A suboptimum response to methotrexate is defined as intolerance, lack of satisfactory efficacy with a dosage of up to 25 mg/week, or a contraindication to the drug.

DMARD, disease-modifying antirheumatic drug; NSAID, nonsteroidal anti-inflammatory drug; mono Rx, monotherapy; combination Rx, combination therapy.

Reprinted with permission from American College of Rheumatology Subcommittee on Rheumatoid Arthritis Guidelines. Guidelines for the Management of Rheumatoid Arthritis. *Arthritis Rheum.* 2002;46:328-346.

Table 1

Disease-Modifying Antirheumatic Drugs (DMARDs)

Generic name (trade name)	Dosage range	Administration schedule	Dosage forms
Hydroxychloroquine (Plaquenil®)	200-400 mg	1-2 doses per day	PO
Sulfasalazine (Azulfidine®)	2000-4000 mg	2-3 doses per day	PO
Methotrexate (Rheumatrex®)	7.5-20 mg	Once weekly	PO, IM, SC, IV
Gold sodium thiomalate (Myochrysine®)	25-50 mg	Every 2-4 weeks	IM
Auranofin (Ridaura®)	3-6 mg	1-2 doses per day	PO
Azathioprine (Imuran®)	50-150 mg	1-2 doses per day	PO, IV
Penicillamine (Cuprimine®)	250-750 mg	2-3 doses per day	PO
Minocycline (Minocin®)	100-200 mg	2 doses per day	PO
Leflunomide (Arava®)	10-20 mg	1-2 doses per day	PO
Etanercept (Enbrel®)	25 mg	Twice weekly	SQ
Infliximab (Remicade®)	3 mg/kg	Weeks 0, 2, and 6, then every 8 weeks	IV
Anakinra (Kineret®)	100 mg	1 dose per day	SQ

Table 2

Drug Therapy with Nonsteroidal Anti-Inflammatory Drugs (NSAIDs)

Generic name (trade name)	Dosage range (mg/d)	Administration schedule (doses/d)	Available dosage forms
Acetic acids			
Diclofenac (Voltaren®)	150-200	3-4	PO, ophth
Diclofenac (Voltaren XR®)	100-200	1-2	PO
Etodolac (Lodine®)	800-1200	3-4	PO
Etodolac (Lodine XL®)	400-1200	1-2	PO
Indomethacin (Indocin®)	100-200	2-3	PO, IV, supp
Indomethacin (Indocin SR®)	75-150	1-2	PO
Nabumetone (Relafen®)	1000-2000	1-2	PO
Tolmetin (Tolectin®)	1600-2000	3-4	PO
Sulindac (Clinoril®)	300-400	2	PO
Propionic acids			
Fenoprofen (Nalfon®)	1600-3200	3-4	PO
Flurbiprofen (Ansaid®)	200-300	2-4	PO
Ibuprofen (Motrin®)	1600-3200	3-4	PO
Ketoprofen (Orudis®)	150-300	3-4	PO
Ketoprofen SR (Oruvail®)	100-200	1	PO
Naproxen (Naprosyn®)	500-1500	2-3	PO
Oxaprozin (Daypro®)	1200-1800	1	PO
Fenamates			
Meclofenamate (Meclomen®)	300-400	3-4	PO
Oxicams			
Piroxicam (Feldene®)	10-20	1	PO
COX-2 selective			
Celecoxib (Celebrex®)	200-400	1-2	PO
Rofecoxib (Vioxx®)	12.5-25	1	PO
Valdecoxib (Bextra®)	10	1	PO

Dosage
- The usual daily dosage needed to achieve anti-inflammatory effects is 3-5 grams per day.

Patient instructions
- Aspirin should be taken with food or milk to decrease gastrointestinal intolerance. Patients should report any dark or black stools, abdominal pain, or swelling to his/her physician immediately.

Adverse drug events
- Aspirin irreversibly inhibits platelet activity and serious bleeding may result. Dyspepsia, gastrointestinal bleeding, tinnitus, hepatitis, and renal damage have been reported.

Drug-drug and drug-disease interactions
- Warfarin: aspirin may enhance the hypoprothrombinemic effects of warfarin.

- Uricosuric agents: the uricosuric effects of agents such as probenecid are antagonized by aspirin.

- Methotrexate: aspirin may displace methotrexate from its protein binding sites thereby increasing serum methotrexate concentrations.

Parameters to monitor
- Complete blood count as well as creatinine should be monitored at least yearly.

Other nonsteroidal anti-inflammatory drugs (NSAIDs)
Mechanism of action
- See aspirin, above

Patient instructions
- See aspirin, above. Studies indicate that the optimal times for taking an NSAID might be after the evening meal and immediately upon waking. Patients with a hypersensitivity to aspirin should not take NSAIDs.

Adverse drug events
- Compared to patients with osteoarthritis, patients with RA on NSAID therapy are at increased risk for a serious complication.
  - *As with aspirin, NSAIDs cause platelet dysfunction. Unlike aspirin, however, this effect is readily reversible with discontinuation of the medication.
  - *All NSAIDs are capable of causing gastrointestinal intolerance and peptic ulceration. Risk factors for the development of peptic ulcer disease include advanced age, history of previous ulcer, concomitant use of corticosteroids or anticoagulants, higher dosage of NSAID, use of multiple NSAIDs, or serious underlying disease. Options to decrease the risk of developing GI ulceration include adding a high-dose H_2 blocker such as Zantac® or a proton pump inhibitor such as Prevacid to the patient's regimen. Prevacid® was recently granted FDA approval for reducing the risk of NSAID-induced gastric ulcers in those patients with a previous risk of ulceration and who continue to require NSAID treatment. Also the agent Cytotec® (misoprostol), an oral prostaglandin analogue, may be added at a dose of 100-200 µg four times daily to prevent ulceration. Misoprostol is available in combination with diclofenac and sold under the trade name Arthrotec®. There is also some evidence that compared to other NSAIDs, ibuprofen, nabumetone, and naproxen carry lower risks of ulceration and GI symptoms. Piroxicam, on the other hand, appears to carry a higher risk of serious GI consequences.
  - *Hepatic failure has been reported with NSAID use.
  - *Renal blood flow can be decreased by NSAIDs, which may lead to permanent renal damage. Prostaglandins are responsible for maintaining the patency of the afferent renal tubule. Inhibition by NSAIDs decreases glomerular filtration pressure, resulting in decreased blood flow. Due to this mechanism, patients with hypertension, severe vascular disease, kidney or liver problems, and those taking diuretics must be monitored closely.
  - *Central nervous system side effects such as dizziness, drowsiness, and confusion may occur with all NSAIDs.
  - *Within the class, there are some drug-specific adverse reactions. Meclofenamate, for example, has a high incidence (>10%) of abdominal cramping and diarrhea. Paradoxically, indomethacin tends to have more severe CNS adverse effects such as headache.

Drug-drug interactions
- See aspirin, above. It appears that ibuprofen may diminish the antiplatelet mechanism of aspirin if it is taken before aspirin or taken daily on a scheduled basis. It is recommended to take aspirin 2 hours before taking ibuprofen.

Cyclooxygenase-2 (COX-2) inhibitors
- COX-1 is the isoenzyme constitutively found in most tissues that produce the prostaglandins PGI_2 and PGE_2, which protect the gastric barrier, and thromboxane A_2, which is responsible for platelet function. COX-2 is the

inducible isoenzyme present at sites of inflammation. COX-2 is also found in the brain, kidneys, and reproductive organs. Celebrex has been shown to lower the incidence of endoscopically-demonstrated gastroduodenal lesions compared to ibuprofen, naproxen, and diclofenac. The same was shown with Vioxx when compared to ibuprofen. It appears that the lower risk for GI complications is eliminated when patients take low-dose aspirin concomitantly.

Celebrex (celecoxib), Vioxx (rofecoxib), and Bextra (valdecoxib)

Mechanism of action
- Each selectively inhibits prostaglandin synthesis by specifically targeting the COX-2 isoenzyme.

Patient instructions
- Patients with a history of allergic reaction to sulfonamides should avoid the use of Celebrex and Bextra.

Adverse drug events
- Although the rates of GI ulceration have been demonstrated to be lower with COX-2 inhibitors compared to traditional NSAIDs, the risk is not completely eliminated. In addition, the risk of dyspepsia, abdominal pain, and nausea is not significantly less with COX-2 inhibitors compared to traditional NSAIDs. It is still unclear whether COX-2 selectivity affects renal function.

Drug-drug interactions
- See above interactions associated with aspirin.

Parameters to monitor
- Complete blood count as well as creatinine should be monitored at least yearly.

Other
- Data from the VIGOR trial comparing Vioxx with naproxen found a higher number of patients with myocardial infarction, although there was not a significant difference in mortality between the groups. It is unclear if this represents a potential risk associated with Vioxx or one that is inherent with all those in the COX-2 class.

Disease-modifying antirheumatic drugs (DMARDs)
- Unlike the NSAIDs, DMARDs have the ability to reduce or prevent joint damage and preserve joint integrity and function. The American College of Rheumatology recommends that the initiation of DMARD therapy not exceed 3 months from the diagnosis of RA in patients who have ongoing joint pain despite adequate treatment with NSAIDs, significant morning stiffness, active synovitis, persistent elevation of ESR or CRP level, or radiographic evidence of joint damage. Unfortunately, all DMARDs tend to lose effectiveness over time. It is rare for a patient to use one medication for longer than 2 years.

Plaquenil (hydroxychloroquine)

Mechanism of action
- May inhibit interleukin-1 release by monocytes, thereby decreasing macrophage chemotaxis and phagocytosis.

Patient instructions
- Beneficial effect may not be seen until 1-6 months of use. The patient should report any changes in vision to their physician immediately.

Adverse drug events
- The most serious potential adverse effect associated with Plaquenil is retinal damage that can lead to vision loss. This is caused by the deposition of the drug in the melanin layer of the cones. A cumulative dose of 800 grams and >70 years of age increases the risk. Plaquenil may also cause rash, abdominal cramping, diarrhea, myopathy, skin pigment changes, and peripheral neuropathy.

Parameters to monitor
- Ophthalmic evaluations should be performed every 6-12 months. It is unnecessary to perform a baseline evaluation if the patient is under 40 years of age. Those patients receiving the drug for over 7 years should have monthly visual field and color vision testing.

Dose
- 6-7.5 mg/kg of lean body weight daily or 200 mg bid (maximum dose).

Azulfidine (sulfasalazine)

Mechanism of action
- The intestinal flora breaks sulfasalazine down to 5-aminosalicylic acid and sulfapyridine, the active moiety in RA. Sulfapyridine likely inhibits endothelial cell proliferation, reactive oxygen species, and cytokines. In addition, it has been shown to slow radiographic progression of RA.

Patient instructions
- Sulfasalazine may produce effects more quickly (within 1 month) than Plaquenil. A coated tablet form may help reduce GI adverse effects.

Adverse drug events
- The most common adverse reactions associated with sulfasalazine include headache, GI intolerance, dysgeusia, rash, leukopenia, and thrombocytopenia.

Drug-drug interactions
- Sulfasalazine may inhibit the absorption of folic acid.

Parameters to monitor
- Patient tests should include baseline CBC, liver function tests, and G6PD levels. Patients should then have a CBC drawn every 2-4 weeks for the first 3 months, then every 3 months thereafter.

Dose
- Begin with 500 mg daily titrated up to 1-3 grams per day divided tid or qid.

Rheumatrex (methotrexate)
Mechanism of action
- Methotrexate inhibits dihydrofolate reductase. It reduces dihydrofolate to tetrahydrofolate, which can be utilized as a carrier of single carbon units for the synthesis of nucleotides and thymidylate. Therefore, methotrexate interferes with DNA synthesis, repair, and cellular replication.

Patient instructions
- Never change the amount of methotrexate you take without first consulting your physician.

Adverse drug events
- *Liver:* Methotrexate may cause liver damage. People with diabetes, liver problems, obesity, psoriasis, and those who are elderly or alcoholic are at higher risk; if LFTs (liver function tests) are greater than three times the upper limit of normal, methotrexate should be discontinued.

- *Bone marrow:* Leukopenia, thrombocytopenia, and pancytopenia are rare but serious adverse events associated with methotrexate therapy

- Pulmonary toxicity occurs in up to 5% of people who take methotrexate. Risk factors for the development of pulmonary toxicity include age, diabetes, rheumatoid involvement of the lungs, protein in the urine, and previous use of sulfasalazine, oral gold, or penicillamine.

- *GI:* Nausea, vomiting, and stomatitis occur with an incidence of 5- 30%

Drug-drug interactions
- Aspirin and other NSAIDs may increase methotrexate concentrations by as much as 30-35 %. Septra may cause additive hematologic abnormalities due to its similar affinity for dihydrofolate reductase.

Parameters to monitor
- CBC, platelet count, AST, albumin, and creatinine should be monitored every 4-8 weeks.

Other
- Taking folate supplements may help to minimize adverse effects like liver toxicity. Folic acid in doses up to 3 mg per day has proven effective and does not diminish methotrexate activity.

Dose
- 7.5 mg to 25 mg *once* weekly

Arava (leflunomide)
Mechanism of action
- Leflunomide inhibits dihydro-orotate dehydrogenase (an enzyme involved in de novo pyrimidine synthesis) and has antiproliferative activity. Several in vivo and in vitro experimental models have demonstrated its anti-inflammatory effect.

Patient instructions
- Leflunomide is under pregnancy category X. Women taking Arava who wish to become pregnant should follow the drug elimination procedure outlined below.

Adverse drug events
- Diarrhea, elevated LFTs, alopecia, hypertension, and rash have been reported with leflunomide therapy.

Drug-drug interactions
- There is an increased risk of liver toxicity when leflunomide is used in conjunction with methotrexate. Rifampin causes a 40% increase in levels of leflunomide's active metabolite, M1.

Parameters to monitor
- It is recommended that liver function tests be monitored at baseline, monthly (initially), and periodically thereafter. If ALT exceeds two times the upper limit of normal, reduce the dose of leflunomide to 10 mg per day.

Kinetics
- After absorption, 80% of the parent compound is converted to the active metabolite, M1, which is responsible for all of leflunomide's activity. Since the half-life is 2 weeks, a loading dose is necessary.

Other
- Begin a drug elimination procedure if a patient decides to become pregnant. It is as follows: 8 grams of cholestyramine three times daily for 11 days; plasma levels of M1 <0.02 mg/L must be verified on two separate occasions at least 14 days apart.

Many randomized controlled trials have established leflunomide as an alternative to methotrexate as monotherapy.

Dose
- 100 mg daily for 3 days (loading dose), then 20 mg daily

Cuprimine (D-penicillamine)
Mechanism of action
- It is currently unknown how penicillamine induces therapeutic effects in RA. It is known, however, that it significantly reduces IgM rheumatoid factor and appears to suppress disease activity.

Patient instructions
- Penicillamine should be taken on an empty stomach and at least 2 hours from any dose of antacids or iron supplements.

Adverse drug events
- *Bone marrow:* Penicillamine may cause thrombocytopenia and leukopenia approximately 6 months into therapy. Rarely, aplastic anemia develops and is associated with its use.

- *Renal:* Proteinuria may occur in up to 32% of patients on penicillamine therapy.

- *Dermatologic:* Skin rash may occur 6-9 months after starting therapy.

- *Other:* Penicillamine causes stomatitis, dysgeusia, and polymyositis.

Drug-drug interactions
- Absorption decreases approximately 70% with concomitant administration of antacids, iron, and zinc. Penicillamine may increase digoxin levels. In addition, penicillamine's chelating effects in combination with oral gold compounds may cause gold from deep tissue compartments to mobilize, which can increase toxicity.

Parameters to monitor
- Patients should have CBC, platelet count, creatinine, and urine dipstick for protein lab testing done before initiating therapy. Afterwards, the patient should have a CBC and urine dipstick for protein every 2 weeks until the dosage is stable, then every 1-3 months.

Other
- It may take up to 1 year for penicillamine to be effective. Note that more than half of the patients who take it withdraw due to side effects.

Dose
- Begin with 125-250 mg daily and increase by 125-250 mg daily every for 8-10 weeks, not to exceed a maximum dose of 750 mg per day.

Gold compounds (gold sodium thiomalate [Myochrysine; given IM] and aurothioglucose [Solganal; given IM], and auranofin [Ridaura; given PO])
Mechanism of action
- The MOA of gold compounds is currently unknown; they appear to suppress the synovitis seen in RA. Current research indicates that they may stimulate specific protective factors such as interleukins 6 and 10.

Patient instructions
- Patients receiving gold therapy should avoid prolonged sun exposure, which may increase the risk of serious rash.

Adverse drug events
IM gold
- Patients may experience an immediate "nitroid reaction," ie, flushing, weakness, dizziness, sweating, syncope, and hypotension. Rash is the single largest adverse effect associated with gold therapy. The rash may range from simple erythema to exfoliative dermatitis. Gold therapy may also cause proteinuria or microscopic hematuria. Rarely, immunologic glomerulonephritis may occur, in which case gold therapy should be permanently discontinued. Leukopenia and thrombocytopenia may occur with a 1-3% incidence.

PO gold
- Adverse reactions are similar to those associated with the IM formulation. However, GI complaints of nausea, diarrhea, emesis, and dysgeusia are higher.

Drug-drug interactions
- Patients receiving concomitant penicillamine therapy may be subject to an increased risk of toxicity associated with gold therapy. The risk of rash is higher when gold therapy is used with hydroxychloroquine.

Parameters to monitor
- At baseline, all patients should have a CBC, platelet count, creatinine, and urine dipstick for protein checked. For patients receiving IM therapy, a CBC, platelet count, and urine dipstick are recommended every 1-2 weeks for first 20 weeks, and then again at the time of each (or every other) injection. Those on oral therapy should have a CBC, platelet count, and urine dipstick for protein every 4-12 weeks.

Other

- Solganal may have a lower rate of injection reactions; its sesame seed formulation slows absorption.

Dosing

IM gold

- 10-mg test dose IM followed by 25-mg test dose on week two, then weekly 50-mg doses until a cumulative dose of 1 gram is achieved. Maintenance regimen: 50 mg every 2 weeks for 3 months or until 1.5 grams is given, then every 3 weeks, then monthly.

PO gold

- 3 mg bid up to 3 mg tid

Anti–tumor necrosis factor therapy (Remicade [infliximab] and Enbrel [etanercept])

Mechanism of action

- Composed of human constant and murine variable regions, infliximab binds specifically to human tumor necrosis factor (TNF).

- Similarly, by binding specifically to TNF, etanercept binds and blocks its interaction with the cell surface's TNF receptors. It is produced via recombinant technology in Chinese hamster ovaries.

Patient instructions

- Patients should not receive live vaccines during treatment. Therapy should be temporarily discontinued in the event of an acute infection.

Adverse drug events

- Therapy has been associated with serious mycobacterial, fungal, and opportunistic infectious complications, eg, sepsis and tuberculosis. Other adverse reactions include rash, headache, nausea, and cough. Although rare, both etanercept and infliximab have been associated with nerve damage that resembles the disease process in multiple sclerosis.

Drug-drug interactions

- Live vaccines

Parameters to monitor

- There are no recommended monitoring parameters at this time.

Other

- Patients should be tested for tuberculosis before initiating therapy. Currently, infliximab is only approved for therapy in combination with methotrexate.

Dose

Remicade

- 3 mg/kg IV initially, at weeks 2 and 6, then every 8 weeks in combination with methotrexate.

Enbrel

- 25 mg SQ twice weekly

Kineret (anakinra)

Mechanism of action

- Kineret blocks the biologic activity of IL-1 by competitively inhibiting IL-1 binding to the interleukin-1 type I receptor (IL-1RI).

Patient instructions

- Kineret is supplied as a single-use, prefilled syringe that should be stored in the refrigerator. Any syringe left unrefrigerated for over 24 hours should be discarded.

Adverse drug events

- Similar to the anti-TNF agents, anakinra increases the risk of serious infections. Injection site reactions are extremely common. Headache, nausea, diarrhea, sinusitis, flu-like symptoms, and abdominal pain have also been reported.

Drug-drug interactions

- Live vaccines

Parameters to monitor

- Patients should have a CBC checked at baseline, then monthly for 3 months, followed by every 3 months for the first year of therapy.

Dose

- 100 mg daily SQ

Other agents

Imuran (azathioprine)

- This agent is a purine analog immunosuppressive agent generally reserved for refractory RA. It is associated with dose-related bone marrow suppression, stomatitis, diarrhea, rash, and liver failure. Patients must have a baseline CBC, creatinine, and liver profile. Patients should then have a CBC and platelet count drawn every 1-2 weeks after any change in dosage and every 1-3 months thereafter. Imuran should not be administered with allopurinol since xanthine oxidase metabolizes 6-mercaptopurine.

Sandimmune (cyclosporine A)

- By blocking T-cell activation, this agent produces powerful immunosuppressive effects and is beneficial as monotherapy in the treatment of RA. Serious adverse effects such as hypertension, nephrotoxicity, glucose intolerance, and hepatotoxicity have limited its use.

Corticosteroids

- Low-dose oral corticosteroids (<10 mg per day of prednisone or the equivalent) and local injections of glucocorticoids are highly effective. Due to their inability to alter the course of RA, these agents are generally considered last-line therapy. They may be useful for acute flare-ups and in patients with significant systemic manifestations of RA. RA is associated with an increased risk of osteoporosis (independent of steroid therapy), and the addition of said agents increases the risk. Patients on glucocorticoids should receive 1500 mg of elemental calcium per day and 400-800 IU of vitamin D per day.

Nondrug Therapy

Surgery/Prosorba
Prosorba column
- A device called the Prosorba column removes inflammatory antibodies from the patient's blood.

Joint surgery
- Patients may have arthroscopy performed to clean out the bone and cartilage fragments that cause pain within the joint capsule. Patients may eventually require complete joint replacement surgery.

Lifestyle modifications
- Mild exercise

- *Diet:* There is some evidence to suggest a moderate increase in daily protein intake may be beneficial in RA.

- *Psychological:* Patients with RA benefit from a formal support group.

2. Osteoarthritis

- Osteoarthritis (OA), a disease that affects the weight-bearing joints of the peripheral and axial skeleton, is the most common form of arthritis in the U.S. OA is also known as degenerative joint disease (DJD).

Incidence

- Based on radiologic evidence, approximately 60-80% of people over the age of 65 have OA. Before the age of 50, men have a higher incidence; however, after the age of 50, women have a higher incidence.

Clinical Presentation

- Pain is a common initial finding in patients with OA. This pain typically worsens with weight-bearing activity and improves with rest of the affected joint.

- Changes in weather and barometric pressure tend to influence the severity of pain.

- Joint stiffness, including morning stiffness, is another common complaint. This stiffness differs from that of RA; it is relatively short in duration, is related to periods of inactivity, and resolves with movement.

- Crepitus is common, especially when the knee joint is involved.

- Joint deformities also occur in OA. Heberden's nodes, Bouchard's nodes, and osteophytes on the DIP and PIP are commonly seen.

Pathophysiology

- Although the causes of OA are not completely understood, biomechanical stresses affecting the articular cartilage and subchondral bone are thought to be the primary factors in the development of OA. In addition, inflammatory, biochemical, and immunologic components play a role. The function of the normal cartilage, ie, to dissipate the force and stress caused by normal weight-bearing activity, is impaired in OA.
  1. Collagen fibers are destroyed and subsequently release proteoglycans. The hydration of the cartilage increases, and the cartilage becomes thick.
  2. Metalloproteinases, which degrade the proteoglycans, are released to initiate the reparation process. This degradation causes an increase in chondrocyte activity.

3. The resulting cartilage is thin because the chondrocyte activity cannot match the rate at which proteoglycan degradation occurs.

4. With this ever-thinning layer of cartilage now exposing bone, the grinding motion stimulates osteoclast/osteoblast activity, thereby causing bone resorption and vascular changes. Ultimately, this leads to the formation of osteophytes.

Diagnostic Criteria

Osteoarthritis of the hip (American College of Rheumatology Classification Criteria)
• See Table 3.

Osteoarthritis of the knee (American College of Rheumatology Classification Criteria)
• See Table 4.

Treatment Principles

• Treatment of patients with OA focuses on symptom control; there are currently no therapeutic options known to change the course of the disease (Tables 5 and 6).

Drug Therapy

• Pain relief is the primary treatment goal for patients with OA. The recommended initial drug of choice is acetaminophen. For those patients that do not respond fully, the addition of an NSAID (see discussion of this class in the RA section) is made.

Table 3

Traditional Means of Diagnosing Osteoarthritis of the Hip

Hip pain and at least two of the following three:
• Erythrocyte sedimentation rate <20 mm/h
• Radiographic femoral or acetabular osteophytes
• Radiographic joint space narrowing

Other criteria:
• Hip pain and radiographic femoral or acetabular osteophytes
or
• Hip pain and radiographic joint space narrowing and erythrocyte sedimentation rate < 20 mm/h

Table 4

Traditional Means of Diagnosing Osteoarthritis of the Knee

Knee pain, radiographic osteophytes, and at least one of the following three:
• Age >50 years
• Morning stiffness ≤30 minutes in duration
• Crepitus on motion

Other criteria:
• Knee pain and radiographic osteophytes
or
• Knee pain and age ≥40 years, morning stiffness ≤30 minutes in duration, and crepitus on motion

Acetaminophen
Mechanism of action
• Acetaminophen centrally inhibits prostaglandin synthesis.

Table 5

Medical Management of Patients with Osteoarthritis of the Hip

Nonpharmacologic therapy
  Patient education
      Self-management programs (eg, arthritis self-help course)
  Health professional social support via telephone contact
  Weight loss (if overweight)
  Physical therapy
      Range-of-motion exercises
      Strengthening exercises
      Assistive devices for ambulation
  Occupational therapy
      Joint protection and energy conservation
      Assistive devices for ADLs and IADLs
  Aerobic aquatic exercise programs

Pharmacologic therapy
  Nonopioid analgesics (eg, acetaminophen)
  Nonsteroidal anti-inflammatory drugs
  Opioid analgesics (eg, propoxyphene, codeine, oxycodone)

ADLs, activities of daily living; IADLs, instrumental ADLs.

Table 6

Medical Management of Patients with Osteoarthritis of the Knee

---

Nonpharmacologic therapy
  Patient education
        Self-management programs (eg, arthritis self-help
          course)
  Health professional social support via telephone contact
  Weight loss (if overweight)
  Physical therapy
        Range-of-motion exercises
        Quadriceps strengthening exercises
        Assistive devices for ambulation
  Occupational therapy
        Joint protection and energy conservation
        Assistive devices for ADLs and IADLs
  Aerobic exercise programs

Pharmacologic therapy
  Intra-articular steroid injections
  Nonopioid analgesics (eg, acetaminophen)
  Topical analgesics (eg, capsaicin and methylsalicylate creams)
  Nonsteroidal anti-inflammatory drugs
  Opioid analgesics (eg, propoxyphene, codeine, oxycodone)

ADLs, activities of daily living; IADLs, instrumental ADLs.

Patient instructions

- Patients with hepatic disease or viral hepatitis are at risk of toxicity from chronic acetaminophen use.

Adverse drug events

- Hepatotoxicity is the most severe side effect associated with acetaminophen therapy. For this reason, patients should not ingest more than 4 grams of acetaminophen per day. Long-term therapy has also been linked to renal failure.

Other

- Acetaminophen is generally considered the initial drug of choice; however, there have been no clinical trials comparing its side effects, potential toxicity, or pain-relieving properties with those of NSAIDs.

Topical agents (capsaicin)
Mechanism of action

- Derived from the pepper plant, capsaicin works by exciting the nociceptive C-afferent neurons, which in turn causes the release of substance P, which is responsible for transmitting pain from the peripheral to the central nervous system.

Patient instructions

- Patients should avoid contact with eyes. It is important to wash hands thoroughly after use.

Adverse drug events

- Patients will experience mild burning and stinging at the site of application.

Other

- Patients usually derive benefit after several weeks of application. Capsaicin is often used in conjunction with oral agents.

Glucosamine sulfate and chondroitin
Mechanism of action

- Glucosamine is found naturally in articular cartilage and acts as a substrate in the synthesis of proteoglycans. Chondroitin, another constituent in the cartilage, attracts and retains water, which provides shock absorption. In addition, chondroitin prevents the breakdown of cartilage and stimulates RNA synthesis of chondrocytes.

Patient instructions

- Patients taking anticoagulants concomitantly may be at increased risk of bleeding.

Adverse drug events

- Adverse events tend to be mild but include dyspepsia and euphoria.

Other

- This combination is available over the counter and has some clinical literature to support its use. The Arthritis Foundation, however, does not currently recognize it as a treatment for OA.

Other agents

- Hyaluronic acid derivatives have been approved by the FDA for the treatment of pain associated with OA of the knee. These agents may be an option after all conventional therapies for OA have been exhausted. The injection of this product into the synovium appears to replenish the viscosity to the space, thus enabling normal tissue to regenerate.

Nondrug Therapy

- See Table 7.

Table 7

Nondrug Therapy for Osteoarthritis

Patient education
Self-management programs (eg, Arthritis Foundation
    Self-Management Program)
Personalized social support through telephone contact
Weight loss (if overweight)
Aerobic exercise programs
Physical therapy (ie, range-of-motion exercises)
Muscle-strengthening exercises
Assistive devices for ambulation
Patellar taping
Appropriate footwear
Lateral-wedged insoles (for genu varum); bracing
Occupational therapy
Joint protection and energy conservation
Assistive devices for ADLs

ADLs, activities of daily living.

3. Gout

- Gout, a systemic disease caused by the build-up of uric acid in the joints, causes inflammation, swelling, and pain. Hyperuricemia is defined as a urate level greater than 8 mg/dL in men and 7 mg/dL in women.

Incidence

- Gout has been known as "the disease of kings and the king of diseases," and can be traced to the time of Hippocrates. Gout occurs in approximately 1% of the population; the vast majority of these are men.

Clinical Presentation

- Pain in one joint of the lower extremity is the most common first symptom of gout. The initial period of pain, usually monarticular and self-limiting, is followed by a period in which the patient is completely asymptomatic.

- Termed *intercritical periods,* the time between acute gouty arthritis attacks may be 3 months to 2 years; the length of time shortens as the disease progresses.

- The first attack is typically at night or in the early morning.

- Gout commonly affects the ankle, heel, knee, wrist, finger, elbow, and instep. The most common site of the initial attack is the first metatarsophalangeal joint, and is known as *podagra*.

- The patient may experience fever, chills, and malaise during an acute gouty arthritis attack. Left untreated, the attack may last 1-2 weeks.

- The skin over the affected joint becomes red, hot, swollen, and tender. As the patient recovers from the attack, local desquamation may occur.

Pathophysiology

- Uric acid is the end product of purine metabolism (Figure 2).

- Xanthine oxidase is the rate-limiting step in the formation of uric acid.

- Uric acid, which serves no known biological function, has a body content of 1-1.2 grams.

Figure 2.

Ribose-uric acid pathway.

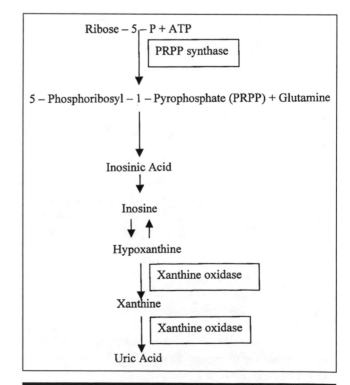

- Approximately 70% of uric acid is excreted via the kidneys.

- At physiologic pH, uric acid primarily exists as monosodium urate salt.

- Approximately 95% of serum uric acid is filtered across the glomerulus. Of this filtered amount, almost 100% is reabsorbed in the early part of the proximal tubule, only to be secreted back into the lumen in the more distal part of the tubule.

- Primary gout is a result of an innate defect in purine metabolism or uric acid excretion.
  * In this case, hyperuricemia may result from uric acid overproduction (in "overproducers"), impaired renal clearance of uric acid (in "underexcreters"), or a combination of both.
  * In rare instances, enzyme defects of either hypoxanthine guanine phosphoribosyltransferase (HGPRT) or phoribosyl-1-pyrophosphate (PRPP) may cause primary gout (Figure 2).

- Secondary gout is associated with increased nucleic acid turnover, decreased renal function, increased purine production, or drug-induced decreased elimination of uric acid.
  * Hematologic disorders that are lymphoproliferative and myeloproliferative in nature are known causes of secondary hyperuricemia.
  * Salicylates such as aspirin may inhibit tubular secretion of uric acid at low doses.
  * All diuretics, with the exception of spironolactone, may cause hyperuricemia.
  * Ethambutol, pyrazinamide, nicotinic acid, ethanol, niacin, and cyclosporine are known to cause an increase in serum uric acid.

- Acute gout attacks are caused by the deposition of monosodium urate crystals (MSU) in the synovium of the joint.

- This deposition results in the stimulation of the body's inflammatory cascade. The MSU crystals undergo phagocytosis by polymorphonuclear leukocytes. These leukocytes, damaged by the sharp crystals, burst and release their contents (interleukin-1, lysosomes, and prostaglandins) into the synovium. This results in the inflammatory reaction, ie, pain, swelling, and erythema.

- If left untreated, deposits of MSU crystals, also known as tophi, lead to joint deformity and disability. Ultimately, patients may develop one of two types of renal disease—urate nephropathy or uric acid nephropathy. Urate nephropathy results from the deposition of MSU crystals in the renal interstitium; uric acid nephropathy results from the deposition of uric acid in the collecting tubules.

Diagnostic Criteria

- The American Rheumatism Association lists the following criteria for the diagnosis of gout:
  * **Definite:** Sodium urate crystals in affected joint appear negatively birefringent when viewed through a polarized light source.
  * **Suggestive:** A minimum of six of the following criteria should be met.
    - More than one attack of arthritis
    - Development of maximum inflammation within 1 day
    - Oligoarthritis attack
    - Redness over joint
    - Painful or swollen first metatarsophalangeal joint
    - Unilateral attack on first metatarsophalangeal joint
    - Unilateral attack on tarsal joint
    - Tophus
    - Hyperuricemia
    - Asymptomatic swelling within a joint
  * It is also important to rule out **pseudogout.** In pseudogout, crystals deposited into the joint synovium cause intense pain and inflammation, but the culprit is calcium pyrophosphate dihydrate, not monosodium urate.

Treatment Goals

- Relieve pain and inflammation

- Reduce serum uric acid concentration

- Prevent recurrent gout attacks

Drug Therapy

- See Table 8.

Acute gouty arthritis attack

- There are three treatments available: colchicine, NSAIDs (indomethacin in particular), and corticosteroids. It is best to avoid treatments that affect serum uric acid concentrations during an acute attack.

Colchicine
Mechanism of action

- Colchicine inhibits the phagocytosis of urate crystals by leukocytes. Colchicine also inhibits the release of

Table 8

Drugs for the Treatment of Gout

Generic name (trade name)	Classification	Normal dose	Comments	Dosage forms
Colchicine	Anti-inflammatory	0.6 mg-1.2 mg PO every 1-2 hours until resolution of symptoms, severe GI symptoms occur, or a max of 8 mg reached	May be used for chronic suppressive therapy; must dose adjust for renal insufficiency	PO, IV
Probenecid (Benemid®)	Uricosuric agent	250 mg-500 mg bid	Avoid salycilates; take with plenty of water	PO
Sulfinpyrazone (Anturane®)	Uricosuric agent	50 mg-200 mg bid	Avoid salycilates; take with plenty of water	PO
Allopurinol (Zyloprim®)	Xanthine oxidase inhibitor	100 mg-300 mg qd	May cause rash; reduce dosage in renal failure	PO
Indomethacin (Indocin)	NSAID	50 mg tid-qid	May cause fluid retention, GI bleeding	PO, IV, supp

chemotactic factor, thus reducing the adhesion of polymorphonuclear leukocytes. The net result makes colchicine an anti-inflammatory agent without analgesic activity.

Patient instructions
- Patients should immediately stop taking colchicine once abdominal cramping and/or diarrhea occurs. Patients should never exceed a total of 8 mg during an acute gouty arthritis attack.

Adverse drug events
- Nausea, bloating, emesis, and diarrhea occur in up to 80% of patients taking colchicine. Rarely, it may cause bone marrow suppression. This effect occurs with a higher incidence in those patients with underlying renal or hepatic dysfunction. When colchicine is given intravenously, possible extravasation may cause local skin necrosis.

Drug-drug and drug-disease interactions
- Patients with active peptic ulcer disease should not take colchicine.

Parameters to monitor
- With long-term therapy, patients should have a serum creatinine test, liver function test, and complete white blood cell count checked periodically.

Dose
- For the treatment of an acute gouty arthritis attack, patients should take 0.6-1.2 mg orally every 2 hours until pain relief is achieved, diarrhea occurs, or a maximum dose of 8 mg is reached. When given intravenously, an initial dose of 2 mg is given fol-

lowed by two additional doses of 1 mg at 6-hour intervals. The dose should never exceed 4 mg.

Other
- Colchicine is most effective when initiated within 12-36 hours of the attack.

Indomethacin
- (Please see review of NSAIDs in RA section.) Indomethacin is the most extensively studied NSAID in the treatment of an acute gouty arthritis attack. Unlike colchicine, indomethacin is effective at any point during the acute attack.

Corticosteroids
- For the treatment of acute gout pain, corticosteroids are effective when given intra-articularly, intra-venously, or orally. Their use is limited to treatment failures of colchicine and NSAIDs. Intramuscular corticotropin (ACTH) is also effective when given (40U) to treat an acute gouty arthritis attack.

Gout prophylaxis (intercritical period)
- Patients with asymptomatic hyperuricemia should not be routinely treated with pharmacologic agents. These patients should undergo a work-up to determine the cause of hyperuricemia. The use of low-dose (0.6-1.2 mg/d) colchicine can prevent subsequent attacks of gout. Patients in the intercritical period (after an acute gouty arthritis attack) are candidates for long-term prophylactic therapy directed at affecting serum uric acid levels. Choice of therapy is based on the patient's pathophysiologic cause of hyperuricemia. Patients are generally classified as "overproducers" or "underexcreters." Placing the patient on a purine-restricted diet

and performing a 24-hour urine collection to measure uric acid concentration may identify overproducers of uric acid. Those patients who excrete more than 600 mg of uric acid are considered overproducers. Once this diagnosis is made, patients are treated with one of two classes of agents: xanthine oxidase inhibitors or uricosurics.

Benemid (probenecid)

Mechanism of action

- Probenecid is a uricosuric agent that promotes the excretion of uric acid by blocking its reuptake at the proximal convoluted tubule.

Patient instructions

- Patients should drink at least 2 liters of water per day in order to decrease the risk of uric acid stone formation. Patients should take probenecid with food if GI intolerance occurs.

Adverse drug events

- Probenecid is generally well-tolerated and is associated with very few adverse side effects. Up to 10% of patients receiving probenecid therapy develop uric acid stones. Probenecid may cause abdominal discomfort, but this is often avoided by taking it with food.

Drug-drug interactions

- Since probenecid prevents the tubular secretion of many weak organic acids, it has potential drug interactions, eg, the penicillins, cephalosporins, nitrofurantoin, and rifampin. Although the interaction between probenecid, penicillins, and cephalosporins has been utilized therapeutically, its interaction with nitrofurantoin reduces nitrofurantoin's effectiveness. Aspirin interferes with uric acid secretion and therefore should never be used in conjunction with probenecid. Additionally, the diuretic effects of furosemide and hydrochlorothiazide are magnified when probenecid is taken concomitantly. Finally, patients receiving sulfonylureas should be monitored closely for hypoglycemia when started on probenecid.

Other

- Patients should never begin uricosuric therapy during an acute gouty arthritis attack due to the risk of exacerbating the attack. Probenecid should not be used in patients with a creatinine clearance less than 50 mL/min.

Anturane (sulfinpyrazone)

Mechanism of action

- Sulfinpyrazone is a uricosuric agent that promotes the excretion of uric acid by blocking its reuptake at the proximal convoluted tubule.

Patient instructions

- Patients should drink at least 2 liters of water per day in order to decrease the risk of uric acid stone formation. Patients should take sulfinpyrazone with food if GI intolerance occurs. Patients who are sensitive to aspirin should not take this agent due to the risk of bronchoconstriction.

Adverse drug events

- Like probenecid, sulfinpyrazone is generally well-tolerated. The most common reported adverse effects are GI discomfort and uric acid stone formation. In addition, rarely it is has been associated with bone marrow suppression and immunoallergic interstitial nephritis.

Drug-drug interactions

- Sulfinpyrazone decreases the effectiveness of nitrofurantoin. When sulfinpyrazone is taken with aspirin, the effect of sulfinpyrazone is lessened.

Parameters to monitor

- Patients should have complete blood work periodically due to the rare risk of bone marrow suppression associated with sulfinpyrazone therapy.

Other

- Patients should never start uricosuric therapy during an acute gouty arthritis attack; it may exacerbate the attack. When increasing the dose of sulfinpyrazone, titrate upward slowly to minimize the risk of uric acid stone formation. Since uricosuric therapy may precipitate an acute gouty arthritis attack, patients should take an NSAID or colchicine for the first 6-12 months of therapy. Patients with a creatinine clearance of less than 50 mL/min should not use sulfinpyrazone.

Zyloprim (allopurinol)

Mechanism of action

- Allopurinol and its metabolite, oxypurinol, inhibit xanthine oxidase formation (XO), which is the rate-limiting step in uric acid synthesis. This facilitates the clearance of the more water soluble precursors of uric acid, oxypurines.

Patient instructions

- Patients should immediately report any signs of rash to their providers. Allopurinol should be taken with food to minimize GI discomfort.

Adverse drug events

- Allopurinol is generally well tolerated; the overall occurrence of adverse effects is less than 1%. Patients should be advised that rash, the most common adverse effect, might occur at any time during therapy. The rash may be as simple as a maculopapular eruption or as serious as the life-threatening Stevens-Johnson syndrome (which is exfoliative *and* erythematous). Rarely, allopurinol may cause alopecia, neutropenia, and hepatitis.

Drug-drug interactions

- The chemotherapeutic agents azathioprine and 6-mercaptopurine are metabolized via the xanthine oxidase pathway; therefore, allopurinol and its metabolite oxypurinol may increase serum levels of these agents. The concomitant administration of ampicillin or amoxicillin with allopurinol increases the risk of rash to approximately 20%.

Parameters to monitor

- Patients should be encouraged to report the first signs of rash to their physicians immediately. Patients should have serum creatinine as well as liver function tests drawn periodically.

Kinetics

- With a half-life of 30 hours, allopurinol is rapidly converted to its active metabolite (oxypurinol). This allows for once-daily dosing.

Other

- To reduce the risk of precipitating an acute gouty arthritis attack, allopurinol should be initiated at a dose of 100 mg per day and increased at 100-mg intervals weekly to an average dose of 300 mg per day. Patients with renal insufficiency require a dose adjustment. Assuming the target dose is 300 mg per day, patients with a creatinine clearance of 10-20 mL/min should receive 200 mg per day. Those with a clearance of less than 10 mL/minute should receive 100 mg per day.

Secondary hyperuricemia

- As discussed earlier, hyperuricemia may be caused by lymphoproliferative and myeloproliferative disorders, as well as their chemotherapeutic treatments (eg, tumor lysis syndrome). It is common to add allopurinol to the prescribed chemotherapeutic regimen to prevent complications of hyperuricemia, eg, an acute gouty arthritis attack. Elitek® (rasburicase) is a newly approved therapeutic agent used to prevent hyperuricemia in children with leukemia, lymphoma, and solid tumor malignancies. Rasburicase is a recombinant urate oxidase enzyme that converts uric acid to allantoin, thereby allowing it to be eliminated. Patients with G6PD deficiency should not use rasburicase.

4. Systemic Lupus Erythematosus

- SLE is a chronic autoimmune inflammatory disorder that can affect any system in the body, including the skin, joints, and internal organs.

Classification

- SLE is broken down into three types: (1) discoid lupus, which affects the skin; (2) drug-induced lupus, which generally resolves after discontinuing the offending medication; and (3) overlap syndrome, in which the patient has features that overlap with another rheumatic disease process.

Clinical Presentation

- Signs and symptoms consistent with SLE include:
  * Malar rash (a butterfly-shaped rash over the cheeks and across the bridge of the nose)
  * Discoid rash (scaly, disk-shaped sores on the face, neck, and/or chest)
  * Photosensitivity
  * Oral ulcers
  * Arthritis
  * Serositis (inflammation of the lining around the heart, lungs, and/or abdomen that causes pain and shortness of breath)
  * Proteinuria
  * Central nervous system problems
  * Antinuclear antibodies (autoantibodies that react against the body's own cells)
  * Anemia
  * Fatigue
  * Fever
  * Skin rash
  * Muscle aches
  * Nausea
  * Vomiting and diarrhea
  * Anorexia
  * Raynaud's phenomenon
  * Weight loss

- Patients typically present with chronic fatigue and depression. Dermatitis and arthritis (in multiple joints) are the most common clinical manifestations. The arthritic pain patients describe is generally out of proportion to the amount of synovitis present. Although it is rare, serious renal abnormalities can occur in patients with SLE. Central nervous system involvement, also rare, can be serious. Lupus-related encephalopathy may occur due to scarring of arterioles in the subcortical white matter. In addition, patients with SLE are at risk of stroke due to the thomboembolic nature of the antiphospholipid antibody.

Pathophysiology

- The exact pathophysiology of SLE remains unknown. It is an autoimmune disease (type III hypersensitivity) in which patients have an overactivity of B cells. The result is hypergammaglobulinemia that ultimately precipitates immune complexes on the vascular membranes, thereby causing activation of complement. Drugs, procainamide being the most predominant, may also cause SLE. Other such medications include phenytoin, chlorpromazine, hydralazine, quinidine, methyldopa, and isoniazid.

Diagnostic Criteria

- See Table 9.

Therapy

- Therapy for each case of SLE is based on the particular symptoms of any given patient. Arthritis is commonly treated with NSAIDs or glucocorticoids. Dermatologic complications can be treated with hydroxychloroquine (see RA section). Thrombocytopenia generally responds to glucocorticoid therapy. Refractory cases may respond to cyclophosphamide therapy and/or splenectomy. Finally, plasmopheresis has been used with some degree of success.

Table 9

Criteria for Diagnosing Systemic Lupus Erythematosus

1. Characteristic rash across the cheek(s)
2. Discoid lesion rash
3. Photosensitivity
4. Oral ulcers
5. Arthritis
6. Inflammation of membranes in lungs, heart, or abdomen
7. Evidence of kidney disease
8. Evidence of severe neurologic disease
9. Blood disorders, including low red blood cell, white blood cell, and platelet counts
10. Immunologic abnormalities
11. Positive antinuclear antibody (ANA)

Note: A patient must experience four of the criteria before a classification of SLE can be made. These criteria, proposed by the American College of Rheumatology, should not be the sole characteristics for diagnosis, however.

5. Key Points

- Rheumatoid arthritis (RA), a highly variable, autoimmune disease characterized by symmetric, erosive synovitis, often affects extra-articular sites.

- RA usually affects diarthrodial joints, eg, the proximal interphalangeal (PIP) joints, metacarpophalangeal (MCP) joints, metatarsophalangeal (MTP) joints, wrists, and ankles. Also commonly involved are the elbows, shoulders, sternoclavicular joints, temporomandibular joints, hips, and knees.

- Morning stiffness is the hallmark of RA.

- According to the American College of Rheumatology, the goals in managing RA are to prevent or control joint damage, prevent loss of function, and decrease pain.

- The American College of Rheumatology recommends the use of DMARDs within 3 months of diagnosis of RA.

- Unlike the NSAIDs, DMARDs have the ability to reduce or prevent joint damage, joint integrity, and joint function. DMARDs carry the risk of various toxicities and they must be monitored on a regular basis.

- Osteoarthritis is the most common form of arthritis in the United States.

- Joint stiffness, a common complaint in osteoarthritis, differs from RA in that it is relatively short in duration and resolves with movement.

- Unlike RA, pain relief is the primary treatment goal in osteoarthritis. The initial drug of choice is acetaminophen.

- Gout, a systemic disease caused by the build-up of uric acid in the joints, causes inflammation, swelling, and pain.

- Primary gout is a result of an innate defect in purine metabolism or uric acid excretion.

- Patients with gout are classified as overproducers or underexcreters based on measuring 24-hour uric acid concentration levels.

- Treatment of an acute gouty arthritis attack involves the use of colchicine, NSAIDs, or glucocorticoids.

- Uricosuric agents and/or xanthine oxidase inhibitors are used to prevent further gout attacks. These agents should not be used during an acute gouty arthritis attack.

- Systemic lupus erythematosus is a chronic autoimmune inflammatory disorder that can affect any system in the body.

- Therapy for SLE is primarily driven by the clinical manifestations of the disease.

6. Questions and Answers

A 45-year-old man presents to his local physician with a complaint of extreme stiffness in the morning that lasts until noon on most days. He also states that he feels "drained" all the time and both of his knees are swollen and painful. Upon examination, the physician documents the presence of rheumatoid nodules. The patient's laboratory work-up is significant for thrombocytopenia and a positive rheumatoid factor. He states that he has been taking over-the-counter ibuprofen at a dose of 200 mg 2-3 times daily without relief.

1. Which of the following represents the best drug therapy option for this patient?
    A. Increase dose of ibuprofen to 800 mg three times daily
    B. Increase dose of ibuprofen and add methotrexate 25 mg twice daily
    C. Increase dose of ibuprofen and add celecoxib 100 mg twice daily
    D. Increase dose of ibuprofen and add leflunomide at a dose of 100 mg daily for 3 days followed by 20 mg daily

2. Which of the following represents the best way to decrease potential liver toxicity with methotrexate while achieving optimal therapeutic benefit?

    A. Add 1-3 mg of folic acid per day to the patient's regimen
    B. Decrease the dose of methotrexate to 25 mg once monthly
    C. Add monthly injections of leucovorin to the patient's regimen
    D. Add leflunomide to the patient's regimen

3. As combination DMARD therapy may be more efficacious in the refractory RA population, which of the following represents the BEST choice for combination therapy?

    A. Arava 20 mg once daily + Rheumatrex 25 mg once weekly
    B. Remicade 3 mg/kg IM + Rheumatrex 25 mg once weekly
    C. Myochrysine IM + Plaquenil 200 mg twice daily
    D. Remicade 3 mg/kg IV + Rheumatrex 25 mg once weekly

4. A physician inquires about the recommended monitoring parameters for patients started on Ridaura. Which of the following represents the most appropriate response?

   A. Baseline ophthalmologic exam, CBC, and serum creatinine, followed by a yearly CBC, serum creatinine, and ophthalmologic exam
   B. Baseline liver function tests, CBC, and albumin, followed by monthly liver function tests
   C. Baseline CBC, serum creatinine, and urine dipstick for protein, followed by a CBC and urine dipstick for protein every 1-2 months
   D. There are no recommended monitoring parameters at this time

5. All of the following represent methods used to decrease the GI toxicity associated with NSAIDs except:

   A. Changing patients from a nonselective cyclooxygenase inhibitor to a type II specific inhibitor such as Celebrex
   B. Adding a proton pump inhibitor such as Prevacid to the patient's NSAID
   C. Adding Cytotec to the patient's NSAID
   D. Instructing the patient to take his/her NSAID at night, when acid secretion is limited

6. Which of the following is(are) true concerning diclofenac?

   I. It is available as an extended release product, Voltaren XR
   II. It is available as an injectable product, Voltaren IM
   III. It is available in combination with misoprostol, Arthotec

   A. I only
   B. I and II only
   C. I, II, and III
   D. I and III only

7. Which of the following would be a contraindication for the use of Enbrel?

   A. Renal insufficiency
   B. Active infection
   C. Persons over the age of 65
   D. Patients with congestive heart failure

8. Regarding therapies designed to target tumor necrosis factor and interleukin-1 in the treatment

of RA, the following statements are correct EXCEPT:

   A. Kineret is packaged as a single-use prefilled syringe that should be kept in the refrigerator.
   B. Patients should have a tuberculin skin test completed before initiating Enbrel or Remicade.
   C. Kineret is a soluble receptor that binds tumor necrosis factor.
   D. Enbrel is approved for use as a single agent.

9. The use of glucocorticoids is associated with numerous adverse effects and long-term consequences. All of the following are initiatives to treat and/or prevent/minimize these adverse effects EXCEPT:

   A. Instruct patients to take the glucocorticoid once daily versus dividing the total daily dose into two to four doses.
   B. Instruct patients on long-term therapy to add 1500 mg of elemental calcium and 400-800 IU of ergocalciferol to their regimen.
   C. Suggest adding a bisphosphonate to their therapy.
   D. Inform patients that stopping glucocorticoid abruptly is contraindicated.

10. A young lady enters your pharmacy and informs you that she is planning on becoming pregnant and would like you to review her medication profile to see if any would be potentially harmful. Upon review of her profile, you notice that she is taking Arava for RA. Which is the most appropriate response?

   A. Arava is a category C drug, and could potentially harm the fetus. She should discuss the risks and benefits of becoming pregnant with her physician first.
   B. Arava is a category X drug, and she should undergo the drug-elimination procedure with cholestyramine before trying to become pregnant.
   C. Arava is a category X drug with no active metabolites and a short half-life; therefore she should discontinue the drug and wait 1-2 weeks before trying to become pregnant.
   D. Arava is a category B drug and the risk of toxicity to the fetus is extremely low.

11. R.Y. is a 67-year-old man with chief complaints of a swollen big left toe and extreme pain. The area is erythematous and tender. Laboratory analysis reveals a uric acid level of 10 mg/dL.

Review of R.Y.'s past medical history reveals hypertension and congestive heart failure. A diagnosis of gout is made. Which is the best choice for the treatment of R.Y.'s acute gouty arthritis attack?

A. Probenecid 500 mg now followed by 500 mg twice daily
B. Indomethacin 50 mg now followed by 50 mg three to four times daily
C. Allopurinol 100 mg once daily
D. Colchicine 0.6 mg every hour until resolution of symptoms, development of diarrhea, or a cumulative dose of 8 mg is reached

12. The following comments are consistent with the diagnosis of gout EXCEPT:

A. The presence of negatively birefringent crystals in the affected synovial joint fluid
B. The presence of calcium pyrophosphate in the affected synovial joint fluid
C. Presence of tophi
D. Presence of hyperuricemia

13. Which of the following best describes Benemid?

A. Like allopurinol, it decreases the body's production of uric acid.
B. Like Anturane, it is a uricosuric agent that aids in the tubular reabsorption of uric acid.
C. It blocks the excretion of uric acid in the urine.
D. Like Anturane, it is a uricosuric agent that blocks reuptake of uric acid at the proximal convoluted tubule.

14. Which of the following represents a therapeutically ineffective combination that should be avoided?

A. Benemid + penicillin G
B. Benemid + aspirin (>2 g per day)
C. Anturane + Macrobid
D. Benemid + colchicine

15. All of the following statements are true regarding Zyloprim EXCEPT:

A. It works to decrease the formation of uric acid by inhibiting xanthine oxidase.
B. It does not require dosage adjustment in patients with renal insufficiency.
C. Skin reactions, including Stevens-Johnson syndrome, have been reported with its use.

D. It should not be used for the treatment of an acute gouty arthritis attack.

16. Which of the following represent potentially dangerous drug interactions with Zyloprim?

I. Amoxicillin
II. Imuran
III. Essidrex

A. I only
B. I and II only
C. I, II, and III
D. III only

17. All of the following are consistent with the diagnosis of osteoarthritis EXCEPT:

A. Presence of morning stiffness that is not associated with immobility and may last for several hours
B. Pain is a common initial finding that typically worsens with weight-bearing activity and subsides with rest
C. It commonly occurs in the knees or the hips
D. Crepitus is common.

18. Which of the following medications is(are) suggested for the treatment of osteoarthritis by the American College of Rheumatology?

I. Tylenol
II. Capsaicin
III. Glucosamine sulfate and chondroitin

A. All of the above
B. II only
C. III only
D. I and II only

19. Concerning treatment of osteoarthritis, which of the following statements is incorrect?

A. Tylenol is generally considered the initial drug of choice.
B. Tylenol is considered safe and effective, and has minimal adverse effects, especially in doses greater than 4 g per day.
C. Muscle-strengthening exercises may be helpful.
D. Hyaluronic acid derivatives have been approved by the FDA for the treatment of pain associated with osteoarthritis.

20. The following medications are considered to be DMARDs EXCEPT:

A. Plaquenil
B. Cuprimine
C. Myochrysine
D. Nalfon

Answers

1. **D.** Although the patient currently has room to increase his dose of NSAID, he is demonstrating signs and symptoms of systemic RA. This indicates that the addition of DMARD therapy is necessary. Methotrexate represents a viable option; however, the dose of 25 mg twice daily is excessive (it should be dosed once weekly). The addition of leflunomide is the best choice.

2. **A.** The addition of folic acid to the methotrexate regimen has been demonstrated to reduce the risk of liver toxicity. Lowering the dose of methotrexate is likely to decrease risk, but is also likely to decrease its effectiveness. Leucovorin, an injectable formulation of folate, is used only to reverse methotrexate toxicity.

3. **D.** Arava plus methotrexate may be a very efficacious combination, but it increases the risk of liver toxicity significantly. Gold therapy in combination with Plaquenil increases the risk of rash. Remicade, only approved for use in combination with Rheumatrex, is given IV and not IM; this combination represents the best choice.

4. **C.** Gold therapy is associated with glomerulonephritis, thrombocytopenia, and leukopenia; therefore, a baseline renal evaluation and periodic testing should occur during the entire course of therapy.

5. **D.** Adding a proton pump inhibitor, Cytotec, or changing to a selective COX-II inhibitor has been demonstrated to lower the risk of significant GI adverse effects. Timing of the dose of an NSAID has never been demonstrated to affect the risk of GI toxicity.

6. **D.** Diclofenac is available as an immediate-release product, an extended-release product, and in combination with misoprostol. It is not available in an injectable formulation.

7. **B.** Due to its effects on tumor necrosis factor, Enbrel may decrease a patient's ability to fight infection. Enbrel is contraindicated in patients with an active infection. Its use should be temporarily discontinued until the acute process has resolved.

8. **C.** Kineret targets interleukin-1, not tumor necrosis factor. Kineret is available as a single-use prefilled syringe. Unlike Remicade, Enbrel is approved as monotherapy.

9. **A.** Patients taking glucocorticoids are at risk of developing osteoporosis. Efforts to minimize this adverse effect include the addition of calcium and vitamin D to the patient's regimen as well as adding a bisphosphonate, eg, Fosamax, to suppress bone resorption. Due to adrenal suppression that occurs with long-term glucocorticoid therapy, patients should taper off the agent.

10. **B.** Since Arava is a teratogenic agent with an active, long half-life metabolite, a drug-elimination procedure should be performed before becoming pregnant.

11. **D.** Both Probenecid and allopurinol may exacerbate an acute gouty arthritis attack and should only be reserved for the prevention of further attacks. Indomethacin is an option for the treatment of an acute gouty arthritis attack; however, due to NSAIDs' tendency to cause fluid retention in the renal tubules, it would not be the ideal agent in a patient with congestive heart failure. Colchicine represents the best option from this list.

12. **B.** The presence of calcium pyrophosphate is consistent with the diagnosis of pseudogout, not gout.

13. **D.** Benemid is a uricosuric agent that blocks reuptake of uric acid at the proximal convoluted tubule. It does not affect the body's ability to produce uric acid. Response B is incorrect because Benemid does not promote the reabsorption of uric acid.

14. **C.** Benemid does prevent the tubular secretion of penicillin. However, this interaction is therapeutically utilized to increase the duration of action of a single dose of penicillin. Although low doses of aspirin may inhibit the tubular secretion of uric acid, larger doses (>2 g per day) do not have the same effect. The combination of Benemid and colchicine (marketed under the trade name Colbenemid) has been therapeutically utilized to prevent the manifestation of an acute gouty arthritis attack.

Finally, a combination of Anturane and Macrobid will inhibit Macrobid from reaching its site of action, thus diminishing its therapeutic efficacy.

15. **B.** Zyloprim must be adjusted in patients with renal insufficiency. Its use has been associated with serious skin reactions that may occur at any point during therapy. Zyloprim should never be used in the treatment of an acute gouty arthritis attack.

16. **B.** The co-administration of amoxicillin and allopurinol increases the risk of rash up to 20%. Imuran is metabolized via xanthine oxidase, whose activity is inhibited by allopurinol. This increases the risk of toxicity associated with Imuran. Although Essidrex may increase uric acid levels, there is no direct drug-drug interaction associated with allopurinol.

17. **A.** The morning stiffness associated with osteoarthritis is usually of short duration, is associated with periods of inactivity, and resolves with movement.

18. **D.** Both Tylenol and capsaicin are effective and recommended by the American College of Rheumatology as treatment options for osteoarthritis. Although there is some clinical data to support its use, glucosamine sulfate and chondroitin are not currently recommended by the American College of Rheumatology.

19. **B.** Tylenol is generally considered to be safe and effective; however, its use is associated with hepatic failure and the rare incidence of renal failure. Patients should be advised to take LESS than 4 g per day to limit the risk of hepatic failure.

20. **D.** Nalfon, also known as fenoprofen, is an NSAID, not a DMARD.

7. References

Rheumatoid arthritis
Boyce EG. Rheumatoid arthritis. In: Herfindal ET, Gourley DR, et al, eds. *Textbook of Therapeutic Drugs and Disease Management*, 7th ed. Baltimore: Lippincott Williams & Wilkins; 2000:641-666.

Goekoop YP, Allaart CF, Breedveld FC, et al. Combination therapy in rheumatoid arthritis. *Curr Opin Rheumatol.* 2001;30:249-254.

Kremer JM. Rational use of new and existing disease-modifying agents in rheumatoid arthritis. *Ann Intern Med.* 2001;134:695-706.

Kwoh CK, Anderson LG, Greene JM, et al. Guidelines for the management of rheumatoid arthritis. *Arthritis Rheum.* 2002;46:328-346.

Sims RW, Kwoh CK, Anderson LG, et al. Guidelines for monitoring drug therapy in rheumatoid arthritis. *Arthritis Rheum.* 1996;39:723-731.

Schuna AA, Schmidt MJ, Pigarelli DW. Rheumatoid arthritis. In: Dipiro JT, Talbert RL, et al, eds. *Pharmacotherapy: A Pathophysiologic Approach*, 4th ed. New York: McGraw-Hill; 1997:1427-1440.

Wolfe F, Rehman W, Lane NE, et al. Starting a disease-modifying antirheumatic drug or a biologic agent in rheumatoid arthritis: Standards of practice for RA treatment. *J Rheumatol.* 2001;28:1704-1711.

Osteoarthritis
Altman RD, Hochberg MC, Moskowitz RW, et al. Recommendations for the medical management of osteoarthritis of the hip and knee. *Arthritis Rheum.* 2000;43:1905-1915.

Boh LE. Osteoarthritis. In: Dipiro JT, Talbert RL, et al, eds. *Pharmacotherapy: A Pathophysiologic Approach*, 4th ed. New York: McGraw-Hill; 1997:1441-1459.

Roberts LJ, Morrow JD. Analgesic-antipyretic and antiinflammatory agents and drugs employed in the treatment of gout. In: Hardman JG, Limbird LE, et al, eds. *Goodman and Gilman's The Pharmacological Basis of Therapeutics*, 10th ed. New York: McGraw-Hill; 2001:687-732.

Whitaker AL, Small RE. Osteoarthritis. In: Herfindal ET, Gourley DR, et al, eds. *Textbook of Therapeutic Drug and Disease Management*, 7th ed. Baltimore: Lippincott Williams & Wilkins; 2000:667-678.

Gout

American College of Rheumatology Fact Sheet 2000. Gout. http://www.rheumatology.org/patients/factsheet/gout.html.

Emmerson BT. The management of gout. *N Engl J Med.* 1996;334:445-451.

Hawkins DW, Rahn DW. Gout and hyperuricemia. In: Dipiro JT, Talbert RL et al, eds. *Pharmacotherapy: A Pathophysiologic Approach*, 4th ed. New York: McGraw-Hill; 1997:1460-1465.

Kelley WN, Schumaker HR, Jr. Gout. In: *Textbook of Rheumatology*, 6th ed. Philadelphia: WB Saunders; 2001.

Maloley PA, Westfall GR. Gout and hyperuricemia. In: Herfindal ET, Gourley DR, et al, eds. *Textbook of Therapeutic Drug and Disease Management*, 7th ed. Baltimore: Lippincott Williams & Wilkins; 2000:679-690.

Terkeltaub RA, Edwards NL, Pratt PW, et al. Gout. In: Klippel JH, ed. *Primer on the Rheumatic Diseases,* 11th ed. Atlanta: Arthritis Foundation; 1998:230-243.

Systemic lupus erythematosus

Burlingame MB, Delafuente JC. Systemic lupus erythematosus. In: Dipiro JT, Talbert RL, et al, eds. *Pharmacotherapy: A Pathophysiologic Approach,* 4th ed. New York: McGraw-Hill; 1997:1378-1392.

Fuller SH, Camara C. Systemic lupus erythematosus. In: Herfindal ET, Gourley DR, et al, eds. *Textbook of Therapeutic Drug and Disease Management*, 7th ed. Baltimore: Lippincott Williams & Wilkins; 2000:691-708.

The Lupus Foundation of America. Lupus. http://www.lupus.org/.

23. Pain Management and Migraines

Elizabeth S. Miller, PharmD
Assistant Professor, Department of Pharmacy
University of Tennessee College of Pharmacy

Contents

1. Pain

Definitions

- *Pain:* any unpleasant sensory and emotional experience associated with actual or potential tissue damage, or defined in terms of such damage or both.

- Chronic pain is a largely unrecognized problem in American society.
  - Currently, about 75 million individuals suffer from some form of chronic benign pain.
  - Between one-third and one-half of chronic pain sufferers have pain severe enough to require daily medication.

Types and Clinical presentation

- Pain can be classified as either acute, chronic benign, or malignant.

- Acute pain is caused by an injury, illness, or surgery.
  - Acute pain responds to medications and usually resolves when the underlying cause has been treated or healed.
  - It is often associated with physiologic symptoms such as tachycardia, hypertension, diaphoresis, and mydriasis.

- Chronic benign pain exists beyond an expected time for healing, typically 3-6 months or more.
  - It is often associated with psychological effects including social isolation, depression, and anxiety.
  - Chronic pain syndromes are often not responsive to traditional analgesics and require the use of adjuvant medications.

- Malignant pain may be acute, chronic, or intermittent and is often related to cancer progression or chemotherapy.

- Pain is also defined by source. Such a classification divides pain into somatic, visceral, and neuropathic pain.

- Somatic pain originates from the skin, muscles, tendons, ligaments, and bones.
  - Somatic pain is localized and described as sharp, stabbing, throbbing, or aching in nature.
  - While somatic pain can be severe, it tends to respond well to treatment with opioids.

- The body's internal organs such as the liver, intestines, or stomach generate visceral pain.

- Visceral pain tends to be poorly localized and more likely to generate referred pain felt some distance away from the actual problem.
  - Opioids are not as effective for visceral pain as they are for somatic pain.

- Neuropathic pain results when the nerves themselves are damaged.
  - Neuropathic pain is typically burning in nature, although it may also be numb, aching, or cause a sensation like an electric shock.
  - Opioid medications are often ineffective for treating neuropathic pain and adjuvant analgesics play a significant role in treatment.

Pathophysiology

- Nociception, the pain sensation, begins when a sensory nerve ending is stimulated and sends repetitive signals to the spinal cord along ascending nerve fibers. An individual nerve does not transmit directly to the brain, but instead connects to secondary nerves in the dorsal horn of the spinal cord. The secondary nerves eventually connect to nerve cells in the brain stem.

- A descending antinociceptive pathway also exists. Neurotransmitters from the descending fibers inhibit the transmission of the pain signal. Opioids chemically resemble these neurotransmitters.

- Chronic pain is not a prolonged version of acute pain. As pain signals are repeatedly generated, neural pathways undergo changes that make them hypersensitive to pain signals and resistant to antinociceptive input.

Diagnostic Criteria

- The individual's self-report of pain is the primary source of information in acute pain.

- Chronic pain assessment should include a detailed history of the pain's intensity and characteristics, a physical examination emphasizing the neurological exam, and a psychosocial assessment (Figure 1).

- The purpose of diagnostic tests, such as x-rays, CT or MRI scans, or laboratory tests differs between chronic benign pain and acute pain or malignant pain.
  - In cancer patients, the major purpose is to visualize the disease progression.
  - In chronic benign pain, the major purpose of diagnostic testing is to rule out the presence of

Figure 1.

Algorithm for comprehensive evaluation and management of chronic pain.

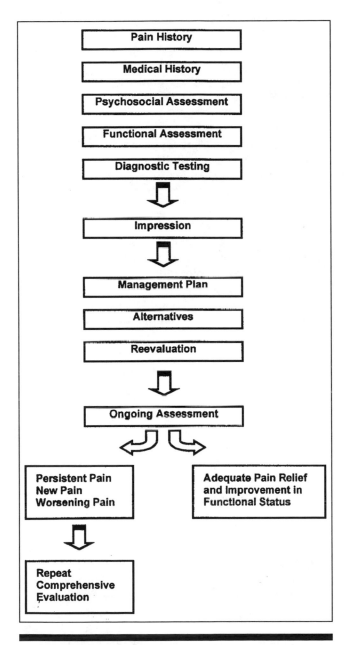

From the Pain Management Center of Paducah, Paducah, KY. Used with permission.

any diseases for which there is a curative treatment.

Goals of Pain Management

Acute pain
- The goal in acute pain management is to provide the patient with pain relief that allows them to rest comfortably and to rehabilitate their surgery or injury. This can be accomplished with short-acting prn medications.

Malignant pain
- A major goal of cancer pain management is to relieve the patient's pain without inducing disabling side effects.

- The World Health Organization has developed a three-step hierarchy for analgesic pain management in cancer pain patients (Figure 2). In general, this includes using nonopioid analgesics as a baseline, supplementing with opioid analgesics as needed, and adding adjunctive medications when appropriate.

- Cancer patients may suffer from constant pain that continues for months or years. For this reason, treat-

Figure 2.

The WHO's three-step hierarchy for analgesic pain management in cancer patients.

Reproduced with permission from WHO, 1996.

ment with long-acting agents is more appropriate than treatment with short-acting medications. However, short-acting agents, referred to as "break-through" or "rescue" doses, are often available in addition to the long-acting medications.

Chronic benign pain
- The goal of chronic benign pain treatment is to restore the patient to the highest degree of function possible.

- Multimodal therapy, the use of several different types of treatment, is usually required. Multimodal therapies include nerve blocks, rehabilitation, physical therapy, pharmacotherapy, acupuncture, and psychotherapy.

- Basic pharmacotherapy follows the World Health Organization guidelines for treating cancer pain (Figure 2). Analgesics are categorized into nonopioid analgesics, opioid analgesics, and adjuvant analgesics.

- Nonopioid analgesics such as acetaminophen and nonsteroidal anti-inflammatory drugs (NSAIDs) relieve all types of mild to moderate pain.
  * Unless contraindicated, all pain patients should be first be given a trial of nonopioid analgesics.
  * Nonopioids and opioids relieve pain via different mechanisms. Thus, combination therapy offers the potential for improved relief with fewer side effects.
  * Nonopioids do not produce tolerance, physical dependence, or addiction.

- Adjuvant analgesics are drugs with a primary indication other than pain. Commonly used analgesic adjuvants include antiepileptic drugs, tricyclic antidepressants, and local anesthetics.

Principles of opioid use
- Opioids have no ceiling effect of analgesia.

- Oral medications should be used whenever possible. Intramuscular injections are painful and should be avoided.

- When patients have constant or near-constant pain, analgesics should be given around the clock. This is often accomplished with the use of long-acting opioid analgesics.

- The use of short-acting opioids as rescue medication is controversial in chronic benign pain. If allowed, doses of rescue medications should range from 10-15% of the total daily long-acting opioid dose.

- Mixed agonist-antagonist opioids are not used in chronic pain. They may induce a withdrawal syndrome in patients tolerant to opioids.

Drug Therapy

Mechanism of action
Opioid receptors
- Morphine and other opioid agonists are thought to produce analgesia by mimicking the action of endogenous opioid peptides that bind at opioid receptors in the antinociceptive pathway.

- Opioid receptors are located in the CNS, pituitary gland, and GI tract. They are abundant in the periaqueductal gray matter of the brain and the dorsal horn of the spinal cord, two areas that are very active in pain reduction.

- When a drug binds to one of these receptors as an agonist, it produces analgesia. When a drug binds to one of these receptors as an antagonist, analgesia and other effects are blocked.

- The three major types of opioid receptor sites involved in analgesia are mu (μ), kappa (κ), and delta (δ).
  * Binding to the μ receptor produces analgesia, sedation, euphoria, respiratory depression, physical dependence, constipation, and other effects.
  * Activation of the κ receptor produces analgesia and respiratory depression. In addition, psychotomimetic effects such as anxiety, strange thoughts, nightmares, and hallucinations are more common.
  * Activation of δ receptors produces analgesia without many adverse events. However, there is no available δ receptor agonist.

Opioid analgesics
- Opioids are classified by activity at the receptor site, ie, they are classified as pure opioid agonists, agonist-antagonists, or pure opioid antagonists.

- Pure opioid agonists primarily activate μ receptors, although they may produce some κ receptor activation (Table 1).
  * Pure opioid agonists are the most clinically useful opioid analgesics.
  * Morphine is the prototypical pure opioid agonist.
  * Methadone is an opioid agonist with additional antagonist activity at the NMDA receptor. The NMDA receptor is believed to be active primarily in chronic pain.

Table 1

Starting Doses for Strong Opioids for Severe Pain in Adults

Generic name	Common product name and strength	Dosing interval (h)	IV starting dose (mg)		Oral starting dose
			IV	Oral	
Pure mu agonists					
Fentanyl (synthetic)	Injection (INJ): Sublimaze® 50 µg/mL Transdermal (TD): Duragesic® 25, 50, 75, 100 µg/h Transmucosal lozenge (LOZ): Actiq® 200, 400, 600, 800, 1200, 1600 µg; Oralet® 100, 200, 300, 400 µg	INJ: 0.5-2 TD: q 2-3 days LOZ: prn	0.1	Not available	Transmucosal: Start with 100 to 200 µg and titrate to effect
Hydromorphone (semisynthetic)	Dilaudid®: Tablet: 2, 4, 8 mg Liquid: 1 mg/mL Injection: 1, 2, 4 mg/mL and HP 10 mg/mL Suppository: 3 mg	PO/PR 3-6; IV 6-8	1.5	7.5	4-8
Levorphanol (semisynthetic)	Levo-Dromoran®: Tablet: 2 mg Injection: 2 mg/mL	PO 6-8 IV 3-4 IM/SC 6-8	2	4	2-4
Meperidine (synthetic)	Demerol®: Tablet: 50 mg Liquid: 10 mg/mL Injection: 25, 50, 75, 100 mg/mL	3-4	75	300	50-150
Methadone (synthetic)	Tablet: Dolophine®/Methadose® 5, 10 mg; Methadose 40 mg dispersible Liquid: Methadone 2, 5, 10 mg/mL; Methadose 10 mg/mL Injection: Methadone 10 mg/mL	3-8	Not available 10 acute; 2-4 chronic	20 acute, 2-4 chronic	5-10
Morphine (natural)	Tablet: MSIR® 15, 30 mg Liquid: Roxanol®/MSIR 2, 4 mg, 20, 100 mg/mL Injection: 0.5, 1, 2, 4, 8, 10, 15, 25, 50 mg/mL Controlled Release: Oramorph SR® 15, 30, 60, 100 mg; MS Contin® 15, 30, 60, 100, 200 mg; Kadian® 20, 30, 50, 60, 100 mg; Avinza® 30, 60, 90, 120 mg	2-4 Oramorph SR 6-8 MS Contin 8-12 Kadian 12-24 Avinza 24	10	30	15-30
Oxycodone (semisynthetic)	Capsule: OxyIR® 5 mg Tablet: Roxicodone® 5, 15, 30 mg Liquid: Roxicodone 1, 20 mg/mL; OxyFAST® 20 mg/mL Oxycodone/acetaminophen tablet: (mg): Percocet® 2.5/325, 5/325, 7.5/325, 10/325; Roxicet® 5/325, 5/500, Tylox® 5/500 Controlled release tablet: OxyContin® 10, 20, 40, 80 mg	3-4 OxyContin 8-12	Not available	20	15-30
Oxymorphone (semisynthetic)	Injection: 1, 1.5 mg/mL Suppository: Numorphan® 5 mg	3-6	1	10 rectal	Not available

- Mixed agonist-antagonists bind as agonists at the κ receptor, producing weak analgesia. They bind as weak antagonists at the µ receptor (Table 2).
  * The result is more dysphoria and psychotomimetic effects with a lower risk of respiratory depression.
- Pentazocine is the prototypical agonist-antagonist opioid.

Table 2

Opioid Dosing for Mild to Moderate Pain in Adults

Generic name	Common product name and strength	Dosing interval (h)	IV starting dose (mg)	Oral starting dose (mg)
Moderate-mild opioids				
Codeine (natural)	Tablet: 15, 30, 60 mg (CII)			
	Codeine/acetaminophen tablet: Tylenol with Codeine® #1 = 300/7.5, #2 = 300/15, #3 = 300/30, #4 = 300/60 mg	4-6	15-30	30-60
	Liquid: 5 mg/mL			
	Injection: 30, 60 mg/mL			
Hydrocodone (semisynthetic)	Hydrocodone/APAP Tablet (mg): Vicodin® 5/500; Vicodin ES® 7.5/750; Lorcet® or Vicodin HP® 10/650; Lortab® 2.5/500, 5/500, 7.5/500, 10/500; Norco® 5/325, 7.5/325, 10/325	4-8	Not available	5-10
	Hydrocodone/ibuprofen tablet (mg): Vicoprofen® 7.5/200			
Propoxyphene (synthetic)	Propoxyphene/acetaminophen tablet (mg): Darvocet N® 50 (50/325), Darvocet N® 100 (100/650)	4-6	Not available	65-130; max 600 mg/day
	Capsule: Darvon® 32, 65 mg			
Agonists-antagonists				
Pentazocine	Pentazocine 50/naloxone 0.5 mg tablet: Talwin NX®		30-60 mg; max	50-100; max
	Pentazocine 12.5/aspirin 325 tablet: Talwin Compound®	3-4	360 mg/day	600 mg/day
	Injection: 30 mg/mL			
Butorphanol	Injection: Stadol® 1, 2 mg/mL	3-4	IV 0.5-2 mg	Not available
	Nasal spray: Stadol NS® 10 mg/mL		NS 1 mg followed by 2nd dose in 60-90 min prn	
Nalbuphine	Injection: Nubain® 10, 20 mg/mL	3-6	10	Not available
Buprenorphine	Injection: Buprenex® 0.3 mg/mL	6-8	0.3-0.6	Not available
Dezocine	Injection: Dalgan® 5, 10, 15 mg/mL	IM 3-6; IV 2-4	5-20 mg IV; 2.5-10 mg IV	Not available
Miscellaneous				
Tramadol	Tablet: Ultram® 50 mg	4-6	Not available	50-100; max
	Tramadol/acetaminophen tablet: Ultracet® 325/37.5 mg			400 mg/day

* Buprenorphine is actually a partial agonist at μ and κ receptors. This opioid has limited efficacy in pain management and is primarily used in detoxification programs.

• Opioid antagonists block the μ and κ receptors (Table 3).
   * These drugs do not produce analgesia. They are used to reverse respiratory and CNS depression caused by overdose with opioid agonists.
   * Naloxone and naltrexone are opioid antagonists.

Opioid analgesic adverse effects
Central nervous system

• Opioids produce a number of CNS effects including sedation, euphoria, dysphoria, changes in mood, and mental clouding. Confusion, disorientation, and cognitive impairment are also possible.

• Chronic sedation can be treated with CNS stimulants such as methylphenidate or dextroamphetamine. Modafinil also promotes daytime wakefulness.

• Mild to moderate muscle jerks are common in patients on high doses of opioids. Myoclonus can be

Table 3

Opioid Antagonists

Generic name	Common product name and strength	Dosing interval (h)	IV starting dose (mg)	Oral starting dose (mg)
Naloxone	Injection: Narcan® 0.02, 0.4, 1 mg/mL	Every 2-3 min	Opioid overdose 0.4-2 mg; postoperative narcotic depression 0.1-0.2 mg	Not available
Naltrexone	Tablet: Trexan®/Revia® 50 mg (approved for alcohol dependence and narcotic addiction)	qd, qod, or q3d		Alcoholism 50 mg qd; narcotic addiction 50 mg qd, 100 mg qod, or 150 mg q3d
Nalmefene	Injection: Revex® 0.1, 1 mg/mL	Every 2-5 min	Opioid overdose 0.5-1 mg; postoperative respiratory depression 0.25 µg/kg	Not available

treated by changing the opioid dose, changing the opioid, or giving low doses of a benzodiazepine.

Neuroendocrine
- Morphine acts in the hypothalamus to inhibit the release of gonadotropin-releasing hormone (GnRH) and corticotropin-releasing factor (CRF), thus decreasing levels of luteinizing hormone (LH), follicle-stimulating hormone (FSH), ACTH, and β-endorphins.

- Changes in hormone levels may cause decreased levels of testosterone and cortisol, disturbances in menstruation, and sexual dysfunction.

- High doses of morphine and related opioids produce convulsions. Most convulsions occur at doses far in excess of those required to produce analgesia.

Respiratory
- Respiratory depression is the most serious opioid-induced adverse effect.

- Opioids depress respiration by a direct effect on the brain stem respiratory centers, making the brain stem less responsive to carbon dioxide.

- The µ receptor is the primary receptor involved in respiratory depression, although activation of the κ receptor also contributes.

- At equianalgesic doses, all of the pure opioid agonists depress respiration to the same degree. The agonist-antagonists have a ceiling effect (ie, a dose beyond which further respiratory depression or analgesia is not produced), but this is usually above recommended doses.

- Opioids depress cough by inducing a direct effect on the cough reflex in the medulla.

Cardiovascular
- Therapeutic doses of many opioids produce peripheral vasodilation, reduced peripheral resistance, and inhibition of the baroreceptor reflexes.

- Peripheral vasodilation results primarily from opioid-induced release of histamine. Orthostatic hypotension and fainting can result.

- The naturally occurring and semisynthetic products are potent histamine releasers. Fentanyl has little propensity to release histamine.

- Recently, methadone has been associated with torsades de pointes, an atypical rapid ventricular tachycardia, at an average daily dose of 400 mg.

Gastrointestinal
- All clinically significant µ agonists produce some degree of nausea and vomiting by direct stimulation of the chemoreceptor trigger zone in the medulla, sensitization of the vestibular system, and slowing of GI motility.

- Nausea and vomiting commonly occurs in ambulatory patients (15-40% of patients with nausea and vomiting are ambulatory). Both can be pretreated with an antiemetic such as promethazine or prochlorperazine.

- Opioids promote constipation by delaying gastric emptying, slowing bowel motility, and decreasing peristalsis. Opioids may also reduce secretions from the colonic mucosa. At its worst, gastrointestinal dysfunction results in ileus, fecal impaction, and obstruction.

- Because transdermal delivery bypasses absorption from the GI tract, constipation has been reported to be less frequent than with other opioids.

- Patients on opiates do not develop tolerance to constipation. All patients taking around-the-clock opioid analgesics should be placed on prophylactic bowel regimens. Bowel regimens include increased fluid and fiber intake, daily stool softeners, and mild laxatives.

- Manage severe constipation with osmotic laxatives such as magnesium citrate and milk of magnesia.

Genitourinary tract
- Opioids increase smooth muscle tone in the bladder and ureters and may cause bladder spasm and urgency.

- An opioid-induced increase in sphincter tone can make urination difficult. Urinary retention is most common in elderly men.

Biliary
- Opioids increase smooth muscle tone in the biliary tract, especially in the sphincter of Oddi, which regulates the flow of bile and pancreatic fluids.

- This can result in a decrease in biliary and pancreatic secretions and a rise in the bile duct pressure. Patients may experience epigastric distress and occasionally biliary spasm.

- All opioids are capable of causing constriction of the sphincter of Oddi and the biliary tract. Although morphine may cause more biliary constriction in animals than other opioids, this has never been shown to be clinically useful in humans.

Skin and eyes
- Therapeutic doses of morphine dilate cutaneous blood vessels, which causes flushing on the face, neck, and upper thorax. Sweating and pruritus may also occur.

- * These changes may be due in part to release of histamine.
- * Histamine release may induce or worsen asthmatic attacks in predisposed patients and can lead to wheezing, bronchoconstriction, and status asthmaticus.

- Skin rash around the transdermal fentanyl patch is a common side effect caused by the patch adhesive.

- Following a toxic dose of μ agonists, miosis is marked and pinpoint pupils are pathognomonic; however, mydriasis occurs when asphyxia intervenes.

Overdose
- Acute overdose with opioids is manifested by respiratory depression, somnolence progressing to stupor or coma, skeletal muscle flaccidity, cold and clammy skin, constricted pupils, and sometimes pulmonary edema, bradycardia, hypotension, and death.

- An opioid antagonist may be given to block opioid receptors and reverse the effects of overdose.

- Antagonist administration may cause a complete reversal of opioid effects and precipitate an acute withdrawal syndrome in persons physically dependent on opioids.

- Antagonists are dosed to patient response every few minutes. If no response is observed after 10 mg, the diagnosis of opioid-induced toxicity should be questioned.

- Infusion may be useful in cases of overdose with long-acting drugs such as methadone. The infusion rate for adults is approximately 100 mL/h (0.4 mg/h).

Tolerance and physical dependence
- Opioids often have their use limited by concerns regarding tolerance, physical dependence and addiction.

- Tolerance can be defined as a state in which a larger dose is required to produce the same response that could formerly be elicited by a smaller dose.

- Tolerance to analgesia is demonstrated by the need for an increased dosage of a drug to produce the same level of analgesia. Tolerance to analgesia develops more slowly than tolerance to other opioid effects.

- Tolerance to adverse effects of opioids occurs after 2-3 weeks of continuous administration. Tolerance to the constipating and neuroendocrine effects of opioids does not occur.

- Physical dependence is the occurrence of a withdrawal syndrome after an opioid is stopped or quickly decreased without titration. Warn patients to avoid abrupt discontinuation of such drugs.

- Addiction is the psychological dependence on the use of substances for psychic effects and is characterized by compulsive use. Consider addiction if patients no longer have control over drug use and continue to use drugs despite the harm they promote.

Pharmacokinetics of Selected Opioids

Morphine
- Compared with other opioids, morphine is relatively insoluble in lipids (ie, in adults, only small amounts of the drug cross the blood-brain barrier).

- Morphine does not accumulate in tissues when given in normal doses, and therefore does not cause increasing toxicity with frequent dosing.

- Morphine is primarily metabolized by glucuronidation during the first pass through the liver. Approximately 50% of morphine is converted by the liver to morphine-3-glucuronide (M3G) and 15% to morphine-6-glucuronide (M6G). The pharmacologic effects of morphine (both analgesia and side effects) are due in part to M6G.

- Much of an oral dose is inactivated during this first pass through the liver; consequently, oral doses need to be much larger than parenteral doses to produce the same analgesic effects.

Fentanyl
- Fentanyl is highly soluble in lipids. It accumulates in skeletal muscle and fat and is slowly released into the blood. Plasma half-life is 3-4 hours after parenteral administration.

- Fentanyl is rapidly metabolized, primarily by dealkylation, to inactive metabolites in the liver. This process is mediated through the cytochrome P450 (CYP450) 3A4 hepatic enzyme system. The presence of inactive metabolites makes it a preferred drug in patients with liver dysfunction.

- It is not used orally because of low oral bioavailability.

Transdermal fentanyl
- The uptake of fentanyl through the skin is relatively slow and constant. The skin does not metabolize the drug and 92% of the dose is delivered into the bloodstream as intact fentanyl. Increased body temperature can accelerate the absorption of fentanyl. Increasing body temperature from 37 to 40°C has been shown to increase absorption by up to 33%.

- Serum fentanyl concentrations are measurable within 2 hours after application of the first patch, and analgesic effects can be observed 8-16 hours after application. This delay is required to establish a reservoir of fentanyl in the stratum corneum of the skin. Steady state is reached after several sequential patch applications.

- After removal of the patch, systemic absorption of residual fentanyl in the skin continues. Serum drug levels fall slowly with a variable half-life of about 17 hours (range, 13-22 hours).

Transmucosal fentanyl citrate
- The absorption pharmacokinetics of fentanyl from the oral transmucosal dosage form is a combination of initial rapid absorption from buccal mucosa and a delayed absorption of fentanyl from the GI tract. Normally 25% of the total dose is available by buccal absorption and 25% is available from the GI tract, making the total bioavailability 50%.

- Analgesia begins in 10-15 minutes, peaks in 20 minutes, and persists for 1-2 hours.

Methadone
- After therapeutic doses, about 90% of methadone is bound to plasma protein and is widely distributed in tissues. Methadone is found in low concentrations in the blood and the brain, with higher concentrations in the kidney, spleen, liver, and lung. Terminal half-life is extremely variable (15-55 hours); therefore accumulation is possible and dosing intervals need to be carefully monitored.

- Methadone is extensively metabolized in the liver, mainly by N-demethylation. This appears to be mediated by several CYP450 enzymes. The major metabolites are excreted in the bile and urine.

- Analgesic efficacy does not correspond to the half-life of the drug. Methadone may be dosed every 3 hours for pain control.

Oxycodone
- Oxycodone is metabolized to noroxycodone, oxymorphone, and their glucuronides via the CYP450

2D6 enzyme system. The major circulating metabolite is noroxycodone. Noroxycodone is reported to be a weaker analgesic than oxycodone. Oxymorphone, although possessing analgesic activity, is present in the plasma only in low concentrations.

Normeperidine

- Normeperidine, a metabolite of meperidine, produces anxiety, tremors, myoclonus, and generalized seizures when it accumulates with repetitive dosing. Patients with compromised renal function are particularly at risk. Naloxone does not reverse this hyperexcitability. For these reasons, meperidine should not be used in patients with renal or CNS disease, for more than 48 hours, or at doses greater than 600 mg/24 hours.

Propoxyphene

- Propoxyphene is appropriate for short-term mild to intermittent pain. It produces a toxic metabolite, norpropoxyphene, with effects similar to normeperidine.

Drug Interactions and Drug-Disease Interactions

Drug interactions

- All drugs with CNS depressant actions (barbiturates, benzodiazepines, alcohol) can intensify sedation and respiratory depression caused by morphine and other opioids.

- Antihistamines, tricyclic antidepressants, and atropine-like drugs can exacerbate morphine-induced constipation and urinary retention.

- Antihypertensive drugs and others that lower blood pressure can exacerbate opioid-induced hypotension.

- The combination of meperidine and a monoamine oxidase inhibitor has produced a syndrome characterized by excitation, delirium, hyperpyrexia, convulsions, and severe respiratory depression. Death has also occurred. Although this syndrome has not been reported with other opioids, combinations containing opioids and monoamine oxidase inhibitors should be avoided.

- Agonists-antagonists can precipitate a withdrawal syndrome if administered to an individual who is physically dependent on a pure opioid agonist.

Cytochrome P450 substrates, inhibitors, and inducers

- CYP450 enzymes metabolize codeine, hydrocodone, fentanyl, methadone, and oxycodone. Although not

well documented, drug interactions through this system may exist.

- Codeine, hydrocodone, and oxycodone require metabolism through CYP450 2D6 to active drug (Table 4). Approximately 7% of Caucasians, 3% of African-Americans, and 1% of Asians are poor metabolizers of CYP2D6; they produce no CYP2D6 or produce undetectable levels of it. Poor metabolizers may experience little to no analgesia from drugs requiring 2D6 for conversion to active metabolites.

- About 5% have multiple copies of the CYP2D6 gene, making them ultrafast metabolizers. The clearance of some opioids may be increased, thus making it necessary to dose the medications more often.

Drug-disease interactions

- In view of their extensive hepatic metabolism, the effects of opioids may be increased in patients with liver disease, particularly those with severe liver failure. Most opioids require dose reduction in severe liver disease.

- Fentanyl, morphine, and methadone require dosing adjustment in renal impairment. Doses of fentanyl and morphine should be reduced 25% when CrCl is 10-50 mL/min and by 50% when CrCl is <10 mL/min. The dosing interval of methadone should be increased to at least every 6 hours when CrCl is 10-50 mL/min and to every 8 hours when CrCl is <10 mL/min.

- Renal impairment slows the clearance of morphine conjugates, resulting in accumulation of the active metabolite M6G (morphine-6-glucuronide). For this

Table 4

CYP2D6 Enzyme Activity

Substrates	Inhibitors	Inducers
Oxycodone	Celecoxib	Carbamazepine
Tramadol	Cimetidine	Ethanol
Hydrocodone	Citalopram	Phenobarbital
Codeine	Sertraline	Phenytoin
Meperidine	Paroxetine	Rifampin
Propoxyphene	Fluoxetine	
Methadone	Propoxyphene	
	Methadone	

reason, dosage reduction may be advisable in the presence of clinically significant renal impairment.

- Methadone appears to be firmly bound to protein in various tissues, including the brain. After repeated administrations, there is gradual accumulation in tissues. The risk of accumulation is more likely in patients with impaired renal or hepatic function, since both organs are involved with the metabolism of methadone.

Patient Counseling

- Respiratory depression is increased by concurrent use of other drugs with CNS depressant activity (eg, alcohol, barbiturates, and benzodiazepines). Outpatients should be warned against the use of alcohol with all other CNS depressants.

- Inform patients about symptoms of hypotension (lightheadedness, dizziness). Minimize hypotension by moving slowly when changing from a supine to an upright position.

Transdermal patch
- The fentanyl transdermal patch must be applied to a clean, nonhairy site on the upper torso. Use only water to clean the area. Do not use soap or alcohol because this can increase the effects of the medication. Do not apply the patch to oily, broken, burned, cut, or irritated skin.

- It must be held in place for a minimum of 30 seconds to ensure adhesion.

- Apply each new patch to a different area of skin to avoid irritation. If a patch comes off or causes irritation, remove it and apply a new patch to a different site.

- To dispose of the patch, fold in half and flush down the toilet.

- Do not cut or damage the patch.

Long-acting opioid formulations
- The long-acting formulations should be swallowed whole (ie, not broken, chewed, or crushed).

- Avinza®, a long-acting morphine capsule formulation, contains fumaric acid. Doses above 1600 mg per day contain a quantity of fumaric acid that has not been demonstrated to be safe, and which may result in serious renal toxicity.

- Kadian® and Avinza (long-acting morphine sulfate) may be opened and the beads ingested with a small amount of applesauce (sprinkle administration). In addition, Kadian is approved for sprinkle administration through a gastrostomy tube.

Oral transmucosal fentanyl citrate lozenge
- The lozenge is used by placing it in the mouth between the cheek and gum. Consumption of the lozenge should take 15 minutes. Another lozenge may be used 30 minutes after the start of the first one. Tell the patient not to bite or chew transmucosal fentanyl citrate.

- To dispose of a finished lozenge, discard the handle in a place that is out of the reach of children and pets. If medicine remains on the handle, place the handle under hot running tap water until the medicine is dissolved. Never leave unused or partly used lozenges where children or pets can get to them.

Parameters to monitor
- Evaluate for pain control 1 hour after opioid administration. If analgesia is insufficient, consider a dosage increase. Patients taking opioids chronically should be evaluated regularly for adequate doses.

- Monitor the patient for respiratory depression. Higher risk for respiratory depression exists in patients who are not tolerant to opioid analgesics. Consider treatment when the respiratory rate is less than 8-12 respirations per minute for 30 minutes or longer despite stimulation and/or if oxygen saturation is less than 90%.

- If a patient is easily arousable, he or she is unlikely to have respiratory depression.

Tramadol

- Tramadol is an analog of codeine that has weak agonist activity at μ opioid receptors. The drug works primarily by blocking uptake of norepinephrine and serotonin, thereby inhibiting monoaminergic spinal activation of pain.

- Tramadol is not a federally controlled substance.

- Tramadol is metabolized to active metabolites by CYP2D6.

- The most common adverse effects are sedation, dizziness, headache, dry mouth, and constipation. Respiratory depression is minimal. Seizures have been reported; avoid its use in patients with seizure disorders or other neurologic disorders.

2. Nonpharmacologic Treatment of Pain

General Principles of Nonpharmacologic Treatment

- Nonpharmacologic strategies used in combination with appropriate drug regimens may improve pain relief by enhancing the therapeutic effects of medications and permitting lower doses to be used.

- Nonpharmacologic interventions should not be a substitute for analgesic use.

Physical Interventions

Physical therapy
- Physical therapy is most commonly used to help restore physical strength and functioning after injury or surgery.

- Physical therapy can also provide pain relief for patients with musculoskeletal pain, some types of neuropathic pain, and sympathetically mediated pain.

- The National Institutes of Health recognize the benefit of acupuncture as an adjunct treatment of painful conditions.

Transcutaneous electrical nerve stimulation (TENS)
- In TENS, a controlled, low-voltage electrical current is applied through electrodes placed on the skin. Theoretically, the current will interfere with the ability of nerves to transmit pain signals to the spinal cord and brain.

- Even after several decades of research, it still is not clear if TENS provides any better pain relief than placebo.

Neurostimulation
- Neurostimulation involves implanting a computerized generator and electrodes near the spinal cord, peripheral nerves, or within the brain.

- Stimulators are most effective for patients with neuropathic pain, and are not very beneficial in other types of pain.

Behavioral Techniques

Biofeedback
- In biofeedback, electrodes connected to amplifiers are placed on the body or scalp. During biofeedback sessions, a therapist helps the patient learn to mentally control and change the signals from the electrodes, which helps the patient gain conscious control over normally unconscious functions.

- Biofeedback is most commonly used to relax muscles and reduce stress.

- Its advantages are that it is noninvasive, inexpensive, and safe; however, usually between 5 and 15 sessions are required before effective control is achieved.

Distraction and relaxation
- Distraction and relaxation assist the patient in refocusing attention on nonpainful stimuli.

- Both are believed to improve mental health, which translates into improved pain control.

3. Migraines

Definition

- Migraine is a chronic neurovascular disorder characterized by recurrent attacks of severe headache and autonomic nervous system dysfunction. Some patients also experience aura with neurologic symptoms.

- An estimated 18% of women and 6% of men experience migraine.

Clinical Presentation and Diagnostic Criteria

- Migraine classification is based on whether an aura of visual or sensory symptoms is present. Migraine with aura is less common than migraine without aura.

- Migraine headache manifests as moderate or severe throbbing pain that is localized in the temple or around the eye. It is accompanied by nausea in 90% of patients and vomiting in about half of patients.

- Photophobia (increased sensitivity to light) and phonophobia (increased sensitivity to sound) also are frequent complaints. A prodrome of mood changes, stiff neck, fatigue, or other symptoms may occur hours or days before the onset of the headache.

Criteria for diagnosing migraine without aura
- At least five headaches lasting 4-72 hours each

- The headaches have at least two of the following four characteristics:
  - Unilateral location
  - Pulsating quality
  - Moderate or severe intensity (inhibits or prohibits daily activities)
  - Aggravation with walking stairs or similar routine physical activity

- During the headache, at least one of the following symptoms occurs: nausea or vomiting, photophobia, or phonophobia.

- Symptoms cannot be consistent with other headache types.

Criteria for diagnosis of migraine with aura
- At least two attacks with three of the following four criteria:

- One or more completely reversible aura symptoms indicating focal cerebral cortical or brain stem dysfunction (or both)
- At least one aura symptom develops gradually (>4 minutes) or two or more symptoms occur in succession
- No aura symptom lasts >60 minutes
- Headache follows aura in <1 hour

- There is no evidence of related organic disease.

Pathophysiology

Migraine and the brain
- The pathogenesis of migraine is unclear and is thought to be multifactorial.

- The vascular theory of migraine theorizes that headache results from abnormal synthesis of vasoactive amines, such as norepinephrine and serotonin, which cause cerebral vasoconstriction followed by compensatory vasodilation.

- The underlying cause of inflammation and dilation is not completely understood. Available data suggest the involvement of both calcitonin gene-related peptide (CGRP) and serotonin (5-HT).

- Serotonin is now recognized as an important mediator of migraine headache.

Treatment Principles

Abortive therapy
- The U.S. Headache Consortium identifies the following goals for successful treatment of acute attacks of migraine:
  - Treat attacks rapidly and consistently without recurrence.
  - Restore the patient's ability to function.
  - Minimize the use of rescue medication.
  - Optimize self-care and reduce subsequent use of resources.
  - Promote cost-effective therapies with minimal adverse effects.

- Successful treatment of migraine depends on early intervention in relation to onset of headache and adequate dosing.

Preventive therapy
- Preventive therapy should be considered in the following situations:
  - Attacks unresponsive to abortive medication
  - Attacks causing substantial disability
  - Attacks occurring twice or more monthly

* Patient is at risk for rebound headache
* Trend in increasing frequency of attacks

- Two-thirds of patients taking preventive medication will have a 50% decrease in frequency of attacks. *Note:* Use of abortive therapies should be limited to 2-3 days per week.

- The goals of migraine preventive therapy are as follows:
  * Reduction of attack frequency, severity, and duration
  * Improve responsiveness to treatment of acute attacks
  * Improve function and reduce disability

Rebound headaches
- Persons who take abortive medications daily can develop drug rebound headaches, or headaches that begin upon discontinuation of a medication.

- Essentially all of the medications, with the possible exception of the triptans, cause rebound headache.

Drug Therapy

Abortive therapy: Nonprescription medications
- Aspirin, acetaminophen, ibuprofen, and other aspirin-like analgesics provide adequate relief of mild to moderate migraines.

Combinations with caffeine
- Combination products containing aspirin, acetaminophen, or both with caffeine are available without a prescription.

- Caffeine has analgesic and possibly anti-inflammatory properties. It may also increase gastric acidity and perfusion, enhancing the absorption of aspirin.

- Excedrin Migraine® (acetaminophen 250 mg, aspirin 250 mg, and caffeine 65 mg) is the only nonprescription preparation that carries a specific indication for migraine relief.

Abortive therapy: Nonspecific prescription medications
- Combination products containing an analgesic, caffeine, and butalbital or codeine are available.
  * The butalbital may be useful for its sedative properties.
  * Excessive use of these products can cause physical dependence and rebound headaches.

- A combination of the vasoconstrictor isometheptene, the sedative dichloralphenazone, and acetaminophen (Midrin) may be useful for mild to moderate migraines and is generally well tolerated.

- It is well recognized that opioids are good analgesics, but there is good evidence only for the efficacy of butorphanol nasal spray for migraine. Although opioids are commonly used, surprisingly few studies of opioid use in headache pain document whether overuse and the development of dependence are as frequent as clinically perceived.

- Given intravenously, the antiemetic metoclopramide may be appropriate as monotherapy for acute attacks, particularly in patients with significant nausea. Chlorpromazine and prochlorperazine may also be considered. Serotonin receptor antagonists (5-HT$_3$) have not been shown to be useful migraine treatments.

Abortive therapy: Ergotamine
Mechanism of action
- In cranial arteries, ergotamine acts directly to promote constriction and reduce the amplitude of pulsations. In addition, the drug can affect blood flow by depressing the vasomotor center. Antimigraine effects are possibly due to agonist activity at serotonin receptor subtypes 5-HT$_{1B}$ and 5-HT$_{1D}$.

- Because of the risk of dependence, ergotamine should not be taken daily on a long-term basis.

- Multiple ingredients are added to ergotamine to enhance efficacy (Table 5). Caffeine enhances vasoconstriction and ergotamine absorption. Pentobarbital provides sedation. The belladonna alkaloids suppress emesis.

Pharmacokinetics
- Oral ergotamine has poor bioavailability due to extensive first-pass metabolism. Sublingual administration may not provide therapeutic blood levels.

- Although the half-life of ergotamine is only 2 hours, pharmacologic effects can be seen for 24 hours after administration.

- The drug is eliminated primarily by hepatic metabolism. Metabolites are excreted in the bile.

Adverse effects
- Ergotamine is well tolerated at usual therapeutic doses.

- The drug can stimulate the chemoreceptor trigger zone to cause nausea and vomiting in about 10% of patients. Concurrent treatment with metoclopramide

Table 5

Agents Used in Migraine Treatment

Drug	Available strengths	Maximum daily dose (weekly maximum)	Dosing instructions
Ergot alkaloids			
Ergotamine	SL tablet: Egomar® 2 mg		
	Tablet: Ergostat® 2 mg, Wigrettes® 2 mg	PO: 6 mg (10 mg)	1 tablet at onset; then 1 every 30 min prn
	Injection: Gynergen® 0.5 mg/mL	INJ: 1 mg per week	IM 125-500 µg, repeated if needed to weekly maximum
	Inhalation: Medihaler-Ergotamine® 9 mg/mL	INH: 820 µg (5.4 mg)	1 inhalation (360 µg) followed by one inhalation after 30-60 min
Ergotamine 1 mg/caffeine 100 mg tablet	Cafergot®, Wigraine®	Ergotamine 6 mg (10 mg)	2 tablets at onset; then 1 every 30 min prn
Ergotamine 0.3 mg/pentobarbital 20 mg/bellafoline 0.1 mg tablet	Bellergal®	Ergotamine 6 mg (10 mg)	2 tablets at onset; then 1 every 30 min prn
Ergotamine 0.6 mg/pentobarbital 40 mg/belladonna 0.2 mg tablet	Bellamine®, Bellamine S®, Bellaspas®, Bellaphen S®, Bellergal S®, Duragal S®	Ergotamine 6 mg (10 mg)	2 tablets at onset; then 1 every 30 min prn
Ergotamine 1 mg/pentobarbital 30 mg/belladonna 0.125 mg/caffeine 100 mg tablet	Cafergot PB®	Ergotamine 6 mg (10 mg)	2 tablets at onset; then 1 every 30 min prn
Ergotamine 1 mg/belladonna 0.1 mg/caffeine 100 mg/phenacetin 130 mg suppository	Wigraine®	Ergotamine 4 mg (10 mg)	Insert 1 at onset; repeat in 1 hour prn
Ergotamine 2 mg/phenobarbital 60 mg/belladonna 0.25 mg/caffeine 100 mg suppository	Cafergot PB, Wigraine PB®	Ergotamine 4 mg (10 mg)	Insert 1 at onset; repeat in 1 hour prn
Ergotamine 2 mg/caffeine 100 mg suppository	Cafergot	Ergotamine 4 mg (10 mg)	Insert 1 at onset; repeat in 1 hour prn
Dihydroergotamine (DHE)	Injection: 1 mg/mL D.H.E. 45®	DHE 2 mg (6 mg IV or 3 mg IM)	0.5-1 mg IV/IM every hour as needed
	Nasal spray: Migranal® 4 mg/mL	DHE 2 mg (6 mg)	Administer one spray (0.5 mg) in each nostril, followed in 15 min by an additional spray in each nostril
Miscellaneous agents			
Isometheptene 65 mg/dichloralphenazone 100 mg/acetaminophen 325 mg capsule	Midrin®	5 capsules within a 12-hour period	2 capsules at once, followed by 1 capsule every hour until headache is relieved

or a phenothiazine antiemetic can help suppress this response.

- Other common side effects include weakness in the legs, myalgia, numbness and tingling in the periphery, angina-like pain, tachycardia, and bradycardia.

Overdose
- Acute or chronic overdose can cause serious toxicity (ergotism).

- Symptoms include ischemia, myalgias, and paresthesias. Ischemia can progress to gangrene.

- The risk of ergotism is highest in patients with sepsis, peripheral vascular disease, and renal or hepatic impairment.

Drug-drug and drug-disease interactions
- Ergotamine should not be combined with selective serotonin receptor agonists due to the risk of a prolonged vasospastic reaction.

- Separate doses of ergotamine and serotonin agonists by at least 24 hours.

- Ergotamine is contraindicated for patients with hepatic or renal impairment, sepsis, coronary artery disease, and peripheral vascular disease.

Patient counseling
- Monitor patients to avoid overuse of the medication.

- Ergotamine and its derivatives are FDA pregnancy category X. They should not be taken during pregnancy due to its ability to promote uterine contractions and cause fetal harm or abortion.

- Teach patients to recognize signs of ergotism. Muscle pain, paresthesias, and cold or pale extremities should be reported immediately.

Dihydroergotamine (DHE)
Mechanism of action
- The action of dihydroergotamine is similar to that of ergotamine. Like ergotamine, dihydroergotamine alters transmission at serotonergic, dopaminergic, and α-adrenergic junctions.

- In contrast to ergotamine, dihydroergotamine causes minimal peripheral vasoconstriction, little nausea and vomiting, and no physical dependence. However, diarrhea is prominent.

- Contraindications are the same as for ergotamine:

coronary artery disease, peripheral vascular disease, sepsis, pregnancy, and hepatic or renal impairment.

- As with ergotamine, do not administer dihydroergotamine within 24 hours of a serotonin agonist.

Pharmacokinetics
- Dihydroergotamine is not active orally due to extensive first-pass metabolism.

- An active metabolite, 8'-hydroxydihydroergotamine, contributes to its therapeutic effects. The half-life of dihydroergotamine plus its active metabolite is about 21 hours.

Abortive therapy: Selective serotonin receptor agonists (triptans)
- The selective serotonin receptor agonists, also known as triptans, are first-line drugs for terminating a migraine attack (Table 6).

- The triptans all activate $5\text{-}HT_{1B}/5\text{-}HT_{1D}$ and to a lesser extent $5\text{-}HT_{1A}$ or $5\text{-}HT_{1F}$ receptors. Triptans have no known affinity for $5\text{-}HT_2$ or $5\text{-}HT_3$ and other 5-HT receptor subclasses, nor do they bind to adrenergic, dopaminergic, muscarinic, or histaminergic receptors.

Pharmacokinetics
- The pharmacokinetics of the different triptans vary somewhat. However, all are generally well tolerated and efficacious at appropriate doses.

- Subcutaneous sumatriptan injection has the fastest onset of action when compared with other triptans. Sumatriptan nasal spray has a slightly slower onset than the injection.

- The onset of the majority of oral triptans, including the dissolving wafers, is similar among the available agents. Rizatriptan may have a slightly faster onset of action at 1-1.5 hours.

- Migraine recurrence rates may be lower with long half-life triptans such as naratriptan and frovatriptan. However, triptans with longer half-lives tend to have a slower onset of action.

Adverse effects
- Triptans are generally well tolerated. Most side effects are mild and transient.

- The triptans differ slightly from one another in terms of tolerability but not in terms of safety.

Table 6

Selective Serotonin Receptor Agonists (Triptans)

Drug	Available strengths	Dosage (maximum daily dose)	Half-life (h)	Onset (min)	Metabolism
Almotriptan (Axert®)	Tablet: 6.25, 12.5 mg	12.5 mg; repeat in 2 hours (25 mg)	3.5	60	CYP450; MAO
Sumatriptan (Imitrex®)	Tablet: 25, 50, 100 mg	50 to 100 mg; repeat in 2 hours. (200 mg)	2.5	60-120	MAO
	Nasal 5, 20 mg	5 or 20 mg; repeat in 2 hours (40 mg)		15-20	
	Injection: 6 mg/mL	6 mg; repeat in 1 hour (12 mg)		10-15	
Eletriptan (Relpax®)	Tablet: 20, 40 mg	20 mg; repeat in 2 hours (80 mg)	5	60	CYP 3A4
Frovatriptan (Frova®)	Tablet: 2.5 mg	2.5 mg: repeat in 2 hours (7.5 mg)	25	60-120	Renal 50%
Rizatriptan (Maxalt®)	Tablet/wafer: 5, 10 mg	5 or 10 mg; repeat in 2 hours (30 mg)	2-3	30	MAO
Zolmitriptan (Zomig®)	Tablet/wafer: 2.5, 5 mg	2.5 or 5 mg; repeat in 2 hours (10 mg)	2.5-4	45	CYP450; MAO
Naratriptan (Amerge®)	Tablet: 1, 2.5 mg	1 or 2.5 mg; repeat in 4 hours (5 mg)	6	60	Renal 70%; CYP450

CYP450, cytochrome p450 hepatic enzyme system; MAO, monoamine oxidase enzyme.

- The most frequent side effects are tingling and paresthesias, and sensations of warmth in the head, neck, chest, and limbs.

- Less frequent effects are dizziness, flushing, and neck pain or stiffness.

Chest symptoms

- About 50% of patients on sumatriptan experience unpleasant chest symptoms usually described as "heavy arms" or "chest pressure" rather than pain.

- These symptoms are transient and not related to ischemic heart disease.

- Possible causes are pulmonary vasoconstriction, esophageal spasm, intercostal muscle spasm, and bronchoconstriction.

Coronary vasospasm

- Rarely, sumatriptan causes angina secondary to coronary vasospasm.

- Electrocardiographic changes have been observed in patients with CAD or Prinzmetal's (vasospastic) angina.

- To reduce the risk of angina, do not give sumatriptan to patients who have risk factors for CAD. These patients include postmenopausal women, men over 40, smokers, and patients with hypertension, hypercholesterolemia, obesity, diabetes, or a family history of CAD.

Other adverse effects

- Mild reactions include vertigo, malaise, fatigue, and tingling sensations.

- Transient pain and redness may occur at sites of SC injection.

- Intranasal administration may cause irritation in the nose and throat as well as an offensive or unusual taste.

Drug-drug and drug-disease interactions
Ergot alkaloids and other triptans

- All triptans and ergot alkaloids cause vasoconstriction. Accordingly, if one triptan is combined with another or with an ergot alkaloid, excessive and prolonged vasospasm could result.

- Do not use triptans within 24 hours of an ergot derivative or another triptan.

- Monoamine oxidase inhibitors (MAOIs) can suppress degradation of triptans, which causes plasma levels to rise and toxicity to result. Furthermore, triptans should not be administered within 2 weeks of stopping an MAOI.

- Triptans are contraindicated for patients with a history of ischemic heart disease, myocardial infarction, uncontrolled hypertension, or other heart disease.

- Do not use triptans during pregnancy

Patient counseling

- Patients should be counseled to contact a physician if pain or tightness in the chest occurs.

- Patients should not exceed daily maximum doses. If migraines occur more than three times a month, prophylactic treatment should be considered.

- Pain at the sumatriptan injection site should last less than 1 hour.

Migraine Prophylactic Therapy (Table 7)

β-Adrenergic blocking agents

- Propranolol is the drug of choice for migraine prophylaxis. This agent can reduce the number and intensity of attacks in about 70% of patients.

- Not all β-blockers are active against migraines. Agents with demonstrated efficacy include propranolol, atenolol, metoprolol, nadolol, and timolol.

- Since not all β-blockers are effective, it would appear that a mechanism other than β-blockade is responsible for the beneficial effects.

Anticonvulsants

- There is good evidence for the efficacy of divalproex sodium and sodium valproate. Adverse events with these therapies are not uncommon and include weight gain, hair loss, tremor, and teratogenic potential, such as neural tube defects.

- Carbamazepine has been shown to be ineffective in migraine prevention. There is limited evidence for moderate efficacy of gabapentin and topiramate.

- Clonazepam has not been shown to be an effective migraine prevention treatment.

Antidepressants

- Amitriptyline has been more frequently studied than the other antidepressants and is the only one with consistent support for efficacy in migraine prevention. There is no evidence for the use of other TCAs such as nortriptyline, protriptyline, doxepin, clomipramine, or imipramine.

Table 7

Selected Migraine Preventive Treatments

Drug	Dose	Selected side effects
β-Adrenergic receptor antagonists		
Propranolol	40-120 mg twice daily	Reduced energy, tiredness, postural
Metoprolol	100-200 mg daily	symptoms
Antidepressants		
Amitriptyline	25-75 mg at bedtime	Drowsiness
Fluoxetine	10-20 mg daily	Headache, nausea, nervousness, insomnia, drowsiness
Serotonin antagonists		
Methysergide	1-6 mg daily (treatment must be discontinued for 1 month every 6 months)	Drowsiness, leg cramps, hair loss, retroperitoneal fibrosis
Calcium channel blockers		
Diltiazem	90-180 mg daily	Headache
Verapamil	160-320 mg daily	Constipation, peripheral edema, cardiac conduction disturbances
Anticonvulsants		
Divalproex	400-600 mg twice daily	Drowsiness, weight gain, tremor, hair loss, hematologic and liver abnormalities, teratogenicity
Gabapentin	900-2400 mg daily	Somnolence, dizziness
Topiramate	25-200 mg daily	Confusion, paresthesias, weight loss

Adapted from Goadsby et al, 2002.

- Drowsiness, weight gain, and anticholinergic symptoms are frequently reported with the TCAs.

- Limited evidence exists that supports using fluoxetine at dosages ranging from 20 mg every other day to 40 mg per day. Controlled trials offer no evidence for the use of fluvoxamine, paroxetine, sertraline, phenelzine, bupropion, mirtazapine, trazodone, or venlafaxine in this manner.

Calcium channel blockers
- Several calcium channel blockers are moderately effective at reducing migraine attacks. These include verapamil, nifedipine, and nimodipine.

- Beneficial effects develop slowly, reaching a maximum in 1-2 months.

- Calcium channel blockers cause side effects in 20-60% of patients. Constipation and orthostatic hypotension are most common. Vascular headache develops in about 25% of patients taking nifedipine.

Methysergide
- Methysergide is an ergot alkaloid used in migraine prophylaxis. It is not effective for aborting an ongoing attack.

- It is more efficacious than propranolol but has significantly more side effects.

- The drug seems to activate serotonin receptors in the CNS. Suppression of pain pathways by this mechanism may explain its usefulness.

- Methysergide causes a number of adverse effects.
  * With long-term therapy, methysergide can cause retroperitoneal, pleuropulmonary, and cardiac fibrosis. Fibrotic changes, although rare, are most serious.
  * Other adverse effects include vascular insufficiency, insomnia, altered mood, depersonalization, hallucinations, nightmares, and GI disturbances such as nausea, vomiting, and diarrhea.
  * Ergot alkaloids, serotonin receptor agonists, β-adrenergic blockers, dopamine, and drugs that inhibit the CYP3A4 subclass of hepatic metabolizing enzymes increase the risk of arterial spasm.

4. Nonpharmacologic Treatment of Migraines

General Principles of Nonpharmacologic Therapies

- Nonpharmacologic approaches may be well suited to patients who have exhibited a poor tolerance or poor response to drug therapy, who have a contraindication to drug therapy, and/or who have a history of long-term, frequent, or excessive use of analgesics or other acute medications.

- Nonpharmacologic interventions may also be useful in patients who are pregnant, are planning to become pregnant, or are nursing.

Treatment Recommendations

- Patients with migraine pain may experience relief from resting or sleeping in a cool, quiet, dark environment. Half of migraine patients experience considerable relief by applying a cold compress to the head.

- Relaxation training, thermal biofeedback combined with relaxation training, electromyographic (EMG) biofeedback, and cognitive-behavioral therapies are somewhat effective in preventing migraine.

- Evidence pertaining to the treatment of migraine with acupuncture is limited and the results are mixed. Similarly, limited evaluation has been conducted with hypnosis, TENS, cervical manipulation, and hyperbaric oxygen.

Trigger Management

- Trigger management is important in preventing migraine attacks. Triggering factors can cause migraine, and if recognized and/or avoided, may impede an impending attack.

- Triggers vary from person to person. Examples of triggers include changes in weather or air pressure, bright sunlight, glare, fluorescent lights, chemical fumes, menstrual cycles, and certain foods such as processed meats, red wine, beer, dried fish, broad beans, fermented cheeses, aspartame, and MSG.

5. Key Points

Pain management

- Opioids relieve pain by mimicking the actions of endogenous opioid peptides at μ, κ, and δ receptors.

- Opioids fall into three categories: pure μ agonists, agonist-antagonists, and pure antagonists. Pure μ agonists are the most pharmacologically useful.

- Addiction is a behavior pattern involving the continued use of a substance for nonmedical reasons despite harm. Physical dependence refers to the occurrence of an abstinence syndrome if the opioid is abruptly discontinued.

- With prolonged use, tolerance develops to analgesia, euphoria, sedation, respiratory depression, and other adverse effects, but not to constipation.

- Opioid overdose induces coma, respiratory depression, and pinpoint pupils. Naloxone and other pure opioid antagonists are used in cases of overdose to reverse most effects of opioids.

- Alcohol and other CNS depressants can intensify opioid-induced sedation and respiratory depression. Tricyclic antidepressants and antihistamines may worsen opioid-induced constipation and urinary retention.

- Hydrocodone, codeine, fentanyl, methadone, and oxycodone are metabolized by the cytochrome P450 system. Thus, drug interactions through the CYP enzymes may exist.

- The liver extensively metabolizes opioids; dose adjustments may be required in liver dysfunction. Fentanyl, morphine, and methadone require dosing adjustments in renal dysfunction.

Migraine

- Migraine results from intracranial vasodilation and perivascular inflammation that is likely mediated by serotonin.

- The goal of abortive therapy is to eliminate headache pain and associated nausea and vomiting. The goal of preventive therapy is to reduce the incidence of migraine attacks.

- Nonopioid analgesics are effective for abortive therapy of mild to moderate pain.

- Opioid analgesics are reserved for severe migraine that has not responded to other drugs.

- Ergotamine is used for abortive therapy but should not be used daily. Overdose with ergotamine can cause ergotism, a serious condition in which generalized constriction of peripheral arteries and arterioles causes severe tissue ischemia.

- Triptans are drugs of choice for abortive therapy of migraines. They activate $5\text{-HT}_{1B}/5\text{-HT}_{1D}$ receptors, thereby causing constriction of cranial blood vessels and suppression of inflammatory neuropeptides.

- Triptans can cause coronary vasospasm and are contraindicated in patients with ischemic heart disease, prior myocardial infarction, and uncontrolled hypertension. If a triptan is combined with another triptan or with an ergot alkaloid, excessive prolonged vasospasms could result. Due to increased triptan toxicity, monoamine oxidase inhibitors (MAOIs) should not be administered concurrently with a triptan or for 2 weeks after MAOI discontinuation.

- Propranolol and divalproex and preferred drugs for prevention of migraines.

6. Questions and Answers

1. Approximately how many people in the United States experience severe chronic pain?

   A. 10 million
   B. 23 million
   C. 40 million
   D. 50 million
   E. 75 million

2. Addiction is currently understood to be

   I. Characterized by compulsive use of drugs
   II. Synonymous with physical dependence on a medication
   III. The use of a substance for psychic effects

   A. I only
   B. III only
   C. I and III only
   D. II and III only
   E. I, II, and III

3. The World Health Organization analgesic hierarchy emphasizes

   A. Concurrent use of nonopioids, opioids, and adjuvant medications
   B. Avoiding opioid use
   C. Reserving opioid use only for severe pain
   D. Using single agents rather than a combination of medications
   E. Using nonopioids only for treatment of mild pain

4. All of the following adverse effects are manifestations of μ opioid agonists except

   A. Constipation
   B. Respiratory depression
   C. Atrial flutter
   D. Nausea
   E. Miosis

5. The preferred route of opioid administration is

   A. Oral
   B. Intravenous
   C. Subcutaneous
   D. Rectal
   E. Intramuscular

6. Which of the following opioids has the longest duration of analgesic effect?

   A. Methadone
   B. Controlled release morphine
   C. Hydromorphone
   D. Transdermal fentanyl
   E. Controlled release oxycodone

7. All of the following opioids are metabolized through the cytochrome P450 hepatic enzyme system except

   A. Hydrocodone
   B. Oxycodone
   C. Morphine
   D. Methadone
   E. Fentanyl

8. The clearance of which opioid may be increased in patients with multiple copies of the CYP2D6 gene?

   A. Methadone
   B. Oxycodone
   C. Fentanyl
   D. Morphine
   E. Hydromorphone

9. Which of the following statements regarding methadone pharmacokinetics is true?

   A. The half-life corresponds to analgesic efficacy.
   B. It is highly plasma protein bound and widely distributed in tissue.
   C. The clearance of methadone is rapid, resulting in frequent dosing.
   D. Methadone has low bioavailability from the GI tract and therefore is not useful when given orally.
   E. Methadone is metabolized by hepatic glucuronidation.

10. Which agent can be used to reverse respiratory effects caused by opioid overdose?

    A. Naloxone
    B. Pentazocine
    C. Buprenorphine
    D. Naltrexone
    E. Tramadol

11. Which of the following opioids is not appropriate for use as an around-the-clock medication in chronic pain?

    A. Morphine
    B. Oxycodone

C. Fentanyl
D. Hydromorphone
E. Methadone

12. Which of the following opioids has a toxic metabolite that can accumulate in renal dysfunction?

   A. Oxycodone
   B. Fentanyl
   C. Meperidine
   D. Hydromorphone
   E. Methadone

Use Case Study 1 to answer Questions 13 and 14.

13. Which of her medications is most likely to worsen opioid-induced constipation?

   A. Paxil
   B. Zocor
   C. Lotensin
   D. Premarin
   E. Elavil

14. The physician recommends changing her opioid to one that is less constipating. Which of the following medications is least likely to cause constipation?

   A. Morphine extended release
   B. Methadone
   C. Oxycodone extended release

Case Study 1

Patient Name:	Mary Martin
Address:	815 Elm Street
Age:	65
Sex:	Female
Allergies:	NKDA

Diagnosis: Chronic low back pain, hypertension, hypercholesterolemia, and chronic constipation.

Medications:

3/3	Paxil® 20 mg qd
3/3	Zocor® 40 mg qd
3/3	Lotensin® 20 mg qd
3/3	Premarin® 0.625 mg
3/3	Morphine sulfate extended release 60 mg bid
3/3	Senokot S®
3/28	Elavil® 50 mg qhs
4/1	Milk of magnesia

D. Transdermal fentanyl patch
E. Hydromorphone

15. The rationale of adding caffeine to a simple analgesic for migraine treatment is to

   I. Decrease the required dose of acetaminophen and aspirin
   II. Cause cerebral arterial vasoconstriction
   III. Increase gastric acidity and perfusion, enhancing aspirin absorption

   A. I only
   B. III only
   C. I and III only
   D. II and III only
   E. I, II, and III

16. Which of the following agents is a selective serotonin agonist?

   A. Sumatriptan
   B. Ketorolac
   C. Dihydroergotamine
   D. Metoclopramide
   E. Caffeine

17. Which is true regarding the adverse effects of ergotamine?

   A. Ergotamine inhibits the chemoreceptor trigger zone to minimize nausea and vomiting.
   B. Ergotamine has minimal risk of dependence.
   C. Muscle weakness is an uncommon side effect of ergotamine.
   D. Angina-like pain reported with the triptans is not seen with ergotamine use.
   E. Overuse of ergotamine can result in ischemia.

18. Which statement about triptans is correct?

   A. There are few contraindications to the use of triptans.
   B. Triptans are contraindicated in ischemic cardiovascular disease.
   C. Triptans are preferred for migraine treatment during pregnancy.
   D. Patients taking ergot alkaloids can use triptans concomitantly.
   E. Triptans are strictly contraindicated in patients with hypertension.

19. Which of the following statements is true regarding the use of opioids for migraines?

A. Opioid use is not associated with rebound headaches.

B. Butorphanol nasal spray is efficacious in migraine abortive therapy.

C. Opioids in combination with butalbital and caffeine do not produce physical dependence.

D. Opioids scheduled around the clock are useful for migraine prophylaxis.

E. Opioids are not commonly prescribed for migraine treatment.

20. Which of the following agents is most likely to cause pulmonary fibrosis?

   A. Methysergide
   B. Amitriptyline
   C. Carbamazepine
   D. Propranolol
   E. Valproic acid

21. Which statement about Midrin is correct?

   I. Midrin can be used concomitantly with over-the-counter products containing acetaminophen.
   II. Midrin dose is limited to 5 capsules per 12 hours.
   III. Midrin may cause sedation.

   A. I only
   B. III only
   C. I and III only
   D. II and III only
   E. I, II, and III

22. Dihydroergotamine differs from ergotamine in which of the following ways?

   A. Lower incidence of nausea and vomiting
   B. Higher incidence of physical dependence
   C. No contraindications for ischemic cardiovascular disease
   D. Higher incidence of diarrhea
   E. It can be administered concomitantly with a triptan

Use Case Study 2 to answer Questions 23 and 24.

23. Which of the following statements is true regarding initiation of prophylactic migraine therapy in Mr. Hunt?

   A. Mr. Hunt is at high risk for rebound headaches due to excessive sumatriptan use.
   B. Mr. Hunt is limiting his sumatriptan use to 3 days per week and is not a candidate for prophylactic treatment.

Case Study 2

Patient Name:	James Hunt
Address:	817 Elm Street
Age:	45
Sex:	Male
Allergies:	NKDA

Diagnosis: Migraine with aura, controlled hypertension

Medications:

1/1	sumatriptan 100 mg tablet	oral	use as directed	#9 tabs
1/1	lisinopril 10 mg tablet	oral	qd	#30 tabs
2/1	sumatriptan 100 mg tablet	oral	use as directed	#9 tabs
2/1	lisinopril 10 mg tablet	oral	qd	#30 tabs
3/1	sumatriptan 100 mg tablet	oral	use as directed	#9 tabs
3/1	lisinopril 10 mg tablet	oral	qd	#30 tabs
3/9	sumatriptan 100 mg tablet	oral	use as directed	#9 tabs
3/14	sumatriptan 100 mg tablet	oral	use as directed	#9 tabs

C. Mr. Hunt is a candidate for prophylactic therapy due to the increasing frequency of attacks.

D. Mr. Hunt requires prophylactic therapy because his hypertension is a contraindication to using abortive therapies.

E. Prophylactic treatment is contraindicated in migraines with aura.

24. Which medication is appropriate to give Mr. Hunt for migraine prophylaxis?

   A. Butorphanol
   B. Propranolol
   C. Dihydroergotamine
   D. Acetaminophen
   E. Hydrocodone

Answers

1. **E.** Currently, about 75 million individuals suffer from some form of chronic benign pain.

2. **C.** Physical dependence is the occurrence of a withdrawal syndrome after an opioid is stopped or quickly decreased without titration. Addiction is the psychological dependence on the use of substances for psychic effects and is characterized by compulsive use.

3. **A.** The WHO analgesic hierarchy involves choosing among three stepped levels of treatment. Mild pain may respond to nonopioid drugs alone. Combing a low-dose opioid with a

nonopioid can relieve pain of moderate severity. More severe pain requires the addition of a higher-dose opioid preparation to the nonopioid. At any step, analgesic adjuvants may be useful.

4. **C.** Atrial flutter is not a documented adverse effect of opioids. However, therapeutic doses of many opioids produce peripheral vasodilation, reduced peripheral resistance, and inhibition of the baroreceptor reflexes. Recently, methadone has been associated with torsades de pointes, an atypical rapid ventricular tachycardia.

5. **A.** Oral medications should be used whenever possible because of convenience, flexibility, and steady serum levels.

6. **D.** Transdermal fentanyl provides analgesia for up to 72 hours. The analgesic effects of methadone do not correlate with its long half-life.

7. **C.** Morphine is metabolized by hepatic glucuronidation.

8. **B.** Oxycodone is metabolized through CYP450 2D6 to active metabolites. Fast metabolizers, those with multiple copies of the CYP450 2D6 gene, would clear oxycodone and its metabolites quickly.

9. **B.** About 90% of methadone is bound to plasma protein and is widely distributed in tissues. Methadone has a long terminal half-life resulting in slow clearance. This half-life does not correspond to analgesic dosing. It is metabolized via the CYP450 enzyme system.

10. **A.** Naloxone is a μ antagonist useful in opioid overdose. Naltrexone is also a μ antagonist, but it is reserved for use in alcoholism and opioid addiction.

11. **D.** Hydromorphone is an opioid with a short half-life with no available long-acting formulation. Thus it is not useful as an around-the-clock medication.

12. **C.** Normeperidine, a metabolite of meperidine, can accumulate with chronic use, renal impairment, and when the dose exceeds 600 mg/24 hours.

13. **E.** The anticholinergic effects of tricyclic antidepressants such as Elavil can exacerbate

opioid-induced constipation and urinary retention.

14. **D.** Because transdermal delivery bypasses absorption from the GI tract, constipation has been reported to be less frequent than with other opioids.

15. **C.** Caffeine has analgesic and possibly anti-inflammatory properties. Therefore reduced doses of acetaminophen and aspirin may be required. Caffeine may also increase gastric acidity and perfusion, enhancing the absorption of aspirin.

16. **A.** Sumatriptan is a selective serotonin agonist.

17. **E.** Adverse effects of ergotamine include nausea and vomiting, physical dependence, muscle weakness, and angina-like pain. Overuse of ergotamine can result in ischemia that may progress to gangrene.

18. **B.** Triptans are contraindicated in pregnancy and ischemic cardiovascular disease. They cannot be used within 24 hours of another triptan or ergot alkaloid.

19. **B.** There is good evidence for the efficacy of butorphanol nasal spray in migraine abortive therapy. Although opioids are commonly used for abortive therapy, they may be associated with rebound headaches and physical dependence.

20. **A.** With long-term therapy, methysergide can cause retroperitoneal, pleuropulmonary, and cardiac fibrosis. Fibrotic changes, although rare, are serious.

21. **D.** Midrin may be useful for mild to moderate migraines. It is generally well tolerated but may cause sedation. Due to its acetaminophen content, use of other acetaminophen products should be limited.

22. **D.** In contrast to ergotamine, dihydroergotamine causes minimal peripheral vasoconstriction, little nausea and vomiting, and no physical dependence. However, diarrhea is prominent.

23. **C.** Prophylactic therapy should be considered since his migraines occur more than twice monthly and there is a trend toward increasing frequency of attacks.

24. **B.** To date, propranolol has shown the most

efficacy for migraine prophylaxis. This agent can reduce the number and intensity of attacks in about 70% of patients. Butorphanol, acetaminophen, dihydroergotamine, and hydrocodone are not approved for migraine prophylaxis.

7. References

Pain

American Pain Society. *Principles of Analgesic Use in the Treatment of Acute Pain and Cancer Pain*, 4th ed. Glenview, Illinois: American Pain Society; 1999.

Baumann TJ. Pain Management. In: DiPiro JT, Talbert PE, Hayes PE, et al, eds. *Pharmacotherapy: A Pathophysiologic Approach*, 4th ed. New York: Elsevier; 1999:1014-1025.

Bonica JJ, ed. *The Management of Pain,* 2nd ed. Philadelphia: Lea & Febiger; 1990.

Brookoff D. Chronic pain: 1. a new disease. *Hosp Pract (Off Ed)*. 2000:35;45-52, 59.

Holdsworth M, Forman W, Killilea T, et al. Transdermal fentanyl disposition in elderly subjects. *Gerontology.* 1994;40:32-37.

Hutchison TA, Shahan DR, eds. DRUGDEX® System. MICROMEDEX, Greenwood Village, Colorado (volume expired 3/2003).

IASP Task Force on Taxonomy. Merskey H, Bogduk N, eds. *Classification of Chronic Pain,* 2nd ed. Seattle: IASP Press; 1994:209-214.

Jacox A, Carr DB. Management of Cancer Pain. Clinical Practice Guideline No. 9. Rockville, Maryland: Agency for Health Care Policy and Research, U.S. Department of Health and Human Services, Public Health Service, 1994:34. AHCPR Publication No. 94-0492.

JCAHO. Pain Assessment and Management. An Organizational Approach. Oakbrook Terrace, Illinois: Joint Commission on Accreditation of Healthcare Organizations; 2000.

National Institute of Health. NIH Consensus Statement on Acupuncture, Vol. 15, No. 5, November 3-5, 1997; available online at http://odp.od.nih.gov/consensus/cons/107/107_statement.htm

NIH American Pain Society. Acupuncture. *Principles of Analgesic Use in the Treatment of Acute Pain and Cancer Pain,* 4th ed. Glenview, IL: American Pain Society; 1999.

Portenoy RK. Opioid therapy for chronic nonmalignant pain: A review of the critical issues. *J Pain Symptom Manage.* 1996;11:203-217.

Practice guidelines for chronic pain management: A report by the American Society of Anesthesiologists Task Force on Pain Management, Chronic Pain Section. *Anesthesiology.* 1997;86:995-1004.

Public policy statement on definitions related to the use of opioids in pain treatment. American Society of Addiction Medicine. *J Addict Dis.* 1998;17:129-133.

The Use of Opioids for the Treatment of Chronic Pain. A consensus statement from the American Academy of Pain Medicine and the American Pain Society. *Clin J Pain.* 1997;13:6.

Turk DC, Melzack R, eds. *Handbook of Pain Assessment,* 2nd ed. New York: Guilford Press; 2001.

World Health Organization. *Cancer Pain Relief: With a Guide to Opioid Availability*, 2nd ed. Geneva: World Health Organization; 1996.

Migraines

Anthony M, Rasmussen BK. Migraine without aura. In: Olesen J, Tfelt-Hansen P, Welch KMA, eds. *The Headaches.* New York: Raven Press; 1993:255-261.

Barbanti P, Fabbrini G, Pesare M, Cerbo R. Unilateral cranial autonomic symptoms in migraine. *Cephalalgia.* 2002;22:256-259.

Cady RK, Schreiber CP. Sinus headache or migraine? Considerations in making a differential diagnosis. *Neurology.* 2002;58(suppl 6):S10-S14.

Campbell JK, Penzien DB, Wall EM. Evidence-based guidelines for migraine headache: behavioural and physical treatments, 2000. Accessed at http://www.aan.com/professionals/practice/guidelines.cfm.

Couch JR. Sinus headache: a neurologist's viewpoint. *Semin Neurol.* 1988;8:298-302.

Diamond M. The role of concomitant headache types and non-headache co-morbidities in the underdiagnosis of migraine. *Neurology.* 2002;58(suppl 6):S3-S9.

Drug Treatments for the Prevention of Migraine Headache. Technical Review 2.3. February 1999. Prepared for the Agency for Healthcare Policy and Research (contract no. 290-94-2025). Available from the National Technical Information Service (NTIS Accession No. 127953).

Goadsby P, Lipton R, Ferrari M. Migraine—current understanding and treatment. *N Engl J Med.* 2002;346:257-270.

Hargreaves RJ, Shepheard SL. Pathophysiology of migraine—new insights. *Can J Neurol Sci.* 1999;26(suppl 3):S12-S19.

Headache Classification Committee of the International Headache Society. Classification and diagnostic criteria for headache disorders, cranial neuralgias and facial pain. *Cephalalgia.* 1988;8(suppl 7):1-96.

Hutchison TA, Shahan DR, eds. DRUGDEX® System. MICROMEDEX, Greenwood Village, Colorado (edition expired 3/2003).

International Headache Society Web site. Revised classification proposal. Accessed at: http://216.25.100.131/members/Sections/members/login/Temp_Frame/frameset_26_06_02.htm.

Kaniecki RG, Totten J. Cervicalgia in migraine: prevalence, clinical characteristics, and response to treatment. Poster presented at 10th Congress of the International Headache Society, New York; 2002.

Lipton RB, Diamond S, Reed M, Diamond ML, Stewart WF. Migraine diagnosis and treatment: results from the American Migraine Study II. *Headache.* 2001;41:638-645.

Lipton RB, Stewart WF, Diamond S, et al. Prevalence and burden of migraine in the United States: data from the American Migraine Study II. *Headache.* 2001;41:646-657.

Matchar DB, Young WB, Rosenberg JH, et al. Evidence-based guidelines for migraine headache in the primary care setting: pharmacological management of acute attacks, 2000. Accessed at http://www.aan.com/professionals/practice/guidelines.cfm.

Ramadan NM, Silberstein SD, Freitag FG, Gilbert TT, Frishberg BM. Evidence-based guidelines for migraine headache in the primary care setting: pharmacological management for prevention of migraine, 2000. Accessed at http://www.aan.com/professionals/practice/guidelines.cfm.

Rasmussen BK, Jensen R, Schroll M, Olesen J. Interrelations between migraine and tension-type headache in the general population. *Arch Neurol.* 1992;49:914-918.

Smith TR. Pitfalls in migraine diagnosis and management. *Clin Cornerstone.* 4(3), 2001. Accessed at http://www.medscape.com/viewarticle/418183.

Snow V, Weiss K, Wall EM, Mottur-Pilson C. Pharmacological management of acute attacks of migraine and prevention of migraine headache. *Ann Intern Med.* 2002;137:840-849.

Spierings ELH, Ranke AH, Honkoop PC. Precipitating and aggravating factors of migraine versus tension-type headache. *Headache.* 2001;41:554-558.

Tepper S, Newman L, Dowson A, et al. The prevalence and diagnosis of migraine in a primary care setting in the United States—insights from the Landmark Study. Poster presented at the Annual Scientific Meeting of the American Headache Society, June 21-23, 2002, Seattle, Washington.

24. Seizure Disorders

Stephanie J. Phelps, PharmD, BCPS
Professor, Departments of Pharmacy and Pediatrics
University of Tennessee College of Pharmacy
Vice-Chair, Professional Experiential Program
University of Tennessee Health Science Center,
 Memphis, Tennessee

Contents

1. Epilepsy

- Neurons become depolarized and repetitively fire action potentials.

- Involuntary and episodic

- Term applied after two unprovoked seizures

- A seizure does not mean a person has epilepsy; however, epilepsy means a person has seizures

- Anticonvulsants *do not* cure epilepsy

Terminology

- *Aura:* a subjective sensation or motor phenomenon that marks a seizure onset and is generally associated with sensations that are localized in a particular region of the brain.

- *Automatisms:* purposeless movement seen with partial seizures

- *Postictal:* symptoms and signs seen after a seizure

Types Of Epilepsy

- There are two main types of epilepsy: partial seizures and generalized seizures.

Complex partial seizures
- Begins in one hemisphere of the brain; unilateral, asymmetric movements; generally associated with an aura and altered consciousness

Drugs of choice
- Carbamazepine; oxcarbazepine

Second-line agents
- Phenytoin, valproic acid, phenobarbital

- Consider all of the newer anticonvulsants (gabapentin, lamotrigine, topiramate, zonisamide, tiagabine, levetiracetam, felbamate)

Generalized seizures
- Begins simultaneously in both brain hemispheres; bilateral movements; *no* aura

Absence seizures
- Type of generalized sezure that has a sudden onset; brief (seconds); blank stare, upward rotation of the eyes, lip smacking (confused for daydreaming); 3

per second spike and wave on EEG; can be precipitated by hyperventilation

Drugs of choice
- Ethosuximide or valproic acid (*if >2 year*)

Primary generalized tonic-clonic seizure (formerly called grand mal)
- There are two phases to this seizure type.

Tonic phase
- Rigid, violent, sudden muscular contractions (stiff or rigid); cry or moan; deviation of the eyes and head to one side; rotation of the whole body and distortion of features; suppression of respiration; fall to the ground, loss of consciousness; tongue biting; involuntary urination

Clonic phase
- Repetitive jerks; cyanosis continues; foam at the mouth; small grunting respirations between seizures, but deep respirations as all muscles relax at end of seizure

Drugs of choice
- Phenytoin, carbamazepine

Second-line agents
- Lamotrigine, valproic acid, phenobarbital, primidone

- Consider topiramate

Juvenile myoclonic epilepsy (JME)
- Myoclonic seizures precede generalized tonic-clonic seizure; generally occur upon awakening; sleep deprivation and alcohol commonly precipitate; lifelong treatment required (valproic acid, lamotrigine, topiramate)

Other less common seizure types
Catamenial epilepsy
- Associated with hormonal changes during menstruation; may be treated with acetazolaminde (Diamox)

Infantile spasms
- Begins in the first 6 months of life; occur in clusters, several times a day; parents describe symptoms that sound like colic; high mortality and morbidity; treated with ACTH or oral steroids

Post-traumatic epilepsy
- Seizures that occur after head trauma; patients may be started on phenytoin for a period of 7 days; if no seizures occur, it should be discontinued

Etiologies For Epilepsy

- Mechanical: birth injuries; head trauma; tumors; vascular abnormalities (stroke)

- Metabolic: electrolyte disturbances; glucose abnormalities; inborn errors of metabolism

- Genetic: JME only

- Other: fever; infection

Medications
- Recreational (alcohol; cocaine/crack; ephedra; narcotics; methylphenidate)

- Carbapenems (imipenem); lindane; local anesthetics (lidocaine); metoclopramide; theophylline; tricyclic antidepressants

- Meperidine: the metabolite normeperidine can cause seizures in patients with renal failure who receive normal doses

- Anticonvulsants that are used for treatment of a non-indicated seizure type (Table 1)

Criteria for Treating Epilepsy

- Almost *no* child should be treated after one seizure

- Treat adults who have structural brain damage, a first seizure that was severe, or those with an occupation that places them at risk of injury should a second seizure occur.

Table 1

Seizures Caused by Anticonvulsants

| Anticonvulsant | Seizure type | | |
	Absence	Generalized tonic-clonic	Myoclonic
Carbamazepine (Tegretol®)			Causes
Ethosuximide (Zarontin®)		Causes	
Phenytoin (Dilantin®)	Causes		
Phenobarbital	Causes		Causes

Principles in the Treatment of Epilepsy

- Monotherapy (1 agent): *always* preferred

- Polytherapy (2 agents): add an anticonvulsant with a different mechanism of action *provided* doses of the first anticonvulsant have been maximized. Begin to slowly reduce the dose of the first drug. This is especially important if the patient has developed side effects or if the patient has not responded to the first anticonvulsant.

- Polytherapy (≥3 agents): although rarely needed, add a third anticonvulsant if: (1) a combination of anticonvulsants is tolerated and significantly reduces seizure frequency or severity, but greater control might be achieved; (2) the two anticonvulsants have been maximized. Reassess response and discontinue unnecessary anticonvulsants as soon as possible.

Reasons for Treatment Failure

- Incorrect diagnosis

- Wrong anticonvulsant selected

- Inappropriate dose, route, or formulation

- Poor patient adherence

- Seizure is refractory to therapy

Patient Counseling Information Applicable to All of the Anticonvulsants

- It is important that you keep a diary of your seizure(s) and keep regular appointments with your doctor, so it can be determined if your medication is working properly and if you are experiencing unwanted side effects.

- The full effects of this medication may not be seen for several weeks. Continue to take the medication unless directed otherwise by your physician.

- Take with food or milk if upset stomach occurs.

- Do not drink alcohol or take CNS depressants or illegal drugs with this medication.

- This medication may cause blurred vision or drowsiness. Do not drive or operate heavy machinery while taking this medication until you have become accustomed to its effects (exception: gabapentin).

- Consult with your physician if you anticipate pregnancy, become pregnant, or plan to breast-feed while taking this medication.

- It is extremely important if you are a woman capable of having children that you take 1 mg of folic acid a day.

- Do not stop taking this medication unless your doctor advises you to do so; some medicines have to be stopped slowly. Let your doctor or pharmacist know if you stop taking this medication.

- Check with your pharmacist or doctor before taking or starting any new medication (prescription, over-the-counter, or herbal product).

- Missed doses: if you miss a dose, take it as soon as you remember unless it is almost time for the next dose. If it is almost time for the next dose, then skip the missed dose and resume your regular schedule. Do not take extra or double doses. If you miss two or more doses contact your physician for further instructions. (See data for each anticonvulsant for additional counseling information.)

- Women of childbearing age who have epilepsy should take 1 mg/d of folic acid.

Mechanisms of Action for the Anticonvulsants

- Anticonvulsants work through a variety of mechanisms including:
  * Enhancement of sodium channel inactivation
  * Reducing current through T-type calcium channels
  * Enhance GABA activity
  * Some possess antiglutamate activity

2. Medications Used to Treat Epilepsy (Tables 2 and 3)

Phenobarbital

- Indications: neonatal seizures, generalized seizures (except absence); other anticonvulsants are more effective in complex partial seizures

Pharmacokinetics
- Bioavailability: excellent

- Protein binding: not clinically important

- Metabolism: liver

- Renal elimination: low; can increase with alkalinization of the urine

- Half-life: long (20-150 hours)

- Reference range: 15-40 mg/L

- Other: Primidone (Mysoline®) is an active anticonvulsant that is metabolized to phenobarbital.

Side effects
- *On initiation:* drowsiness, dizziness, light headedness, incoordination, headaches, or nervousness

- *With chronic therapy:*
  * Hyperactivity, primarily in children; however, rarely necessitates discontinuation of therapy
  * Cognition: lower memory and concentration abilities, slightly lowers IQ
  * Folate deficiency causing megaloblastic anemia
  * Vitamin K–deficient hemorrhagic disease: administer vitamin K to mother before delivery and to her newborn

- *Severe life-threatening:*
  * Hepatic failure: discontinue phenobarbital if liver function tests increase to >3 times above normal
  * Stevens-Johnson syndrome: discontinue phenobarbital if signs or symptoms of a severe rash develop; refer patient to physician

- Teratogenic (phenobarbital syndrome): developmental delay, short noses, low nasal bridges, low-set ears, wide mouths, protruding lips, distal digital hypoplasia. *The American College of Obstetricians and Gynecologists advocates phenobarbital as the anticonvulsant of choice in pregnancy.*

Table 2

Anticonvulsants: Dosage Forms, Normal Maintenance Doses, and Dosing Interval

Generic name	Trade name	Dosage form	Adult oral maintenance dose[1]	Interval[2]
Carbamazepine	Tegretol®	Suspension (100 mg/5 mL)	800-1200 mg/d	Suspension: qid
		Chewable tablet (100 mg)		Chewable tablet: tid-qid
		Tablet (200 mg)		Tablet (200 mg): bid
		Extended-release tablet (Tegretol XR®: 100, 200, 400 mg)		Extended-release tablet: bid
		Controlled-release tablet (Tegretol CR®: 200, 400 mg)		Controlled-release tablet: bid
	Carbitrol®	Extended-release capsule (200, 300 mg)		Extended-release capsule: bid
		Syrup (250 mg/5 mL)		
Ethosuximide	Zarontin®	Capsule (250 mg)	25-1500 mg/d	bid
Fosphenytoin	Cerebyx®	Injection (150 mg/2 mL; 750 mg/10 mL) 150 mg of fosphenytoin = 100 mg phenytoin	Not applicable	
Phenobarbital	Barbital®	Elixir (15 mg/5 mL, 20 mg/5 mL)	3-120 mg/d	bid-tid
	Luminal®	Tablet (8, 15, 16, 30, 32, 60, 65, 100 mg)		
	Solfoton®	Capsule (16 mg); powder for injection (120 mg); injection (30, 60, 65, 130 mg/mL)		
Phenytoin	Dilantin®	Suspension (125 mg/5 mL); chewable tablet (50 mg); prompt-release capsule (30, 100 mg); extended-release capsule (30, 100 mg); injection (50 mg/mL)	100-600 mg/d	qd-tid
Primidone	Mysoline®	Suspension (250 mg/5 mL); tablet (50, 125, 250 mg); chewable tablet (125 mg)	250-750 mg/d	tid-qid
Valproic acid				
Sodium valproate	Depacon®	Injection (100 mg/mL)	250-4000 mg/d	bid-tid
Divalproex sodium	Depekene®	Syrup (250 mg/5 mL)		
	Depekene	Gel capsule (125, 250 mg)		
	Depakote Sprinkles®	Capsule (125 mg)		
	Depakote®	Delayed-release tablet (125, 250, 500 mg)		
	Depakote ER®	Extended-release tablet (250, 500 mg)		qd

[1]With the exception of fosphenytoin and the intravenous dosage forms, these anticonvulsants are begun at low doses and slowly titrated to a dose that will control the patient's seizures.

[2]Interval may either decrease or increase in the presence of medications that induce or inhibit metabolism, respectively.

Drug-drug interactions: (inducer)
- Drugs that increase the serum concentration or effect of phenobarbital: chloramphenicol, felbamate, ketoconazole, methylphenidate, valproic acid

- Drugs that decrease the anticonvulsant effect of phenobarbital: phenytoin

- Phenobarbital may increase the serum concentration or effect of: alcohol, caffeine, MAO inhibitors

- Phenobarbital may decrease the serum concentration or effect of: rifampin, birth control pills, corticosteroids, cyclophosphamide, cyclosporine, delavirdine, griseofulvin, haloperidol, lamotrigine, metronidazole, propranolol, quidinine, ritonavir, saquinavir, theophylline, and warfarin

Table 3

Dosage Forms, Normal Maintenance Doses, and Dosing Intervals for the Newer Anticonvulsants

Generic name	Trade name	Dosage form	Oral maintenance dose[1]	Interval[2]
Felbamate	Felbatol®	Suspension (500 mg/5 mL), tablet (400, 600 mg)	1200-3600 mg/d	tid-qid
Gabapentin	Neurontin®	Capsules (100, 300, 400 mg), suspension (50 mg/mL)	900-3600 mg/d[3]	tid
Lamotrigine	Lamictal®	Chewable tablet (5, 25 mg), tablet (25, 100, 150, 200 mg)	50-400 mg/d	qd-bid
Levetiracetam	Keppra®	Tablet (250, 500, 750 mg)	1000-3000 mg/d	bid
Oxcarbazepine	Trileptal®	Tablet (150, 300, 600 mg)	600-2400 mg/d	bid
Tiagabine	Gabitril®	Tablet (4, 12, 16, 20 mg)	4-56 mg/d	bid-qid
Topiramate	Topamax®	Sprinkle capsule (15, 25 mg), tablet (25, 100, 200 mg)	50-1600 mg/d[4]	bid
Zonisamide	Zonegran®	Capsule (100 mg)	100-600 mg/d	qd

[1]With the exception of gabapentin, these anticonvulsants are begun at low doses and slowly titrated over weeks to a dose that will control the patient's seizures.

[2]Interval may either decrease or increase in the presence of medications that induce or inhibit metabolism, respectively.

[3]Much larger doses have been given.

[4]Doses >400 mg are no more effective than doses ≤400 mg. Typical maintenance dose in epilepsy is 200-400 mg/d.

Patient counseling specific to this medication

- This medication decreases the effectiveness of birth control pills. Use a backup birth control method to prevent pregnancy while taking phenobarbital.

Phenytoin

- Indications: all seizure types *except* absence and febrile seizures

Pharmacokinetics

- Bioavailability: slow, variable, decreased in children, and formulation-dependent

- Protein binding: very high (90-95%)

- Metabolism: liver (90%)

- Renal elimination: low (<5%)

- Half-life: phenytoin exhibits capacity-limited or saturable (ie, Michaelis-Menten) pharmacokinetics

- Reference range: 10–20 mg/L

Side effects

- *Upon initiation:* nausea, vomiting, drowsiness, and dizziness

- *With chronic therapy:*
  * Peripheral neuropathy
  * Hydantoin facies (thickening of subcutaneous tissues, enlargement of nose and lips)
  * Acne, hirsutism, and gingival hyperplasia (suggest good oral hygiene)
  * Osteomalacia (treat with vitamin D if alkaline phosphates increase and 25-hydroxycholecalciferol decreases)
  * Vitamin K–deficient hemorrhagic disease: administer vitamin K to mother before delivery and to newborn
  * Folate deficiency causing megaloblastic anemia

- *Severe life-threatening:*
  * Hepatic failure: discontinue if liver function test increase >3 times above normal
  * Stevens-Johnson syndrome: discontinue if signs or symptoms suggest a severe rash; notify physician

- Teratogenic (fetal hydantoin syndrome): craniofacial anomonalies, broad nasal bridges, short upturned noses, low set and prominent ears, distal digital hypoplasia, intrauterine growth restriction

Drug-drug interactions

- Drugs that increase the serum concentration or effect of phenytoin: acute alcohol use, amiodarone, chloramphcnicol, chlordiazepoxide, diazepam, disulfiram, estrogens, felbamate, H_2 antagonists (eg, cimetidine), halothane, isoniazid, methylphenidate, phenothiazines, phenylbutazone, salicylates, succinimides, sulfonamides (sulfadiazine, sulfamethoxazole, and sulfisoxazole), tolbutamide, trazodone, warfarin, zidovudine

- Drugs that decrease the effect of phenytoin: antacids, bleomycin, cisplatin, nevirapine, rifampin, ritonavir, vinblastine, zidovudine, and the herbals shankhapushpi, kava kava and valerian

- Phenytoin may increase the serum concentration or effect of valproic acid.

- Phenytoin may decrease the serum concentration or effect of phenobarbital.

Drug-nutrient interactions
- Patients receiving tube feedings and oral phenytoin at the same time may have a significant decrease in absorption of phenytoin. If possible, discontinue feeding 2 hours before and after a dose of phenytoin.

Patient counseling specific to phenytoin
- Do not break, crush or chew capsule before swallowing; swallow whole. Shake suspension well.

- This medication may alter your gums. Brush and floss daily, and have regular visits with your dentist.

- Contact your physician immediately if skin rash occurs.

- May decrease the effectiveness of birth control pills

- Missed doses: *Once daily dosing:* If it has been <12 hours since the scheduled time, take as soon as possible. If >12 hours have passed, skip the missed dose and go back to your regular schedule. *Divided dosages:* Take missed dose as soon as possible, even if it means taking two doses, then return to the regular schedule. Contact your physician or pharmacist if you missed two or more doses.

Carbamazepine

- Indications: most widely used anticonvulsant in adults and children; drug of choice for complex partial seizures; effective in most generalized seizures; ineffective in absence seizures and febrile seizures

Pharmacokinetics
- Bioavailability: good; dispense in moisture-proof containers because studies show decreased bioavailability with high humidity (ie, medicine cabinets)

- Protein binding: not important

- Metabolism: hepatic metabolism is extensive

- Renal elimination: low

- Half-life: about a day if used as monotherapy; about 12 hours if given with >1 anticonvulsant

- Reference range: 4-12 mg/L (monotherapy = 8-12 mg/L; polytherapy = 4-8 mg/L)

Other
- Carbamazepine is metabolized to a 10,11 carbamazepine epoxide, which is both effective as an anticonvulsant and capable of causing toxicity

- Carbamazepine is one of a few drugs that can induce its own metabolism (ie, autoinduction). Mean time to onset is 21 days (range: 17-31 days)

Side effects
- *Upon initiation:* dose-related, transient, and reversible rash that rarely cause the drug to be discontinued; nausea, vomiting, drowsiness, and dizziness

- *With chronic therapy:*
    * SIADH (hyponatremia and water retention)
    * Osteomalacia (treat with vitamin D if alkaline phosphates increase and 25-hydroxycholecalciferol decreases)
    * Vitamin K–deficient hemorrhagic disease: administer vitamin K to mother before delivery and to newborn
    * Folate deficiency causing megaloblastic anemia

- *Severe life-threatening:*
    * Direct hepatotoxicity (*FDA Black Box Warning*): <1 month; fever; rash; fatalities may occur even if drug is discontinued; stop carbamazepine if liver function tests increase >3 times above normal
    * Aplastic anemia (*FDA Black Box Warning*): recommended to discontinue carbamazepine if WBC <2000-3000 or neutrophils <1000-1500

- Teratogenic (fetal carbamazepine syndrome): epicanthal folds; short nose, long philtrum, hypoplastic nails, microcephaly, developmental delay

Drug-drug interactions

- Drugs that increase the serum concentration or effect of carbamazepine: erythromycin, cimetidine, lithium, propoxyphene

- Drugs that decrease the anticonvulsant effect of carbamazepine: phenobarbital, primidone, phenytoin

- Carbamazepine may increase the serum concentration or effect of felbamate; felbamate will increase concentration of the 10,11 epoxide metabolite and cause toxicity

- Carbamazepine may decrease the serum concentration or effect of: cyclosporine, doxycycline, haloperidol, oral contraceptives, theophylline

Patient counseling

- Shake suspension well.

- Do not use with monoamine oxidase inhibitors.

Valproic Acid

- Indications: all types of generalized and partial seizures. Along with ethosuximide this is the drug of choice for absence seizures. *Do not* use in children <2 years of age.

Pharmacokinetics

- Bioavailability: excellent

- Protein binding: high

- Metabolism: hepatic

- Reference range: 50-150 mg/L

Side effects

- *Upon initiation:* nausea and vomiting

- *With chronic therapy:*
  * Weight gain: at times significant enough to warrant discontinuing the medication
  * Alopecia: partial or total (to prevent/treat supplement with zinc and selenium)
  * Tremor: dose-dependent (treat by decreasing the dose, discontinuing the drug, or adding propranolol)
  * Thrombocytopenia: dose-dependent decrease in platelets
  * Elevations in liver enzymes: may be transient and responds to discontinuation of valproic acid

- *Severe life-threatening:*
  * Fatal hepatotoxicity (*FDA Black Box Warning*): most common in children <2 years of age who have severe epilepsy and are receiving multiple anticonvulsants
  * Fatal hemorrhagic pancreatitis (*FDA Black Box Warning*)

- Teratogenic (*FDA Black Box Warning*): fetal valproate syndrome): craniofacial anomonalies, small inverted noses, shallow philtrum, flat nasal bridge, long upper lip, congenital liver disease, and spina bifida. There is an association between folic acid deficiency and spina bifida, so all women with epilepsy who are of childbearing years should be on daily folic acid (1 mg).

Drug-drug interactions

- Drugs that increase the serum concentration or effect of valproic acid: felbamate, phenytoin, salicylates

- Drugs that decrease the anticonvulsant effect of valproic acid: carbamazepine, felbamate, lamotrigine, phenytoin, phenobarbital, primidone

- Valproic acid may increase the serum concentration or effect of: amitriptyline, carbamazepine, ethosuximide, felbamate, lamotrigine, phenobarbital, primidone, zidovudine

- Valproic acid may decrease the serum concentration or effect of: phenytoin

Patient counseling

- You may take this medication with food or milk to reduce stomach irritation. Do not take with carbonated drinks.

- Valproic acid capsules: swallow whole with water only; do not break, chew, or crush.

- Divalproex sodium delayed-released capsules: swallow whole or sprinkle the contents on a small amount of cool, soft food (eg, applesauce or pudding) and swallow without chewing immediately after preparation.

- Divalproex sodium delayed-release tablets: swallow the tablets whole; do not break, chew, or crush.

- Valproic acid syrup: you may mix the syrup with any liquid or add it to a small amount of food.

- Report any sore throat, fever, fatigue, bleeding, or bruising that is severe or persists to patient's physician.

- Your doctor may monitor your liver function with blood tests every 1-2 weeks initially, and periodically thereafter.

- Missed dose: *do not* double dose. *Once daily:* Take as soon as possible, but do not take if you don't remember until the next day. *Multiple doses:* If you remember within 6 hours, take your remaining doses for that day at equally spaced intervals. If you miss two or more consecutive doses, contact you physician for further instructions.

Felbamate (Rarely Used)

Indications: Lennox-Gastaux syndrome, tonic-clonic (grand mal), tonic-myoclonic, and refractory partial seizures with or without secondary generalization

Pharmacokinetics
- 50% renally eliminated

Side effects
- *With chronic therapy:* weight loss significant enough to warrant discontinuing the medication

- *Severe life-threatening:*
    * Hepatotoxicity: (*FDA Black Box Warning*)
    * Aplastic anemia: (*FDA Black Box Warning*)

Drug-drug interactions
- Inhibitor and inducer: If a patient on carbamazepine has symptoms of toxicity and their carbamazepine serum concentration is low they likely have an increased concentration of the active metabolite (10,11 epoxide). Reduce the dose of carbamazepine.

Patient counseling
- Patient or legal guardian should sign a consent form before taking this medication.

- Your doctor may monitor your liver function with blood tests every 1-2 weeks initially, and periodically thereafter and may also do urine test.

Gabapentin

- Indications: partial seizures. This drug is used most often for peripheral neuropathies and not epilepsy.

Pharmacokinetics
- Bioavailability: poor

- Renal elimination: 100%

Side effects
- *Severe life-threatening:* None

Drug-drug interactions
- No interactions that affect metabolism; aluminum- and/or magnesium-containing antacids may decrease the absorption; not a true drug interaction, but combination with carbamazepine may cause dizziness (reduce the dose of carbamazepine).

Patient counseling
- Food may decrease the extent of absorption.

- If you take antacids, wait at least 2 hours before taking gabapentin.

- Missed dose: Take as soon as possible. If <2 hours until the next dose, take the missed dose and then take the next dose 1-2 hours later, resuming your normal regimen. If you miss more than one dose, call your pharmacist or doctor for instructions.

Lamotrigine

- Indications: partial seizures; primary and secondary generalized tonic-clonic seizures; absence, atypical absence, atonic, myoclonic seizures; and seizures associated with Lennox-Gaustaut syndrome

Pharmacokinetics
- None unique

Side effects
- *Severe life-threatening:*
    * Skin rash (*FDA Black Box Warning*): may lead to Stevens-Johnson syndrome. *Must* titrate a patient to a maintenance dose very slowly. This is especially true if they are also receiving valproic acid.

Drug-drug interactions
- Drugs that increase the serum concentration or effect of lamotrigine: valproic acid

- Drugs that decrease the anticonvulsant effect of lamotrigine: carbamazepine, phenytoin, phenobarbital, primidone

- Lamotrigine may increase the serum concentration or effect of: none

- Lamotrigine may decrease the serum concentration or effect of: valproic acid

- Not a true drug-drug interaction, but the combination with carbamazepine may cause dizziness (reduce the dose of carbamazepine)

Patient counseling

- Notify your physician *immediately* if a skin rash occurs.

- Women of childbearing years with epilepsy should take 1 mg of folic acid.

Topiramate

- Indications: indicated as adjunctive therapy for adults and pediatric patients ages 2-16 years with partial onset seizures, or primary generalized tonic-clonic seizures, and in patients 2 years of age and older with seizures associated with Lennox-Gastaut syndrome.

Pharmacokinetics
- Elimination: primarily renal

Side effects
- *Upon initiation:* drowsiness; dizziness; difficulty with concentration; loss of appetite; mood changes; paresthesias; oligohidrosis (rare): monitor use in children in hot climates

- *With chronic therapy:*
  * Kidney stones (patients with a history of kidney stones should be adequately hydrated)
  * Word finding difficulties/CNS effects
  * Significant weight loss

- *Severe life-threatening:* None

Drug-drug interactions
- Drugs that increase the serum concentration or effect of topiramate: CNS depressants (alcohol, morphine, codeine), carbonic anhydrase inhibitors (acetazolamide)

- Drugs that decrease the anticonvulsant effect of topiramate: phenobarbital, phenytoin, valproic acid

- Topiramate may increase the serum concentration or effect of: metformin

- Topiramate may decrease the serum concentration or effect of: oral contraceptives, valproic acid

Patient counseling
- If using the Topamax sprinkle capsules, sprinkle the contents on a small amount of cool, soft food (eg, applesauce or yogurt) and swallow immediately without chewing.

- Drink plenty of fluids

- Consult your physician if you anticipate pregnancy,

become pregnant, or plan to breast-feed while taking this medication.

Tiagibine

- Indications: partial seizures

Pharmacokinetics:
- Protein binding: high

- Hepatically cleared

Side effects
- *Severe life-threatening:* none

Drug-drug interactions
- Drugs that increase the serum concentration or effect of tiagabine: valproic acid

- Drugs that decrease the anticonvulsant effect of tiagabine: carbamazepine, phenobarbital, primidone, phenytoin

- Tiagabine may increase the serum concentration or effect of: none

- Tiagabine may decrease the serum concentration or effect of: valproic acid

Patient counseling
- None unique

Zonisamide

- Indications: partial seizures

Side effects
- *Chronic therapy:* (very similar to topiramate)
  * Inability to sweat (unique to zonisamide)
  * Kidney stones
  * Weight loss
  * Reversible or irreversible psychosis (rare)

- *Severe life-threatening:*
- Oligohidrosis (may not sweat) (*FDA Bold Warning*): Children taking may not sweat as needed and could develop hyperthermia. Warn of the need to be aware of getting overheated and to drink plenty of water.

Drug-drug interactions
- Drugs that decrease the effect of zonisamide: carbamazepine, phenobarbital, phenytoin, valproic acid

Patient counseling

- Drink plenty of fluids to help prevent kidney stones.

- Contact your doctor if your child is not sweating as usual.

Levetiracetam

- Indications: partial seizures

Side effects
- *Upon initiation:* dizziness, fatigue, sedation

- *With chronic therapy:* None

- *Severe life-threatening:* None

Drug-drug interactions
- No significant ones noted to date

Patient counseling
- None

3. Other Issues

Nondrug Treatment of Epilepsy

- Ketogenic diet

- Vagal nerve stimulator

- Surgical correction

Withdrawal of Anticonvulsants

- Over half of patients who remain seizure free for 2 years can have their anticonvulsant successfully withdrawn. Virtually all who are seizure-free for 4 years can be successfully withdrawn.

- Unless the patient is experiencing a severe or life-threatening adverse effect *never* abruptly discontinue an anticonvulsant; taper slowly over 2-6 months.

Status Epilepticus

- A seizure that lasts longer than 30 minutes or ≥2 discrete seizures between which there is incomplete recovery of consciousness.

- Status epilepticus is a medical emergency.

- See Table 4 for suggested order of therapies.

Benzodiazepines
- First-line agents; *diazepam or lorazepam are drugs of choice*

Phenytoin (intravenous)
- Can only be mixed with normal saline.

- Loading dose: if an individual is not already receiving phenytoin, give 15-20 mg/kg. Because phenytoin contains propylene glycol and is in itself cardiotoxic, do not infuse faster than 50 mg/min.

- Maintenance dose: If the maintenance dose is to be given every 12 hours, give the first dose 12 hours after the end of the loading dose. If the maintenance dose is to be given every 24 hours, give the first dose 24 hours after the end of the loading dose.

- Not only is the bioavailability of phenytoin reduced, but its alkaline pH precludes its administration by the IM route.

Table 4

Time Frame for the Treatment of Status Epilepticus

As soon as possible	• Assess cardiorespiratory status; insert oral airway and administer oxygen as needed • Place secure IV and start infusion of normal saline • Obtain medical history; perform neurological examination • Obtain the following test: If the patient has been on anticonvulsants as an outpatient, obtain blood for serum drug concentrations; chemistry panel including electrolytes, glucose, BUN, and urine drug screen • Administer 25 g of glucose and 100 mg of thiamine IV
If still seizing:	• Administer either diazepam or lorazepam up to maximum dosage until seizure stops
<30 minutes *If still seizing:*	• Load with IV phenytoin (provided patient not on phenytoin at home or has low serum concentrations) and begin maintenance doses • Monitor blood pressure and EEG
30-60 minutes	• If seizures persist give loading dose of IV phenobarbital or begin a continuous infusion of midazolam
1 hour	• Begin medically-induced coma • Adjust EEG to burst-suppression • Avoid hypotension during infusion of the barbiturate

Fosphenytoin

• Phenytoin prodrug which is converted to phenytoin within minutes after infusion.

• Can be admixed with any IV solution

• Must be dose in PE (phenytoin equivalents): 1 mg of phenytoin = 1.5 mg of fosphenytoin

• Can be given at a rate of 150 mg/min (three times faster than phenytoin)

Phenobarbital

• May cause respiratory depression/arrest (likelihood may be increased if benzodiazepines have been given)

• Sedation may eliminate the ability to perform an accurate neurologic assessment.

Midazolam

• Continuous infusion due to short half-life

Medically-induced coma

• Usually achieved with pentobarbital

• Use for severe refractory status epilepticus

• Give loading dose (20-40 mg/kg) over 1-2 hours, followed by continuous infusion (1-4 mg/kg per hour).

• If hypotension occurs, begin dopamine or slow the rate of infusion.

• Titrate to burst suppression (isoelectric) on EEG.

Other therapies used for refractory status epilepticus

• Propofol

• Magnesium

• Lidocaine

• IV immune globulin

Febrile Seizures

• A benign seizure occurring in the absence of CNS infection in a child with fever

• Most common seizure disorder in childhood

- Age of onset: 4 months to 5 years (peak at 14-18 months)

- Risk factors (≥2 of the following):
  * A first- or second-degree relative with a history of a febrile seizure
  * Developmental delay
  * Delayed discharge (>28 days) from a newborn center
  * Day care attendance

- Risk for developing epilepsy:
  * The development of epilepsy is rare.
  * About 15% of children who have a complex febrile seizure will develop epilepsy.

- There are two types of febrile seizures:
  * Simple febrile seizure:
    • Benign
    • A primary generalized seizure
    • Last <15 minutes
    • Does not recur within 24 hours
  * Complex febrile seizure:
    • Focal (involves an arm, leg, or face on one side only or eye deviation towards one side)
    • Prolonged (>15 min) and/or recurring within 24 hours of the initial seizure

Acute treatment of a simple or complex partial seizure
- Seizure control: drugs of choice for prolonged febrile seizure are ***rectally administered benzodiazepines*** (rectal diazepam [Valium®] or lorazepam [Ativan®])

- Diastat®: commercially available as a gel of diazepam to be given rectally

Prophylaxis for a simple or complex partial seizure
- If temperature is >38C° give acetaminophen.

- Daily anticonvulsants are ***not*** indicated for the prevention of recurrent febrile seizures.

Maintenance therapy:
- ***Not*** generally used

- An anticonvulsant (ie, phenobarbital) may be considered after a complex febrile seizure if epilepsy is suspected.

- Carbamazepine and phenytoin are ***not*** effective in the prevention of recurrent febrile seizures

4. Key Points

- Phenytoin can only be mixed with normal saline and should not be given faster than 50 mg/min.

- Gabapentin is not associated with any significant drug interactions.

- As of January 2003, the following anticonvulsants carry a "black box" warning: carbamazepine (aplastic anemia, hepatic failure), valproic acid (liver failure, teratogenicity, pancreatitis), felbamate (aplastic anemia, hepatic failure), and lamotrigine (serious rash). Zonisamide and topiramate have recently been reported to cause oligohidrosis and hyperthermia.

- The drug of choice for absence seizures is ethosuximide. Valproic acid may also be given to those ≥2 years of age.

- Carbapenems (eg, imipenem) and normeperidine (a metabolite of meperidine that accumulates in renal failure) may cause seizures.

- Carbamazepine undergoes autoinduction (ie, induces it own metabolism) and phenytoin has capacity-limited or saturable (ie, Michaelis-Menten) pharmacokinetics.

- Because of the potential for severe life-threatening liver toxicity, valproic acid is generally not used in a patient ≤2 years of age.

- There is an association between folic acid deficiency and spina bifida; hence all women and especially those with epilepsy who are of childbearing years should be on daily folic acid (1 mg).

- Unless a patient is experiencing a life-threatening adverse effect, an anticonvulsant should not be abruptly discontinued.

- Topiramate may cause significant weight loss and valproic acid may cause significant weight gain.

- Topiramate and zonisamide may cause kidney stones.

5. Questions and Answers

1. Which of the following is true regarding phenytoin?

   A. The maximum rate of intravenous administration is 50 mg/min.
   B. If intravenous access can't be established, phenytoin can be given IM.
   C. Because phenytoin contains propylene glycol it is soluble is any IV fluid.
   D. It is an inhibitor of the cytochrome P450 system.
   E. A major limitation to the use of the product in pediatric patients is the lack of a commercially available liquid formulation.

2. A 50-kg patient with no history of epilpesy presents in status epilepticus. They are given an adequate dose of lorazepam and are about to be given a loading dose of intravenous phenytoin. Assuming a phenytoin Vd of 0.6 L/kg, what dose of phenytoin should be given to achieve a serum phenytoin concentration of ~16-18 mg/L?

   A. 18 mg/kg
   B. 500 mg
   C. 30 mg/kg
   D. 50 mg
   E. 5 g

3. Which of the following is true regarding a patient with refractory status epilepticus who is placed in a medically-induced coma with a barbiturate?

   A. If the patient is mechanically ventilated, the barbiturates with induce respiratory arrest.
   B. The goal of a coma that is medically-induced with a barbiturate is to induce burst suppression (isoelectric) on EEG.
   C. If hypotension develops, the patient should be given nitroprusside.
   D. The barbiturates are not associated with drug interactions.
   E. A major problem with this type of therapy is kidney failure.

4. Which of the following is associated with autoinduction?

   A. Phenobarbital
   B. Phenytoin
   C. Carbamazepine
   D. Gabapentin
   E. Levetiracetam

5. Which of these agents reduces the likelihood of congenital malformations in epileptic women receiving valproate?

   A. Folic acid
   B. Vitamin B_{12}
   C. Gingko biloba
   D. Iron
   E. Selenium

6. A 33-year-old woman is being started on an anticonvulsant. The woman is already slightly overweight and is very concerned about the effects of the various medications on her weight. Which of the following is true regarding anticonvulsants and their effect on weight?

   I. Valproic acid increases weight.
   II. Topiramate decreases weight.
   III. Phenytoin increases weight.

   A. I
   B. I and II
   C. II
   D. III
   E. I, II, and III

7. A 24-year-old with complex partial seizures is currently controlled with valproic acid, gabapentin, and topiramate. She calls your pharmacy to ask if any of her medications can cause nosebleeds since she has had 1-2 in the past week. You refer her to her LMD, where her platelet count is reported to be 95,132/mm^3. Which of the following is true?

   A. None of her anticonvulsants cause thrombocytopenia.
   B. Valproate can cause a dose-related thrombocytopenia.
   C. Gabapentin has inhibited the metabolism of topiramate, and the elevated concentration of topiramate is responsible for the thrombocytopenia.
   D. Gabapentin can cause idiosyncratic thrombocytopenia.
   E. Topiramate can cause thrombocytopenia.

8. A patient has hypertension, diabetes mellitus, and chronic renal failure (serum Cr 6.8), and has developed seizures. Which of the following anticonvulsants would require dosage adjustment in this patient?

A. Gabapentin, topiramate
B. Lamotrigine, felbamate
C. Phenobarbital, gabapentin
D. Phenytoin, valproic acid
E. Phenobarbital, levetiracetam

9. Which of the following anticonvulsants is metabolized to phenobarbital?

   A. Ethosuximide
   B. Primidone
   C. Zonisamide
   D. Levetiracetam
   E. Carbamazepine

10. A 7-year-old on valproic acid for partial complex seizures with secondary generalization that are refractory to phenobarbital, phenytoin, carbamazepine, and gabapentin, continued to have seizures and was started on lamotrigine 2 weeks ago. Today he presents with a diffuse maculopapular erythematous rash with lesions on the lips. Which of the following is correct?

    A. A rash associated with lamotrigine generally occurs within the first few days; hence the rash is not associated with an anticonvulsant.
    B. The patient should be given diphenhydramine and the lamotrigine should be continued.
    C. Lamotrigine should be discontinued.
    D. The rash is secondary to a drug interaction between gabapentin and carbamazepine.
    E. All of the anticonvulsants are associated with life-threatening rash. In order to prevent status epilepticus associated with abrupt discontinuation of the anticonvulsants, the medications should be slowly discontinued.

11. A new anticonvulsant has just been approved by the FDA. Its bioavailability is >95% and it is highly protein bound to alpha$_1$-acid glycoprotein. It undergoes extensive hepatic metabolism by CYP 2C9. Less than 5% is excreted unchanged in the urine. It is known to inhibit CYP 3A4. A patient on this anticonvulsant has developed significant depression and is being started on an antidepressant that is 93% bound to albumin and is a potent inhibitor of CYP 2C19. The antidepressant is metabolized by CYP 3A4 to an active metabolite that is hepatically cleared by CYP 2C9. The neurologist wants to know if any drug interactions may occur that would necessitate reduction in drug dosage.

    A. No drug interactions should occur in this patient.
    B. The dose of the anticonvulsant should be reduced because of a potential protein binding interaction that would increase the serum concentration of the anticonvulsant.
    C. The dose of the anticonvulsant should be increased.
    D. The dose of the antidepressant should be reduced.
    E. Because of an interaction in the gut that decreased bioavailability, the dose should be increased.

12. Which of the following are not associated with any drug-drug interactions?

    I.   Gabapentin
    II. Carbamazepine
    III. Levetiracetam

    A. I
    B. II
    C. I and III
    D. II and III
    E. I and II
    F. III

13. A 42-year-old woman has been successfully treated with valproic acid for years, but she has experienced some undesirable side effects. She is slowly titrated onto a new anticonvulsant and the valproic acid is slowly discontinued. She presents to the ED with severe flank pain and is diagnosed with a kidney stone. Which of the following may have precipitated her current situation?

    A. Gabapentin
    B. Lamotrigine
    C. Levetiracetam
    D. Topiramate
    E. Levetiracetam

14. Which of the following drugs carries a black box warning?

    I.   Carbamazepine
    II. Felbamate
    III. Levetiracetam

    A. II
    B. III
    C. I
    D. I and II
    E. II and III

15. Which of the following carries a black box warning for pancreatitis?

   A. Carbamazepine
   B. Felbamate
   C. Zonisamide
   D. Valproic acid
   E. Phenytoin

16. What is the drug of choice for absence seizures in a child <2 years of age?

   A. Phenytoin
   B. Phenobarbital
   C. Ethosuximide
   D. Valproic acid
   E. Primidone

17. Diastat is given by which of the following routes?

   A. Rectally
   B. Intramuscular
   C. Intravenously
   D. Intranasally
   E. Subcutaneously

18. Which of the following is true?

   A. Febrile seizures must be accompanied by a CNS infection.
   B. Complex febrile seizures last >15 minutes.
   C. Most children who have a febrile seizure go on to develop epilepsy.
   D. The drug of choice for a simple febrile seizure is carbamazepine.
   E. Simple febrile seizures should never be treated.

19. Which of the following anticonvulsants are available in a liquid, chewable tablet, and intravenous formulation?

   I. Carbamazepine
   II. Phenytoin
   III. Valproic acid

   A. II
   B. III
   C. I
   D. I and II
   E. I, II, and III

20. Patients should be told to drink plenty of fluid when taking which of the following?

   A. Carbamazepine
   B. Topiramate
   C. Levetiracetam
   D. Gabapentin
   E. Phenytoin

21. Which of the following medications may cause seizures in an adult patient with renal failure?

   A. Meperidine
   B. Phenobarbital
   C. Carbamazepine
   D. Lamotrigine
   E. Theophylline

22. Which of the following is associated with Michaelis-Menten pharmacokinetics?

   A. Carbamazepine
   B. Valproic acid
   C. Topiramate
   D. Phenytoin
   E. Phenobarbital

23. A patient on this medication should be made aware of the importance of good oral hygiene.

   A. Felbamate
   B. Phenytoin
   C. Zonisamide
   D. Phenobarbital
   E. Levetiracetam

Answers

1. **A.** Because phenytoin contains propylene glycol and is itself cardiotoxic, the IV formulation should not be infused faster than 50 mg/min. Phenytoin is extremely alkaline (pH ~13). Not only is IM administration associated with tissue damage, it is erratically absorbed. Phenytoin can only be admixed with normal saline, is an inducer, and is also available as a suspension and a chewable tablet.

2. **B.** The equation for calculation of a loading dose is as follows: dose = Cp desired x Vd. So Cp desired is ~17 x (0.6 L/kg x 50 kg) ≈ 510 mg.

3. **B.** The goal is to produce a "flat" EEG. If the patient is mechanically ventilated, the effect of a medication on respiration is not a factor in its administration. Although pentobarbital may cause hypotension if given too rapidly, nitroprusside is a vasodilator used to treat

hypertension. The barbiturates are known inducers. Coma that is medically-induced with a barbiturate does not cause kidney failure.

4. **C.** Carbamazepine induces it own metabolism, with peak effects seen about 21 days after beginning the medication or following an increase in dosage. Phenobarbital and phenytoin are inducers. Gabapentin and levetiracetam are not cleared hepatically.

5. **A.** Many of the anticonvulsants can cause folic acid deficiency. There is an association between folic acid deficiency and spina bifida; hence all women with epilepsy who are of childbearing years should receive supplemental folic acid every day (1 mg).

6. **B.** Topiramate can cause significant weight loss and valproate can cause significant weight gain. Phenytoin does not significantly affect weight.

7. **B.** Valproic acid can cause clinically significant thrombocytopenia. Gabapentin is not associated with any drug interaction that affects metabolism, and it does not cause a decrease in platelets. Topiramate does not cause thrombocytopenia.

8. **A.** Gabapentin and topiramate would require dosage adjustment since they are renally eliminated.

9. **B.** Primidone (Mysoline) is an active anticonvulsant, but it is also metabolized to phenobarbital.

10. **C.** Lamotrigine has a black box warning for severe rash. Since this patient has a diffuse rash *and* lesions on the lips, the lamotrigine should be discontinued. Because the incidence of severe rash may be higher in children than adults, current practice would be to discontinue lamotrigine and not "treat through" the rash with diphenhydramine. Gabapentin does not interact with lamotrigine. However, the combination of valproic acid and lamotrigine is associated with a higher incidence of rash. While abrupt discontinuation of an anticonvulsant may induce status epilepticus, an anticonvulsant may be abruptly discontinued in the face of a life-threatening event.

11. **D** is correct because the new anticonvulsant inhibits CYP 3A4 and the antidepressant is metabolized by this enzyme.

12. **C.** At this time, neither gabapentin nor levetiracetam are associated with significant drug-drug interactions. The absorption of gabapentin may be reduced by concurrent administration of aluminum- and/or magnesium-containing antacids; hence antacids should be given 2 hours before or after a dose of gabapentin. Carbamazepine is an inducer that is associated with numerous drug-drug interactions.

13. **D.** Both topiramate and zonisamide may cause kidney stones. Individuals with a history of kidney stones should not be prescribed this drug.

14. **D.** Both carbamazepine and felbamate are associated with aplastic anemia and hepatic failure. Levetiracetam has no black box warning.

15. **D.** Valproic acid may cause fatal hemorrhagic pancreatitis.

16. **C.** Although valproic acid is extremely effective and is frequently used as monotherapy for absence seizures, it should not be given to a patient ≤2 years of age.

17. **A.** Diastat is commercially available as a gel form of diazepam that is given rectally.

18. **B.** Unlike simple febrile seizures that last a brief period, complex febrile seizures are prolonged (>15 minutes) and/or recurring within 24 hours of the initial seizure. Febrile seizures must occur in the absence of CNS infection in a child with fever. Most febrile seizures are benign and children do not go on to develop epilepsy. Carbamazepine is ineffective in febrile seizures.

19. **A.** Only phenytoin is available as a liquid (125 mg/5 mL), chewable tablet (50 mg), and in an intravenous dosage form. Carbamazepine is not available in an IV dosage form and valproic acid is not available as a chewable tablet.

20. **B.** Because topiramate may cause kidney stones, patients should be encouraged to drink plenty of fluids. This would also be true for zonisamide.

21. **B.** Normeperidine, a metabolite of meperidine, can accumulate in patients with renal failure who receive normal doses and cause seizures. The other agents listed are not eliminated renally in adults.

22. **D.** Phenytoin has capacity-limited or saturable (ie, Michaelis-Menten) pharmacokinetics.

23. **B.** Phenytoin may cause gingival hyperplasia (ie, overgrowth of the gums). Hence patients should be instructed to brush and floss daily, and have regular visits with the dentist.

6. References

American Academy of Neurology. Quality Standards Subcommittee. Practice Parameter: A guideline for discontinuing antiepileptic drugs in seizure-free patients—summary statement. *Neurology.* 1996;47:660-702.

Anderson GD. A mechanistic approach to antiepileptic drug interactions. *Ann Pharmacother.* 1998;32:554-563.

Baumann RJ, Duffner PK. Treatment of children with simple febrile seizures: the AAP practice parameter. American Academy of Pediatrics. *Pediatr Neurol.* 2000;23:11-17.

Brunbech L, Sabers A. Effect of antiepileptic drugs on cognitive function in individuals with epilepsy: a comparative review of newer versus older agents. *Drugs.* 2002;62:593-604.

Carroll MC, Yueng-Yue KA, Esterly NB, et al. Drug-induced hypersensitivity syndrome in pediatric patients. *Pediatrics.* 2001;108:485-492.

Commission on antiepileptic drugs, International League Against Epilepsy. Guidelines for therapeutic monitoring on antiepileptic drugs. *Epilepsia.* 1993;34:585-587.

Deckers CL, Knoester PD, de Haan GJ, et al. Selection criteria for the clinical use of the newer antiepileptic drugs. *CNS Drugs.* 2003;17:405-421.

Johannessen SI, Battino D, Berry DJ, et al. Therapeutic drug monitoring of the newer antiepileptic drugs. *Ther Drug Monit.* 2003;25:347-463.

Perucca E. The clinical pharmacokinetics of the new antiepileptic drugs. *Epilepsia.* 1999;40(suppl 9):S7-S13.

Working Group on Status Epilepticus. Treatment of convulsive status epilepticus: Recommendations of the Epilepsy Foundation of America's Working Group on Status Epilepticus. *JAMA.* 1993;270: 854-859.

25. Psychiatric Disease

Melissa L. Tucker, PharmD
Assistant Professor of Psychopharmacology,
  Department of Pharmacy
University of Tennessee College of Pharmacy
Director of Pharmacy
Memphis Mental Health Institute, Memphis, Tennessee

1. Schizophrenia

Schizophrenia is a psychiatric disorder characterized by a profound disruption in perception, cognition, and emotion.

Epidemiology

- Approximately 1% of the U.S. adult population has schizophrenia

- 200,000 new cases are reported yearly

- No gender or racial differences

- Earlier onset in males (average age, 18-24) than females (average age, late 20s to early 40s)

Types and Classifications

Paranoid
- Prominent preoccupation with hallucinations (usually auditory) and one or more delusions

Disorganized
- Disorganized speech and behavior
- Blunted, flat, or inappropriate affect

Catatonic
- Psychomotor disturbances that may involve catalepsy or stupor, excessive motor activity, rigid posture, mutism, peculiar or repetitive movements, and/or echolalia or echopraxia

Undifferentiated
- Hallucinations/delusions are present but without prominent paranoid, disorganized, or catatonic symptoms

Residual
- Hallucinations/delusions are not prominent, but there is continued evidence of an ongoing disturbance (flat affect, poverty of speech, or avolition)

Clinical Presentation

- The onset of schizophrenia is typically characterized by deterioration in occupational and social situations over a period of 6 months or more

Symptoms
- Hallucinations (auditory, visual, tactile, olfactory, and/or gustatory)
- Delusions (usually persecutory and/or grandiose)

- Disorganized thoughts and/or speech

- Impaired cognition, attention, concentration, judgment, and motivation

- Symptoms are commonly referred to as *positive* (hallucinations, delusions), *negative* (flat affect, avolition, anhedonia, poverty of thought), or *disorganized* (disorganized speech and/or behavior)

- Most patients fluctuate between acute episodes and remission, but complete remission without any symptoms is uncommon

Associated features
Morbidity
- There are many comorbid disease states (mental and medical), eg, substance abuse is found in 60-70% of persons with schizophrenia

Mortality
- Shortened life expectancy

- Increased risk of suicide (10% commit suicide)

- Risk factors for suicide:
    * Male gender, social isolation, comorbid psychiatric disorders, unemployed, <30 years of age

Etiology (Most Likely Multifactorial)

Genetic

Neurobiologic

Developmental
- Season of birth, viral, traumatic

DSM-IV Diagnostic Criteria

- Two or more of the following symptoms prevail for at least 1 month:
    * Hallucinations
    * Delusions
    * Disorganized speech
    * Grossly disorganized or catatonic behavior
    * Negative symptoms
    * Anhedonia
    * Flat affect
    * Avolition

- Significant social dysfunction
    * Signs of the disturbance are continuous and persist for 6 months
    * Schizoaffective disorders and mood disorders, mental retardation, substance abuse, and other

causative medical disorders have been ruled out.

Treatment Principles and Goals

- All antipsychotics are equally effective if used properly

- Clozapine is the only agent proven effective in treating refractory schizophrenia

- Basis for choosing an antipsychotic medication
  * Past history of response (patient's response or a family member's response to a medication)
  * Side effect profile of the antipsychotic

- Therapy with a trial of antipsychotics (at least 4-6 weeks at recommended doses)

- Do everything possible to simplify the drug regimen

- Consider depot preparations in situations of poor compliance

Drug Therapy (Tables 1 and 2)

Mechanism of action
- These drugs block postsynaptic dopamine-2 receptors. They share anticholinergic, antihistaminic, and alpha-blocking properties.

Other conventional agents (not commonly used)
- Perphenazine (Trilafon®), thiothixene (Navane®), trifluoperazine (Stelazine®), and loxapine (Loxitane®)

Management of adverse effects
Sedation
- Level of sedation depends on the drug used; low-potency drugs in this class are more sedating than high-potency drugs

- Sedation effects are worse initially, but become more tolerable over time

Orthostasis
- Severity depends on the drug used; low-potency formulations promote more orthostasis than high-potency formulations

Table 1

Typical (Conventional or Older) Antipsychotics

Drug and form	Potency	Dosage range	Equivalent oral dose	Clinical pearls
Chlorpromazine (Thorazine®) 10, 25, 50, 100, 200 mg tabs; 30, 75, 150, 200, 300 mg SR caps; 10 mg/5 mL syrup; 30 mg/mL, 100 mg/mL concentrate; 25 mg, 100 mg rectal supp.; 25 mg/mL injection	Low	50-2000 mg/d	100 mg	First antipsychotic used clinically; contributed to deinstitutionalization of many patients in the 1950s; 100 mg of chlorpromazine is equivalent to 2 mg of haloperidol
Thioridazine (Mellaril®) 10, 15, 25, 50, 100, 150, 200 mg tabs; 25 mg/5 mL, 100 mg/5 mL susp.; 30 mg/mL, 100 mg/mL concentrate	Low	50-800 mg/d	100 mg	Pigmentary retinopathy at daily doses >800 mg/d; black box warning: QT prolongation
Fluphenazine (Prolixin®) 1, 2.5, 5, 10 mg tabs; 25 mg/mL decanoate injection; 2.5 mg/mL injection; 2.5 mg/5 mL elixir; 5 mg/mL concentrate	High	1-65 mg/d (PO); 12.5-75 mg IM (decanoate) every 2 weeks	2 mg	Decanoate injection given every 2 weeks; immediate-release injection, 5-10 min onset
Haloperidol (Haldol®) 0.5, 1, 2, 5, 10, 20 mg tabs; 2 mg/mL concentrate; 50, 100 mg/mL decanoate injection; 5 mg/mL injection	High	1-100 mg/d (PO); 50-300 mg IM (decanoate) every 4 weeks	2 mg	Decanoate injection given every 4 weeks; immediate-release injection, 5-10 min onset

Table 2

Adverse Effects of Typical Antipsychotic Medications

Drug	EPS	Sedation	Orthostasis	Weight gain	Anticholinergic
Chlorpromazine	+	+++	+++	+++	+++
Thioridazine	+	+++	+++	+++	+++
Fluphenazine	++++	+	+	+	+
Haloperidol	++++	+	+	+	+

EPS, extrapyramidal symptoms.

• Especially problematic in elderly patients

Weight gain
• Very prominent in this population
• Use low doses; appropriate diet and exercise is encouraged to offset weight gain

Anticholinergic
• Severity depends on the drug used; low-potency drugs of this type are more sedating than high-potency ones

• Dry mouth, blurred vision, constipation, and/or urinary hesitancy may occur

• Use high-potency agents in patients bothered by anticholinergic side effects

Extrapyramidal symptoms (EPS)
• Most likely attributed to an imbalance in dopamine and acetylcholine; antipsychotics cause a hypo-dopaminergic state

Dystonic reactions
• Usually occur within 24-96 hours of initiating or changing dose

• Present as painful, involuntary muscle spasms in skeletal muscles (most commonly in the facial/neck muscles; may also occur in back, arm, and leg muscles)

• Treatment: Benztropine (Cogentin®) 1-2 mg IM or diphenhydramine (Benadryl®) 25-50 mg IM every 30 minutes until relieved

• Prophylaxis with oral therapy is usually initiated

Akathisia
• Usually occurs within a few weeks of initiating antipsychotic therapy

• Described as a subjective feeling of discomfort usually seen as motor restlessness of the legs (inability to stand still or sit still)

• Treatment: Lipophilic β-blockers (eg, propranolol), benzodiazepines, clonidine, and anticholinergics

Pseudoparkinsonism
• Usually occurs within months to years of therapy

• Resembles Parkinson's symptoms (eg, cogwheel rigidity, bradykinesia, tremor, shuffling gait)

• Treatment: Amantadine (Symmetrel®) 100 mg bid or anticholinergics

Other adverse effects
Tardive dyskinesia (TD)
• Irreversible drug-induced movement disorder that occurs after years of antipsychotic therapy

• Due to long-term suppression of dopamine

Triad of symptoms
* Choreoathetosis: splayed, writhing fingers
* Oral/buccal movements: grimacing, bruxism, lip-smacking
* Protrusion of tongue

• Only treatment is prevention (ie, only use lowest effective dose of antipsychotic)

• Various therapies (vitamin E, lecithin, and vitamin B$_6$) may help alleviate symptoms

- Monitor for TD by administering the Abnormal Involuntary Movement Scale (AIMS) to all patients taking antipsychotics

Neuroleptic malignant syndrome (NMS)
- Low incidence, high mortality

- Thought to be due to dopamine blockade

Clinical presentation
   * Rapid progression (<24 hours)
   * Body temperature >104° F
   * Lead-pipe rigidity
   * Hypertension
   * Diaphoresis
   * Increased HR
   * Incontinence
   * Increased LFTs, CPK, WBC

- Treatment: emergency room STAT, discontinue antipsychotic, administer supportive therapy (cooling blankets, hydration), bromocriptine (dopamine agonist), dantrolene (smooth muscle relaxant)

Endocrine and metabolic effects
- Amenorrhea, galactorrhea, and/or gynecomastia due to hyperprolactinemia
   * Dopamine regulates prolactin release; when dopamine is blocked, prolactin is elevated

- Weight gain

- Decreased glucose tolerance

Dermatologic effects
(especially in long-term therapy)
- Allergy to medication, photosensitivity, pigmentation problems

Hypothalamic effects
- Temperature dysregulation, ie, sensitivity to extreme temperatures

Cardiac effects
- QT prolongation possible

- More common with thioridazine (black box warning)

- Recommendation: obtain ECG for all patients on antipsychotics

Ophthalmologic effects
- Pigmentary retinopathy is associated with daily thioridazine doses >800 mg; melanin deposits on cornea and may lead to blindness

Atypical (newer) antipsychotics (Table 3)
- No universally accepted definition of "atypical"
   * Less severe side effects (little or no EPS, minimal to no prolactin increase, less risk of TD)
   * More effective for negative symptoms than conventional medications
   * Decreased affinity for the dopamine receptor

Mechanism of action
- These drugs are weak dopamine and dopamine-2 receptor blockers that block serotonin and α-adrenergic, histaminic, and muscarinic receptors in the central nervous system

Treatment strategies

Acute schizophrenia
- Decrease danger to self and/or others

- May use haloperidol or fluphenazine (immediate-release) 5-10 mg IM and lorazepam 2 mg IM q4h prn for psychosis/agitation; an anticholinergic may also be needed (eg, benztropine or diphenhydramine for EPS)

Maintenance
- Start an atypical antipsychotic at recommended dose or continue conventional agent (if it was effective for patient before hospital admission)

- Positive symptoms will respond first

- Monitor for side effects; emphasize compliance

- Lifelong therapy is usually needed

- Use lowest effective dose to decrease risk of side effects (eg, TD)

Noncompliance and alternative dosing
Haloperidol decanoate (Haldol-D®)
- Conversion from PO to IM: PO daily dose x 10 = IM dose every 4 weeks
   * **Example:** 20 mg daily dose x 10 = 200 mg every 4 weeks
   * Reaches steady state in 8-12 weeks

Fluphenazine decanoate (Prolixin-D®)
- Conversion from PO to IM: 1 mg PO = 1.25 mg IM
   * **Example:** 20 mg daily dose x 1.25 mg = 25 mg IM every 2 weeks
   * Reaches steady state in approximately 6 weeks

Depot administration technique
- Both medications are suspended in sesame seed oil

Table 3

Atypical Antipsychotics

Drug	Usual dose	Adverse effects	Clinical pearls
Clozapine (Clozaril®) 25, 100 mg tabs *Note:* Indicated for refractory schizophrenia only	12.5 mg titrated up to 300-900 mg/d	Sedation; weight gain; hypersalivation; seizure risk (>600 mg/d); agranulo-cytosis; no EPS or TD	Weekly CBC w/differential required; WBC <3500 or ANC <1500 *must* discontinue; if stable CBC w/differential for 6 months, may go to biweekly
Risperidone (Risperdal®) 0.25, 0.5, 1, 2, 3, 4 mg tabs; 1 mg/mL concentrate	1 mg bid up to 4-6 mg/d; max dose 16 mg/d	Dose-related EPS (>8 mg/d); +/– weight gain; +/– sedation; prolactin elevation; orthostasis	Available in concentrate; don't mix with teas or colas; used commonly in dementia (0.25-1 mg)
Olanzapine (Zyprexa®) 2.5, 5, 7.5, 10, 15, 20 mg tabs Zyprexa Zydis® (disintegrating olanzapine tabs) 5, 10, 15, 20 mg	10-20 mg/d; higher doses have been reported	Sedation; weight gain; possible dose-related EPS	Olanzapine is also indicated for acute manic episodes of bipolar disorder; Zydis useful for patients who are unable to swallow or are "cheeking" meds
Quetiapine (Seroquel®) 25, 100, 200, 300 mg tabs	75-800 mg/d; higher doses have been reported	Sedation; orthostasis	Low EPS risk
Ziprasidone (Geodon®) 20, 40, 60, 80 mg caps; 20 mg/mL injection	20-160 mg/d (PO); 20 mg IM x 1 dose (may repeat in 4 h; max IM daily dose 40 mg)	+/– Sedation; +/– weight gain; QT prolongation warning in package insert	Only atypical with IM formulation (as of April 2003); use caution with other meds that prolong QT interval
Abilify (Aripiprazole®) 10, 15, 20, 30 mg tabs	10-30 mg/d	Possible insomnia; +/– weight gain	Released to market November 2002; qd dosing benefit

(they are very viscous; ensure no allergy to sesame seed oil)

- Must administer in gluteal or deltoid muscle with a 16- or 18-gauge needle

2. Bipolar Disorder

Bipolar disorder (manic-depressive illness) is a recurrent mood disorder with a lifetime prevalence of 0.8-1.6%

- Associated with significant morbidity and mortality

- Incidence is equal in women and men

- Onset is usually between the ages of 18 and 44

- The first episode for women is usually marked by a depressive episode; for men, a manic episode

Types and Classifications

Bipolar I
- Characterized by the occurrence of manic episodes and major depressive episodes

Bipolar II
- Characterized by the occurrence of hypomanic episodes and major depressive episodes

Cyclothymia
- Defined as numerous episodes of hypomania and depressive episodes that cannot be classified as major depressive episodes; diagnosis requires that cyclothymia occur for at least a 2-year period

Clinical Presentation

(see *DSM-IV* for complete diagnostic criteria)

Mania
- Characterized by heightened mood (euphoria), flight of ideas, rapid or pressured speech, grandiosity, increased energy, decreased need for sleep, irritability, and impulsivity

- Judgment is significantly impaired, eg, increased risk-taking behavior

- Marked impairment in social and/or occupational functioning

- Psychotic features are usually present; hospitalization is needed

- Changes in sleeping patterns (especially insomnia) commonly initiate manic episodes

Hypomania
- Less severe form of mania

- Usually does not cause marked impairment in social and/or occupational functioning

- Many patients find this state highly desirable because they experience a great sense of well-being and feel productive, creative, and/or confident

Dysphoric (or mixed) mania
- Characterized by manic and depressive features, mood variability, and mood lability

- Symptoms usually include agitation, insomnia, suicidal ideation, psychosis, and appetite disturbances

Major depression
- See section on depression

Rapid cycling
- Patient experiences >4 mood episodes in a year

- Mood episodes may occur in any combination

- Rapid cycling primarily occurs in women (70-90%)

- Usually poor prognosis

Etiology

- Unknown

- Leading hypothesis supports genetic etiology

- Other theories include neurotransmitter involvement, circadian rhythm, and kindling hypothesis

Clinical Course

- Mean age of onset is 21 years

- First episode for women is usually depression; for men, mania

- Untreated episodes may last from weeks to months

- High mortality rate due to suicide

- Comorbid substance abuse is very common (60-70%)

Treatment Principles and Goals

Acute
- Control the current episode (slow patient down, reduce harm to self and/or others)

Maintenance
- Prevent or minimize future episodes

- Maintain drug therapy and reduce adverse effects

- Prevent drug interactions

- Educate patient and family about disorder

- Provide adequate follow-up services (including substance abuse treatment)

- Maximize patient's functional status and quality of life

Drug Therapy (Table 4)

Lithium
Indications
- Acute treatment and prophylaxis of manic episodes associated with bipolar disorders; effective for both the manic and depressive components

Table 4

Mood Stabilizers

Drug and form	Usual dose	Adverse effects	Clinical pearls
Lithium (Lithobid®, Eskalith CR®) 150, 300, 600 mg caps; 300 mg, 450 mg (CR) tabs; 300 mg (SR) tabs; syrup, as citrate 300 mg/5 mL (Cibalith-S®)	Starting: 900-1200 mg in divided doses; titrate to desired response/level	Tremor; polydipsia/polyuria; nausea/diarrhea; weight gain; hypothyroidism; mental dulling	Many drug interactions; toxicity is a concern (pregnancy category D); monitor blood levels—acute: 0.6-1.2 mEq/L; maintenance: 0.8-1.0 mEq/L
Divalproex sodium (Depakote®) 125, 250, 500 mg tabs; 250, 500 mg (ER) tabs	Starting: 500 mg; bid-tid or 15 mg/kg; max dose 60 mg/kg per day	GI upset; sedation, tremor; weight gain; alopecia; transient elevation in LFTs	Black box warnings: hepatoxicity; hemorrhagic pancreatitis; teratogenicity (pregnancy category D); monitor blood levels—50-125 µg/mL
Carbamazepine (Tegretol®) (see text for contraindications) 200 mg tabs; 100 mg chew tabs; 100, 200, 400 mg ER tabs; 100 mg/5 mL susp.	Starting: 200 mg bid; increase to 800-1200 mg/d (tid-qid doses); usual range 400-1600 mg/d	Ataxia; dizziness; sedation; slurred speech; aplastic anemia	Many drug interactions (pregnancy category C); monitor blood levels—4-12 µg/mL

Mechanism of action
- Unknown

- Various theories: lithium facilitates gamma-aminobutyric acid function, alters cation transport across cell membranes in nerve and muscle cells, and/or influences reuptake of 5-HT and/or norepinephrine (NE)

Contraindications
- Renal disease, severe cardiovascular disease, history of leukemia, first trimester of pregnancy, hypersensitivity to lithium

Precautions
- Use with caution in patients with thyroid disease, sodium depletion, patients receiving diuretics, or dehydrated patients

Monitoring (baseline/follow-up)
Thyroid panel

- Lithium may cause hypothyroidism; baseline and TSH every 6-12 months or as clinically indicated

SCr/BUN
- Lithium is 100% renally eliminated; baseline and every 3 months for patients with renal dysfunction; every 12 months otherwise or as clinically indicated

CBC w/differential
- Lithium may cause leukocytosis and may reactivate leukemia; baseline and every month for 3 months, then as clinically indicated

Electrolytes
- In the event of hyponatremia, lithium toxicity may occur

ECG
- Lithium causes flattened or inverted T waves, which is reversible; baseline and every 6-12 months or as clinically indicated

Urinalysis
- Lithium may decrease specific gravity

Pregnancy test
- Lithium may cause cardiovascular defects (eg, Ebstein's anomaly)

Lithium level
- Reaches steady-state levels in 4-5 days ($t_{1/2}$ = ~24 h); obtain level 8-2 hours post-dose (acute: 0.6-1.2 mEq/L; maintenance: 0.8-1.0 mEq/L); draw level weekly for 4 weeks then monthly for 3 months or as clinically indicated

Drug Interactions (Table 5)

Toxicity concerns
Mild toxicity (serum levels 1.5-2.0 mEq/L)
- GI upset (nausea/vomiting/diarrhea), muscle weak-

ness, fatigue, fine hand tremor, difficulty with concentration and memory

Moderate toxicity (serum levels 2.0-2.5 mEq/L)
• Ataxia, lethargy, nystagmus, worsening confusion, severe GI upset, coarse tremors, increased deep tendon reflexes

Severe toxicity (serum levels >3.0 mEq/L)
• Severely impaired consciousness, coma, seizures, respiratory complications, death

Treatment of toxicity
• Discontinue lithium and initiate gastric lavage

• Correct electrolyte and fluid imbalances

• Monitor neurologic changes

• Give supportive care

• Give dialysis if indicated

Patient information
• Monitoring serum lithium levels routinely is important; maintain a steady salt and fluid intake; do not crush or chew extended or slow-release dosage forms

Divalproex sodium
Indication (as related to bipolar disorder)
Acute manic episodes
• *Note:* Considered first-line treatment; unlabeled use for prophylaxis of manic episodes; effective for

rapid cyclers and patients with dysphoric mood; helpful in the management of agitation/aggression

Mechanism of action
• Unknown, but divalproex sodium is thought to increase GABA or mimic its action at the postsynaptic receptor site

Contraindications
• Hepatic dysfunction

• Pregnancy
  * Valproic acid may cause neural tube defects; if benefit outweighs risk, supplement with 4-5 mg/d of folic acid to decrease risk of fetal damage

• Hypersensitivity to divalproex sodium

• Patients <2 years old

Monitoring
• Valproic acid level reaches steady state in 3-5 days ($t_{1/2}$ = 9-16 h); 50-125 μg/mL optimal

• Draw level weekly for 2-3 weeks, then every 3 months or as clinically indicated

LFTs
• Baseline and every month for 6 months, then every 6 months or as clinically indicated

• Divalproex sodium is hepatically eliminated; black box warning for hepatotoxicity

CBC with differential
• Baseline and every month for 6 months, then every 6 months or as clinically indicated

• Valproic acid may cause thrombocytopenia.

Drug interactions
• CYP2C19 enzyme substrate; CYP2C9 and -2D6 inhibitor, weak CYP3A3/4 inhibitor

• Carbamazepine, lamotrigine, and phenytoin
  * Increased sedative effects with phenobarbital and benzodiazepines

Patient information
• Take with food to avoid GI upset; take a multivitamin with selenium and zinc if alopecia (hair loss) occurs

• Important to monitor VPA levels routinely

Table 5

Drug Interactions with Lithium

Increase level of lithium	Decrease level of lithium
NSAIDs	Theophylline
ACE inhibitors	Caffeine
Fluoxetine	Pregnancy
Metronidazole	Osmotic diuretics (mannitol, urea)
Diuretics (eg, thiazides)	
Sodium depletion	
Low sodium diet	
Excessive exercise/sweating	
Vomiting/diarrhea	
Salt deficiency	

Carbamazepine (CBZ)
- Considered second-line therapy for acute and pro-phylactic treatment of bipolar disorder

Mechanism of action
- Unknown

Monitoring
- CBC with differential, electrolytes, LFTs, SCr/BUN, ECG (if age >40 or pre-existing heart disease)

- CBZ is an autoinducer; monitor levels routinely, especially during first few months of therapy

- 4-12 µg/mL = optimal

Contraindications
- History of previous bone marrow depression, hyper-sensitivity to CBZ

Drug interactions
- CYP2C8 and 3A3/4 enzyme substrate

- CYP1A2, 2C, and 3A3/4 inducer

- CBZ may induce the metabolism of benzodi-azepines, clozapine, corticosteroids, oral contracep-tives, VPA, warfarin, phenytoin, and tricyclic antide-pressants (plus others)

- Cimetidine, clarithromycin, diltiazem, propoxy-phene, verapamil, metronidazole, and lamotrigine (plus others) inhibit CBZ

Other therapies
Antipsychotics (conventional and atypical)
- Usually used as adjunctive therapy in patients who may be psychotic or overly aggressive/agitated

- Atypical medications are usually favored over con-ventional ones due to lower incidence of side effects

- Olanzapine (Zyprexa) has an indication for acute mania (other drugs are also being used)

Gabapentin (Neurontin®)
- May be useful as adjunctive therapy for bipolar disorder

- No significant drug interactions

- No required drug serum level monitoring

- Renally eliminated

- Mild adverse effects (sedation, ataxia, fatigue)

Lamotrigine (Lamictal®)
- May be especially useful in the depressed phase of bipolar disorder

- Titration of dose is required to monitor for signs/symptoms of severe and potentially life-threat-ening skin rashes (co-administration with VPA increases risk)

Other drug interactions
- CBZ, phenytoin, and phenobarbital decrease lamot-rigine concentrations

- Adverse effects: nausea, headache, tremor/anxiety, and sedation

Oxcarbazepine (Trileptal®)
- Structurally similar to CBZ (keto-analogue of CBZ)

- At times utilized as a mood stabilizer in some patients with bipolar disorder, but further studies needed

- No autoinduction problems, no drug serum levels to monitor

- Appears to have fewer drug-drug interactions than CBZ

Topiramate (Topamax®)
- May be useful for treatment of bipolar disorder, but further studies needed
- Doses are usually lower than those indicated for treating seizure disorders

- May cause weight loss.

Calcium channel blockers
- Usually reserved as last-line therapy

- Only variable information is available about using verapamil for mania (other CCBs may be effective)

- Not routinely utilized

- Possible for use in pregnancy

3. Major Depression

Major depression is a prevalent and serious illness in the U.S.

- Affects 10-14 million people of all ages

- Treatable but grossly undertreated

- Most cases go unrecognized, which may be due to the social stigma surrounding depression

- Several myths contribute to the problem of under-treatment (eg, personal weakness, inability to handle life's problems)

Epidemiology

- Lifetime prevalence rate is 17%
  * 1 out of 4 females (10-24%)
  * 1 out of 8 males (5-12%)

- Most common between the ages of 25-44 years

Risk factors
- Family history

- Female gender

- Previous depressive episode

- Previous suicide attempt

- Comorbid medical or substance abuse disorder

Etiology

- Unknown

- Many different hypotheses
  * Dysregulation of neurotransmitters
  * Decreased concentration of certain neurotransmitters
  * Genetic basis for disorder

Clinical Presentation

Physical findings
- Fatigue

- Pain (ie, headaches, back pain, GI upset)

- Sleep disturbances (usually insomnia)

- Appetite disturbances (usually decreased appetite)

- Psychomotor retardation or agitation

Emotional symptoms
- Anhedonia

- Depressed mood for most of the day

- Hopelessness/helplessness

- Inappropriate feelings of guilt and worthlessness

- Anxiety/worry

- Suicidal ideation

Cognitive symptoms
- Decreased ability to concentrate

- Indecisiveness

Laboratory studies
- There are no diagnostic laboratory tests for depression, but the following lab work should be conducted to rule out other medical illnesses that may manifest as depressive symptoms:
  * CBC with differential
  * TFTs
  * Rapid plasma reagin (RPR) (test for syphilis)
  * Urine drug screen (UDS)

- Medical conditions that may contribute to the development or worsening of depression:
  * MI, CVA, Parkinson's, MS, SLE, HIV, RA, thyroid abnormalities, DM, cancer, vitamin deficiency

- Possible drug-induced causes of depression should also be ruled out:
  * Corticosteroids, oral contraceptives, propranolol, clonidine, methyldopa

Prognosis

- 70% of patients are responsive to antidepressant therapy

- Following the first episode, 50-60% of patients will have another episode; following the second episode, 70-80% will have a third; following the third, 90% will have another

- If untreated, an episode may resolve spontaneously within 6 to 24 months

- Approximately 15% of patients will commit suicide

* Risk factors for suicide: Male gender, >50 years old, unemployed status, recent loss of job/spouse, social isolation, presence of a weapon, comorbid substance abuse
* *Note:* Males are more likely to commit suicide; females are more likely to attempt suicide; males commonly use more violent means (eg, firearms, hanging) of suicide than females (eg, slashing of wrists, drug overdoses)

Diagnostic Criteria (*DSM-IV*)

* At least five symptoms (see clinical presentation section above) must be present mostly every day for a 2-week period and represent a change from previous functioning; at least one of the symptoms must be depressed mood or anhedonia

Treatment Principles and Goals

* Improve patient's ability to function and quality of life

* Reduce or eliminate target symptoms with an antidepressant

* Incorporating psychotherapy is optimal

* Prevent relapse

* All antidepressants are equally effective in a given population
    * Response varies from person to person
    * Each differs in side effect and drug interaction profiles
    * None are "speed" or "uppers"

Basis for choosing an agent
* Past history of a patient's response or a family member's response to certain agent(s)

* Side effect profile and how it relates to any given patient's situation

Monitoring parameters
First week
* Patient should demonstrate decreased anxiety
* Trend towards normalization of appetite and sleep pattern

Second to third week
* Increase in energy

* *Note:* There is an increased risk for suicide at this time because the patient has the energy to carry out any ideations.

* Improvement in concentration and memory

* Improvement in somatic symptoms

Four to six weeks
* Improvement in mood

* Decreased suicidal ideation

* Increased libido

Duration of therapy
Acute phase
* Duration is usually 6-12 weeks or the length of time needed to stabilize depressive symptoms

Maintenance phase
* Maintain therapeutic doses of antidepressant

* Usually 1-year duration; may taper antidepressant for a period of time and monitor for signs of relapse

* Goal is to prevent relapse

Prophylaxis
* Chronic antidepressant therapy may be necessary for certain patients

* Those with a first-degree relative with bipolar disorder or recurrent depression

* Onset before age 20 or after age 60

* Recurrence within 1 year after medication discontinuation

* Severe, sudden, or life-threatening depression

Drug Therapy (Table 6)

Tricyclic antidepressants
Mechanism of action
* TCAs increase the synaptic concentration of 5-HT and/or norepinephrine in the CNS, ie, TCAs inhibit the presynaptic neuronal membrane's reuptake of 5-HT and/or NE.

Other information about TCAs
* Doses may be titrated to full dose range over 1-3 weeks

* Many patients are dosed half-strength due to sedative effects; however, for patients with insomnia, the sedating effects may be helpful.

* Deadly in overdose (blocks sinoatrial node in heart)

Table 6

Tricyclic Antidepressants (TCAs)

Drug and form	Indications	Initial dose (mg/d)	Dose range (mg)
Amitriptyline (Elavil®) 10, 25, 50, 75, 100, 150 mg tabs; 10 mg/mL injection (pregnancy category D)	Depression; chronic & neuropathic pain; migraine prophylaxis; peripheral neuropathy	50-75	75-300
Nortriptyline (Pamelor®, Aventyl®) 10, 25, 50, 75 mg caps; 10 mg/5 mL injection (pregnancy category D)	Depression; chronic pain	25-50	40-200
Imipramine (Tofranil®) 75, 100, 125, 150 mg pamoate capsule (Tofranil-PM®); 10, 25, 50 mg tabs; 12.5 mg/mL injection (pregnancy category D)	Depression; childhood enuresis; chronic & neuropathic pain	50-75	75-300
Doxepin (Sinequan®) 10, 25, 50, 75, 100, 150 mg caps; 10 mg/mL concentrate; 5% cream (pregnancy category C)	Depression; anxiety; unlabeled: chronic & neuropathic pain	75 (in divided doses)	75-300
Clomipramine (Anafranil®) 25, 50, 75 mg (pregnancy category C)	Obsessive-compulsive disorder; depression; panic attacks; chronic pain	25-100 mg qd, titrated up for 1-2 weeks	Usual effective dose 200-250 mg/d; max dose 250 mg due to dose-related increased risk of seizure
Desipramine (Norpramin®) 10, 25, 50, 75, 100, 150 mg tabs (pregnancy category C)	Depression; chronic pain; unlabeled: peripheral neuropathy	50-75	75-300

- Drug serum levels are not commonly utilized in guiding therapy, but monitoring may be useful in patients taking amitriptyline, desipramine, imipramine, or nortriptyline

Adverse effects
- Orthostatic hypotension, tachycardia, sedation, anticholinergic effects, arrhythmias (prolonged QT interval), weight gain, sexual dysfunction

- Tertiary amines (eg, amitriptyline, imipramine, doxepin, and clomipramine) have more intense adverse effects compared to secondary amines (eg, nortriptyline, desipramine)

Contraindications
- Concomitant use of MAOI within the last 14 days, pregnancy, lactation, and narrow angle glaucoma

Precautions
- Use with caution in patients with cardiac conduction disturbances, seizure disorders, hyperthyroidism, and renal or hepatic impairment. Avoid abrupt withdrawal in patients with prolonged use

Drug interactions
- Increase in TCAs increases the levels of SSRIs (selective serotonin reuptake inhibitors), cimetidine, diltiazem, verapamil, labetalol, propoxyphene, quinidine, haloperidol, and methylphenidate

- Decrease in TCA level affects CBZ, phenytoin, and barbiturate metabolism

- Administration with MAOIs may cause serotonin syndrome

- Monitoring BP, pulse, ECG changes, and mental status changes is prudent; drug serum monitoring may be useful for amitriptyline, desipramine, imipramine, and nortriptyline

Monoamine oxidase inhibitors (MAOIs) (Table 7)
Mechanism of action
- MAOIs increase the synaptic concentration of NE, 5-HT, and DA by inhibiting the breakdown enzyme, monoamine oxidase

- *Notes:* May be useful for patients who do not respond to other antidepressants and/or to treat atypical depression; MAOIs are rarely utilized due to the need for dietary restrictions, side effect profile, and potentially dangerous interactions with other medications

Adverse effects
- Orthostatic hypotension, weight gain, sexual dysfunction, anticholinergic effects, and hypertensive crisis

Contraindications
- Renal or hepatic dysfunction, CVD, concomitant sympathomimetic therapy (eg, pseudoephedrine, ephedra); MAOIs cannot be used within 5 weeks of fluoxetine or within 2 weeks of any other SSRI

Precautions
- Drug-food interaction with tyramine-containing foods (eg, red wine, aged cheeses, and marmite)

Drug interactions
- TCAs, SSRIs, sympathomimetics, and meperidine

Selective serotonin reuptake inhibitors (Table 8)
Mechanism of action
- These agents selectively inhibit the reuptake of 5-HT

- *Notes:* All SSRIs should be tapered upon discontinuing treatment (over 2-4 weeks), except fluoxetine; side effects with abrupt withdrawal include flu-like symptoms, dizziness, nausea, tremor, anxiety, and palpitations

Adverse effects
- GI complaints, nervousness, insomnia, headache, fatigue, and sexual dysfunction, but safer in over-dose compared to TCAs

Drug interactions
- TCAs, MAOIs, and SSRIs (variable depending on which SSRI; escitalopram and citalopram reportedly have fewer drug interactions)

Other classes of antidepressant medication
Venlafaxine (Effexor®, Effexor XR®)

Mechanism of action
- Inhibits the reuptake of 5-HT and NE (and also DA at higher doses); it is frequently referred to as a serotonin-norepinephrine inhibitor (SNRI); anticholinergic and antihistaminic effects are negligible; as dose increases, NE and DA reuptake are more pronounced

Adverse effects
- GI upset, anxiety, insomnia, headache, elevation in BP possible (use with caution in patients with uncontrolled hypertension); XR formulation is available to minimize GI upset; other side effects are similar to those with SSRIs; withdrawal symptoms may occur if abruptly discontinued

- *Notes:* Indicated for both generalized anxiety disorder (GAD) and major depression; not recommended in patients with uncontrolled HTN or recent MI or CV disorders; there are no known significant drug interactions

Bupropion (Wellbutrin®, Wellbutrin SR®, Zyban®)
Mechanism of action
- Bupropion, an inhibitor of NE and DA reuptake (effects on 5-HT reuptake are minimal) is referred to as a norepinephrine-dopamine reuptake inhibitor (NDRI)

Adverse effects
- GI upset, insomnia, anxiety, headache, and psychosis (rare); it is associated with less sexual dysfunction than SSRIs and other classes; it decreases the seizure threshold (see Notes section).

Table 7

Monoamine Oxidase Inhibitors

Drug	Initial dose	Dose titration	Dose range
Phenelzine (Nardil®) 15 mg tabs	15 mg tid (>16 years old)	Increase by 15 mg/week	60-90 mg/d
Tranylcypromine (Parnate®) 10 mg tabs	30 mg/d in divided doses	Increase by 10 mg/d every 1-3 weeks	30-60 mg/d

Table 8

Selective Serotonin Reuptake Inhibitors

Drug and Form	Initial Dose	Usual Dose	Clinical Pearls
Citalopram (Celexa®) 10, 20, 40 mg tabs; 10 mg/5 mL syrup	10 mg	20-40 mg/d; max dose 60 mg/d	Used in geriatric patients; fewer drug interactions
Escitalopram (Lexapro®) 5, 10, 20 mg tabs	10 mg	10-20 mg/d	S-isomer of citalopram; 40 mg Celexa = 10 mg Lexapro
Fluvoxamine (Luvox®) 50, 100 mg tabs	50 mg	100-300 mg/d	Available in generic; primarily used for OCD drug interactions
Paroxetine (Paxil®) 10, 20, 30, 40 mg tabs; 10 mg/5 mL susp.	10-20 mg	10-40 mg; max dose 50 mg/d	Least-activating SSRI
Paxil CR® 12.5, 25, 37.5 mg tabs	12.5-25 mg	25-37.5 mg	CR formulation associated with fewer side effects; 10 mg Paxil = 12.5 mg Paxil CR
Fluoxetine (Prozac®) 10, 20, 40 mg caps; 10 mg tabs; 20 mg/5 mL syrup	10-20 mg	20-80 mg/d	Longer $t_{1/2}$, so tapering unnecessary
Sertraline (Zoloft®) 25, 50, 100 mg tabs; 20 mg/mL concentrate	25-50 mg	50-100 mg/d; max dose 200 mg/d	Used in geriatric patients; fewer drug interactions

---

Drug interactions
- Cimetidine and ritonavir inhibit bupropion metabolism; CBZ induces bupropion metabolism

- *Notes:* There is an increased risk of seizure with bupropion, especially in patients with a seizure disorder, eating disorder, or electrolyte imbalance; maximum single dose is 150 mg; maximum daily dose is 450 mg (400 mg SR); titrate dose slowly to minimize seizure risk; bupropion is marketed as Zyban for smoking cessation

Trazodone (Desyrel®)
Mechanism of action
- Inhibits 5-HT reuptake and blocks 5-HT$_{2A}$ receptors

Adverse effects
- Extremely sedating, orthostatic hypotension, and priapism; there are no anticholinergic or cardiotoxic effects

Drug interactions
- Fluoxetine and ritonavir inhibit trazodone metabolism

- *Notes:* Due to excessive sedation, trazodone is not clinically used as an antidepressant; rather, it is commonly used in combination with other antidepressants; such a combination may cause insomnia (usually dosed 25-150 mg HS for insomnia)

Nefazodone (Serzone®)
Mechanism of action
- Inhibits 5-HT and NE uptake and blocks 5-HT$_{2A}$ receptors

Adverse effects
- GI upset, sedation, dry mouth, constipation, lightheadedness; it is associated with minimal sexual dysfunction and/or orthostatic hypotension

Drug interactions
- Potent inhibitor of CYP3A4 isoenzyme; use with caution with drugs metabolized via this enzyme (eg, buspirone, HMG-CoA reductase inhibitors, alprazolam, triazolam, and digoxin); ritonavir inhibits nefazodone metabolism

- Notes: Usually dosed bid due to short half-life; there is a black box warning for hepatotoxicity

Mirtazapine (Remeron®, Remeron Soltab®)
(15 and 30 mg tabs)
Mechanism of action
- Antagonizes presynaptic α_2 autoreceptors and heteroreceptors that prevent the release of 5-HT and NE

(resulting in increased 5-HT and NE in the synapses); it antagonizes $5\text{-}HT_{2A}$ and $5\text{-}HT_3$ receptors, resulting in less GI upset and less anxiety

Adverse effects

- Sedation, increased appetite, weight gain, constipation; elevation in LFTs, increase in TGs; there is a small risk of agranulocytosis or neutropenia

- *Notes:* May be useful in geriatric patients since it causes increased appetite, is sedating, and there are no significant drug interactions

Psychostimulants

- Methylphenidate has been used to treat depression (especially in the geriatric population) and has been shown to increase activity level as well as improve mood symptoms; it may cause GI upset, insomnia, and CV effects; use with caution in anxious or psychotic patients; it inhibits TCA metabolism

Nonpharmacologic Treatments

- Psychotherapy is especially useful combined with drug therapy

Electroconvulsive therapy (ECT)

- Very safe and effective for treating depression

- Believed to physically "reset" receptors in the brain

- Usually reserved for refractory or psychotic patients

Procedure

- Patient is anesthetized and paralyzed in an outpatient setting
- Patient is monitored via EEG during procedure, and a seizure is induced for 30-90 seconds

Acute treatment

- Administered every other day for 6-9 treatments

- Maintenance treatment is variable for each patient, but ECT is usually administered monthly after acute treatment

Adverse effects

- Short-term memory loss, confusion on the day of treatment

Relative contraindications

- Increases intracranial pressure, and therefore is not recommended in patients with recent MI, intracerebral hemorrhage, or cerebral lesions

4. Anxiety Disorders

Anxiety disorders are serious, debilitating mental illnesses that include a group of conditions that share extreme anxiety as the primary mood disturbance.

Epidemiology

- Affects approximately 19 million adults in the U.S.

- No racial or cultural differences; gender differences depend on specific anxiety disorder

- Significant comorbidity with other psychiatric illnesses, eg, substance abuse

Types and Classifications

Generalized anxiety disorder (GAD)
- Characterized by unprovoked excessive worry and tension; anxiety usually consumes the patient's day, thereby affecting social and occupational functioning; physical complaints (eg, GI upset, headache, muscle tension, tremors, insomnia, and/or fatigue) are common; incidence is higher in females than males

Panic disorder with or without agoraphobia (PD)
- Characterized by feelings of terror that suddenly strike without warning and usually last for approximately 10-15 minutes

Physical symptoms
- Increased HR, sweating, tremors, shortness of breath, chest pain, and/or dizziness); patient feels as if death is imminent

- Agoraphobia (fear of open or public places) usually develops later in the illness, especially if PD is not treated; agoraphobic patients associate panic attacks with certain places and occasions, so they avoid going out and remain at home; agoraphobia is more prevalent in females than males

Obsessive-compulsive disorder (OCD)
- Characterized by intrusive, recurrent, and repetitive thoughts that severely interfere with the patient's social and occupational functioning (eg, preoccupation with contamination, order, counting, cleanliness, and/or safety)

- Compulsions (eg, repetitive washing of hands, checking and rechecking) are acts that must be performed in an attempt to decrease the anxiety felt about the obsessions. There is equal male-female prevalence.

Social anxiety disorder (SAD)
- Characterized by feelings of anxiety in social situations (eg, speaking in front of others, social gatherings); patients feel as though everyone is staring and judging them; affected persons usually do not seek treatment and will instead self-medicate with alcohol; there is equal male-female prevalence

Simple (or specific) phobias
- Defined as specific fears (eg, heights, dogs, mice, spiders, and needles) that cause an extreme anxiety response; affected persons usually do not seek treatment and instead will avoid situations that involve the phobia

Treatment
- Exposure therapy to the perceived threat is common therapy; incidence in females is greater than in males

Posttraumatic stress disorder (PTSD)
- Characterized by severe anxiety that is caused by an event outside of normal human experience (eg, war, rape, and natural disasters); symptoms include vividly reliving the event to the extent that anxiety symptoms (ie, flashbacks, nightmares/night terrors, extreme mood changes, feelings of fright) commonly occur; PTSD is often associated with strong guilt feelings, impaired relationships, social withdrawal, and personality changes; there is a greater prevalence in females than males

Anxiety due to a medical disorder
- Anxiety is likely to be related to evidence of a medical condition (eg, CHF, hyperthyroidism, COPD)

Substance-induced anxiety disorder
- Anxiety symptoms are likely to be a direct result of use of an agent (eg, amphetamines, toxin, and medication); symptoms may also occur with intoxication or withdrawal

Associated features
- High comorbidity with other psychiatric illnesses (especially depression)

- High comorbidity with alcohol/substance abuse

- Associated with chronic medical illnesses (eg, chronic pain syndromes, long-term illnesses, GI stress, headaches

Etiology
- Presently unknown

- Most current evidence suggests the cause is primarily biologic (imbalance of GABA, 5-HT, NE) with genetic predisposition

Drug Therapy

Benzodiazepines (BZDs) (Table 9)
- Most commonly utilized anxiolytics

Mechanism of action
- BZDs potentiate the actions of GABA by increasing the influx of chloride ions into neurons; it is hypothesized that through their effects on neurons mediated by receptor complexes, BZDs reduce neuronal firing and thus the symptoms of anxiety

- *Notes:* Rate of absorption varies with BZDs; the more lipophilic compounds (ie, alprazolam, diazepam, chlorazepate, and flurazepam) are rapidly absorbed and result in quicker onset of action; the less lipophilic BZDs are chlordiazepoxide, clonazepam, and lorazepam

Adverse effects
- Sedation, dizziness, confusion, blurred vision, diplopia, syncope, residual daytime sedation, reduced psychomotor and cognitive dysfunction

Metabolism
- Lorazepam, oxazepam, and temazepam (LOT) are conjugated and are preferred in patients with hepatic dysfunction and elderly patients

Drug interactions
- BZDs metabolized by CYP3A4 (eg, alprazolam, diazepam, and triazolam) have decreased clearance if taken concomitantly with CYP3A4 inhibitors (eg, ketoconazole, erythromycin, and nefazodone); BZDs are deadly in overdose if taken concomitantly with alcohol

Clinical pearls
- May cause a paradoxical reaction in children, cognitively impaired elderly patients, mentally retarded patients, and post–head injury patients

- Never abruptly discontinue BZDs as this may precipitate status epilepticus; always taper dose to avoid seizure risk and withdrawal symptoms

- In elderly patients, the BZDs of choice are those that are conjugated (LOT); there is an increased risk of falls in this population

Table 9

Benzodiazepines

Drug	Time to peak plasma concentration (h)	Half-life (h)	Usual daily dose (mg/d)	Metabolic pathway
Alprazolam (Xanax®)	1-2	12-15	0.5-4	Oxidation
Chlordiazepoxide (Librium®)	2-4	5-30	5-200	Oxidation
Clonazepam (Klonopin®)	1-2	18-50	1-3	Nitro reduction
Clorazepate (Tranxene®)	1-2	Not significant	15-60	Oxidation
Diazepam (Valium®)	0.5-2	20-80	2-40	Oxidation
Estazolam (ProSom®)	2	10-24	0.5-2	Oxidation
Flurazepam (Dalmane®)	0.5-2	Not significant	15-30	Oxidation
Halazepam (Paxipam®)	1-3	7-14	80-160	Oxidation
Lorazepam (Ativan®)	1-6	10-20	2-6	Conjugation
Oxazepam (Serax®)	2-4	5-20	30-120	Conjugation
Prazepam (Centrax®)	6	1.2	20-60	Oxidation
Quazepam (Doral®)	2	25-41	7.5-30	Oxidation
Temazepam (Restoril®)	2-3	10-40	15-30	Conjugation
Triazolam (Halcion®)	1	1.5-5	0.125-0.5	Oxidation

- Best to avoid in pregnancy (especially first trimester) due to risk of cleft palate; BZDs are also present in breast milk and should be avoided in nursing women

- Abuse potential is great; BZDs are not recommended for patients with substance abuse issues

- Tolerance is common and increasing doses are needed to control anxiety levels

Buspirone (BuSpar®)
Mechanism of action
- Poorly understood; 5-HT$_{1A}$ is a partial agonist and buspirone reportedly stimulates presynaptic 5-HT1A receptors; in addition, the agent has a moderate affinity for D$_2$ receptors

- Does not interact with the BZD-GABA receptor complex

- Onset of anxiolytic effect is longer than BZD (2-3 weeks)

Adverse effects
- GI upset, headache, nervousness

- Possible benefits over BZDs

- Usually less sedating than BZDs

- Little to no psychomotor or cognitive impairment

- Has not been associated with withdrawal symptoms, abuse, or physical dependence

- Not cross-tolerant with BZDs or alcohol

Antidepressants as treatment for anxiety disorders
- TCAs are usually used third-line due to side effects and danger of overdose; clomipramine is effective for OCD

- MAOIs are usually used third-line due to side effects and drug/food interactions

- SSRIs are usually used first-line for many anxiety disorders (especially in patients with comorbid depression and substance abuse problems)

- Venlafaxine is especially useful in patients with anxiety and comorbid depression

- Titrate doses of antidepressants slowly to decrease risk of initial anxiety symptoms; ultimately, higher doses are commonly utilized for anxiety disorders

Other classes of drugs used to treat anxiety disorders
- β-Blockers (eg, propranolol, atenolol) ease peripheral symptoms of anxiety and may be useful for use in panic disorders and SAD

• Hydroxyzine reduces anxiety and is often used in patients with substance abuse issues

Nonpharmacologic Treatment

• Supportive psychotherapy (individual, group, family)

• Cognitive behavioral therapy (CBT)
  * Focuses on coping with the fear of the symptoms of anxiety

• Relaxation techniques

• Exercise and/or lifestyle modifications (reduce caffeine and simple sugars)

5. Eating Disorders

Anorexia Nervosa (AN)

Characteristics
• A refusal to maintain body weight at or above a minimal, normal weight for age and height (less than 15% of expected body weight)

• Intense fear of gaining weight or becoming fat, although underweight

• Disturbance in self-perception of body weight, size, proportion, and attractiveness

• Amenorrhea for at least three consecutive cycles

Types
• Restricting and binge eating/purging types

Bulimia Nervosa (BN)

Characteristics
• Recurrent episodes of binge eating (often followed by intense feelings of guilt); patient may consume as much as 5000-20,000 calories over 2-8 hours

• Recurrent and inappropriate compensatory behavior in order to prevent weight gain

• Average of 2 binges/week for 3 months

• Person's self evaluation is primarily influenced by body shape and weight

Types
• Purging (vomiting, abuse of laxatives/diuretics) and nonpurging (excessive exercise, fasting)

Binge Eating Disorder

Characteristics
• Recurrent episodes of binge eating (patients usually obese)

• Eating when not physically hungry; eating more rapidly than normal; feeling disgusted with oneself

• Marked distress is present regarding binge eating

• Binge eating episodes occur, on average, at least 2 days/week for 6 months

Etiology and Prevalence

- The etiology is essentially unknown, but there are various theories (genetic predisposition, environmental/societal issues, chemical imbalance in the brain)

- There is usually a defined event or situation that begins the disorder (eg, a significant stressor such as starting college, divorce, or death of a loved one)

- Most commonly seen in Caucasian, middle- to upper-class females

Age of onset
- Anorexia nervosa: 13-20 years old
    * Male-to-female ratio, 1:10-20

- Bulimia nervosa: 16-18 years old
    * Male-to-female ratio, 1:10

Medical Complications and Signs of Disease

- Eating disorders produce states of semistarvation and noticeable malnutrition, especially in anorexia; in bulimia, patients are more difficult to identify because they are commonly of normal body weight

- Dehydration

- High incidence of comorbid anxiety, depression, OCD, and substance abuse

- Dental caries/enamel erosion due to stomach acid exposure

- Calluses on dorsum of hand and/or fingers due to induction of vomiting

- Mortality rate ~10% from starvation (primarily due to electrolyte imbalances), arrhythmia, or suicide

- Long-term complications: Endocrine/metabolic, cardiovascular, renal, gastroenterologic, hematologic, pulmonary, musculoskeletal, immunologic, dermatologic

Treatment

- Psychotherapy is the mainstay of treatment; therapy can be individual, group, family, supportive, cognitive-behavioral, or insight-oriented

- Primary objectives: Define and examine extent of problem; patient learns to accept condition; treatment results in a reconstruction of self-identity and self-confidence

- Dietary intake is slowly normalized with goal of restoring normal body weight; nutritional counseling is utilized

- Distorted ideas about caloric intake and body shape are corrected

- Relapse prevention focuses on developing and using coping mechanisms and avoiding high-risk situations

Drug therapy
Antidepressants
- SSRIs are primarily utilized and may be more effective for patients with bulimia

- Ideal treatment includes both psychotherapy and pharmacotherapy.

6. Key Points

Schizophrenia

- Patients with schizophrenia have positive (hallucinations, delusions), negative (flat affect, avolition, anhedonia, poverty of thought), and disorganized (speech, behavior) symptoms; positive symptoms usually respond to drug therapy first

- Antipsychotics (conventional or atypical) are essential treatment for schizophrenia; conventional agents (low-potency: chlorpromazine, thioridazine) are more often used than high-potency agents (haloperidol, fluphenazine)

- Low-potency agents have more sedation, orthostatic hypotension (OH), and anticholinergic (AC) side effects and less extrapyramidal symptoms (EPS) compared to high-potency agents; high-potency agents have more EPS and less sedation, OH, and AC effects

- Extrapyramidal symptoms consist of dystonic reactions (to be remedied by diphenhydramine 25-50 mg IM or benztropine 1-2 mg IM every 30 minutes until resolution), akathisia (to be treated with lorazepam, clonidine, or propranolol), and pseudoparkinsonism (ameliorated by amantadine or benztropine)

- Atypical medications (risperidone, olanzapine, quetiapine, ziprasidone, and aripiprazole) are considered first-line treatment because they have fewer adverse effects than conventional medications and appear to be more beneficial for negative symptoms

- Clozapine is the only agent proven effective for refractory schizophrenia

- Consider depot preparations in situations of poor compliance

Bipolar disorder

- The acute treatment for bipolar disorder focuses on slowing the patient down and reducing harm to self and others; maintenance treatment focuses on prevention and/or reducing the number of future episodes

- A mood stabilizer is an essential component in the treatment of bipolar disorder; first-line mood stabilizers include lithium and divalproex sodium (or valproic acid)

- The risk of lithium side effects and toxicity can be prevented by monitoring the patient for signs and symptoms of problems and by obtaining regular blood level readings

- Other drug therapies that may be used to treat the patient with bipolar disorder include atypical antipsychotics, gabapentin, carbamazepine, oxcarbazepine, topiramate, and lamotrigine (especially if depressed)

Major depression

- All antidepressants are equally effective in a given population

- Response varies from person to person; antidepressants differ in side effect and drug interaction profiles; none are "speed" or "uppers"

- Choice of agent depends on the history of response of other family members to certain antidepressants (if available) and the particular side effect profile (as it relates to any given patient)

- First-line agents include SSRIs, bupropion, and venlafaxine; second-line agents may include mirtazapine and nefazodone; third-line agents may include TCAs and MAOIs

- Reduce or eliminate target symptoms with an antidepressant; incorporating psychotherapy is optimal

- The goal of treatment of depression is to improve the patient's ability to function and his or her quality of life

Anxiety disorders

- Anxiety disorders are serious, debilitating mental illnesses that have extreme anxiety as the primary mood disturbance

- Various drug therapies include benzodiazepines, buspirone, antidepressants (especially SSRIs and venlafaxine), β-blockers, and hydroxyzine

- Nonpharmacologic therapy of anxiety disorders is an important aspect of care (eg, supportive therapy, cognitive behavioral therapy, relaxation techniques, and exercise/lifestyle modifications)

Eating disorders

- Anorexia nervosa is characterized by a refusal to maintain body weight (at or above a minimal normal weight for age and height), an intense fear of gaining weight, a disturbance in self-perception of body weight, and amenorrhea for at least three consecutive cycles

- Bulimia nervosa is characterized by recurrent episodes of binge eating, recurrent and inappropriate compensatory behavior in order to prevent weight gain, an average of two binges/week for 3 months, and self-evaluation that is primarily influenced by body shape and weight

- Eating disorders most commonly occur in young, Caucasian, middle- to upper-class females

- Medical complications and comorbid psychiatric disorders (eg, anxiety, depression, and substance abuse) are extremely common in this population

- Medications such as antidepressants may be helpful in treating eating disorders (especially bulimia); optimal therapy should include psychotherapy in combination with drug therapy

7. Questions and Answers

Select the single best response for Questions 1 through 4.

1. SJ is a 30-year-old WF with a 10-year history of schizophrenia. Her current therapy includes haloperidol 10 mg PO bid. The psychiatrist wants to convert her to haloperidol decanoate. What would be the appropriate equivalent monthly dose of haloperidol decanoate?

   A. 100 mg
   B. 10 mg
   C. 500 mg
   D. 200 mg
   E. 12.5 mg

2. BT reports to the nursing station with his head pulled sharply to the side and rear. He complains of severe pain in his neck and back area. The most appropriate diagnosis and treatment would be:

   A. Akathisia; propranolol 20 mg IM until resolution
   B. Dystonic reaction; diphenhydramine 50 mg IM every 30 minutes until resolution
   C. Tardive dyskinesia; physical therapy
   D. Dystonic reaction; lorazepam 2 mg IM every 30 minutes until resolution
   E. None of the above

3. Negative symptoms in schizophrenia could include all of the following except:

   A. Flat affect
   B. Anhedonia
   C. Avolition
   D. Persecutory delusions
   E. Poverty of thought

4. A 48-year-old BM arrives at the ED seeking his "nerve pill." He has a 27-year history of paranoid schizophrenia with multiple hospitalizations. In recent years, he has been effectively maintained on fluphenazine 10 mg PO bid. He now states that he feels "really bad today." His arms and jaws are stiff, his temperature is 104°F, his BP is 176/110, and his WBC is 19,000. LFTs and CPK are ordered STAT. While you await the test results, you would:

A. Discontinue oral fluphenazine and begin quetiapine

B. Discontinue oral fluphenazine

C. Continue oral fluphenazine and add bromocriptine

D. Discontinue oral fluphenazine and give fluphenazine decanoate 25 mg IM STAT

E. Do nothing; labs need to be evaluated first

For Questions 5 through 8, one or more of the answers given may be correct. Answer each question as follows:

A. I only
B. II only
C. I and III only
D. II and III only
E. I, II, and III

A 25-year-old WM has been increasingly disruptive at home. He has been claiming that he is the President of the United States and has been staying awake all night planning bills for Congress. He has been argumentative and threatening with his friends and family. Though he appears extremely tired physically, he is constantly active.

5. The psychiatrist has decided to initiate Eskalith CR 450 mg bid in this patient. Which of the following lab tests will need to be performed for this patient before starting this drug therapy regimen?

I. Pregnancy test
II. Thyroid function tests
III. SCr

6. As the pharmacist on the treatment team, you alert the patient's family to the common side effects of lithium, which include:

I. Polyuria
II. Alopecia
III. Elevated hepatic enzymes

7. Which of the following statements are correct regarding the treatment bipolar disorder?

I. Lithium and divalproex sodium are considered first-line therapy options for mood stabilization.
II. When treating a patient with lithium, the WBC and ANC must be monitored due to lithium's propensity to cause agranulocytosis.
III. Patients diagnosed with bipolar I disorder exhibit intermittent cycles of mania and major depression.

8. Which of the following therapies have been used for the treatment of bipolar disorder?

I. Olanzapine
II. Topiramate
III. Calcium channel blockers

Select the single best response for Questions 9 through 16.

9. Insomnia, GI upset, and headache are common side effects of which of the following antidepressants?

A. Phenelzine
B. Amitriptyline
C. Fluoxetine
D. Trazodone
E. Both B and C

10. A 29-year-old depressed BF has shown little improvement with tranylcypromine treatment so the psychiatrist decides to change her medication to fluoxetine. What is your recommendation for the switch?

A. Gradually decrease tranylcypromine dosage over a 4-week period and then start fluoxetine
B. Wait 2 weeks after stopping tranylcypromine and then begin fluoxetine
C. Over 6 weeks, gradually decrease tranylcypromine dosage as you gradually increase the fluoxetine dosage
D. Wait 5 weeks after stopping tranylcypromine before initiating fluoxetine
E. Maintain tranylcypromine dosage and start fluoxetine; stop the tranylcypromine when the fluoxetine has achieved therapeutic level

11. Which of the following has been shown to induce or worsen depression?

A. Oral contraceptives
B. Amoxicillin
C. Thiamine
D. Methylphenidate
E. Phenelzine

12. Which of the following is correct regarding electroconvulsive therapy (ECT)?

A. For maximum effectiveness, seizures should last 5-10 minutes
B. Contraindicated in patients with COPD
C. Effective treatment for pregnant females with major depression

D. Memory loss for 1-2 week period duration is common

E. ECT may cause amenorrhea in female patients

13. A 33-year-old waitress is experiencing symptoms of anxiety, including night terrors and mood lability. She reports no past psychiatric history but admits that these symptoms started about 2 weeks after armed and masked gunman robbed her restaurant. She is most likely experiencing:

A. LSD
B. PTSD
C. GAD
D. OCD

14. A new patient presents to your clinic. He reports that it took him 3 hours to get ready for this appointment and that he returned home several times in order to check to see if the door was locked. During the interview, he straightens up your desk, making sure all square items are at right angles to each other. He would most likely be diagnosed as:

A. PTSD
B. PCP
C. OCD
D. GAD

15. Which of the following statements regarding the use of SSRIs in anxiety disorders is most accurate?

A. SSRIs are not usually effective in the treatment of anxiety.
B. SSRI doses for anxiety should be started lower than initial doses for depression.
C. SSRIs should only be used after a failed treatment trial with benzodiazepines.
D. SSRIs may be used on a prn basis when anxiety symptoms emerge.

16. Which of the following statements are not correct regarding benzodiazepines?

A. Potentiate the effect of gamma-aminobutyric acid
B. Highly lipophilic
C. Cross tolerant with alcohol
D. Similar pharmacologic action to buspirone
E. Risk of seizure if abruptly discontinued

For Questions 17 through 20, one or more of the following answers given are correct. Answer each question as follows:

A. I only
B. II only
C. I and III only
D. II and III only
E. I, II, and III

17. Which of the following is true regarding anorexia nervosa?

I. Anorexia nervosa (AN) is characterized by recurrent and inappropriate compensatory behavior in order to prevent weight gain.
II. Patients with AN generally appear to be of normal weight for age and height.
III. AN patients have an intense fear of gaining weight or becoming fat, although they are underweight.

18. What *DSM-IV* criteria for AN are diagnostic for this type of eating disorder?

I. Absence of at least three consecutive menstrual cycles
II. Sunken eyes with dark circles underneath
III. Binge eating/purging episode occurs at least once in past 6 months

19. Which of the following is true regarding bulimia nervosa (BN)?

I. The individual may consume 5000-20,000 calories in a single binge episode that may last as long as 2-8 hours.
II. The two specific types of bulimic patients are purging type and nonpurging type.
III. There is an average of two binges/week for 3 consecutive months.

20. Patients with AN may demonstrate which of the following characteristics?

I. Kleptomania
II. Laxative/diuretic abuse
III. Amenorrhea

Answers

1. **D.** The patient is on haloperidol 10 mg bid. Therefore, to convert to the decanoate injection, the total oral daily dose is multiplied by 10. The dose would be Haldol-D 200 mg IM every 4 weeks.

2. **B.** The patient is experiencing a dystonic reaction, which can be treated with either benztropine 1-2 mg IM or diphenhydramine 25-50 mg IM every 30 minutes until resolved. The dystonic reaction is thought to occur due to an imbalance in dopamine and acetylcholine in the nigrostriatal region of the brain.

3. **D.** Delusions are fixed and false beliefs are evident. Both symptoms are referred to as "positive" for patients with schizophrenia.

4. **B.** The symptoms that the patient is displaying appear to be the result of neuroleptic malignant syndrome (NMS). All neuroleptics have the propensity to cause this rare but deadly adverse effect. The first step in treating NMS is to discontinue the offending agent, offer supportive therapy, a dopamine agonist, and (commonly) a skeletal muscle relaxant.

5. **D.** Initiation of lithium requires several baseline labs tests: Pregnancy test (if patient is of childbearing age); ECG and BP to assess CV status; thyroid function tests to rule out euthyroid goiter or hypothyroidism; SCr/BUN (lithium is 100% renally eliminated); and CBC with differential to evaluate for leukocytosis. Electrolytes should also be evaluated (decreased Na can increase lithium levels).

6. **A.** Common side effects that occur with the initiation of lithium include polyuria, polydipsia, tremor, and GI upset. Common side effects that may occur later in therapy include weight gain and mental dulling. Elevated hepatic enzymes and alopecia are side effects that may occur with divalproex sodium.

7. **C.** Agranulocytosis is a side effect that is monitored weekly with clozapine therapy for 6 months. After 6 months, monitoring can be done every 2 weeks for the duration of therapy.

8. **E.** All of the therapies listed have been used for mood stabilization in bipolar disorder.

9. **C.** SSRIs commonly cause insomnia, GI upset, anxiety, headache, and sexual dysfunction. Phenelzine, amitriptyline, and trazodone cause sedative effects.

10. **D.** Due to fluoxetine's long half-life, 5 weeks should pass before initiating MAOI therapy. If fluoxetine is not cleared from the body by the time the MAOI is started, there is a risk of developing serotonin syndrome.

11. **A.** Many medications can cause or worsen depression, eg, antihypertensives (reserpine, methyldopa, propranolol, clonidine), antiparkinsonian agents (levodopa, carbidopa, amantadine), hormone agents (estrogens, progesterone), corticosteroids, cycloserine, and the anticancer agents vinblastine and vincristine.

12. **C.** ECT is a safe and effective therapy for pregnant females and patients with COPD. Relative contraindications include increased intracranial pressure, recent MI, recent intracerebral hemorrhage, and cerebral lesions. Memory loss is a common side effect, but usually only on the day of treatment and perhaps the following day. The induced seizure lasts 30-90 seconds and is monitored by EEG. Additionally, ECT does not cause amenorrhea in female patients.

13. **B.** The patient experienced a violent and frightening episode 2 weeks before her symptoms. The symptoms of re-experiencing the event, night terrors, and mood lability are common in patients with PSTD.

14. **C.** The patient is displaying signs and symptoms of OCD (eg, a long time is spent getting ready, there is checking behavior, and preoccupation with rearranging items to 90-degree angles). These activities are time consuming and limit his social and occupational functioning.

15. **B.** Because SSRIs can be activating and may initially cause symptoms of anxiety, it is important to "start low and go slow" with these agents when utilized for anxiety disorders.

16. **D.** Buspirone's mechanism of action is agonism of $5\text{-}HT_{1A}$ receptors. Buspirone also possesses moderate affinity for D_2 receptors. It does not interact with the BZD-GABA receptor complex like the BZDs. The BZDs cross the blood-brain barrier and are cross-tolerant with alcohol. If abruptly discontinued, seizures can result.

17. **C.** Patients with AN refuse to maintain body weight at or above a minimal, normal weight for age and height (less than 15% of expected body weight). Patients with AN may respond to antidepressants, but psychotherapy is usually more effective. AN is most commonly seen in Caucasian, middle- to upper-class females.

18.   **A.** *DSM-IV* criteria list the refusal to maintain body weight at or above a minimal, normal weight for age and height (less than 15% of expected body weight, an intense fear of gaining weight or becoming fat although underweight), disturbance in self-perception of body weight (ie, size, proportion, attractiveness), and amenorrhea for at least three consecutive cycles.

19.   **E.** All of the answers are correct regarding BN.

20.   **D.** Patients with AN commonly reduce weight by reducing food intake. Many patients use other ways to lose weight such as excessive exercise, laxative and/or diuretic use, substance abuse, and self-induced vomiting. Amenorrhea ensues as a result of estrogen deficiency; it may occur before weight loss.

8. References

American Psychiatric Association. *Diagnostic and Statistical Manual of Mental Disorders*, 4th ed, Text Revision. Washington: American Psychiatric Association; 2000.

Bennett JA, Dunayevich E, McElroy SL, et al. The new mood stabilizers and the treatment of bipolar disorder. *Drug Benefit Trends*. 2000;12:3-16.

Botts SR, Raskind J. Gabapentin and lamotrigine in bipolar disorder. *Am J Health-Syst Pharm*. 1999;56:1939-1944.

Canales PL, Cates M, Wells BG. Anxiety disorders. In: Herfindal ET, Gourley DR, eds. *Textbook of Therapeutics: Drug and Disease Management*, 7th ed. Philadelphia: Lippincott Williams & Wilkins; 2000:1185-1202.

Cohen LJ, Jermain DM, Clarke SO, et al. Psychiatric Pharmacy Practice Specialty Certification Examination Review Course. Course presented at ASHP Psychiatric Clinical Specialists Meeting, Denver, CO, 2001 Mar 31-Apr 1.

DeVane CL. Keeping depression at bay. *Drug Topics*. 2001;15:49-58.

Easson WM, Rock NL. *Psychiatry Specialty Board Review*. New York: Brunner/Mazel; 1991.

Fuller MA, Sajatovic M, eds. *Drug Information for Mental Health,* 1st ed. Cleveland: Lexi-Comp; 2001.

Jacobson JL, Jacobson AM, eds. *Psychiatric Secrets*. Philadelphia: Hanley & Belfus; 1996.

Kane JM. Drug therapy: Schizophrenia. *N Engl J Med*. 1996;334:34-41.

Kane JM, McGlashan TH. Treatment of schizophrenia. *Lancet*. 1995;346:820-825.

Mandl DL, Iltz JL. Obesity and eating disorders. In: Herfindal ET, Gourley DR, eds. *Textbook of Therapeutics: Drug and Disease Management*, 7th ed. Philadelphia: Lippincott Williams & Wilkins; 2000:1271-1287.

McElroy SL, Keck PE. Pharmacologic agents for the treatment of acute bipolar mania. *Biol Psychiatry*. 2000;48:539-557.

McEvoy JP, Scheifler PL, Frances A. The expert consensus guideline series. Treatment of schizophrenia. *J Clin Psychiatry.* 1999;60(suppl 11):3-80.

National Institute of Mental Health. Anxiety disorders. Bethesda, MD: NIH publication no. 00-3879; 2000.

National Institute of Mental Health. Pamphlet on eating disorders. Washington: U.S. Department of Health and Human Services; NIH publication no. 94-3477; 1994.

Norton J. Oxcarbazepine in mood disorders. *Hosp Pharm.* 2001;36:1254-1256.

Post RM. Rapid cycling: clinical presentation and treatment approaches. New research presented at the 155th Annual Meeting of the American Psychiatric Association. Philadelphia; May 2002.

Practice guideline for the treatment of patients with major depressive disorder (revision). American Psychiatric Association Practice Guidelines. *Am J Psychiatry.* 2000;157(4 Suppl):1-45.

Practice guideline for the treatment of patients with bipolar disorder (revision). American Psychiatric Association Practice Guidelines. *Am J Psychiatry.* 2002;159(suppl):1-50.

Practice guideline for the treatment of patients with schizophrenia. American Psychiatric Association Practice Guidelines. *Am J Psychiatry.* 1997;154(suppl 4):1-63.

Risby E, Donnigan D, Nemeroff CB. Pharmacotherapeutic considerations for psychiatric disorders: Depression. *Formulary.* 1997;32:46-59.

Sachs GS, Printz DJ, Kahn DA, et al. The expert consensus guideline series. Medication treatment of bipolar disorder 2000. *Postgraduate Med.* 2000;4:1-104.

Stahl SM. *Psychopharmacology of Antidepressants.* London: Martin Dunitz; 1998.

Stahl SM. *Psychopharmacology of Antipsychotics.* London: Martin Dunitz; 1999.

Stimmel GL. Mood disorders. In: Herfindal ET, Gourley DR, eds. *Textbook of Therapeutics: Drug and Disease Management*, 7th ed. Philadelphia: Lippincott Williams & Wilkins; 2000:1203-1216.

Stimmel GL. Schizophrenia. In: Herfindal ET, Gourley DR, eds. *Textbook of Therapeutics: Drug and Disease Management*, 7th ed. Philadelphia: Lippincott Williams & Wilkins; 2000:1217-1227.

Substance Abuse and Mental Health Services Administration and National Institute of Mental Health. Mental Health: A Report from the Surgeon General. www.surgeongeneral.gov/Library/MentalHealth/home.html (accessed 2003 Mar 12)

26. Common Dermatologic Disorders

James C. Eoff, PharmD, BSPh
Executive Associate Dean and Professor,
 Department of Pharmacy
University of Tennessee College of Pharmacy

Contents

1. Acne (Acne Vulgaris)

- Acne is an inflammatory disorder of the pilosebaceous glands, which occurs most commonly during the teenage years, at or soon after puberty.

- It may reappear later or begin in adults who had clear skin in their teens, more commonly in women than men.

Classification and Clinical Presentation

Type I (comedonal)
- A mild form, with primarily noninflammatory lesions (open and closed comedones) and relatively few superficial inflammatory lesions with no scarring

Type II (papular)
- A moderate form, with multiple papules on the face and trunk, with minimal scarring

Type III (pustular)
- An advanced form that can lead to moderate scarring

Type IV (nodulocystic)
- The most severe and destructive form with multiple deep inflammatory lesions or nodules (often called cysts) that leads to extensive scarring

Pathophysiology

- Increased sebum production by androgenic hormones at onset of puberty

- Obstruction of hair follicle opening due to increasing adherence and production of epithelial cells, producing closed comedones (whiteheads) progressing ultimately to open comedones (blackheads)

- Increased growth of a primary microorganism on the skin and in the sebaceous ducts, *Propionibacterium acnes* (*P acnes*), a gram-positive anaerobic rod that produces enzymes, including lipases

- Inflammation due to the enzymatic breakdown of triglycerides into free fatty acids, which causes the influx of polymorphonuclear leukocytes, ultimately resulting in pustule formation

Treatment Principles

Type I (comedonal)
- Topical nonprescription medications

  * Benzoyl peroxide is usually the first line of therapy

Type II (papular)
- Topical antibiotics and/or topical retinoids

Type III (pustular)
- Oral antibiotics in addition to topical medications

Type IV (nodulocystic)
- Isotretinoin

Topical Therapy

Nonprescription agents
- Benzoyl peroxide (most effective OTC agent)

- Benzoyl peroxide products 2.5, 5, and 10%:
  * Clearasil® maximum strength vanishing cream
  * Exact® vanishing cream
  * Neutrogena® oil-free acne mask
  * Noxzema® anti-acne lotion
  * Oxy-10®
  * Benzac®
  * Panoxyl®
  * Zapzyt® gel

Mechanism of action
- Destroy the anaerobic *P acnes* due to release of oxygen

- Exfoliant effect, causing peeling of the outer layers of the skin

- *P acnes* does not become resistant to benzoyl peroxide; therefore, it can be used concurrently with topical antibiotics to prevent resistance (eg, using BP for one course of therapy, alternating with a course of topical antibiotic therapy)

Patient counseling
- Use with caution with sensitive skin.

- Do not allow contact with eyes, lips, or mouth

- Avoid unnecessary sun exposure and/or use sunscreen

Adverse effects
- May cause redness, dryness, burning, itching, peeling, and swelling

- May bleach hair or dyed fabrics

Other nonprescription agents
- Sulfur (3-8%)
  - * SAStid® soap: precipitated sulfur 10% (keratolytic and antibacterial action)

- Salicylic acid (0.5-2%)
  - * Clearasil Clearstick®, Neutrogena® Oil Free Acne Wash®, Noxzema®, Stridex®: irritant effect, keratolytic, and increases rate of turnover of epithelial cells

- Resorcinol
  - * Keratolytic (usually combined with sulfur)

- Combinations:
  - * Sulfur and resorcinol: Clearasil®, Acnomel®

- Medicated soaps and cleansers: alcohol, acetone, other degreasing lotions

Topical antimicrobial therapy:
- See Table 1.

Clindamycin
Mechanism of action
- Suppresses growth of *P acnes*

- May directly reduce free fatty acid concentrations on the skin

Patient counseling
- Contact physician if no improvement within 6 weeks

- Discontinue medication and contact physician if severe diarrhea and/or abdominal cramps or pain develop

Adverse effects
- Contact dermatitis or hypersensitivity

- Dry or scaly skin or peeling

- Rarely: pseudomembranous colitis (severe abdominal cramps, pain, bloating, and severe diarrhea)

Erythromycin
Mechanism of action
- Suppress growth of *P acnes*

Patient counseling
- Wait at least 1 hour before applying any other topical acne medication

- Avoid contact with eyes, mouth, nose and other mucous membranes

- While improvement is generally expected within 4 weeks, some patients do not respond for 8-12 weeks

Adverse effects
- More common: dry or scaly skin, irritation, and itching

- Less common: stinging, peeling, and redness

Retinoids
- See Table 2.

Mechanism of action
- Retinoids are chemically related to vitamin A.

- Retinoids normalize follicular keratinization, heal comedones, decrease sebum production, and decrease inflammatory lesions.

Patient counseling
- Do not use astringents, drying agents, abrasive scrubs, or harsh soaps concurrently, and only use mild soap once or twice daily.

Table 1

Topical Antimicrobials

Generic name	Trade name	Form
Clindamycin	Cleocin-T®	Liquid
Erythromycin	Theramycin Z®	Liquid
	Benzamycin® 2%	Gel
	Emgel® 2%	Gel

Table 2

Retinoids

Generic name	Trade name	Form and strength
Tretinoin	Retin-A®	0.015%, 0.05%, 0.1% cream; 0.1% gel, 0.05% lotion
	Renova®	0.05% cream
	Avita®	0.025% cream and gel
Adapalene	Differin®	0.1% gel
Tazarotene	Tazorac®	0.05%, 0.1% gel
Alitretinoin	Panretin®	0.1% gel

- Apply every other night to adjust to drying effect for the first 2 weeks.

- Apply nightly after 2 weeks

- May take up to 2-3 months before skin improves

- Use sun block on face before sun exposure due to increased sensitivity

Adverse drug effects
- May irritate skin and cause redness dryness and scaling

- Tazarotene is the most irritating retinoid.

- Adapalene appears to be least irritating and is preferred for sensitive skin

Azelaic acid 20%
- Trade names Azelex® and Finevin®

Mechanism of action
- Suppresses growth of *P acnes*

- Improves inflammatory and noninflammatory lesions

- Normalization of keratinization leading to anticomedonal effect

Patient counseling
- If sensitivity develops, discontinue use.

- Keep away from mouth, eyes, and mucous membranes

- Other topical medications must be used at different times during the day

Adverse drug effects
- Temporary skin irritation (pruritus and burning) may occur upon initiation of therapy

Systemic Therapy

Antimicrobials
- See Table 3.

General
- Useful for type 2 (papular) acne and type 3 (pustular) acne

- After 6-8 weeks, dosage may be increased if necessary

Table 3

Oral Antimicrobials

Generic name	Trade name	Dosage and form
Tetracycline	Achromycin®, Sumycin®	500 mg qd or bid caps
Erythromycin	E.E.S.®, Erythrocin®	250-500 qd or bid tabs
Doxycycline	Vibramycin®	100 mg qd caps/tabs
Minocycline	Minocin®	50 mg bid caps

- If the first antibiotic was ineffective after increasing the dosage, a second antibiotic is prescribed

- After 6 months to 1 year of therapy, the antibiotic dose may be tapered if continued at all

Mechanism of action
- Suppresses growth of *P acnes* in sebaceous duct

- Possible direct anticomedonal effect

Patient counseling, adverse drug effects, and drug interactions
- See chapter on antimicrobials

Isotretinoin
- Trade name Accutane®, 10-, 20-, and 40-mg capsules

General
- For patients with severe, nodulocystic, draining acne who have not responded to systemic antibiotic therapy or who have required more than 3 years of systemic antibiotic therapy

- Over 90% effective in producing an acne-free state for years following a 4- to 5-month course of therapy

- Originally held in reserve for severe cases of nodulocystic acne, but may also be indicated as first-line treatment for severe acne that results in scarring

Mechanism of action
- Reduces sebum production (up to 90% inhibition)

- Decreased production of microcomedones, possibly by decreasing cohesiveness of follicular epithelial cells

- Possible anti-inflammatory effect

Patient counseling
- Should be taken with food and best absorbed with a fatty meal

- Can take the dose divided twice daily or the entire dose with the evening meal

- Effects are gradual, and acne may worsen during the first month of therapy; however, improvement usually begins by the sixth week of therapy

- Use lip balm to treat cheilitis and moisturizers to treat dry skin

Adverse drug effects
- ***Teratogenic: Absolutely contraindicated in pregnancy***
    * Causes significant birth defects.
    * Females of childbearing potential, **must** take measures to avoid pregnancy during the course of isotretinoin therapy.
    * Females should be tested for pregnancy before initiation of therapy and told to use two methods of contraception for at least 1 month prior to initiation of therapy, and 1 month after discontinuation of therapy.

Side effects and toxicity
- Most common (90-100%):
    * Cheilitis (chapped lips)
    * Dry mouth
    * Dry skin
    * Pruritus

- Common (30-40%):
    * Dry nose, leading to nasal crusting and epistaxis
    * Dry eyes, leading to conjunctivitis and problems with contact lenses
    * Muscular soreness or stiffness

- Less common (10-25%):
    * Headaches
    * Hyperlipidemia (primarily elevation of triglycerides, which may lead to attack of pancreatitis)

- Rare (less than 5%):
    * Decreased night vision
    * Thinning of hair
    * Easily injured skin
    * Peeling of palms and soles
    * Skin rash and skin infections

- Very rare (<1%):
    * Acute depression: very rare, but reversible if detected early

* Pseudotumor cerebri (benign intracranial hypertension with visual disturbances)

- Treatment of most common side effects:
    * Cheilitis: frequent use of lip balm
    * Dry skin: skin lubrication with moisturizers
    * Nosebleeds: lubricate the nostrils with petrolatum
    * Muscular soreness or stiffness: mild OTC analgesic/anti-inflammatory agents

Monitoring parameters
- Lipid panel

- Liver function tests (elevations are common during initiation of therapy, but usually return to normal during treatment)

- Complete blood counts

- Pregnancy testing for women prior to use of drug

Dosing
- 1 mg/kg per day (may start out 0.5 mg/kg per day for the first month before increasing) taken once or twice daily with food; best absorbed with a fatty meal

- Goal: a total dose of 120-150 mg/kg over 4-5 months

- Longer courses of 6-8 months may be required.

Other
- Approximate 20% relapse within 1 year, and up to 40% within 3 years after discontinuation of therapy

- Repeat therapy for 4-6 months is acceptable and effective

Oral corticosteroids
- Commonly known as "prom pills"

- Can temporarily suppress acne with a 7- to 10-day course of prednisone 20 mg daily

- Rapidly effective when a brief course is necessary to cause prompt improvement (eg, important social event such as wedding, prom, etc)

- Systemic corticosteroids used continuously may actually cause or worsen acne

- Topical corticosteroids have **no** value in the treatment of acne, and the high potency topical corticosteroids will aggravate acne and should never be used on the face of acne patients

2. Fungal Skin Infections

- Tinea are skin infections known as ***dermatomycoses*** caused by the fungi *Trichophyton, Microsporum,* and *Epidermophyton.*

Classification

- Tinea pedis (athlete's foot)

- Tinea capitis (ringworm of the scalp)

- Tinea cruris (jock itch)

- Tinea corporis (ringworm of the skin)

- Tinea unguium (onychomycosis; fungal infection of toenails or fingernails)

Pathophysiology

- The fungi invade dead cells of the stratum corneum of skin, hair, and nails, digesting keratin

- Unlike *Candida*, they cannot exist on unkeratinized mucous membranes

- More common in immunosuppressed patients

Treatment Principles and Goals

- Tinea pedis: self-treat topically initially; if ineffective, add orals

- Tinea capitis: oral systemic therapy

- Tinea cruris: self-treat topically initially; if ineffective, add orals

- Tinea corporis: self-treat topically initially; if ineffective, add orals

- Tinea unguium: oral systemic therapy

Drug Therapy

OTC treatment
- Terbinafine 1% (Lamisil AT®) cream and spray
   * Most effective OTC antifungal agent

- Miconazole 2% (Micatin®)

- Clotrimazole 1% (Lotrimin AF®, Desenex AF®)

- Tofnaftate 1% (Tinactin®, Aftate®, Blis-To-Sol®, Dr. Scholl's Fungi Solution®)

- Undecylenic acid 10-25% (Cruex®, Desenex®)

Prescription treatment
* See Table 4.

Topicals
- Newer antifungals are initially applied only once daily, and recurrences can be prevented by once- or twice-weekly applications.

Systemic therapy
- Occasionally topical therapy is not effective for tinea pedis, tinea cruris, and tinea corporis, and systemic therapy is required.

- Systemic antifungal therapy is required for tinea capitis (ringworm of the scalp) and tinea unguium (fungal infections of the fingernails and toenails):
   * Griseofulvin
   * Ketoconazole
   * Fluconazole
   * Itraconazole
   * Terbinafine

- See chapter on antimicrobials for discussion of systemic antifungals.

Table 4

Prescription Topical Antifungals

Generic name	Trade name
Econazole	Spectazole® cream, Ecostatin® cream
Naftifine	Naftin® gel, cream
Ciclopirox	Loprox® gel, cream, lotion; Penlac® solution
Butenafine	Mentax® cream

3. Hair Loss (Alopecia)

- Male pattern baldness (androgenic alopecia) is the gradual and progressive loss of hair in males as they age.

Clinical Presentation

- Onset and progression varies greatly

- Distinct pattern of progressive hair loss in the frontotemporal areas and crown with sparing of the occiput

- Hair loss limited to scalp

- Miniaturization of hair is seen, where normal thick terminal hairs are converted to very fine vellus hairs

Pathophysiology

- Alopecia is primarily due to two factors:
  * Heredity (genetic)
  * Testostcrone, which promotes growth of hair in the beard, axillae, pubis, and other parts of body, does not promote the growth of scalp hair, and actually contributes to premature loss because it is converted by the enzyme 5-α-reductase to dihydrotestosterone, which binds preferentially to receptors in the hair follicles on the scalp causing them to produce progressively thinner hair, until the follicles eventually cease activity altogether.

Treatment Principles and Goals

- Although there is no cure, there are two drugs available for the treatment of androgenic alopecia:
  * Minoxidil (Rogaine®; available OTC)
  * Finasteride (Propecia®; by prescription only)

- In the early stages, topical minoxidil or oral finasteride may reverse the gradually decreasing diameter of the hair shaft

- Any hair growth stimulation is temporary and only lasts as long as therapy continues; if therapy is discontinued, new hair growth is lost within 1 year

- Early hair loss occurring recently in younger men is more likely to respond than later hair loss at an older age or when hair loss is not recent

- Alopecia of the crown in men responds better than hair loss in the frontotemporal area

Drug Therapy

Minoxidil
- OTC: trade name Rogaine® 2% and Rogaine Extra Strength® 5%

Mechanism of action
- Probably increased cutaneous blood flow directly to hair follicles due to vasodilation

- Possible stimulation of resting hair follicles (telogen phase) into active growth (anagen phase)

- Possible stimulation of hair follicle cells

Patient counseling
- Apply 1 mL twice daily (approximately one 60-mL bottle each month).

- May be applied without shampooing hair

- Use at least 4 hours before bedtime to avoid oil on pillows and bed linens

- Absorbed over a 4-hour period, so do not swim, shampoo, or walk in rain for 4 hours.

- Wash hands immediately after application to prevent unwanted absorption.

- Do not inhale mist as systemic absorption is possible.

- Do not use on infected, irritated, inflamed, or sunburned skin.

- Discontinue use immediately and contact physician if chest pain, increased heart rate, faintness or dizziness, or swollen hands or feet occur.

- Women should avoid 5% strength (no better results than 2%); women have greater incidence of increased growth of facial hair with 5% solution.

- Generally takes 4-6 months before any benefit occurs.

- No effects within 8 months for women and 12 months for men indicate therapeutic failure and treatment should be discontinued.

- Must continue using to maintain new hair growth.

Adverse drug effects
- Scalp dermatitis is common, producing dryness, pruritus, and flaking or scaling.

- Hypertrichosis (excessive hair growth) on areas other than scalp (chest, forearms, ear rim, back, face, arms, etc)

- Some women report unwanted facial hair growth when applied to scalp, primarily with 5% solution.

- May rarely produce systemic side effects (chest pain, increased heart rate, faintness or dizziness)

- Contraindicated in patients less than age 18 years

- Contraindicated in women who are pregnant or breastfeeding

Finasteride
- Trade name: Propecia® 1 mg

- Originally approved in 1992 for the treatment of enlarged prostate glands (benign prostatic hypertrophy) in a 5-mg dose (Proscar®)

- 1-mg daily dose approved for ***men only*** as prescription treatment for androgenic alopecia

- Effectiveness: over a 2-year period, may halt the progressive hair loss of androgenic alopecia

Mechanism of action
- Inhibits the enzyme 5-α-reductase, which is responsible for the conversion of testosterone to the more powerful dihydrotestosterone (DHT), which is the main androgen responsible for androgenic hair loss

Patient counseling
- May be taken with or without food

- Take for at least 3 months to see if effective

- Improvement lasts only as long as treatment continues (new hair will be lost with 1 year of stopping treatment).

Adverse drug effects
- Gynecomastia (breast enlargement and tenderness) reported from 2 weeks to 2 years following initial therapy; usually reversible when therapy is discontinued.

- Hypersensitivity (skin rash, swelling of lips)

- Decreased libido, erectile dysfunction, and ejaculatory dysfunction, which are reversible when the drug is discontinued

- Contraindicated in women of childbearing age, due to abnormalities of the external genitalia in male fetuses; and also not effective in postmenopausal women.

4. Dry Skin

- Refers to lack of moisture or sebum in the stratum corneum

- Most commonly occurring in the winter (also known as "winter rash")

- More common in older adults

Clinical Presentation

- Flaking and scaling

- Xerosis and roughness

- Pruritus

- Loss of skin elasticity

Pathophysiology

- Dry skin is due to inadequate moisture retention in the stratum corneum, which is caused by the following factors:
  * Decreased sebum production and decreasing moisture binding capacity of skin in elderly patients
  * Low humidity causes the skin to lose water, and become dry and hardened
  * Overexposure to sunlight
  * Excessive cleansing and bathing removes lipids and other skin components
  * Chronic skin diseases which impair moisture retention of skin (psoriasis, scleroderma, ichthyosis, and contact dermatitis)

Treatment Principles and Goals

- Increasing moisture level of the stratum corneum by increasing cell hydration and binding capacity, which improves skin permeability and restores elasticity

Drug Therapy

Emollients and moisturizing agents (petrolatum; mineral oil [Lubriderm® Bath and Shower Oil])
- Increase relative moisture content of the stratum corneum

- Produce a general soothing effect by reducing frictional heat and perspiration

Humectants (glycerin [Corn Husker's® Lotion], propylene glycol, phospholipids)
- Hygroscopic agents that increase hydration of the stratum corneum

Keratin-softening agents
- Urea (10-30%) (Aquacare®, Carmol®)
  * Improves the skin's moisture-binding capacity
  * Keratolytic at higher concentrations
  * May cause irritation and burning

- Lactic acid (2-5%) (LactiCare®, Lowila®)
  * Increases skin hydration by controlling the rate of keratinization
  * Markedly hygroscopic

- Allantoin (Alphosyl®, Psorex®, Tegrin®)
  * Relieves dry skin by disrupting keratin structure (less effective than urea)
  * Desensitizes many skin-sensitizing drugs as a protectant

Antipruritic agents
- Camphor and menthol provide cooling sensation.

- Local anesthetics (benzocaine, pramoxine, etc)

- Colloidal oatmeal (Aveeno®)
  * **Caution:** colloidal oatmeal can cause extremely slippery bathtub.

- Systemic antihistamines (H_1-receptor antagonists): limited effectiveness

Hydrocortisone
- Reduces inflammatory response that accompanies dry skin conditions

- Although HC does not directly increase skin hydration, it does prevent itching associated with dry skin and inhibits dehydration.

- Ointment better than cream for dry skin

- Must use sparingly

- Do not use more than 5 to 7 days for dry skin pruritus

Astringents
- Aluminum acetate 0.1-0.5% (Burrow's solution)

- Hamamelis water (witch hazel)

Protectants
- Zinc oxide

Nondrug Recommendations and Therapy

- Bathing less frequently

- Reduce use of soap to a minimum and only where necessary

- Lubricate skin immediately after bathing (eg, application of bath oil after bathing and before drying)

- Use extrafatted soaps such as Basis®

Use combination products to treat dry skin:
- * Alpha Keri® Moisture Rich Cleansing Bar: mineral oil, lanolin oil, glycerin
- * Aveeno® Bath Treatment Moisturizing Formula: colloidal oatmeal and mineral oil
- * Jergens® Advanced Therapy Dry Skin Care Lotion: dimethicone, lanolin, cetyl alcohol, isopropyl myristate, glycerin
- * Keri® Original Dry Skin Lotion: mineral oil, lanolin oil, glyceryl stearate, propylene glycol
- * Moisturel® Lotion: petrolatum, dimethicone, cetyl alcohol, glycerin
- * Neutrogena® Body Oil: isopropyl myristate, sesame oil
- * Pacquin® Plus Dry Skin Hand and Body Cream: lanolin anhydrous, cetyl alcohol, glycerin
- * Sardo® Bath Oil: mineral oil, isopropyl palmitate
- * Vaseline® Dermatology Formula Lotion: white petrolatum, mineral oil, dimethicone, glyceryl stearate, cetyl alcohol, glycerin

5. Dermatitis

- Nonspecific term to describe a variety of inflammatory dermatologic conditions characterized by erythema

- A general term to describe any eczematous rash of unknown etiology that can't be classified among the major endogenous dermatoses

- *Eczema* and ***dermatitis*** are often used interchangeably

Types and Classification

- Several of the major classifications or types of dermatitis are:
  - * Atopic dermatitis (atopic eczema)
  - * Chronic dermatitis (hand dermatitis)
  - * Contact dermatitis (irritant and allergic)

Clinical Presentation

Atopic dermatitis (atopic eczema)
- Occurs primarily in infants and children

- May disappear before adulthood

- Cause unknown; possibly genetic

- Usually seen on face, knees, elbows, and neck

- Frequently seen with asthma, allergic rhinitis, and urticaria

- Exacerbating factors: soaps, detergents, chemicals, temperature changes, molds, allergens

Chronic dermatitis (hand dermatitis or hand eczema)
- Stubborn itchy rash referred to as eczema that occurs in certain persons with sensitive or irritable skin.

- Skin very dry and easily irritated by overuse of soaps, detergents, and/or rough woolen clothing.

- Exacerbated by very hot or very cold weather

- Probably genetically determined

- No permanent cure

- Usually can control by enhancing skin hydration

with emollients and moisturizers, and using hydro-cortisone cream to relieve itching

Contact dermatitis
Irritant contact dermatitis (chemical contact dermatitis)
- Caused by exposure to irritating substances producing mechanical or chemical trauma

- Examples: soap, solvents, paints, abrasive cleansers, cosmetics, lubricants, antiseptics, cacti, rose hips, thorns, peppers, tobacco

- Not a sensitization, but direct toxicity to skin tissue

Allergic contact dermatitis
- Process of sensitization with reaction on elicitation

- Over 50% of all dermatitis is allergic contact dermatitis.

- Examples: benzocaine, zinc pyrithione (ZPT), neomycin, sodium bisulfite, perfumes, many cosmetics, skin lubricants, antiseptic creams, rubber and epoxy glues, poison ivy and oak, and many other common substances

Treatment Principles and Goals

- Treated by applying a corticosteroid:
  * Ointments and creams are more lubricating than solutions, lotions, or gels
  * Ointments should be recommended if skin is dry
  * Lotions or gels should be recommended for a weeping, eczematous dermatitis
  * Lotions, solutions, and gels are also easier to use in hairy areas of the body

- Patient should apply small amounts of corticosteroid cream or ointment and massage in gently but thoroughly

- Apply the moderate- and high-strength cortisones only once daily

- Improvement should begin within one week

- Avoid excess soap, keep skin lubricated with moisturizers

- Treat itching with camphor, menthol, phenol, or local anesthetics

- Occasionally with severe cases (less than 5%) may have to use systemic corticosteroids for 1-2 weeks.

Drug Therapy

Topical corticosteroids (see Table 5).

Adverse effects
- Striae may result in skin folds.

- Thinning of epidermis where subcutaneous vessels become visible

- The more potent types can cause or aggravate acne or rosacea on the face.

- Percutaneous absorption leading to systemic effects: (see chapter on endocrine diseases for complete list of systemic adverse effects)
  * Hyperglycemia
  * Glycosuria
  * Hypothalamic-pituitary-adrenal (HPA) axis suppression which could pose a threat in case of surgery, systemic illness, or trauma/injury

- Percutaneous absorption leading to systemic effects most likely with:
  * The higher potency (HP) types of agents
  * Inflamed skin, and also in infants and children
  * Long-term use and/or use over a large area of the skin
  * Occlusion markedly increases absorption of topical corticosteroids and should therefore be used cautiously in limited areas and reserved for severe, resistant lesions.

Topical antipruritics
- Local anesthetics (benzocaine up to 20% and pramoxine 1%)

- Benzyl alcohol

- Colloidal oatmeal (Aveeno)

- Others (camphor, menthol, phenol)

Emollients
- Petrolatum

- Lanolin

- Mineral oil

Oral corticosteroids
- Corticosteroids are the only systemic anti-inflammatory agents effective.

Oral antihistamines
- Very limited effectiveness, possibly antipruritic

Table 5

Topical Corticosteroids Classified by Relative Potency

Relative potency	Generic name	Trade name	Strength
Low	Hydrocortisone (OTC)	Cortaid®, Cortizone®	1% = OTC
		Allercort®, Hytone®, Synacort®, Emo-Cort®	2.5% = Rx only
Medium	Desonide	Tridesilon Des Owen®	0.05%
	Fluocinolone acetonide	Synalar®	0.01-0.025%
	Flurandrenolide	Cordran®	0.025-0.05%
	Hydrocortisone butyrate	Locoid®	0.1%
	Hydrocortisone valerate	Westcort®	0.2%
	Triamcinolone acetonide	Aristocort®	0.025%
High	Betamethasone valerate	Valisone®, Dermobet®	0.1%
	Fluocinolone	Synalar®, Synemol®	0.025%
	Triamcinolone acetonide	Aristocort®	0.1%
Very high	Desoximetasone	Topicort®	0.25%
	Diflorasone diacetate	Maxiflor®	0.05%
	Fluocinonide	Lidex®	0.01-0.05%
	Halcinonide	Halog®	0.1%
Ultra-high	Betamethasone dipropionate	Diprosone®, Maxivate®	0.05%
	Betamethasone dipropionate (in optimized vehicle)	Diprolene AF®	0.05%
	Clobetasol propionate	Temovate®	0.05%
	Diflorasone diacetate	Psorcon®	0.05%
	Halobetasol propionate	Ultravate®	0.05%

6. Poison Ivy, Poison Oak, and Poison Sumac Allergy (Rhus Dermatitis)

- Allergic reaction to sap (urushiol) of some plants of the genus *Rhus* (poison ivy, poison oak, and poison sumac)

- The most common form of allergic contact dermatitis

- Direct contact with leaves, roots, or branches is not required to get rash; can reach skin indirectly from clothing, a pet, or burning (volatilization)

- *Rhus* allergy is acquired; individuals are not born with it

- Most persons are sensitized to *Rhus* because it is such a common plant; however, some people are never allergic to it

- No effective way to desensitize a person with allergy to rhus plants

Types and Classification

Mild
- Localized patches of pruritus and erythema, followed by appearance of vesicles and papules on the upper and/or lower extremities

Moderate
- Extensive pruritus and irritation, with severe vesicles and appearance of bullae and edematous swelling

Severe
- Extreme pruritus, irritation, severe vesicle and bullae formation

- Extensive involvement, widespread over the body and/or face

- Extensive edema of extremities and/or face

- Eye, genitalia, or mucous membrane involvement

Clinical Presentation

- Not contagious

- Fluid in blisters does not spread rash

- Rash appears after a latent period that varies from 4 hours to 10 days, depending on an individual's sensitivity and the amount of plant contact

- When more rash appears after treatment has begun, these are areas with a longer latent period

- Symptoms may last from 5-21 days following initial rash.

- Secondary infections can occur if scratching excoriates the skin and the abrasion become infected

Treatment Principles and Goals

- Self-limited: mild cases will clear without treatment within 7-14 days.

- Prevent itching and excessive scratching and possible secondary skin infections.

Treatment options
- Mild cases: topical antipruritics, such as calamine, camphor, menthol, phenol, or local anesthetics to prevent itching and topical HC cream or ointment

- Moderate cases: topical high-potency corticosteroids for small areas

- Severe cases: systemic corticosteroids daily up to 2 weeks
    * Severe rash needs systemic corticosteroids to ease the misery and disability
    * Usually needed during early severe stages because remedies applied to skin may not penetrate deeply enough

Therapy

OTC topical therapy
- Astringents/protectants: compresses, soaks, or wet dressings will dry the oozing, reduce the weeping, aid in removal of crusts, and soothe the skin
    * Aluminum acetate solution 1:40 ratio (Burrow's solution)
    * Aluminum sulfate (Domeboro® powder)
    * Calamine lotion
    * Others: aluminum hydroxide gel, kaolin, zinc acetate, zinc carbonate, zinc oxide

- Local anesthetics (benzocaine up to 20% and pramoxine 1%, benzyl alcohol)
    * Caladryl® lotion: calamine and pramoxine 1%
    * Ruli® calamine spray: calamine, benzocaine, and camphor
    * Ivarest® 8-Hour Medicated Cream: calamine and diphenhydramine 2%
    * Ivy Dry® Cream: benzyl alcohol, camphor, menthol, zinc acetate

- 1% Hydrocortisone products

- Colloidal oatmeal (Aveeno) provides temporary skin protection from exposures

- Cool compresses

Prescription topical therapy
- Topical medium- to high-potency corticosteroids (see section on allergic contact dermatitis)

Prescription systemic corticosteroid therapy
- See section on allergic contact dermatitis and the chapter on endocrine disorders for complete details

- Use of systemic corticosteroids is the only therapy that will actually reduce the severity and duration of the allergic response

- Effects of oral corticosteroids are dramatic (can take up to 40-100 mg prednisone for 2 or 3 weeks if necessary); however, many patients clear up quickly with a corticosteroid "dosepak" (eg, Aristocort®, Decadron®, or Medrol®)

- Extremely severe cases or large scale rash may require parenteral dose of corticosteroid (100 mg prednisone equivalent)

Other recommendations
Prevention
- Avoidance: "leaves of three, let it be"

- Removal: washing with soap and water within 15 minutes of exposure may reduce the extent and duration of dermatitis

- Bentoquatam 5% solution: Ivy Block® lotion
    * An organoclay
    * Only barrier product approved by the FDA
    * Patient instructions: apply 15 minutes before possible plant contact; reapply every 4 hours

Scaly Dermatoses

- There are three common forms of scaly dermatoses: dandruff, seborrhea, and psoriasis

Dandruff

- Dandruff is a chronic, noninflammatory scalp condition resulting in excessive scaling of the scalp epidermis.

- It is a common condition affecting 20% of the population.

- It is not a serious disorder, but can be cosmetically unsightly.

Clinical presentation
- Scaling and pruritus, causing white flakes to accumulate on the scalp

Pathophysiology
- Increased epidermal cell turnover rate of approximately twice normal (time reduced from 25-30 days to 13-15 days) prevents complete keratinization of desquamated cells due to unknown reasons.

- May be related to increased *Pityrosporum ovale*, a fungal scalp organism

Treatment
- Routine shampooing with mild hypoallergenic shampoo is essential.

Cytostatic agents
- Cytostatic agents suppress cell turnover; goal is to reduce epidermal rate of turnover of scalp cells
  * Zinc pyrithione (ZPT) (0.3-2%) (Head and Shoulders®, X-Seb®, Zincon®); mechanism of action: antifungal effect and/or reducing cell turnover rate
  * Selenium sulfide 1% (Selsun Blue® 1%; Selsun® $2^1/_2$%); mechanism of action: reduce the cell rate turnover and/or inhibit growth of *P ovale*
  * Coal tar (Balnetar®, Denorex®, Estar®, Ionil T®, Polytar®, Tegrin®); mechanism of action: coal tar reduces the number and size of epidermal cells
  * Patient instructions: contact time with cytostatic agents is very important for effectiveness; advise patients to rub shampoo in well and leave in up to 5 minutes before rinsing out.

Keratolytics
- Salicylic acid (1.8-3%) (Ionil®, Sebucare®)
  * Ability to lower the pH of tissues, increasing the water concentration of epidermal cells, which softens and destroys the stratum corneum. Causes upper skin layer to become inflamed and soft, followed by desquamation. This keratolytic action removes the scales of dandruff.

- Sulfur (2-5%) (Sulfoam®, Sulray®)
  * Possibly exerts an antifungal effect
  * Usually found in combinations with salicylic acid

- Combination sulfur and salicylic acid: Meted® and Sebulex®

Antifungals
- Ketoconazole (1%) shampoo (Nizoral AD®)
  * Active against *P ovale*
  * Use twice weekly, or every 3 or 4 days
  * Stress adequate contact time for a minimum of 3 minutes
  * Adverse effects include itching, stinging, or irritation

Seborrhea (Seborrheic Dermatitis)

- Seborrhea is a chronic inflammatory skin disease in areas of greatest sebaceous gland activity, on the scalp and other hairy areas such as the face, trunk, armpits, and groin.

Clinical presentation
- Scaling rash accompanied by pruritus

- Yellowish, greasy scales unlike the dry scale of dandruff

- Inflammatory, often accompanied by erythema

- Fluctuates in severity and characterized by exacerbations and remissions

- Most commonly occurs on the face, eyebrows, and eyelashes, but not on the extremities

- Aggravated and worsened by nervous stress and poor health

- Not contagious

- Persists for life; no cure, but can control

Pathophysiology

- Accelerated cell turnover rate of approximately 3 times normal rate; probably as few as 9-10 days

- Higher cell turnover rate than dandruff, but less than psoriasis

- *Pityrosporum ovale* may be causative, but this is not universally accepted.

Treatment

- Similar to treatment for dandruff, but more difficult to treat (overuse of selenium can make scalp oily and actually exacerbate seborrhea)

- Topical corticosteroids are used to control itching and inflammation (up to 7 days) (Cortaid®, others)

- Add the topical antifungal ketoconazole 1% shampoo (Nizoral AD®)
    * Active against *Pityrosporum ovale*
    * Use twice weekly, every 3 or 4 days
    * Stress adequate contact time; leave in for at least 3 minutes
    * Adverse effects include itching, stinging, or irritation

"Cradle cap" (infantile seborrheic dermatitis)

- Seborrhea of the scalp in newborns or infants

- Most common in first few months of life

- Most common on top of head; may be due to poor washing

- Probably not related to fungal infection

- Treatment:
    * Massage with oils
    * Nonmedicated shampoos
    * Use milder keratolytics (Meted, Sebulex) 2 or 3 times per week

Psoriasis

- Psoriasis is a chronic inflammatory papulosquamous erythematous skin disease.

- It is marked by the presence of silvery scales with sharply delineated edges.

- Lesions are usually localized, but can gradually grow to cover large areas.

- It can have significant physiological and psychological effects.

- It affects 1-3% of the population.

Classification

Type I
- Early age of onset, family history, increased frequency of human lymphocyte antigen

Type II
- Develops later in life, no family history

Pathophysiology

- Hyperproliferative skin condition resulting from skin cell turnover rate of approximately 10-20 times normal; skin cells of psoriatic plaque reach the outermost layer in 3-4 days.

- Genetic predisposition, as well as exposure of skin to trauma or triggering factors such as stressful incidents

Clinical presentation

- Plaque most common and known as *psoriasis vulgaris*

- Plaque known also as scales; silvery on top and pink to red beneath

- May be found anywhere on the body, but more likely on scalp, sacral area, extensor surfaces of knees and elbows (less common on face)

- Borders of plaque are sharp with inflammation surrounding the plaque

- Chronic condition; varies from mild forms of the disease to very severe with such extensive coverage that it hinders social and work life

- Marked by spontaneous exacerbations and remissions

Treatment

Topicals
- Topical corticosteroids

- Coal tar: contained in Denorex®, DHS®, Ionil T®, MG217®, Neutrogena T®, Pantene Pro-V®, Polytar®, Tegrin®, X-Seb T Plus®

- Keratolytics: salicylic acid and sulfur

- Combinations: Sebutone® (salicylic acid, sulfur, and coal tar)

- Retinoids: tretinoin, adapalene, tazarotene, alitretinoin

- Anthralin: Anthraforte®, Anthranol®, Dritho-Scalp®

- Calcipotriene: Dovonex® (a vitamin D$_3$ analog)

Systemic treatment
- Oral corticosteroids

- Antimetabolites (eg, methotrexate and cyclosporine)

- Psoralens (combined with UV light therapy)

- Acitretin: Soriatane® (reserved for severe and extensive psoriasis)

- Retinoids (eg, etretinate)

Other
- Ultraviolet light therapy
  * Following coal tar applications
  * Concurrent with oral psoralens

8. Pediculosis

- Head lice is the primary or most common form

- Very common, especially in schoolchildren

- Lice are transmitted by direct contact with the head of an infected individual or through fomites (inanimate objects capable of transmitting disease, eg, sharing combs, brushes, headwear)

- Most common in August and September, after long holidays and/or summer camps

- Body lice is a less common form that usually occurs in individuals who do not change clothing often (eg, homeless)

- Pubic lice (crab lice) is transferred through sexual contact and is found primarily in pubic areas, but also can affect armpits

Classification

- There are three types of human pediculosis:
  * Head lice: *Pediculus humanus* capitis
  * Body lice: *Pediculus humanus* corporis (same species as head lice)
  * Pubic lice: *Pthirus pubis* (crab louse is a different species)

Clinical Presentation

- Pruritus is the most common symptom.

- Often symptomatic, diagnosis is made visually by seeing live lice

- Difficult to locate or visualize the flat, gray-brown adult lice; the nits (larvae) firmly attached to hair may be more visible

Drug Therapy

Synergized pyrethrins (0.17-0.33%; A-200®, Barc®, End-Lice®, Lice-Enz®, Pronto®, R&C® shampoo, Rid®, Triple X®)
- Natural chemical derived from chrysanthemums which is synergized by addition of 2-4% piperonyl butoxide (petroleum derivative)

Mechanism of action
- Blocks transmission of nerve cell impulses in lice, causing paralysis

Patient counseling

- Wash and dry hair and apply for 10 minutes.

- Use lice/nit comb to remove dead lice and nits following rinsing.

- Treat all family members

- Avoid contact with the eyes, mouth, and nose

- Do not use on irritated or inflamed scalp.

- Treatment should be repeated in 1 week to 10 days

Adverse drug effects

- Irritation, erythema, itching

Permethrin 1% (Nix® Cream Rinse); permethrin 5%, prescription-only strength (Acticin®, Elimite® Cream)

- Synthetic chemical derivative of pyrethrin

- 1% OTC-strength approved only for head lice; however, it is effective against pubic lice

- 5% Prescription-strength is approved for scabies (mites) infestation

- Patients prefer because of single-application effectiveness

Mechanism of action

- Blocks transmission of nerve cell impulses in lice, causing paralysis

Patient information

- Applied to washed hair and scalp

- Leave on hair for 10 minutes, then rinse

- After rinsing, comb with lice comb to remove lice and nits

- *One-time* treatment (*do not* repeat in 10 days)

- Recommend that all family members be treated

Adverse effects

- Scalp irritation, pruritus, and stinging

- Contraindicated in patients allergic to chrysanthemums

- Contraindicated in children under 2 years of age

Lindane (Kwell® shampoo, cream, lotion; prescription only)

- Former name was gamma benzene hexachloride

- Effective against pediculosis capitis and pubis and scabies (caused by *Sarcoptes scabiei*)

- Drug currently unavailable for use in the U.S.

Adverse effects

- Lindane is absorbed significantly through the skin and has been reported to have significant neurotoxic effects, especially in infants and children.

- CNS effects reported: convulsions, dizziness, incoordination, restlessness, irritability

- Other effects: rapid heartbeat, muscle cramps, vomiting

- The OTC medications are considered much safer, especially in children

Nondrug recommendations

- Change clothing daily.

- Treat infested clothes and shower daily.

- All household contacts should be inspected and treated if necessary.

- All bed linens and clothes should be dry cleaned or washed in hot water cycle and dried on heated air cycle for at least 20 minutes.

- Wash hairbrushes, combs, and toys in hot water for at least 10 minutes.

- Treat surrounding environment (bedding, pillows, carpets, draperies, furniture) with A-200® Control Spray or Rid® Control Spray

9. Warts

- Warts (verrucae) are harmless skin growths resulting from an infectious disease caused by the human papilloma virus (HPV).

Classification

- Common warts (verruca vulgaris) on fingers, hands, knees

- Common flat warts (verruca plana) on face, hands, legs

- Plantar warts (verruca plantaris) on the soles of the feet

- Anogenital warts (verruca genitalia) on the ano-genital area

Clinical Presentation

- Warts are contagious, and may spread on the body.

- Warts are more common in children and immuno-compromised patients.

- Warts on the face or hands protrude.

- Warts occurring on the pressure areas such as the bottom of the feet (plantar warts) grow inward from the pressure of standing and walking, are often painful, and may be confused with corns.

Treatment Principles and Goals

- Warts can be eliminated by:
  * Direct application of the following caustics: salicylic acid, formalin, lactic acid, trichloroacetic acid, podophyllin
  * Freezing with liquid nitrogen (cryotherapy); cryotherapy is preferable for warts on the face, elbows, and knees.
  * Surgery

OTC drug therapy

- Only FDA-approved OTC medication is salicylic acid (SA)

- Use topical salicylic acid preparations on a daily basis until wart is removed

- Since warts are contagious, use special care in washing hands before and after treatment, and use a separate towel for drying other parts of the body.

- Do not use salicylic acid on irritated, broken, or infected skin.

- If wart remains after 12 weeks of continuous treatment, see a dermatologist or podiatrist.

- Salicylic acid products contraindicated in patients with diabetes and other patients with poor circulation because reduced sensation in the foot delays awareness of skin breakdown, allowing possible development of infection that can lead to sepsis.

- Refer diabetics to a physician or podiatrist for removal of warts.

OTC salicylic acid products
- Salicylic acid 17% in flexible collodion vehicle:
  * Compound W®, Duofilm®, Wart-Off®, Off-Ezy® Wart Remover Kit

- Salicylic acid 40% imbedded in pads or discs:
  * Clear Away® discs, Dr. Scholl's Clear Away®, Compound W® One Step Pads

10. Corns and Calluses

- Corns and calluses are excessive growth of the upper keratinized layer of the skin.

- They are more common in women.

- Diabetics have an increased incidence of calluses on their feet due to the loss of sensation, preventing them from noticing the pressure that would otherwise be uncomfortable.

Classification

- Hard corns (heloma durum): corns overlying a bony prominence such as the toes or bottom of the heel

- Soft corns (heloma molle; interdigital corns): corns between the toes (especially the fourth and fifth)

- Calluses (callosities): superficial patches of hornified epidermis; flattened, but thickened with no central core

Clinical Presentation and Pathophysiology

- Caused by excessive growth of the upper keratinized layer of the skin (hyperkeratoses), due to friction or pressure, usually from improper or tight-fitting shoes

Treatment

- The only FDA-approved OTC medication is salicylic acid formulated in flexible collodion, plasters, disks, or pads.

Mechanism of action
- Salicylic acid produces a keratolytic action, increasing hydration and lowering the pH of the outer skin, which initially softens, then destroys the outer layer of skin.

Patient counseling
- Do not apply to irritated, infected, or reddened skin.

- If discomfort persists after using 14 days, see physician or podiatrist.

- Contraindicated in diabetics

Adverse drug effects
- Salicylic acid products are contraindicated in patients with diabetes and other patients with poor circulation because reduced sensation in the foot delays awareness of skin breakdown, allowing possible development of infection that can lead to sepsis.

- Refer diabetics to physician or podiatrist for removal of corns or calluses.

OTC salicylic acid (SA) corn and callus products
- Freezone® Corn and Callus Remover 13.6% SA

- Freezone® One Step Corn Remover 40% SA

- Mediplast® 40% SA plaster, cut to size

- Mosco® Corn and Callus Remover 17.6% SA

- Off-Ezy® Corn and Callus Remover 17% SA

- One Step® Callus Remover 40% SA

- Dr. Scholl's® Corn and Callus Remover Liquid 12.6% SA

- Dr. Scholl's® Corn or Callus Cushion Gel 40% SA

- Dr. Scholl's® One Step Corn or Callus Remover Disc 40% SA

11. Key Points

Acne

- Acne occurs primarily in the teenage years due to the increase of androgens during puberty that produces increased activity of the sebaceous glands.

- Isotretinoin (Accutane) is the drug of choice for nodulocystic acne (type IV acne), which if left untreated will lead to extensive scarring.

- Isotretinoin (Accutane) is contraindicated in pregnancy due to the high incidence of serious birth defects.

- The most common side effects of isotretinoin (Accutane) are cheilitis (dry, chapped lips), dry skin, and dry eyes.

Fungal infections of the skin

- The most efficacious nonprescription topical antifungal in terbinafine (Lamisil).

- Systemic antifungal therapy is required for treatment of tinea captis (ringworm of the scalp) and tinea unguium (fungal infection of the toenails).

Hair loss

- Androgenic alopecia, predominantly seen in males, is due to the conversion of testosterone to dihydrotestosterone, which binds to the hair follicles causing them to produce progressively thinner hair.

- In the treatment of androgenic alopecia, minoxidil (Rogaine) should be applied and left on the scalp for 4 hours for maximum effects.

- Finasteride (Propecia) decreases the effect of androgens on hair follicles by inhibiting 5-α-reductase, which prevents the conversion of testosterone to dihydrotestosterone.

Dry skin

- Dry skin occurs primarily in older adults due to decreased sebum production and decreased moisture binding capacity of the skin.

- Products containing urea and lactic acid improve the skin's moisture binding capacity, thereby increasing skin hydration.

Dermatitis

- Contact dermatitis, whether irritant or allergic, is initially treated with topical corticosteroid products.

- The absorption and subsequent adverse systemic effects of topical corticosteroids is increased with (1) occlusion, (2) in infants skin, (3) with the use of high-potency agents, and (4) with long-term use.

Poison ivy and oak

- Poison ivy, poison oak, and poison sumac are examples of allergic contact dermatitis, and are the result of contact with the sap of plants of the genus *Rhus*.

- Severe cases of poison ivy, poison oak, or poison sumac require systemic corticosteroids to relieve symptoms, decrease the severity of the rash, and shorten the course of the disorder.

Scaly dermatoses

- The cytostatic agents that suppress cell rate turnover, zinc pyrithione (ZPT; Head and Shoulders) and selenium sulfide (Selsun Blue), are the primary agents of choice for treatment of dandruff.

- Seborrhea usually requires topical corticosteroids and/or the topical antifungal ketoconazole for effective treatment.

- Psoriasis is a chronic inflammatory disease characterized by inflammation and silvery scales (known as plaques) with sharp delineated edges.

- Treatment of advanced psoriasis may require systemic corticosteroids and/or antimetabolites in addition to topical treatments in order to effectively manage the disease.

Pediculosis

- Head lice (*Pediculus humanus* capitis) occur most commonly in elementary schoolchildren in the months of August and September.

- Permethrin (Nix) is the nonprescription agent of choice for treatment of head lice (*Pediculus humanus* capitis) because it usually does not have to be repeated in 7-10 days as do other available nonprescription pediculicidal agents (synergized pyrethrins).

Corns and warts

- Nonprescription products for the treatment of corns and warts contain salicylic acid.

- Self treatment for corns or warts with OTC agents is not recommended for diabetic patients due to reduced sensation in their feet which delays awareness of possible development of infections, and can lead to sepsis.

- Warts result from an infection of the human papilloma virus, and therefore are contagious and may spread on the body.

- Warts may be eliminated by surgery, freezing with liquid nitrogen (cryotherapy), or the direct application of caustics (eg, salicylic acid, formalin, lactic acid, trichloroacetic acid, or podophyllin).

12. Questions and Answers

1. Initial treatment of mild to moderate acne would include which of the following?

   I. Topical antimicrobials
   II. Topical retinoids
   III. Isotretinoin

   A. I only
   B. II only
   C. III only
   D. I and II
   E. I, II, and III

2. Acne is due to

   I. Increased sebum production
   II. Obstruction of hair follicle opening
   III. Inflammation

   A. I only
   B. II only
   C. III only
   D. I and II
   E. I, II, and III

3. Patients using topical retinoids such as tretinoin (Retin-A®) should be counseled

   I. To use sunblock before exposure to sunlight
   II. Not to use it with astringents, drying agents, or abrasive soaps
   III. That rapid improvement occurs within 2 or 3 days of starting therapy

   A. I only
   B. II only
   C. III only
   D. I and II
   E. I, II, and III

4. The most common side effects of isotretinoin (Accutane®) include which of the following?

   I. Cheilitis (dry chapped lips)
   II. Acute depression
   III. Decreased night vision

   A. I only
   B. II only
   C. III only
   D. I and II
   E. I, II, and III

5. Which of the following is an important contraindication and precaution to the use of isotretinoin (Accutane®)?

   A. Hypertension
   B. Migraines
   C. Allergic rhinitis
   D. Pregnancy
   E. Streptococcal infections

6. Which of the following is the most efficacious nonprescription topical antifungal?

   A. Tolnaftate (Tinactin®)
   B. Terbinafine (Lamisil®)
   C. Miconazole (Micatin®)
   D. Undecylenic Acid (Cruex®)
   E. Clotrimazole (Lotrimin AF®)

7. Which of these fungal infections may be treated effectively with the use of topical antifungal agents?

   I.   Tinea capitis (ringworm of the scalp)
   II. Tinea unguium (fungal infection of the nails)
   III. Tinea corporis (ringworm of the skin)

   A. I only
   B. II only
   C. III only
   D. I and II
   E. I, II, and III

8. Tinea pedis is also known as

   A. Athlete's foot
   B. Jock itch
   C. Onychomycosis
   D. Ringworm of the scalp
   E. Ringworm of the skin

9. The treatment of choice for tinea unguium (fungal infection of the nails) would be

   A. Clotrimazole
   B. Miconazole
   C. Undecylenic acid
   D. Griseofulvin
   E. Tolnaftate

10. All of the following are true regarding androgenic alopecia EXCEPT

    A. It is predominantly seen in males.
    B. It is due to the conversion of testosterone to dihydrotestosterone, which binds to the hair

follicles causing them to produce progressively thinner hair.
    C. Hair growth stimulation is temporary and only lasts as long as therapy.
    D. Hair loss in the frontotemporal area responds to treatment better than hair loss of the crown.
    E. Early hair loss occurring recently in young males is more likely to respond than later hair loss at an older age.

11. All of the following are true regarding the patient instructions for the proper use of minoxidil EXCEPT

    A. It should be applied and left on the scalp for 4 hours for maximum effects
    B. The patient should not swim, shampoo, or walk in rain during the application of minoxidil.
    C. Do not use on infected, irritated, inflamed, or sunburned skin.
    D. The patient must continue therapy to maintain effectiveness.
    E. Women with alopecia should use the 5% strength of minoxidil rather than the 2% strength.

12. Adverse effects of Minoxidil include which of the following?

    I.   Hypertrichosis
    II. Dermatitis and pruritus of the scalp
    III. Hepatic damage

    A. I only
    B. II only
    C. III only
    D. I and II
    E. I, II, and III

13. The mechanism of action of finasteride (Propecia®) to reduce male baldness is

    A. A direct effect on hair follicles to deepen hair roots
    B. Inhibition of the enzyme 5-α-reductase, which blocks the conversion of testosterone to dihydrotestosterone
    C. Increased cutaneous blood flow to the hair follicles on the scalp due to vasodilation
    D. Increased cutaneous blood flow to the hair follicles on the scalp due to opening the potassium channel
    E. Increased development of new hair follicles on the scalp

14. All of the following are true regarding finasteride EXCEPT

   A. It is contraindicated in females of childbearing age.
   B. It was originally approved for treatment of benign prostatic hypertrophy.
   C. Improvement lasts only as long as treatment continues (new hair will be lost within 1 year of stopping treatment).
   D. It must be taken on an empty stomach for complete absorption.
   E. Two percent of men report reversible sexual dysfunction while taking it.

15. All of the following regarding dry skin are true EXCEPT

   A. It occurs primarily in older adults.
   B. It occurs most commonly in the summer months.
   C. It is caused by decreasing sebum production and decreased moisture binding capacity of the skin.
   D. Flaking, scaling, xerosis, and pruritus are common manifestations of dry skin.
   E. Excessive cleansing and bathing removes lipids and worsens dry skin.

16. All of the following statements are true regarding the treatment of dry skin EXCEPT

   A. Hydrocortisone should only be used for short-term therapy of dry skin to relieve itching.
   B. Urea-containing products improve the skin's moisture binding capacity.
   C. Lactic acid is a keratolytic agent which removes the upper epidermal skin cells and relieves the itching of dry skin.
   D. Emollients and moisturizers are helpful in the treatment of dry skin, especially when applied immediately after bathing.
   E. While colloidal oatmeal may be helpful in the treatment of dry skin, patients should be cautioned about prevention of falls due to slippery bathtubs.

17. The agent of choice for the initial treatment of contact dermatitis, whether irritant or allergic, is

   A. Topical antihistamines
   B. Oral antihistamines
   C. Topical corticosteroids
   D. Local anesthetics
   E. Coal tar products

18. An increase in topical corticosteroid systemic absorption with subsequent systemic side effects may be seen in which of the following?

   I. Occlusion
   II. Infant's skin
   III. Long-term use of high-potency agents

   A. I only
   B. II only
   C. III only
   D. I and II
   E. I, II, and III

19. All of the following are true regarding poison ivy EXCEPT

   A. It is an example of allergic contact dermatitis.
   B. It is the result of contact with the sap of plants of the genus *Rhus*.
   C. The treatment of choice is desensitization.
   D. It may be caused by direct or indirect contact (eg, with clothing or pets).
   E. Skin eruptions may occur from several hours up to 10 days following contact with the plants.

20. The treatment of choice for severe or extensive cases of poison ivy or poison oak is

   A. Local anesthetics such as benzocaine
   B. Bentoquatam (Ivy Block®)
   C. Camphor and menthol antipruritics
   D. Colloidal oatmeal
   E. Systemic corticosteroids

21. Which of the following agents for treatment of dandruff are cytostatic agents that suppress cell rate turnover?

   I. Zinc pyrithione (Head and Shoulders®)
   II. Selenium sulfide (Selsun Blue®)
   III. Salicylic acid (Ionil®)

   A. I only
   B. II only
   C. III only
   D. I and II
   E. I, II, and III

22. All of the following statements are true regarding seborrhea EXCEPT

   A. It is a chronic inflammatory skin disease seen in areas of greatest sebaceous gland activity.

    B. It fluctuates in severity and is worsened by stress and poor health.

    C. Moderate to severe cases require topical corticosteroids and/or the topical antifungal ketoconazole for effective treatment.

    D. It is called "cradle cap" when it occurs in infants.

    E. It most commonly occurs on the extremities, legs, and arms.

23. Which of the following are characteristic of psoriasis?

    I. Chronic inflammation
    II. Silvery scales (know as plaques) with sharply delineated edges
    III. Spontaneous exacerbations and remissions

    A. I only
    B. II only
    C. III only
    D. I and II
    E. I, II, and III

24. Treatment of advanced psoriasis may require topical therapy combined with which of the following systemic agents?

    I. Corticosteroids
    II. Antimetabolites such as methotrexate
    III. Antralin

    A. I only
    B. II only
    C. III only
    D. I and II
    E. I, II, and III

25. All of the following are true statements regarding head lice (*Pediculus humanus* capitis) EXCEPT

    A. It occurs most commonly in elementary schoolchildren.

    B. It occurs most commonly in the springtime months of April and May.

    C. It is transmitted by direct contact.

    D. Pruritus is the most common symptom.

    E. Head lice is the most common type of pediculosis infestation.

26. All of the following statements are true regarding treatment of pediculosis with synergized pyrethrins (piperonyl butoxide and pyrethrins) EXCEPT

    A. All family contacts should be inspected and treated if necessary.

    B. Apply after washing and drying the hair and leave on overnight.

    C. Remove dead lice and nits after treatment with a lice/nit comb.

    D. Treatment should be repeated in 7-10 days.

    E. Avoid contact with the eyes, nose, and mouth.

27. The most effective nonprescription agent for treatment of head lice (*Pediculus humanus* capitis) is which of the following agents?

    A. Permethrin (Nix®)
    B. Synergized pyrethrins (A-200®)
    C. Lindane (Kwell®)
    D. Ketoconazole
    E. Salicylic acid

28. Nonprescription products for the treatment of corns and warts contain which of the following agents?
    A. Salicylic acid
    B. Ketoconazole
    C. Lactic acid
    D. Acetylsalicylic acid
    E. Hydrocortisone

29. All of following are true statements regarding corns EXCEPT

    A. They are excess growth of the upper keratinized layer of skin.

    B. Salicylic acid is available in pads, disks, or flexible collodion for removal of corns.

    C. Self treatment for corns or warts with OTC agents is not recommended for diabetic patients due to their reduced sensation in the feet, which delays awareness of development of infections and may lead to sepsis.

    D. They are contagious and may spread on the body.

    E. They are usually caused by pressure or friction from improper or tight-fitting shoes.

30. All of the following are true regarding warts EXCEPT:

    A. They result from infection with the human papilloma virus.

    B. They are contagious.

    C. They may spread on the body.

    D. Plantar warts are located on the fingers, hands, and knees.

    E. They are more common in children and immunocompromised patients.

31. Warts may be eliminated by which of the following procedures?

I. Surgery
II. Freezing with liquid nitrogen (cryotherapy)
III. The direct application of caustics (eg, salicylic acid)

    A. I only
    B. II only
    C. III only
    D. I and II
    E. I, II, and III

Answers

1. **D.** Topical antimicrobials and/or topical retinoids are the agents of choice for mild to moderate acne. Isotretinoin (Accutane®) is reserved for nodulocystic acne (type IV acne), which if left untreated will lead to extensive scarring.

2. **E.** Acne is primarily due to hormonal changes occurring at or near puberty which increase sebum production, obstruct the hair follicle opening, and breaking down of triglycerides to free fatty acids due to enzymes from *P acnes* which causes inflammation.

3. **D.** Topical retinoid therapy will sensitize skin to ultraviolet light rays; therefore, patients should use sunblock prior to sun exposure. Patients using topical retinoids should use only mild soaps for cleansing the face, and avoid astringents, drying agents, and abrasive soaps. Improvement will usually occur within 2-3 weeks after initiation of therapy.

4. **A.** Cheilitis (dry chapped lips), along with dry skin and dry eyes, are the most common side effects of isotretinoin therapy.

5. **D.** Isotretinoin (Accutane®) is contraindicated in pregnancy due to the high incidence of serious birth defects.

6. **B.** Terbinafine (Lamisil®) is the most effective nonprescription topical antifungal.

7. **C.** Topical antifungal agents are the first line of therapy against tinea corporis (ringworm of the skin). However, systemic antifungal therapy is usually required for treatment of tinea capitis (ringworm of the scalp) and tinea unguium (fungal infection of the nails).

8. **A.** Tinea pedis is also known as athlete's foot.

9. **D.** Treatment of choice for tinea unguium (fungal infection of the nails) is a systemic antifungal agent such as griseofulvin. Topical therapy is generally not effective for fungal infections of the nails.

10. **D.** Hair loss in the crown responds to treatment better than hair loss of the frontotemporal areas.

11. **E.** Women with alopecia should **only** use the 2% strength of minoxidil. Studies indicate there is no greater degree of effectiveness with the 5% and the incidence of adverse effects including increased growth of facial hair is much greater in women using the 5% preparation.

12. **D.** Common adverse effects of minoxidil include hypertrichosis (increased hair growth in areas other than the scalp) and dermatitis and pruritus of the scalp. Systemic side effects with topical minoxidil are rare and do not include hepatic damage.

13. **B.** The mechanism of action of finasteride to reduce male baldness is blocking the conversion of testosterone to dihydrotestosterone by inhibiting the enzyme 5-α-reductase.

14. **D.** Finasteride does **not** have to be taken on an empty stomach. It may be taken with or without food. Finasteride was originally approved for treatment of benign prostatic hypertrophy. Improvement of alopecia lasts only as long as treatment continues, is contraindicated in females of childbearing age, and 2% of men report reversible sexual dysfunction.

15. **B.** Dry skin occurs most commonly in the winter months and is often referred to as "winter rash."

16. **C.** Lactic acid is used in the treatment of dry skin, not as a keratolytic agent, but as an agent which increases skin hydration.

17. **C.** Topical corticosteroids are the agents of choice for the initial treatment of irritant or allergic contact dermatitis. If the condition is severe or widespread, oral corticosteroids may be useful. Oral or topical antihistamines have minimal effect in the course of the treatment of contact dermatitis, possibly producing some antipruritic effect, but not affecting the course of the disorder.

18. **E.** Topical corticosteroid systemic absorption is increased with occlusion, long-term use, use of high-potency agents, and on an infant's skin. Systemic corticosteroid adverse effects may be severe and include adrenocortical suppression.

19. **C.** Desensitization has no place in the treatment of poison ivy, and most studies indicate desensitization is not an effective method to prevent poison ivy.

20. **E.** The treatment of choice for severe or extensive cases of poison ivy or poison oak is systemic corticosteroids. Topical agents are limited in effectiveness and do not alter the course of the disease.

21. **D.** Zinc pyrithione (Head and Shoulders®) and selenium sulfide (Selsun Blue®) are cytostatic agents used in the treatment of dandruff that suppress cell rate turnover. Salicylic acid is a keratolytic agent.

22. **E.** Seborrhea most commonly occurs on the face, especially eyebrows and eyelashes, but not on the extremities.

23. **E.** Psoriasis is a chronic inflammatory disease marked by silvery scales (known as plaques) with sharp delineated edges and is marked by spontaneous exacerbations and remissions.

24. **D.** Treatment of advanced psoriasis may require both topical therapy combined with either oral corticosteroids or antimetabolites such as methotrexate.

25. **B.** Head lice (*Pediculus humanus* capitis) occurs most commonly in the months of August and September.

26. **B.** Synergized pyrethrins should be applied after washing and drying the hair and left on 10 minutes, *not* overnight.

27. **A.** Permethrin (Nix®) does not have to be repeated in 7-10 days like the other available nonprescription pediculicidal agent, synergized pyrethrins (A-200®). Lindane (Kwell®) is not available over the counter and significant neurologic toxicities have been reported with its use.

28. **A.** Nonprescription products for the treatment of corns and warts contain salicylic acid as the active therapeutic agent.

29. **D.** Corns are *not* contagious and may *not* spread on the body. Corns are an excess growth of the upper keratinized layer of skin, usually caused by pressure or friction from improper or tight-fitting shoes. Salicylic acid is available OTC for removal of corns in pads, disks, or flexible collodion. Self treatment for corns or warts with OTC agents is not recommended for diabetic patients due to their reduced sensation in the feet, which delays awareness of the development of infections which could lead to sepsis.

30. **D.** Plantar warts are not located on the fingers, hands, or knees. Plantar warts are located on the soles of the feet.

31. **E.** Warts may be eliminated by surgery, freezing with liquid nitrogen (cryotherapy), or the direct application of caustics (eg, salicylic acid).

13. References

Arndt KA. *Manual of Dermatologic Therapeutics,* 5th ed. Boston: Little, Brown; 1995.

Arndt KA, Wintroub BU, Robinson JK, et al, eds. *Primary Care Dermatology*. Philadelphia: WB Saunders; 1997.

Berardi RR, et al, eds. *The Handbook of Nonprescription Drugs*, 13th ed. Washington: American Pharmaceutical Association; 2002.

Burnham TH, ed. *Drug Facts and Comparisons*. St. Louis: Facts and Comparisons, Inc.; 2003.

Champion RH, Burton JL, Burns DA, eds. *Textbook of Dermatology*, 6th ed. Oxford, England: Blackwell Scientific Publications; 1998.

DiPiro JT, et al, eds. *Pharmacotherapy: A Pathophysiologic Approach,* 4th ed. Stamford, CT: Appleton & Lange; 1999.

Epstein E. *Common Skin Disorders*, 5th ed. Philadelphia: WB Saunders; 2001.

Freedberg IM, Eisen AZ, Wolff K, et al. *Dermatology in General Medicine*, 5th ed. New York: McGraw-Hill; 1999.

Fitzpatrick JE. *Dermatology Secrets in Color*, 2nd ed. Philadelphia: Hanley and Belfus; 2001.

Habif TP, Campbell JL, Quitadamo MJ. *Skin Disease: Diagnosis and Treatment*. St. Louis: Mosby; 2001.

Herfindal T, Gourley D, eds. *Textbook of Therapeutics,* 6th ed. Baltimore: Williams & Wilkins; 2000.

Nonprescription drug therapy; guiding patient self-care. St. Louis: Facts and Comparisons, Inc; 2003.

Odom RB, James WD, Berger TG, eds. *Andrew's Diseases of the Skin: Clinical Dermatology*. Philadelphia: WB Saunders; 2000.

Pray WS. *Nonprescription Product Therapeutics*. Hagerstown, MD: Lippincott Williams & Wilkins; 1999.

Top OTC/HBC Brands in 2002. *Drug Topics*. 2003;145:33-34.

Wolverton SE, ed. *Comprehensive Dermatologic Drug Therapy*. Philadelphia: WB Saunders; 2001.

27. Nonprescription Medications

Andrea Franks, PharmD, BCPS
Assistant Professor, Departments of Pharmacy
 and Family Medicine
University of Tennessee College of Pharmacy

Contents

1. Cough, Cold, and Allergy

The Common Cold

Etiology
- Usually viral, most commonly rhinoviruses

- Transmitted via hand-to-hand contact followed by touching eyes or nasal mucosa

Pathophysiology
- Release of numerous inflammatory mediators, primarily cytokines

Clinical presentation
- Sore throat, nasal symptoms, watery eyes, sneezing, cough, malaise, low-grade fever

- High fever and myalgias more characteristic of influenza

- Gradual onset with slow progression

- Duration: 1-2 weeks

Treatment
- Nonprescription drug treatment (symptomatic):
    * Decongestants for nasal congestion
    * Antihistamines for excess nasal discharge
    * Analgesics for related pain or headaches
    * Local anesthetic lozenges/sprays for sore throat (pharyngitis)

- Nondrug therapy:
    * Humidifiers
    * Increase fluid intake
    * Rest

Allergic Rhinitis

Etiology
- Exposure to allergens and development of nasal symptoms
    * Perennial
    * Seasonal

Pathophysiology
- Complex, involving numerous mediators (primarily histamine) and cell types (mast cells)

Clinical presentation
- Nasal: congestion, rhinorrhea, nasal pruritus, sneezing, post-nasal drip

- Ocular: itching, lacrimation, redness, irritation

- General: headache, malaise, mood swings, irritability

Treatment
- Avoidance: avoid offending allergens
    * Limit outside exposure during high pollen times
    * Avoid indoor and outdoor mold
    * Avoid dust, especially in bedroom
    * Avoid pet dander, especially cats

Pharmacotherapy for allergic rhinitis
- Mild allergies
    * Antihistamine as needed

- Moderate allergies
    * Nasal congestion: antihistamine plus decongestant
    * Ocular symptoms: ophthalmic antihistamine

- Chronic allergies
    * Cromolyn (Nasalcrom)
    * Not useful taken PRN
    * Dosage: one spray every 4-6 h up to 4-6 times daily

- Severe allergies
    * Nasal corticosteroids: prescription only

- Very severe allergies
    * Systemic corticosteroids: prescription only
    * Adverse effects with chronic use

Immunotherapy (allergy shots)
- If pharmacotherapy fails to relieve symptoms

Drug Therapy for Treatment of Common Cold and Allergies

Antihistamines (Table 1)
Pharmacology
- H_1 receptor antagonists

- First-generation: nonselective, sedating

- Second-generation: peripherally selective, nonsedating

Side effects
- Sedation

- Anticholinergic effects (primarily with first-generation antihistamines)

- Dry mouth

Table 1

Selected Nonprescription Antihistamine Products

Generic name (trade name)	Adult dosage/max in 24 h
Chlorpheniramine (Chlortrimeton®)	4 mg q4-6h/ 24 mg
Brompheniramine (Dimetane®)	4 mg q4-6h/24 mg
Diphenhydramine (Benadryl®)	25-50 mg q6h/200 mg
Clemastine (Tavist®)	1.34 mg bid/2.68 mg
Triprolidine (in Actifed®)	2.5 mg q6h/10 mg
Loratadine (Claritin®, Alavert®)	10 mg qd

- Dry eyes

- Urinary retention

- Constipation

- Paradoxical stimulation in some children

Precautions and contraindications
- Counsel patients not to drive or operate heavy machinery

- Avoid use with alcohol

- Prostatic hyperplasia

- Narrow-angle glaucoma

Prescription products
- Second-generation antihistamines: low incidence of sedation; no anticholinergic effects
    * Azatadine (Optimine® 1 mg bid)
    * Cetirizine (Zyrtec® 5-10 mg qd)

* Desloratadine (Clarinex® 5 mg qd)
* Fexofenadine (Allegra® 60 mg bid or 180 mg qd)

Oral decongestants (Table 2)
Pharmacology
- α-adrenergic agonists, vasoconstrictors

- Constricts blood vessels to decrease blood supply to nasal mucosa and decrease mucosal edema

- No effect on histamine or allergic mediated reaction

Side effects
- Products relatively safe with no dependence

- Can be used long term

- Most common side effects
    * Nervousness
    * Irritability
    * Restlessness
    * Insomnia

- Less common side effects
    * Increased heart rate
    * Increased blood pressure
    * Irregular HR
    * Palpitations

Precautions and contraindications
- Hypertension: generally accepted with mild or well controlled hypertension; should not use with uncontrolled hypertension

- Heart disease (arrhythmias) increase heart rate

- Diabetes: minimal effect on blood sugar level

Table 2

Selected Nonprescription Oral Decongestant Products

Generic name	Products	Comments	Side effects	Adult dosage (maximum daily dose)
Phenylephrine	Combination products	Weakest oral decongestant	+	10 mg q4h (60 mg)
Pseudoephedrine	Sudafed	Less CNS stimulation	++	60 mg q6h (240 mg)
Phenylpropanolamine	Withdrawn 12/2002	Increased risk of hemorrhagic stroke	+++	25 mg q4h (150 mg)
Ephedrine	Combination products for asthma	Used as bronchodilator due to β agonist activity	++++	12.5-25 mg q4h (150 mg)

- Hyperthyroidism: more sensitive to sympatho-mimetics

- Enlarged prostrate: exacerbates BPH by constricting smooth muscle of bladder neck

- Narrow angle glaucoma: dilation increases intraocular pressure

- MAO inhibitors interact with decongestants to increase blood pressure.

Topical decongestants
Pharmacology
- α-Adrenergic agonists act locally as vasoconstrictors

- Constrict blood vessels, decrease blood supply to nose, decrease mucosal edema

- No effect on histamine or allergy-mediated reaction

Side effects
- Minimal systemic absorption results in few side effects.

- Local effects may include burning, nasal irritation, sneezing.

Precautions and contraindications
- Rhinitis medicamentosa (rebound congestion) may occur if duration of use >3-5 days.

Topical decongestant dosage forms
- Sprays
    * Simplest dosage delivery
    * Large surface area covered
    * Imprecise dosing, contamination of bottle

- Drops
    * Preferred for use in small children
    * Cover small surface area
    * Pass to larynx, where they may be swallowed and result in systemic effects

- Nasal inhaler
    * Requires unobstructed airway to deliver drug to nasal mucosa
    * Sympathomimetic amines; also contain camphor and menthol
    * Loses efficacy after 2-3 months
    * Propylhexedrine (Benzedrex® inhaler)
    * Levodesoxyephedrine (Vicks® inhaler)

Select products
- Short-acting: phenylephrine (Neo-Synephrine®, Dristan®, Vicks, Sinex®)

- Intermediate-acting: naphazoline (Privine®)

- Long-acting: xylometazoline (Otrivin®)

- Longest-acting: oxymetazoline (Afrin®, Duration®, NeoSynephrine 12-hour)

Nasal saline solution
- Very safe

- Good for use in infants and children

- Can be used with oral decongestants

- Saline drops (Ayr®, NaSal®)

- Saline sprays (Ayr, NaSal, Ocean Spray®, HuMist®)

Cromolyn (Nasalcrom®)
- Role in therapy: prevention and treatment of allergic symptoms

- Pharmacology: mast cell stabilizer; prevents the mast cells from releasing mediators

- Dosage: one spray each nostril q4-6h up to 4-6 times daily

- Onset of action: approximately 1 week, 2-3 weeks for maximal effect

- Not efficacious if taken prn; must be taken on a scheduled basis

- Side effects: nasal irritation, nasal burning, stinging, sneezing, cough, unpleasant taste

Analgesics
- Role in therapy: for pain, fever, and headaches associated with cold, flu, or allergies

- Aspirin (mostly replaced now by acetaminophen and NSAIDs)

- Acetaminophen (APAP)

- Nonsteroidal anti-inflammatory drugs (NSAIDs)
    * Ibuprofen
    * Ketoprofen
    * Naproxen

Selected cold, allergy, and sinus products
Decongestant/analgesic
- Advil® Cold & Sinus (pseudoephedrine 30 mg, ibuprofen 200 mg)

- Tylenol® Sinus, Maximum Strength (pseudoephedrine 30 mg, APAP 500 mg)

- Sinutab® Maximum Strength (pseudoephedrine 30 mg, APAP 500 mg)

Antihistamine/decongestant/analgesic
- Alka-Seltzer Plus® Cold Medicine (APAP 250 mg, chlorpheniramine 2 mg, phenylephrine 5 mg)

- Tylenol Allergy Sinus (APAP 500 mg, chlorpheniramine 2 mg, pseudoephedrine 30 mg)

Antihistamine/decongestant (short-acting)
- Actifed® Cold and Allergy Tablets (triprolidine 2.5 mg, pseudoephedrine 60 mg)

- Benadryl® Allergy and Sinus Tablets (diphenhydramine 25 mg, pseudoephedrine 60 mg)

Antihistamine/decongestant (long-acting)
- Drixoral® Cold and Allergy 12 Hour Relief (pseudoephedrine 120 mg, dexbrompheniramine 6 mg)

- Claritin D® 12 Hour (loratadine 5 mg, pseudoephedrine 120 mg)

- Claritin D 24 Hour (loratadine 10 mg, pseudoephedrine 240 mg)

Cough

Pathophysiology
- Important defense mechanism to rid the airways of mucus, foreign bodies

- May be acute (<3 weeks duration) or chronic (>3 weeks duration)

Causes
- Upper respiratory infection (viral or bacterial)

- Sinusitis

- Rhinitis

- Asthma, chronic obstructive pulmonary disease (COPD)

- Gastroesophageal reflux disease (GERD)

- Congestive heart failure

- Drug-induced cough
  * ACE inhibitors
  * β-Blockers

Cough characteristics
- Productive

- Nonproductive

Treatment
Antitussives/cough suppressants
Narcotic
- Codeine
  * Gold standard antitussive
  * Available in some states without prescription
  * Mechanism of action: centrally-mediated suppression of cough threshold
  * Adult dose: 10-20 mg q4h (120 mg/d maximum)
  * Role in therapy: used primarily for night cough
  * Side effects: sedation, nausea, constipation

Nonnarcotic
- Dextromethorphan (DM)
  * ***Only*** category 1 OTC nonnarcotic antitussive
  * Mechanism of action: centrally-mediated suppression of cough threshold
  * Adult dosage: 10-30 mg q4-8h (120 mg/d maximum)
  * Role in therapy: nonproductive cough
  * Side effects: drowsiness, gastrointestinal effects
  * Drug interactions: MAO inhibitors

- Diphenhydramine
  * Category II antitussive
  * Mechanism of action: centrally-mediated suppression of cough center, anticholinergic
  * Adult dosage: 25 mg q4h (75 mg/d maximum)

- Benzonatate (Tessalon Perles®)
  * Prescription only
  * Anesthetizes stretch receptors in respiratory passages, lungs
  * Adult dose: 100-200 mg tid
  * Side effects: sedation, bronchospasm

Expectorant
Guaifenesin (Robitussin®, Mucinex®, Humibid®)
- ***Only*** category I OTC expectorant

- Mechanism of action: thins mucus to enhance clearance

- Adult dosage:
  * Immediate-release 200-400 mg q4h (maximum 2400 mg/d)
  * Extended-release: 600-1200 mg q12h (maximum 2400 mg/d)

- Role in therapy: productive cough

- Side effects: gastrointestinal discomfort

- Patient education: increase fluid intake

Topical antitussives
Volatile oils
- Only camphor and menthol are FDA-approved.

- Mechanism of action: local anesthetic effect in nasal mucosa

- Product availability: lozenge, ointment, steam inhalation

- Patient education: ointment and solution toxic if ingested

Selected cough products
- Expectorant: guaifenesin
    * Immediate-release: Robitussin Syrup (100 mg/5 mL)
    * Extended-release: Mucinex® (600 mg or 1200 mg) Humibid Sprinkle® (300 mg)

- Cough suppressant: dextromethorphan
    * Benylin® Adult Cough Formula Liquid (15 mg/5 mL)
    * Delsym – Extended Release Suspension (30 mg/5 mL)

- Expectorant/cough suppressant:
    * Robitussin DM Cough Control (guaifenesin 100 mg, dextromethorphan 15 mg/5 mL)

- Expectorant/decongestant:
    * Robitussin PE (guaifenesin 100 mg, pseudoephedrine 30 mg/5 mL)

- Expectorant/decongestant/cough suppressant:
    * Robitussin Cough & Cold (guaifenesin 100 mg, pseudoephedrine 30 mg, dextromethorphan 15 mg/5 mL)

- Other combination products:
    * Vick's Nyquil® Hot Therapy Powder (pseudoephedrine 60 mg, doxylamine 125 mg, acetaminophen 1000 mg, dextromethorphan 30 mg)
    * Theraflu® Maximum Nighttime, Flu, Cold, & Cough Medicine (acetaminophen 1000 mg, pseudoephedrine 60 mg, dextromethorphan 30 mg, chlorpheniramine 4 mg)

Sore Throat Remedies

- Saline gargle

- Sprays, lozenges:
    * Benzocaine: Chloraseptic® lozenges, Cepacol® lozenges
    * Dyclonine: Cepacol Spray
    * Phenol: Chloraseptic Gargle
    * Menthol: Halls®

2. Constipation

Clinical Presentation

- Difficult or infrequent passage of stools

- Patient may complain of abdominal or rectal fullness

Etiology

- Inadequate fluid intake

- Inadequate fiber intake

- Lack of physical exercise

- Diseases:
    * Neurologic disease
        - Parkinson's disease
        - Multiple sclerosis
        - Cerebrovascular disease
    * Gastrointestinal disease
        - Irritable bowel syndrome
        - Hemorrhoids
        - Masses (polyps, tumors)
    * Diabetes
    * Hypothyroidism

- Drug-induced constipation:
    * Antacids containing aluminum or calcium
    * Anticholinergics
    * Phenothiazines
    * Tricyclic antidepressants
    * Opiates (codeine, morphine)
    * Antihistamines, especially in children
    * ACE inhibitors
    * Calcium channel blockers (especially verapamil)
    * Sucralfate
    * Iron

Treatment

Nondrug therapy
- Increase fluid intake

- Increase dietary fiber

- Exercise

- Establish good bowel habits

Drug therapy
Bulk-forming laxatives
Pharmacology
- Mechanism of action
    * Natural or semisynthetic hydrophilic polysaccharide derivatives
    * Absorb water to soften stool and increase bulk to facilitate elimination and peristalsis
    * Effects may not be seen for 2-3 days

- Role in therapy:
    * Safest, most natural therapy for constipation
    * Most often recommended for chronic use

- Drug interactions:
    * May bind digoxin, warfarin, and other drugs
    * Calcium complexes may bind with tetracycline, inhibiting its absorption
    * Recommend to separate doses from other medications

- Side effects:
    * Potential for allergic reaction/anaphylaxis
    * Inhalation of powder reported to cause bronchospasm
    * Caution diabetics about sugar content of some products

Selected products
- Psyllium seed (plantago seed): Metamucil®, Perdiem®

- Methylcellulose: Citrucel®
    * Synthetic cellulose derivative

- Carboxymethyl cellulose sodium

- Calcium polycarbophil: Fibercon®

- Malt soup extract: Maltsupex®

Emollient laxatives (stool softeners)
Pharmacology
- Act as surfactants, absorbing water into the stool

- Effects may take 2-3 days

- May cause systemic absorption of mineral oil, therefore contraindicated

- Often used in combination products

- Useful for patients who should avoid straining
    * Rectal surgery
    * Postpartum
    * Recent myocardial infarction

Selected products

- Docusate sodium: Colace®, Correctol®, Ex-Lax®

- Docusate calcium: Surfak®

- Docusate potassium: Dialose®

Stimulant laxatives

- Stimulate bowel motility via localized mucosal irritation

- Increase secretion of fluids into bowel

- Can cause cramping

- Cathartic colon with chronic use
  * Impaired colon function

Anthraquinones

- Pharmacology:
  * Absorbed into bloodstream with action on large intestines
  * Onset of effects: 6-12 hours
  * Dose at bedtime

- Side effects:
  * Discoloration of urine
  * Stimulant habituation
  * Melanosis coli
    • Dark pigmentation of colonic mucosa

- Precautions and contraindications:
  * Contraindicated in breastfeeding

- Select products:
  * Senna (Senokot®, Ex-Lax)
    • More abdominal cramping
  * Cascara sagrada (Nature's Remedy®)
  * Casanthranol
    • Considered mild stimulant laxative
    • Synthetic compound
    • Usually in combination with docusate

Diphenylmethanes

- Bisacodyl (Dulcolax® tablets or suppositories, Correctol)
  * Minimal systemic absorption
  * Only stimulant compatible with breastfeeding
  * Enteric coated: do not crush or take with antacids
  * Onset of effects varies with route of administration
    • Rectal: 15-60 minutes
    • Oral: 6-8 hours
  * Also available in suppository form

Phenolphthalein (removed from market 1998)

Stimulant oils (castor oil)
  * Acts on small intestine
  * Strong cathartic: may induce fluid/electrolyte disturbances
  * Most rapid *oral* laxative (onset: 30 minutes to 1 hour)
  * Contraindicated in pregnancy (may induce labor)

Dangers of chronic stimulant laxative use
- Laxative habit
- Cathartic colon
- Melanosis coli
- Loss of fluids on electrolytes
- Cramping pains

Hyperosmotic laxative (glycerin)
Pharmacology
- Osmotic effect and local irritant stimulates bowel movement
- Onset of action usually within 30 minutes
- Glycerin suppositories safe for infants

Selected products
- Glycerin suppositories
- Fleet Babylax®

Saline and osmotic laxatives
Pharmacology
- Nonabsorbable cations create osmotic gradient to pull water into intestine
- Onset varies with route of administration:
  * Rectal: 5-30 minutes
  * Oral: 30 minutes to 4 hours
- 20% of magnesium may be absorbed systemically
- Contraindicated in patients with impaired renal function (magnesium- or phosphate-containing), congestive heart failure, or hypertension (sodium-containing)

Selected products
- Magnesium hydroxide (milk of magnesia)
- Magnesium citrate (citrate of magnesia)
- Magnesium sulfate (epsom salts)

- Sodium phosphate (Fleets Oral Solution)

Lubricant laxatives
Pharmacology
- Soften the feces by emulsifying contents of intestinal tract

- Onset of action: 6-8 hours

- May decrease absorption of fat-soluble vitamins and some drugs

- Contraindicated in children and elderly patients due to risk of aspiration and lipid pneumonitis

- Do not administer with stool softeners

Selected products
- Mineral oil: liquid petrolatum

- Olive oil: "sweet oil"

- Combination products:
  * Softener-stimulants
    - Peri-Colace: docusate sodium and casanthranol
    - Senokot-S: docusate sodium and senna

Enemas
- Fleet Enema (monobasic and dibasic sodium phosphates)

- Oil retention

- Soap suds

- Warm tap water

Lactulose
- Chronulac, Duphalac, Cephulac

- Prescription only

- Nonabsorbed disaccharide, metabolized by bacteria in gastrointestinal tract to produce acetic and formic acid; it then exerts osmotic effect

Special patient populations
Pregnancy
- Hormonal changes cause smooth muscle relaxation early in pregnancy.

- Enlarged uterus compresses colon.

- Recommend only bulk forming laxatives or stool softeners.

3. Diarrhea

Clinical Presentation

- Abnormal increase in frequency of stools and stool looseness

- May be acute (<14 days) or chronic (>4 weeks)

Etiology

Acute infectious diarrhea
Viral
- Norwalk virus (adults and children)

- Rotaviruses (young children)

Bacterial
- Food-borne illness

- Contaminated water

- Traveler's diarrhea

Protozoal

Drug-induced diarrhea
- Antibiotics

- Laxatives

- Antacids

- Cytotoxic agents

Diet-induced diarrhea
- Allergies

- Spicy foods

- High carbohydrate load

- Lactose intolerance

Complications

- Dehydration (especially in infants, elderly)

- Electrolyte abnormalities

Nondrug Treatment

- Oral rehydration therapy (ORT; eg, Pedialyte)
  * Rehydration
  * Maintenance

- Avoid fatty foods, spicy foods, high sugar content

Drug Therapy

Loperamide (Imodium AD®)
- Pharmacology: synthetic opioid antagonist slows gastrointestinal motility

- Dosage: 4 mg initially, then 2 mg after each loose stool; <16 mg/d

Side effects
- Well-tolerated

- Constipation

- Dizziness

- Dry mouth

Precautions and contraindications
- Product information recommends use in children >2 years old, but the American Academy of Pediatrics does *not* recommend in children <6 years old.

- Should not be used if patient has bloody or black stool; consult physician before use if patient has fever, mucus in stool, or a history of liver disease.

Adsorbents
- Pharmacology: nonselective absorption of toxins, bacteria, water

Side effects
- Constipation

- Bloating

Precautions and contraindications
- Do not use in children age <2 years.

Drug interactions
- May absorb other drugs from gastrointestinal tract (digoxin, antibiotics)

- Separate doses to avoid drug interactions

Selected products
- Attapulgite

- Kaolin-pectin

- Polycarbophil

Bismuth subsalicylate (BSS)
Pharmacology
- Reacts with stomach acid to form salicylic acid and bismuth oxychloride

- Reduces frequency of diarrhea

- Improves stool consistency

- Direct antimicrobial effect, therefore effective in traveler's diarrhea

Side effects
- Salicylate toxicity (tinnitus)

- Bismuth toxicity (neurotoxicity)

- Gray-black discoloration of tongue and/or stool

Precautions and contraindications
- Contraindicated in aspirin allergy

- Contraindicated in children/teens with viral illness (Reye's syndrome)

- Contraindicated if history of GI bleeding, or on warfarin

4. Nausea and Vomiting

Definitions

- Nausea refers to the sensation that one is about to vomit.

- Vomiting is the forceful expulsion of gastric contents through the mouth.

Physiology

- Vomiting is coordinated by the vomiting center in the medulla.

- Stimuli from the peripheral nervous system and within the central nervous system act on the vomiting center

- Responding to these impulses, the vomiting center stimulates the abdominal muscles, stomach, and esophagus to induce vomiting.

Etiology

Irritation of chemoreceptor trigger zone (CTZ)
- Drug-induced:
  * Cancer chemotherapy
  * Narcotics
  * Theophylline
  * Digoxin
  * Antibiotics
  * Drug withdrawal (opiates, sedatives)

- Metabolic disorders:
  * Ketoacidosis
  * Uremia
  * Pregnancy
  * Electrolyte imbalances

Vestibular disorders
- Motion sickness

- Vestibular inflammation
  * Otitis interna
  * Meniere's syndrome

Central nervous system disorders
- Psychogenic

- Migraine headache

- Increased intracranial pressure

Gastrointestinal tract disorders
- Obstruction

- Gastroparesis

- Gastroenteritis

- Viral or bacterial infection

- Locally irritating drugs
  * Alcohol
  * NSAIDs
  * Antibiotics

Complications

- Dehydration

- Electrolyte imbalance

- Aspiration

- Malnutrition

- Acid-base disturbances

Treatment

Nonprescription antiemetics (Table 3)
Antihistamines
- Cross blood-brain barrier to depress vestibular excitability

Phosphorated carbohydrate solution (Emetrol®)
- Hyperosmolar solution

- Mixture of levulose (fructose), dextrose (glucose), and phosphoric acid

- Buffered to a pH of 1.5

- Reduces gastric muscle contraction through an unknown direct effect

- Must not be diluted (raises the pH)

Bismuth salts (Pepto-Bismol®)
- Available as nonprescription suspension, caplet, and chewable tablet

- See diarrhea section for additional information.

Histamine$_2$-receptor antagonists (H$_2$ antagonists)
- May provide symptomatic relief by inhibiting gastric acid secretion

Table 3

Nonprescription Drugs of Choice for Prevention of Motion Sickness

Generic name (trade name)	Adult dosage (max daily dose)	Children age 6-12 (max daily dose)	Children age 2-6 (max daily dose)
Dimenhydrinate (Dramamine®)	50-100 mg q4-6h (400 mg)	25-50 mg q6-8h (150 mg)	12.5-25 mg q6-8h (75 mg)
Diphenhydramine	25-50 mg q4-6h (300 mg)	12.5-25 mg q4-6h (150 mg)	6.25 mg q4-6h (37.5 mg)
Cyclizine	50 mg q4-6h (200 mg)	25 mg q6-8h (75 mg)	Not recommended
Meclizine (Bonine®)	25-50 mg qd (50 mg)	Not recommended	Not recommended

- Potential drug interactions with cimetidine

- Side effects:
  * Headache
  * Constipation
  * Diarrhea

- See peptic ulcer disease section for additional information on H_2 antagonists.

Antacids
- May treat nausea, dyspepsia, and stomach upset associated with excessive intake of food or drink

- Combinations of magnesium hydroxide, sodium salts, aluminum hydroxide, calcium carbonate, and magnesium carbonate

- Usual adult dosage: 15 mL 30 minutes after meals and at bedtime

- Side effects:
  * Constipation
  * Diarrhea
  * Sodium overload

- Drug interactions:
  * May decrease absorption of some medications
  * Administer other medications 1-2 hours before or after antacids

Special patient populations
Pregnancy
- Nausea may be associated with pregnancy, especially during the first trimester.

- Recommend nonpharmacologic therapy initially:
  * Small, frequent meals
  * Avoid rich, fatty foods
  * Snack on salty crackers or pretzels

- Refer to primary care provider if considering pharmacologic therapy
  * Pyridoxine 25 mg tid
  * Antihistamines
  * Prescription antiemetics

5. Pain and Fever

Pathophysiology of Pain

- Nociceptors are peripheral pain receptors.

- Nociceptors send pain stimuli to the spinal cord via afferent, nociceptive nerves.

- Impulses then pass to the brain via dorsal root ganglia.

Pathophysiology of Fever

- Core temperature is the temperature of the blood surrounding the hypothalamus.

- The thermoregulatory center in the anterior hypothalamus controls body temperature via physiologic and behavioral mechanisms.

- Pyrogens, fever-producing substances, increase the thermoregulatory set point, raising the body temperature.

Treatment

Acetaminophen (Table 4)
Pharmacology
- Exerts analgesic and antipyretic activity via central inhibition of prostaglandin synthesis

- Does not have peripheral anti-inflammatory activity

Side effects
- Generally well tolerated

- Hepatotoxicity

Drug interactions
- Alcohol: increases risk of hepatotoxicity

- Warfarin: higher doses may enhance hypoprothrombinemic effect of warfarin

Precautions and contraindications
- Increased risk of hepatotoxicity with doses >4 g/d

- Pre-existing liver disease

- Chronic alcohol use

- Fasting

Special patient populations
- Accepted in pregnancy and breastfeeding

Salicylates
Pharmacology
- Inhibit peripheral prostaglandin synthesis

- Reduce pain, inflammation, and fever

- Acetylated salicylates (eg, aspirin) inhibit platelet aggregation

- Nonacetylated salicylates (eg, prescription salsalate, choline magnesium trisalicylate) do not have significant antiplatelet activity

Side effects
- Gastritis

- Gastric ulcers/bleeding

Table 4

Selected Analgesic/Antipyretic Products

Generic name (trade name)	Adult dosage (max daily dosage)	Pediatric dosage (max daily dosage)
Acetaminophen (Tylenol®, Tempra®)	650-1000 mg q4-6h (4000 mg)	10-15 mg/kg q4-6h (5 doses/day)
Aspirin (Bayer®)	650-1000 mg q4-6h (4000 mg)	10-15 mg/kg q4-6h (80 mg/kg per day)
Ibuprofen (Motrin®, Advil®)	200-400 mg q4-6h (1200 mg OTC)	5-10 mg/kg q6-8h (40 mg/kg per day)
Naproxen (Aleve®)	220-440 mg q8-12h (660 mg)	Not recommended <12 years old; >12 years old: use adult dosage
Ketoprofen (Orudis®)	12.5-25 mg q6-8h (75 mg)	Not recommended <16 years old; >16 years old: use adult dosage

- Allergy and hypersensitivity:
  - Rare (<1 %) in the general population
  - Higher risk in individuals with asthma, nasal polyps

- Reye's syndrome:
  - Potentially fatal illness associated with salicylate use in children/teens with concurrent viral illness (influenza, varicella-zoster)

Drug interactions
- Alcohol: enhances gastrointestinal toxicity

- Methotrexate: salicylates displace methotrexate from protein binding sites

- Warfarin: salicylates enhance hypoprothrombinemic effects of warfarin

Precautions and contraindications
- Bleeding disorders

- Hemophilia

- Peptic ulcer disease

- Children/teenagers with viral illness (Reye's syndrome)

- Gout

Special patient populations
- Avoid in third trimester of pregnancy

Nonsteroidal anti-inflammatory drugs (NSAIDs)
Pharmacology
- Peripheral inhibition of prostaglandin synthesis

- Analgesic, antipyretic, anti-inflammatory activity

Side effects
- Gastrointestinal effects, including bleeding

- Rash

- Photosensitivity

- High incidence of cross-reactivity in individuals with aspirin allergy

Drug interactions
- Warfarin: increased bleeding risk

- Alcohol: increased risk of gastrointestinal bleeding

- Methotrexate: decreased methotrexate clearance

- Antihypertensives:
  - ACE inhibitors: decreased hypotensive effects, hyperkalemia
  - β-blockers: decreased hypotensive effects
  - Potassium-sparing diuretics: hyperkalemia

- Digoxin: decreased renal clearance, risk of digoxin toxicity

Precautions and contraindications
- Alcohol: increased risk of GI bleeding

- Renal impairment

- Congestive heart failure

Special patient populations
- Ibuprofen, naproxen compatible with breastfeeding

- Avoid NSAIDs in third trimester of pregnancy

6. Ophthalmic Disorders

Dry Eye

* *Definition:* tear film instability caused by a deficiency of any component of the tear film

* *Clinical presentation:* ocular discomfort, blurred vision, desire to rub the eyes, burning or redness

Etiology
* Aqueous tear deficiency

* Exposure to dry air

* Keratoconjunctivitis sicca

* Sjögren's syndrome

* Blepharitis

* Vitamin A deficiency

* Allergic conjunctivitis

* Contact lenses

* Drug-induced

Nonpharmacologic treatment
* Avoid known irritants

* Use cool-mist humidifier/warm-steam vaporizer

Pharmacologic treatment
* See Table 5

Loose Foreign Material in the Eye

* *Symptoms:* irritation, inflammation, involuntary tearing, uncontrollable blinking, discomfort

* *Etiology:* dirt, an eyelash, or particles solubilized or suspended by the tears

Treatment
Eyewashes
* Isotonic, buffered solutions of sterile water

Key points
* Eyewashes should not be used if the patient has open wounds near the eye.

* Contact lens wearers should remove their lenses prior to using eyewashes, if possible.

* Use of eye cups should generally be avoided.

Redness Caused by Minor Irritation

* Common causes: airborne pollutants (gasses or smoke), chlorinated water, infectious diseases, glaucoma

Table 5

Pharmacologic Treatment of Dry Eyes

Product	Common preparations	Comments
Artificial tears: act as demulcents to mimic mucin; use twice daily is suggested		
Cellulose derivatives (carboxymethylcellulose)	Bion Tears®, Celluvisc®, Clear Eyes CLR®	Enhanced duration compared to other products; tend to form dry crusts which may be easily washed off with warm water
Polyvinyl alcohol (glycerin, propylene glycol, polyethylene glycols, polysorbate 80)	Moisture Eyes®, Hypo Tears®, Murine Tears®, Tears Plus®	Shorter duration; no crust formation
Povidone and dextran 70	AquaSite®	Can cause transient stinging/burning
Ocular emollients: ointments have longer contact; more likely to cause blurred vision		
Lanolin, mineral oil, petrolatum, white ointment, white wax or yellow wax	Moisture Eyes PM®, Lacri-Lube SOP®, Refresh PM®, Stye®	

Treatment
Ophthalmic vasoconstrictors (ocular decongestants; Table 6)

- Constrict blood vessels of the conjunctiva

- 1-2 drops in affected eye up to four times daily

- Contraindicated in patients with narrow-angle glaucoma (causes mydriasis)

- Avoid use in contact lens wearers

- Can cause a rebound hyperemia, especially with overuse

- Can cause tachycardia, aggravate arrhythmias if absorbed systemically

Allergic Conjunctivitis

- *Symptoms:* chronic, recurring itching; eyes that are slightly red, tearing, burning, with little discharge

- *Etiology:* animal hair, pollen, ragweed, or other plants

- *Treatment:* combination products containing ophthalmic vasoconstrictor and ocular antihistamine

- Naphazoline + pheniramine or antazoline (Naphcon A, Ocuhist, Opcon-A, Vasocon-A)

- 1-2 drops in affected eye(s) up to four times daily

- *Warnings:* should be avoided in patients with heart disease, high blood pressure, enlarged prostate, or narrow-angle glaucoma

Conditions Requiring Referral to a Physician or Eye Care Specialist

Corneal edema
- *Symptoms:* foggy vision, haloes around lights, photophobia, irritation, foreign-body sensation, extreme pain

- *Causes:* prolonged contact lens wearing, infection, glaucoma, iritis

Treatment
- Referral to eye care specialist

- Sodium chloride (2-5%)

- 1-2 drops in affected eye(s) every 3-4 hours

Foreign body in the eye
- Metal shavings, wood splinters, or dust

- Improper removal may lead to permanent damage

Ocular trauma
- Automobile accidents, sports injuries

Chemical exposure
- Remove contact lenses

- Flush immediately with lukewarm water for at least 15 minutes

- Do *not* place drops in the eyes.

Table 6

Ophthalmic Vasoconstrictors

Product	Common preparations	Key points
Phenylephrine	Prefrin Liquifilm Relief®	Can precipitate angle-closure glaucoma
Naphazoline	Clear Eyes®, Clear Eyes ACR®, Bausch & Lomb Sensitive Eyes®	Ocular decongestant of choice
Tetrahydrozoline	Visine®, Visine AC®, Visine Advanced Relief®	Less likely to alter pupil size; may cause stinging upon instillation
Oxymetazoline	Visine LR®	Relatively free of ocular or systemic side effects

7. Otic Disorders

Impacted Cerumen

Cerumen-softening agents
- Instill in ear

- Follow with warm water irrigation using otic syringe
    * Carbamide peroxide in anhydrous glycerin + alcohol
        - Debrox®, Murine® Earwax Removal System
        - Softens ear wax and facilitates removal
    * Hydrogen peroxide/water
        - 1:1 solution of warm water: 3% hydrogen peroxide
        - Not effective drying agent
    * Olive oil (sweet oil)
    * Glycerin
        - Emollient and humectant

Water Clogged Ears

- 95% isopropyl alcohol in 5% anhydrous glycerin
    * Swim Ear® Drops
    * Only FDA-approved ear drying aid

- Compounded 50:50 acetic acid 5%: isopropyl alcohol 95%
    * Recommended by American Academy of Otolaryngology

Boils

- Infected hair follicles in the ear canal

- Usually self-limiting

- Apply warm compress

8. Home Monitoring and Testing Devices

Diabetes

- See diabetes chapter

Fertility Prediction Tests

Basal thermometry
- Temperatures taken orally, rectally, and vaginally.

- Taken every morning before arising

- Results are plotted graphically.

- Resting temperatures usually below normal for first part of reproductive cycle.

- Temps closer to normal after ovulation.

- Temp results plotted against time to assess spikes (ovulation).

- Very user-dependent

Bioself® Fertility Indicator
- Digital temp readings

- Must input first day of menses into device.

- Calculates user's average cycle length.

- Predicts user's most fertile period.

- Each morning indicator displays prediction (90% effective).

- Indicates if nonfertile phase, conception possible, or most fertile.

- Can obtain printout via modem download

Ovulation prediction kits
- Test contains antibodies that bind to LH in urine.

- LH surge is detected by difference in color or color intensity from one day to the next.

- Early morning urine collection recommended.

- User must know the length of the last three cycles before using.

- Testing usually begins 2-4 days prior to ovulation (based on average of last three cycles).

Clear Plan Easy Fertility Monitor

- Measures both LH and E3G (estrogen component)

- Tests 20 consecutive days to establish baseline in first month

- Tests 10-20 days per month

- Peak time identified by meter.

Fertility microscopes

- Reusable microscope that analyzes saliva changes to predict ovulation

- OVU-Tec Fertility Detector®, Cycle View®

- Do not use within 2 hours of smoking, drinking, or eating.

Male fertility testing

- Fertil MARQ®

- Determines if sperm concentration is adequate

- Two tests needed to confirm

- Test sample color is compared to known control color sample

Pregnancy detection

- Early testing is very important.

- Detects levels of hCG in urine (within 1-2 weeks after conception)

- Antibodies designed to react with hCG in shape of straight line, check, or plus sign.

- If pregnant, color is produced

- Pregnancy tests are 98-100% accurate; however, human error decreases that rate to 50-75% (Table 7)

Important tips for patients using pregnancy tests

- Encourage use of first morning urine to test (hCG more concentrated)

- If not first morning urine sample, restrict fluids 4-6 hours before urine collection.

- Use only supplied collection devices.

- Try to test sample immediately after collection (if not, allow refrigerated samples to come to room temperature).

Table 7

Causes of Error in Home Pregnancy Testing

False positives	False negatives
Miscarriage within previous 8 weeks	Test performed first day of a missed cycle
Childbirth within previous 8 weeks	Refrigerated urine not allowed to come to room temperature
Use of fertility medications (Pergona®l, Profasi®)	Use of wax cups or soap residues in household containers

- If negative, wait 1 week and retest if no cycle yet.

- If positive, contact ob/gyn immediately and start prenatal vitamins.

Urinary Tract Infection Tests

- Tests for nitrites in urine

- Specific for gram-negative organisms only

- AZO® Test Strips: test for both nitrites and leukocyte esterase (*discontinued*)

- False-negative: vegetarian diet, vitamin C, tetracycline

- False-positive: phenazopyridine

Colorectal Cancer

- ColoCARE® Stool Blood Test

- EZ-Detect® Hidden Blood in the Stool

- Colorimetric assay for hemoglobin

- Blue-green color indicates positive test

- More likely to detect lower GI problems

- Uses biodegradable paper that is placed in the toilet bowl after bowel movement

- Ingestion of red meat or vitamin C may cause false-positive

Hypercholesterolemia

Cholestrak® Home Cholesterol Test
- Tests for total cholesterol only

- Results available without need for lab

Biosafe® Cholesterol Collection Kit
- Fingerstick blood placed on small collection card

- Sample mailed to Biosafe Lab

- Results for whole lipid profile given

- Results reviewed by licensed MD before being sent to patient

Home Access® Instant Cholesterol Test
- Fingerstick blood sample sent to Home Access lab

- Results reviewed by "professionals" and patient given counseling

- May be the least expensive versus other tests

BioScanner 2000®
- Potential to test full lipid panel, glucose, and ketones

- Stores results

- Reusable

Hypertension

Mercury column devices
- Blood pressure reference standard

- Routine home discouraged because they are cumbersome; risk of mercury poisoning

- Requires good eyesight and hearing

Aneroid devices
- Most accurate and reliable (except mercury column)

- Light, portable, affordable

- Many come with attached stethoscope

- Requires good eyesight and hearing for effective use (large-print devices available)

Digital devices
- Less accurate than aneroid devices

- Semiautomatic (manually inflated)

- Fully automatic (autoinflating)

Acquired Immunodeficiency Syndrome (AIDS)

Home Access and Home Access Express
- Tests for antibodies to HIV virus

- Can take 3 weeks to 6 months before antibodies are detectable

- Fingerstick blood sample placed on the specimen card

- Mailed to lab within 10 days

- Home Access: results in 7 days

- Home Access Express: results in 3 days

Illicit Drug Use Testing

PDT-90 (hair testing)
- Not subject to tampering like urine

- Subject must have used drugs for longer periods

- Collect as close to scalp as possible (from crown)

- Results reported as low, medium, high (not THC)

- Do not collect from hairbrush

- Samples mailed from home to independent lab

- Results obtained anonymously by phone

- Tests for marijuana, cocaine, opiates, methamphetamine, PCP

Urine testing
- Is subject to tampering

- Detects use of drugs from several hours to 2-3 days prior to test

- Results reported as positive or negative; not quantified

- Results available within 2-3 business days

- Products: Dr. Brown's®, Parent's Alert®

Hepatitis C

Home Access® Hepatitis C Check
- Apply blood to card, allow to dry for 30 minutes prior to mailing

- Results available in 4-10 business days

9. Smoking Cessation

Unless the patient has contraindications, pharmacotherapy should be offered to all patients attempting to quit smoking (Table 8).

First-line agents (reliably increase long-term smoking abstinence rates):
- * Nicotine gum (Nicorette®, generic) OTC
- * Nicotine patch (Habitrol®, Nicotrol®, Nicoderm CQ®) OTC
- * Nicotine inhaler (Nicotrol® inhaler)
- * Nicotine nasal spray (Nicotrol® NS)
- * Bupropion SR (Zyban®)

Second-line agents (if fail/cannot tolerate first-line):
- * Clonidine
- * Nortriptyline

Combination nicotine replacement therapy
- Combining the nicotine patch with a self-administered form of nicotine replacement therapy (either the nicotine gum or nicotine nasal spray) is more efficacious than a single form of nicotine replacement. Combined treatment should be recommended if the patient is unable to quit using a single type of first-line pharmacotherapy.

Side effects of nicotine replacement therapy (NRT)
- Insomnia/sleep disturbances

- Patch: local irritation
  - * 50% of patients
  - * Usually resolves by rotating site
  - * Treat with hydrocortisone cream or triamcinolone cream

- Nasal spray
  - * Nasal irritation

Contraindications and precautions for nicotine replacement therapy (NRT)
- Cardiovascular disease
  - * <2 weeks post-MI
  - * Serious arrhythmias
  - * Serious/worsening angina

- Esophagitis, peptic ulcer disease (gum)

- Seek medical advice if pregnant or breastfeeding

- Do not smoke while using NRT.

- Allergies, asthma, sinus conditions (nasal spray)

Table 8

The "5 A's" Clinicians Should Use to Assist Patients in Smoking Cessation

Ask about tobacco use.	Identify and document tobacco use status for every patient at every visit.
Advise to quit.	In a clear, strong, and personalized manner urge every tobacco user to quit.
Assess willingness to make a quit attempt.	Is the tobacco user willing to make a quit attempt at this time?
Assist in quit attempt.	For the patient willing to make a quit attempt, use counseling and pharmacotherapy to help him or her quit.
Arrange follow-up.	Schedule follow-up contact, preferably within the first week after the quit date.

10. Natural and Herbal Products

Complementary and alternative medicine (CAM) definitions:

* *Conventional treatment*: medical practices widely accepted and practiced by the mainstream medical community
* *Complementary therapy*: therapy used *in addition* to conventional treatment(s)
* *Alternative*: therapy used *instead of* conventional treatment(s)

Dietary Supplement and Health Education Act of 1994 (DSHEA)

Definition of a dietary supplement: "A product intended to supplement the diet that . . . contains one or more of the following dietary ingredients: a vitamin, mineral, herb or other botanical, amino acid; a dietary substance for use by man to supplement the diet by increasing the total daily intake, or a concentrate, metabolite, constituent, extract, or combination of these ingredients" (Table 9).

Table 9

Drugs versus Dietary Supplements

Drug	**Dietary supplement**
Active ingredient identified	May not identify active ingredient
Safety and efficacy proven by manufacturer	No proof of efficacy required; FDA must provide proof if unsafe
Purity and contents regulated	No standards for quality or purity
Claims to treat/cure/prevent disease	No claims to treat/cure/prevent specific disease

Regulation of dietary supplements:
* FDA: regulates labeling, safety, and manufacturing
* FTC: regulates advertising

Herbal Natural Products

Ginkgo biloba (dried leaf extract)
* Common uses:
    * Enhance memory and concentration
    * Intermittent claudication
    * Vertigo and tinnitus
    * Impotence (in combination with papaverine)

* Proposed mechanisms:
    * Increases blood flow
    * Antioxidant
    * Inhibits platelet aggregation

Dosage
* Recommend standardized product, 120-240 mg/d divided bid or tid

Side effects
* Mild: GI distress, headache, dizziness

* Serious: spontaneous bleeding has been reported (eg, subdural hematomas, subarachnoid hemorrhage)

Drug interactions
* Drugs (aspirin, ticlopidine, clopidogrel, dipyridamole, warfarin) or herbs (garlic, ginseng) with antiplatelet or anticoagulant activity

Contraindications
* Ginkgo should be discontinued prior to surgery to avoid potential bleeding complications.

St. John's wort (*Hypericum perforatum*)
* Common uses:
    * Depression

* Anxiety

* Proposed mechanism:
  * Inhibition of dopamine, serotonin, and norepinephrine reuptake
  * Decreased IL-6 concentrations

Dose
* Product standardized to 0.3% hypericin, 300 mg tid

Side effects
* Mild GI distress, dizziness, fatigue, insomnia, itching, dry mouth, hypertension

* Photosensitivity: recommend sun avoidance or sunscreen

Drug interactions
* Numerous, potentially serious

* Antidepressants (SSRIs, TCAs):
  * Similar mechanisms
  * Serotonin syndrome

* CYP 3A4 inducer significantly decreases levels of:
  * Cyclosporine
  * Indinavir

* Decreases levels of digoxin

* Oral contraceptives (increases metabolism of estradiols)

Asian ginseng
* Common uses:
  * Fatigue
  * Enhance concentration

* Proposed mechanism:
  * **Suppresses** and **stimulates** CNS
  * Corticosteroid activity
  * Hypoglycemic activity

Dosage
* 1-2 grams of crude root or 100-300 mg of ginseng extract tid

Side effects
* Hypertension

* Euphoria, restlessness, nervousness, insomnia

* Rash

* Edema

* Diarrhea

Contraindications
* Hypertension

* Antipsychotic drugs

* Ginseng should be discontinued prior to surgery to avoid potential bleeding complications.

Precautions
* Heart disease

* Diabetes

* Hypotension

Drug interactions
* Risk with anticoagulants and antiplatelet agents (aspirin, ticlopidine, clopidogrel, dipyridamole, warfarin), other herbs (ginkgo, garlic)

* Stimulants (including caffeine)

* Antipsychotics

* Diabetes drugs

Garlic (*Allium sativum L.*)
* Common uses:
  * Lower cholesterol
  * Prevent atherosclerosis

* Proposed mechanisms:
  * Inhibits platelet aggregation
  * Free radical scavenger
  * Stimulates fibrinolysis
  * Lowers cholesterol and lipid levels by inhibition of HMG-CoA reductase

Dosage
* 4 grams of fresh minced garlic bulb, 600-900 mg/d (100 mg garlic powder tablets); or 2-5 mg allicin daily

Side effects
* Malodorous breath, smell of garlic may permeate the skin

* GI discomfort, heartburn, gas

* Dermatitis, allergic reactions

Drug interactions
- Anticoagulants and antiplatelet agents (aspirin, ticlopidine, clopidogrel, dipyridamole, warfarin, ginkgo, ginseng)

- Saquinavir AUC decreased by 50% in healthy volunteers

Contraindication
- Garlic should be discontinued prior to surgery to avoid potential bleeding complications.

Echinacea purpurea
- Common uses:
  * Colds and other respiratory tract infections
  * Topical use for poorly healing wounds and chronic ulcerations

- Proposed mechanisms:
  * Stimulates the immune system
  * Increases white blood cells

Dosage
- One capsule (contains 900-1000 mg powdered herb) tid

- Dosing should begin at the onset of viral symptoms.

- Continue treatment until 24-48 hours after symptoms abate

Side effects
- Allergic reactions can occur

- Tolerance: limit use to 6-8 weeks at a time

Disease interactions
- Autoimmune disorders (immune system stimulation)

- Potentially severe allergic response, including anaphylaxis, in individuals with asthma or allergies to members of the daisy family (ragweed, daisies, chrysanthemums, marigolds)

Drug interactions
- Immunosuppressive agents

Saw palmetto (*Serenoa repens*)
- Common uses:
  * Benign prostatic hyperplasia

Proposed mechanism
  * Inhibits 5α-reductase and dihydrotestosterone (DHT) binding to androgen receptors
  * Antiandrogenic

Dosage
- Fluid extracts 1:1 = 1-2 mL bid, 1:2 = 2-4 mL bid

- Dry extract 4:1 (w/w) (~25% fatty acids) = 400 mg bid

- Product with 80-90% fatty acids, dose of 160 mg bid

- Take with morning and evening meals to decrease GI upset

- Treatment usually lasts for 3 months.

Side effects
- Rarely: GI upset, headache, hypertension
- Urinary tract symptoms (urine retention, dysuria)

- Impotence

Precautions
- Recommend thorough prostate exam and discussion with physician before starting treatment.

Kava-kava (root)
- Common uses:
  * Anxiety/stress

- Proposed mechanism:
  * Possibly binds at GABA receptors
  * Possibly dopamine antagonist

Dosage
- 100 mg 2-3 times a day

Side effects
- Similar to alcohol (adversely affects motor reflexes and judgment for driving and/or operating heavy machinery) but does not act as a CNS depressant

- Mydriasis

- Extrapyramidal symptoms

- Kava dermopathy: yellow, flaking, scaly skin, eye redness

- Liver failure leading to transplantation or death (Table 10)

Drug interactions
- L-dopa: decreased effectiveness

- Barbiturates, benzodiazepines, alcohol: additive sedative effects

Table 10

Natural Products Associated with Serious Toxicity

Common name	Promoted for	Associated with
Blue cohosh	Uterotonic, diuretic	Vasoconstriction, GI spasms
Comfrey	Gout, arthritis, infections	Obstruction of blood flow to the liver possibly resulting in death
Chinese weight loss preparations (*Aristolochia fangchi* mistaken for *Stephania tetrandra*)	Primarily weight loss	Kidney cancer, referred to as "Chinese-herb nephropathy"
Ephedra/ma huang	Weight loss, energy, decongestion	Hypertension, arrhythmias, seizures, stroke, myocardial infarction, *death*
Kava-kava	Stress reduction	Liver failure
Licorice root	Peptic ulcers, expectorant	Pseudoaldosteronism
Yohimbe	Aphrodisiac	Weakness, paralysis, anxiety, *death* (overdose)

Contraindications
• Pre-existing liver disease

• Regular alcohol ingestion

Precautions
• Do not take for >4 weeks

• Discontinue immediately if jaundice occurs.

Ma huang (ephedra)
• Common uses:
  * Diseases of the respiratory tract with mild bronchospasm
  * No evidence supports ephedra as an effective weight loss product.

• Proposed mechanism:
  * Sympathomimetic stimulant (α_1, β_1, β_2 stimulation)

Dosage
• Use should not be recommended

Side effects
• Palpitations, tachycardia

• Insomnia, anxiety

• Anorectic (exploited in weight loss products)

• Serious adverse effects:
  * ***Death***
  * Hypertension
  * Arrhythmia

  * Myocardial infarction
  * Stroke

Contraindications
• Anxiety and restlessness

• Hypertension

• Diabetes (hyperglycemic effects)

• Heart disease

• Thyroid disease

• Glaucoma

Drug interactions
• β-Blockers

• Other CNS stimulants (eg, caffeine, theophylline)

• Cardiac glycosides

• MAO inhibitors (risk of hypertensive crisis)

Nonherbal Natural Products

S-adenosylmethionine (SAMe)
• Common uses:
  * Depression
  * Osteoarthritis

• Proposed mechanisms:
  * Depression: methyl donor to catecholamines (increased norepinephrine, dopamine)

* Anti-inflammatory: enhances the synthesis of proteoglycans in chondrocytes

Dosing
• Depression: 800-1600 mg/d divided tid-qid

• Arthritis: 200 mg tid (range 400-1200 mg/d)

Side effects
• Generally mild: gas, vomiting, diarrhea, nausea

• Patients with bipolar disorder may experience switch to mania.

Melatonin
• Common uses:
    * Sleep disorders
    * Reset sleep-wake cycle (jet lag)

• Proposed mechanism:
    * Mimics endogenous release of melatonin from the pineal gland
    * Concentrations increase significantly 1-2 hours before sleep

Dosage
• Insomnia: 0.1-1 mg at bedtime

• Jet lag: 3-5 mg for 3 days before and after departure

Side effects
• Infertility

• Headache

• Confusion

• Possible immune stimulant

Drug interactions
• Benzodiazepines: enhanced anxiolytic effects

Dehydroepiandrosterone (DHEA)
• Common uses:
    * Depression
    * General anti-aging effects
    * Osteoporosis
    * Antidiabetogenic

• Proposed mechanisms:
    * Adult concentrations of DHEA fall to about 20% of maximum by 70 years of age
    * Sex hormone precursor
    * Increased secretion of IL-2
    * Inhibits platelet aggregation
    * Enhanced fibrinolysis

Dosage
• ~50 mg/d is average

Side effects
• Oily skin, acne, hirsutism

• Abnormal menses

• Headache

• Abnormal aggressiveness

Contraindications
• Patients with hormone-sensitive tumors (eg, breast cancer, prostate cancer)

Glucosamine
• Common uses:
    * Osteoarthritis

• Proposed mechanism:
    * Serves as a precursor to glycosaminoglycans, which make up cartilage and synovial fluid
    * May help regenerate cartilage and replete synovial fluid

Dosage
• 500 mg tid (with meals) glucosamine sulfate for 6-8 weeks

Side effects
• Mild GI effects: nausea, heartburn

• Little known about long-term use

• Diabetes: may worsen insulin resistance (case reports)

11. Sleep Aids and Stimulants

Insomnia

Nonpharmacologic treatment of insomnia
- Establish regular waking and sleeping schedule.

- Exercise regularly.

- Do not nap during the daytime.

- Avoid caffeine, especially after noon.

- Avoid large meals close to bedtime.

- Participate in a relaxing activity at bedtime (eg, reading, hot bath)

Pharmacologic treatment of insomnia: nonprescription products (Table 11)
Antihistamines
- Diphenhydramine

- Doxylamine

Pharmacology
- Block histamine-1 and muscarinic receptors

Role in therapy
- Antihistamines should be used for short-term management of occasional insomnia in conjunction with good sleep hygiene.

Dosage
- Diphenhydramine 25-50 mg 30-60 minutes before bedtime (elderly, 25 mg)

- Do not exceed 7-10 days of therapy (to avoid tolerance).

Side effects
- Sedation, especially the next morning

- Anticholinergic effects
    * Dry mouth/eyes
    * Constipation
    * Urinary retention
    * Confusion (elderly)

Contraindications and precautions
- Benign prostatic hyperplasia (BPH)

- Dementia

- Narrow-angle glaucoma

Drowsiness

Nonpharmacologic treatment of drowsiness
- Good sleep hygiene preferable to drug therapy (see insomnia section, above).

Pharmacologic treatment of drowsiness
Caffeine
- The only FDA-approved nonprescription stimulant

- Acts as CNS stimulant

- Physical dependence can develop.

- 50-200 mg: increased alertness, decreased fatigue

- >200 mg: nervousness, insomnia, irritability

- Precautions
    * Peptic ulcer disease
    * Cardiac dysrhythmias
    * Anxiety disorders

- Special patient populations
    * Pregnancy: restrict to <300 mg caffeine per day to minimize risk of low birth weight
    * Breastfeeding: 1% of caffeine crosses into breast milk; peak effect 1 hour after consumption. Minimize caffeine use in breastfeeding, especially in infants.

Table 11

Selected Nonprescription Products for Insomnia

Drug or combination	Trade name
Doxylamine	Unisom Nighttime Sleep Aid Tablets®
Diphenhydramine	Nytol®, Sominex®
Diphenhydramine + acetaminophen	Tylenol PM®, Unisom Pain Relief®
Diphenhydramine + aspirin	Bayer PM®

12. Key Points

Cough, cold, and allergy
- Nonprescription drug therapy for the common cold includes symptomatic management using decongestants (nasal congestion), antihistamines (excess nasal discharge), analgesics (headache), and local anesthetic lozenges or sprays (pharyngitis)

- Nonprescription treatment of allergies includes systemic antihistamines (sedating or nonsedating), ocular antihistamines, decongestants (if nasal congestion), and cromolyn (scheduled, not as needed).

- Cough can be relieved by a product containing a cough suppressant (dextromethorphan). An expectorant (guaifenesin) should be recommended to enhance clearance of mucus.

Constipation
- Diet and lifestyle changes should always be recommended to prevent or treat constipation (increase in fiber and fluid intake, exercise).

- Bulk-forming laxatives and stool softeners are the safest products to prevent and treat constipation, and can be used chronically.

- Stimulant laxatives should be used only occasionally to avoid laxative dependence or other complications.

Diarrhea
- Loperamide, adsorbents, or bismuth subsalicylate may be recommended to treat diarrhea.

- Maintaining adequate hydration is very important, especially in young children and the elderly.

Nausea and vomiting
- Nonprescription treatment options for nausea and vomiting include antihistamines (meclizine, dimenhydrinate) and phosphorated carbohydrate solution (Emetrol).

- Histamine-2 receptor antagonists (cimetidine, ranitidine) or bismuth salts (Pepto-Bismol) may relieve gastric discomfort or indigestion.

Pain and fever
- Pain and fever may be treated with aspirin and other salicylates, nonsteroidal anti-inflammatory drugs (NSAIDs), or acetaminophen.

- Aspirin and NSAIDs inhibit platelet aggregation. Nonacetylated salicylates and acetaminophen do not have antiplatelet activity.

- Salicylates and NSAIDs can cause gastropathy, including gastritis, gastric ulcers, and gastric bleeding. They may decrease the effectiveness of some antihypertensives, and may have deleterious effects on kidney function.

- Acetaminophen does not have anti-inflammatory activity, and can be hepatotoxic in excessive doses (>4 g/d), or when used concurrently with alcohol.

Ophthalmic products
- Dry eyes can be treated with artificial tears or ocular emollients.

- Ophthalmic vasoconstrictors (ocular decongestants) cause vasoconstriction in the conjunctiva to treat redness. Naphazoline is the ocular decongestant of choice. Ocular decongestants are contraindicated in narrow-angle glaucoma, due to the potential to cause rebound.

- Combination products containing an ophthalmic vasoconstrictor and ocular antihistamine should be recommended for allergic conjunctivitis (naphazoline + pheniramine or antazoline).

Otic products
- Impacted cerumen can be treated with cerumen-softening agents (carbamide peroxide in anhydrous glycerin + alcohol; hydrogen peroxide + water).

- Water-clogged ears may be managed with the commercial preparation of isopropyl alcohol + anhydrous glycerin, or compounded acetic acid + isopropyl alcohol.

Home monitoring and testing devices
- Home tests are available for:
  * Blood glucose monitoring (diabetes)
  * Fertility and ovulation
  * Pregnancy
  * Urinary tract infection
  * Colorectal cancer
  * Blood pressure monitoring
  * Acquired immunodeficiency syndrome (AIDS)
  * Illicit drug use
  * Hepatitis C

Smoking cessation
- First-line agents for pharmacotherapy in smoking cessation:

* Nicotine gum (Nicorette, generic) OTC
* Nicotine patch (Habitrol, Nicotrol, Nicoderm CQ) OTC
* Nicotine inhaler (Nicotrol inhaler)
* Nicotine nasal spray (Nicotrol NS)
* Bupropion SR (Zyban)

• Contraindications for nicotine replacement therapy:
  * Cardiovascular disease
    • <2 weeks post-MI
    • Serious arrhythmias
    • Serious/worsening angina
  * Esophagitis, peptic ulcer disease (gum)
  * Seek medical advice if pregnant or breast-feeding
  * Do not smoke while using NRT.
  * Allergies, asthma, sinus conditions (nasal spray)

Natural and herbal products
• Herbal products that should be discontinued prior to surgery: ginkgo, garlic, ginseng

• St. John's wort: takes several weeks to see effect; potential for serious drug interactions.

Sleeping aids
• Ethanolamine antihistamines (diphenhydramine, doxylamine) should be used for short-term management of occasional insomnia in conjunction with good sleep hygiene.

Stimulants
• Caffeine, a CNS stimulant, is the only FDA-approved nonprescription stimulant.

• The recommended dosage of 50-200 mg may increase alertness and decrease fatigue.

• Doses exceeding 200 mg may cause nervousness, insomnia, and/or irritability.

13. Questions and Answers

1. The primary advantage of recommending dextromethorphan instead of codeine is:

   A. It is twice as effective as codeine in suppression of cough.
   B. It has less dependence potential.
   C. It has peripheral rather than central action.
   D. It is less expensive.
   E. It is much longer acting than codeine.

2. All of the following statements regarding guaifenesin are correct EXCEPT:

   A. It is the only FDA-approved OTC expectorant.
   B. It requires large amounts of water to be effective.
   C. It is available OTC as Robitussin.
   D. It may cause an decrease in platelet aggregation and an increase in bleeding time.
   E. It is available in some prescription cough and cold formulations.

3. All of the following statements regarding diphenhydramine are true EXCEPT:

   A. It is less likely to cause drowsiness compared to other OTC antihistamines.
   B. It is the active ingredient in some OTC products for insomnia.
   C. It is available OTC under trade name of Benadryl.
   D. A small percentage of children may exhibit a paradoxical CNS stimulant effect.
   E. Elderly patients may experience delirium or confusion with diphenhydramine.

4. All of the following statements about the routine use of oral decongestants in treating the common cold are true EXCEPT:

   A. Phenylpropanolamine has been removed from all OTC cold and allergy products.
   B. They are relatively safe with no dependence.
   C. They are absolutely contraindicated in patients with patients with controlled diabetes and mild hypertension.
   D. The most common side effects are nervousness and insomnia.
   E. They cannot be used in patients on MAO inhibitor antidepressants.

5. All of the following are correct generic and trade name combinations EXCEPT:

   A. Chlor-Trimeton = chlorpheniramine
   B. Dimetane = diphenhydramine
   C. Claritin = loratadine
   D. Nasalcrom = cromolyn
   E. Zyrtec = cetirizine

6. Which of the following is *not* a side effect of loperamide?

   A. Sedation
   B. Dizziness
   C. Dry mouth
   D. Drowsiness
   E. Insomnia

7. Which of the following is *not* an adverse effect of Pepto-Bismol?

   A. Anticholinergic effects, dry mouth, and dry eyes
   B. Tinnitus
   C. Cross-sensitivity to aspirin allergy
   D. Grayish-black tongue
   E. Dark stools

8. Which of the following drugs exhibits analgesic and antipyretic properties, but *not* peripheral anti-inflammatory properties?

   A. Ibuprofen
   B. Sodium salicylate
   C. Acetaminophen
   D. Magnesium salicylate
   E. Naproxen

9. Which drug does *not* interact with NSAIDs?

   A. Methotrexate
   B. Warfarin
   C. Antihypertensive agents
   D. Diphenhydramine
   E. None of the above

10. Mary is a 32-year-old female with asthma and serious aspirin sensitivity. She comes to the pharmacist seeking assistance selecting a nonprescription product for aches and pains. Which of the following should the pharmacist recommend for Mary?

    A. Ibuprofen
    B. Naproxen
    C. Acetaminophen

D. A and B only
E. All of the above

11. Nonprescription antiemetics are primarily useful for preventing which type nausea?

    A. Nausea due to alterations in the vestibular apparatus
    B. Nausea due to drugs acting centrally on the chemo-receptor trigger zone
    C. Nausea due to visceral pain
    D. Nausea due to cortical stimulation from smells or sight
    E. Nausea due to afferent impulses from the gastrointestinal tract

12. A mother requests advice for her 6-month-old who has been constipated the last 2 days after beginning cereal feedings. Which of the following agents would be the best laxative agent to recommend?

    A. Dulcolax
    B. Fletcher's Castoria
    C. Mineral oil
    D. Glycerin suppositories
    E. Milk of magnesia

13. All of the following statements about stool softeners are true EXCEPT:

    A. They are not safe to use in pregnancy.
    B. The onset of action is usually between 1 and 2 days.
    C. They are useful in patients with constipation who have hemorrhoids.
    D. Extra water helps their effectiveness.
    E. They are often combined with mild stimulant laxatives.

14. All of the following statements about bisacodyl are true EXCEPT:

    A. It should *not* be taken concurrently with antacids.
    B. It can be crushed or chewed if needed.
    C. It should *not* be recommended in pregnancy.
    D. It is available in oral tablet and suppository dosage forms.
    E. It is the active ingredient in Doxidan.

15. Which of the following ethanolamine antihistamines are available in OTC products for insomnia?

    A. Diphenhydramine

B. Doxylamine
C. Loratadine
D. A and B
E. All of the above

16. Baby Matthew is 1 year old and weighs 24 lb. He has a fever of 102°F, is irritable, seems uncomfortable, and isn't sleeping well. His mother is confused by the assortment of fever relief products. You recommend acetaminophen. Which product and dosage do you recommend?

A. Tylenol Infant Drops 80 mg/0.8 mL; give 1.6 mL q4-6h
B. Tylenol Children's Liquid 160 mg/5 mL; give 2 tsp. q6-8h
C. Advil Infant Drops 50 mg/1.25 mL; give 1.25 mL q4-6h
D. Motrin Children's Suspension 100 mg/5 mL; give 2.5 mL q6-8h
E. Tylenol Infant Drops 80 mg/0.8 mL; give 3.2 mL q4-6h

17. The next morning, baby Matthew's mother comes back to your pharmacy. Her pediatrician recommended alternating the maximum dose ibuprofen with the acetaminophen, and she is asking for help selecting an ibuprofen product and dosage. Which do you recommend?

A. Advil Infant Drops 50 mg/1.25 mL; give 0.625 mL q8h
B. Motrin Children's Suspension 100 mg/5 mL; give 2 tsp. q4h
C. Motrin Infant Drops 50 mg/1.25 mL; give 2.5 mL q6h
D. Advil Children's Chewable Tablet 50 mg; give one tablet q8h
E. Advil Children's Chewable Tablet 50 mg; $^1/_2$ tablet q4h

18. Which of the following tests does *not* require a blood sample?

A. Cholesterol test
B. Ovulation prediction tests
C. HIV tests
D. Hepatitis C test
E. Accu-chek Advantage

19. B.R. is a 62-year-old obese male who has been diagnosed by his physician with benign prostatic hyperplasia (BPH). Which of the following herbal remedies might be used to treat his symptoms?

A. Ginseng
B. Echinacea
C. DHEA
D. Garlic
E. Saw palmetto

20. Which of the following products should be discontinued prior to surgery?

A. Ginkgo biloba
B. Gentian root
C. Glutamine
D. Glucosamine
E. Folic Acid

Answers

1. **B.** Although there have been reports of limited recreational abuse of dextromethorphan, its potential for dependence/addition is significantly less than that of codeine.

2. **D.** Guaifenesin does *not* have any effects on platelet aggregation or bleeding time. It is the only FDA-approved OTC expectorant, works better with increased fluid intake, and is included in Robitussin products.

3. **A.** Diphenhydramine, an ethanolamine, is the most sedating OTC antihistamine.

4. **C.** Systemic decongestants are not recommended in individuals with uncontrolled diabetes or hypertension due to their sympathomimetic effects. They are contraindicated with MAOIs, and can commonly cause nervousness or insomnia. Phenylpropanolamine was removed from the market in 2000.

5. **B.** Dimetane contains brompheniramine.

6. **E.** Dizziness, dry mouth, and drowsiness are common side effects of loperamide.

7. **A.** Common adverse effects of Pepto-Bismol include tinnitus and grayish-black tongue or stools. It does contain a salicylate, therefore should not be used in individuals with aspirin allergy.

8. **C.** Acetaminophen is a centrally-acting antipyretic and analgesic, but does not exhibit peripheral anti-inflammatory activity. Salicylates and other NSAIDs do.

9. **D.** NSAIDs can significantly decrease

methotrexate clearance, enhance the effect of warfarin, and blunt the hypotensive effect of hypertensive medications. There is no known interaction with diphenhydramine.

10. **C.** All NSAIDs and aspirin-containing products should be avoided in individuals with aspirin sensitivity. Acetaminophen can be recommended in this setting.

11. **A.** Nonprescription antiemetics are anti-histamines that exert their effect by inhibiting histamine in neural centers controlling vomiting, salivation, and vestibular excitability, making them especially well-suited for motion sickness.

12. **D.** Glycerin suppositories are safe for infants. The other agents should not be used in this patient population.

13. **A.** Stool softeners are safe to use in pregnancy, and usually exert their effect within 1-2 days. Stool softeners are recommended for individuals in whom hard stools or straining could cause pain or complications (eg, hemorrhoids, postoperatively, postpartum, post-MI). Increased fluid intake enhances their effectiveness. They are frequently used in combination products containing stimulant laxatives.

14. **B.** Because bisacodyl is an enteric-coated product, it should not be taken with antacids, or be crushed, chewed, or broken. It should not be used in pregnancy. It is available in both oral tablets and rectal suppositories.

15. **D.** Both diphenhydramine and doxylamine are ethanolamines used in sleeping aids. Loratadine is a nonsedating antihistamine.

16. **A.** The pediatric dosage of acetaminophen is 10-15 mg/kg q4-6h.

    24 lb x kg/2.2 lb = 10.9 kg x 10-15 mg/kg
    = 109 – 163.5 mg

    Tylenol Infant Drops 80 mg/0.8 mL;
    1.6 mL = 160 mg acetaminophen

17. **C.** The pediatric dosage of ibuprofen is 5-10 mg/kg q6-8h.

    24 lb x kg/2.2 lb = 10.9 kg x 5-10 mg/kg
    = 54.5 – 109 mg

    Motrin Infant Drops 50 mg/1.25 mL;
    2.5 mL = 100 mg ibuprofen

18. **B.** Cholesterol, HIV, hepatitis C, and blood glucose tests all require a blood sample. Most ovulation prediction tests use urine.

19. **E.** Saw palmetto may have some efficacy in treating BPH, although the patient should be evaluated by a physician to rule out prostate cancer.

20. **A.** Ginkgo biloba has antiplatelet activity, and should therefore be withheld prior to surgical procedures.

14. References

Berardi RR, ed. *Handbook of Nonprescription Drugs: An Interactive Approach to Self Care,* 13th ed. Washington: American Pharmaceutical Association; 2002.

Eisenberg DM, et al. Trends in alternative medicine use in the United States, 1990-1997. *JAMA.* 1998;280:1569-1575.

Fiore MC, Bailey WC, Cohen SJ, et al. Treating Tobacco Use and Dependence. Clinical Practice Guideline. Rockville, MD: U.S. Department of Health and Human Services; Public Health Service: June 2000.

Pray WS. *Nonprescription Product Therapeutics,* 1st ed. Baltimore: Lippincott Williams & Wilkins; 1999.

Robbers JE, Tyler VE. *Tyler's Herbs of Choice: The Therapeutic Use of Phytomedicinals.* New York: The Hayworth Herbal Press; 1999.

Scott GN, Elmer GW. Update on natural product-drug interactions. *Am J Health-Syst Pharm.* 2002;59:339-347.

28. Asthma and Chronic Obstructive Pulmonary Disease

Timothy H. Self, PharmD
Professor, Department of Pharmacy
University of Tennessee College of Pharmacy

Contents

1. Asthma

Definition

- Asthma is a chronic inflammatory disorder of the airways in which many cells and cellular elements play a role, in particular mast cells, eosinophils, T lymphocytes, neutrophils, and epithelial cells. In susceptible individuals, this inflammation causes recurrent episodes of wheezing, breathlessness, chest tightness, and cough, particularly at night and in the early morning. Asthma affects over 15 million Americans, and is the most common cause of missed school days for children. Mortality due to asthma is increasing; death rates are greatest in inner-city African-Americans and Hispanics.

Types and Classifications

- *Childhood-onset (atopic):* positive family history of asthma, allergy to tree or grass pollen, house dust mites, household pets, and molds (extrinsic asthma)

- *Adult-onset:* usually a negative family history and negative skin tests to common aeroallergens (intrinsic asthma)

- Classification of severity is shown in Figure 1 (this classification is extremely important in defining treatment options; see Figure 2).

Clinical Presentation

- Episodic wheezing, coughing, chest tightness, shortness of breath; worse at night, early morning, and with exercise

Pathophysiology

- Inflammatory airway disease; also a disease with bronchospasm

- Common triggers of symptoms include aeroallergens, respiratory viral illness, exercise (especially in cold, dry air), environmental smoke, fumes, cats

- Drug-induced asthma includes that due to aspirin, NSAIDs, and β-blockers (low-dose β_1 selective agents okay if concurrent post MI or CHF and do not have severe asthma; COX-2 inhibitors may be okay in aspirin-sensitive asthma)

- Complex interaction among inflammatory cells (eg, mast cells, eosinophils, lymphocytes), mediators (eg, leukotrienes), and cytokines (eg, IL-4, IL-5)

- The result is airway inflammation (mucus and swelling in the lining of the airways) and airway hyperreactivity

- *Early phase* response to inhaling an aeroallergen occurs immediately; *late phase* response occurs 4-12 hours later

- Asthma is commonly worsened by poorly controlled concurrent allergic rhinitis, sinusitis, and GERD; it may also worsen in the premenstrual or perimenstrual period.

Diagnostic Criteria

- The main basis for diagnosis is a detailed history of episodic symptoms that are typically worse at night-time/early morning and associated with common triggers.

- Reversible airway obstruction (improvement in pulmonary function tests [FEV_1] of >12% after inhaling a short-acting β_2 agonist)

- Exclude alternate diagnoses

Treatment Principles and Goals

- Optimal long-term management of asthma includes four major areas, including objective assessment and monitoring, environmental control, pharmacologic therapy, and patient education as a partnership.

- Treatment goals are shown in Figure 1; a stepwise approach to managing asthma is shown in Figures 2 and 3.

Drug therapy for acute exacerbations in asthma
- See Table 1 for long-term control medications, Table 2 for quick-relief medications, and Figure 4 for management of asthma exacerbations.

Monitoring

- Optimal management for the great majority of patients will result in a dramatic reduction in symptoms (including nocturnal and early morning symptoms), as well as reduced acute care visits, lost work or school days, and the need for quick-relief medications.

- Monitoring peak expiratory flow (PEF) using a peak flow meter at home is required ("green zone" is 80-100% of personal best value; "yellow zone" is 50-79% of personal best, and indicates consultation with a health care professional is advisable; and "red

Figure 1.

Classification of asthma severity.

Goals of Asthma Treatment

- Prevent chronic and troublesome symptoms (e.g., coughing or breathlessness in the night, in the early morning, or after exertion)
- Maintain (near) "normal" pulmonary function
- Maintain normal activity levels (including exercise and other physical activity)
- Prevent recurrent exacerbations of asthma and minimize the need for emergency department visits or hospitalizations
- Provide optimal pharmacotherapy with minimal or no adverse effects
- Meet patients' and families' expectations of and satisfaction with asthma care

Classify Severity of Asthma

Clinical Features Before Treatment*

	Symptoms**	Nighttime Symptoms	Lung Function
STEP 4 Severe Persistent	- Continual symptoms - Limited physical activity - Frequent exacerbations	Frequent	- FEV_1 or PEF $\leq 60\%$ predicted - PEF variability $>30\%$
STEP 3 Moderate Persistent	- Daily symptoms - Daily use of inhaled short-acting beta$_2$-agonist - Exacerbations affect activity - Exacerbations ≥ 2 times a week; may last days	>1 time a week	- FEV_1 or PEF $>60\% - <80\%$ predicted - PEF variability $>30\%$
STEP 2 Mild Persistent	- Symptoms >2 times a week but <1 time a day - Exacerbations may affect activity	>2 times a month	- FEV_1 or PEF $\geq 80\%$ predicted - PEF variability 20–30%
STEP 1 Mild Intermittent	- Symptoms ≤ 2 times a week - Asymptomatic and normal PEF between exacerbations - Exacerbations brief (from a few hours to a few days); intensity may vary	≤ 2 times a month	- FEV_1 or PEF $\geq 80\%$ predicted - PEF variability $<20\%$

* The presence of one of the features of severity is sufficient to place a patient in that category. An individual should be assigned to the most severe grade in which any feature occurs. The characteristics noted in this figure are general and may overlap because asthma is highly variable. Furthermore, an individual's classification may change over time.

** Patients at any level of severity can have mild, moderate, or severe exacerbations. Some patients with intermittent asthma experience severe and life-threatening exacerbations separated by long periods of normal lung function and no symptoms.

PEF, peak expiratory flow; FEV_1, forced expiratory volume in 1 second.

Reproduced from NIH Expert Panel Report 2.

Figure 2.

Stepwise approach for managing infants and young children (≤5 years of age) with acute or chronic asthma.

Classify Severity: Clinical Features Before Treatment or Adequate Control		Medications Required To Maintain Long-Term Control
	Symptoms/Day **Symptoms/Night**	**Daily Medications**
Step 4 Severe Persistent	Continual Frequent	■ **Preferred treatment:** – High-dose inhaled corticosteroids **AND** – Long-acting inhaled beta₂-agonists **AND, if needed,** – Corticosteroid tablets or syrup long term (2 mg/kg/day, generally do not exceed 60 mg per day). (Make repeat attempts to reduce systemic corticosteroids and maintain control with high-dose inhaled corticosteroids.)
Step 3 Moderate Persistent	Daily > 1 night/week	■ **Preferred treatments:** – **Low-dose inhaled corticosteroids and long-acting inhaled beta₂-agonists** **OR** – **Medium-dose inhaled corticosteroids.** ■ Alternative treatment: – Low-dose inhaled corticosteroids and either leukotriene receptor antagonist or theophylline. .... If needed (particularly in patients with recurring severe exacerbations): ■ Preferred treatment: – Medium-dose inhaled corticosteroids and long-acting beta₂-agonists. ■ Alternative treatment: – Medium-dose inhaled corticosteroids and either leukotriene receptor antagonist or theophylline.
Step 2 Mild Persistent	> 2/week but < 1x/day > 2 nights/month	■ **Preferred treatment:** – **Low-dose inhaled corticosteroid (with nebulizer or MDI with holding chamber with or without face mask or DPI).** ■ Alternative treatment (listed alphabetically): – Cromolyn (nebulizer is preferred or MDI with holding chamber) OR leukotriene receptor antagonist.
Step 1 Mild Intermittent	≤ 2 days/week ≤ 2 nights/month	■ No daily medication needed.

Quick Relief
 All Patients
	■ Bronchodilator as needed for symptoms. Intensity of treatment will depend upon severity of exacerbation.
	   – Preferred treatment: Short-acting inhaled beta₂-agonists by nebulizer or face mask and space/holding chamber
	   – Alternative treatment: Oral beta₂-agonist
	 ■ With viral respiratory infection
	   – Bronchodilator q 4–6 hours up to 24 hours (longer with physician consult); in general, repeat no more than once every 6 weeks
	   – Consider systemic corticosteroid if exacerbation is severe or patient has history of previous severe exacerbations
	 ■ Use of short-acting beta₂-agonists >2 times a week in intermittent asthma (daily, or increasing use in persistent asthma) may indicate the need to initiate (increase) long-term control therapy.

⬇ **Step down**
 Review treatment every 1 to 6 months; a gradual stepwise reduction in treatment may be possible.

⬆ **Step up**
 If control is not maintained, consider step up. First, review patient medication technique, adherence, and environmental control.

Note
- The stepwise approach is intended to assist, not replace, the clinical decisionmaking required to meet individual patient needs.
- Classify severity: assign patient to most severe step in which any feature occurs.
- There are very few studies on asthma therapy for infants.
- Gain control as quickly as possible (a course of short systemic corticosteroids may be required); then step down to the least medication necessary to maintain control.
- Provide parent education on asthma management and controlling environmental factors that make asthma worse (e.g., allergies and irritants).
- Consultation with an asthma specialist is recommended for patients with moderate or severe persistent asthma. Consider consultation for patients with mild persistent asthma.

Goals of Therapy: Asthma Control
- Minimal or no chronic symptoms day or night
- Minimal or no exacerbations
- No limitations on activities; no school/parent's work missed
- Minimal use of short-acting inhaled beta₂-agonist (< 1x per day, < 1 canister/month)
- Minimal or no adverse effects from medications

Reproduced from National Institutes of Health 2002, Guidelines for the Diagnosis and Management of Asthma.

Figure 3.

Stepwise approach for managing asthma in adults and children >5 years of age: Treatment.

Classify Severity: Clinical Features Before Treatment or Adequate Control			Medications Required To Maintain Long-Term Control
	Symptoms/Day **Symptoms/Night**	**PEF or FEV₁** **PEF Variability**	**Daily Medications**

Step 4
Severe Persistent
	Continual
	Frequent
		≤ 60%
		> 30%
			■ **Preferred treatment:**
			  – **High-dose inhaled corticosteroids**
			    AND
			  – **Long-acting inhaled beta₂-agonists**
			    AND, if needed,
			  – Corticosteroid tablets or syrup long term (2 mg/kg/day, generally do not exceed 60 mg per day). (Make repeat attempts to reduce systemic corticosteroids and maintain control with high-dose inhaled corticosteroids.)

Step 3
Moderate Persistent
	Daily
	> 1 night/week
		> 60% – < 80%
		> 30%
			■ **Preferred treatment:**
			  – **Low-to-medium dose inhaled corticosteroids and long-acting inhaled beta₂-agonists.**
			■ Alternative treatment (listed alphabetically):
			  – Increase inhaled corticosteroids within medium-dose range
			    OR
			  – Low-to-medium dose inhaled corticosteroids and either leukotriene modifier or theophylline.
			
			If needed (particularly in patients with recurring severe exacerbations):
			■ **Preferred treatment:**
			  – **Increase inhaled corticosteroids within medium-dose range and add long-acting inhaled beta₂-agonists.**
			■ Alternative treatment:
			  – Increase inhaled corticosteroids within medium-dose range and add either leukotriene modifier or theophylline.

Step 2 Mild Persistent	> 2/week but < 1x/day > 2 nights/month	≥ 80% 20–30%	■ **Preferred treatment:** – **Low-dose inhaled corticosteroids.** ■ Alternative treatment (listed alphabetically): cromolyn, leukotriene modifier, nedocromil, OR sustained release theophylline to serum concentration of 5–15 mcg/mL.
Step 1 Mild Intermittent	≤ 2 days/week ≤ 2 nights/month	≥ 80% < 20%	■ No daily medication needed. ■ Severe exacerbations may occur, separated by long periods of normal lung function and no symptoms. A course of systemic corticosteroids is recommended.

Quick Relief All Patients	■ Short-acting bronchodilator: 2–4 puffs **short-acting inhaled beta₂-agonists** as needed for symptoms. ■ Intensity of treatment will depend on severity of exacerbation; up to 3 treatments at 20-minute intervals or a single nebulizer treatment as needed. Course of systemic corticosteroids may be needed. ■ Use of short-acting beta₂-agonists >2 times a week in intermittent asthma (daily, or increasing use in persistent asthma) may indicate the need to initiate (increase) long-term control therapy.

⬇ **Step down**
Review treatment every 1 to 6 months; a gradual stepwise reduction in treatment may be possible.

⬆ **Step up**
If control is not maintained, consider step up. First, review patient medication technique, adherence, and environmental control.

Goals of Therapy: Asthma Control
- Minimal or no chronic symptoms day or night
- Minimal or no exacerbations
- No limitations on activities; no school/work missed
- Maintain (near) normal pulmonary function
- Minimal use of short-acting inhaled beta₂-agonist (< 1x per day, < 1 canister/month)
- Minimal or no adverse effects from medications

Note
- The stepwise approach is meant to assist, not replace, the clinical decisionmaking required to meet individual patient needs.
- Classify severity: assign patient to most severe step in which any feature occurs (PEF is % of personal best; FEV₁ is % predicted).
- Gain control as quickly as possible (consider a short course of systemic corticosteroids); then step down to the least medication necessary to maintain control.
- Provide education on self-management and controlling environmental factors that make asthma worse (e.g., allergens and irritants).
- Refer to an asthma specialist if there are difficulties controlling asthma or if step 4 care is required. Referral may be considered if step 3 care is required.

Reproduced from National Institutes of Health 2002, Guidelines for the Diagnosis and Management of Asthma.

Table 1

Long-term asthma control medications

Generic name	Trade name	Usual dosage range	Dosage form	Schedule[1]
Inhaled corticosteroids				
Beclomethasone HFA 40 µg/puff; 80 µg/puff	QVAR®	80-480 µg/day	MDI	bid
Budesonide 200 µg/inhalation	Pulmicort®	1-3 inhalations/day	Turbuhaler	bid
Budesonide 0.25 & 0.5 mg	Respules®	0.5-2.0 mg/day	Nebulized	bid
Flunisolide 250 µg/puff	Aerobid®	1-8 puffs/day	MDI	bid
Fluticasone 44, 110, 220 µg/puff	Flovent®	88-660 µg/day	MDI	bid
Fluticasone	Flovent Rotadisk®	100-500 µg/day	DPI	bid
Fluticasone-salmeterol combination (each dose: 50 µg salmeterol + 100, 250, or 500 µg fluticasone)	Advair Diskus® (Advair 100, 250, 500)	1 inhalation	DPI	bid
Triamcinolone 100 µg/puff	Azmacort®	4-20 puffs/day	MDI/spacer	bid
Leukotriene modifiers				
Montelukast	Singulair®	4 mg (age 2-5 y)	Chewable tab	HS
		5 mg (age 6-14 y)	Chewable tab	HS
		10 mg (adult) tablet	Tablet	HS
Zafirlukast	Accolate®	20-40 mg/day tablet	Tablet	bid
Zileuton	Zyflo®	2400 mg/day tablet	Tablet	qid
Mast cell stabilizers				
Cromolyn	Intal®	1-4 puffs MDI	MDI	qid
	Intal®	20 mg	Nebulizer soln	qid
Nedocromil	Tilade®	1-4 puffs MDI	MDI	qid
Long-acting inhaled β_2 _agonists_				
Formoterol	Foradil Aerolizer®	1 inhalation DPI	DPI	bid
Salmeterol	Serevent Diskus®	1 inhalation DPI	DPI	bid
Methylxanthines				
Theophylline (numerous products)	Uniphyl®	10 mg/kg per day[2] up to 300 mg max in adults to start; aim for 5-15 µg/mL steady state	Tablet	Daily; 5 or 6 pm

MDI, metered dose inhaler, DPI, dry powder inhaler (breath-activated).

[1]Usual schedule (some patients do well on once daily dosing).

[2]Complex, high-risk drug to dose; see references cited for details; do not use unless competent in dosing and monitoring serum theophylline concentrations.

zone," or <50% of personal best, indicates a written action plan should be implented, and there is no quick response, immediate medical attention should be sought).

• Spirometry in the physician's office

Table 2

Quick-relief asthma medications

Generic name	Trade name	Usual dosage[1]	Dosage form	Schedule
Short-acting inhaled β_2 agonists[2]				
Albuterol	Proventil®, Ventolin®	2 puffs	MDI	q4h prn
		2.5 mg	Nebulizer soln.	q4h prn
Pirbuterol	Maxair Autohaler®	2 puffs	MDI	q4h prn
Anticholinergics				
Ipratropium	Atrovent®	2 puffs	MDI	q6h
		0.25 mg	Nebulizer soln.	q6h
Ipratropium with albuterol	Combivent®	2 puffs	MDI	q6h
		3 mL	Nebulizer soln.	q6h
Systemic corticosteroids[3]				
Methylprednisolone	Medrol®	1 mg/kg per day	Tablets	Daily
Prednisone		1 mg/kg per day	Tabs/liquid	Daily
Prednisolone		1 mg/kg per day	Tablets	Daily

[1]Usual dosage for routine home use (dose in emergency department is higher/more frequent).

[2]For prevention of exercise-induced asthma, inhale 2 puffs 5-15 minutes before exercise. Increasing use indicates poor asthma control; increase anti-inflammatory therapy and reassess environmental control (good asthma control is indicated by infrequent need for quick-relief therapy).

[3]Short courses are used for <2 weeks.

Mechanism of Action

(Section on mechanism of action from NIH Expert Panel Report 2.)

Long-term control medications

Corticosteroids

- Anti-inflammatory: block late reaction to allergen and reduce airway hyperresponsiveness; inhibit cytokine production, adhesion protein activation, and inflammatory cell migration and activation

- Reverse β_2-receptor downregulation: inhibit microvascular leakage

Cromolyn and nedocromil

- Anti-inflammatory: block early and late reaction to allergen; interfere with chloride channel function; stabilize mast cell membranes and inhibit activation and release of mediators from eosinophils and epithelial cells

- Inhibit acute response to exercise, cold dry air, and SO_2

Long-acting β_2-agonists

- Bronchodilation: smooth muscle relaxation following adenylate cyclase activation and increase in cyclic AMP, producing functional antagonism of bronchoconstriction

- In vitro, inhibit mast cell mediator release, decrease vascular permeability, and increase mucociliary clearance

- Compared to short-acting inhaled β_2-agonist, salmeterol (but not formoterol) has slower onset of action (15-30 minutes) but longer duration (>12 hours)

Methylxanthines

- Bronchodilation: smooth muscle relaxation from phosphodiesterase inhibition and possibly adenosine antagonism

- May affect eosinophilic infiltration into bronchial mucosa as well as decrease T-lymphocyte numbers in epithelium

- Increases diaphragm contractility and mucociliary clearance

Leukotriene modifiers

- Leukotriene receptor antagonist; selective competitive inhibitor of LTD_4 and LTE_4 receptors
- 5-Lipoxygenase inhibitor

Figure 4.

Management of asthma exacerbations: Emergency department and hospital-based care.

PCO$_2$, partial pressure of carbon dioxide; PEF, peak expiratory flow; FEV$_1$, forced expiratory volume in 1 second.
Reproduced from NIH Expert Panel Report 2.

Quick-relief medications
Short-acting inhaled β₂ agonists
- Bronchodilation: smooth muscle relaxation following adenylate cyclase activation and increase in cyclic AMP, producing functional antagonism of bronchoconstriction

Anticholinergics
- Bronchodilation: competitive inhibition of muscarinic cholinergic receptors

- Reduces intrinsic vagal tone to the airways; may block reflex bronchoconstriction secondary to irritants or to reflux esophagus

- May decrease mucus gland secretion

Patient Instructions and Counseling

- Patient education is absolutely essential for optimal asthma management.

- Emphasize the necessity to take controller/preventer medications *EVERY DAY*, even when the patient feels well and is having no breathing problems.

- Instruct the patient regarding the dangers of overuse of short-acting inhaled β₂ agonists (if inflammation is worsening, see a physician if the usual dose does not give quick relief).

- Demonstrate the correct use of the MDI, the MDI plus spacer, and the DPI, and then *OBSERVE* the patient using the devices (most patients do not perform well initially; the devices can be difficult to use at first; see Figure 4).

- Demonstrate correct use of peak flow meters and OBSERVE the patient using them (see Table 3); explain about the green, yellow, and red zones (including the written action plan).

- Teach how to prevent exercise-induced asthma.

- Be sure patients receive influenza vaccination every fall.

Adverse Drug Effects

(Section on adverse drug effects from NIH Expert Panel Report 2.)
Long-term control medications
Corticosteroids
- Cough, dysphonia, oral thrush (candidiasis)

Table 3

Directions for use of peak flow meter[1]

1. Stand while using the meter.

2. Position the indicator at the bottom of the scale.

3. Hold the peak flow meter so your fingers do not block the opening.

4. Inhale as deeply as possible, place mouthpiece well into your mouth, and make sure your lips form a tight seal around it.

5. Blow out as fast and as hard as possible![2] BLAST! Emphasize to the patient that the maneuver is highly effort dependent.

6. Repeat steps 2-5 two more times, and record the highest of the three readings along with the date and time.

[1]If a short acting inhaled β₂ agonist is required in the early morning, remember to check the peak expiratory flow before using the drug, and record the value; then repeat PEF testing 15 minutes later.
[2]Do not accelerate air with your tongue (ie, use a spitting motion). This incorrect maneuver will give false elevation in PEF.

- In high doses, systemic effects may occur, although studies are not conclusive, and the clinical significance of these effects (eg, adrenal suppression, osteoporosis, growth suppression, skin thinning and easy bruising) has not been established .

- Short-term use: reversible abnormalities in glucose metabolism, increased appetite, fluid retention, weight gain, mood alteration, hypertension, peptic ulcer, and rarely aseptic necrosis of the femur

- Long-term use: adrenal axis suppression, growth suppression, dermal thinning, hypertension, diabetes, Cushing's syndrome, cataracts, muscle weakness, and in rare instances, impaired immune function

- Consideration should be given to coexisting conditions that could be worsened by systemic corticosteroids, such as herpes virus infections, varicella, tuberculosis, hypertension, peptic ulcer, and strongyloidiasis.

Cromolyn and nedocromil
- Fifteen to 20 percent of patients complain of an unpleasant taste from nedocromil.

Figure 5.

Steps for using an inhaler.

Please demonstrate your inhaler technique at every visit.

1. Remove the cap and hold inhaler upright.
2. Shake the inhaler.
3. Tilt your head back slightly and breathe out slowly.
4. Position the inhaler in one of the following ways (A or B is optimal, but C is acceptable for those who have difficulty with A or B. C is required for breath-activated inhalers):

A. Open mouth with inhaler 1 to 2 inches away.

B. Use spacer/holding chamber (that is recommended especially for young children and for people using corticosteroids).

C. In the mouth. Do not use for corticosteroids.

D. NOTE: Inhaled dry powder capsules require a different inhalation technique. To use a dry powder inhaler, it is important to close the mouth tightly around the mouthpiece of the inhaler and to inhale rapidly.

5. Press down on the inhaler to release medication as you start to breathe in slowly.
6. Breathe in slowly (3 to 5 seconds).
7. Hold your breath for 10 seconds to allow the medicine to reach deeply into your lungs.
8. Repeat puff as directed. Waiting 1 minute between puffs may permit second puff to penetrate your lungs better.
9. Spacers/holding chambers are useful for all patients. They are particularly recommended for young children and older adults and for use with inhaled corticosteroids.

Avoid common inhaler mistakes. Follow these inhaler tips:
- Breathe out *before* pressing your inhaler.
- Inhale *slowly.*
- Breathe in through your mouth, not your nose.
- Press down on your inhaler at the *start* of inhalation (or within the first second of inhalation).
- Keep inhaling as you press down on inhaler.
- Press your inhaler only *once* while you are inhaling (one breath for each puff).
- Make sure you breathe in evenly and deeply.

NOTE: Other inhalers are becoming available in addition to those illustrated above. Different types of inhalers may require different techniques.

Reproduced from NIH Expert Panel Report 2.

Long-acting β_2 agonists
- Tachycardia, skeletal muscle tremor, hypokalemia, prolongation of QTc interval in overdose

- A diminished bronchoprotective effect may occur within 1 week of chronic therapy. Clinical significance has not been established.

Methylxanthines
- Dose-related acute toxicities include tachycardia, nausea and vomiting, tachyarrhythmias (SVT), central nervous system stimulation, headache, seizures, hematemesis, hyperglycemia, and hypokalemia.

- Adverse effects at usual therapeutic doses include insomnia, gastric upset, aggravation of ulcer or reflux, increase in hyperactivity in some children, and difficulty in urination in elderly males with prostatism.

Leukotriene modifiers (updated from 1997 NIH Guidelines)
- Montelukast and zafirlukast are usually well tolerated.

- Zileuton can cause liver dysfunction.

Quick-relief medications
Short-acting inhaled β_2-agonists
- Tachycardia, skeletal muscle tremor, hypokalemia, increased lactic acid, headache, hyperglycemia; the inhaled route, in general, causes few systemic adverse effects; patients with preexisting cardiovascular disease, especially the elderly, may have adverse cardiovascular reactions with inhaled therapy.

Anticholinergics
- Drying of mouth and respiratory secretions, increased wheezing in some individuals, blurred vision if sprayed in eyes

Corticosteroids
- Short-term use: reversible abnormalities in glucose metabolism, increased appetite, fluid retention, weight gain, mood alteration, hypertension, peptic ulcer, and rarely aseptic necrosis of femur

- Consideration should be given to coexisting conditions that could be worsened by systemic corticosteroids, such as herpes virus infections, varicella, tuberculosis, hypertension, peptic ulcer disease, and strongyloidiasis.

Drug-Drug and Drug-Disease Interactions

- For zafirlukast, administration with meals decreases bioavailability; take at least 1 hour before or 2 hours after meals.

- Zileuton and zafirlukast may increase the effect of warfarin and increase theophylline levels.

- Well known inducers of cytochrome P450 (carbamazepine, phenobarbital, phenytoin, and rifampin) are documented to decrease the effect of systemic corticosteroids.

- Examples of drugs that may increase the effect of systemic corticosteroids include erythromycin, clarithromycin, itraconazole, oral contraceptives, and conjugated estrogen.

Parameters to Monitor

- Refill record for daily controller/preventer meds and quick-relief meds

- Reduction in symptoms (including nocturnal and early morning symptoms)

- ED visits and hospitalizations; unscheduled office visits

- Need for "bursts" of systemic corticosteroids

- Lost work or school days, and the need for quick-relief medications

- Peak expiratory flow (PEF) using a peak flow meter at home

- If also have rhinitis or GERD, monitor refills to ensure optimal control (if rhinitis and GERD are not well controlled, asthma control will likely suffer)

Kinetics

- Theophylline is no longer used extensively in asthma, but when it is used, knowledge of its kinetics is essential due to its high risk.

- Other drugs, disease states, smoking, age, and diet can all affect theophylline kinetics and dose requirements (see Table 4).

- Therapeutic serum theophylline concentrations are 5-15 µg/mL (***NOT*** the old recommendation of 10-20 µg/mL; see latest NIH Guidelines [1997 and 2002]).

Table 4.

Factors Affecting Serum Theophylline Levels

Factor	Decreases Theophylline Concentrations	Increases Theophylline Concentrations	Recommended Action
Food	↓ or delays absorption of some sustained-release theophylline (SRT) products	↑ rate of absorption (fatty foods) products	Select theophylline preparation that is not affected by food.
Diet	↑ metabolism (high protein)	↓ metabolism (high carbohydrate)	Inform patients that major changes in diet are not recommended while taking theophylline.
Systemic, febrile viral illness (e.g., influenza)		↓ metabolism	Decrease theophylline dose according to serum concentration level. Decrease dose by 50 percent if serum concentration measurement is not available.
Hypoxia, cor pulmonale, and decompensated congestive heart failure, cirrhosis		↓ metabolism	Decrease dose according to serum concentration level.
Age	↑ metabolism (1 to 9 years)	↓ metabolism (<6 months, elderly)	Adjust dose according to serum concentration level.
Phenobarbital, phenytoin, carbamazepine	↑ metabolism		Increase dose according to serum concentration level.
Cimetidine		↓ metabolism	Use alternative H$_2$ blocker (e.g., famotidine or ranitidine).
Macrolides: TAO, erythromycin, clarithromycin		↓ metabolism	Use alternative antibiotic or adjust theophylline dose.
Quinolones: ciprofloxacin, enoxacin, pefloxacin		↓ metabolism	Use alternative antibiotic or adjust theophylline dose. Circumvent with ofloxacin if quinolone therapy is required.
Rifampin	↑ metabolism		Increase dose according to serum concentration level.
Ticlopidine		↓ metabolism	Decrease dose according to serum concentration level.
Smoking	↑ metabolism		Advise patient to stop smoking; increase dose according to serum concentration level.

* This list is not all-inclusive; for discussion of other factors, see package inserts.

Reproduced from NIH Expert Panel Report 2.
TAO, triacetyloleandomycin.

- Elimination half-life in an otherwise healthy non-smoking adult is about 8 hours, but in a smoker about 4 hours, and in a small child (>1 year) about 4 hours.

- Neonates have greatly prolonged elimination half-life.

- Elimination half-life in decompensated heart failure or cirrhosis is about 24 hours.

- Volume of distribution is about 0.5 L/kg.

- High fat meals may cause "dose dumping" for some products (check product literature).

Other

- MDIs should be stored at room temperature, between 59 and 86°F; if left in car in freezing or near-freezing temperatures, aerosol particles will be too large to inhale into lungs.

- MDIs should be "primed" (release one dose) only with first use, or if it is a prn agent used only once every few weeks (frequent priming is unnecessary and wastes expensive medications).

- MDI dust cap should be left on inhaler when not in use! Check mouthpiece for foreign objects before inhaling!

Non-Drug Therapy

- An essential component of optimal asthma management is environmental control.

- Without good control of the environment at home, school, and work, drug therapy will often be inadequate.

- Have the patient identify known asthma triggers, and help the patient identify potential triggers not yet realized (do not forget someone smoking at home or work!).

2. Chronic Obstructive Pulmonary Disease (COPD)

Definition

- COPD is characterized by airflow limitation that is not fully reversible. The airflow limitation is usually both progressive and associated with an abnormal inflammatory response of the lungs to noxious particles or gases. COPD is a major cause of death and suffering in the U.S. and around the world. It is the fourth leading cause of chronic morbidity and mortality in the U.S.

Types and Classifications (Table 5)

- Some clinicians still refer to chronic bronchitis and emphysema in characterizing different levels of COPD (eg, emphysema patients have destructive damage to the alveolar walls whereas chronic bronchitis is associated with chronic productive cough).

Clinical Presentation

- Shortness of breath

- Cough and sputum production

- Usually a history of cigarette smoking for several years

- In the more severe form, respiratory failure and heart failure

Pathophysiology

- Usually caused by long-term smoking (may also be caused by exposure to other noxious particles and gases)

- Chronic inflammation throughout the airways but via different inflammatory cells and mediators than those that cause asthma (thus the response to inhaled corticosteroids is much less than is seen with asthma)

- Imbalance of proteinases and antiproteinases in the lung

- Rare hereditary cause of emphysema is α_1 antitrypsin deficiency.

- Pathologic changes are found in the central and peripheral airways as well as the alveoli and pulmonary vasculature.

Table 5

Classification of COPD by Severity

Stage	Characteristics
0: At Risk	• Normal spirometry • Chronic symptoms (cough, sputum, production)
I: Mild COPD	• FEV_1/FVC <70% • FEV_1 ≥80% predicted • With or without chronic symptoms (cough, sputum production)

II: Moderate COPD	• FEV_1/FVC <70%
	• 50% ≤ FEV_1 <80% predicted
	   (IIA: 50% FEV_1 <80% predicted)
	   (IIB: 30% FEV_1 <50% predicted)
	• With or without chronic symptoms (cough, sputum production, dyspnea)

III: Severe COPD	• FEV_1/FVC <70% • 30% ≤ FEV_1 < predicted or FEV_1 <50% predicted plus respiratory failure or clinical signs of right heart failure
IV: Very severe COPD	FEV_1/FVC <70% FEV_1 <30% predicted or FEV_1 <50% predicted plus chronic respiratory failure

FEV_1, forced expiratory volume in 1 second; FVC, forced vital capacity.
Respiratory failure defined as arterial partial pressure of oxygen (PaO_2) less than 8.0 kPa (60 mm Hg) with or without arterial partial pressure of CO_2 ($PaCO_2$) greater than 6.7 kPa (50 mm Hg) while breathing air at sea level.
From Pauwels et al, 2001.

- Mucus hypersecretion

- Ciliary dysfunction

- Airflow limitation

- Lung hyperinflation

- Gas exchange abnormalities

- Secondary pulmonary hypertension

- Cor pulmonale

Diagnostic Criteria

- History of cigarette smoking or exposure to other noxious particles or fumes

- Chronic cough and sputum production

- Spirometry (reduced FEV_1; see Table 5 for classification of severity)

- Rule out other lung diseases.

Treatment Principles and Goals

- Prevent disease progression.

- Relieve symptoms.

- Improve exercise tolerance.

- Improve health status.

- Prevent and treat complications.

- Prevent and treat exacerbations.

- Reduce mortality.

- Bronchodilators are central to the symptomatic treatment of COPD; these agents will increase exercise capacity without necessarily improving the FEV_1.

- Inhaled bronchodilators are preferred to oral bronchodilators for initial therapy; the specific choice of agent depends on patient response.

- Long-acting inhaled β_2 agonists are effective and more convenient for maintenance therapy.

- Anticholinergics currently available (ipratropium) are a logical second (or first) choice for maintenance therapy.

- Short-acting inhaled β_2 agonists are preferred for prn use in patients already receiving long-acting agents and anticholinergics.

- Theophylline is logical step 3 agent for maintenance therapy in patients who are not optimally controlled with β_2 agonists and anticholinergics.

Therapy at each stage (per GOLD Guidelines)
- For each stage, avoid risk factors (eg, smoking cessation) and receive influenza vaccine each autumn. Also, give pneumococcal vaccine per current guidelines.

Stage 0: At risk
- No recommended treatment

Stage I: Mild COPD
- As-needed short-acting bronchodilator

Stage II: Moderate COPD
Stage IIA
- Regular treatment with one or more bronchodilators, rehabilitation, inhaled corticosteroids only if significant symptoms and lung function response

Stage IIB
- Regular treatment with one or more bronchodilators, rehabilitation, inhaled corticosteroids only if significant symptoms and lung function response OR if repeated exacerbations

Stage III: Severe COPD
- Regular treatment with one or more bronchodilators

- Inhaled corticosteroids if significant symptoms and lung function responses or if repeated exacerbations

- Treatment of complications

- Long-term O_2 therapy if respiratory failure

Stage IV: Very severe COPD
- Same treatments as for stage III and consider surgical treatment

Drug therapy for acute exacerbations of COPD
- Inhaled albuterol and/or ipratropium

- Systemic corticosteroids (eg, prednisone 40 mg daily for 10 days)

- Oral antibiotics for purulent sputum (typically trimethoprim-sulfamethoxazole [Septra®], amoxicillin, or doxycyline)

- O_2

Monitoring
- Spirometry: FEV_1

- Symptoms of dyspnea, cough, sputum production, change in sputum color and volume

- PaO_2

- Exercise tolerance/fatigue

Long-term drug therapy
- See content under asthma for specific drugs

Nondrug therapy
- The most important nondrug therapy is smoking cessation (ie, beyond nicotine replacement therapy and bupropion, support groups, and counseling).

- Oxygen therapy

- Nutritional support

- Psychosocial support

- Pulmonary rehabilitation

3. Key Points

Asthma

- Asthma is primarily an inflammatory airway disease.

- It is undertreated, resulting in much unnecessary suffering and economic loss.

- Managing patients via the principles of the NIH Guidelines has been clearly shown to reduce ED visits and hospitalizations and improve patient quality of life.

- Optimal long-term management includes objective assessment, environmental control, drug therapy, and patient education working as a partnership.

- Patients with persistent asthma need daily controller therapy (anti-inflammatory agents).

- Inhaled corticosteroids are the most efficacious agents to control asthma.

- Inhaled long-acting inhaled β_2 agonists are indicated with inhaled corticosteroids for patients with moderate persistent or severe persistent asthma.

- Short-acting inhaled β_2 agonists are the agents of choice for quick relief of symptoms.

- Pharmacists should teach patients how to use inhalers (MDI, MDI-spacer, DPI) by demonstrations and *OBSERVATION* of the patient.

- Pharmacists should instruct patients on how to use peak flow meters, including color-coded zone management with a written action plan.

- Patients must clearly understand the purpose of daily controller/preventer meds vs. quick-relief meds.

Chronic obstructive pulmonary disease
(Taken directly from GOLD Workshop Summary 2001)

- The overall approach to managing stable COPD should be characterized by a stepwise increase in treatment, depending on the severity of the disease.

- For patients with COPD, health education can play a role in improving skills, ability to cope with the illness, and health status. It is effective in accomplishing certain goals, including smoking cessation.

- None of the existing medications for COPD has been shown to modify the long-term decline in lung function that is the hallmark of this disease. Therefore, pharmacotherapy for COPD is used to improve symptoms and/or decrease complications.

- Bronchodilator medications are central to the symptomatic management of COPD. They are given on an as-needed basis or on a regular basis to prevent or reduce symptoms.

- The principal bronchodilator treatments are β_2 agonists, anticholinergics, theophylline, and a combination of one or more of these drugs. Inhaled therapy is preferred.

- Combining bronchodilators may improve efficacy and decrease the risk of side effects compared to increasing the dose of a single bronchodilator.

- Regular treatment with inhaled glucocorticosteroids should only be prescribed for symptomatic COPD patients with a documented spirometric response to glucocorticosteroids or for those with an FEV_1 <50% predicted and repeated exacerbations requiring treatment with antibiotics and/or oral glucocorticosteroids.

- Chronic treatment with systemic glucocorticosteroids should be avoided because of an unfavorable benefit-to-risk ratio.

- All COPD patients benefit from exercise training programs, improving with respect to both exercise tolerance and symptoms of dyspnea and fatigue.

- The long-term administration of oxygen (>15 hours per day) to patients with chronic respiratory failure has been shown to increase survival.

4. Questions and Answers

1. Asthma is primarily due to which underlying problem?

   A. Pulmonary fibrosis
   B. Infection
   C. Inflammation
   D. Bronchospasm
   E. Granulomas

2. Which objective measure for routine monitoring asthma is available at home?

   A. PEF
   B. FEV_1
   C. FVC
   D. O_2 saturation
   E. PD20

3. Which device requires slow inhalation?

   A. Diskus
   B. Turbuhaler
   C. Aerolizer
   D. MDI
   E. Rotadisk

4. How many seconds is optimal for breath holding after inhaling from an MDI?
   A. 4
   B. 5
   C. 15
   D. 2
   E. 10

5. When using a peak flow meter, what percentage of the personal best value is the yellow zone?

   A. <50
   B. <60
   C. 50-79
   D. 60-89
   E. 40-60

6. What are the trade names for long-acting inhaled β_2 agonists?

   A. Foradil and Serevent
   B. Pulmicort and Flovent
   C. Aerobid and Combivent
   D. Maxair and Atrovent
   E. Flovent and Ventolin

7. Which disease states decrease theophylline elimination and often result in reduced dosage requirements?

   A. Hepatitis
   B. Heart failure (decompensated)
   C. Hypertension
   D. A, B, and C
   E. A and B

8. Which drug(s) are preferred for long-term treatment of moderate persistent asthma?

   A. Budesonide + formoterol
   B. Fluticasone + salmeterol
   C. Beclomethasone + ipratropium
   D. A or B
   E. B or C

9. What is the drug of choice for quick relief of asthma symptoms?

   A. Atrovent
   B. Serevent
   C. Foradil
   D. Azmacort
   E. Proventil

10. For patients with asthma or COPD exacerbations not responding adequately to inhaled bronchodilators, what is the agent of choice to add to manage the acute exacerbation?

    A. Fluticasone
    B. Budesonide
    C. Cromolyn
    D. Theophylline
    E. Prednisone

11. Which drug may increase serum theophylline concentrations?

    A. Clarithromycin
    B. Hydrochlorothiazide
    C. Carbamazepine
    D. Rifampin
    E. Phenytoin

12. Which side effect of inhaled corticosteroids is reduced by spacer devices?

    A. Hoarseness
    B. Decreased bone density
    C. Thinning of skin
    D. Oropharyngeal candidiasis
    E. Cataracts

13. The therapeutic range for theophylline per the NIH Guidelines for asthma management is:

   A. 5-15 μg/mL
   B. 8-12 μg/mL
   C. 10-20 μg/mL
   D. 15-25 μg/mL
   E. 10-15 μg/mL

14. Which asthma controller drug is given HS?

   A. Accolate
   B. Singulair
   C. Zyflo
   D. Intal
   E. Tilade

15. When it is not well controlled, which disease state may worsen asthma?

   A. Coronary artery disease
   B. GERD
   C. Diabetes
   D. Hypertension
   E. Arthritis

16. Which class of drugs is only indicated in COPD patients who have frequent exacerbations?

   A. Long-acting inhaled β_2 agonists
   B. Anticholinergics
   C. Short-acting inhaled β_2 agonists
   D. Inhaled corticosteroids
   E. Methylxanthines

The next two questions relate to Case Study 1.

17. Which class of drugs is preferred in Mr. Johnson for optimal control of asthma?

   A. Anticholinergics
   B. Inhaled corticosteroids
   C. Methylxanthines
   D. Mast cell stabilizers
   E. Oral corticosteroids

18. What is an appropriate alternative to Lopressor in Mr. Johnson?

   A. An ACE inhibitor
   B. Propranolol 40 mg bid
   C. Clonidine
   D. Hydralazine
   E. Atenolol 200 mg daily

The next two questions relate to Case Study 2.

19. What concerns should the pharmacist have in this situation regarding theophylline?

   A. Cirrhosis is well documented to decrease elimination of theophylline
   B. The mg/kg dose is too low
   C. Mrs. Adams should be on a q12h product
   D. Uniphyl should be dosed in the morning, not evening
   E. Long-acting inhaled β_2 agonists increase theophylline clearance

20. The patient has a friend who has COPD and has told her about Combivent. Mrs. Adams wants to know the opinion of the pharmacist. You would say:

   A. I'll call your doctor and suggest a new Rx for Combivent.
   B. Combivent is a third line drug for COPD. I would not use it now.

Case Study 1: Medication Profile

Patient Name:	Thomas Johnson
Address:	5689 Washington St.
DOB:	9-15-55
Drug Allergies:	aspirin sensitivity
Height:	5'10" Weight: 75 kg
Diagnosis:	(1) asthma (childhood onset, moderate persistent)
	(2) allergic rhinitis
	(3) hypertension

Medications:

Date	Rx #	MD	Drug & Strength	Quantity	Sig	Refills
3/16	94385	Betts	Accolate 20 mg	60	1 bid	3
3/16	94386	Betts	albuterol MDI	1	2 puffs q4h	6
3/16	94387	Betts	Flonase	1	bid as dir.	3
3/25	95523	T. Jones	Lopressor 50 mg	60	1bid	6
3/27	95734	Betts	albuterol MDI	1	2 puffs q4h	5

Pharmacist Notes: 3/16—discussed proper use of MDI and observed patient use. Coached Mr. Johnson to inhale slowly (he was inhaling fast); he used the MDI correctly for the other steps.

Case Study 2: Medication Profile

Patient Name:	Mrs. S.T. Adams	
Address:	7129 James Ave.	
DOB:	1-6-37	
Drug Allergies:	sulfonamides	
Height:	5'3"	Weight: 55 kg
Diagnosis:	(1) COPD—53 pack-year Hx smoking	
	(quit 2 years ago)	
	(2) cirrhosis	

Medications:

Date	Rx #	MD	Drug & Strength	Quantity	Sig	Refills
2/18	84389	Jones	Serevent Diskus	1	1 bid	6
2/18	84390	Jones	albuterol MDI	1	2 puffs q4h prn	6
2/18	84391	Jones	Atrovent MDI	1	2 puffs q6h	6
2/18	84392	Jones	Uniphyl 600 mg	30	1 qd 6 PM	2

Pharmacist Notes: 2/18—discussed proper use of Diskus and observed patient use; taught Mrs. Adams to inhale deeply and rapidly (she was inhaling slowly for only <2 seconds). Also observed use of MDI (she forgot to exhale gently before pressing down on MDI).

C. Combivent is a good drug, but I want to talk to your doctor about starting a medicine called Flovent.

D. Since you have a prescription for Atrovent and for Serevent, your doctor has correctly prescribed prn albuterol. You do not need Combivent.

E. I think Foradil Aerolizer would be better for you.

21. Which drug is best for long term management of mild persistent asthma?

   A. Cromolyn
   B. Montelukast
   C. Nedocromil
   D. Theophylline
   E. Budesonide

22. Which total daily dose of prednisone is best for home management of an acute exacerbation of asthma in a 60-kg adult?

   A. 5 mg
   B. 60 mg
   C. 10 mg
   D. 20 mg
   E. 7.5 mg

23. Which drug is most likely to cause an asthma exacerbation in a patient sensitive to aspirin?

   A. Ibuprofen
   B. Acetaminophen
   C. Rofecoxib
   D. Salsalate
   E. Sodium salicylate

24. Which type of inhaler does not work well in very cold temperatures?

   A. Diskus
   B. Turbuhaler
   C. Aerolizer
   D. MDI
   E. Rotahaler

Answers

1. **C.** Although asthma certainly does have a bronchospastic component, it is primarily due to inflammation, so good control of inflammation dramatically reduces bronchospasm. A good indicator of disease control is the rare need for short-acting inhaled β_2 agonists.

2. **A.** Peak flow meters are inexpensive and relatively easy to use. Good measurement of peak expiratory flow (PEF) requires appropriate technique, and if good technique is used, patients have valuable objective evidence of asthma control (or exacerbation).

3. **D.** Dry powder inhalers currently available require rapid inhalation. MDIs require slow inhalation to minimize impaction of aerosol in the mouth and throat.

4. **E.** Ten seconds is best; there is no need to hold longer. Four to five seconds is okay if 10 seconds is uncomfortable.

5. **C.** The yellow zone is 50-79%, which indicates suboptimal control (the red zone is <50%, which indicates to start the crisis action plan and seek medical attention).

6. **A.** Foradil (formoterol) and Serevent (salmeterol).

7. **E.** Hepatitis and decompensated heart failure both can dramatically reduce theophylline clearance.

8. **D.** (A. budesonide + formoterol **OR** B. fluticasone + salmeterol) See Figures 2 and 3.

9. **E.** Atrovent is also a quick-relief agent, but it is not as efficacious in asthma and has a slower onset than albuterol and other short-acting inhaled β_2 agonists.

10. **E.** Prednisone or other systemic corticosteroids (eg, methylprednisolone) are well documented to be efficacious in asthma and COPD acute exacerbations.

11. **A.** Clarithromycin is documented to increase serum concentrations. Hydrochlorothiazide does not affect serum theophylline concentrations and the remaining choices are all documented to decrease serum theophylline concentrations.

12. **D.** Oropharyngeal candidiasis or thrush is correct. The other side effects are not reduced by spacers.

13. **A.** The currently accepted range for asthma is 5-15 µg/mL (***NOT*** the old range of 10-20 µg/mL). There is no benefit in exceeding 15 µg/mL, and many patients receive benefit at lower doses.

14. **B.** Since asthma is a disease of circadian rhythm and is worse between 2 AM and 6 AM, it is best to give this once-daily drug at bedtime.

15. **B.** GERD can worsen asthma if it is not properly treated. The exact mechanisms are debated, but there is excellent documentation that asthma improves if this condition is well managed.

16. **D.** This class of drugs should NOT be used routinely in COPD patients with mild disease. In moderate disease, inhaled corticosteroids are only indicated if there are frequent exacerbations. Remember: in asthma, inhaled corticosteroids are the best agents for long-term control; but in COPD their role is limited.

17. **B.** Inhaled corticosteroids is correct (see Figures 2 and 3 for treatment choices). The pharmacist should share the NIH Guidelines with Mr. Johnson's prescriber to help ensure optimal care.

In addition, the pharmacist should educate the patient regarding the purpose of the meds and proper use of inhalers (eg, should observe the patient using the device).

18. **A.** An ACE inhibitor should be efficacious with few side effects (monitor for cough). β-Blockers should be avoided in Mr. Johnson unless he is post MI or had CHF (in which case use a low dose of a β_1-selective blocker and monitor carefully).

19. **A.** Cirrhosis is well documented to decrease elimination of theophylline. Ensure a check of a steady state theophylline level (peak) and anticipate dose reduction (usually 50% dose reduction in liver disease).

20. **D.** Since the patient has prescriptions for Atrovent and Serevent, the doctor has correctly prescribed prn albuterol (patient does not need Combivent). Using Combivent would mean scheduling a short-acting and long-acting β_2 agonist, which would bring little benefit and increase the chance for side effects such as tremor and nervousness. If there was no long-acting β_2 agonist prescribed, then Combivent would be logical.

21. **E.** Budesonide is an inhaled corticosteroid, the class of drugs recommended to treat even mild persistent asthma.

22. **B.** Sixty milligrams is an appropriate dose. If it is started as soon as the patient is in the red zone and not responding quickly to short-acting inhaled β_2 agonists, usually only a few days of treatment will be required (usually <1 week).

23. **A.** Ibuprofen has the same mechanism of action as aspirin and will predictably trigger symptoms in an aspirin-sensitive patient (ie, increased production of leukotrienes). COX-2 inhibitors are likely to be safe (rofecoxib was proven safe in one excellent study). Acetaminophen is the choice agent for minor pain in these patients.

24. **D.** MDIs release large aerosol particles that do not penetrate deeply into the lungs in cold temperatures. Dry powder inhalers are okay.

5. References

Asthma

Busse WW, Lemanske RF. Asthma. *N Engl J Med.* 2001;344:350-362.

Hendeles L, Jenkins J, Temple R. Revised FDA labeling guideline for theophylline oral dosage forms. *Pharmacotherapy.* 1995;15:409.

Knorr B, Matz J, Bernstein JA, et al. Montelukast for chronic asthma in 6- to 14-year-old children. *JAMA.* 1998;279:1181-1186.

National Institutes of Health. *Expert Panel Report 2. Guidelines for the Diagnosis and Management of Asthma, 1997.* NIH publication no. 97-4051.

National Institutes of Health. *Guidelines for the Diagnosis and Management of Asthma—Update on Selected Topics 2002.* NIH publication no. 02-5075. Also published in *J Allergy Clin Immunol.* 2002;110:S141-S219; available online at www.nhlbi.nih.gov/guidelines/asthma/asthsumm.htm

Pauwels R, Lofdahl CG, Postma DS, et al. Effect of inhaled formoterol and budesonide on exacerbations of asthma. Formoterol and Corticosteroids Establishing Therapy (FACET) International Study Group. *N Engl J Med.* 1997;337:1405; erratum in *N Engl J Med.* 1998;338:139.

Self TH, Finch CK. Studies demonstrating improved outcomes in patients with asthma: A 10 year review. *Am J Manag Care.* 2001;7:187-196.

Shannon M. Life threatening events after theophylline overdose: a 10-year prospective analysis. *Arch Intern Med.* 1999;159:989.

Shapiro G, Lumry W, Wolfe J, et al. Combined salmeterol 50 mcg and fluticasone propionate 250 mcg in the Diskus device for the treatment of asthma. *Am J Respir Crit Care Med.* 2000;161:527.

Weiss KB, Sullivan SD. The health economics of asthma and rhinitis. I. Assessing the economic impact. *J Allergy Clin Immunol.* 2001;107:3.

Chronic Obstructive Pulmonary Disease

Calverley P et al. Combined salmeterol and fluticasone in the treatment of COPD: a randomized controlled trial. *Lancet.* 2003;361:449-56.

Dahl R, Greefhorst LA, Nowak D, et al. Inhaled formoterol dry powder versus ipratropium bromide in COPD. *Am J Respir Crit Care Med.* 2001;164:778-784.

Mahler D, Donohue JF, Barbee RA, et al. Efficacy of salmeterol xinafoate in the treatment of COPD. *Chest.* 1999;115:957-965.

Pauwels RA, Buist AS, Calverley PM et al and the GOLD Scientific Committee. Global strategy for the diagnosis, management, and prevention of chronic obstructive pulmonary disease. NHLBI/WHO Global Initiative for Chronic Obstructive Lung Disease (GOLD) Workshop summary. *Am J Respir Crit Care.* Med 2001;163:1256-76; website: www.goldcopd.com.

Pauwels R, Lofdahl CG, Laitinen LA, et al. Long term treatment with inhaled budesonide in persons with mild COPD who continue smoking. European Respiratory Society Study on Chronic Obstructive Pulmonary Disease. *N Engl J Med.* 1999;340:1948-1953.

Rigotti NA. Treatment of tobacco use and dependence. *N Engl J Med.* 2002;346:506-512.

29. Infectious Disease

Joyce E. Broyles, PharmD, BCNSP
Associate Professor, Department of Pharmacy
University of Tennessee College of Pharmacy

Contents

1. General Principles of Infectious Disease

Note: Please note that several infectious disease topics are addressed in other chapters of this review. They are: HIV/AIDS in Chapter 31, common colds in Chapter 27, and otitis media in Chapter 33. For additional information about specific anti-infective agents, please see Chapter 30.

Diagnosis

- Diagnosis of most infectious diseases consists of: (1) isolation and identification of microorganisms, (2) assessment of patient signs and symptoms, and (3) analysis of other laboratory data.

Isolation of organisms
- To identify the causative agent of the disease, samples should be taken from appropriate body sites prior to the initiation of anti-infective therapy. Higher predictive value comes from organisms isolated from normally sterile body sites (blood, urine, spinal fluid), than from normally bacteriologically colonized areas such as skin or fecal material.

Identification of organisms
- Organisms should be Gram stained as soon as is practical to determine cell morphology and guide empiric therapy. After the species of organism is determined, standardized concentrations of antibiotics are exposed to the isolated organism to determine what concentrations inhibit growth. The lowest concentration that prevents microbial growth after 18-24 hours is called the minimum inhibitory concentration (MIC). Breakpoint concentrations of antibiotics are defined as susceptible, intermediate, or resistant. These concentrations are determined by considering tissue concentrations with normal dosing and population distribution of the organism and determine if the antibiotic can be used for therapy.

- Physical signs and symptoms of infection such as fever, redness, swelling, pain, and cough must be considered both for initial diagnosis and assessment of antibiotic effectiveness.

Laboratory tests
- White blood cell (WBC) count. In the initial stage of infection, the neutrophil count may increase above normal, and immature neutrophil forms (bands) may appear.

- Inflammatory markers such as C-reactive protein,

erythrocyte sedimentation rate, and tumor necrosis factor may increase during infection.

- Laboratory tests may not be reliable in patients who are elderly, malnourished, neonatal, or severely infected.

Treatment Strategies

- Anti-infective agents should only be used when a significant infection has been diagnosed, is strongly suspected, or where indication for prophylactic therapy exists.

Prophylactic therapy
- Anti-infective therapy is directed to prevent infection. Common uses of prophylactic therapy are after exposure to infection, such as tuberculosis, or before surgical intervention in areas of high bacterial inoculum, such as bowel surgery.

- Empiric therapy. Usually broad-spectrum in nature, the therapy is directed toward all common pathogens associated with a disease state.

- Culture-guided therapy. Characterized by a narrower spectrum than empiric therapy, therapy covers only the specific organism isolated that is sensitive to the therapy. This approach is preferred due to increased cost-effectiveness and decreased bacterial resistance from unnecessary antibiotic exposure.

Choice of Anti-Infective Agent

- The clinician must answer several questions to determine optimal anti-infective therapy, or to review the appropriateness of others decisions. These include:
  * Is an antibiotic indicated on the basis of the clinical findings?
  * Have appropriate specimens been obtained, examined, and sent for culture?
  * What organisms are most likely to be causing the infection?
  * If several antibiotics are available to treat this likely or known organism, which agent is best for the patient? Patient allergies and concurrent disease states will be of consideration.
  * Is an antibiotic combination appropriate? A combination of drugs should be given only when clinical experience has shown such therapy to be more effective than single-agent therapy in a particular setting. Such multiple-agent regimens can increase the risk of toxic drug effects, and occasionally may result in drug antagonism and loss of effectiveness. However, some combinations of anti-infective

agents have demonstrated increased effectiveness that is greater than their individual effectiveness combined, a phenomenon known as synergy. An example of this is the combination of aminoglycosides with cell wall inhibitors such as penicillin in many gram-positive organisms.

* What is the best route of administration? This will depend on the overall plan for the patient. Oral therapy is preferred for outpatient therapy, and many intravenous anti-infectives have oral forms with similar pharmacokinetic profiles.

* What is the appropriate dose and dose interval? Regimen design should take into account patient size, renal/hepatic function, the disease state to be treated, and pharmacodynamic considerations of the agents used.

* Will initial therapy need modification after culture data are returned?

* What is the optimal duration of therapy, and is the development of resistance during prolonged therapy likely to occur?

Lack of Therapeutic Effectiveness

• When anti-infective therapy fails, careful analysis of possible causes should be made prior to changing the regimen. Factors associated with therapeutic failure include: misdiagnosis of the infection, improper drug regimen, inappropriate choice of antibiotic agent, microbial resistance, and situations in which antibiotic therapy may not be effective without additional interventions, such as surgical drainage.

2. Common Bacterial, Fungal, and Viral Infections

Meningitis

• Meningitis is defined as an inflammation of the meninges that is identified by an abnormal number of white blood cells in the cerebrospinal fluid.

Causative agents
• A wide variety of organisms are associated with this disease, including many gram-positives and gram-negatives.

Clinical presentation
• Patients may present with fever, headache, photophobia, neck rigidity, diarrhea, vomiting, and altered mental status. Infants may present with a bulging anterior fontanelle.

Diagnostic criteria
• Analysis of the cerebrospinal fluid may be diagnostic of the infective agent. Bacterial agents are associated with a large increase in WBCs, increased CSF protein, and decreased CSF glucose. Fungal and viral agents exhibit smaller increases in CSF WBCs, smaller increases in CSF protein, and limited decreases in CSF glucose.

Treatment
• Empiric treatment is usually determined by the age of the patient. Due to limited antibiotic penetration by many agents, the highest safe antibiotic doses are generally used. Table 1 summarizes empiric therapy for meningitis.

Endocarditis

• Endocarditis is an infection of the endocardium, the membrane lining the heart chamber and valves.

Causative agents
• Most patients have previous damage to the heart, such as artificial valve placement, prior to infection. The most common organisms are *Streptococcus* and *Staphylococcus* species.

Clinical presentation
• Patients present with low-grade fever, fatigue, and weakness. A diagnostic finding is the presence of splinter hemorrhages and petechiae.

Diagnostic criteria
• There is no specific laboratory test for this infection; most present with elevated ESR or CRP. Visual-

Table 1

Empiric Treatment of Meningitis

Age of patient	Most likely organism(s)	Empiric treatment
Newborn to 1 month	Gram negative enterics (E coli) Group B streptococci *Listeria monocytogenes*	Ampicillin and aminoglycoside **or** Cefotaxime **or** Ceftriaxone
1 month to 4 years	*Haemophilus influenzae* *Neisseria meningitidis* *Streptococcus pneumoniae*	Cefotaxime or ceftriaxone **and** Vancomycin
5-29 years	*Neisseria meningitidis* *Streptococcus pneumoniae* *Haemophilus influenzae*	Cefotaxime or ceftriaxone **and** Vancomycin
30-60 years	*Streptococcus pneumoniae* *Neisseria meningitidis*	Cefotaxime or ceftriaxone **and** Vancomycin
>60 years	*Streptococcus pneumoniae* Gram-negative enterics (*E coli*) *Listeria monocytogenes*	Ampicillin and aminoglycoside/vancomycin **or** Cefotaxime **or** Ceftriaxone

ization of the vegetations on the surface of the heart is often diagnostic of the disease.

Treatment
• According to American Heart Association guidelines, treatment varies by causative organism and the presence of prosthetic devices (which requires longer therapy) (Table 2).

Acute/Chronic Bronchitis

• Bronchitis is an inflammation of the bronchioles, often associated with bronchopneumonia. Chronic bronchitis is largely associated with heavy smoking.

Causative agents
• Viral infections account for half of all cases. *Mycoplasma pneumoniae, Streptococcus pneumoniae, Haemophilus influenzae, Moraxella catarrhalis* and *Chlamydia pneumoniae* are common bacterial pathogens.

Clinical presentation
• Patients present with history of acute productive cough, low-grade fever, and a clear chest x-ray.

Diagnostic criteria
• Sputum cultures are usually not useful in diagnosis due to multiple etiologies, and most physicians prescribe from physical findings.

Treatment
• Treatment is controversial for most acute illnesses due to the large percentage of viral cases. Chronic cases are treated, but due to multiple antibiotic treatments, bacterial resistance can easily develop (Table 3).

Pneumonia

• Pneumonia is an inflammation of the lung parenchyma characterized by consolidation of the affected part, filling of the alveolar air spaces with exudates, inflammatory cells, and fibrin. Distribution may be lobar, segmental, or lobular. If associated with bronchitis (see above), it is termed bronchopneumonia.

Causative agents
• Multiple bacterial etiologies are possible, depending on predisposing conditions (Table 4).

Clinical presentation
• Typically, the onset of illness is abrupt or subacute, with fever, chills, dyspnea, and productive cough

Table 2

Therapy for Endocarditis

Organism	Therapy	Duration (wk)
Penicillin-susceptible streptococci	Penicillin G alone **or**	4
	Penicillin G with gentamicin **or**	2
	Ceftriaxone alone **or**	4
	Vancomycin (if allergic to penicillin)	4
Streptococci relatively resistant to penicillin	Penicillin G alone **or**	4
	Penicillin G with gentamicin **or**	2
	Vancomycin (if allergic to penicillin)	4
Staphylococcus without prosthetic material (methicillin-sensitive)	Nafcillin or oxacillin	4-6
	(3-5 days of gentamicin may be added)	4-6
	Cefazolin (with or without gentamicin)	4-6
	Vancomycin (if allergic to penicillin)	4-6
Staphylococcus without prosthetic material (methicillin-resistant)	Vancomycin (if allergic to penicillin)	4-6

predominating. On physical examination, the patient is tachypneic and tachycardiac, frequently with chest wall retractions and grunting respirations. The complete blood count usually reflects a leukocytosis with a predominance of polymorphonuclear cells.

Diagnostic criteria
- Sputum culture may be useful in identification of some pathogens. However, difficulty in obtaining deep sputum cultures, and problems in culturing some organisms (such as *Legionella*) makes positive identification of the organism difficult.

Treatment
- Varies by age groups.

Table 3

Treatment for Acute and Chronic Bronchitis

Illness	Treatment (7-10 days usual duration)
Acute (rare; for severe disease only)	Erythromycin, clarithromycin, azithromycin (drugs used for treatment of chronic disease may be used; see below)
Chronic	Amoxicillin, amoxicillin-clavulanate, trimethoprim-sulfamethoxazole, erythromycin, clarithromycin, azithromycin, doxycycline, cefuroxime, cefaclor, cefprozil

Tuberculosis

- Tuberculosis is a communicable infectious disease caused by *Mycobacterium tuberculosis*. It can produce silent, latent infection as well as active infection. Although infection of any tissue or organ with *Mycobacterium tuberculosis* is possible, the usual site of infection is pulmonary.

Clinical presentation
- Tuberculosis can present with generalized symptoms of weight loss, fever, and night sweats with persistent cough productive of sputum. Latent disease is defined by a positive PPD test, in absence of other symptoms.

Diagnostic criteria
- Diagnosis is often made by a combination of chest x-ray, which often shows patchy or nodular infiltrates in the apical areas of the upper lobes or the superior segment of the lower lobes, and positive PPD skin test. Patients with severe HIV disease may not react to the standard PPD skin test. Sputum or lung biopsy may be acid-fast stained to reveal the organism. Due to the extended time period needed to grow the organism, sensitivities to anti-infective agents may take weeks to months to determine.

Treatment
- See Table 5.

Table 4

Empiric Treatment for Pneumonia

Age or type	Usual organisms	Empiric treatment(s)
Neonatal	Group B streptococci, *Listeria monocytogenes, Escherichia coli*	Ampicillin **and** gentamicin **or** cefotaxime **and** gentamicin
1-3 months	*Chlamydia trachomatis, Bordetella*	Erythromycin, clarithromycin, cefuroxime
3 months to 5 years	*Streptococcus pneumoniae, C trachomatis*	Clarithromycin, cefuroxime, cefotaxime
5-18 years	*Mycoplasma pneumoniae, S pneumoniae, Chlamydia pneumoniae*	Clarithromycin, erythromycin, cefuroxime
Adult, community acquired	*S pneumoniae, Haemophilus influenzae, Klebsiella pneumoniae, M pneumoniae*	***Ambulatory:*** oral macrolide (azithromycin, clarithromycin, erythromycin) or fluoroquinolone (levofloxacin, gatifloxacin or moxifloxacin) ***Hospitalized:*** cefotaxime or ceftriaxone with or without macrolide, or fluoroquinolone alone (levofloxacin, gatifloxacin or moxifloxacin)
Adult, hospitalized acquired	*K pneumoniae, Enterobacter aerogenes, Serratia* spp, *Acinetobacter* spp, *Pseudomonas aeruginosa, Staphylococcus aureus*	Aminoglycoside (tobramycin, amikacin or gentamicin) plus one of the following: cefotaxime, ceftriaxone, cefepime, ticarcillin/-clavulanic acid, piperacillin-tazobactam, meropenem, or imipenem; vancomycin to be added if MRSA suspected
Adult, aspiration	Mouth anaerobes	***Uncomplicated:*** penicillin G, clindamycin ***Hospital-acquired:*** ticarcillin-clavulanic acid, piperacillin-tazobactam

Infectious Diarrhea

- Diarrhea is defined as an increase in frequency and/or liquidity of stool compared with a patient's normal stool.

Causative agents
- Many disease states, drugs, and infectious organisms have been associated with diarrhea.

Clinical presentation
- Patient may present with several of the following symptoms: fever, chills, nausea, vomiting, and abdominal cramping.

Diagnostic criteria
- Etiology is often determined by patient history and physical examination. Due to the nature of the disease, cultures are not often diagnostic, except for determination of carrier states.

Table 5

Treatment of Tuberculosis

Disease stage	Treatment	Duration
Latent (probably isoniazid sensitive)	Isoniazid	9 months (6 months possible except for children and HIV+ persons)
Latent (probably isoniazid resistant)	Rifampin + pyrazinamide	2 months
Active disease	Isoniazid + rifampin + pyrazinamide	2-4 months

Treatment (Table 6)
- Supportive care (hydration, antipyretics, antiemetics) is useful. Antimotility agents are discouraged due to the potential to cause toxic megacolon. Antibacterial therapy is reserved for severe presentations or patients with risk factors.

Skin and Soft Tissue Infections

- Bacterial infection of the skin can be classified as direct infection of the skin (cellulitis) or secondary infection of a wound or incision.

Causative agents
- Cellulitis is usually an infection of a single organism. Most common are *Streptococcus pyogenes* and *Staphylococcus aureus*. Secondary infections may be polymicrobial, including both anaerobic and aerobic organisms.

Clinical presentation
- These infections are characterized by erythema and edema of the skin.

Diagnostic criteria
- Diagnosis is usually made from physical examination. Cultures are not usually diagnostic.

Treatment
- Treatment is empiric, based on likely organisms (Table 7).

Urinary Tract Infections

- Infections of the urinary tract represent a wide variety of clinical syndromes including urethritis, cystitis, prostatitis, and pyelonephritis.

Causative agents
- Most common agents are gram-negative facultatively anaerobic rods (coliforms). Hospitalized catheterized patients may also acquire *Pseudomonas* and *Staphylococcus* species.

Clinical presentation
- Lower urinary tract infections tend to present with dysuria, urgency, frequency, nocturia, and suprapu-

Table 6

Treatment of Infectious Diarrhea

Symptoms	Organism	Treatment
Violent presentation 1-6 hours after eating high-protein foods (eggs)	*Staphylococcus aureus*	Supportive
Indolent presentation with mild fever after eating meat, vegetables, or eggs	*Bacillus cereus*	Supportive
Mild to severe presentation 8-16 hours after eating canned products	*Clostridium perfringens*	Supportive
Mild to severe presentation with mild fever; may be associated with meat/egg contamination or contamination of other foods with contaminated water	*Escherichia coli*	Supportive, if outpatient; if hospitalized, fluoroquinolones or trimethoprim-sulfamethoxazole (TMP-SMX)
Mild to severe presentation with mild fever, chills, and cramping; associated with contamination of other foods with contaminated water; carrier state possible	*Salmonella* spp	Treatment only if febrile (fluoroquinolones or TMP-SMX)
Bloody mucoid diarrhea with fever and cramps	*Shigella* spp	TMP-SMX
Mild indolent presentation, often thought to be "flu"; transmitted by contaminated water	*Campylobacter*	Macrolides or fluoroquinolones
Severe presentation with fever and abdominal pain associated with seafood ingestion	*Yersinia enterocolitica*	Fluoroquinolones
Mild presentation with fever and abdominal pain associated with seafood ingestion	*Vibrio parahaemolyticus*	Tetracycline or fluoroquinolones
Severe, explosive presentation associated with contaminated water	*Vibrio cholerae*	Tetracycline or fluoroquinolones
Mild to severe presentation associated with travel, 6-10 days after exposure, with cramping and low-grade fever	*Escherichia coli*	Mostly supportive; severe prophylactic regimens

Table 7

Treatment of Infections of the Skin and Soft Tissues

Infection	Organisms	Treatments
Cellulitis	Group A streptococcus; *Staphylococcus aureus*	***Outpatient:*** dicloxacillin, cefadroxil, cephalexin, erythromycin ***Inpatient:*** cefazolin, erythromycin ***Severe cases:*** vancomycin
Diabetic foot infections	*Proteus* spp, *Escherichia coli*, *S aureus*, *Bacteroides fragilis*, anaerobic streptococci	Clindamycin or cephalexin ***Severe cases:*** ticarcillin-clavulanic acid or other beta-lactamase inhibitor; vancomycin may be needed if MRSA
Decubitus ulcers	Gram-negative bacilli, *Pseudomonas aeruginosa*, anaerobes	As for diabetic foot infections, above

bic heaviness or pain. Fever is rare. Upper urinary tract infections tend to present with flank pain and fever.

Diagnostic criteria
- Key to the diagnosis of urinary tract infections is the ability to demonstrate significant numbers of organisms present in an appropriately drawn urine sample. In general, higher numbers of organisms ($>10^5$ cells/mL) are needed to diagnose UTIs in females than males ($>10^3$ cells/mL), due to the fact that more organisms are able to ascend the shorter female urethra. In addition, the presence of WBCs in the urine sample may be a significant clue for infection.

Treatment
- A variety of antibacterials may be useful for the treatment of urinary tract infections (Table 8). These include: fluoroquinolones, cephalosporins, TMP-

SMX, and doxycycline. Fluoroquinolones are especially useful for treatment of prostatitis. Length of therapy varies according to the severity of disease.

Bacterial Venereal Diseases (Gonorrhea and Syphilis)

- Venereal diseases are diseases which can be transmitted via sexual intercourse. This section covers only the major bacterial venereal diseases, gonorrhea and syphilis. Additional viral venereal diseases will be covered in sections below (ie, herpes and hepatitis), or in other chapters (HIV, Chapter 31).

Causative agents
- Syphilis is caused by an infection with the spirochete *Treponema pallidum*, while gonorrhea is caused by the gram-negative coccus *Neisseria gonorrhoeae*.

Table 8

Treatment of Urinary Tract Infections

Diagnosis	Organisms	Treatments
Acute uncomplicated cystitis	*E coli, Staphylococcus saprophyticus*	TMP-SMX x 3 days **or** Quinolone x 3 days
Acute pyelonephritis	*E coli, Proteus mirabilis, Klebsiella pneumoniae, Enterococcus*	Quinolone x 14 days **or** TMP-SMX x 14 days; if severe, parenteral therapy with quinolone, extended-spectrum penicillin plus aminoglycoside should be used
Prostatitis	*E coli, Proteus* spp, *K pneumoniae*	Quinolone x 4-6 weeks **or** TMP-SMX x 4-6 weeks

Clinical presentation

- Primary syphilis presents as a painless lesion or chancre appearing at the site of infection around 21 days after exposure. These lesions persist for about 8 weeks before spontaneously disappearing. Secondary syphilis develops 2-6 weeks after the onset of the primary stage. It is characterized by a variety of rashes and flu-like symptoms. These symptoms disappear without treatment within 4-10 weeks. Untreated patients will develop symptoms of tertiary syphilis within 2-25 years after infection. These include general paresis, nerve deafness, progressive dementia, and aortic insufficiency.

- Gonorrhea, in contrast, presents as a urethritis within 2-3 days of exposure. Dysuria, urinary frequency, and purulent discharge are common. The majority of infected patients become asymptomatic without treatment within 6 months. About 15% of infected women will develop pelvic inflammatory disease, which can be an indirect cause of infertility.

Diagnostic criteria

- Since *T pallidum* cannot be grown in culture, dark-field or indirect fluorescent antibody microscopic examination is used in conjunction with serologic testing for diagnosis. The most common tests are the Venereal Disease Research Laboratory (VDRL) and the rapid plasma reagin (RPR) tests. Gonorrhea is diagnosed by Gram stain and culture of infected secretions. Alternative methods of diagnosis include enzyme immunoassay and DNA probes. Patients should be screened for the presence of other venereal diseases.

Treatment

- Due to the potential of both diseases to cause significant morbidity to infants born to infected mothers, diagnosis and treatment of pregnant women is of concern. The two organisms differ sharply in resistance to anti-infective agents. *Treponema pallidum* is sensitive to penicillin and has not developed any significant resistance. *Neisseria gonorrhoeae* has not only developed significant resistance to penicillin, but fluoroquinolones as well, leaving third-generation cephalosporins as the major treatment modality (Table 9). Patients diagnosed with gonorrhea should also receive therapy against chlamydial infection (usually doxycycline 100 mg bid x 7 days or azithromycin 1 g once). All sexual partners must also be treated.

Sepsis

- Sepsis has been defined by the American College of Chest Physicians as the systemic inflammatory response syndrome (SIRS) produced in response to infection. SIRS has been defined as requiring two of the following criteria: T >38°C or <36°C; HR >90 bpm; RR >20 breaths/min or $PaCO_2$ <32 torr; WBC >12,000 cells/mm^3 or <4000 cells/mm^3, or >10% immature (band) forms.

Causative agents

- Sepsis may be caused by a variety of organisms, including gram-negative and gram-positive organisms, as well as fungi. Most cases occur in the setting of hospitalized patients and reflect the organisms and resistance pattern of the institution.

Clinical presentation

- In the early phase, the patient may have fever or hypothermia, rigors, chills, tachycardia, tachypnea, hyperglycemia, and lethargy, progressing to hypotension, hypoglycemia, myocardial depression, oliguria, leukopenia, and pulmonary edema leading to multisystem organ failure.

Table 9

Treatment for Syphilis and Gonorrhea

Type	Syphilis	Gonorrhea
Uncomplicated adult presentation	Benzathine penicillin G 2.4 million units IM x 1	Ceftriaxone 125 mg IM x 1 **or** Spectinomycin 2 g IM q12h x 2
Infant born of untreated mother	Penicillin G 50,000-75,000 U/kg q12h x 10-21 days	Cefotaxime 25 mg/kg q12h x 7 days
Disseminated infections	***Secondary/latent disease:*** benzathine penicillin G 2.4 million units IM q week x 3 ***Tertiary disease:*** penicillin G 2-4 million units q4h for 10-14 days	Ceftriaxone 1 g qd x 10 days

Diagnostic criteria
- In addition to physical signs and symptoms, cultures of blood, urine, and sputum may yield clues for antibacterial therapy.

Treatment
- Local organisms and sensitivities will determine anti-infective therapy. Initial therapy should be broad, covering all likely organisms, until culture results are obtained. The *Medical Letter* suggests the following regimens for life-threatening sepsis in adults: cefotaxime, ceftriaxone, cefepime, ticarcillin-clavulanic acid, piperacillin-tazobactam, meropenem, or imipenem with an aminoglycoside (tobramycin, gentamicin, or amikacin). If gram-positive organisms are suspected, vancomycin may be added to the regimen.

Systemic Febrile Syndromes Spread by Ticks (Lyme Disease, Rocky Mountain Spotted Fever, Ehrlichiosis, Tularemia)

- These diseases are similar in transmission and natural history. The organisms responsible for these infections are *Rickettsia*, known for their intracellular growth in host cells. As such, they cannot be grown in culture media, and serologic tests are used for diagnosis. Patients present with fever, rash, and flu-like symptoms, with a history of tick exposure.

Treatment
- See Table 10

Systemic Fungal Infections

- Fungal infections fall into two categories: primary, able to cause infection in both healthy and immunocompromised patients, and opportunistic, able to cause infection only in immunocompromised patients. Many fungal infections have a pulmonary focus, due to the aerosol spread of mold spores. Due to increasing use of antibacterial agents and the increase in immunocompromised patients, the incidence of fungal infection is rising.

Clinical presentation
- Patients present with a gradual onset of general malaise, fever, and weakness, unrelieved by antibacterial therapy. Pulmonary infection presents with pneumonia-like symptoms.

Diagnostic criteria
- Diagnosis is made from patient history, cultures (usually blood, sputum, and biopsy of lesions), and serologic tests.

Treatment
- Treatment is often empiric, until the organism is isolated (Table 11). Due to the relatively slow culture of most fungi, and the lack of commercial testing against antifungal agents, patient response is used to determine resistance to therapy.

Viral Infections (Hepatitis, Influenza, Herpes Simplex Family)

Note: Antiviral therapy is not curative, but decreases the level of virus so that a patient's immune system can handle the infection.

Hepatitis
- Hepatitis is a general term referring to a generalized inflammation of the liver. Etiologies may be viral or chemical.

Causative agents
- Five viruses (hepatitis types A-E) have been identified as causative agents for hepatitis. Syndromes may be either acute or chronic.

Clinical presentation
- Patients present with a history of anorexia, nausea, fatigue, and malaise. This usually progresses to fever, right upper quadrant pain, dark urine, light

Table 10

Treatment of Tick-Borne Diseases

Disease	Causative agent	Primary treatment	Alternative treatment
Lyme disease	*Borrelia burgdorferi*	Doxycycline	Cefuroxime
Rocky Mountain spotted fever	*Rickettsia rickettsii*	Doxycycline	Chloramphenicol
Ehrlichiosis	*Ehrlichia phagocytophila*	Doxycycline	Tetracycline
Tularemia	*Francisella tularensis*	Gentamicin or tobramycin	Chloramphenicol; possibly ciprofloxacin

Table 11

Treatment of Systemic Fungal Infections

Disease	Organism	Treatment(s)
Invasive pulmonary disease	*Aspergillosis* spp	Amphotericin B, itraconazole, caspofungin, voriconazole
Cutaneous, pulmonary or extrapulmonary	*Blastomyces dermatitidis*	Itraconazole, amphotericin B, fluconazole
Bloodstream infection	*Candida albicans*	Fluconazole, amphotericin B
Primary pulmonary disease	*Coccidioides immitis*	Itraconazole, fluconazole
Meningitis	*Cryptococcus neoformans*	Amphotericin B + flucytosine, fluconazole
Pulmonary, disseminated, or localized	*Histoplasma capsulatum*	Itraconazole (moderate disease); amphotericin B (severe disease)

colored stools, and worsening of systemic symptoms. Some patients have no symptoms, and little hepatic damage.

Diagnostic criteria
• In addition to physical signs, laboratory tests are remarkable for elevations in AST, ALT, and serum bilirubin.

Treatment
• Treatment is dependent upon the viral strain and type of presentation (Table 12). Standard therapies have not been established for hepatitis A, D, or E.

Influenza
• Influenza is an acute respiratory viral infection.

Causative agents
• Three viruses, influenza A, B, and C, are responsible for most infections.

Clinical presentation
• Patients present with sudden onset of chills, fever, severe prostration, headache, muscle aches, and a cough that usually is dry and may be followed by secondary bacterial infections.

Diagnostic criteria
• Diagnosis is from patient physical signs and symptoms.

Therapy
• Therapy may be either prophylactic or treatment and is determined by viral strain in the community (Table 13). Currently, no therapies exist for influenza C infections.

**Herpes simplex family
(herpes, cytomegalovirus [CMV], chickenpox/shingles)**
• The herpes simplex family is responsible for three serious viral infections: herpes genital infections, cytomegalovirus infections in the immunocompromised, and varicella-zoster infections (chickenpox/shingles).

Causative agents
• Each disease is caused by a slightly different herpes virus.

Table 12

Treatment for Hepatitis

Organism	Presentation	Therapy
Hepatitis B	Chronic	Lamivudine + interferon alfa-2b
Hepatitis C	Chronic	Interferon alfa-2b + ribavirin
Hepatitis C	Acute	Interferon alfa-2b

Table 13

Treatment for Influenza

Organism	Treatment type	Therapy
Influenza A	Prophylaxis	Oseltamivir, rimantadine, amantadine
Influenza A	Treatment	Zanamivir, oseltamivir, rimantadine, amantadine
Influenza B	Prophylaxis	Oseltamivir
Influenza B	Prophylaxis	Zanamivir, oseltamivir

Clinical presentation

- Varies by disease:
  - * Genital herpes presents with flu-like symptoms of fever, headache, malaise, and myalgias, in addition to development of painful pustular or ulcerative lesions on the external genitalia.
  - * CMV usually presents as retinitis, colitis, or esophagitis.
  - * Varicella zoster presents with flu-like symptoms with pustular rash located on body dermatomes.

Diagnostic criteria

- Mostly from signs and symptoms, although tissue samples may be examined for the presence of the virus by immunofluorescence.

Treatment

- Depends upon viral and disease state; treatment is summarized in Table 14.

3. Key Points

- The hallmark of initial anti-infective therapy is to target the specific organisms associated with the disease.

- Conversely, after the identification of the organism causing the disease, anti-infective therapy should be narrowed to cover that specific organism.

- Therapy should reflect not only the best anti-infective agent for the organism, but also should reflect aspects of the patient's condition (eg, renal function, concurrent disease states).

- Combination anti-infective therapy should be reserved for documented clinical efficacy, therapeutic failure on monotherapy, and polymicrobial infection.

- Clinical signs of infection should be followed to determine patient response to therapy.

- Empiric therapy of meningitis is age specific, reflecting the age-specific nature of the common pathogens.

- Endocarditis therapy is specific to the organism isolated. The presence of a prosthetic valve increases the time for therapy.

- Many cases of bronchitis are viral in etiology, making routine antibiotic therapy controversial.

- Empiric pneumonia therapy reflects both coverage of age-related organisms and organisms associated with patient-specific risk factors.

Table 14

Treatment of Herpes Virus Infections

Organism	Disease	Treatment
Herpes simplex	Initial episode	Acyclovir
	Reoccurrence	Famciclovir
	Chronic suppression	Valacyclovir
	Immunocompromised	Acyclovir
	Resistant to acyclovir	Foscarnet
Cytomegalovirus	Retinitis, colitis, esophagitis	Ganciclovir, valganciclovir, foscarnet, cidofovir, fomivirsen
Varicella zoster	Chickenpox, shingles	Acyclovir
Varicella zoster	Immunocompromised, resistant to acyclovir	Foscarnet

- Diarrhea therapy should be mainly supportive, with careful use of anti-infectives and antimotility agents.

- Diagnosis of urinary tract infections varies by numbers of organisms found in the urine. Higher numbers ($>10^5$ cells/mL) are needed to diagnose UTIs in females than are needed in males ($>10^3$ cells/mL), due to the higher numbers of organisms able to ascend the shorter female urethra.

- A frequently overlooked aspect of treatment of bacterial venereal disease is treatment of sexual partners.

- Initial therapy of sepsis should be broad in scope, covering all likely organisms, until results of cultures are obtained.

- Due to the long doubling time of most fungi, and the difficulty in obtaining sensitivity to specific antifungal agents, patient response is used to determine resistance to therapy.

- Antiviral therapy is not curative, but decreases the level of virus so that a patient's immune system can handle the infection.

4. Questions and Answers

1. The lowest concentration of anti-infective that prevent microbial growth is called

   A. Minimum bactericidal concentration
   B. Minimum bacteriostatic concentration
   C. Minimum inhibitory concentration
   D. Minimum inhibiting concentration
   E. Minimum schillings concentration

2. Laboratory markers of infections, such as C-reactive protein, white blood count, and erythrocyte sedimentation rate may not be accurate in which patient populations?

   I. Elderly patients
   II. Patients with chronic obstructive pulmonary disease
   III. Malnourished patients

   A. I only
   B. II only
   C. I and III only
   D. II and III only
   E. I, II, and III

3. The hallmark of empiric therapy is

   A. Coverage of the most common pathogen associated with the infection
   B. Coverage of the common pathogens associated with the infection
   C. Coverage of all possible pathogens associated with the infection
   D. Coverage of polymicrobial pathogens associated with the infection
   E. Coverage of all viral organisms associated with the infection

4. When two anti-infective therapies together produce a greater effect than the effects of each added together, this is termed

   A. Commensalism
   B. Synergy
   C. Antagonism
   D. Additive
   E. Interacting

5. Analysis of the cerebrospinal fluid may give valuable clues to the identity of the pathogen in meningitis. Given the following results, what would be indicative of a fungal infection?

I.   Increase in WBCs
II. Decreased glucose
III Increased protein

A. I only
B. II only
C. I and III only
D. II and III only
E. I, II, and III

6. Empiric therapy for meningitis for patients up to 1 month of age includes

A. Vancomycin and ampicillin
B. Aminoglycoside and ampicillin
C. Ceftriaxone and vancomycin
D. Vancomycin and aminoglycoside
E. Ampicillin and ceftriaxone

7. When treating penicillin-allergic patients for endocarditis, _____ may be used for therapy.

A. Vancomycin
B. Erythromycin
C. Cefazolin
D. Meropenem
E. Nafcillin

8. Patients presenting with acute bronchitis without risk factors should be treated empirically with

A. Supportive care
B. Clarithromycin
C. Cefuroxime
D. Ciprofloxacin
E. Erythromycin

9. The most common organism(s) associated with community-acquired pneumonia in adults are

A. *Chlamydia pneumoniae, Mycoplasma pneumoniae, Haemophilus influenzae*
B. *Streptococcus pneumoniae, Haemophilus influenzae, Chlamydia pneumoniae*
C. *Mycoplasma pneumoniae, Chlamydia pneumoniae, Streptococcus pneumoniae*
D. *Mycoplasma pneumoniae, Streptococcus pneumoniae, Haemophilus influenzae*
E. *Chlamydia pneumoniae, Staphylococcus aureus, Haemophilus influenzae*

10. Empiric therapy for patients with hospital-acquired pneumonia should include

A. Tobramycin and gentamicin

B. Cefotaxime and cefepime
C. Vancomycin and gentamicin
D. Gentamicin and cefepime
E. Cefepime and vancomycin

11. Treatment of latent tuberculosis infections where isoniazid-resistant strains of *Mycobacterium tuberculosis* are predominant should include

A. Rifabutin and pyrazinamide
B. Rifampin and pyrazinamide
C. Isoniazid, rifampin, and pyrazinamide
D. Isoniazid, rifabutin, and pyrazinamide
E. Ethambutol and rifampin

12. The use of antimotility agents in infectious diarrhea is

A. Discouraged, due to the potential to cause toxic megacolon
B. Encouraged, due to increased cure rates
C. Discouraged, due to increased reinfections
D. Encouraged, due to decreased reinfections
E. Discouraged, due to lack of efficacy

13. Cellulitis is usually associated with

A. *Staphylococcus aureus*
B. *Streptococcus bovis*
C. *Peptostreptococcus boydii*
D. *Escherichia coli*
E. *Klebsiella pneumoniae*

14. The best empiric regimen to treat prostate infection is

A. Ciprofloxacin for 10 days
B. TMP-SMX for 10 days
C. Ciprofloxacin and TMP-SMX for 10 days
D. Ciprofloxacin for 4-6 weeks
E. TMP-SMX for 4-6 weeks

15. Tertiary syphilis in adults should be treated with

A. Benzathine penicillin 2.4 million units x 1
B. Penicillin 50,000 U/kg q12h x 10-21 days
C. Penicillin 4 million units q4h x 10-14 days
D. Benzathine penicillin 2.4 million units q week x 3
E. Penicillin 150,000 U/kg q12h x 10-21 days

16. *Candida albicans* infections may be treated with

A. Itraconazole
B. Amphotericin B
C. Voriconazole

D. Caspofungin
E. Ketoconazole

17. The antiviral agent with the widest spectrum of activity against influenza is:

   A. Zanamivir
   B. Rimantadine
   C. Amantadine
   D. Oseltamivir
   E. Amantadine

18. Herpes infections resistant to acyclovir may be treated with

   A. Famciclovir
   B. Valacyclovir
   C. Foscarnet
   D. Ganciclovir
   E. High-dose acyclovir

19. The only organism below that can be easily cultured is

   A. *Treponema pallidum*
   B. *Mycobacterium tuberculosis*
   C. *Rickettsia rickettsii*
   D. *Ehrlichia phagocytophila*
   E. *Francisella tularensis*

20. Anti-infective therapy should always be used with infectious diarrhea caused by which organism?

   A. *Escherichia coli*
   B. *Vibrio cholerae*
   C. *Staphylococcus aureus*
   D. *Salmonella*
   E. *Bacillus cereus*

21. J.B. is an 18-year-old WF who just gave birth to her first child. Since she presented without any prenatal care or history, a full prenatal panel of tests including a vaginal swab was taken. Two days after birth, she complained of a purulent vaginal discharge and low-grade fever. Blood cultures were negative, but the vaginal swab revealed the presence of gram-negative cocci. WBCs are elevated at 13,000 cells/mm^3. What is the probable infection that JB has?

   A. Herpes simplex
   B. Gonorrhea
   C. Syphilis
   D. Urinary tract infection
   E. Food poisoning

22. What should be done for J.B. and her baby?

   A. Both mother and child should be treated
   B. Neither mother nor child should be treated
   C. The child should be treated, but the mother should not
   D. The mother should be treated, but the child should not
   E. Mother, child, and partner should be treated

23. L.B. is a 45-year-old white female presenting to the ER with a fever of 103°F, flank pain, dysuria, urgency, and frequency. Her laboratory is significant for an increased WBC of 18,000 mm3/mL and 3% immature forms (bands). Her urinalysis revealed >105 cells/mL of gram-negative rods. What does L.B. have?

   A. Herpes simplex
   B. Gonorrhea
   C. Syphilis
   D. Urinary tract infection
   E. Food poisoning

24. What therapy would be useful for L.B.?

   A. Oral quinolone
   B. IV quinolone
   C. Oral penicillin
   D. IV carbapenem
   E. IV vancomycin

Answers

1. **C.** The minimum inhibitory concentration determines the level of anti-infective to which dosing regimens may be set.

2. **C.** Each of these groups of patients may not be able to respond with appropriate laboratory markers of infections, due to limited reserves or deletion of inflammatory factors.

3. **B.** Coverage of common pathogens associated with the infection increases the probability of curing the infection without increasing anti-infective exposure to other organisms, increasing the possibility of resistance.

4. **B.**

5. **E.** Although fungal CNS infections show relatively slight changes in WBCs, protein, and glucose compared to bacterial infections, the trend is similar.

6. **E.** This regimen covers the most likely organism(s) for meningitis in this age group: gram-negative enterics, such as *E coli*, group B streptococci, and *Listeria monocytogenes*.

7. **A.** Vancomycin covers all gram-positive organisms associated with endocarditis, with no cross-sensitivity to penicillin.

8. **A.** Since half of bronchitis infections are caused by a viral etiology, antibacterial therapy for low-risk patients should not be attempted, with the exception of severe presentation.

9. **D.** Chlamydia pneumoniae is not a pathogen associated with adult pneumonia.

10. **D.** Empiric therapy for hospital-acquired pneumonia should have an aminoglycoside and one other gram-negative agent, such as cefepime. Vancomycin can be added if MRSA is suspected.

11. **B.** Latent infections are usually treated with isoniazid alone. In the case of isoniazid-resistant TB, rifampin and pyrazinamide are effective at treating latent infections. The three-drug regimens are used to treat active disease.

12. **A.** Use of such agents increase the chance of intestinal perforation and increases the length of symptoms.

13. **A.** Most cellulitis infections are associated with *Staphylococcus aureus* and *Streptococcus pyogenes*.

14. **D.** Prostate infections are difficult to treat, requiring 4-6 weeks of therapy. Although TMP-SMX is a reasonable choice to treat most prostate infections, ciprofloxacin is preferred due to its ability to concentrate in prostate fluid.

15. **C.** Due to the organism load of tertiary syphilis, high doses of penicillin G are needed for clinical cure. B and E are congenital syphilis doses for neonates.

16. **B.** Voriconazole and caspofungin have activity against *Candida*, but have not yet been tested in a variety of settings. Ketoconazole and itraconazole should not be used for serious *Candida* infections. Amphotericin B and fluconazole are currently recommended for *Candida*.

17. **D.** Oseltamivir may be used for either treatment or prophylaxis against both influenza A and B.

18. **C.** Foscarnet has activity against acyclovir-resistant herpes.

19. **B.** *Mycobacterium tuberculosis*, although very slow growing, can be grown on culture media. The remaining organisms cannot be grown without use of cell culture techniques, forcing the clinician to rely on serum testing and direct staining for identification of the organism.

20. **B.** *Staphylococcus* and *Bacillus* diarrhea is an intoxication, not caused by a living organism. Both *Salmonella* and *E coli* diarrheas should not be treated unless severe, or signs of systemic infection are present. *Vibrio cholerae* causes a severe diarrhea requiring anti-infective treatment.

21. **B.** Given the lack of prenatal care, physical signs and symptoms, and presence of gram-negative cocci, J.B. most probably has gonorrhea.

22. **E.** Mother, partner, and child should be treated. J.B. and her partner should receive ceftriaxone 125 mg IM x 1 and treatment for concurrent chlamydial infection (doxycycline 100 mg bid x 7 days). The child should receive cefotaxime 25 mg/kg q12h x 7 days. Both mother and child should be screened for additional sexually transmitted diseases.

23. **D.** Given the clinical presentation and laboratory, L.B. has a severe urinary tract infection. The presence of systemic symptoms (fever and chills) suggests an upper urinary tract infection or pyelonephritis.

24. **B.** Given the severity of disease, parenteral therapy would be reasonable for initial therapy. Since the Gram stain of the urine revealed gram-negative rods, either a quinolone or extended-spectrum penicillin in combination with an aminoglycoside would be reasonable empiric therapy until the organism was identified and sensitivities obtained.

5. References

Many general references will provide basic information concerning anti-infective therapy. A good brief yearly review of antibacterial and antiviral therapies is published by *The Medical Letter* (www.medletter. com). Listed here are recent practice guidelines in areas of infectious disease.

Endocarditis
Wilson WR, Karchmer AW, Dajani AS, et al. Antibiotic treatment of adults with infective endocarditis due to streptococci, enterococci, and staphylococci, and HACEK microorganisms. *JAMA.* 1995;274:1706-1713.

Pneumonia
Bartlett JG, Dowell SF, Mandell LA, et al. Practice guidelines for the management of community-acquired pneumonia in adults. Infectious Diseases Society of America. *Clin Infect Dis.* 2000;31:347-382.

Tuberculosis
Horsburgh CR, Feldman S, Ridzon R. Practice guidelines for the treatment of tuberculosis. *Clin Infect Dis.* 2000;31:633-639.

Infectious diarrhea
Diagnosis and management of food borne illnesses: a primer for physicians. *MMWR Recomm Rep.* 2001;50(RR-2):1-69.

Guerrant RL, Van Gilder T, Steiner TS, et al. Practice guidelines for the management of infectious diarrhea. *Clin Infect Dis.* 2001;32:331-351.

Urinary tract infections
Warren JW, Abrutyn E, Hebel JR, et al. Guidelines for antimicrobial treatment of uncomplicated acute bacterial cystitis and acute pyelonephritis in women. Infectious Diseases Society of America (IDSA). *Clin Infect Dis.* 1999;29:745-758.

Sexually transmitted diseases
Centers for Disease Control and Prevention. Diseases characterized by urethritis and cervicitis. Sexually transmitted diseases treatment guidelines. *MMWR Recomm Rep.* 2002;51(RR-6):30-42.

Centers for Disease Control and Prevention. Diseases characterized by genital ulcers. Sexually transmitted diseases treatment guidelines. *MMWR Recomm Rep.* 2002;51(RR-6):11-25.

Centers for Disease Control and Prevention. Vaccine preventable STDs. Sexually transmitted diseases treatment guidelines. *MMWR Recomm Rep.* 2002;51(RR-6):59-64.

Sepsis
American College of Chest Physicians/Society of Critical Care Medicine Consensus Conference. Definitions for sepsis and organ failure and guideline for the use of innovative therapies in sepsis. *Crit Care Med.* 1992;20:864-874.

Practice guidelines for evaluating new fever in critically ill adult patients. *Crit Care Med.* 1998;26:392-408.

Tick-borne disease
Wormser GP, Nadelman RB, Dattwyler RJ, et al. Practice guidelines for the treatment of Lyme disease. *Clin Infect Dis.* 2000;31(Suppl 1):1-14.

Fungal infections
Chapman SW, Bradsher RW, Campbell GD, Pappas PG, Kauffman CA. Practice guidelines for the management of patients with blastomycosis. Infectious Diseases Society of America. *Clin Infect Dis.* 2000;30:679-683.

Rex JH, Walsh TJ, Sobel JD, et al. Practice guidelines for the treatment of candidiasis. Infectious Diseases Society of America. *Clin Infect Dis.* 2000;30:662-678.

Saag MS, Graybill RJ, Larsen RA, et al. Practice guidelines for the management of cryptococcal disease. Infectious Diseases Society of America. *Clin Infect Dis.* 2000;30:710-718.

Stevens DA, Kan VL, Judson MA, et al. Practice guidelines for diseases caused by *Aspergillus.* Infectious Diseases Society of America. *Clin Infect Dis.* 2000;30:696-709.

Viral infections
Association for Genitourinary Medicine (AGUM), Medical Society for the Study of Venereal Disease (MSSVD). 2002 National guideline for the management of genital herpes. London: AGUM, MSSVD; 2002.

Association for Genitourinary Medicine (AGUM), Medical Society for the Study of Venereal Disease (MSSVD). 2002 National guideline on the management of the viral hepatitides A, B, and C. London: AGUM, MSSVD; 2002.

Bridges CB, Fukuda K, Uyeki TM, Cox NJ, Singleton JA. Prevention and control of influenza. Recommendations of the Advisory Committee on Immunization Practices (ACIP). *MMWR Recomm Rep.* 2002;51(RR-03):1-31.

30. Anti-Infective Agents

Ronald L. Braden, PharmD
Associate Professor, Department of Pharmacy
University of Tennessee College of Pharmacy
Clinical Pharmacy Specialist–Critical Care
Veterans Affairs Medical Center, Memphis, Tennessee

Contents

1. Aminoglycosides

Aminoglycosides are antibiotics active against most aerobic gram-negative bacteria and select aerobic gram-positive bacteria, but they are not effective against most anaerobic bacteria. Aminoglycosides are primarily used in serious infections due to their significant toxicity. The most commonly used aminoglycosides include amikacin, kanamycin, gentamicin, neomycin, netilmicin, streptomycin, and tobramycin.

Mechanism of Action

* Aminoglycosides inhibit bacterial protein synthesis through binding to the 30S ribosomal subunit, thereby irreversibly inhibiting bacterial RNA synthesis. Aminoglycosides are bactericidal.

Spectrum of Activity

* Amikacin is a semisynthetic parenteral aminoglycoside with the broadest antimicrobial activity of the class, and it frequently possesses activity against bacteria resistant to other aminoglycosides.

* Kanamycin is a minimally absorbed oral aminoglycoside used to decrease bacterial content of the bowel. Kanamycin has been used for preoperative bowel preparation and as an adjunct in hepatic encephalopathy.

* Gentamicin is a parenteral aminoglycoside which is more active against *Acinetobacter, Serratia,* and enterococci than tobramycin.

* Neomycin: see kanamycin.

* Netilmicin is a parenteral aminoglycoside which may be the least ototoxic aminoglycoside.

* Streptomycin is a parenteral aminoglycoside active against enterococci, streptococci, mycobacteria, and some gram-negative anaerobes. Streptomycin is used as an adjunct agent only because many bacterial isolates are resistant to streptomycin monotherapy. Streptomycin should only be administered by IM injection.

* Tobramycin is a parenteral aminoglycoside that is more active against *Pseudomonas* than gentamicin.

Adverse Drug Events

* Nephrotoxicity is demonstrated by an increase in blood urea nitrogen (BUN) and serum creatinine.

The nephrotoxicity is usually manifest as nonoliguric renal failure and may cause potassium, calcium, and magnesium wasting. Nephrotoxicity may occur in 10-25% of patients receiving aminoglycosides and is usually reversible upon discontinuation of the agent. Risk factors include:
* Pre-existing renal dysfunction
* Prolonged duration of therapy
* Concomitant use of other nephrotoxic agents
* Possibly elevated trough concentrations:
  * Gentamicin and tobramycin <2 µg/mL
  * Amikacin < 8 µg/mL

* Neuromuscular blockade is an uncommon but potentially serious toxicity. Risk factors include:
  * Concomitant use of neuromuscular blocking agents
  * Myasthenia gravis
  * Hypocalcemia
  * Elevated peak serum concentrations

* Ototoxicity is due to eighth cranial nerve damage demonstrated by auditory and vestibular symptoms. Auditory symptoms include tinnitus and loss of high-frequency hearing. Vestibular toxicity is demonstrated by dizziness, nystagmus, vertigo, and ataxia. The incidence of ototoxicity is not clearly known since profound high-frequency hearing loss can occur prior to detection.

Pharmacokinetics

* Aminoglycosides are renally eliminated.
  * $t_{1/2}$ = 2.5-2.7 hours (normal renal function)
  * $t_{1/2}$ = ~69 hours (anephric clearance)
  * Vd = 0.27-0.3 L/kg (IBW)

Target serum concentrations (traditional dosing; Table 1)
  * Amikacin peak = 15-30 µg/mL
  * Amikacin trough = <5 µg/mL
  * Gentamicin and tobramycin peak = 4-10 µg/mL
  * Gentamicin and tobramycin trough = <2 µg/mL

Extended interval dosing
  * Amikacin trough = <3 µg/mL
  * Gentamicin and tobramycin = <1 µg/mL

Table 1

Aminoglycosides

Generic name	Trade name	Dosage forms	Normal dose	Elimination
Amikacin	Amikin®	IV, IM	15 mg/kg per day	Renal
Gentamicin	Garamycin®	IV, IM	3 mg/kg per day conventional dose, 7 mg/kg per day extended interval	Renal
Kanamycin		IV, PO	15 mg/kg per day	Renal
Neomycin		PO	50-100 mg/kg per day	Renal
Netilmicin		IV, IM	3-6 mg/kg per day	Renal
Streptomycin		IM	15 mg/kg per day	Renal
Tobramycin		IV, IM	3 mg/kg per day conventional dose, 7 mg/kg per day extended interval	Renal

Note: Use ideal body weight for all aminoglycoside dosing.

2. Penicillins

Mechanism of Action

- Penicillin binding proteins (PBPs) make up the cell wall. When penicillin binds to these PBPs, it is able to inhibit cell wall synthesis in the bacteria, causing cell wall lysis and ultimately cell death.

- Bactericidal (they inhibit bacterial cell wall synthesis).

- They are known as β-lactam antibiotics because their chemical structure consists of a β-lactam ring adjoined to a thiazolidine ring.

- Penicillinase-resistant penicillins: Substitutions to the β-lactam ring sterically inhibit penicillinase.

Spectrum of Activity and Dosing

See Tables 2 and 3.

Adverse Drug Events

- Allergic/hypersensitivity reaction in 3-10% of patients. Rash (4-8%) to anaphylaxis (0.01-0.05%) can occur within 10-20 minutes; IV > PO.

- GI: nausea and vomiting with PO use

- Neurologic reactions (seizures) are seen with high doses of penicillin given to patients with renal insufficiency.

- Hypokalemia, hypernatremia (carboxypenicillins; carbenicillin > ticarcillin).

- Increased transaminases: oxacillin, nafcillin, carbenicillin.

- Cholestatic jaundice: ureidopenicillins

- Hematologic reactions (hemolytic anemia)

- Interstitial nephritis

Drug-Drug Interactions

- Probenecid increases blood levels of natural penicillins and may be given with them for this purpose.

- Aminoglycosides: either incompatible or synergism.

- Oral contraceptives: concomitant use may decrease the effectiveness of oral contraceptives and increase incidence of breakthrough bleeding.

Table 2

Spectrum of Activity of the Penicillins

Category	Spectrum
Natural penicillins	Effective against all viridans streptococci, S pyogenes, and 60% of S pneumoniae, mouth anaerobes and Clostridium perfringens (gas gangrene) Because natural penicillins are readily hydrolyzed by penicillinases (β-lactamases), they are ineffective against S aureus and other organisms that resist penicillin Penicillin G is 5-10 times more active than penicillin V against gram-negative organisms and some anaerobic organisms
Penicillinase-resistant penicillins	Methicillin-sensitive staphylococci, streptococci (not enterococci species)
Aminopenicillins	Greater penetration of outer membrane of gram-negative rods and higher affinity for PBPs Cover most enterococci, Listeria, Proteus mirabilis Cover 60% of Streptococcus pneumoniae, Haemophilus influenzae, Escherichia coli, some Salmonella and Shigella
Carboxypenicillins and ureidopenicillins	Spectrum like ampicillin, but less gram-positive coverage; covers Proteus (including P vulgaris), Klebsiella (not ticarcillin), Enterobacter, Pseudomonas (piperacillin > ticarcillin); add an aminoglycoside for synergy for serious gram-negative infections Ureidopenicillins possess better in vitro activity against Pseudomonas and other gram-negative organisms Ureidopenicillins have in vitro activity against streptococci, enterococci, most Enterobacteriaceae, Pseudomonas, and many anaerobes, including Bacteroides fragilis, Fusobacterium, Clostridium, and peptostreptococci; β-lactamase–producing staphylococci and H influenzae are resistant to the ureidopenicillins
β-Lactamase inhibitors (clavulanic acid, sulbactam, and tazobactam)	Active against some chromosomally produced β-lactamases of S aureus, H influenzae, Moraxella catarrhalis, Bacteroides, E coli, and other Enterobacteriaceae Not active against the chromosomally produced beta-lactamases of Enterobacter, Citrobacter, Serratia, and Pseudomonas
Amoxicillin-clavulanic acid	H influenzae, M catarrhalis, Klebsiella pneumoniae, MSSA, anaerobes
Ticarcillin-clavulanic acid	More activity against H influenzae, M catarrhalis, Klebsiella pneumoniae, MSSA, anaerobes
Piperacillin-tazobactam	More gram-positive, gram-negative, and anaerobic coverage than ticarcillin-clavulanic acid; monotherapy treatment failures against Pseudomonas

Other characteristics

- Nafcillin and oxacillin: primarily biliary excretion, therefore do not have to adjust for renal dysfunction.

- Penicillin G benzathine: repository drug formulation. Given IM, insoluble salt allows slow drug absorption from the injection site, and therefore it has a longer duration of action (12-24 h).

Table 3

Dosing of Penicillins

Type and generic name	Trade name	Elimination route	Administration route	Common doses
Natural penicillins				
Penicillin G	Pfizerpen®	Renal	IV, IM, PO	2-4 million units IV q4h
Penicillin G procaine	Wycillin®	Renal	IM	300,000-600,000 U/d
Penicillin G benzathine	Bicillin LA®	Renal	IM	Strep throat: 1.2 million units; syphilis: 2.4 million units
Penicillin V (phenoxymethyl penicillin)	Pen-Vee K®; Veetids®	Renal	PO	250-500 mg PO bid-qid (250 mg bid for prophylaxis)
Penicillinase-resistant penicillins				
Methicillin[1]	Staphcillin®	Renal	IV, IM	1-2 g IV q4-6h
Oxacillin	Prostaphilin®, Bactocill®[1]	Hepatic	PO, IV, IM	1-2 g IV q4-6h
Nafcillin	Nafcil®, Unipen®	Hepatic	IV, IM	1-2 g IV q4-6h
Cloxacillin	Cloxapen®	Renal	PO	200-500 mg q6h
Dicloxacillin	Dynapen®, Dycill®	Renal	PO	250-500 mg PO q6h
Aminopenicillins				
Ampicillin	Omnipen®, Principen®	Renal	PO, IM, IV	1-2 g IV q6h
Amoxicillin	Amoxil®, Trimox®	Renal	PO	250-500 mg PO q8h
Bacampicillin	Spectrobid®	Renal	PO	400-800 mg q12h
Carboxypenicillins				
Carbenicillin	Geopen®	Renal	IM, IV	1-5 g q4-6h
Ticarcillin	Ticar®	Renal	IV, IM	3-4 g IV q4-6h
Ureidopenicillins				
Azlocillin	Azlin®	Renal	IV, IM	2-4 g IV q4-6h
Mezlocillin	Mezlin®	Renal	IV, IM	1-3 g q4-6h
Piperacillin	Pipracil®	Renal	IV, IM	3-4 g IV q4-6h
Penicillin plus β-lactamase inhibitors				
Amoxicillin-clavulanic acid	Augmentin®	Renal	PO	250-500 mg PO tid, 500-875 mg PO bid
Ampicillin-sulbactam	Unasyn®	Renal	IV, IM	1.5 g or 3g IV q6-8h
Piperacillin-tazobactam	Zosyn®	Renal	IV	3.375 g IV q6h
Ticarcillin-clavulanic acid	Timentin®	Renal	IV	3.1 g IV q4-6h

[1]Discontinued in the United States.

3. Cephalosporins

Cephalosporins are beta-lactam antibiotics that are structurally and pharmacologically similar to penicillins.

Mechanism of Action

- Cephalosporins are bactericidal agents. Antimicrobial activity is achieved via inhibition of mucopeptide synthesis in the bacterial cell wall, which results in the formation of defective cell walls and subsequent cell lysis and cell death.

Spectrum of Activity

- Cephalosporins are broad-spectrum antimicrobial agents; however, the spectrum of activity varies greatly among the individual agents. Thus cephalosporins are grouped into four broad classes, or generations, according to their antimicrobial coverage (Table 4).

First-generation (cefadroxil, cefazolin, cephalexin)
- Gram-positive activity is extensive, including many strains of *Staphylococcus aureus* and *Staphylococcus epidermidis* in addition to *Streptococcus pyogenes* (group A beta-hemolytic streptococci), *Streptococcus agalactiae* (group B streptococci), and *Streptococcus pneumoniae*. First-generation agents are inactive against enterococci, methicillin-resistant staphylococci (MRSA/MRSE), and *Listeria monocytogenes*.

- Gram-negative activity is limited, although some strains of *Escherichia coli*, *Klebsiella pneumoniae*, *Proteus mirabilis*, and *Shigella* may display susceptibility. First-generation agents are inactive against *Haemophilus influenzae*, *Pseudomonas*, *Enterobacter*, *Citrobacter*, *Serratia*, other *Proteus* spp, and anaerobes such as *Bacteroides fragilis*.

Second-generation (cefaclor, cefamandole, cefotetan, cefoxitin, cefprozil, cefuroxime, cefmetazole, loracarbef)
- Gram-positive activity is similar to that of first-generation agents.

- Gram-negative activity of second-generation agents is generally more extensive than that of first-generation agents, including some strains of *Acinetobacter*, *Citrobacter*, *Enterobacter*, *Neisseria*, *Proteus*, and *Serratia*, in addition to *E coli* and *Klebsiella*. Second-generation agents are active against *Haemophilus influenzae*, and some (cefotetan, cefoxitin, cefamandole) also have anaerobic activity. Second-generation agents are inactive against *Pseudomonas*.

Third-generation (cefixime, cefoperazone, cefotaxime, ceftizoxime, ceftriaxone)
- Gram-positive activity is decreased versus first- and second-generation agents.

- Gram-negative activity is extensive, including *Enterobacter*, *Citrobacter*, *Serratia*, *Neisseria*, and *Haemophilus*. Some third-generation agents are active against *Pseudomonas* (ceftazidime, cefoperazone). Anaerobic coverage varies among individual agents.

Fourth-generation (cefepime)
- Gram-positive activity is increased versus third-generation agents. Cefepime is inactive against MRSA, enterococci, and *Listeria*.

- Gram-negative activity is extensive, including enhanced activity against *Pseudomonas* and Enterobacteriaceae that produce inducible β-lactamases.

- The extended spectrum of activity of cefepime is attributed to a more rapid penetration of the outer membrane of gram-negative bacteria. Cefepime is also more resistant to inactivation by β-lactamases.

Adverse Drug Events

- Hypersensitivity: fever, rash, pruritus, urticaria, anaphylaxis, hemolytic anemia

- Gastrointestinal effects: nausea, vomiting, diarrhea

- Nephrotoxicity (rare)

- Seizures: potential risk with high doses in patients with renal impairment

- *Clostridium difficile* colitis

- Bleeding/hypoprothrombinemia (cefoperazone, cefmetazole, cefotetan): this is due to the presence of an N-methylthiotetrazole (NMTT) side chain in the structure of these agents and can be prevented or reversed with administration of vitamin K.

- Blood dyscrasias (rare)

Drug-Drug Interactions

- Disulfiram-like reactions have been reported with ingestion of alcohol during treatment with cephalosporin antibiotics.

- Probenecid competitively inhibits tubular secretion of cephalosporins, resulting in higher serum concentrations.

Drug-Disease Interactions

- All cephalosporins (except cefoperazone) require dosage adjustments in patients with renal insufficiency.

Monitoring Parameters

- Serum concentration monitoring is not necessary.

Table 4

Cephalosporins

Generic name	Trade name	Dosage forms	Dose	Elimination	Notes
First-generation (more gram-positive than gram-negative activity)					
Cefadroxil	Duricef®, Ultracef®	PO	1-2 g/d	Renal	
Cefazolin	Ancef®, Kefzol	IV	250-1000 mg q8h	Renal	
Cephalexin	Keflex®	PO	250-500 mg q6h	Renal	
Cephapirin	Cephadyl®	IV, IM	500-2000 mg q4-6h	Renal	
Cephradine	Anspor®, Velosef®	PO, IV	250-500 mg q6h	Renal	
Second-generation (enhanced gram-negative activity vs. first-generation drugs)					
Cefaclor	Ceclor®	PO	250-500 mg q8h	Renal	
Cefmetazole	Zefazono®	IV	2 g q6-12h	Renal	NMTT side-chain
Cefonicid	Monocid®	IV	1-2 g/d	Renal	
Cefotetan	Cofotan®	IV, IM	1-2 g q12h	Renal	Anaerobic activity, NMTT side-chain
Cefoxitin	Mefoxin®	IV	1-2 g q6-8h	Renal	Anaerobic activity
Cefprozil	Cefzil®	PO	250-500 mg q12-24h	Renal	Anaerobic activity
Cefuroxime	Ceftin®, Zinacef®	IV, IM	750-1500 mg q8h	Renal	
Cefamandole	Mandole®	IV	500-1000 mg q4-8h	Renal	NMTT side-chain
Loracarbef	Lorabid®	PO	200 mg q12h	Renal	Anaerobic activity
Third-generation (more gram-negative than gram-positive activity; CSF penetration)					
Cefixime	Suprax®	PO	400 mg/d	Renal	
Cefdinir	Omnicef®	PO	300 mg q12h	Renal	
Cefoperazone	Cefobid®	IV	2-4 g q12h	Hepatic	NMTT side-chain
Cefotaxime	Claforan®	IV	1-2 g q6-8h	Renal	
Cefpodoxime	Vantin®	PO	100-400 mg q12h	Renal	Anaerobic activity
Ceftazidime	Fortaz®, Tazicef®	IV, IM	1-2 g q8-12h	Renal	Antipseudomonal activity
Ceftibuten	Cedax®	PO	400 mg/d	Renal	
Ceftizoxime	Cefizox®	IV	1-2 g q8-12h	Renal	
Ceftriaxone	Rocephin®	IV, IM	1-2 g/d	Renal	
Fourth-generation (gram-positive and gram-negative activity)					
Cefepime	Maxipime®	IV, IM	1-2 g q12h	Renal	Antipseudomonal activity

[1]Discontinued in the United States.

- Patients should be monitored for clinical response and resolution of infection.

Patient Instructions and Counselling

- Verify that the patient is not allergic to penicillins. Cross-sensitivity with penicillins has been reported in up to 10% of patients receiving cephalosporins. A thorough history should be obtained in any patient with a previous hypersensitivity reaction to any β-lactam antibiotic. In general, cephalosporins should be avoided in these patients.

Other

- Bacterial resistance to cephalosporins may result via production of β-lactamases.

4. Gram-Positive Antibiotics (Table 5)

Linezolid

- Linezolid is a synthetic oxazolidine antibiotic.

Mechanism of action
- Linezolid binds to the 23S ribosomal subunit of the 50S RNA subunit which inhibits bacterial translation.

Spectrum of activity
- Linezolid is bacteriostatic against enterococci and staphylococci and bactericidal against streptococci. Linezolid is active against *Enterococcus faecium* isolates, including VRE, while most *Enterococcus faecalis* isolates are resistant.

Adverse drug effects
- Hematologic effects including myelosuppression (anemia, leukopenia, pancytopenia, and thrombocytopenia) have been reported. Hematologic effects appear to be reversible upon discontinuation of the agent.

- Monoamine oxidase inhibition: linezolid is a weak MAO inhibitor, but caution should be exercised in patients receiving vasopressors.

Quinupristin-Dalfopristin

- Quinupristin-dalfopristin is a semisynthetic streptogramin antibiotic. The combination acts synergistically against gram-positive bacteria.

Mechanism of action
- Quinupristin inhibits late phase protein synthesis, while dalfopristin inhibits early phase protein synthesis through binding to the 50S subunit of bacterial RNA.

Spectrum of activity
- Quinupristin-dalfopristin is bactericidal against staphylococci and streptococci and bacteriostatic against *Enterococcus faecium*, including VRE. Quinupristin-dalfopristin is not active against *Enterococcus faecalis*.

Adverse drug effects
- Thrombophlebitis and severe injection site reactions are common, and some sources recommend administration via a central venous catheter only.

- Hyperbilirubinemia has been reported in up to 25% of patients receiving the agent.

- Arthralgias and myalgias are common, some requiring discontinuation of the agent.

Vancomycin

- Vancomycin is a glycopeptide antibiotic.

Mechanism of action
- Vancomycin binds to the bacterial cell wall, inhibiting peptidoglycan synthesis. This binding occurs at a site different from that of the penicillins. Vancomycin may also inhibit RNA synthesis.

Spectrum of activity
- Vancomycin is active against most gram-positive bacteria including staphylococci (including MRSA), streptococci, enterococci, *Corynebacterium*, and *Clostridium* (including *C difficile*). Vancomycin is bactericidal against all susceptible isolates except enterococci (bacteriostatic). Vancomycin acts synergistically with aminoglycosides against enterococci.

Adverse drug effects
- Nephrotoxicity is manifested by an increase in serum creatinine and BUN. The incidence of nephrotoxicity is not well described, but appears to be low in the absence of concomitant nephrotoxic agents. Renal dysfunction is normally reversible upon discontinuation of the agent, but may be irreversible.

- Ototoxicity is induced by eighth cranial nerve damage and has been reported to cause permanent hearing loss. Vancomycin rarely causes vestibular toxicity. The incidence of ototoxicity appears to be low in the absence of concomitant ototoxic agents.

- Thrombophlebitis is common and requires frequent IV site rotation.

- Histamine release or "red-man syndrome" is a reaction most commonly associated with rapid IV infusion. Histamine reactions can be minimized by slow IV infusion, not to exceed 500 mg/30 min.

Monitoring
- Vancomycin trough concentrations should be monitored in patients with pre-existing renal dysfunction or patients with increased serum creatinine or BUN during therapy. Vancomycin peak concentrations are not routinely required, but may be monitored in patients with serious infections, central nervous system infections, or those patients not responding to therapy.

Table 5

Gram-Positive Antibiotics

Generic name	Trade name	Dosage forms	Dose	Elimination	Notes
Linezolid	Zyvox®	IV, PO	600 mg q12h	Renal	
Quinupristin-dalfopristin	Synercid®	IV	7.5 mg/kg q8h	Hepatic	
Vancomycin	Vancocin®	IV, PO	500 mg q6h or 1 g q12h IV; 125-250 mg PO q6h	Renal	Adjust dose per serum concentrations

Pharmacokinetics

- Vancomycin is renally eliminated.
    * $t_{1/2}$ = 6 hours (normal renal function)
    * $t_{1/2}$ = 7-10 days (anephric patients)
    * Vd = 0.7 L/kg (TBW)
    * Peak concentration = 20-40 µg/mL
    * Trough concentration = 5-10 µg/mL

5. Fluoroquinolones (Table 6)

Quinolones are broad-spectrum antibacterial agents

Mechanism of Action

- Fluoroquinolones are bactericidal agents. The mechanism of action of these agents is not understood entirely, but antimicrobial activity is known to involve inhibition of bacterial DNA topoisomerase and subsequent disruption of bacterial DNA replication.

Spectrum of Activity

- Gram-positive activity includes many strains of staphylococci. Streptococcal activity is variable, and streptococcal resistance to quinolones is increasingly common. Newer fluoroquinolones (sparfloxacin, gatifloxacin, clinafloxacin, moxifloxacin) generally demonstrate superior gram-positive coverage versus older agents (ciprofloxacin, ofloxacin, levofloxacin). Fluoroquinolones have limited enterococcal activity and are inactive against MRSA.

- Gram-negative activity is extensive, including *Escherichia coli, Klebsiella, Enterobacter, Citrobacter, Proteus, Salmonella,* and *Shigella* in addition to *Moraxella catarrhalis* and *Haemophilus influenzae.* Activity against *Pseudomonas aeruginosa* and *Stenotrophomonas maltophilia* varies among individual agents.

- Anaerobic coverage is poor.

- Atypical coverage varies among individual agents. All fluoroquinolones are highly active against *Legionella.* Newer agents have more reliable coverage of *Mycoplasma pneumoniae* and *Chlamydia pneumoniae.*

Table 6

Fluoroquinolones and Nonfluorinated Quinolones

Generic name	Trade name	Dosage forms	Normal dose	Elimination	Notes
Fluoroquinolones					
Ciprofloxacin	Cipro®	IV	400 mg q12h	Renal	Less gram-positive activity, enhanced antipseudomonal activity vs other fluoroquinolones
		PO	500 mg q12h		
Enoxacin	Penetrex®	PO	200-400 mg q12h	Renal	
Gatifloxacin	Tequin®	IV, PO	400 mg q24h	Renal	
Levofloxacin	Levaquin®	IV, PO	500 mg q24h	Renal	
Lomefloxacin	Maxaquin®	PO	400 mg/d	Renal	
Moxifloxacin	Avelox®	PO	400 mg qd	Hepatic	
Norfloxacin	Noroxin®	PO	400 mg bid	Hepatic	
Ofloxacin	Floxin®	PO, IV	100-400 mg/d	Renal	
Sparfloxacin	Zagam®	PO	200 mg q24h	Renal	Enhanced anaerobic activity
Trovafloxacin	Trovan®	IV alatrofloxacin	300 mg q24h	Hepatic/fecal	Gram-negative, gram-positive, atypicals, anaerobes; rarely used due to hepatotoxicity
		PO	200 mg q24h		
Nonfluorinated quinolones					No gram-positive activity; effective only in GU and GI tracts
Cinoxacin	Cinoxacin®/Cinobac®	PO	500 mg bid	Renal	
Nalidixic acid	NegGram®	PO	1 g q6h	Renal	

Adverse Drug Events

- GI: nausea, dyspepsia

- CNS: headache, dizziness, insomnia

- CV: QT prolongation (avoid use in patients with pre-existing QT prolongation)

- Endocrine: hypoglycemia or hyperglycemia

- GU: crystalluria (at high doses with alkaline pH)

- Other: arthropathy, tendinitis, photosensitivity

- Rare: rash, urticaria, leukopenia, hepatotoxicity (trovafloxacin)

Drug-Drug Interactions

- Ciprofloxacin increases theophylline levels. Concomitant use should be avoided, or theophylline levels should be monitored during treatment. Risk of theophylline toxicity is less with other fluoroquinolones.

- Antacids, sucralfate, and divalent or trivalent cations (Ca, Mg, Fe) significantly decrease the absorption of fluoroquinolones. These agents should not be administered for at least 2 hours after each dose of a fluoroquinolone.

- Fluoroquinolones may enhance the effects of oral anticoagulants. PT and INR should be monitored if concomitant therapy cannot be avoided.

- Agents that increase the QT interval (cisapride, class IA or III antiarrhythmics) increase the risk of torsades de pointes. Concomitant use of fluoroquinolones with these agents should be avoided.

Drug-Disease Interactions

- Dosage adjustments should be made for renally-cleared fluoroquinolones when CrCl is less than 40 mL/min.

Monitoring Parameters

- Serum concentrations are not monitored.

- The patient should be monitored for clinical response/resolution of infection.

Kinetics

- Quinolones display concentration-dependent activity and have a post-antibiotic effect against most susceptible organisms.

- Fluoroquinolones have a large volume of distribution and achieve high tissue concentrations in the lung, gallbladder, kidney, prostate, and genital tract.

Patient Instructions and Counselling

- Fluoroquinolones should be avoided in children or pregnant or nursing women due to risk of cartilage erosion in growing bone tissue.

- Do *NOT* take antacids, multivitamins, or other calcium, magnesium, or iron supplements for at least 2 hours after each dose.

6. Macrolides (Table 7)

Mechanism of Action

- Macrolides are bacteriostatic against susceptible organisms. The agents bind to the 50S RNA subunit, thereby inhibiting RNA synthesis.

Spectrum of Activity

- Macrolides, or erythromycins, are active principally against gram-positive organisms including penicillin-resistant streptococci. The macrolides are also effective against *Chlamydia, Mycoplasma, Ureaplasma,* spirochetes, and mycobacteria.

Adverse Drug Events

- Gastrointestinal effects: erythromycins stimulate GI motility, leading to abdominal pain and cramping, nausea, vomiting, and diarrhea. Clarithromycin appears to be the least stimulating to the GI tract.

- Local effects: erythromycin lactobionate is reported to cause venous irritation and thrombophlebitis. The agent should be diluted in at least 250 mL and infused over 30-60 minutes to decrease the venous irritation.

- Cardiac effects: QT interval prolongation and torsades de pointes has been rarely reported with erythromycins. Adequate dilution and slow IV infusion appears to decrease this reaction.

- Ototoxicity: erythromycin has been rarely reported to be ototoxic in doses of 4 g/d or more.

Table 7

Macrolides

Generic name	Trade name	Dosage forms	Normal dose	Elimination	Notes
Azithromycin	Zithromax®	PO, IV	250 mg/d	Hepatic	PO dose = IV dose
Clarithromycin	Biaxin®, Biaxin XL®	PO	250 mg bid	Renal	XL = qd dosing
Erythromycin	Various	PO	250-500 mg q6h	Hepatic	Erythromycin base, ethyl succinate, and stearate
		IV	500-1000 mg q6h	Hepatic	Erythromycin lactobionate

7. Tetracyclines (Table 8)

Mechanism of Action

- Bacteriostatic: inhibit bacterial protein synthesis by reversible binding on the 30S ribosomal subunit and blocking the attachment of transfer RNA to an acceptor site on the messenger RNA ribosomal complex.

Spectrum of Activity

- Tetracyclines are the drugs of choice for infections caused by the following organisms:
  * Respiratory infections: atypical pneumonia (*Mycoplasma pneumoniae, Chlamydia pneumoniae*)
  * Genital infections: *Chlamydia trachomatis*, granuloma inguinale
  * Systemic infections: relapsing fever (*Borrelia recurrentis*), *Vibrio* (*V cholerae, V vulnificus*, and *V parahaemolyticus*)
  * Other infections: methicillin-resistant *Staphylococcus aureus* and *S epidermidis* (minocycline) when vancomycin or other agents are not considered appropriate, *Pasteurella multocida, Mycobacterium marinum, Yersinia pestis, Helicobacter pylori* (in combination with bismuth subsalicylate and metronidazole or clarithromycin)
  * Prophylaxis: mefloquine-resistant *Plasmodium falciparum* malaria

- Doxycycline:
  * *Mycobacterium fortuitum* and *M chelonae*
  * *Streptococcus pneumoniae*

- *Pseudomonas* and *Proteus* organisms are now resistant to tetracyclines

- Used in the treatment of *Propionibacterium acnes*

Patient Instructions and Counseling

- Administering the drug with food can minimize GI distress.

Adverse Drug Events

- Photosensitivity reactions (may be less frequent with doxycycline and minocycline).

- Generally contraindicated during pregnancy, breast-feeding, and in children younger than 8 years because of their association with tooth discoloration and interference with bone growth.

- Hepatotoxicity, specifically acute fatty necrosis, may occur in pregnant women and in patients with renal impairment.

- Minocycline use:
  * Vestibular side effects (dizziness, ataxia, nausea, and vertigo)
  * Skin and mucous membrane pigmentation
  * Lupus-like symptoms
- GI intolerance (diarrhea, nausea, anorexia)

- Cross-sensitivity within the tetracycline group is common.

- IV tetracyclines may cause phlebitis.

Drug-Drug and Drug-Disease Interactions

- Milk, antacids, iron supplements, and probably other substances with calcium, magnesium, aluminum, and iron decrease tetracycline GI absorption considerably and should be ingested at least several hours before or after administration of tetracycline.

- Although doxycycline and minocycline absorption may be less affected by these divalent and trivalent cations, avoiding administration within 1 to 2 hours after ingestion of interfering foods is wise.

- Anticonvulsants (eg, barbiturates, carbamazepine, and phenytoin) induce hepatic microsomal metabolism of tetracyclines and therefore decrease tetracycline serum concentrations.

- If given with cholestyramine or colestipol, may bind tetracycline and reduce GI absorption.

- Oral contraceptive efficacy may be decreased with concurrent use of tetracyclines.

- May potentiate warfarin-induced anticoagulation, therefore monitor PT and INR.

- Demeclocycline antagonizes the action of antidiuretic hormone (ADH).

Table 8

Tetracyclines

Generic name	Trade name	Dosage forms	Common doses	Primary mode of elimination
Demeclocycline	Declomycin®	PO	300 mg- 1 g/d	Renal
Doxycycline	Vibramycin® and others	PO	100-200 mg q12h	Renal
Methacycline		PO, IV	150 mg q6h to 300 mg q12h	Hepatic
Minocycline	Minocin®	PO, IV	100-200 mg q12h	Hepatic
Oxytetracycline	Terramycin®	PO, IM	250-500 mg q6h, 250-500 mg qid, or 300 mg/d in 1 or 2 divided doses	Renal
Tetracycline	Achromycin V®, Sumycin®, Tetracyn®, and others	PO, IV, IM	1-2 g/d	Renal

8. Sulfonamides (Table 9)

Sulfonamides are synthetic derivatives of sulfanilamide. Sulfonamide utility has decreased over time due to the development of resistance.

Mechanism of Action

- Sulfonamides interfere with bacterial folic acid synthesis by competitively inhibiting p-aminobenzoic acid utilization. Sulfonamides are bacteriostatic.

Spectrum of Activity

Gram-positive bacteria
- Staphylococci (MSSA and MRSA); streptococci (not enterococci); *Bacillus anthracis*; *Clostridium perfringens*; *Nocardia*

Gram-negative bacteria
- *Enterobacter*; *E coli*; *Klebsiella*; *Proteus*; *Salmonella*; *Shigella*

Other organisms
- *Chlamydia trachomatis*; *Toxoplasma gondii*; *Plasmodium*

Adverse Drug Effects

- Hypersensitivity reactions appear to be cross-reactive with other sulfonamides, diuretics (including acetazolamide and thiazides), and sulfonylurea antidiabetic agents.

- Dermatologic reactions include rash, urticaria, and Stevens-Johnson syndrome.

Table 9

Sulfonamides

Generic name	Trade name	Dosage forms	Dose	Elimination	Notes
Sulfadiazine		IV, PO	2-4 g/d	Renal	
Sulfamethizole	Urobiotic®	PO	0.5-1 g q6h	Renal	
Sulfamethoxazole	Septra®	IV, PO	1-3 g/d	Hepatic	Combined with trimethoprim (Septra)
Sulfisoxazole	Gantrisin®	IV, PO	2-8 g/d	Renal	

9. Miscellaneous Antibiotics (Table 10)

Clindamycin

Clindamycin is a semi-synthetic antibiotic derived from lincomycin.

Mechanism of action

- Clindamycin inhibits the 50S subunit thereby inhibiting RNA synthesis. Clindamycin is either bacteriostatic or bactericidal depending on the serum concentration of the agent and the MIC of the organism.

Spectrum of activity

- Clindamycin is active against most aerobic gram-positive and most anaerobic gram-negative bacteria. Clindamycin has no activity against aerobic gram-negative bacteria.

Adverse drug effects

- Adverse GI effects occur frequently with all forms of clindamycin, and include nausea, vomiting, diarrhea, abdominal pain, and tenesmus. Clindamycin has induced *C difficile* enterocolitis.

- IV administration can lead to thrombophlebitis, erythema, and pain and swelling at the IV site. IM administration has caused pain, induration, and sterile abscesses.

- Clindamycin has caused transient leukopenia, neutropenia, eosinophilia, thrombocytopenia, and agranulocytosis. These effects are usually reversible upon discontinuation of the drug.

Imipenem-Cilastatin

Imipenem is a semi-synthetic carbapenem beta-lactam antibiotic. Cilastatin prevents renal metabolism of imipenem by dehydropeptidases.

Mechanism of action

- Imipenem binds to penicillin-binding proteins similarly to beta-lactams, thereby inhibiting peptidoglycan synthesis. Imipenem is bactericidal in susceptible isolates. Cilastatin competitively inhibits dehydropeptidase, an enzyme present on the brush border of the proximal renal tubule which hydrolyzes imipenem. Cilastatin has no antibacterial activity.

Spectrum of activity

- Imipenem is a very broad-spectrum antibiotic with activity against most gram-positive and gram-nega-

tive aerobes and anaerobes, as well as activity against some *Mycobacterium* and *Chlamydia* spp.

Adverse drug effects

- GI adverse effects are the most common ADRs reported with imipenem. The effects include nausea, vomiting, diarrhea (including *C difficile* enterocolitis), gastroenteritis, abdominal pain, glossitis, papillary hypertrophy, staining of the teeth, heartburn, pharyngeal pain, and taste abnormalities.

- Eosinophilia, leukopenia, neutropenia, agranulocytosis, hemolytic anemia, and thrombocytopenia have been reported.

- Seizures have been reported in approximately 0.4% of patients receiving imipenem. Risk factors include:
  * History of seizures or head trauma
  * High doses
  * Renal dysfunction

Meropenem

Similar to imipenem with the following differences:
  * Decreased CNS toxicity
  * No hydrolysis by dehydropeptidases

Table 10

Miscellaneous Antibiotics

Generic name	Trade name	Dosage forms	Dose	Elimination	Notes
Clindamycin	Cleocin®	IV, PO	300 mg q6h PO; 600-900 mg q8h IV	Hepatic	PO only for *C difficile*
Imipenem-cilastatin	Primaxin®	IV, IM	250 mg q6h; 500 mg or 1 g q6h or q8h depending on whether the organism is fully or moderately susceptible	Renal	
Meropenem	Merrem®	IV	500-2000 mg q8h	Renal	

10. Antifungal Agents (Table 11)

Amphotericin B

Amphotericin B is a polyene antifungal agent used in the treatment of potentially life-threatening systemic fungal infections.

Mechanism of action
- Amphotericin B binds to ergosterol in the fungal cell wall, leading to increased permeability and cell death. Amphotericin B is fungistatic.

Spectrum of activity
- *Aspergillus, Coccidioides, Cryptococcus, Histoplasma, Mucor*

- *Candida*, including *C albicans, C dubliniensis, C glabrata, C krusei, C parapsilosis,* and *C tropicalis*; *C lusitaniae* exhibits variable sensitivity.

Adverse drug effects
- Infusion reactions: fever, chills, hypotension, rigors, pain, thrombophlebitis, anaphylaxis

- Renal and electrolyte effects: nephrotoxicity is the major dose-limiting toxicity.
    * Hypokalemia, hypocalcemia, hypomagnesemia
    * Usually reversible upon discontinuation of the agent
    * Renal tubular acidosis and nephrocalcinosis are possible

- Hematologic effects: normocytic, normochromic anemia secondary to decreased erythropoietin production

- Hepatic effects: increased AST, ALT, alkaline phosphatase, bilirubin

Amphotericin B lipid formulations
- Amphotericin B cholesterol sulfate complex (Amphotec®), Amphotericin B lipid complex (Abelcet®), and Amphotericin B liposomal (Ambisome®) formulations are available for the treatment of severe fungal infections in patients who fail or are intolerant of conventional amphotericin B. The lipid formulations may decrease toxicity ~20-30%.

Caspofungin

Caspofungin is approved for the treatment of aspergillosis in patients refractory to or intolerant of other therapies.

Adverse drug effects
- Hepatic effects: increased AST, ALT

- Sensitivity reactions: histamine-release reactions such as rash, pruritus, and anaphylaxis

- Infusion reactions: fever, thrombophlebitis, nausea, vomiting, myalgias

Fluconazole

Fluconazole is a synthetic triazole antifungal and is fungistatic.

Mechanism of action
- The azole antifungals appear to inhibit fungal CYP 450 14-α-desmethylase, thereby decreasing ergosterol concentrations in susceptible fungi.

Spectrum of activity
- *Candida krusei, C glabrata, C lusitaniae,* and *C tropicalis* are commonly resistant.

Table 11

Antifungal Agents

Generic name	Trade name	Dosage forms	Normal dose	Elimination	Notes
Amphotericin B	Fungizone®	IV	0.5-1 mg/kg per day	Unknown	Dose should not exceed 1.5mg/kg/d
Caspofungin	Cancidas®	IV	50 mg/d	Hepatic	
Fluconazole	Diflucan®	IV, PO	100-800 mg/d	Renal	
Flucytosine	Ancobon®	PO	50-150 mg/kg per day	Renal	
Griseofulvin	Fulvicin P/G®	PO	500 mg	Hepatic	
Itraconazole	Sporanox®	IV, PO	200-600 mg/d	Hepatic	
Ketoconazole	Nizoral®	PO, topical	200-400 mg bid	Hepatic	Requires acid environment for dissolution and absorption
Nystatin	Mycostatin®	Topical		Fecal	
Terbinafine	Lamisal®	PO	250 mg/d	Hepatic	Pulse therapy also effective
Voriconazole	Vfend®	IV, PO	200 mg q12h PO; 4-6 mg/kg q12h IV	Renal	

Adverse drug effects
- GI effects: nausea, vomiting, abdominal pain, and diarrhea

- Hepatic effects: cholestasis, increased AST, ALT, and GGTP, hepatic necrosis, and rarely severe hepatic dysfunction

- Hemolytic effects: eosinophilia, anemia, leukopenia, neutropenia, and thrombocytopenia

- Nervous system effects: dizziness, headache, somnolence, coma, and seizures are rare

Flucytosine

Mechanism of action
- Flucytosine appears to enter fungal cells, where it is converted to 5-FU. Flucytosine is either fungistatic or fungicidal depending on the concentration of the agent.

Spectrum of activity
- Active against most strains of *Candida* and *Cryptococcus*

Adverse drug effects
- GI effects: GI hemorrhage, ulcerative colitis due to the antiproliferative effects, anorexia, abdominal pain, nausea, vomiting, and diarrhea

- Hepatic effects: increased AST, ALT, and bilirubin

- Renal effects: increased serum creatinine, BUN, and crystalluria

- Nervous system effects: confusion, hallucinations, psychosis, headache, parkinsonism, paresthesias, peripheral neuropathy, hearing loss, and vertigo

- Sensitivity reactions: erythema, pruritus, urticaria, rash, and toxic epidermal necrolysis

Griseofulvin

Mechanism of action
- Griseofulvin disrupts the fungal cell's mitotic spindle structure, thereby inhibiting the metaphase of cell division. Griseofulvin is fungistatic.

Spectrum of activity
- *Trichophyton, Microsporum,* and *Epidermophyton*

Adverse drug effects
- Nervous system effects: headache, fatigue, dizziness, paresthesias of the hands and feet after prolonged therapy

- GI effects: epigastric pain, nausea, vomiting, flatulence, and diarrhea

- Renal effects: proteinuria and nephrosis

- Sensitivity reactions: rash, urticaria, erythema multiforme, angioedema, serum sickness, photosensitivity, and lupus-like reactions

Itraconazole

Itraconazole is a synthetic triazole antifungal.

Spectrum of activity
- Effective in aspergillosis, blastomycosis, histoplasmosis, oropharyngeal and esophageal candidiasis, sporotrichosis, onychomycosis, coccidioidomycosis, and cryptococcosis.

Adverse drug effects
- GI effects: nausea, vomiting, diarrhea, abdominal pain, dyspepsia, dysphagia, flatulence, gastritis, ulcerative stomatitis

- Dermatologic and sensitivity reactions: rash, pruritus, urticaria, angioedema, Stevens-Johnson syndrome
- Nervous system reactions: headache, dizziness, tremor, neuropathy

- Cardiovascular effects: congestive heart failure, peripheral edema, pulmonary edema, prolonged QT interval, ventricular dysrhythmias, and death

- Hepatic effects: increased AST, ALT

- Electrolyte and metabolic effects: hypokalemia, adrenal insufficiency, gynecomastia

Ketoconazole

Ketoconazole is a synthetic imidazole antifungal.

Spectrum of activity
- Blastomycosis, candidiasis, coccidioidomycosis, histoplasmosis, dermatophytosis

Adverse drug effects
- GI effects: nausea, vomiting, abdominal pain, GI bleeding

- Hepatic effects: increased AST, ALT, alkaline phosphatase

- Endocrine and metabolic effects: gynecomastia, decreased cortisol production

- Dermatologic and sensitivity reactions: pruritus, rash, dermatitis, purpura

- Nervous system effects: headache, dizziness, lethargy, photophobia, abnormal dreams

Nystatin

Mechanism of action
- Nystatin binds to fungal sterols. Nystatin is fungistatic.

Spectrum of activity
- Cutaneous and mucocutaneous candidiasis

Adverse drug effects
- Mild nausea and diarrhea

Terbinafine

Terbinafine is a synthetic allylamine antifungal.

Mechanism of action
- Interferes with sterol biosynthesis

Spectrum of activity
- *Trichophyton, Microsporum, Epidermophyton, Aspergillus, Blastomycosis,* and yeasts

Adverse drug effects
- Hepatic effects: hepatitis, hepatic failure

- Dermatologic and sensitivity reactions: anaphylactoid reactions, Stevens-Johnson syndrome, and erythema multiforme

Voriconazole

Voriconazole is a synthetic triazole antifungal.

Spectrum of activity
- Aspergillosis

Adverse drug effects
- Hepatic effects: hepatitis, cholestasis, fulminant hepatic failure

- Dermatologic and sensitivity reactions: anaphylactoid reactions, pruritus, rash, Stevens-Johnson syndrome, and photosensitivity

11. Antitubercular Agents (Table 12)

Aminosalicylic Acid (PAS)

Mechanism of action
* Aminosalicylic acid inhibits folic acid synthesis similarly to the sulfonamides and is bacteriostatic.

Spectrum of activity
* Aminosalicylic acid is active against *Mycobacterium tuberculosis* only.

Adverse drug events
* Gastrointestinal effects: nausea, vomiting, abdominal pain, diarrhea, and anorexia

* Vitamin and mineral absorption: vitamin B_{12}, folic acid, and iron malabsorption have been rarely reported

* Hypersensitivity reactions: fever, skin eruptions, joint pain, and leukopenia have been reported

Capreomycin

Mechanism of action
* The exact mechanism of action of capreomycin is unknown. The agent is bacteriostatic against susceptible isolates.

Spectrum of activity
* Capreomycin is active against the following *Mycobacterium* species: *M tuberculosis, M bovis, M kansasii,* and *M avium.*

Adverse drug events
* Renal effects: nephrotoxicity is exhibited in up to 30% of patients receiving the agent. It is manifest as acute tubular necrosis which is usually reversible upon discontinuation of the agent.

* Ototoxicity: this is experienced by up to 30% of patients; eighth cranial nerve damage results which can produce irreversible hearing loss.

* Hepatic effects: elevated liver function tests have been noted when used in conjunction with other hepatotoxins.

* Hypersensitivity reactions: fever, urticaria, and skin eruptions have been noted.

Cycloserine

Mechanism of action
* Cycloserine is structurally similar to d-alanine and inhibits cell wall synthesis by competing for incorporation into the bacterial cell wall.

Spectrum of activity
* Cycloserine is active against the following *Mycobacterium* species: *M tuberculosis, M bovis, M avium,* and some *M kansasii* isolates.

Adverse drug events
* CNS effects: headache, vertigo, confusion, psychosis, and seizures

Ethambutol

Mechanism of action
* Ethambutol appears to inhibit bacterial cellular metabolism and is bacteriostatic.

Table 12

Antitubercular Agents

Generic name	Trade name	Dosage forms	Normal dose	Elimination	Notes
Aminosalicylic acid	Paser®	PO	150 mg/kg per day	Renal	Max dose 12 g/d
Capreomycin	Capastat®	IM	15 mg/kg per day	Renal	Max dose 1 g/d
Cycloserine	Seromycin®	PO	15-20 mg/kg per day	Renal	Max dose 1 g/d
Ethambutol	Myambutol®	PO	15-25 mg/kg per day	Hepatic	
Ethionamide	Trecator-SC®	PO	500-1000 mg per day	Hepatic	
Isoniazid	Various	PO	5-10 mg/kg per day	Hepatic	Max dose 300 mg/d
Pyrazinamide	Various	PO	15-30 mg/kg per day	Hepatic	Max dose 2 g/d
Rifampin	Various	PO, IV	10-20 mg/kg per day	Hepatic	Max dose 600 mg/d

Spectrum of activity

- Ethambutol is active against the following *Mycobacterium* species: *M tuberculosis, M bovis,* and some isolates of *M kansasii* and *M avium.*

Adverse drug events

- Ocular effects: optic neuritis with decreased visual acuity, central and peripheral scotomas, and loss of red-green color discrimination have been noted. These effects are usually reversible upon discontinuation of the agent.

Ethionamide

Mechanism of action

- Ethionamide appears to inhibit cell wall synthesis by an unidentified mechanism. The agent is bactericidal or bacteriostatic depending on tissue concentrations of the agent.

Spectrum of activity

- Ethionamide is active against the following *Mycobacterium* species: *M tuberculosis, M bovis, M kansasii,* and some *M avium* isolates.

Adverse drug events

- Hepatic effects: hepatitis is a rare complication.

Isoniazid (INH)

Mechanism of action

- INH appears to inhibit cell wall synthesis of susceptible isolates and is therefore active against actively dividing cells only. INH is bactericidal or bacteriostatic depending on tissue concentrations of the agent.

Spectrum of activity

- INH is active against the following *Mycobacterium* species: *M tuberculosis, M bovis,* and some strains of *M kansasii.*

Adverse drug events

- CNS effects: peripheral neuritis and rarely seizures, encephalopathy, and psychosis have been reported.

- Hepatic effects: increases in bilirubin, AST, and ALT are noted in up to 20% of patients receiving this agent. INH has lead to fulminant hepatitis and death.

- Hematologic effects: agranulocytosis, eosinophilia, thrombocytopenia, and hemolytic anemia have been reported.

Pyrazinamide (PZA)

Mechanism of action

- *Mycobacterium tuberculosis* converts PZA to pyrazinoic acid which possesses antitubercular activity.

Spectrum of activity

- PZA is active against *Mycobacterium tuberculosis* only.

Adverse drug events

- Hepatic effects: increased liver enzymes are common and fulminant hepatitis has been reported.

- Gout: PZA inhibits renal excretion of uric acid and may induce or worsen gout.

Rifampin

Mechanism of action

- Rifampin inhibits RNA synthesis in susceptible isolates.

Spectrum of activity

- Rifampin is active against the following *Mycobacterium* species: *M tuberculosis, M bovis, M kansasii,* and some *M avium* isolates.

- Rifampin also has activity against many gram-positive and gram-negative organisms.

Adverse drug events

- GI effects: nausea, vomiting, diarrhea, and abdominal pain may require discontinuation of the agent. *C difficile* colitis has been reported with rifampin.

- CNS effects: headache, dizziness, mental confusion, and psychosis have been reported.

- Hepatic effects: increased bilirubin, AST, and ALT are common. Fulminant hepatitis has been reported.

- Hematologic effects: thrombocytopenia, leukopenia, and hemolytic anemia have been reported rarely.

- Renal effects: renal insufficiency and interstitial nephritis have been reported.

12. Key Points

Aminoglycosides
- Aminoglycoside antibiotics exhibit concentration-dependent bacterial killing.

- Aminoglycoside antibiotics are reserved for severe infections or for use against multidrug resistant bacteria.

- Aminoglycoside antibiotic dosing should be pharmacokinetically tailored for each patient to optimize the therapeutic effect and minimize toxicity.

Penicillins
- Penicillin antibiotics exhibit time-dependent bacterial killing.

- All penicillins except nafcillin and oxacillin are renally eliminated and require dosage adjustments in renal dysfunction.

Cephalosporins
- Cephalosporin antibiotics exhibit time-dependent bacterial killing.

- First-generation cephalosporins: gram-positive activity is extensive, but gram-negative activity is limited.

- Second-generation cephalosporins: gram-positive activity is similar to that of first-generation agents, but gram-negative activity is generally more extensive than that of first-generation agents.

- Third-generation cephalosporins: gram-positive activity is decreased versus first- and second-generation agents, but gram-negative activity is extensive.

Gram-positive antibiotics
- Linezolid and quinupristin-dalfopristin are clinically effective against MRSA, MRSE, and VRE.

- Vancomycin is a broad-spectrum gram-positive antibiotic that should be pharmacokinetically tailored for each patient to maximize therapeutic benefit and minimize toxicity.

Fluoroquinolones
- Quinolone antibiotics exhibit concentration-dependent bacterial killing similar to the aminoglycosides.

- The later generation quinolones possess improved gram-positive activity, including against resistant streptococci.

Macrolides
- Erythromycins are primarily active against gram-positive bacteria including penicillin-resistant streptococci.

Tetracyclines
- Tetracyclines are drugs of choice for atypical pneumonias.

Sulfonamides
- Sulfonamides are primarily urinary anti-infectives whose utility has decreased due to the development of resistance.

Miscellaneous antibiotics
- Clindamycin is an effective anaerobic antibiotic as well as an effective gram-positive aerobic antibiotic with activity against many MRSA isolates.

- The carbapenem antibiotics possess a very broad spectrum of activity and should be restricted to appropriate indications to minimize development of resistance.

Antifungal agents
- Amphotericin B, caspofungin, fluconazole, itraconazole, and voriconazole are effective against systemic fungal infections.

- Imidazole antifungal agents are potent inhibitors of hepatic metabolism, thereby decreasing the elimination of numerous agents.

Antitubercular agents
- Isoniazid, rifampin, and streptomycin exhibit the lowest incidence of resistance.

- Isoniazid, rifampin, and pyrazinamide are the agents of first choice.

13. Questions and Answers

1. Which of the following statements regarding aminoglycoside antibiotics is/are true?

I. Aminoglycoside antibiotics are bactericidal against most susceptible isolates.
II. Aminoglycoside antibiotics exhibit concentration-dependent bacterial killing.
III. Aminoglycoside antibiotics should be reserved for serious infections.

   A. I only
   B. I and II
   C. I and III
   D. II and III
   E. I, II, and III

2. Which of the following statements most accurately characterize aminoglycoside toxicity?

I. Ototoxicity due to eighth cranial nerve damage
II. Nephrotoxicity exhibited as acute tubular necrosis
III. Bone marrow suppression

   A. I only
   B. II only
   C. III only
   D. I and II
   E. II and III

3. Which of the following statements best characterize aminoglycoside antimicrobial activity?

I. Active against most aerobic gram-negative bacteria
II. Active against most anaerobic gram-negative bacteria
III. Active against most fungal isolates

   A. I only
   B. II only
   C. II only
   D. I and II
   E. II and III

4. Which of the following antifungals is/are effective against systemic infections?

I. Amphotericin B
II. Fluconazole
III. Nystatin

   A. I only
   B. II only
   C. III only
   D. I and II
   E. I and III

5. Which of the following statements is/are true about amphotericin B–induced nephrotoxicity?

I. Nephrotoxicity is the major dose limiting toxicity.
II. Nephrotoxicity is usually reversible upon discontinuation of the drug.
III. Amphotericin B lipid formulations decrease nephrotoxicity by 20-30%.

   A. I only
   B. II only
   C. I and II
   D. II and III
   E. I, II, and III

6. Which of the following statements best describe the drug interactions noted with the imidazole antifungals?

I. Increased elimination of warfarin
II. Decreased elimination of warfarin
III. Increased metabolism of the oral contraceptives

   A. I only
   B. II only
   C. III only
   D. II and III
   E. I, II, and II

7. Linezolid is best described by which of the following statements?

I. Linezolid is bacteriostatic against staphylococci
II. Linezolid is bactericidal against staphylococci
III. Linezolid is a weak MAO inhibitor

   A. I only
   B. II only
   C. I and III
   D. II and III
   E. I, II, and III

8. Linezolid possesses activity against which of the following bacteria?

I. MRSA
II. *Enterococcus faecium*
III. *Enterococcus faecalis*

A. I only
B. II only
C. III only
D. I and II
E. I and III

9. Quinupristin-dalfopristin is best described by which of the following statements?

I. Exhibits activity against MSSA
II. Exhibits activity against MRSA
III. Exhibits activity against streptococci

A. I only
B. II only
C. III only
D. I and II
E. I, II, and III

10. Vancomycin is best described by which of the following statements?

I. Exhibits activity against MRSA
II. Exhibits activity against *Enterobacter*
III. Exhibits activity against *Clostridium difficile*

A. I only
B. II only
C. III only
D. I and II
E. I and III

11. Vancomycin toxicity is best described by which of the following statements?

I. Nephrotoxicity exhibited as acute tubular necrosis that is seldom reversible
II. Ototoxicity that is commonly exhibited as vestibular toxicity
III. Histamine release or "red-man syndrome" which is associated with rapid IV infusion

A. I only
B. II only
C. III only
D. I and II
E. II and III

12. Which of the following statements best describe appropriate vancomycin monitoring?

I. Trough serum concentrations should be routinely monitored in patients with pre-existing renal dysfunction.
II. Peak serum concentrations should be routinely

monitored in patients with pre-existing renal dysfunction.
III. Serum concentration monitoring is of no benefit in vancomycin monitoring.

A. I only
B. II only
C. III only
D. I and II
E. II and III

13. Clindamycin exhibits antibacterial activity against which of the following micro-organisms.

I. Aerobic gram-positive bacteria
II. Anaerobic gram-negative bacteria
III. Aerobic gram-negative bacteria

A. I only
B. II only
C. III only
D. I and II
E. I and III

14. Which statements best describe the carbapenem antibiotics?

I. Exhibit activity against most gram-positive and gram-negative aerobes and anaerobes
II. Meropenem induces seizures more commonly than imipenem
III. Cilastatin exhibits activity against most gram-positive aerobes

A. I only
B. II only
C. III only
D. I and II
E. II and III

15. Which of the following statements best describe the penicillins?

I. Exhibit concentration-dependent bacterial killing
II. Exhibits time-above-MIC-dependent bacterial killing
III. Exhibits excellent MRSA activity

A. I only
B. II only
C. III only
D. I and II
E. II and III

16. Which of the following penicillins require dosage adjustment in renal dysfunction?

I. Ampicillin
II. Nafcillin
III. Oxacillin

A. I only
B. II only
C. III only
D. I and II
E. II and III

17. Which of the following statements best describe the cephalosporins?

I. Exhibit concentration-dependent bacterial killing
II. Exhibit time-above-MIC-dependent bacterial killing
III. Exhibit excellent MRSA activity

A. I only
B. II only
C. III only
D. I and II
E. II and III

18. Which of the following statements best describe the antibacterial activity of the cephalosporins?

I. First-generation cephalosporins: gram-positive activity is extensive, but gram-negative activity is limited.
II. Second-generation cephalosporins: gram-positive activity is similar to that of first-generation agents, but gram-negative activity is generally more extensive than that of first-generation agents.
III. Third-generation cephalosporins: gram-positive activity is decreased versus first- and second-generation agents, but gram-negative activity is extensive.

A. I only
B. II only
C. III only
D. All of the above
E. None of the above

19. Which of the following statements best describe the antibacterial activity of the quinolones?

I. Exhibit concentration-dependent bacterial killing
II. Exhibit time-above-MIC-dependent bacterial killing
III. Exhibit extensive anaerobic activity

A. I only
B. II only

C. III only
D. I and III
E. II and III

20. Which statements best describe the important patient counseling points for the quinolones?

I. Avoid use in children and pregnant or nursing women due to the risk of cartilage erosion in growing bone tissue.
II. Do not take within 2 hours of antacids, multivitamins, calcium, magnesium, or iron supplements.
III. Take with a full glass of water and remain sitting or upright for 2 hours to avoid esophageal irritation.

A. I only
B. II only
C. III only
D. I and II
E. II and III

21. Which of the following statements best describe the sulfonamides?

I. Interferes with B_{12} synthesis by competitively inhibiting PABA utilization
II. Drugs of choice for *C difficile* colitis
III. Primarily urinary anti-infectives whose utility has decreased due to the development of resistance

A. I only
B. II only
C. III only
D. I and II
E. I, II, and III

22. Which of the following statements best describe the tetracyclines?

I. Exhibit bacteriostatic activity
II. Are the drugs of choice for atypical pneumonia
III. Tetracycline is contraindicated in children less than 8 years old

A. I only
B. II only
C. III only
D. I and II
E. I, II, and III

23. Which of the following statements best describe the macrolides?

I. Primarily effective against gram-positive aerobic bacteria
II. Effective against penicillin-resistant streptococci
III. Ineffective against penicillin-resistant streptococci

A. I only
B. II only
C. III only
D. I and II
E. I and III

24. Which antitubercular agent(s) exhibit the lowest incidence of resistance?

I. Isoniazid
II. Rifampin
III. Streptomycin

A. I only
B. II only
C. III only
D. I and II
E. I, II, and III

25. Which of the following combination regimens is considered the agents of first choice?

I. Isoniazid, rifampin, and streptomycin
II. Isoniazid, rifampin, and pyrazinamide
III. Isoniazid, ethambutol, and cycloserine

A. I only
B. II only
C. III only
D. All of the above
E. None of the above

Answers

1. **E.** Aminoglycoside antibiotics are bacteriocidal against most susceptible isolates, exhibit concentration-dependent bacterial killing, and are usually reserved for serious infections due to toxicity.

2. **D.** Ototoxicity is due to eighth cranial nerve damage and may be irreversible. Nephrotoxicity is exhibited as an acute tubular necrosis that is usually reversible and seldom requires dialysis. Neuromuscular blockade is the third most common toxicity noted with the aminoglycosides.

3. **A.** Aminoglycosides are active against most aerobic gram-negative and selected aerobic

gram-positive bacteria. They have no activity against anaerobic bacteria, or fungi.

4. **D.** Amphotericin B, caspofungin, fluconazole, itraconazole, and voriconazole are effective against systemic fungal infections.

5. **E.** Acute renal dysfunction is the most common dose-limiting amphotericin B toxicity, the renal dysfunction is usually reversible and seldom requires dialysis, and lipid formulations decrease toxicity by ~20-30%.

6. **B.** The imidazole antifungals decrease hepatic clearance of numerous hepatically metabolized medications, thereby increasing their activity and risk for toxicity.

7. **C.** Linezolid is bacteriostatic against staphylococci and enterococci. It is bacteriocidal against *Streptococcus* species only. The agent is a weak MAO inhibitor.

8. **D.** Linezolid is active against MSSA, MRSA and *Enterococcus faecium* (VRE). *Enterococcus faecalis* isolates are resistant.

9. **E.** Quinupristin-dalfopristin is active against MSSA, MRSA, streptococci and *Enterococcus faecium* (VRE). *Enterococcus faecalis* isolates are commonly resistant.

10. **E.** Vancomycin is active against aerobic gram-positive bacteria only; it has no clinically significant gram-negative activity. Vancomycin is the second-line drug of choice for *C difficile* colitis.

11. **C.** Vancomycin nephrotoxicity is uncommon and is exhibited as acute tubular necrosis which is commonly reversible and seldom requires dialysis. Ototoxicity is due to eighth cranial nerve damage which exhibits as high-frequency hearing loss, seldom affecting the vestibular system. The histamine or red-man reaction is most commonly infusion rate–related.

12. **A.** Vancomycin serum concentration monitoring is not required in patients responding well to therapy and with normal renal function. Vancomycin trough concentrations should be assessed in patients with pre-existing renal dysfunction, worsening renal function, or those not responding to therapy.

13. **C.** Clindamycin exhibits activity against aerobic

gram-positive bacteria and anaerobic gram-positive and gram-negative bacteria. It has no clinically significant aerobic gram-negative activity.

14. **A.** Carbapenems are active against most aerobic and anaerobic gram-positive and gram-negative bacteria. Imipenem is more likely to induce seizures, and cilastatin inhibits the metabolism of imipenem but has no antibacterial activity.

15. **B.** Penicillins exhibit time-dependent bacterial killing and have no activity against MRSA.

16. **A.** All penicillins with the exception of nafcillin and oxacillin require dosage adjustment in renal dysfunction.

17. **B.** Cephalosporins exhibit time-dependent bacterial killing and have no activity against MRSA.

18. **D.** First-generation cephalosporins exhibit extensive gram-positive activity, but limited gram-negative activity. Second-generation cephalosporins maintain gram-positive activity similar to the first-generation agents, but their gram-negative activity is generally improved. Third-generation cephalosporins exhibit decreased gram-positive activity, but gram-negative activity is significantly improved.

19. **A.** Quinolones exhibit concentration-dependent bacterial killing similar to the aminoglycosides. They possess good aerobic gram-positive and gram-negative activity, but have limited anaerobic activity.

20. **D.** Quinolones have been shown to decrease cartilage formation in beagle pups, but this effect in humans is somewhat controversial. Their use in children should be reserved for serious infections to avoid the risk. Quinolones are bound to divalent cations and should not be coadministered. They do not cause significant esophageal irritation.

21. **C.** Sulfonamides interfere with folic acid metabolism by inhibiting PABA utilization. They have no activity against *C difficile* colitis, and are primarily relegated to urinary anti-infectives due to resistance.

22. **C.** Tetracyclines are bacteriostatic. They are drugs of choice for atypical pulmonary pathogens, and should not be administered to children less that 8 years old to avoid permanent tooth staining and potential deposition into bone.

23. **C.** Erythromycins are primarily gram-positive aerobic antibiotics with good activity against most penicillin-resistant *Streptococcus* isolates.

24. **E.** Isoniazid, rifampin and streptomycin exhibit the lowest incidence of MTB resistance.

25. **B.** Isoniazid, rifampin and pyrazinamide are considered agents of first choice due to a low incidence of resistance and acceptable tolerability profile. Ethambutol is commonly added to the regimen in areas of increased resistance.

14. References

Alvarez-Elcoro S, Enzler, MJ. The macrolides: Erythromycin, clarithromycin, and azithromycin. *Mayo Clin Proc.* 1999;74:613-634.

Cunha BA, ed. *Antibiotic Therapy, Part I*. The Medical Clinics of North America. Philadelphia: WB Saunders; 2000.

Cunha BA, ed. *Antibiotic Therapy, Part II*. The Medical Clinics of North America. Philadelphia: WB Saunders; 2001.

Edson RS, Terrell CL. The aminoglycosides. *Mayo Clin Proc.* 1999;74:519-528.

Hardman JG, Limbird LE, Molinoff PB, et al, eds. *Goodman and Gilman's The Pharmacological Basis of Therapeutics*, 9th ed. New York: McGraw-Hill; 1996.

Hellinger WC, Brewer, NS. Carbapenems and monobactams: Imipenem, meropenem, and aztreonam. *Mayo Clin Proc.* 1999;74:420-434.

Kucers A, Bennett NM, eds. *Use of Antibiotics: A Comprehensive Review with Clinical Emphasis*, 4th ed. Philadelphia: Lippincott Williams & Wilkins; 1998.

Kasten MJ. Clindamycin, metronidazole, and chloramphenicol. *Mayo Clin Proc.* 1999;74:825-834.

Mandell GL, Bennett JE, Dolin R, eds. *Principles and Practice of Infectious Diseases*, 5th ed. Philadelphia: Churchill Livingstone; 2000.

Marshall WF, Blair, JE. The cephalosporins. *Mayo Clin Proc.* 1999;74:187-195.

Patel R. Antifungal agents. Part I. Amphotericin B preparations and flucytosine. *Mayo Clin Proc.* 1998;73:1205-1225.

Reese RE, Betts RF, eds. *A Practical Approach to Infectious Diseases*, 4th ed. Boston: Little, Brown and Company; 1996.

Smilack JD. The Tetracyclines. *Mayo Clin Proc.* 1999;74:727-730.

Smilack, JD. Trimethoprim-sulfamethoxazole. *Mayo Clin Proc.* 1999;74:730-734.

Terrrell CL. Antifungal agents. Part II. The azoles. *Mayo Clin Proc.* 1999;74:78-100.

Van Scoy RE, Wilkowske CJ. Antimycobacterial therapy. *Mayo Clin Proc.* 1999;74:1038-1048.

Walker RC. The fluoroquinolones. *Mayo Clin Proc.* 1999;74:1030-1037.

Wilhelm MP. Vancomycin. *Mayo Clin Proc.* 1999;74:928-935.

Wright AJ. The penicillins. *Mayo Clin Proc.* 1999;74:290-308.

31. Human Immunodeficiency Virus and the Acquired Immunodeficiency Syndrome

Camille W. Thornton, PharmD, BCPS
Assistant Professor, Department of Pharmacy
University of Tennessee College of Pharmacy

Contents

1. Overview

- The *human immunodeficiency virus (HIV)* is a retrovirus that depletes the helper T lymphocytes (CD4 cells), resulting in continued destruction of the immune system and subsequent gradual development of opportunistic infections and malignancies.

- The *acquired immunodeficiency syndrome (AIDS)* is HIV with a CD4 count less than 200 cells/mm³ or a history of opportunistic infection (eg, unexplained fever for more than 2 weeks, thrush, *Pneumocystis carinii* pneumonia, toxoplasmosis, cryptococcal meningitis, histoplasmosis, and *Mycobacterium avium*).

Epidemiology

- At the end of 2002, these were the global estimates of children and adults with HIV/AIDS:
    * People living with HIV/AIDS: 42 million
    * New HIV infections in 2002: 5 million
    * Deaths due to HIV/AIDS in 2002: 3.1 million
    * Cumulative number of deaths due to HIV/AIDS: 28 million

- Complete current world epidemiology can be found at www.unaids.org.

- At the end of 2001, these were the estimates of children and adults with HIV/AIDS in the U.S.:
    * People living with HIV/AIDS: 506,154
    * New HIV infections in 2001: 35,575
    * Deaths due to HIV/AIDS in 2001: 8998
    * Cumulative number of deaths due to HIV/AIDS: 467,918

- Complete current United States epidemiology can be found at: www.cdc.gov/hiv/stats/hasrlink.htm.

Subtypes
- HIV-1: most commonly found in the U.S.

- HIV-2: most commonly found in Africa

Clinical Presentation

- Opportunistic infection

- Patient not ill but has tested as HIV-positive

- Acute retroviral syndrome:
    * 50-90% of patients acutely infected with HIV experience some of the symptoms

    * Symptoms generally appear 2-4 weeks after virus exposure
    * Duration of the clinical syndrome is ~14 days (the range is a few days to >10 weeks).
    * The disease is not readily recognized in the primary care setting because its symptoms are similar to those of the flu, mononucleosis, and other common illnesses.

Pathophysiology

- A retrovirus that replicates in and destroys CD4 cells

- The result is a chronically deteriorating immune system leading to opportunistic infections and eventual death.

- Seroconversion typically occurs ~3 weeks after the acute infection (the range is from 2 weeks to 6 months).

- Antibodies generally appear within 3 months of infection (the range is from 2 weeks to 6 months).

- Transmission is via infected blood or hazardous body fluids:
    * Unprotected sexual contact with an infected person
      • Multiple partners increase risk.
      • Ongoing or past medical history of sexually transmitted disease increases risk.
    * Sharing needles and/or syringes with an infected person
    * Transfusions of infected blood or blood clotting factors (U.S. began screening the blood supply in 1985)
    * Vertical transmission (infected mother to infant)
    * Breastfeeding
    * Occupational exposure is rare.
    * Household contact is rare.

Diagnostic Criteria

- Enzyme linked immunosorbent assay (ELISA):
    * Initial screening test for detection of anti-HIV antibodies
    * False positive results can occur in patients with:
      • Collagen vascular diseases
      • Chronic hepatitis
      • Other chronic diseases

- Western blot:
    * All positive ELISA tests must be confirmed by a Western blot.

* Specificity and sensitivity of the Western blot is >99%.
* Western blot tests for anti-HIV antibodies.

• Other diagnostic tests (all should be confirmed by Western blot):
  * OraQuick® Rapid HIV-1 antibody test
  * OraSure® HIV-1
  * Sentinel® HIV-1 Urine electroimmunoassay
  * Home Access® HIV-1 test
  * p24 antigen

Monitoring Tools

Viral load
• Measures amount of virus in blood

• Can assess disease progression and evaluate the efficacy of antiretroviral therapy

• Two assays are available:
  * RT-PCR® by Roche Amplicor
  * bDNA® by Chiron (not FDA approved)
    • [bDNA 3.0 tests are equal to RT-PCR tests except at the lower end of the range; at <1500 copies/mL, RT-PCR levels are approximately two times higher than those obtained by bDNA 2.0.])

• Lower limit of detection is 400 copies/mL (ultrasensitive limits would be 20-50 copies/mL).

• A minimally significant change in viral load is considered to be a threefold or $0.5 \log_{10}$ increase or decrease.

• Acute illness and immunizations can cause increases in HIV RNA for 2-4 weeks; viral load testing should not be performed during this time.

• Baseline viral loads are established by averaging two viral loads (that do not differ by $>0.5 \log_{10}$) taken 2-4 weeks apart.

• Monitoring viral load of patients *not* on antiretroviral therapy should occur every 3-4 months.

CD4 cell count
• Indicates extent of immune system damage and risk of developing opportunistic infections

• Normal $CD4^+$ cell counts are 800-1200 cell/mm^3.

• $CD4^+$ cell counts should be measured every 3-6 months in patients on or off antiretroviral therapy.

• A significant change in $CD4^+$ cells is considered to be a 30% increase or decrease from baseline.

Treatment Principles and Goals

Goals of therapy
• Maximal and durable suppression of viral load

• Restoration and/or preservation of immunologic function

• Improvement in quality of life

• Reduction of HIV-related morbidity and mortality

• Factors involved in achieving goals of therapy:
  * Adherence to the antiretroviral regimen
  * Rational sequencing of drugs
  * Preservation of future treatment options
  * Use of resistance testing in selected clinical settings

• See Table 1 for indications for the initiation of antiretroviral therapy in the chronically HIV-1 infected patient.

• Benefits of early therapy:
  * Control of viral replication is easier to achieve and maintain.
  * Delay or prevention of immune system compromise
  * Lower risk of resistance with complete viral suppression
  * Possible decreased risk of HIV transmission (undetectable viral loads decrease risk of transmission)

• Risks associated with early therapy:
  * Drug-related reduction in quality of life (side effects)
  * Treatment is lifelong (ie, the earlier the patients start, the longer they will be on therapy).
  * Current treatments do not cure HIV.
  * Earlier development of drug resistance (if viral suppression is suboptimal)
  * Limitation of future antiretroviral treatment options

• Benefits of delaying therapy:
  * Avoid negative effects on quality of life (ie, inconvenience, side effects).
  * Avoid drug-related adverse events.
  * Delay in development of drug resistance
  * At a later date, the number of available and future drug options is likely to have increased

Table 1

Indications for the Initiation of Antiretroviral Therapy in the Chronically HIV-1 Infected Patient

Clinical category	CD4+ cell count	Plasma HIV RNA	Recommendation
Symptomatic (AIDS, severe symptoms)	Any value	Any value	Treat
Asymptomatic, AIDS	<200/mm^3	Any value	Treat
Asymptomatic	>200/mm^3 but <350/mm^3	Any value	Treatment should generally be offered though controversy exists
Asymptomatic	>350/mm^3	Viral load >55,000 copies/mL	Some experts would recommend initiating therapy, recognizing that the 3-year risk of developing AIDS in untreated patients is >30%, and some would defer therapy and monitor CD4+ cell counts more frequently
Asymptomatic	>350/mm^3	Viral load <55,000 copies/mL	Many experts would defer therapy and observe, recognizing that the 3-year risk of developing AIDS in untreated patients is <15%

and will be available to the patient when his or her HIV disease risk is higher.

- Risks of delaying therapy:
  * Possible risk of irreversible immune system depletion
  * Possible greater difficulty in suppressing viral replication
  * Possible increased risk of HIV transmission

- See Table 2 for antiretroviral agents recommended for initial treatment of established HIV infection

Indications for Consideration of Changing Antiretroviral Therapy

- Failure to suppress plasma HIV RNA to undetectable levels (<50 copies/mL) within 4-6 months of initiating a therapy

- Repeated detection of virus in plasma following initial suppression to undetectable levels

- Consider genotyping and/or phenotyping to assist in identifying drugs for next regimen if:
  * Adherent to failing regimen for the previous 4-6 weeks
  * Viral load above 1000 copies/mL

- Persistently declining CD4+ T cell numbers as measured on at least two separate occasions

- Clinical deterioration

- Never change just one medication in a failing regimen (ie, use at least two new drugs, and preferably an entirely new regimen).

- Change one medication in a successful regimen if a patient is experiencing intolerable side effects or if there is overlapping toxicity with other medications (see Table 3).

- If possible, a new regimen should consist of a different combination of medications from Table 2.

- Avoid changing from ritonavir to indinavir or vice versa since high-level cross-resistance is likely.

- Avoid changing within the NNRTIs to remedy drug failure; high level cross-resistance is likely.

Table 2

Antiretroviral Regimens for Treatment of HIV Infection in Antiretroviral Naïve Patients

		No. of pills per day
NNRTI-based regimens		
Preferred regimens	Efavirenz + lamivudine + zidovudine *or* tenofovir *or* stavudine[1] (except for pregnant women or women with pregnancy potential)	3-5 pills/day
Alternative regimens	Efavirenz + lamivudine + didanosine (except for pregnant women or women with pregnancy potential)	3-5 pills/day
	Nevirapine + lamivudine + (zidovudine or stavudine or didanosine)	4-6 pills/day
PI-based regimens		
Preferred regimens	**Kaletra® (lopinavir + ritonavir) + lamivudine + zidovudine *or* stavudine**	8-10 pills/day
Alternative regimens	Amprenavir + ritonavir[2] + lamivudine + zidovudine *or* stavudine	12-14 pills/day
	Indinavir + lamivudine + zidovudine *or* stavudine	8-10 pills/day
	Indinavir + ritonavir[2] + lamivudine + zidovudine *or* stavudine	8-12 pills/day
	Nelfinavir[3] + lamivudine + zidovudine *or* stavudine	6-14 pills/day
	Saquinavir (sgc or hgc)[4] + ritonavir[2] + lamivudine + zidovudine *or* stavudine	14-16 pills/day
Triple NRTI regimen (as an alternative to PI- or NNRTI-based regimens)		
Alternative regimens	Abacavir + lamivudine + zidovudine *or* stavudine	2-6 pills/day

NNRTI, non-nucleoside reverse transcriptase inhibitor; NRTI, nucleoside reverse transcriptase inhibitor; PI, protease inhibitor.

[1]Preliminary 96-week data comparing stavudine + lamivudine vs. tenofovir + lamivudine revealed higher incidence of lipodystrophy and lipid abnormalities in the stavudine group.

[2]Low-dose 100-400 mg ritonavir.

[3]Nelfinavir 625 mg tablet (soon to be available).

[4]Sgc, soft gel capsule; hgc, hard gel capsule.

Table 3

HIV-Related Drugs with Overlapping Toxicities

Bone marrow suppression	Peripheral neuropathy	Pancreatitis	Nephrotoxicity	Hepatotoxicity	Rash	Diarrhea	Ocular effects
Cidofovir	Didanosine	Co-trimoxazole	Adefovir	Fluconazole	Abacavir	Didanosine	Didanosine
Co-trimoxazole	Isoniazid	Didanosine	Aminoglycosides	Isoniazid	Amprenavir	Clindamycin	Ethambutol
Cytotoxic	Stavudine	Lamivudine	Amphotericin B	Itraconazole	Co-trimoxazole	Nelfinavir	Rifabutin
chemotherapy	Zalcitabine	(children)	Cidofovir	Ketoconazole	Dapsone	Ritonavir	Cidofovir
Dapsone		Pentamidine	Foscarnet	NRTIs	NNRTIs	Lopinavir/	
Flucytosine		Ritonavir	Indinavir	NNRTIS	Sulfadiazine	ritonavir	
Ganciclovir		Stavudine	Pentamidine	PIs		Tenofovir	
Hydroxyurea				Rifabutin			
Interferon alfa				Rifampin			
Primaquine							
Pyrimethamine							
Ribavirin							
Rifabutin							
Sulfadiazine							
Trimetrexate							
Zidovudine							

2. Drug Therapy

Nucleoside Reverse Transcriptase Inhibitors (NRTIs) (Table 4)

Mechanism of action
- Interfere with HIV viral RNA-dependent DNA polymerase, resulting in chain termination and inhibition of viral replication

Class toxicities (monitor for signs and symptoms)
- Lactic acidosis

- Severe hepatomegaly with steatosis

- Most patients should be dose-adjusted for renal impairment (exception: abacavir).

- Most are not affected by food (except didanosine).

- Low pill burden as a class; few drug interactions

- Do not use zidovudine with stavudine due to antagonism.

- Do not use didanosine with stavudine during pregnancy due to increased risk of lactic acidosis and liver damage.

- Two combination products are available:
  * Combivir® (zidovudine 300 mg + lamivudine 150 mg)
  * Trizivir® (zidovudine 300 mg + lamivudine 150 mg + abacavir 300 mg)

- No special storage requirements are necessary for drugs in this class.

- The "D" drugs (ddI-didanosine, d4T-stavudine, ddC-zalcitabine) can cause pancreatitis and peripheral neuropathy; when used together, this effect can be additive.

- The "D" drugs are more closely associated with lactic acidosis.

- Therapy with zalcitabine has the highest incidence of peripheral neuropathy and is contraindicated with didanosine, stavudine, and lamivudine.

- Usually use two in combination with 1 NNRTI or 1 PI

Table 4

Characteristics of Nucleoside Reverse Transcriptase Inhibitors (NRTIs)

Generic name [trade name]	Zidovudine (AZT, ZDV) [Retrovir®]	Lamivudine (3TC) [Epivir®]	Abacavir (ABC) [Ziagen®]	Didanosine (ddI) [Videx®, Videx EC®]
Form	100 mg caps; 300 mg tabs; 10 mg/mL IV and oral solution	150 mg tabs; 10 mg/mL oral solution	300 mg tabs; 20 mg/mL oral solution	125, 200, 250, 400 mg EC caps (preferred formulation); 25, 50, 100, 150, 200 mg chewable/dispersible buffered tabs; 100, 167, 250 mg buffered powder for oral solution
Dosing recommendations	**300 mg q12h** or 200 mg q8h	**150 mg q12h;** <50 kg: 2 mg/kg q12h	**300 mg q12h**	>60 kg: **400 mg qd** (caps or two 200 mg tabs) *or* 200-250 mg q12h; <60 kg: 250 mg qd *or* 125-167 mg q 12 h
Food effect	Take without regard to meals	Take without regard to meals	Take without regard to meals	Take ½ h before or 2 h after meals
Adverse events	Bone marrow suppression: **anemia and/or neutropenia;** subjective complaints: GI intolerance, headache, insomnia, asthenia; rare: myopathy, hepatitis, cardiomyopathy	Minimal toxicity	**Hypersensitivity reaction;** fever, rash, N/V, malaise or fatigue, loss of appetite; respiratory symptoms may also be component (sore throat, cough, SOB)	**Pancreatitis, peripheral neuropathy,** nausea, diarrhea
Drug interactions	Ribavirin, d4T (competitive inhibition of AZT); increased toxicity with high doses of ganciclovir, PCP treatment doses of TMP-SMX, medications that can cause bone marrow suppression	No clinically significant drug interactions	Alcohol increases ABC levels by 41%	Increased levels and/or side effects: tenofovir, hydroxyurea, alcohol; methadone decreases ddI levels; buffer in tabs may decrease absorption of meds that need acidic environment (eg, azoles, quinolones, tetracyclines, indinavir, ritonavir delavirdine); increased toxicity with d4T when used in pregnancy
Monitoring	CBC, platelets, LFTs	None necessary	For signs and symptoms of hypersensitivity	CBC, LFTs, amylase, uric acid

Bold type highlights the most common dosing and important side effects. **(continued)**

Monitor all for signs and symptoms of pancreatitis, peripheral neuropathy and lactic acidosis.

Combivir is AZT 300 mg + 3TC 150 mg, 1 tab q 12 hours. Trizivir is AZT 300 mg + 3TC 150 mg + ABC 300 mg, 1 tab q 12 hours.

Table 4

Characteristics of Nucleoside Reverse Transcriptase Inhibitors (NRTIs) (continued)

Generic name [trade name]	Stavudine (d4T) [Zerit®, Zerit XR®]	Zalcitabine (ddC) [Hivid®]	Tenofovir (TDF) [Viread®]	Emtricitabine (FTC) [Emtriva®]
Form	15, 20, 30, 40 mg caps; 75, 100 mg extended-release caps; 1 mg/mL oral solution	0.375, 0.75 mg tabs	300 mg tabs	200 mg tabs
Dosing recommendations	>60 kg: **40 mg q12h** or 100 mg qd (XR); <60 kg: 30 mg q12h or 75 mg qd (XR)	**0.75 mg q8h**	**300 mg qd** for CrCl ≥60 mL/min; not recommended for patients with CrCl <60 mL/min	**200 mg qd**
Food effect	Take without regard to meals	Take without regard to meals	Increased bioavailability when taken with food	Take without regard to meals
Adverse events	**Pancreatitis; peripheral neuropathy; hyperlipidemia;** lactic acidosis + ascending motor weakness	**Pancreatitis; peripheral neuropathy;** oral aphthous ulcers	**Diarrhea, N/V,** asthenia, headache, flatulence	**N/V, diarrhea,** pharyngitis, infection, asthenia
Drug interactions	Antagonism with AZT, do not use together; increased toxicity with ddI when used in pregnancy	Increased side effects, concomitant use not recommended with: didanosine, stavudine, lamivudine	Increased levels and side effects of didanosine; increased levels of: cidofovir, ganciclovir, valganciclovir	Chemically related to 3TC, do not use together; cross-resistance with 3TC; no other clinically significant drug interactions identified to date
Monitoring	Signs and symptoms of lactic acidosis with muscle weakness; monitor lipids	CBC, LFTs, amylase	Renal function	None necessary

Bold type highlights the most common dosing and important side effects.
Monitor all for signs and symptoms of pancreatitis, peripheral neuropathy, and lactic acidosis.
Tenofovir is a nucleotide reverse transcriptase inhibitor: it requires fewer phosphorylations to become activated.
Emtricitabine should be available summer of 2003 (name brand may change).
Use caution with ddI, d4T, and ddC when used with other drugs that can cause peripheral neuropathy or pancreatitis.

Non-Nucleoside Reverse Transcriptase Inhibitors (NNRTIs) (Table 5)

Mechanism of action
• Bind to reverse transcriptase at a different site than the NRTIs, resulting in inhibition of HIV replication

• Class toxicities include rash and hepatic toxicity.

• One-step mutation confers class resistance.

• All should be dose-adjusted for hepatic impairment.

• Most are not affected by food (except efavirenz).

• Efavirenz is contraindicated in pregnancy (it is teratogenic in monkeys).

• Usually, use one in combination with two NRTIs.

• No special storage requirements are necessary for drugs in this class.

Drug interactions
• See Tables 6, 7 and 8.

Table 5

Characteristics of Non-Nucleoside Reverse Transcriptase Inhibitors (NNRTIs)

Generic name [trade name]	Efavirenz (EFV) [Sustiva®]	Nevirapine (NVP) [Viramune®]	Delavirdine (DLV) [Rescriptor®]
Form	50, 100, 200 mg caps; 600 mg tabs	200 mg tab; 10 mg/mL oral suspension	100, 200 mg tabs
Dosing recommendations	**600 mg hs**	**200 mg qd x 14 d, then 200 mg q12h**	**400 mg q8h**
Food effect	Avoid taking after high fat meals	Take without regard to meals	Take without regard to meals
Adverse events	**CNS side effects:** abnormal dreams, confusion, abnormal thinking, impaired concentration, depersonalization, hallucinations, somnolence; rash, increased LFTs; teratogenic in monkeys	**Rash, increased LFTs, hepatitis**	**Rash, increased LFTs,** headaches
Drug interactions	CYP 450 3A4, 2C19 inhibitor and 3A4 inducer (see Tables 6, 7, and 8)	CYP 3A4 inducer (see Tables 6, 7, and 8)	CYP 450 3A4, 2D6 inhibitor; separate dosing with ddI or antacids by 1 hour (see Tables 6, 7, and 8)
Monitoring	CNS side effects, rash, LFTs	Rash, LFTs (at 2 and 4 weeks, then every 3-6 months)	Rash, LFTs (at 1 month, then every 3-6 months)
Additional information	Lowest incidence of rash in the class; contraindicated in patients with psychiatric history; CNS side effects generally occur during first 2-4 weeks, then resolve	Dose is titrated do decrease incidence of rash; investigational dosage: 400 mg qd; fulminant hepatic toxicity has occurred with just one dose; rash has been associated with Stevens-Johnson syndrome	Rash has been associated with Stevens-Johnson syndrome

Bold type highlights the most common dosing and important side effects.

Table 6

Drugs That Should Not Be Used with NNRTIs

Drug category	Nevirapine	Delavirdine	Efavirenz
Calcium channel blocker	None	None	None
Cardiac	None	None	None
Lipid-lowering agents	None	Simvastatin, lovastatin	None
Antimycobacterial	Insufficient data	Rifampin, rifabutin	None
Antihistamine	None	Astemizole, terfenadine	Astemizole, terfenadine
Gastrointestinal drugs	None	Cisapride, H_2 blockers, proton pump inhibitors	Cisapride
Psychotropic	None	Midazolam, triazolam	Midazolam, triazolam
Ergot alkaloids (vasoconstrictor)	None	Ergotamine derivatives	Ergotamine derivatives

Table 7

Drug Interactions with NNRTIs Requiring Dose Modifications or Cautious Use

Drugs affected	Nevirapine (NVP)	Delavirdine (DLV)	Efavirenz (EFV)
Antifungals			
Ketoconazole (keto)	Levels: keto decreased 63%, NVP increased 15-30%; dose: not recommended	No data	No data
Antimycobacterials			
Rifampin	Levels: NVP decreased 37%; dose: not recommended	Levels: DLV decreased 96%; contraindicated	Levels: EFV decreased 25%; no dose adjustment
Rifabutin	Levels: NVP decreased 16%; no dose adjustment*	Levels: DLV decreased 80%, rifabutin increased 100%; dose: Not recommended	Levels: EFV unchanged, rifabutin decreased 35%; dose: increase rifabutin dose to 450-600 mg qd or 600 mg 2-3 x per wk,[1] EFV dose standard
Clarithromycin (clarithro)	Levels: NVP increased 26%, clarithro decreased 30%; no dose adjustment	Levels: clarithro increased 100%, DLV increased 44%; dose adjust for renal failure	Levels: clarithro decreased 39%; alternative recommended
Oral contraceptives	Levels: ethinyl estradiol decreased 20%; use alternative or additional methods	No data	Levels: ethinyl estradiol increased 37%; use alternative or additional methods
Lipid-lowering agents			
Simvastatin, lovastatin	No data	Levels: potential for large increase in statin levels; avoid concomitant use	No data
Anticonvulsants			
Phenobarbital, phenytoin, carbamazepine	Unknown; use with caution; monitor anticonvulsant levels	Unknown, but may decrease DLV levels substantially; monitor anticonvulsant levels.	Unknown; use with caution; monitor anticonvulsant levels
Methadone	Levels: NVP unchanged, methadone decreased significantly; titrate methadone dose to effect	No data	Levels: methadone decreased significantly; titrate methadone dose to effect
Miscellaneous	No data	May increase levels of dapsone, warfarin, and quinidine; sildenafil: potential for increased concentrations; do not exceed 25 mg in a 48-h period	Monitor warfarin when used concomitantly

[1]These recommendations apply to regimens that do not include PIs, which can substantially increase rifabutin levels.

Table 8

Drug Interactions Involving PIs and NNRTIs: Effect of Drug On Levels and Dose

Drug affected	Nevirapine (NVP)	Delavirdine (DLV)	Efavirenz (EFV)
Indinavir (IDV)	Levels: IDV decreased 28%; dose: IDV 1000 mg q8h, NVP standard	Levels: IDV increased >40%; dose: IDV 600 mg q8h, DLV standard	Levels: IDV decrease 31%; dose: IDV 1000 mg q8h, EFV standard
Ritonavir (RTV)	Levels: RTV decreased 11%; dose RTV, NVP standard	Levels: RTV increased 70%; dose RTV: no data, DLV standard	Levels: RTV increased 18%, EFV increased 21%; dose RTV 600 mg q12h, EFV standard
Saquinavir (SQV)	Levels: SQV decreased 25%; dose: no data	Levels: SQV increased 5x; dose: SQV 800 mg q8h, DLV standard (monitor LFTs)	Levels: SQV decreased 62%, EFV decreased 12%; co-administration not recommended
Nelfinavir (NFV)	Levels: NFV increased 10%; dose NFV, NVP standard	Levels: NFV increased 2x, DLV decreased 50%; dose: no data (monitor for neutropenic complications)	Levels: NFV increased 20%; dose: NFV, EFV standard
Amprenavir (APV)	No data	No data	Levels: APV AUC decreased 36%; dose: APV 1200 mg q8h as single PI, or 1200 mg + RTV 200 mg q12h, EFV standard
Lopinavir/ritonavir (LPV/r)	Levels: LPV C_{min} decreased 55%; dose: consider LPV/r 533/133 mg q12h in PI-experienced patients, NVP standard	Levels: LPV levels expected to increase; dose: insufficient data	Levels: LPV AUC decreased 40%; dose: consider LPV/r 533/133 mg q12h in PI-experienced patients, EFV standard
Nevirapine (NVP)	—	No data	Levels: EFV AUC decreased 22%; dose: insufficient data
Delavirdine (DLV)	No data	—	No data

Protease Inhibitors (PIs) (Table 9)

Mechanism of action
- PIs inhibit protease, which then prevents the cleavage of HIV polyproteins and subsequently induces the formation of immature noninfectious viral particles.

- All should be dose-adjusted for hepatic impairment.

- Most should be taken with food (except APV, IDV).

- High pill burden as a class.

- Ritonavir is the most potent inhibitor in the class and is primarily used for intensification of other PIs.

- Goals of intensification:
  * Decrease pill burden.
  * Decrease frequency of doses (ie, decrease from q8h to q12h).

- Indinavir, amprenavir, lopinavir/ritonavir, and nelfinavir are less potent inhibitors of CYP450; saquinavir is the least potent inhibitor.

- Class toxicities:
  * Lipodystrophy
  * Hyperglycemia
  * Hyperlipidemia
  * Hypertriglyceridemia
  * Bleeding in hemophiliacs
  * Osteonecrosis and avascular necrosis of the hips
  * Osteopenia and osteoporosis

- PI monitoring (baseline is 4-6 weeks after starting PI and every 3-6 months thereafter):
  * Glucose
  * LFTs
  * Total cholesterol panel (particularly triglycerides)
  * GI side effects

Table 9

Characteristics of Protease Inhibitors (PIs)

Generic name [trade name]	Lopinavir + ritonavir (LPV/r) [Kaletra®]	Nelfinavir (NFV) [Viracept®]	Ritonavir (RTV) [Norvir®]	Indinavir (IDV) [Crixivan®]
Form	133.3 mg lopinavir + 33.3 mg ritonavir caps; 80 mg lopinavir + 20 mg ritonavir per mL oral solution	250, 625 mg tabs; 50 mg/g oral powder	100 mg caps; 600 mg/7.5 mL oral solution	200, 333, 400 mg caps
Dosing recommendations	400 mg lopinavir + 100 mg ritonavir q12h	1250 mg q12h; 750 mg q8h	100-400 mg with other PIs for intensification; 600 mg q12h	800 mg q8h
Food effect	Take with food	Take with food	Take with food	Take 1 h before or 2 h after meals; may take with skim milk or lowfat meal
Adverse events	GI intolerance, asthenia, increased LFTs, PI class side effects	Diarrhea	GI intolerance, paresthesias, hepatitis, pancreatitis, asthenia, taste perversion; increased LFTs, CPK, uric acid	Nephrolithiasis, GI intolerance, increased indirect bilirubinemia, headache, asthenia, blurred vision, dizziness, rash, metallic taste, thrombocytopenia, alopecia
Drug interactions	CYP450 3A4 inhibitor, weak inducer, see Tables 10, 11, and 12	CYP450 3A4 inhibitor, weak inducer, see Tables 10, 11, and 12	CYP450 3A4 inhibitor, weak inducer; see Tables 10, 11, and 12	CYP450 3A4 inhibitor; see Tables 10, 11, and 12
Storage	Refrigerated caps stable until date on label; stable for 2 months at room temperature	Room temperature	Refrigerated caps stable until date on label; stable for 1 month at room temprature	Room temperature
Additional information	Oral solution contains 42% alcohol	Needs 500 kcal of food for absorption; take after eating; boosting not effective	Primary role is in intensification of other PIs; most potent CYP450 inhibitor in the class	Patients should drink ≥48 oz of H_2O daily to reduce incidence of kidney stones; boosted indinavir increases incidence of kidney stones, removes the food restriction, and reduces frequency to q12h; additional monitoring: signs and symptoms of kidney stones, indirect bilirubin, platelets

Bold type highlights the most common dosing and important side effects.

* Signs and symptoms of bone pain (particularly hip pain)
* Signs and symptoms of fat redistribution

• Usually used in combination with two NRTIs

• All are CYP450 3A4 inhibitors (ie, drug interactions are typical of CYP450 3A4 inhibitors)

• Entry inhibitors include Enfuvirtide (T20), Fuzeon™
  * Mechanism of action: binds to gp41 on HIV surface, which inhibits HIV binding to CD4 cell.
  * Dose: 90 mg SQ q12h
  * Side effects: injection site reactions, headache, fatigue, insomnia, peripheral neuropathy, depression, pancreatitis, poor appetite, asthenia, myalgia, constipation

Table 9

Characteristics of Protease Inhibitors (PIs) (continued)

Generic name [trade name]	Amprenavir (APV) [Agenerase®]	Saquinavir (SQV) SQV-hard gel cap (HGC) [Invirase®]	Saquinavir (SQV) SQV-soft gel cap (SGC) [Fortovase®]	Atazanavir (TAZ) [Reyataz®]
Form	50, 150 mg caps, 15 mg/mL oral solution	200 mg caps		200 mg caps
Dosing recommendations	>50 kg: 1200 mg q12h (caps) or 1400 mg q12h (oral solution); <50 kg: 20 mg/kg q12h (caps) or 1.5 mL/kg q12h (oral solution)	400 mg q12h with 400 mg ritonavir; invirase not recommended otherwise	1200 mg q 8 h	400 mg q day
Food effect	Avoid taking around a high fat meal	No food effect when taken with ritonavir	Take with large meal	Take with food
Adverse events	GI intolerance, rash, oral paresthesias, increased LFTs; sulfonamide, caution in patients with history of sulfa allergy	GI intolerance, headache, increased LFTs		Increased bilirubinemia, GI intolerance, headaches, peripheral neuropathy, rash, microscopic hematuria, uric acid crystals in urine
Drug interactions	CYP450 3A4 inhibitor, weak inducer; see Tables 10, 11, and 12	CYP450 3A4 inhibitor; see Tables 10, 11, and 12		CYP450 3A4 inhibitor; see Tables 10, 11, and 12
Storage	Room temperature	Room temperature	Refrigerated caps stable until date on label; stable for 3 months at room temperature	Room temperature
Additional information	Caps and solution are not equivalent; max dose of caps is 2400 mg/d; max dose of oral solution is 2800 mg/d; oral solution contains propylene glycol[1]; 2400 mg of caps contain 1744 IU vitamin E; can boost with ritonavir, but overall pill burden is minimally affected	Very poor bioavailability but more predictable levels when boosted with RTV	Higher bioavailability and is the preferred formulation in single-PI regimens; boosting with RTV results in erratic levels and is not recommended	Will be available summer of 2003; reduced incidence of hyperlipidemia; additional monitoring: bilirubin, urinalysis

Bold type highlights the most common dosing and important side effects.

[1]Contraindicated in pregnant women, children <4 years old, patients with hepatic or renal failure, and patients treated with disulfiram or metronidazole.

- Generally reserved for deep salvage regimens

- Preferably should be used with at least two other active drugs

- Resistance develops quickly with less potent regimens and in cases of poor adherence.

- No known significant drug interactions to date

- Take without regard to meals.

- Store at room temperature; reconstituted form should be stored in the refrigerator, where it will be stable for 24 hours.

Table 10

Drugs That Should Not Be Used with PIs

Drug category	Indinavir	Ritonavir	Saquinavir	Nelfinavir	Amprenavir	Lopinavir/ ritonavir	Atazanavir
Calcium channel blockers	None	Bepridil	None	None	Bepridil	None	Bepridil
Cardiac	None	Amiodarone, flecainide, propafenone, quinidine	None	None	None	Flecainide, propafenone	None
Lipid-lowering agents	Simvastatin, lovastatin	Simvastatin, lovastatin	Simvastatin, lovastatin	Simvastatin, lovastatin	Simvastatin, lovastatin	Simvastatin, lovastatin	Simvastatin, lovastatin
Antimycobacterial	Rifampin	None	Rifampin, rifabutin	Rifampin	Rifampin	Rifampin	Rifampin
Antihistamine	Astemizole, terfenadine	Astemizole, terfenadine	Astemizole, terfenadine	Astemizole, terfenadine	Astemizole, terfenadine	Astemizole, terfenadine	Astemizole, terfenadine
Gastrointestinal drugs	Cisapride	Cisapride	Cisapride	Cisapride	Cisapride	Cisapride	Cisapride
Neuroleptic	None	Clozapine, pimozide	None	None	None	Pimozide	None
Psychotropic	Midazolam, triazolam	Midazolam, triazolam	Midazolam, triazolam	Midazolam, triazolam	Midazolam, triazolam	Midazolam, triazolam	Midazolam, triazolam
Ergot alkaloids (vasoconstrictor)	Ergot derivatives	Ergot derivatives	Ergot derivatives	Ergot derivatives	Ergot derivatives	Ergot derivatives	Ergot derivatives
Herbs & miscellaneous	St. John's wort, grapefruit juice	St. John's wort, grapefruit juice	St. John's wort, grapefruit juice	St. John's wort, grapefruit juice	St. John's wort, grapefruit juice	St. John's wort, grapefruit juice	St. John's wort, grapefruit juice

Counseling

- All patients should be counseled on the importance of adherence.
  - * >95% adherence is necessary to decrease the incidence of resistance.

- Patients should be given tools to facilitate adherence to complicated regimens (eg, pill boxes, calendars, pagers, etc).

- Patients should be counseled on class side effects, especially any that are unique to particular drugs they are taking.

Table 11

Drug Interactions with PIs Requiring Dose Modifications or Cautious Use

Drugs affected	Indinavir (IDV)	Ritonavir (RTV)	Saquinavir (SQV)
Antifungals			
Ketoconazole (keto)	Levels: IDV increased 68%; dose: IDV 600 mg tid	Levels: keto increase 3 x; dose: use with caution; do not exceed 200 mg keto daily	Levels: SQV increase 3 x; dose: standard
Antimycobacterials			
Rifampin	Levels: IDV decreased 89%; contraindicated	Levels: RTV decrease 35%; dose: no data; increased liver toxicity possible	Levels: SQV decreased 84%; contraindicated, unless using RTV + SQV, then use rifampin 600 mg qd or 2-3 x per week
Rifabutin	Levels: IDV decreased 32%, rifabutin increased 2 x; dose: reduce rifabutin to 150 mg qd or 300 mg 2-3 x per week; increase IDV to 1000 mg q8h	Levels: rifabutin increase 4 x; dose: decrease rifabutin to 150 mg qod or dose 3 x per week; RTV: standard	Levels: SQV decreased 40%; no dose adjustment unless using RTV + SQV, then use rifabutin 150 mg 2-3 x per week
Clarithromycin (clarithro)	Levels: clarithro increased 53%; no dose adjustment	Levels: clarithro increased 77%; dose adjust for renal insufficiency	Levels: clarithro increased 45%, SQV increased 177%; no dose adjustment
Oral contraceptives	Levels: norethindrone increased 26%, ethinyl estradiol increased 24%; no dose adjustment	Levels: ethinyl estradiol decreased 40%; use alternative or additional method	No data
Lipid-lowering agents			
Simvastatin, lovastatin	Levels: potential for large increase in statin levels; avoid concomitant use	Levels: potential for large increase in statin levels; avoid concomitant use	Levels: potential for large increase in statin levels; avoid concomitant use
Anticonvulsants			
Phenobarbital, phenytoin, carbamazepine	Carbamazepine markedly decreases IDV AUC; consider alternative agent	Unknown, use with caution; monitor anticonvulsant levels	Unknown, but may decrease SQV levels substantially; monitor anticonvulsant levels
Methadone	No change in methadone levels	Methadone decrease 37%; monitor and titrate dose if needed	No data
Miscellaneous	Grapefruit juice reduces IDV levels by 26%, separate; sildenafil AUC increased 2- to 11-fold; do not exceed 25 mg in a 48-h period	Desipramine increased 145%, reduce dose; theophylline decreased 47%, monitor levels; sildenafil AUC increased 2- to 11-fold; do not exceed 25 mg in a 48-h period; potential for many drug interactions	Grapefruit juice increased SQV levels; dexamethasone decreased SQV levels; sildenafil AUC increased 2- to 11-fold; do not exceed 25 mg in a 48-h period

(continued)

Table 11

Drug Interactions with PIs Requiring Dose Modifications or Cautious Use (continued)

Drugs affected	Nelfinavir (NFV)	Amprenavir (APV)	Lopinavir/ritonavir (LPV/r)
Antifungals			
Ketoconazole (keto)	No dose adjustment necessary	Levels: APV increased 31%, keto increased 44%; combination under investigation	Levels: LPV AUC decreased 13%, keto increased threefold; combination under investigation
Antimycobacterials			
Rifampin	Levels reduced 82%; contra-indicated	Levels: APV AUC reduced 82%; avoid concomitant use	Levels: LPV AUC reduced 75%; avoid concomitant use
Rifabutin	Levels: NFV reduced 32%, rifabutin increased 2 x; dose: decrease rifabutin to 150 mg qd or 300 mg 2-3 x per week, increase NFV dose to 1000 mg q8h	Levels: APV AUC reduced 15%, rifabutin increased 193%; dose: APV dose standard; reduce rifabutin to 150 mg qd or 300 mg 2-3 x per week	Levels: Rifabutin AUC increased threefold; dose: decrease rifabutin to 150 mg qod, LPV/r dose standard
Clarithromycin (clarithro)	No data	Levels: APV AUC increased 18%; no dose adjustment	No data
Oral contraceptives	Levels: norethindrone reduced 18%, ethinyl estradiol decreased 47%; use alternative or additional method	Levels: potential for metabolic interactions; use alternative or additional method	Levels: ethinyl estradiol reduced 42%, use alternative or additional method
Lipid-lowering agents			
Simvastatin, lovastatin, atorvastatin, pravastatin	Atorvastatin AUC increased 74%, use with caution; simvastatin AUC increased 505%, not recommended; potential for large increase in lovastatin AUC, not recommended	Levels: Potential for large increase in statin levels; avoid concomitant use with lovastatin and simvastatin	Contraindicated with simvastatin and lovastatin; atorvastatin AUC increased 5.88-fold, use with caution and monitoring; pravastatin AUC increased 33%; no dose adjustment necessary
Anticonvulsants			
Phenobarbital, phenytoin, carbamazepine	Unknown, but may decrease NFV levels substantially; monitor anticonvulsant levels	Unknown, but may decrease APV levels substantially; monitor anticonvulsant levels	Unknown, but may decrease LPV levels substantially; monitor anticonvulsant levels
Methadone	NFV may reduce methadone levels, monitor and titrate dose if needed	No data	Methadone AUC reduced 53%, monitor and titrate dose if needed
Sildenafil	Sildenafil AUC increased 2- to 11-fold; do not exceed 25 mg in a 48-h period	Sildenafil AUC increased 2- to 11-fold; do not exceed 25 mg in a 48-h period	Sildenafil AUC increased 2- to 11-fold; do not exceed 25 mg in a 48-h period

Table 12

Drug Interactions Involving PIs: Effect of Drug On Levels and Dose

Drug affected	Ritonavir	Saquinavir	Nelfinavir	Amprenavir	Lopinavir/ritonavir
Indinavir (IDV)	Levels: IDV increased 2-5 x; dose: IDV 400 + RTV 400 mg q12h, or IDV 800 + RTV 100-200 mg q12h	Levels: SQV increased 4-7 x; dose: insufficient data	Levels: IDV increased 50%, NFV increased 80%; dose: limited data for IDV 1200 mg + NFV 1250 mg q12h	Levels: APV AUC increased 33%; dose: no change	Levels: IDV AUC and C_{min} increased; dose: IDV 600 mg q12h, LPV/r standard
Ritonavir (RTV)	—	Levels: SQV increase 20 x; dose: SQV 400 mg + RTV 400 mg q12h	Levels: NFV increased 1.5 x; dose: RTV 400 + NFV 500-750 mg q12h	Levels: APV AUC increased 2.5-fold; dose: limited data for APV 600-1200 + RTV 100-200 mg q12h	Lopinavir is co-formulated with ritonavir as Kaletra
Saquinavir (SQV)	—	—	Levels: SQV increased 3-5 x, NFV increased 20%; dose: standard NFV, SQV 800 mg q8h or 1200 mg q12h	Levels: APV AUC reduced 32%; dose: insufficient data	Levels: SQV AUC and C_{min} increased; dose: SQV 800 mg q12h, LPV/r standard
Nelfinavir (NFV)	—	—	—	Levels: APV AUC increased 1.5-fold; dose: insufficient data	No data
Amprenavir (APV)	—	—	—	—	Levels: APV AUC and C_{min} increased; dose: APV 600-750 mg q12h, LPV/r standard

Table 13

ACTG 076 Guidelines: Dosing of AZT for Prevention of Vertical Transmission

Antepartum	Initiation at 14-34 weeks gestation and continued throughout pregnancy
	A. PACTG 076 regimen: AZT 100 mg 5 times daily
	B. Acceptable alternative regimens:
	       AZT 200 mg 3 times daily
	       or
	       AZT 300 mg 2 times daily

Intrapartum	During labor, AZT 2 mg/kg IV over 1 hour, followed by a continuous infusion of 1 mg/kg/h IV until delivery
Postpartum	Oral administration of AZT to the newborn: AZT syrup 2 mg/kg every 6 hours for the first 6 weeks of life, beginning 8-12 hours after birth

Antiretroviral Therapy in the HIV-Infected Pregnant Woman

- Highly active antiretroviral therapy (HAART) should be offered if the patient is not already receiving treatment.
  - Efavirenz should be avoided.
  - Avoid combining stavudine and didanosine.
  - Consider starting treatment after the first trimester.

- Continue current combination regimens (preferably with zidovudine) if the patient is already receiving therapy (decreases the risk of transmission from 30% to 2.5%).

- Zidovudine alone can decrease risk of transmission when taken during pregnancy. Mother should also receive IV zidovudine during labor; the infant should receive 6 weeks of zidovudine (Table 13)

- Single-dose nevirapine at onset of labor in women who have had no prior antiretroviral therapy

- Single dose nevirapine, given once to the infant between 48-72 hours old, has been shown to decrease transmission rate (transmission rate at 6 weeks = 12%).

Postexposure Prophylaxis (PEP) (Table 14)

- Use universal precautions.

- The most common infectious exposure is needlesticks or cuts (1 in 300 risk).

- The risk with mucous membrane exposure is much lower (1 in 1000 risk).

- There have been 52 documented cases of occupationally-acquired HIV infection.

Table 14

Prevention or Postexposure Prophylaxis Treatment Options

Small volume, short duration *and* high HIV titer exposure *or* Large volume or less severe percutaneous *and* low HIV titer exposure	AZT 200 mg PO q8h or 300 mg PO q12h *plus* 3TC (lamivudine) 150 mg PO q12h
Large volume or less severe percutaneous *and* high HIV titer exposure *or* More severe percutaneous *and* low or high HIV titer exposure	AZT 200 mg PO q8h or 300 mg PO q12h + 3TC (lamivudine) 150 mg PO q12h + Indinavir 800 mg q8h *or* Nelfinavir 750 mg PO q8h or 1250 mg q12h

- Postexposure prophylaxis can reduce HIV infection by about 80%.

- Start therapy within 1-2 hours of exposure.

- Length of therapy is 4 weeks.

Opportunistic Infections

- Only two opportunistic infections require primary prophylaxis:
  * *Pneumocystis carinii* pneumonia (PCP)
    - When CD4$^+$ cells fall below 200/mm^3
    - Treatment of choice is trimethoprim-sulfamethoxazole (TMP-SMX) DS PO qd (see Table 15 for alternatives).
  * *Mycobacterium avium* complex bacteremia (MAC)
    - When CD4$^+$ cells fall below 50/mm^3

- Treatment of choice is mg PO every week.

- All other primary prophylax patient is antigen-positive a sure to the causing factor.

- All other opportunistic infections are treated when the patient is diagnosed.

- After treatment patients receive suppressive therapy.

- Some primary and secondary prophylaxis could possibly be discontinued with immune reconstitution (undetectable viral load and an increase in CD4 cells in response to HAART therapy; see Table 15).

Table 15

Opportunistic Infections

Pathogen	Indication	First choice	Alternative regimens	Comments
Pneumocystis carinii (PCP)	**Prophylaxis:** CD4$^+$ <200/mm^3; thrush; unexplained fever ≥2 weeks; history of PCP	TMP-SMX DS qd; TMP-SMX SS PO qd	Dapsone 100 mg PO qd; atovaquone 1500 mg qd; aerosolized pentamidine 300 mg q mo; TMP-SMX DS q MWF; others	Primary and secondary prophylaxis can possibly be stopped for PCP upon immune reconstitution (patients on HAART with CD4$^+$ greater than 200/mm^3 for >3 mo)
Pneumocystis carinii (PCP)	**Acute infection**	TMP 15 mg/kg/d + SMX 75 mg/kg/d PO or IV x 21 d in 3-4 divided doses (typical oral dosage is TMP-SMX DS 2 tabs q8h)	TMP 15 mg/kg/d PO + dapsone 100 mg PO qd x 21 d; atovaquone 750 mg suspension PO with meal bid 21 days; pentamidine 4 mg/kg/d IV x 21 d (severe cases); clindamycin 600 mg IV q8h or 300-450 mg PO q6h + primaquine 30 mg base PO/d x 21 d; trimetrexate 45 mg/m^2 IV/d + folinic acid 20 mg/m^2 PO or IV q6h	Patients with P$_{O_2}$ <70 mm Hg or A-a gradient >35 mm Hg should receive a corticosteroid taper; treatment is for 21 d
Candida	**Treatment**	**Oropharyngeal (thrush):** clotrimazole oral troches 10 mg 5 x/d for 10-14 d; nystatin 500,000 U gargled 5x/d for 10-14 d; **esophagitis:** fluconazole 200-400 mg qd x 2-3 wk	**Thrush:** fluconazole 100 mg qd; amphotericin B oral susp 1-5 mL qid swish & swallow; ampho B 0.3-.05 mg/kg/d IV; itraconazole 200 mg qd (caps) or 100 mg qd (susp); **esophagitis:** ketoconazole 200 mg qd; itraconazole 200 mg qd (caps) or 100 mg qd (susp)	**Thrush:** treat for 10-14 d; CD4$^+$ <500/mm^3 increases risk; **esophagitis:** treat for 2-3 wk; CD4$^+$ <500/mm^3 increases risk

(continued)

Table 15

Opportunistic Infections (continued)

Pathogen	Indication	First choice	Alternative regimens	Comments
Candida	Maintenance	**Thrush**: cotrimazole (dose as above); nystatin (dose as above); fluconazole 100 mg qd or 200 mg 3x/wk; **esophagitis**: fluconazole 100-200 mg qd	**Thrush**: itraconazole 200 mg qd (caps) or 100 mg qd (susp); ketoconazole 200 mg qd; **esophagitis**: ketoconazole 200 mg qd; itraconazole 200 mg qd (caps) or 100 mg qd (susp)	**Thrush**: most patients relapse within 3 mo in absence of immune reconstitution; options are treatment of each episode or maintenance: **esophagitis**: maintenance therapy is generally needed to prevent relapse
Candida	Primary prophylaxis	Not recommended; efficacy of fluconazole is established for AIDS patients with CD4 counts <100/mm^3; not done because no survival benefit was found, the cost was high, and there is risk of azole-resistant infections		
Cryptococcal meningitis	Treatment	Amphotericin B 0.7-1.0 mg/kg/d IV with or w/o flucytosine 100 mg/kg/d x 10-14 d, **then** fluconazole 400 mg/d for 8-10 wk	Fluconazole 400-800 mg/d PO with or w/o flucytosine 100 mg/kg/d PO x 6-10 wk	CD4$^+$ <100/mm^3 increases risk; spread through inhalation of soil contaminated with bird droppings; fluconazole is superior to itraconazole
Cryptococcal meningitis	Maintenance	Fluconazole 200 mg qd	Amphotericin B 0.6-1 mg/kg 1-3x/wk; fluconazole 400 mg qd; itraconazole 400 mg qd (caps) or 200 mg oral susp qd	Primary and secondary prophylaxis can possibly be stopped for cryptococcosis upon immune reconstitution (patients on HAART with CD4$^+$ >100-200/mm^3 for >6 mo)
Cryptococcal meningitis	Primary prophylaxis	Not generally recommended	Fluconazole 200 mg qd; itraconazole 200 mg PO or 100 mg oral susp qd	**Indications for primary prophylaxis**: antigen-positive high-risk patients (CD4$^+$ <100/mm^3 and work with soil)
Toxoplasmosis	Treatment	Pyrimethamine PO 100-200 mg; loading dose then 50-100 mg/d + folinic acid PO 10 mg/d + sulfadiazine PO 1-2 g q6h for at least 6 wk	Pyrimethamine + folinic acid + clindamycin 900-1200 mg IV q6h or 300-450 mg PO q6h; pyrimethamine + folinic acid + azithromycin 1200-1500 mg/d or clarithromycin 1 g bid or atovaquone 750 mg with food qid; azithromycin 900 mg PO x 2 first day, then 1200 mg/d x 6 wks, then 600 mg/d	Spread through raw or undercooked meat (lamb, beef, and pork) and by contact with infected cat feces; may require dexamethasone if significant cerebral edema is present
Toxoplasmosis	Suppressive therapy	Pyrimethamine PO 25-75 mg/d + folinic acid PO 10 mg/d + sulfadiazine PO 0.5-1 g q6h	Pyrimethamine + folinic acid + clindamycin	May be able to discontinue when CD4 >200/mm^3 for >3 mo and viral load <5000 copies/mL
Toxoplasmosis	Primary prophylaxis	Not generally recommended	TMP-SMX DS qd	**Indications for primary prophylaxis**: positive IgG serology plus CD4+ <100/mm^3

Table 15

Opportunistic Infections (continued)

Pathogen	Indication	First choice	Alternative regimens	Comments
Histoplasmosis	**Treatment**	Amphotericin B 0.7-1.0 mg/kg/d IV for 3-14 d; itraconazole 200 mg PO tid x 3 d, then 200 mg PO bid or oral suspension 100 mg bid x 12 weeks	Fluconazole 800 mg/d	Spread through inhalation of dust particles; found in soils heavily contaminated by avian or bat feces; the Ohio and Mississippi River valleys are endemic areas in the U.S.
Histoplasmosis	**Maintenance therapy**	After amphotericin: itraconazole 200 mg PO tid x 3 d; then 200 mg bid x 12 weeks, then 200-400 mg qd indefinitely	Amphotericin B 1.0 mg/kg weekly; fluconazole 800 mg/d	Itraconazole is superior to fluconazole; No data for discontinuation
Histoplasmosis	**Primary prophylaxis**	Not generally recommended	Itraconazole 200 mg PO qd; fluconazole 200 mg PO qd	**Indications for primary prophylaxis**: antigen positive and live in endemic area or if at high risk (CD4+ <100/mm^3 and work with soil)
Mycobacterium avium complex (MAC)	**Treatment**	Clarithromycin 500 mg PO bid + ethambutol 15 mg/kg/d PO with or w/o rifabutin 300 mg PO qd	Azithromycin + ethambutol with or w/o rifabutin	Treatment is indefinite without immune reconstitution; may be discontinued when MAC treatment is >1 y, CD4 >100/mm^3 for 3-6 months, and patient is asymptomatic
Mycobacterium avium complex (MAC)	**Primary prophylaxis:** generally recommended at CD4 counts <50/mm^3	Azithromycin 1200 mg PO q week; clarithromycin 500 mg PO bid	Rifabutin; azithromycin + rifabutin	May be able to discontinue when CD4 >100/mm^3 for >6 mo with substantial suppression of viral load
Cytomegalovirus retinitis	**Treatment**	Intraocular ganciclovir release device[1] (Vitrasert®) q 6 months + oral ganciclovir 1.0-1.5 g PO tid; valganciclovir 900 mg PO bid x 21 d; foscarnet IV x 14-21 d; ganciclovir IV x 14-21 d; cidofovir IV q wk x 2 wk	Intraocular injections of foscarnet; fomivirsen intravitreal injection	Oral ganciclovir should not be used as sole induction therapy
Cytomegalovirus retinitis	**Maintenance**	Ganciclovir 1000 mg PO tid; valgancyclovir 900 mg PO qd; ganciclovir IV q 5-7 d/wk; foscarnet IV/d; cidovovir IV q 2 wk; intraocular ganciclovir release device (Vitrasert®) q 6 mo + oral ganciclovir 1.0-1.5 g PO tid		Lifelong maintenance therapy is required for retinitis in patients without immune recovery (CD4 >100-150/mm^3 for greater than 6 mo)
Cytomegalovirus retinitis	**Primary prophylaxis**	Not generally recommended unless positive serology and CD4 count <50/mm^3	Ganciclovir PO 1 g tid	

[1]Intraocular device does not protect contralateral eye and does not protect against systemic infection with cytomegalovirus.

3. Prevention

- Abstain from sex with an infected person.

- Ask about the sexual history of current and future sex partners.

- Reduce the number of sex partners to minimize the risk of HIV infection.

- Always use a latex condom from start to finish during any type of sex (vaginal, anal, or oral).

- Use only water-based lubricants.

- Avoid alcohol, illicit drugs, and sharing of needles (or syringes, cookers, or other drug paraphernalia).

- Do not share personal items such as toothbrushes, razors, or any devices used during sex. Such items may be contaminated by blood, semen, or vaginal secretions.

- Do not donate blood, plasma, sperm, body organs, or tissues if you are infected with HIV or have engaged in sex or needle-sharing behaviors that are risk factors for infection with HIV.

4. Hematologic Complications

Anemia

Causes
- HIV infection of marrow progenitor cells

- Drug-induced marrow suppression (AZT, ganciclovir, amphotericin, ribavirin, pyrimethamine, interferon, TMP-SMX)

Treatment
- See Figure 1.

Figure 1.

Guidelines for the treatment of anemia in the HIV patient.

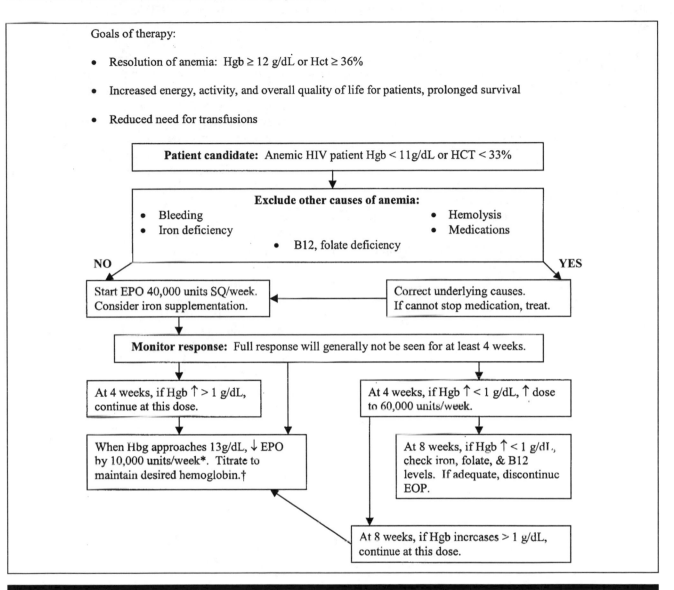

EPO, erythropoietin.

*If Hgb >15 g/dL at any point, hold EPO and restart when Hgb <12 g/dL, using dose reduced by 10,000 U/week.

†During the dose adjustment phase, Hgb should be monitored every 2-4 weeks. Allow at least 4 weeks to assess response to dose changes.

5. Key Points

- The human immunodeficiency virus (HIV) is a virus that destroys the immune system.

- The acquired immunodeficiency syndrome (AIDS) is caused by HIV and is defined as a CD4+ cell count less than 200/mm^3 or the presence of an opportunistic infection.

- The acute retroviral syndrome occurs in 50-90% of patients within the first 2-4 weeks of infection with HIV.

- The viral load indicates the amount of virus in the body and is an indication of how well antiretroviral medications are working.

- The CD4+ cell count refers to the status of the immune system and how at-risk a patient is for developing an opportunistic infection.

- Nucleoside reverse transcriptase inhibitors (NRTIs), non-nucleoside reverse transcriptase inhibitors (NNRTIs), protease inhibitors (PIs), and entry inhibitors are the currently available classes of medications used to treat HIV.

- Prevention of vertical transmission occurs by treating the mother with highly active antiretroviral therapy (HAART; preferred) or zidovudine alone.

- *Pneumocystis carinii* pneumonia (PCP) requires primary prophylaxis at CD4$^+$ cell counts <200/mm^3. TMP-SMX is the preferred treatment.

- *Mycobacterium avium* complex (MAC) requires primary prophylaxis at CD4$^+$ cell counts <50/mm^3. Azithromycin is the preferred drug.

- All other opportunistic infections require treatment followed by secondary prophylaxis.

6. Questions and Answers

1. C.T. is a 23-year-old HIV-positive female who presents to the ER with shortness of breath and a fever. Physical exam reveals a temperature of 102°F, HR of 100 bpm, and decreased breath sounds in the left lower lobe of lungs. Chest x-ray is positive for infiltrates in the left lung. She is diagnosed with PCP pneumonia. She has no previous history of opportunistic infections and is not on any medications at this time (she has not been seen by a health care provider in over a year). Her CD4$^+$ count is 13 cells/mm^3 and viral load is 70,198 copies/mL. What is the treatment of choice for C.T.'s PCP?

   A. TMP-SMX DS 2 tabs PO q8h for 21 days, then 1 tab PO qd
   B. Azithromycin 500 mg PO on day one, then 250 mg PO qd indefinitely
   C. Doxycycline 100 mg PO bid for 7 days, then 100 mg PO qd
   D. Clarithromycin 500 mg PO bid for 10 days, then 250 mg PO qd
   E. Vancomycin 1 g IV q12h for 10 days, then TMP-SMX DS PO qd

2. Should C.T. receive any other prophylaxis against opportunistic infections?

   A. Yes, against MAC: Zithromax® 1200 mg PO q week
   B. Yes, against thrush: Diflucan® 100 mg PO qd
   C. Yes, against toxoplasmosis: Bactrim DS® 1 tab PO q M, W, and F
   D. Yes, against CMV: Valcyte® 450 mg PO q M, W, and F
   E. No

3. Six weeks later C.T. presents to the HIV clinic for follow-up. Her CD4$^+$ count is 12 cells/mm^3 and viral load is 40,202 copies/mL. Should C.T. be started on HIV therapy?

   A. Yes, her CD4$^+$ cell count is <200 cells/mm^3 and she has had an opportunistic infection
   B. Yes, her viral load is greater than 55,000 copies/mL
   C. Yes, her Western blot was positive for HIV
   D. Yes, all patients with HIV should be treated as soon as the diagnosis is made
   E. No

4. C.T. wishes to be started on HIV therapy. Which

of the following would be an appropriate regimen?

A. Zidovudine + efavirenz + nelfinavir
B. Zidovudine + stavudine + indinavir
C. Zalcitabine + didanosine + amprenavir
D. Zidovudine + lamivudine + lopinavir/ritonavir
E. Nelfinavir + indinavir + amprenavir

5. HIV can be transmitted by:

A. Unprotected sexual contact with an infected person
B. Sharing needles or syringes with an infected person
C. Infected mother to infant (vertical transmission)
D. Transfusion of blood (before 1985)

6. M.J. is 13 weeks pregnant and just tested positive for HIV. Her viral load is 22,434 copies/mL and her CD4$^+$ cell count is 425 cells/mm^3. M.J. wishes to receive treatment for her HIV. Which of the following would be an appropriate regimen for M.J.?

A. Zidovudine + stavudine + indinavir
B. Zidovudine + lamivudine + nevirapine
C. Zidovudine + lamivudine + efavirenz
D. Stavudine + didanosine + nelfinavir
E. No treatment is necessary

7. Which of the following antiretroviral medications has shown efficacy as monotherapy in decreasing the vertical transmission of HIV?

A. Efavirenz
B. Nelfinavir
C. Zidovudine
D. Zalcitabine
E. Stavudine

8. R.C. is a nurse in the emergency room. She has just been stuck with a needle that was used for an HIV-positive patient with a known high viral load. Which of the following is true concerning postexposure prophylaxis?

I. The regimen should be started within 2 hours of exposure
II. R.C. will only need to be treated with zidovudine
III. R.C. will need to be treated with a combination of zidovudine + lamivudine + nelfinavir

IV. Treatment will continue for 4 weeks

A. I, III, and IV
B. II only
C. II, III, and IV
D. I, IV
E. I, II, and IV

9. The CD4$^+$ cell count relates to:

I. The activity of the virus
II. The status of the immune system
III. How at-risk a patient is for acquiring an opportunistic infection
IV. When the patient was infected
V. Time to death in treated patients

A. IV, V
B. I, II, and III
C. II, III
D. II, III, and IV
E. I, II, V

10. The viral load relates to:

A. The activity of the virus and efficacy of antiretroviral therapy
B. The status of the immune system
C. When the patient was infected
D. How at-risk a patient is for acquiring an opportunistic infection
E. Time to death in a treated patient

11. S.J. presents to the ER with extreme flank pain with nausea and vomiting. He is diagnosed with a kidney stone. His past medical history is positive for HIV and diabetes. His medications include indinavir, stavudine, didanosine, dapsone, and metformin. Which of his medications might have caused his kidney stone?

A. Indinavir
B. Stavudine
C. Didanosine
D. Metformin
E. Dapsone

12. L.L. comes to clinic today with a chief complaint of burning and tingling in his feet that started about 1 month ago. His current medications include nelfinavir, stavudine, lamivudine, sertraline, and gemfibrozil. Which medication(s) might be causing this problem?

A. Nelfinavir
B. Stavudine
C. Lamivudine
D. Sertraline
E. Gemfibrozil

13. S.E. presents to the ER with a 2-day history of extreme nausea, vomiting, and abdominal pain. Labs reveal elevations in amylase and lipase and a diagnosis of pancreatitis is made. His medications include nevirapine, tenofovir, didanosine, and amitriptyline. Which of his medications could have caused his pancreatitis?

A. Nevirapine
B. Tenofovir
C. Didanosine
D. Amitriptyline
E. All of the above

14. Which of the following HIV medications has a 5% incidence of a hypersensitivity reaction?

A. Efavirenz
B. Ritonavir
C. Zidovudine
D. Abacavir
E. Lamivudine

15. C.J. is starting efavirenz, zidovudine, lamivudine, and TMP-SMX today. What should C.J. be counseled about concerning efavirenz?

A. Anemia
B. CNS side effects
C. Neutropenia
D. Renal toxicity
E. Kidney stones

16. Which of the following can cause hepatotoxicity and requires monitoring of liver enzymes at baseline, 2 weeks, 4 weeks, 6 weeks, and every 3-6 months thereafter while the patient is on the medication?

A. Zidovudine
B. Zalcitabine
C. Lopinavir
D. Amprenavir
E. Nevirapine

17. Which of the following can cause hyperglycemia, hyperlipidemia (particularly elevations in triglycerides), and lipodystrophy?

A. Amprenavir
B. Delavirdine
C. Didanosine
D. Abacavir
E. Lamivudine

18. Lactic acidosis and hepatic steatosis has been reported with which of these antiretroviral medications?

A. Nevirapine
B. Efavirenz
C. Stavudine
D. Saquinavir
E. Nelfinavir

19. The mechanism of action of nucleoside reverse transcriptase inhibitors is to:

A. Directly inhibit reverse transcriptase
B. Prevent entry of the proviral DNA into the nucleus of the CD4$^+$ cell
C. Cause chain termination, resulting in a defective copy of proviral DNA
D. Prevent entry of HIV into the CD4$^+$ cell
E. Prevent cleavage of the newly formed polypeptide chains into a viable HIV

20. The mechanism of action of non-nucleoside reverse transcriptase inhibitors is to:

A. Prevent cleavage of the newly formed polypeptide chains into viable HIV
B. Prevent entry of HIV into the CD4$^+$ cell
C. Prevent entry of the proviral DNA into the nucleus of the CD4$^+$ cell
D. Directly inhibit reverse transcriptase
E. Cause chain termination, resulting in a defective copy of proviral DNA

21. The mechanism of action of protease inhibitors is to:

A. Cause a defective copy of proviral DNA to be made
B. Prevent entry of the proviral DNA into the nucleus of the CD4$^+$ cell
C. Prevent cleavage of the newly formed polypeptide chains into a viable HIV
D. Prevent entry of HIV into the CD4$^+$ cell
E. Directly inhibit reverse transcriptase

22. Which of the following nucleoside reverse transcriptase inhibitor combinations is acceptable?

A. Stavudine + zidovudine
B. Zalcitabine + stavudine
C. Zidovudine + lamivudine
D. Zalcitabine + didanosine
E. Zalcitabine + delavirdine

23. Which of the following opportunistic infections are the only ones requiring primary prophylaxis?

A. PCP and MAC
B. PCP and toxoplasmosis
C. MAC and histoplasmosis
D. MAC and CMV
E. PCP and thrush

24. The antifungal of first choice for maintenance therapy after treatment of cryptococcal meningitis is:

A. Itraconazole
B. Fluconazole
C. Ketoconazole
D. Amphotericin B
E. Terbinafine

25. The first-choice antifungal for treatment of histoplasmosis is:

A. Itraconazole
B. Fluconazole
C. Ketoconazole
D. Caspofungin
E. Terbinafine

Answers

1. **A.** The treatment of choice for PCP is TMP-SMX in patients who are not allergic to sulfa medications. Duration of treatment is for 21 days. Since this patient's CD4$^+$ cell count is below 200 cells/mm^3 and she has had PCP, she will require secondary prophylaxis once treatment is completed. Preferred prophylaxis is once-daily TMP-SMX DS.

2. **A.** This patient's CD4$^+$ cell count is below 50 cells/mm^3; therefore she requires primary prophylaxis against MAC. Zithromax is the drug of choice. Prophylaxis against other opportunistic infections is generally not required.

3. **A.** Current guidelines state that any patient who has had an opportunistic infection or a CD4$^+$ cell count less than 200 cells/mm^3 should start treatment for HIV. This patient has had both.

4. **D.** Most regimens contain two NRTIs and either one PI or one NNRTI. **A** includes one NRTI, one NNRTI and one PI. **E** includes three PIs. Zidovudine and stavudine competitively inhibit each other and would not be used in the same regimen (thus **B** is incorrect). Zalcitabine is contraindicated with didanosine, stavudine, and lamivudine, due to increased toxicity (which makes **C** incorrect).

5. **E.** All items are important risk factors for transmission of HIV. Breastfeeding, history of STDs, occupational exposure to HIV-infected fluids (rare), and household exposure to HIV infected fluids (rare) are also risk factors.

6. **B.** All HIV-positive pregnant women should receive treatment for HIV to decrease the risk of transmission to their offspring. Zidovudine and stavudine competitively inhibit each other and should not be used together. Efavirenz is teratogenic and should not be used in pregnancy. Stavudine and didanosine together are contraindicated in pregnancy due to increased risk of lactic acidosis and liver damage.

7. **C.** Zidovudine and neviripine are the only HIV medications that can reduce vertical transmission when used as monotherapy. Most practitioners treat with combination therapy due to the increased risk of resistance with monotherapy and how this has an impact on future choices of drug regimen.

8. **A.** The approved regimens for postexposure prophylaxis are zidovudine and lamivudine with or without nelfinavir or indinavir. Treatment should continue for 4 weeks and should start within 2 hours of exposure.

9. **C.** CD4$^+$ cell count describes the status of the immune system (ie, how at-risk a patient is for acquiring an opportunistic infection).

10. **A.** Viral load relates to the activity of the virus and efficacy of antiretroviral therapy. The goal of therapy is an undetectable viral load (<50 copies/mL).

11. **A.** Indinavir can cause kidney stones. Patients should drink at least 48 ounces of water a day to decrease the risk of developing a kidney stone.

12. **B.** All the "D" drugs, d4T (stavudine), ddI (didanosine), and ddC (zalcitabine), can cause peripheral neuropathy and pancreatitis.

13. **C.** All the "D" drugs, d4T (stavudine), ddI (didanosine), and ddC (zalcitabine), can cause peripheral neuropathy and pancreatitis.

14. **D.** Abacavir has a 5% incidence of hypersensitivity. Symptoms can include rash, fever, stomach symptoms, throat symptoms, or flu-like symptoms.

15. **B.** Efavirenz can cause CNS side effects such as dizziness, trouble sleeping, drowsiness, trouble concentrating, and/or unusual dreams during the first 2-4 weeks of treatment.

16. **E.** All NNRTIs can cause hepatotoxicity. There have been rare reports of hepatotoxicity after just one dose of nevirapine. Liver enzymes should be monitored at baseline, 2 weeks, 4 weeks, 6 weeks, and every 3-6 months thereafter.

17. **A.** Class side effects of PIs include hyperglycemia, hyperlipidemia, lipodystrophy, increased bleeding in hemophiliacs, and possibly osteoporosis or osteopenia.

18. **C.** Class side effects of NRTIs include lactic acidosis and hepatic steatosis.

19. **C.** NRTIs affect reverse transcriptase by causing chain termination, resulting in a defective copy of proviral DNA.

20. **D.** NNRTIs affect reverse transcriptase by directly inhibiting reverse transcriptase, resulting in less proviral DNA being made.

21. **C.** PIs prevent cleavage of the newly formed polypeptide chains into viable HIV, resulting in an immature virus that is unable to infect other $CD4^+$ cells.

22. **C.** Stavudine is contraindicated with zidovudine due to competitive inhibition. Zalcitabine is contraindicated with other NRTIs that may cause peripheral neuropathy (eg, stavudine and didanosine). Delavirdine is an NNRTI.

23. **C.** PCP requires primary prophylaxis when the $CD4^+$ cell count falls below 200 cells/mm³. The preferred medication is TMP-SMX. MAC requires primary prophylaxis when the $CD4^+$ cell count falls below 50 cells/mm³. The preferred medication is azithromycin.

24. **B.** Generally, cryptococcal meningitis is initially treated with amphotericin B during the induction phase, and then fluconazole for the consolidation phase and maintenance therapy.

25. **A.** Histoplasmosis is generally initially treated with amphotericin B or itraconazole for induction therapy, and then itraconazole for maintenance therapy.

7. References

Bartlett JG, Gallant JE. *2003 Medical Management of HIV Infection*. Baltimore: Johns Hopkins University Press; 2000:357-360.

Carr A, Miller J, Law M, Coopoer DA. A syndrome of lipoatrophy, lactic acidaemia, and liver dysfunction associated with HIV nucleoside analog therapy: Contribution to protease inhibitor–related lipodystrophy syndrome. *AIDS*. 2000;14:F25-F32.

Carr A, Samars K, Thorisdottir A, et al. Diagnosis, prediction, and natural course of HIV-1 protease inhibitor associated lipodystrophy, hyperlipidaemia, and diabetes mellitus: a cohort study. *Lancet*. 1999;353:2093-2099.

Centers for Disease Control and Prevention, Perinatal HIV Guidelines Working Group. Public Health Service Task Force recommendations for the use of antiretroviral drugs in pregnant women infected with HIV-1 for maternal health and for reducing perinatal HIV-1 transmission in the United States. *MMWR Morb Mortal Wkly Rep*. 1998;47:1-30.

Centers for Disease Control and Prevention. 1993 revised classification system for HIV infection and expanded surveillance case definition for AIDS among adolescents and adults. *MMWR Morb Mortal Wkly Rep*. 1992;41:1-19.

Chaisson RE, Keruly JC, Moore RD. Association of initial CD4 cell count and viral load with response to highly active antiretroviral therapy. JAMA. 2000;284: 3128-3129.

Chesney MA. Factors affecting adherence to antiretroviral therapy. *Clin Infect Dis*. 2000;30(suppl 2):S171-176.

Current United States epidemiology figures can be located at www.cdc.gov/hiv/stats/hasrlink.htm.

Current world epidemiology figures can be found at www.unaids.org.

Finzi D, Hermankova M, Pierson T, et al. Identification of a reservoir for HIV-1 in patients on highly active antiretroviral therapy. *Science*. 1997;278:1295-1300.

Furret H, Egger M, Opravil M, et al. Discontinuation of primary prophylaxis against *Pneumocystis carinii* pneumonia in HIV-1 infected adults treated with combination antiretroviral therapy. Swiss HIV Cohort Study. *N Engl J Med*. 1999;340:1301-1306.

Guidelines for postexposure prophylaxis can be located as a living document on the web at www.aidsinfo.nih.gov, which is updated 3-4 times a year.

Guidelines for prevention and treatment and medications used for the treatment of HIV can be located as a living document at www.aidsinfo.nih.gov, which is updated 3-4 times a year.

Guidelines for prophylaxis and treatment of opportunistic infections can be located as a living document at www.aidsinfo.nih.gov, which is updated 3-4 times a year.

Guidelines for prevention of vertical transmission can be located as a living document at www.aidsinfo. nih.gov, which is updated 3-4 times a year.

Hoen B, Dumon B, Harzic M, et al. Highly active antiretroviral treatment initiated early in the course of symptomatic primary HIV-1 infections: Results of the ANRS 053 trial. *J Infect Dis*. 1999;180:1342-1346.

Mellors JW, Munoz A, Giorgi JV, et al. Plasma viral load and CD4$^+$ lymphocytes as prognostic markers of HIV-1 infections. *Ann Intern Med*. 1997;126:946-954.

Report of the NIH panel to define principles of therapy of HIV infection. *MMWR Morb Mortal Wkly Rep*. 1998;47(RR-5):1-41.

1999 USPHS/IDSA guidelines for the prevention of opportunistic infections in persons infected with human immunodeficiency virus. *MMWR Morb Mortal Wkly Rep*.1999;48(RR-10):1-67.

Sperling RS, Shapiro DE, Coombs RW, et al. Maternal viral load, zidovudine treatment, and the risk of transmission of human immunodeficiency virus type 1 from mother to infant. Pediatric AIDS Clinical Trials Group Protocol 076 Study Group. *N Engl J Med*. 1996;335:1621-1629.

Update: Provisional Public Health Service recommendations for chemoprophylaxis after occupational exposure to HIV. *MMWR Morb Mortal Wkly Rep*.1996;45:468-480.

Vittinghoff E, Scheer S, O'Malley P, et al. Combination antiretroviral therapy and recent declines in AIDS incidence and mortality. *J Infect Dis*. 1999;179:717-720.

32. Immunization

Stephan L. Foster, PharmD, RPh
Associate Professor, Department of Pharmacy
University of Tennessee College of Pharmacy

Contents

1. Introduction

Definitions

Immunity: A naturally or artificially-acquired state resulting in an individual being resistant or relatively resistant to the occurrence or effects of a foreign substance. This is the mechanism the body develops for protection from infectious disease. This is usually very specific to a single organism or to a group of closely related organisms.

Antigen: A live or inactivated substance capable of evoking antibody production. Antigens can be a live organism, such as bacteria or viruses, or an inactivated or killed organism or portion of an organism. A live organism generally evokes the most effective immune response.

Antibody: A protein evoked by an antigen which acts to eliminate that antigen.

Mechanisms for Acquiring Immunity

Active immunity: Protection produced by an individual's own immune system. Immunity acquired in this manner has a delayed onset and is usually permanent. Active immunity may be acquired by having an active disease or by vaccination. B lymphocytes (B cells) circulate in the blood and bone marrow for many years. Re-exposure to the antigen causes the cells to replicate and to produce antibody. These cells are also called memory B cells.

Passive immunity: Protection produced by an animal or human and transferred to another. Immunity acquired in this manner has a rapid onset and usually has a brief duration. This is the type of immunity an infant receives from his or her mother. All types of blood products contain varying amounts of antibody. Immune globulins and hyperimmune globulins are also used to induce passive immunity. One source of passive immunity is antitoxins, which contain antibodies against a known toxin.

2. Vaccines

Vaccination is the process of producing active immunity via use of vaccines. The immunological response is similar to natural infection, with a lower risk than that of the disease itself.

Classification of Vaccines

Live, attenuated vaccines: Vaccines produced by modifying a virus or bacteria to produce immunity. These vaccines usually do not produce disease, however they may. When this occurs the disease is usually much milder than the natural disease. These vaccines must replicate to be effective. These vaccines also require special handling, such as protection from heat and light, to keep them alive. Circulating antibody from another source may destroy the vaccine virus and cause vaccine failure. (Table 1).

Inactivated vaccines: Vaccines composed of all or a fraction of a virus or bacterium. These fractions include subunits (subvirions), bacterial cell-wall polysaccharides, conjugated (attached to a protein carrier) bacteria cell-wall polysaccharides, or inactivated toxins (toxoids). The bacteria or virus is inactivated using heat and/or chemicals. Inactivated vaccines are not alive and cannot replicate, therefore they are unable to induce disease. Inactivated antigens are not affected by circulating antibody (Table 2).

Table 1

Live Vaccines Available in the United States, 2003

Measles
Mumps
Rubella
Typhoid fever
Varicella
Yellow fever
Vaccinia (smallpox)

Table 2

Inactivated Vaccines Available in the United States, 2003

Anthrax
Diphtheria
Haemophilus influenzae type b
Hepatitis A
Hepatitis B
Influenza
Japanese encephalitis
Meningococcal A, C, Y, W-135
Pertussis, acellular
Pneumococcal polysaccharide
Pneumococcal conjugate
Rabies
Tetanus toxoid
Typhoid injectable

Vaccination Schedules

Vaccination schedules are available for children, adolescents, and adults (see Figures 1 and 2). The schedules indicate the most ideal times to administer vaccines. Additional catch-up schedules are available for children and adolescents who are behind in their vaccinations.

Intervals between doses of the same vaccine in a series are described in the tables.
- The minimum interval in a series for most vaccines is 4 weeks. Decreasing the interval may interfere with antibody response and protection.
- Usually the last dose in a series is separated from the previous dose by four to six months.
- Increasing the interval does not affect vaccine effectiveness. You never need to restart a series except for oral typhoid vaccine.

Administration of Multiple Vaccines

There are no contraindications to the simultaneous administration of any vaccines. Inactivated and live vaccines may be given in any combination at the same time.

Live vaccines must be separated from the administration of antibodies, such as blood products and immune globulins. Inactivated vaccines are not affected by circulating antibody.

If two live vaccines are not given at the same time, a four-week minimal interval must be observed. This is not true for two inactivated vaccines or an inactivated plus a live vaccine.

Vaccine Adverse Reactions

Vaccine adverse reactions are any untoward side effects caused by a vaccine.

- Local reactions are the most common type of adverse reaction. These include pain, swelling, and redness at the site of injection. These usually occur within minutes to hours of the injection and are usually mild and self-limiting. Occasionally, severe local reactions occur and are known as hypersensitivity reactions.

- Systemic adverse reactions include fever, malaise, myalgias, and headache. Systemic adverse reactions are more common following live vaccines, and are similar to a mild case of the disease.

- Allergic reactions are reactions to the vaccine antigens or some component of the vaccine. While rare, these reactions may be life-threatening.

- Vaccine Adverse Events Reporting System (VAERS) is a CDC-monitored surveillance system, which should be notified within 30 days of an adverse event that requires medical attention.

Contraindications and Precautions

A contraindication is a condition that increases the risk of an adverse reaction or decreases the effect of a vaccine.

A precaution is a condition that might possibly increase the risk of an adverse event or decrease the effect of a vaccine.

Figure 1.

Recommended adult immunization schedule—United States, 2003

	For all persons in this group	Catch-up on childhood vaccinations	For persons with medical / exposure indications
Age Group ▶ **Vaccine ▼**	**19-49 Years**	**50-64 Years**	**65 Years and Older**
Tetanus, Diphtheria (Td)*	1 dose booster every 10 years [1]		
Influenza	1 dose annually for persons with medical or occupational indications, or household contacts of persons with indications [2]	1 annual dose	
Pneumococcal (polysaccharide)	1 dose for persons with medical or other indications. (1 dose revaccination for immunosuppressive conditions) [3,4]		1 dose for unvaccinated persons [3] 1 dose revaccination [4]
Hepatitis B*	3 doses (0, 1-2, 4-6 months) for persons with medical, behavioral, occupational, or other indications [5]		
Hepatitis A	2 doses (0, 6-12 months) for persons with medical, behavioral, occupational, or other indications [6]		
Measles, Mumps, Rubella (MMR)*	1 dose if measles, mumps, or rubella vaccination history is unreliable; 2 doses for persons with occupational or other indications [7]		
Varicella*	2 doses (0, 4-8 weeks) for persons who are susceptible [8]		
Meningococcal (polysaccharide)	1 dose for persons with medical or other indications [9]		

Footnotes to Figure 1.

[1]*Tetanus and diphtheria (Td)*—A primary series for adults is 3 doses: the first 2 doses given at least 4 weeks apart and the 3rd dose, 6-12 months after the second. Administer 1 dose if the person had received the primary series and the last vaccination was 10 years ago or longer. MMWR 1991;40 (RR-10):1-21. The ACP Task Force on Adult Immunization supports a second option: a single Td booster at age 50 years for persons who have completed the full pediatric series, including the teenage/young adult booster. Guide for Adult Immunization. 3rd ed. ACP 1994:20.

[2]*Influenza vaccination*—Medical indications: chronic disorders of the cardiovascular or pulmonary systems including asthma; chronic metabolic diseases including diabetes mellitus, renal dysfunction, hemoglobinopathies, immunosuppression (including immunosuppression caused by medications or by human immunodeficiency virus [HIV]), requiring regular medical follow-up or hospitalization during the preceding year; women who will be in the second or third trimester of pregnancy during the influenza season. Occupational indications: health-care workers. Other indications: residents of nursing homes and other long-term care facilities; persons likely to transmit influenza to persons at high-risk (in-home caregivers to persons with medical indications, household contacts and out-of-home caregivers of children birth to 23 months of age, or children with asthma or other indicator conditions for influenza vaccination, household members and caregivers of elderly and adults with high-risk conditions); and anyone who wishes to be vaccinated. *MMWR* 2002;51(RR-3):1-31.

[3]*Pneumococcal polysaccharide vaccination*—Medical indications: chronic disorders of the pulmonary system (excluding asthma), cardiovascular diseases, diabetes mellitus, chronic liver diseases including liver disease as a result of alcohol abuse (eg, cirrhosis), chronic renal failure or nephrotic syndrome, functional or anatomic asplenia (eg, sickle cell disease or splenectomy), immunosuppressive conditions (eg,

Figure 2.

Recommended childhood and adolescent immunization schedule—United States, 2003

Vaccine ▼ / Age ▶	Birth	1 mo	2 mos	4 mos	6 mos	12 mos	15 mos	18 mos	24 mos	4-6 yrs	11-12 yrs	13-18 yrs
			range of recommended ages			catch-up vaccination				preadolescent assessment		
Hepatitis B[1]	HepB #1	only if mother HBsAg (-)								HepB series		
		HepB #2				HepB #3						
Diphtheria, Tetanus, Pertussis[2]			DTaP	DTaP	DTaP		DTaP			DTaP	Td	
Haemophilus influenzae Type b[3]			Hib	Hib	Hib	Hib						
Inactivated Polio			IPV	IPV		IPV				IPV		
Measles, Mumps, Rubella[4]						MMR #1				MMR #2	MMR #2	
Varicella[5]						Varicella				Varicella		
Pneumococcal[6]			PCV	PCV	PCV	PCV				PCV	PPV	
Hepatitis A[7]										Hepatitis A series		
Influenza[8]						Influenza (yearly)						

Vaccines below this line are for selected populations

This schedule indicates the recommended ages for routine administration of currently licensed childhood vaccines, as of December 1, 2002, for children through age 18 years. Any dose not given at the recommended age should be given at any subsequent visit when indicated and feasible. ▓ Indicates age groups that warrant special effort to administer those vaccines not previously given. Additional vaccines may be licensed and recommended during the year. Licensed combination vaccines may be used whenever any components of the combination are indicated and the vaccine's other components are not contraindicated. Providers should consult the manufacturers' package inserts for detailed recommendations.

congenital immunodeficiency, HIV infection, leukemia, lymphoma, multiple myeloma, Hodgkin's disease, generalized malignancy, organ or bone marrow transplantation), chemotherapy with alkylating agents, anti-metabolites, or long-term systemic corticosteroids. Geographic/other indications: Alaskan Natives and certain American Indian populations. Other indications: residents of nursing homes and other long-term care facilities. *MMWR* 1997;47(RR-8):1-24.

[4]***Revaccination with pneumococcal polysaccharide vaccine***—One time revaccination after 5 years for persons with chronic renal failure or nephrotic syndrome, functional or anatomic asplenia (eg, sickle cell disease or splenectomy), immunosuppressive conditions (eg, congenital immunodeficiency, HIV infection, leukemia, lymphoma, multiple myeloma, Hodgkin's disease, generalized malignancy, organ or bone marrow transplantation), chemotherapy with alkylating agents, anti-metabolites, or long-term systemic corticosteroids. For persons 65 and older, one-time revaccination if they were vaccinated 5 or more years previously and were aged less than 65 years at the time of primary vaccination. *MMWR* 1997;47(RR-8):1-24.

[5]***Hepatitis B vaccination***—Medical indications: hemodialysis patients, patients who receive clotting-factor concentrates. Occupational indications: health-care workers and public-safety workers who have exposure to blood in the workplace, persons in training in schools of medicine, dentistry, nursing, laboratory technology, and other allied health professions. Behavioral indications: injecting drug users, persons with more than one sex partner in the previous 6 months, persons with a recently acquired sexually-transmitted disease (STD), all clients in STD clinics, men who have sex with men. Other indications: household contacts and sex partners of persons with chronic HBV infection, clients and staff of institutions for the developmentally disabled, international travelers who will be in countries with high or intermediate prevalence of chronic HBV infection for more than 6 months, inmates of correctional facilities. MMWR 1991;40 (RR-13):1-25. (www.cdc.gov/travel/diseases/hbv.htm)

[6]***Hepatitis A vaccination***—For the combined HepA-HepB vaccine use 3 doses at 0, 1, 6 months. Medical indications: persons with clotting-factor disorders or chronic liver disease. Behavioral indications: men who have sex with men, users of injecting and noninjecting illegal drugs. Occupational indications: persons working with HAV-infected primates or with HAV in a research laboratory setting. Other indications: persons traveling to or working in countries that have high or intermediate endemicity of hepatitis A. MMWR 1999;48 (RR-12):1-37. (www.cdc.gov/travel/diseases/ hav.htm)

Footnotes to Figure 1 (continued).

[7]Measles, mumps, rubella vaccination (MMR)—Measles component: Adults born before 1957 may be considered immune to measles. Adults born in or after 1957 should receive at least one dose of MMR unless they have a medical contraindication, documentation of at least one dose or other acceptable evidence of immunity. A second dose of MMR is recommended for adults who:

- are recently exposed to measles or in an outbreak setting
- were previously vaccinated with killed measles vaccine
- were vaccinated with an unknown vaccine between 1963 and 1967
- are students in post-secondary educational institutions
- work in health care facilities
- plan to travel internationally

Mumps component: 1 dose of MMR should be adequate for protection. Rubella component: Give 1 dose of MMR to women whose rubella vaccination history is unreliable and counsel women to avoid becoming pregnant for 4 weeks after vaccination. For women of child-bearing age, regardless of birth year, routinely determine rubella immunity and counsel women regarding congenital rubella syndrome. Do not vaccinate pregnant women or those planning to become pregnant in the next 4 weeks. If pregnant and susceptible, vaccinate as early in postpartum period as possible. MMWR 1998;47 (RR-8):1-57.

[8]Varicella vaccination—Recommended for all persons who do not have reliable clinical history of varicella infection, or serological evidence of varicella zoster virus (VZV) infection; health-care workers and family contacts of immunocompromised persons, those who live or work in environments where transmission is likely (eg, teachers of young children, day care employees, and residents and staff members in institutional settings), persons who live or work in environments where VZV transmission can occur (eg, college students, inmates and staff members of correctional institutions, and military personnel), adolescents and adults living in households with children, women who are not pregnant but who may become pregnant in the future, international travelers who are not immune to infection. Note: Greater than 90% of U.S.-born adults are immune to VZV. Do not vaccinate pregnant women or those planning to become pregnant in the next 4 weeks. If pregnant and susceptible, vaccinate as early in postpartum period as possible. MMWR 1996;45 (RR-11):1-36, *MMWR* 1999;48(RR-6):1-5.

[9]Meningococcal vaccine (quadrivalent polysaccharide for serogroups A, C, Y, and W-135)—Consider vaccination for persons with medical indications: adults with terminal complement component deficiencies, with anatomic or functional asplenia. Other indications: travelers to countries in which disease is hyperendemic or epidemic ("meningitis belt" of sub-Saharan Africa; Mecca, Saudi Arabia for the Hajj). Revaccination at 3-5 years may be indicated for persons at high risk for infection (eg, persons residing in areas in which disease is epidemic). Counsel college freshmen, especially those who live in dormitories, regarding meningococcal disease and the vaccine so that they can make an educated decision about receiving the vaccination. *MMWR* 2000;49(RR-7):1-20. Note: The AAFP recommends that colleges should take the lead on providing education on meningococcal infection and vaccination and offer it to those who are interested. Physicians need not initiate discussion of the meningococcal quadrivalent polysaccharide vaccine as part of routine medical care.

Contraindications include:
- An anaphylactic reaction to any previous dose of vaccine or to any of its components
- Pregnancy for live vaccines and selected inactivated vaccines
- Immunosuppression for live vaccines and selected inactivated vaccines
- Active, untreated tuberculosis and live vaccines
- Encephalopathy within 7 days of previous DTaP or DTP

Precautions include:
- Acute moderate to severe illness
- Recent administration of an antibody containing blood products and live vaccines
- DTP or DTaP: unstable or evolving neurological disorder
- MMR: history of thrombocytopenia or thrombocytopenic purpura
- High fever, shock, persistent crying, seizure, or Guillain-Barré syndrome due to previous dose of DTP or DTaP

Vaccine Management

- Maintain cold-chain during shipping
- Follow manufacturers' recommendation for shipping
- Non-frozen vaccines must not freeze during transport
- Refrigerate or freeze depending upon vaccine immediately upon arrival
- Utilize proper refrigerators
  * Monitor temperatures daily
  * Do not store vaccines in refrigerator door

- Inventory management
  * Rotate stock
  * Follow manufacturers guidelines for shelf life
  * Check expiration dates

- Follow manufacturers' directions for reconstitution

3. Diseases and Vaccines

Pneumococcal Disease

- *Streptococcal pneumonia:* 90 known serotypes of gram-positive bacteria with polysaccharide capsule
- Primary serious diseases include pneumonia, sepsis, and meningitis.

Rates of disease
- Highest rates in children less than 2 years of age
- Other children at high risk include those with asplenia, patients with HIV, American Indian-Alaskan Natives, African Americans, and day-care attendees.
- The elderly have fatality rates of 30-60% (those over the age of 50).
- Pneumococcal disease is one of the leading causes of vaccine-preventable diseases, with 20,000 to 40,000 deaths every year.
- Pneumococcal bacteria are common respiratory tract inhabitants, with estimated asymptomatic carriage rates varying from 5–70%.
- Transmission is through direct person-to-person droplet contamination or autoinoculation by carriers.
- Clinical features include abrupt onset, fever, otitis media, shaking chills, productive cough, pleuritic chest pain, dyspnea, hypoxia, tachypnea, headaches, lethargy, vomiting, irritability, nuchal rigidity, seizures, coma, and death.
- Resistance to antibiotics is up to 35% in certain areas of the country and rising.

23-Valent polysaccharide vaccine (Pneumovax-23® by Merck)
- Ineffective in children less than 2 years old
- Effective against 88% of serotypes causing bacteremic disease

Indications
- Adults over the age of 65
- Everyone over age 2 with chronic disease

Dose
- 0.5 mL IM or SC
- Revaccination (2-dose maximum)
  * Patients at high risk of disease if >5 years since previous dose
  * Everyone 65 years and older who received initial dose under the age of 65 and if >5 years since previous dose

- Adverse reactions include pain, swelling, and redness at injection site and slight to moderate systemic reactions such as fever and myalgias.

7-Valent conjugated polysaccharide vaccine (Prevnar® by Wyeth)
- Effective against 86% of serotypes causing bacteremic disease, 83% of serotypes against meningitis, and 65% of serotypes causing otitis media

Indications
- Routine vaccination for all children less than 2 years of age
- Children 24-59 months of age with high-risk medical conditions

Dose:
- 0.5 mL IM at 2, 4, 6, and 12-15 months of age (see schedules for catch-up recommendations)
- Revaccination not recommended but high-risk children should receive 23-valent polysaccharide vaccine after 2 years of age.
- Adverse reactions include pain, swelling, and redness at injection site, difficulty in moving limb (rare) and slight to moderate systemic reactions such as fever and myalgias.

Influenza

- RNA virus of orthomyxovirus family
- Antigenic drift: Frequent minor changes in the antigenic structure of the virus. This can reach epidemic proportions, but not every year. This is what requires yearly adjustments in vaccine formulations. All three types (A, B, C,) can undergo drifts.
- Antigenic shift: Major change in one or both of the major antigens in influenza A, resulting in a different subtype. This can result in major pandemics in all ages.

Influenza A
- Subtypes based upon two surface antigens: hemagglutinin and neuraminidase.
- Four types of hemagglutinin (H1, H2, H3, and H5) cause disease in humans and cause virus attachment to cells.
- Two types of neuraminidase cause disease in humans (N1 and N2) and have a role in viral penetration of cells.
- Causes moderate to severe disease in all ages and can be transmitted in other animals

Influenza B
- No subgroups
- Causes milder disease and effects primarily children
- Only affects humans

Influenza C
- Rarely reported and many cases are subclinical

Influenza disease

- Major serious complications in all types include pneumonia, Reye's syndrome (progressive neurological symptoms associated with aspirin use in children), myocarditis, worsening of chronic bronchitis, and death.
- Rates of disease highest in the elderly (>65), children less than 2 years of age, and persons of any age with medical conditions.
- Influenza is one of the leading causes of vaccine-preventable disease, with 20,000 to 40,000 deaths during epidemics. Pandemics could result in the deaths of over 400,000 people.
- Influenza virus penetrates the respiratory epithelial cells and destroys the host.
- Virus is shed in respiratory secretions for 5-10 days and transmission is through direct person-to-person droplet contamination or contact. The incubation period is approximately 2 days (range 1-5 days).
- Clinical features include abrupt onset, fever, myalgias, sore throat, nonproductive cough, and headache.
- Disease peaks between December and March in Northern Hemisphere, but may occur earlier or later. Year-round cases may be seen in tropical climates.

Influenza vaccine (Fluviron® by Evans and Fluzone® by Aventis-Pasteur)

- Inactivated, split-virus vaccine
- Contains 3 vaccine components (2 type A viruses and 1 type B)
- Vaccines are named according to the virus' type/geographic origin/strain sequence number/year of isolation (hemagglutinin neuraminidase for type A only): For example, A/Panama/2007/99(H3N2) or B/Hong Kong/330/2001.
- Effective in up to 90% of healthy adults, 50-60% of the elderly, and 30-40% of the frail elderly

Indications

- Adults over the age of 50
- Everyone over age 6 months with chronic disease
- People who may infect others, including contacts of patients with diseases, and health care workers
- Pregnancy in second or third trimester
- Patients 6 months to 18 years of age on chronic aspirin therapy
- Anyone who wishes to decrease the likelihood of influenza disease

Dose

- 6-35 months: 0.25 mL IM (repeat in 1 month if first time); 3-8 years: 0.5 mL (repeat in 1 month if first time); >8 years: 0.5 mL
- Fluviron® by Evans indicated for age ≥4 years
- Revaccination yearly

- Contraindications include severe allergic reactions to previous dose and egg allergy.
- Adverse reactions include pain, swelling, and redness at injection site and slight to moderate systemic reactions such as fever, myalgias, chills, and malaise. Severe neurologic reactions are rare.

Tetanus

- Exotoxin produced by *Clostridium tetani*, a gram-positive anaerobic rod that may develop a highly resistant spore. These spores are widely spread in soil, animal intestines and feces, skin surfaces, and infected plants.
- Disease is characterized by generalized rigidity and convulsive spasms of skeletal muscles. Usually involves muscles of face (lockjaw) and neck. Spasms may last 3-4 weeks and complete recovery may take months.
- Enters body through contamination of wound. Spores germinate in anaerobic environment. Toxins are released and transported through body.
- Incubation period is usually 8 days (range, 3-21 days).
- Transmission risk factors include puncture wounds, surgery, burns, minor wounds, dental infections, animal bites, injection drug use, diabetes, and approximately 10% of cases are due to an unknown cause.
- Tetanus is not contagious person-to-person.
- Tetanus occurs in the U.S. at a rate of 0.02-0.05 per 100,000 per year. The case fatality rate is approximately 10%.
- Complications include: laryngospasm, fractures, hypertension, nosocomial infections, pulmonary embolism, aspiration, and death.
- Wound management recommendations may include tetanus immune globulin (see Table 3).

Tetanus toxoid vaccine

- Usually combined with diphtheria toxoid, and for children, pertussis vaccine
- Toxoid is formaldehyde-inactivated toxin adsorbed to aluminum.

Dose

- Pediatric dose: 0.5 mL IM of DT or DTaP given at 2, 4, 6, and 15-18 months of age. Booster dose should be given at 4-6 years.
- Adolescent and adult dose: Booster dose of 0.5 mL Td given at 11-12 years and every 10 years thereafter if the primary series is complete
- Revaccination every 10 years
- Adverse reactions include pain, swelling (nodule may form) and redness at injection site and systemic reactions are uncommon. An exaggerated (Arthus-

Table 3

CDC Guidelines for Tetanus Wound Management

Vaccination history	Clean minor wounds		All other wounds	
	Td[1]	TIG[2]	Td	TIG
Unknown or <3	Yes	No	Yes	Yes
Three or more	No[3]	No	No[4]	No

[1]Td, tetanus-diphtheria vaccine.
[2]TIG, tetanus immune globulin.
[3]Yes, if >10 years since last dose.
[4]Yes, if >5 years since last dose.

type) reaction with extensive painful swelling from shoulder to elbow can occur at injection site and is thought to be caused by too frequent injections.

Diphtheria

- Toxin produced by *Corynebacterium diphtheriae,* an aerobic gram-positive bacterium. This bacterium must be infected by a virus that carries a genetic code for toxin production.
- The most common presentation of diphtheria is characterized by early, nonspecific URI symptoms that develop into pharyngitis. Two to three days later, a bluish-white membrane starts to form that can cover the entire soft palate. The membrane can turn dark if bleeding occurs and manipulation of the membrane can result in bleeding. Airway obstruction may occur.
- Other sites of infection may include the larynx or the skin.
- Other complications may include myocarditis, neuritis with paralysis, respiratory failure and death (overall case fatality rate of 5-10%).
- Asymptomatic human carriers are the source of most infections.
- Incubation period is usually 2-5 days (range, 1-10 days)
- Treatment of acute disease is with antitoxin and antibiotics.

Diphtheria toxoid vaccine
- Combined with tetanus toxoid, and for children, pertussis vaccine. Single toxoid antigen is not available.
- Toxoid is formaldehyde-inactivated toxin adsorbed to aluminum.
- Pediatric version of combination (DT or DTaP) contains 3-4 times as much antigen as the adult version (Td).

Dose
- Pediatric dose: 0.5 mL IM of DT or DTaP given at 2, 4, 6, and 15-18 months of age. Booster dose should be given at 4-6 years.
- Adolescent and adult dose: Booster dose of 0.5 mL Td given at 11-12 years and every 10 years thereafter if the primary series is complete.
- Revaccination every 10 years.
- Adverse reactions include pain, swelling (nodule may form) and redness at injection site; systemic reactions are uncommon. An exaggerated (Arthus-type) reaction with extensive painful swelling from shoulder to elbow can occur at injection site and is thought to be caused by too frequent injections of the tetanus antigen component of the combination vaccines.

Pertussis

- Pertussis, or whooping cough, is caused by *Bordetella pertussis,* an aerobic, gram-negative rod. The bacteria produces multiple antigenic products that are responsible for the clinical disease. The bacteria produces toxin that paralyzes the respiratory cilia and causes inflammation of the respiratory tract.
- The presentation of pertussis is in three stages. The first stage is a catarrhal stage with nonspecific URI symptoms. After 1-2 weeks the paroxysmal stage with the characteristic cough and inspiratory whoop begins and lasts up to 6 weeks. Recovery is gradual and the cough usually resolves in 2-3 weeks.
- The presentation in older children and adults may be much milder and present with a persistent mild cough that lasts up to 7 days and may appear to be similar to other upper respiratory infections.
- Complications may include pneumonia, encephalopathy, seizures, and death (overall case fatality rate of 0.2%).
- Asymptomatic human carriers are the source of most infections.
- Incubation period is usually 7-10 days (range, 14-21 days).
- Treatment of acute disease includes supportive care, antibiotics, and prophylaxis of contacts.
- Transmission is human-to-human by the respiratory route. Pertussis is highly contagious with attack rates of 80% in susceptible contacts.

Pertussis vaccine
- Combined with tetanus toxoid and diphtheria toxoid for children. Single toxoid antigen is not available.
- Whole cell vaccine was developed in the 1930s, but is no longer available in the United States.
- Acellular pertussis vaccine was first licensed in 1991 and has fewer side effects than the whole cell vaccine.

Dose
- Pediatric dose: 0.5 mL IM of DTaP given at 2, 4, 6, and 15-18 months of age. Booster dose should be given at 4-6 years.
- Pertussis vaccine is not recommended for anyone 7 years of age or older due to adverse effects.
- Adverse reactions include pain, swelling (nodule may form) and redness at injection site and systemic reactions are uncommon. An exaggerated (Arthus-type) reaction with extensive painful swelling from shoulder to elbow can occur at injection site and is thought to be caused by too frequent injections of the tetanus antigen component of the combination vaccines.

Hepatitis B

- Hepatitis B is caused by a DNA virus and causes one of the most common infections worldwide. There are an estimated 200-300 million chronic carriers of hepatitis B worldwide.
- The clinical course is similar to that of all other types of viral hepatitis, with symptoms of malaise, weakness, anorexia, nausea, jaundice, abdominal pain, headache, and dark urine. Malaise and fatigue may last for weeks to months after all other symptoms disappear.
- Fulminant hepatitis occurs in 1-2% of all cases, with mortality rates of 60-90%.
- Complications are usually related to chronic infections with hepatitis B virus, and include chronic hepatitis, cirrhosis, liver failure, and hepatocellular carcinoma. Twenty-five percent of all carriers develop chronic, active hepatitis.
- The risk of becoming a carrier following infection ranges from 6-50%.
- Incubation period is usually 7-10 days (range, 14-21 days).
- There is no specific, effective treatment of acute disease.
- Transmission is human-to-human by exposure of body fluids by parenteral or mucosal contact. Hepatitis B is a common sexually transmitted disease. Perinatal transmission is a significant mode of infection.

Hepatitis B vaccine
- First vaccine was a plasma-derived vaccine released in 1981 and removed from the market in 1992.
- Current vaccine is hepatitis B surface antigen (HBsAg) produced using recombinant DNA technology; it was first released in 1986. Two products are currently marketed: Recombivax HB® (Merck) and Engerix-B® (Glaxo SmithKline). Although the antigen contents are different, the two vaccines are interchangeable.

Dose
- Pediatric dose: The usual dose is 0.5mL IM given at birth, 2 months, and 6 months.
- Indications include all infants, all adolescents, and high-risk adults (eg, multiple sex partners, STDs, injection drug use, dialysis, hemophilia, others).
- The usual adult dose is 1.0 mL given at 0, 2, and 6 months.
- Adolescents aged 11-15 years may be given a two-dose series separated by 4 months. This is only approved for Recombivax HB.
- Booster doses should not be given.
- Adverse reactions include pain, swelling (nodule may form) and redness at injection site; systemic reactions are uncommon. An exaggerated (Arthus-type) reaction with extensive painful swelling from shoulder to elbow can occur at the injection site, and is thought to be caused by too frequent injections of the tetanus antigen component of the combination vaccines.

Haemophilus influenzae type b (Hib)

- *Haemophilus influenzae* is a gram-negative coccobacillus, whose outer shell consists of a polyribosyl-ribitol phosphate (PRP) polysaccharide capsule. There are six distinctly different types of *H. influenzae*, labeled a-f; however, type b is responsible for 95% of human disease.
- The organism enters through the nasopharynx and may cause disease or may colonize the nasopharynx, creating an asymptomatic carrier.
- The most common clinical infections caused by Hib are meningitis, epiglottitis, pneumonia, arthritis, and cellulitis. Meningitis accounts for 50-65% of all clinical disease and results in a mortality of 2-5% and neurological sequelae in 15-30% of cases. Other diseases caused by *Haemophilus influenzae* include otitis, sinusitis, and bronchitis; however, these are usually due to nontypable (unencapsulated) strains.
- Hib is primarily a disease of children, with a peak at age 6-7 months and rarely attacks after the age of 5 years.
- Treatment of acute disease includes hospitalization, intravenous antibiotics, and prophylaxis of contacts.
- Transmission is human-to-human by respiratory droplet spread to susceptible individuals.

Haemophilus influenzae vaccine
- The incidence of Hib disease has decreased by more than 99% since the introduction of vaccine.
- The first vaccine licensed (1985-1988) was a pure polysaccharide vaccine that was ineffective in children less than 18 months of age.
- Current vaccines are polysaccharide vaccine conjugated to protein carriers. The specific carriers vary by manufacturer (see Table 4).

Table 4

Haemophilus influenzae **Type B Vaccines**

Vaccine	Protein carrier	Manufacturer	Age indications
PRP-D (ProHIBit®)	Diphtheria toxoid	Connaught	≥18 months
HbOC (HibTITER®)	Mutant diphtheria toxoid	Lederle-Praxis	≥6 weeks
PRP-T (ActHIB® or OmniHIB®)	Tetanus toxoid	Aventis Pasteur	≥6 weeks
PRP-OMB (PedvaxHIB®)	Meningococcal group B outer membrane protein	Merck & Co	≥6 weeks

- PRP-D (ProHIBit®) is not indicated for children less than 18 months of age. All other brands [HbOC (HibTITER®), PRP-T (ActHIB® or OmniHIB®), PRP-OMB (PedvaxHIB®)] are indicated for infants ≥6 months of age.
- Doses given before 6 weeks of age may inhibit the production of antibodies to subsequent doses; therefore the vaccines are contraindicated in children less than 6 weeks of age.

Dose

- The usual dose for the vaccines approved for infants is 0.5 mL IM given at 2 months, 4 months, and 6 months. A booster dose is recommended for children 12-15 months of age. If PRP-OMB (PedvaxHIB) is used for the pediatric series, the 6-month dose should be omitted.
- The catch-up series for Hib vaccine varies by age and manufacturer. Consult the package insert for complete dosing information.
- Vaccination of children >59 months of age is not indicated unless there are certain medical indications. These include persons with asplenia, immunodeficiency conditions, and those undergoing immunosuppressive therapy.
- Combination vaccines of Hib vaccine and hepatitis B vaccine (COMVAX® by Merck) and Hib vaccine and DTaP (TriHIBit® by Aventis Pasteur) are available. TriHIBit is not approved for the initial pediatric series (2, 4, and 6 months) and can only be used for a dose at ≥12 months of age when a previous dose of Hib was given ≥2 months earlier, and TriHIBit will be the last dose in the Hib series. COMVAX must not be administered before 6 weeks of age.
- Adverse reactions include pain, swelling and redness at the injection site; systemic reactions are uncommon.

Hepatitis A

- Hepatitis A is caused by an RNA virus and is the most common hepatitis infection in the United States.
- The clinical course is similar to all other types of viral hepatitis, with symptoms of malaise, weakness, anorexia, nausea, jaundice, abdominal pain, headache, and dark urine. Malaise and fatigue usually lasts for 2 weeks; however, symptoms may last or reoccur for up to 6 months.
- Fulminant hepatitis A is rare, but can occur. The incidence increases with age greater than 40 years.
- While serious complications are not as common as with hepatitis B, morbidity and its associated costs (health care costs and lost work days) are significant.
- There is no risk of becoming a chronic carrier.
- The incubation period averages 28 days (range, 15-50 days).
- Treatment of acute disease is supportive.
- Transmission is human-to-human by the fecal-oral route of exposure.
- Exposure of an unimmunized person to hepatitis A requires the administration of immune globulin intramuscular (IGIM) as well as beginning the hepatitis A vaccine series.

Hepatitis A vaccine—two inactivated whole virus vaccines: Havrix® by GlaxoSmithKline and VAQTA® by Merck and Co.

- Both vaccines are available in pediatric and adult formulations
- Hepatitis A vaccine is not indicated for children <2 years of age
- The two vaccines use different potency measurements, but the volume and schedule of the dose is the same

Dose

- Children and adolescents 2-8 years old are given 0.5 mL and repeated in 6-12 months (Havrix®) or 6-18 months (VAQTA®), for a total of 2 doses
- Adults over 18 years old are are given 1.0 mL and repeated in 6-12 months, for a total of 2 doses
- A combination product with hepatitis B and hepatitis A (Twinrix® by GlaxoSmithKline) is available and is given at 0, 1, and 6-12 months. This product is intended for persons ≥18 years of age
- Adverse reactions include pain, redness, and swelling at the injection site. Mild systemic reactions are rare

Meningococcal

- Meningococcal disease is caused by *Neisseria meningitidis*, a gram-negative bacteria with a polysaccharide capsule.
- The clinical diseases caused by *Neisseria meningitidis* include meningitis, sepsis, pneumonia, myocarditis, and urethritis. It is one of the leading causes of meningitis in the United States.
- The types of *Neisseria meningiditis* that cause over 95% of disease are serogroups A, B, C, W-135, and Y.
- There are approximately 2500-3000 cases per year with an incidence rate of 2 cases per 100,000 people. The incidence in college freshmen that live in dormitories is approximately 4 cases/100,000.
- There is a carrier state that increases in incidence during epidemics.
- Parts of the world, including parts of Africa and Asia, have a high rate of disease.
- Treatment of acute disease is with antibiotics.

Meningococcal vaccine (Menomune® by Aventis Pasteur)

- This is a polysaccharide vaccine effective against serogroups A, C, W-135, and Y. The vaccine does not protect against serogroup B, a common cause of infection.
- Indicated for persons over the age of 2 years.
- Those who should be vaccinated include military personnel, freshmen college students living in dormitories, those with anatomic or functional asplenia, and travelers to the "meningitis belt" of sub-Saharan Africa. Evidence of immunization is required for religious pilgrimages to Saudi Arabia for the Islamic Hajj. Vaccine may also be useful during an outbreak

Dose

- Dose is 0.5 mL given subcutaneously.
- Booster dose after 3-5 years may be needed.

- Adverse reactions include pain, swelling (nodule may form) and redness at the injection site and mild systemic reactions, such as fever, headaches, and malaise.

Polio

- There are three poliovirus types identified as P1, P2, and P3.
- The virus enters the mouth and replicates in the gastrointestinal tract. From the GI tract, the virus enters the bloodstream and infects the cells of the central nervous system.
- Up to 95% of all infections are asymptomatic; however, these persons may transmit the infection to others.
- Approximately 4-8% of infections are mild with nonspecific symptoms of upper respiratory infection, gastroenteritis, and influenza-like symptoms.
- One to two percent of infections present as nonparalytic aseptic meningitis, which typically resolves in 2-10 days.
- Flaccid paralysis occurs in less than 1% of those infected.
- Incubation period is usually 6-20 days (range, 3-35 days).
- Treatment of acute disease includes supportive care.
- Transmission is person to person by the fecal-oral route.

Polio vaccine (IPOL® by Aventis Pasteur)

- The current vaccine available in the United States is an inactivated, trivalent injectable vaccine (IPV).
- Use of oral polio vaccine (OPV) was discontinued in the United States due to the elimination of wild-type polio disease and because yearly cases of vaccine-associated paralytic paralysis (VAPP) were reported.

Dose

- Pediatric dose: 0.5 mL IM given at 2, 4, 6-18 months, and 4-6 years of age.
- Routine vaccine or booster doses for adults are not recommended.
- Adverse reactions include minor pain, swelling, and redness at the injection site; systemic reactions are uncommon.

Measles, Mumps, and Rubella

Measles

- Measles is a viral infection whose main presentation is a maculopapular rash.
- The virus is shed through the nasopharynx.
- Ten to twelve days after exposure, the prodrome phase begins, with progressive fever, cough, coryza, and conjunctivitis.

- Two to four days after the prodrome begins, a maculopapular rash begins on the face and head and gradually spreads throughout the body.
- The rash lasts 3-5 days then gradually fades.
- The incubation period is 10-12 days.
- Transmission is person to person through large respiratory droplets.
- Measles is highly contagious.
- Complications may include pneumonia, otitis, encephalitis, and death.

Mumps

- Mumps is a viral infection with a presentation of parotitis in 30-40% of cases.
- The virus is shed through the nasopharynx.
- Fourteen to eighteen days after exposure, the prodrome phase begins, with headache, malaise, myalgias, and low-grade fever.
- Two days after the prodrome begins is when the parotitis begins.
- Symptoms start to decrease after 1 week and disappear after 10 days.
- The incubation period is 14-18 days (range, 14-25 days).
- Transmission is person to person through large respiratory droplets.
- Complications can include orchitis, oophoritis, pancreatitis, and deafness.

Rubella

- Rubella is a viral infection with up to 20-50% of cases subclinical and inapparent.
- The virus is shed through the nasopharynx.
- A 1-5 day prodrome phase begins after incubation, with headache, malaise, myalgias, lymphadenopathy, low-grade fever, and URI symptoms. This phase is rare in children.
- Fourteen to seventeen days after exposure, a maculopapular rash appears, first on the face, and then descending to cover the rest of the body.
- The rash disappears after about 3 days.
- The incubation period is 14 days (range, 12-23 days).
- Transmission is person to person through large respiratory droplets.
- Complications may include arthritis, arthralgias, encephalitis, and hemorrhaging.
- The major complication is congenital rubella syndrome, which occurs in the offspring of a woman who had rubella during pregnancy. Babies born with CRS have major birth defects that can affect many organs.

Measles-mumps-rubella vaccine (MMRII® by Merck)

- The current vaccine available in the United States is a live, attenuated vaccine against all three diseases.

Dose

- Pediatric dose: 0.5 mL IM given at 12 months of age
- A second dose is recommended at 4-6 years of age to produce immunity in those who did not respond to the first dose.
- This vaccine is contraindicated in pregnancy. Pregnancy should be avoided for 4 weeks following vaccination.
- Serologic testing may be necessary to document immunity to rubella.
- Vaccination with the combination product should be used when one or more of the vaccines are needed unless a contraindication exists for an antigen component of the vaccine.
- Adverse reactions include minor pain, swelling and redness at the injection site, and systemic reactions that mimic a mild case of the diseases.

Varicella (Chickenpox)

- Chickenpox is a viral infection caused by the herpes zoster virus.
- The primary infection is called chickenpox and the recurrent disease is herpes zoster (called shingles).
- The virus enters through the respiratory tract and replicates in the nasopharynx and regional lymph glands.
- The incubation period is 14-16 days (range, 10-21 days).
- A prodromal phase may precede the rash with a slight fever and malaise.
- The rash progresses from a macule to a papule to a vesicle before it crusts over.
- The rash appears in several waves that last 2-3 days each.
- The rash first appears on the face and then the trunk (where most of the rash occurs), and the extremities.
- Recurrent disease (herpes zoster) appears to be related to aging and immunosuppression.
- Recurrent disease usually presents as an outbreak of lesions along a dermatome that is usually unilateral. Neuralgia and intense pain may be present.
- Transmission is person to person by infected respiratory secretions.
- Complications may include pneumonia, secondary bacterial infections, CNS infections and symptoms, and Reye's syndrome if a child is taking aspirin.

Varicella Vaccine (Varivax® by Merck)

- The current vaccine available in the United States is a live, attenuated vaccine.

Dose
- Pediatric dose: 0.5 mL IM given at 12-18 months of age
- The adult dose (age >13 years) is 2 doses of 0.5 mL each separated by 4-8 weeks.
- This vaccine is contraindicated in pregnancy and pregnancy should be avoided for 4 weeks following vaccination.
- Other contraindications include immunosuppressive disease or patients receiving immunosuppressive therapy, and those receiving antibody-containing blood products.
- Adverse reactions include minor pain, swelling and redness at the injection site and systemic reactions that mimic a mild case of the diseases, including a mild generalized rash.
- The vaccine must be stored frozen at +5°F (−15°C). The diluent used to reconstitute the vaccine should be stored at room temperature.

4. Key Points

- The two types of vaccine antigens include live viruses and inactivated viruses or bacterial components.
- There are two types of immunity: active and passive.
- Adverse effects of inactivated vaccines include pain at the injection site and mild systemic symptoms (mild fever). Adverse effects of live vaccines mimic a mild case of the disease.
- Live vaccines should be avoided during pregnancy.
- Influenza viruses undergo shifts and drifts, which accounts for the need for yearly vaccine changes.
- Wound management must include evaluation for the need for tetanus toxoid and tetanus immune globulin.
- Diphtheria toxoid and tetanus toxoid should always be given together, unless there is a contraindication to one of the components. If there is a need for one, then there is a need for both.
- The adult dosage form of tetanus-diphtheria vaccine is Td, which contains $1/3$ the dose of the pediatric form of DT or DTaP when combined with pertussis vaccine. Children 7 years old and older do not receive the pediatric version of DT or DTaP.
- Hepatitis B vaccine is now recommended for all infants, starting at birth, as well as all adolescents. Other indications include adults with high-risk occupations or behaviors.
- Hepatitis A vaccine is recommended for travel to most parts of the world.
- Inactivated polio vaccine (IPV) is the only polio vaccine recommended for use in the U.S. Oral polio vaccine (OPV) is not recommended due to the high incidence of vaccine-associated paralytic polio (VAPP).
- A second dose of MMR vaccine is recommended at 4-6 years of age to produce immunity in those who did not respond to the first dose.

5. Questions and Answers

1. A 62-year-old patient presents to your pharmacy for a refill of his insulin. It is October and he asks you to review his immunization status with him. About which adult vaccine do you need to ask his status?

I.   Influenza vaccine
II. Pneumococcal vaccine
III. Meningococcal vaccine
IV. Hepatitis A vaccine
V.   Diphtheria-tetanus (dT) vaccine

   A. I only
   B. I and II only
   C. III and IV only
   D. I, III, and V only
   E. I, II, and V only

2. The patient in question 1 states that he received his pneumococcal vaccine 2 years ago. When should he receive another?

   A. Never
   B. Every year
   C. In 5 years
   D. When he reaches the age of 67
   E. When he reaches the age of 65

3. Which of the following describes the current injectable influenza vaccine used in the United States.

   A. Inactivated virus
   B. Live attenuated virus
   C. Conjugated vaccine
   D. Toxoid
   E. Toxin

4. Indications for meningococcal vaccine include:

I.   All adolescents
II. Travel to the "meningitis belt" of sub-Saharan Africa
III. Asplenia
IV. Pilgrimage to Saudi Arabia for the Islamic Hajj
V.   College freshmen living in dormitories

   A. I only
   B. II, III, and V only
   C. I, II, and III only
   D. II, III, IV, and V only
   E. All of the above

5. At what age does one switch from DTaP to dT.

   A. 2 years
   B. 5 years
   C. 7 years
   D. 10 years
   E. DTaP can be used in all age groups

6. Which of the following vaccines has BOTH a polysaccharide and a conjugated vaccine on the U.S. market?

   A. Influenza
   B. Meningococcal vaccine
   C. *Haemophilus influenzae* type B vaccine
   D. Hepatitis vaccine
   E. Pneumococcal vaccine

7. Which polio vaccine schedule is recommended in the United States?

   A. Four doses of IPV
   B. Four doses of OPV
   C. Four doses of IPV plus a booster at 18 years of age
   D. Two doses of OPV and 2 doses of IPV
   E. Polio vaccine is no longer recommended in the United States.

8. Hepatitis B vaccine is a:

   A. Polysaccharide vaccine
   B. Recombinant hepatitis B surface antigen vaccine
   C. Live vaccine
   D. Conjugate vaccine
   E. A toxoid

9. An 18-year-old, healthy student is told that she needs to come to the pharmacy for her routine vaccinations prior to starting college. She will be living in the dormitory at school. She has not received any vaccines since grade school. Which of the following vaccines are indicated?

I.   MMR
II. Varicella if she has had not previous vaccination or varicella vaccination
III. Meningococcal vaccine
IV. Pneumococcal vaccine
V.   dT if she has not received one for 10 years

   A. All of the above
   B. I and II only
   C. I, II, III, and IV only
   D. I, III, and V only

E. I, II, III, and V only

10. The patient in question 9 is exposed to a patient with hepatitis A 1 month later. She should receive the following vaccines.

A. Hepatitis A vaccine series only
B. Hepatitis B vaccine series only
C. Hepatitis A vaccine series plus IGIM
D. Hepatitis A vaccine plus hepatitis B vaccine series
E. IGIM only

11. Which of the following are high-risk groups that should be targeted for annual influenza vaccination?

A. Persons aged 5 to 49 years
B. Persons with diabetes
C. Patients aged 21-49 with hypertension
D. Pregnant women in their first trimester
E. Healthy teenagers

12. Which complication of rubella infection is the most significant health problem?

A. Congenital rubella syndrome
B. Secondary infection
C. Patent ductus arteriosus
D. Diarrhea
E. Arthritis

13. Which of the following is a valid contraindication to the receipt of a live-virus vaccine?

A. Taking antibiotics
B. Recent administration of antibody-containing blood products
C. Age over 12 months
D. Allergies to penicillin
E. A parent or sibling living in the same household with a cold

14. The most common adverse reaction to an inactivated vaccine is:

A. Rash
B. Severe headache
C. Injection site reactions
D. Rhinorrhea
E. Stomach pain

15. The only vaccine recommended at birth is:

A. DTaP

B. IPV
C. Hib
D. Pneumococcal conjugate vaccine
E. Hepatitis B

16. A 32-year-old female is injured in an automobile accident and her spleen is removed. Which of the following vaccines is NOT routinely recommended for asplenic adult patients:

A. Pneumococcal vaccine
B. Meningococcal vaccine
C. IPV
D. *Haemophilus influenzae* type B vaccine
E. Yearly influenza vaccines

17. If a second dose of a vaccine were given too soon (before the minimal interval time period) the correct course of action is:

A. Restarting the entire series
B. Do not count that dose and repeat it after the minimal time period has passed since the incorrect dose
C. Do not worry about it and continue with the next dose as scheduled
D. Draw antibody titers to confirm immunity
E. Double the next dose

18. Which of the following groups of children are NOT at increased risk for pneumococcal disease?

A. Children with mild asthma
B. Children of Native Alaskan descent
C. Children of African-American descent
D. Children with sickle cell disease
E. Children infected with the HIV virus

19. Which of the following statements are true concerning *Haemophilus influenzae* type b vaccine (Hib)?

I. Hib is recommended for all infants without contraindications
II. Standard dosing for Hib vaccine is 2, 4, 6, and 12-18 months of age
III. The 6-month dose is omitted if PedvaxHIB is used for the first 2 doses
IV. ProHIBit is indicated for use only >18 months
V. Hib vaccine is not routinely recommended for children aged 5 years and older

A. Only I is correct
B. Only I, II, and III are correct
C. Only II, III, and IV are correct

D. Only I, II, III, and V are correct
E. All are correct

20. Which of the following vaccines available in the United States is a live, attenuated virus vaccine?

   A. Polio (IPV)
   B. *Haemophilus influenzae* vaccine (Hib)
   C. Influenza vaccine
   D. Varicella Vaccine
   E. Pneumococcal Vaccine

Answers

1. **E.** Routine vaccinations in the adult are a yearly influenza vaccine, dT vaccine every 10 years, and a single pneumococcal vaccine for patients with select chronic illnesses (such as diabetes). Meningococcal and hepatitis vaccines are recommended only for certain indications.

2. **D.** Routine revaccination with pneumococcal vaccine is not recommended. Revaccination is recommended for select high-risk groups and everyone 65 years and older who received an initial dose under the age of 65 and if >5 years have elapsed since the previous dose.

3. **A.** Influenza vaccine is an attenuated, split virus vaccine.

4. **D.** Meningococcal vaccine is not routinely recommended for any age group.

5. **C.** DTaP is indicated for children under the age of 7. Due to adverse effects in children age of seven and older, dT is used.

6. **E.** Polysaccharide pneumococcal vaccine (23-valent) is indicated for those over the age of 2 years and conjugated polysaccharide vaccine (7-valent) is approved for ages 2 months to 7 years.

7. **A.** OPV is no longer recommended in the United States and vaccination with IPV will continue until poliovirus is eradicated worldwide.

8. **B.**

9. **E.** Pneumococcal vaccine is not recommended for a healthy individual until the age of 65.

10. **C.** The hepatitis A vaccine will not protect an individual who has previously been exposed to the virus. IGIM, a source of antibodies (short-term protection), will help to protect immediately, and the vaccine will protect against future exposures (long-term protection).

11. **B.** High-risk groups targeted for influenza vaccination beginning in October include persons aged >50 years, persons at increased risk [age >6 months with chronic pulmonary disease (eg, emphysema, COPD), cardiovascular disease (eg, CHF, post-MI, heart anomalies), metabolic disease (eg, diabetes), renal dysfunction, hemoglobinopathies (eg, sickle cell), and immunosuppression (eg, HIV infection, chemotherapy)], residents of long-term care facilities, people 6 months to 18 years old on aspirin chronically, pregnant women in the second or third trimesters, hospital and outpatient employees, nursing home employees with patient contact, home health care providers working with high-risk persons, household members of high-risk persons, and persons desiring to avoid influenza infection.

12. **A.** Complications of rubella may include arthritis, arthralgias, encephalitis, and hemorrhaging; however, the major complication is congenital rubella syndrome, which occurs in the offspring of a woman who had rubella during pregnancy. Babies born with CRS have major birth defects that can affect many organs.

13. **B.** Live virus vaccines will be killed if there has been recent administration of antibodies. The length of time that must separate these two products depends on the dose and type of antibody-containing blood product being used.

14. **C.** Local reactions are the most common type of adverse reaction, and include pain, swelling, and redness at the site of injection. These usually occur within minutes to hours of the injection and are usually mild and self-limiting. Systemic adverse reactions include fever, malaise, myalgias, and headache, and are more common following live vaccines.

15. **E.** All of the other listed vaccines are first given at 2 months of age. Hepatitis B vaccine is recommended at birth to decrease the incidence of hepatitis B in infants of hepatitis B–infected mothers.

16. **C.** Asplenic patients require protection against the encapsulated bacteria (pneumococcus, meningococcus, and *Haemophilus*), as well as common viral infections. Previous series

completions of routine vaccines, such as measles, varicella, and polio, are adequate for protection. Td vaccines should be repeated every 10 years.

17. **B.** The minimal interval in a series for most vaccines is 4 weeks. Decreasing the interval may interfere with antibody response and protection. Usually the last dose in a series is separated from the previous dose by 4-6 months. Increasing the interval does not affect vaccine effectiveness. You never need to restart a series except for oral typhoid vaccine.

18. **A.** Rates of pneumococcal disease are highest in children <2 years of age, those with asplenia, patients with HIV, American Indian-Alaskan Natives, African-Americans, and day care attendees. Mild asthma is not considered a high-risk disease for pneumococcal infection.

19. **E.** While all of the answers are correct, HIB vaccine may be indicated for children over the age of 5 with certain chronic conditions. This vaccine is relatively complicated to use since recommendations vary among manufacturers. Please consult package inserts before administering.

20. **D.** Varicella and measles-mumps-rubella vaccines are the only routinely administered live vaccines in the U.S. Other non-routinely administered live vaccines include oral typhoid vaccine, vaccinia (smallpox) vaccine, and yellow fever vaccine. The majority of vaccines are inactivated or killed vaccines.

6. References

Advisory Committee on Immunization Practices. General recommendations on immunizations. *MMWR Morb Mortal Wkly Rep.* 2000;49(RR-2):1-36.

Advisory Committee on Immunization Practices. Poliomyelitis prevention in the United States: updated recommendations. *MMWR Morb Mortal Wkly Rep.* 2000;49(RR-5):1-22.

Advisory Committee on Immunization Practices. Prevention and control of influenza. *MMWR Morb Mortal Wkly Rep.* 2003; 52(RR-8):1-34.

Advisory Committee on Immunization Practices. Prevention and control of meningococcal disease and meningococcal disease and college students. *MMWR Morb Mortal Wkly Rep.* 2000;49(RR-5):1-20.

Advisory Committee on Immunization Practices. Prevention of hepatitis A through active or passive immunization. *MMWR Morb Mortal Wkly Rep.* 1999;48(RR-12):1-37.

Advisory Committee on Immunization Practices. Prevention of pneumococcal disease. *MMWR Morb Mortal Wkly Rep.* 1997;46:1-24.

Advisory Committee on Immunization Practices. Preventing pneumococcal disease among infants and young children. *MMWR Morb Mortal Wkly Rep.* 2000;49(RR-9):1-38.

Advisory Committee on Immunization Practices. Prevention of varicella. *MMWR Morb Mortal Wkly Rep.* 1996;45(RR-11):1-36.

Advisory Committee on Immunization Practices. Prevention of varicella: updated recommendations of the ACIP. *MMWR Morb Mortal Wkly Rep.* 1999;48(RR-6):1-5.

Advisory Committee on Immunization Practices. Revised ACIP recommendation for avoiding pregnancy after receiving a rubella-containing vaccine. *MMWR Morb Mortal Wkly Rep.* 2001;50:1117.

Advisory Committee on Immunization Practices. Update: recommendations to prevent hepatitis B virus transmission—United States. *MMWR Morb Mortal Wkly Rep.* 1999;48(RR-12):1-37.

Advisory Committee on Immunization Practices. Update: vaccine side effects, adverse reactions, contraindications, and precautions. *MMWR Morb Mortal Wkly Rep.* 1996;45(RR-12):1-35, errata 1997;46:227.

Advisory Committee on Immunization Practices. Use of diphtheria toxoid-tetanus toxoid-acellular pertussis vaccine as a five dose series. *MMWR Morb Mortal Wkly Rep.* 2000;49(RR-13):1-8; erratum 2000; 49(47):1074.

Centers for Disease Control and Prevention. *Epidemiology and Prevention of Vaccine-Preventable Diseases,* 7th ed. CDC; 2003.

Centers for Disease Control and Prevention. National Immunization Website: http://www. cdc.gov/nip

Grabenstein JD. *Immunofacts: Vaccines and Immunologic Drugs,* Revision 26. St. Louis: Facts and Comparisons; May 2002.

Plotkin SA, Orenstein WA, ed. *Vaccines*, 3rd ed. Philadelphia: WB Saunders; 1999.

33. Pediatrics

Catherine M. Crill, PharmD, BCPS, BCNSP
Assistant Professor, Departments of Pharmacy and Pediatrics
University of Tennessee College of Pharmacy

Contents

1. Special Drug Therapy Considerations in Pediatric Patients

Pediatric Age Definitions

Preterm: <36 weeks gestation
Term: ≥36 weeks gestation
Neonate: <1 month
Infant: 1 month to 1 year
Child: 1 to 11 years
Adolescent: 12 to 16 years

Absorption

Gastric pH

- Infants may be considered to be in a relative state of achlorhydria; however, they are capable of producing sufficient gastric acid with stimuli (eg, in response to histamine or pentagastric challenge, enteral feeding, or stress).

- Gastric acid production reaches adult values by approximately 3 years of age.

Implications for drug therapy
   * Increased bioavailability of basic drugs
   * Decreased bioavailability of acidic drugs
   * Increased bioavailability of acid-labile drugs (eg, penicillin)

Gastric emptying time in pediatric patients

- Gastric emptying time (GET) is longer than it is for adults.
   * GET is inversely related to postconceptional age

- Irregular and unpredictable peristalsis

- Decreased motility

- Premature neonates have longer GET than term neonates and have a greater incidence of gastro-esophageal reflux (GER)

- Related to type of feeding (formula-fed infants exhibit longer transit time than breastfed infants)

- Approaches adult function by 7 to 9 months
   * Stomach muscles are mature at 7 months
   * Stomach muscles are completely innervated at 9 months

Implications for drug therapy
   * Erratic absorption of sustained release products (eg, theophylline)

   * The rate of absorption in small intestine, where most drugs are absorbed, is slower; peak drug concentrations are lower than for adults.

Pancreatic enzymes and bile salts
- Low levels of amylase and lipase

- Low intraluminal bile acid concentrations and synthesis

- Decreased proteolytic ability

Implications for drug therapy
- Erratic absorption of drugs requiring pancreatic enzymes for hydrolysis (eg, chloramphenicol)

- Decreased absorption of lipid-soluble drugs

- Decreased fat absorption from enteral feedings

- Decreased absorption of fat-soluble vitamins

GI mucosa
- Decreased functional integrity of intestinal mucosa

- Surface area of gastric mucosa is small compared to that of intestinal mucosa (most drugs absorbed from small intestine)

Other absorption routes
Skin
   * Absorption via skin is inversely related to thickness of stratum corneum and directly related to hydration of skin.
   * Neonates (particularly premature) have increased skin hydration.
   * The stratum corneum of preterm infants is immature and ineffective as an epidermal barrier.
   * Premature neonates may develop drug toxicity if drug is administered via dermal route.

Buccal route
- Not typically used in pediatric patients.

Intramuscular route
   * Drug delivery is restricted by volume of medication and the pain associated with administration. Results are variable in premature neonates due to (1) blood flow and vasomotor instabilities and (2) insufficient muscle mass and tone, contraction, and oxygenation.

Rectal administration
- Effective for drug delivery in older infants and children.

Administration via intraosseous route (IO route)
  * This vessel-rich marrow (up to 5 years of age) is a great site for drug delivery to systemic circulation. It may be an acceptable route in emergency situations for children over 5 years of age (vessel-rich marrow is then replaced by yellow marrow).

Distribution

Protein binding
- Decreased albumin and α_1-acid glycoprotein concentrations

- Lower binding capacity

- Qualitative differences in neonatal plasma proteins

- Competitive binding by endogenous substances (unconjugated bilirubin, free fatty acids)

- Risk of kernicterus (hypoalbuminemia, unconjugated hyperbilirubinemia, displacement by highly protein-bound drugs or free fatty acids)

- Exhibit adult-like binding by 3 to 6 months of age; adult concentrations of albumin and α_1-acid glycoprotein achieved at 10 to 12 months

Differences in body composition
- Altered vascular and tissue perfusion

- Brain and liver are largest organs in children.

- Total body water greater in neonates and infants

- Extracellular fluid volume greater in neonates and infants

- Relative lack of adipose tissue in neonates and infants (adipose level increases into adulthood)

Implications for drug therapy in neonates and infants
- Increased free fraction of drugs

- Increased potential of drug displacement by endogenous substances

- Potential risk of kernicterus with physiologic jaundice (unconjugated hyperbilirubinemia)

- Hydrophilic drugs, which parallel water in the body (eg, aminoglycosides), exhibit greater volume of distribution.

- Lipophilic drugs (eg, diazepam) parallel body fat and will exhibit smaller volume of distribution.

Liver Metabolism

Phase I reactions (nonsynthetic): Oxidation, reduction, hydrolysis, and hydroxylation
  * Hepatic cytochrome P450 system is responsible for most phase I reactions.
  * Capacity of isoenzymes in the P450 system at birth is 20-70% of adult capacity and increases with postnatal age.
  * Full capacity for reduction at birth
  * Hydrolysis is most developed at birth, followed by the processes of oxidation and hydroxylation.
  * Benzyl alcohol, a preservative present in certain medications, can accumulate in neonates due to underdeveloped alcohol dehydrogenase. Gasping syndrome (ie, metabolic acidosis, respiratory failure, seizures, neurologic deterioration and CV collapse) can result.

Phase II reactions (synthetic): Conjugation with glycine or glutathione, glucuronidation, sulfation, methylation, and acetylation
  * Sulfation pathway is the most developed at birth.
  * Glucuronidation begins around 2 months of age (it reaches adult capacity by 3 years of age).
  * Assumptions about substances primarily metabolized by glucuronidation (ie, morphine, bilirubin, chloramphenicol):
    - Potentially toxic in neonates
    - May exhibit long half-lives (eg, toxicity with chloramphenicol)
    - May require greater dosing in infants (eg, morphine conjugated to its more active metabolite)
    - May be metabolized by another pathway in infants (eg, acetaminophen is primarily metabolized via sulfation in infants)
  * Methylation is functional in infants but not significantly expressed in adults. (Methylation is responsible for the conversion of theophylline to caffeine).

Implications for drug therapy
- For drugs undergoing phase I and II reactions, metabolism is reduced and half-life prolonged in infants and neonates.

- Insufficiency of one pathway may lead to metabolism via another.

- Drug metabolism, slower in the neonate, increases between 1 and 5 years of age and is similar to drug metabolism in adults after puberty.

Renal Elimination

- Renal blood flow is only 5-6% of cardiac output at birth, compared to 15-25% in adults (12 mL/min versus 140 mL/min).

- Glomerular filtration rate is lower at birth and reaches adult values by 1 to 5 months of age in term infants.

- Tubular secretion is low at birth and reaches adult values by 7 months of age in term infants.

- Renal elimination is affected by prematurity and postconceptional age; it increases with maturity.

Estimation of creatinine clearance in pediatric patients
- Altered by differences in renal blood flow, glomerular filtration, tubular secretion, and muscle mass

- May be affected by the presence of maternal serum creatinine over the first week of life (ie, false underestimation of creatinine clearance)

- Schwartz equation may be used for calculation of creatinine clearance

    $$CrCl \ (mL/min/1.73m^2) = k \times (length \ in \ cm)/SCr$$

k = proportionality constant that changes with age and sex (see Table 1)

Other Pediatric Drug Issues

- Digoxin-like immunoreactive substance (DLIS) produced in infants and may interfere with digoxin assays and falsely elevate concentrations.

- Di(2-ethylhexyl)phthalate (DEHP), a plasticizer contained in IV bags, is shown to have an effect on the male reproductive system. Pediatric patients at highest risk of DEHP exposure are neonates on ECMO, those receiving parenteral and enteral nutrition, and those receiving plasma exchange transfusions.

- Polyethylene glycol (PEG), an additive used to promote stability in certain IV medications, can cause hyperosmolarity in infants.

Table 1

Proportionality Constant for Calculation of Creatinine Clearance Using Schwartz Equation[1]

Age	k
Low birth weight ≤1 year	0.33
Full term ≤1 year	0.45
2-12 years	0.55
13-21 years (female)	0.55
13-21 years (male)	0.70

[1]From Schwartz et al, 1987.

2. Specific Infections and Disease States in the Pediatric Population

Otitis Media

Otitis media is an inflammatory process of the middle ear.

Classification
- Acute otitis media is an inflammation of the area behind the eardrum (tympanic membrane) in the chamber called the middle ear. It is accompanied by the presence of fluid in the middle ear (effusion) and by the rapid onset of signs or symptoms of ear infection.

- Recurrent otitis media is the diagnosis if three episodes of acute otitis media occur within a 6-month period or 4 episodes occur within a year.

- Otitis media with effusion is fluid in the middle ear (effusion) without the associated signs or symptoms of acute infection.

Clinical presentation
- Signs and symptoms include fever, otalgia (often manifested as ear tugging or pulling), otorrhea (discharge from the ear), changes in balance or hearing, irritability, difficulty sleeping, lethargy, anorexia, vomiting, and diarrhea.

- Associated findings may be runny nose, congestion, and/or cough.

Pathophysiology
Eustachian tube dysfunction
  * The infant's eustachian tube is shorter and more horizontal compared to the adult ear.

* This prevents drainage of middle ear secretions into the nasopharynx and promotes pooling of secretions in the middle ear

- Anatomic abnormalities (eg, cleft palate, adenoid hypertrophy)

- Immature immune system or altered host defenses

- Viral infections, allergies

- Risk factors include male gender; Native American, Canadian Eskimo, or Alaskan descent; family history of acute otitis media or respiratory tract infection; early age of first episode (earlier age is associated with greater severity and recurrence); daycare environment; parental smoking; children not breastfed.

- Complications include mastoiditis, meningitis, subdural empyema, hearing loss, and delayed speech and language development.

Microbial pathogens
Viral
- Up to 50% of cases of acute otitis media may be viral in origin.

Bacterial
- *Streptococcus pneumoniae* is responsible for 40-50% of bacterial otitis media. Resistance is becoming an increasing problem; bacterial resistance occurs primarily through alteration in penicillin-binding protein (decreased affinity for binding sites).

- *Haemophilus influenzae* (primarily nonencapsulated/nontypable strains) is responsible for 20-30% of bacterial otitis media cases. Bacterial resistance occurs via beta-lactamase production.

- *Moraxella catarrhalis* is responsible for 10-15% of bacterial otitis media; almost all strains are beta-lactamase–producing.

Diagnostic criteria
- Clinical presentation (ie, signs and symptoms consistent with infection)

- Presence of middle ear disease
    * Otoscopic examination determines color, translucency, position
        - Redness or opacity of membrane, absence of light reflection, or bulging membrane
    * Pneumatic otoscopic examination determines mobility of tympanic membrane (ie, presence or absence of effusion)
        - Membrane will not move briskly with positive and negative pressure if effusion is present
    * Tympanocentesis (ie, needle inserted through tympanic membrane to withdraw fluid) allows for culture and identification of pathogen.

Treatment principles and goals
- Control pain

- Eradicate infection

- Prevent complications

- Avoid unnecessary antibiotic therapy

- Improve compliance

- Eliminate presence of effusion

- Prevent recurrence

Drug therapy
- Many episodes of otitis media will have spontaneous resolution; however, since there is a risk of developing complications from untreated otitis media, antimicrobials remain the mainstay of therapy.

First-line therapy
- Amoxicillin is the drug of choice for uncomplicated acute otitis media
    * Excellent in vitro activity against *S pneumoniae* and most *H influenzae*
    * Optimal pharmacodynamic profile of available agents; reaches good concentrations in middle ear fluid
    * Excellent safety and efficacy profile with narrow spectrum of activity
    * Palatable and inexpensive
    * May overcome drug-resistant *S pneumoniae* with higher doses (ie, achieves greater concentrations in middle ear fluid).
    * Does not eradicate beta-lactamase–producing organisms

- For penicillin-allergic patients, azithromycin, trimethoprim-sulfamethoxazole, or erythromycin-sulfisoxazole may be substituted; however, resistance appears to be increasing with these agents.

- Second-line therapy agents are amoxicillin-clavulanate, cefuroxime axetil, IM ceftriaxone, and clindamycin.

- Other antimicrobial agents include cephalosporins (cefprozil, cefpodoxime, cefaclor, loracarbef, ceftibuten), and macrolides (erythromycin, clarithromycin, azithromycin). Fluoroquinolones (ciprofloxacin, ofloxacin, levofloxacin) are thought to be effective, but they are not approved for use in pediatric patients.

Dosing issues and drug resistance (Table 2)
• Amoxicillin
    * Standard dose: 40-45 mg/kg per day
    * High dose: 80-90 mg/kg per day

• Amoxicillin-clavulanate
    * Standard dose versus high dose while maintaining clavulanate dose of <10 mg/kg per day (to prevent diarrhea).
    * If using high dose, use newer formulation with higher ratio of amoxicillin to clavulanate (7:1 formulation), or give additional amoxicillin to standard amoxicillin-clavulanate (4:1 formulation).

• IM ceftriaxone
    * Single dose versus three daily doses

Duration of therapy
• Standard 10-day course

• Shorter course (1-5 days)
    * Advantages are improved compliance, decreased adverse effects of drug therapy, decreased risk of bacterial resistance, and lower costs.
    * Disadvantages are delayed or no cure,

increased risk of complications from untreated acute otitis media, and there is greater risk of recurrence.
    * Not appropriate for:
      • Children <2 years of age
      • Those in day care
      • Those with underlying diseases
      • Those with a history of recurrent otitis media

Other therapy
• Antipyretics (acetaminophen, ibuprofen)
    * Use acetaminophen with caution in high doses (hepatotoxicity)
    * Use ibuprofen with caution in patients with vomiting, diarrhea, and poor fluid intake (dehydration predisposes to ibuprofen-induced renal insufficiency)
    * Avoid alternating antipyretic therapy. Encourage parents to choose one agent, inform them of any adverse effects, and educate them about symptoms of these effects (ie, hepatotoxicity or renal insufficiency).

• Topical analgesics include an otic solution, antipyrine-benzocaine (Auralgan®).

• Topical antimicrobials may have a place in therapy, particularly with ruptured membranes (fluoroquinolone otic suspensions [Floxin®, Cipro HC®]).

• Antihistamines/decongestants are ineffective at eliminating effusion or relieving symptoms. Use only if indicated for other signs or symptoms.

Table 2

Drug-Resistant *S Pneumoniae* Therapeutic Working Group Recommendations

	No antibiotics in last 30 days	Antibiotics in last 30 days
First-line therapy	Amoxicillin: standard dose (low-risk patients); high dose (high-risk[1] patients)	High-dose amoxicillin; high-dose amoxicillin-clavulanate; cefuroxime axetil
Failure[2] at day 3	High-dose amoxicillin-clavulanate; cefuroxime axetil; IM ceftriaxone	IM ceftriaxone in 3 daily doses; clindamycin[3]; tympanocentesis
Failure[2] at days 10-28	Same as above (choose different regimen)	High-dose amoxicillin-clavulanate; cefuroxime axetil; IM ceftriaxone in 3 daily doses; tympanocentesis

[1]High-risk: age <2 years, antimicrobials within last 90 days, day care attendance.
[2]Treatment failures: lack of clinical improvement in pain, fever, tympanic membrane findings. With documented treatment failure, provide an agent that is effective against beta-lactamase–producing organisms and drug-resistant *S pneumoniae*.
[3]Clindamycin is not effective against *H influenzae* and *M catarrhalis*.
From Dowell et al, 1999.

Patient instructions and counseling
- Complete entire course of prescribed antibiotics

- Shake bottle well before administering dose. Follow labeling regarding temperature for storage of medication.

- Contact physician if patient develops a rash, has difficulty breathing, or if symptoms persist after 72 hours of initiating therapy.

Adverse drug events
- Gastrointestinal: nausea and diarrhea

- Hypersensitivity: rash, anaphylaxis

Drug interactions
- Macrolides, particularly erythromycin and clarithromycin

Nondrug therapy
- Local heat

- Tympanostomy tubes decrease recurrent episodes, restore hearing, and relieve discomfort. Risks include anesthesia and permanent tympanic membrane scarring.

- Immunization and immunoprophylaxis
  * Pneumococcal conjugate vaccination should provide some protection against strains responsible for majority of bacterial otitis media.
  * *H influenzae* type B vaccination is of no benefit in otitis media (note that most strains causing otitis media are nontypable and not prevented by vaccination).

Recurrent otitis media
- Prophylaxis with half therapeutic dosing of amoxicillin or sulfisoxazole may be initiated in high-risk patients.

- Duration of no more than 3-6 months.

- Active disease on prophylaxis
  * Discontinue prophylactic agent and begin therapy with broad-spectrum agent.
  * Concern is with emergence of resistant organisms

Otitis media with effusion
- Inform parents about environmental factors (eg, parental smoking)

- Monitor for signs of hearing impairment

- Hearing evaluation at 3 months
  * Hearing in normal range or unilateral impairment:
    - Observation/antibiotic
  * Bilateral effusion and bilateral hearing impairment:
    - Antibiotics followed by bilateral tympanostomy tube placement

Otitis Externa

Otitis externa is an inflammation of the outer ear canal, also referred to as swimmer's ear.

Clinical presentation
- Itching, pain, otic exudate, and hearing impairment

Pathophysiology
- Presence of moisture in the ear canal

- Disruption of the integrity of the ear canal

- Most common organisms are *Pseudomonas aeruginosa* and *Staphylococcus aureus*.

- Other pathogens include fungi and *Bacillus* and *Proteus* species

- Therapy consists of antibiotic/steroid otic preparations: neomycin/polymyxin/hydrocortisone (Cortisporin Otic®), neomycin/colistin/hydrocortisone (Coly-Mycin S Otic®), fluoroquinolone otic preparations (ciprofloxacin; Cipro HC®; ofloxacin; Floxin®), acetic acid and hydrocortisone otic preparations (VoSol HC Otic®), or oral analgesics.

- Preventive measures include drying ears after exposure to moisture, using drops containing isopropyl alcohol with or without acetic acid to reduce pH, and avoiding cotton swabs.

- Application of otic drops (see APhA Special Report, 1994):
  1. Wash hands before and after administration.
  2. Warm otic drops to room temperature by holding bottle in hands for several minutes. Avoid instilling cold or hot drops into the ear canal.
  3. Shake the bottle if indicated on the label.
  4. Tilt the child's head to the side or have the child lie down.
  5. Pull the child's ear backward and upward and instill the drops in the ear canal. Do not put the dropper bottle inside the ear canal (to remain free from contamination it should not come into contact with the ear).

6. Press gently on the small flap over the ear to push the drops into the canal.

7. Have the child remain in the same position for the period of time indicated in the labeling. If this is not possible, place a cotton ball gently into the ear to prevent the drops from draining out of the ear canal.

8. Wipe excess medication from the outside of the ear.

Cystic Fibrosis

Cystic fibrosis is an autosomal recessive disease of exocrine gland function resulting in abnormal mucus production.

Genetic classification
- Cystic fibrosis is the result of a gene mutation on the long arm of chromosome 7. The protein encoded by this gene, the cystic fibrosis transmembrane regulator (CFTR), is a channel involved in the transport of water and electrolytes.

Defects in processing
  * The most common genetic mutation involves a 3-base-pair deletion at position 508 (ΔF_{508}).
  * Patients homozygous for ΔF_{508} are pancreatic insufficient.
  * Prognosis not as good as for those who are pancreatic sufficient.

- Defect in protein production, regulation, and conduction

Clinical presentation
Pulmonary complications
- Initial manifestations of chronic cough, wheezing, hyperinflation of lungs, or lower respiratory tract infections

- Patients present with hypoxia, clubbing, labored breathing, acute respiratory exacerbations (fever, sputum production, increased oxygen requirements, dyspnea), changes in forced vital capacity (FVC), forced expiratory volume (FEV), and residual volume, and the development of a chronic obstructive picture as the disease progresses.

Gastrointestinal complications
- Poor digestion of proteins and fats, resulting in foul-smelling steatorrhea; distal intestinal obstruction (commonly manifested as vomiting of bilious material, abdominal distension and pain)

- Infants may have meconium ileus, gastroesophageal reflux

Other
- Cirrhosis and cholelithiasis

- Pancreatic function

- Insulin insufficiency, diabetes mellitus

- Malnutrition

- Nasal polyps and sinusitis, anemia, arthritis, osteopenia, and osteoporosis

Pathophysiology
- Defect in the chloride transport channel in secretory epithelial cells

Normal physiology
- Chloride transported out of blood followed by sodium and water

Cystic fibrosis
- Decreased chloride and water secretion and increased sodium absorption leads to thick, dehydrated secretions and mucus

- Exocrine gland involvement: pancreas, hepatobiliary ducts, gastrointestinal tract and the lungs (secretions build up and block airways and pancreatic and hepatobiliary exocrine flow)

Pulmonary system
- Initial obstruction of small airways with mucus plugging results in bronchiolitis and persistence of bacteria.

- Early bacterial pathogens: *Staphylococcus aureus* and *Haemophilus influenzae* present in younger patients

- Later bacterial pathogens: *Pseudomonas aeruginosa* is the primary pathogen in late childhood

- Other bacterial pathogens: *Proteus* and *Klebsiella* species, *Stenotrophomonas maltophilia*, and *Burkholderia cepacia*

- Possible viral pathogens

- Chronic pulmonary infection and inflammation progress to large airway and eventual chronic obstructive disease

Pancreatic system
- Pancreatic enzyme insufficiency (trypsin, chymotrypsin, lipases, amylase) and decreased bicar-

bonate secretion (necessary for optimal pancreatic enzyme activity)
  * Maldigestion of fats and proteins and fat-soluble vitamin deficiency

- Insulin insufficiency (resistance and decreased secretion) leads to glucose intolerance (occurs later in disease process and may be associated with increased morbidity)

Biliary system
- Biliary cirrhosis or fatty infiltration may lead to portal hypertension, development of bleeding varices, hypersplenism, and may lead to cholelithiasis.

Sweat glands
- High concentration of sodium and chloride in sweat (representing the failure of sweat glands to reabsorb sodium and chloride)

Reproductive system
- Male infertility common due to bilateral absence of vas deferens

- Female infertility due to abnormal cervical mucus

Diagnostic criteria
- Laboratory confirmation of CFTR dysfunction via sweat chloride analysis (ie, administration of pilocarpine)
  1. Sweat is collected and electrolytes are measured.
  2. Chloride of 60 mEq/L or more is diagnostic (values of up to 80 mEq/L have been seen in non-CF patients)
  3. Measurement of 50-60 mEq/L is indeterminate and tests may need to be repeated.

- Presence of clinical characteristics of cystic fibrosis

Treatment goals
- Halt or decrease disease progression

- Maintain normal growth and development and nutrition status

- Maintain pulmonary function

- Optimize drug therapy for pharmacokinetic differences in cystic fibrosis patients

Drug therapy (Table 3)
Antibiotic therapy in acute exacerbations
  Antibiotic selection
- Empiric therapy initially and then treat based on sputum culture and sensitivity.

- IV administration of two antibiotics for 14-21 days in combination with aggressive therapy for clearance of secretions.

- Coverage for *Staphylococcus aureus*, *Haemophilus influenzae*, and *Pseudomonas aeruginosa*

- Double coverage of antibiotics when *Pseudomonas* species are suspected, with antipseudomonal penicillin (piperacillin, mezlocillin, piperacillin-tazobactam, ticarcillin-clavulanate, ticarcillin, aztreonam, meropenem, or imipenem) or cephalosporin (ceftazidime) and an aminoglycoside.
  * Tobramycin plus ticarcillin or piperacillin (*P aeruginosa*)
  * Tobramycin plus ceftazidime (*P aeruginosa*)
  * Oxacillin or nafcillin (methicillin-sensitive *S aureus*)
  * Vancomycin (methicillin-resistant *S aureus*)

- *Burkholderia* and *Stenotrophomonas* species are commonly resistant. Follow culture and sensitivity results. Antibiotics that may be effective include trimethoprim-sulfamethoxazole, chloramphenicol, ceftazidime (*B cepacia*), doxycycline, and piperacillin (*S maltophilia*)

- Other agents: ciprofloxacin

Antibiotic therapy and chronic suppression
- Chronic inhaled antibiotic therapy with tobramycin (TOBI)
  * Significant improvement in FEV_1, decreased hospitalizations, and decreased need for IV antibiotics
  * Decreased systemic concentrations (ie, less resistance) and high pulmonary concentrations
  * Therapy is expensive

Oral antibiotic therapy
  * Fluoroquinolones are the only oral antibiotics with good coverage against *Pseudomonas*.

Patient instructions and counseling
- Compliance with therapeutic regimens

Pancreatic enzyme supplementation
  * Give immediately before or during snacks and meals.
  * Capsule contents may be opened and sprinkled on applesauce or other acidic carrier; contents should not be crushed or chewed.

Aminoglycosides
  * Monitor urine output.

Table 3

Drug Therapy for Cystic Fibrosis

Therapeutic category	Indication and mechanism of action	Comments
Pancreatic enzymes Capsule (Cotazym®, Ku-Zyme®) Microencapsulated (Cotazym-S®, Creon®, Pancrease®, Pancrelipase®, Protilase®, Ultrase®, Zymase®) Tablet (Ilozyme®, Viokase®) Powder (Viokase®)	Supplementation or replacement of pancreatic enzymes (treatment of malabsorption syndrome) Aids in digestion of proteins, carbohydrates, and fats	Products differ by enzyme content (units of lipase, protease, amylase) and dosage form Primary enzyme component is lipase Dose is typically whole dose with meals; half dose with snacks Adequate replacement decreases bowel movements and improves stool consistency
Fat-soluble vitamins	Supplementation of fat-soluble vitamins A, D, E, and K	May be dosed individually, through the use of 1 or 2 multivitamins daily, or with a water-miscible combination preparation
Nebulization therapy	Liquefaction of pulmonary secretions	Can be accomplished with normal saline or sterile water with or without other therapies[1]
N-acetylcysteine (Mucomyst®)	Lowers mucus viscosity through sulfhydryl group, which opens the disulfide bond in mucoproteins	Bad taste and odor; significant efficacy has not been documented
Recombinant human DNase (dornase alfa, Pulmozyme®)	DNA in mucus contributes to viscosity; mechanism of action is through cleavage of DNA (thereby decreasing mucus viscosity)	Expensive; reduces viscosity, improves pulmonary function; may decrease respiratory exacerbations
Ursodeoxycholic acid (ursodiol, Actigall®)	Bile acid that suppresses hepatic synthesis and secretion of cholesterol; inhibits intestinal cholesterol absorption; solubilizes cholesterol	Aids in dissolution of stones with cholelithiasis
Bronchodilators (β_2-agonists, theophylline)	Bronchodilator in reversible or obstructive airway disease	May be of benefit for patients with component of reactive airway disease; should use β_2-agonist before theophylline because of pharmacokinetic issues Response (improvement in FEV_1) should be documented before initiating long-term therapy
Antibiotics	Treat infection	Altered pharmacokinetics may affect and complicate therapy
Ibuprofen	Nonsteroidal anti-inflammatory; controls airway inflammation	Not used routinely; may have an effect on slowing pulmonary disease High dosages needed to achieve good concentrations (requires therapeutic drug monitoring)
Corticosteroids	Anti-inflammatory	Not used routinely; positive effects on pulmonary function but negative effects on growth and development, glucose sensitivity, and bone health

[1]Other therapies include N-acetylcysteine and recombinant human DNase.

- Use ibuprofen with caution if dehydration, diarrhea, and/or decreased oral intake is present.

Adverse drug events
Aminoglycosides
- Nephrotoxicity and ototoxicity

Ibuprofen
- Renal insufficiency

Fluoroquinolones
- Arthropathy

Drug interactions
- Pancreatic enzymes and acid suppression therapy may decrease inactivation of enzymes by gastric acid, thereby reducing dose requirement.

Parameters to monitor
Clinical status
- Fever, activity level

- Pulmonary function (as indicated by FEV_1, FVC, residual volume, chest radiography)

Pharmacokinetic considerations
Aminoglycosides
  * Increased clearance and larger Vd (necessitating greater dosing); concentration-dependent killing and postantibiotic effect against gram-negative organisms
  * Higher doses (10 mg/kg per day)
  * Peak concentrations from 8-12 µg/mL
  * Trough concentrations of less than 2 µg/mL

Beta-lactams
  * No change or increased clearance
  * No change or increased Vd
  * No postantibiotic effect or concentration-dependent killing

Fluoroquinolones
  * Concentration-dependent killing
  * Postantibiotic effect against gram-negative organisms

Nondrug therapy
Pulmonary percussion therapy and postural drainage
- Purpose is to clear mucus and secretions from pulmonary system

- Conducted once or twice per day and up to five times daily or more

- Percussion usually conducted after nebulization therapy with or without bronchodilator or mucolytic

- Therapy with hand-held devices or oscillatory vests

Transplantation
- Lung transplantation

- Liver-lung transplantation if there is liver involvement

Attention Deficit Hyperactivity Disorder

According to *DSM-IV*, ADHD is a behavioral disorder of childhood onset (by the age of 7 years) characterized by symptoms of inattentiveness and impulsive or hyperactive behavior.

Classification (*DSM-IV*)
- Combined type: criteria for inattention, hyperactivity, and impulsivity are met

- Predominantly inattentive type: criteria for inattention are met, but not for hyperactivity and impulsivity

- Predominantly hyperactive, impulsive type: criteria for inattention are not met and criteria for hyperactivity and impulsivity are met

- Not otherwise specified

Clinical presentation
Inattention
- Child has difficulty paying attention, daydreams frequently, is easily distracted and disorganized, and loses things frequently

Hyperactivity
- Child has difficulty staying seated, talks too much

Impulsivity
- Child acts and speaks out without thinking; child interrupts others frequently

Pathophysiology
- Imbalance in catecholamine neurotransmission (specifically between dopamine and norepinephrine)

Genetic basis
- Dopamine transmitter (DAT-1), dopamine D_2 and D_4 receptors (dopamine and norepinephrine are potent agonists of the D_4 receptor)

Diagnostic criteria must be met for accurate diagnosis

- Based on *DSM-IV* criteria of six or more of the criteria for inattention and/or hyperactivity and impulsivity for at least 6 months "to a degree that is maladaptive and inconsistent with developmental level"

- Some impairment was present before 7 years of age

- Impairment is present in at least two settings (eg, home and school)

- Evidence of clinically significant impairment in functioning

- Symptoms not related to other illness (eg, schizophrenia, mood disorder)

Treatment goals

- Educate the patient and family

- Improve functioning and behavior

- Achieve effective drug therapy with minimal side effects

Drug therapy (Table 4)
Patient counseling

- Advise patients and caregivers of the need to store medications away from other children or siblings secondary to potential for lethal overdose (tricyclic antidepressants) and potential for abuse (stimulants)

Adverse drug effects

- Stimulants cause anorexia, abdominal pain, headache, insomnia, jitteriness, social withdrawal, transient motor tics, weight loss (not height-dependent).

- Methylphenidate is contraindicated in seizure disorder according to package insert (ie, it lowers seizure threshold).

- Tricyclics carry cardiotoxicity risk (sudden death). Patients should undergo ECG testing prior to initiation of therapy and periodically throughout therapy.

- Bupropion may lower the seizure threshold. Seizures are associated with high doses and previous history of seizure disorders. Minimize risk by dividing daily dose or by using the extended release formulation.

- Atomoxetine is associated with increased heart rate and increased diastolic blood pressure.

Drug interactions
Methylphenidate

- MAO inhibitors (severe hypertension)

- Caffeine may enhance stimulant effects.

- Methylphenidate may inhibit metabolism of phenytoin, phenobarbital, warfarin, and tricyclics.

Tricyclics

- Multiple pharmacodynamic and pharmacokinetic drug interactions

- Increased plasma concentrations of tricyclics. Potential toxicity when certain antidepressants are added to regimen (fluoxetine, sertraline, fluvoxamine, paroxetine) as well as with cimetidine, methylphenidate, diltiazem, quinidine, and verapamil

- Decreased concentrations of tricyclics may be seen with concomitant administration of carbamazepine and phenytoin

- Increased therapeutic effect and potential toxicity with MAO inhibitors

- Increased CNS depressant effects with alcohol and sedatives

Recommendations for therapy and monitoring
Efficacy of therapy

- Assess behavior changes and evaluate feedback from teachers and parents.

Stimulants

- Begin with a low dose and titrate upward to optimal functioning ability.

- May need to decrease dose due to side effects or if no further improvement is seen with larger dose

- No therapeutic drug monitoring or ECG monitoring

- If one stimulant fails, the patient should be tried on another stimulant; children who fail two stimulants can be tried on a third type of stimulant.

Tricyclics

- Initial and periodic ECGs

Pharmacokinetic considerations

- Methylphenidate does not distribute well into adipose tissue (dose on milligram basis instead of milligrams per kilogram)

Table 4

Drug Therapy for Attention Deficit Hyperactivity Disorder

Therapeutic category	Mechanism of action	Comments
Stimulants (first-line therapy)		
Short-acting methylphenidate (Ritalin®, Methylin®)	Reuptake blockade of catecholamines (norepinephrine and dopamine) in presynaptic nerve endings	Do not give after 4 PM; may cause insomnia
Intermediate-acting methylphenidate (Ritalin SR®, Metadate ER®, Methylin ER®)		Spansules may be opened and contents sprinkled on applesauce
Long-acting methylphenidate (Concerta®, Metadate CD®, Ritalin LA®)		Adderall® can be crushed Drug holidays (eg, summer is a good time to see if patient is outgrowing disease)
Short-acting amphetamine (Dexedrine®, Dextrostat®)		Not addictive in children with ADHD, but some parents or siblings may abuse child's medications
Intermediate-acting amphetamine (Adderall®, Dexedrine® Spansule)		Methylphenidate is not labeled for use in children <6 years of age
Long-acting amphetamine (Adderall-XR®)		Amphetamines are not labeled for use in children <3 years of age
Antidepressants (second-line therapy)		
Tricyclics (imipramine, desipramine)	Reuptake blockade of norepinephrine and serotonin presynaptically	May use tricyclics in patients who fail to respond or are intolerant to stimulants Drug of choice in ADHD with depression Longer duration of action No rebound or wearing off effect Rapid onset in ADHD; effect can be noticed in 3-4 days Taper patient off over 2 to 3 weeks
Bupropion (Wellbutrin®, Wellbutrin SR®)	Indirect dopamine agonist and noradrenergic effects	May induce seizures
Other agents (not currently supported by most recent AAP Guidelines, 2001)		
D-threo-enantiomer of racemic methylphenidate, dexmethylphenidate (Focalin®)	Blockade of dopamine and norepinephrine in presynaptic nerve endings	D-enantiomer thought to be the more active enantiomer
Atomoxetine (Strattera®)	Noradrenergic specific reuptake inhibitor	New nonstimulant agent
Clonidine	α_2 Noradrenergic agonist	Good drug to use with ADHD and coexisting conditions such as sleep disturbances
Pemoline (Cylert®)	Blockade of dopamine and norepinephrine in presynaptic nerve endings	Onset in 2-3 weeks; rarely used now secondary to association with fatal hepatic failure (not dose- or time-related); patients present with malaise, nausea and vomiting, lethargy, elevated LFTs

Nondrug Therapy

- Behavioral techniques (ie, positive reinforcement, time-out, response cost, token economy)

- Environmental modifications

- Classroom management

Conjunctivitis

Conjunctivitis is an inflammation of the conjunctiva of the eye.

Classification
- Bacterial, viral, or allergic

Clinical presentation
- Conjunctivitis is characterized by redness of the eye, itching, ocular discharge, foreign body sensation, and crusting of the eye and eyelid. Patient may have alteration in vision due to presence of discharge.

Pathophysiology
Conjunctivitis of newborn
- Inflammation of the conjunctiva within the first month of life (causative agents include topical antimicrobial agents; bacteria, primarily *Neisseria gonorrhoeae*, *Chlamydia trachomatis*, *Staphylococcus aureus*, *S epidermidis*, *Streptococcus pneumoniae*, *Escherichia coli* and other gram-negative bacteria; viruses, primarily herpes simplex)

Bacterial (outside of first month of life)
- Most commonly *S aureus*, *S epidermidis*, *S pneumoniae*, and *Haemophilus influenzae* (also gonococcal and chlamydial)

- Treated with antibiotic therapy

Viral
- "Pink eye" is contagious. Adenovirus is the most common causative agent.

- Commonly preceded by a cold or sore throat or exposure to another person with viral conjunctivitis

- May also see herpes simplex (corneal involvement may yield permanent visual damage)

Allergic
- Caused by exposure to dander, pollen, or topical eye preparation

- Most patients will exhibit itching of the eye.

Diagnostic criteria
- Based on patient's symptoms

Treatment goals
- Eliminate or avoid the allergen (allergic conjunctivitis).

- Treat the underlying infection (bacterial conjunctivitis).

- Decrease severity and provide symptomatic relief (all forms).

Drug therapy
Neonatal
- Preventive medicine includes prophylaxis after delivery with antibacterial ophthalmic ointment (erythromycin, tetracycline, silver nitrate, povidone-iodine)

- Onset day 1: no treatment (secondary to prophylaxis after delivery)

- Onset day 2-4 (*N gonorrhoeae*): penicillin G or ceftriaxone for 7 days

- Onset day 3-10 (*C trachomatis*): oral + ointment erythromycin for 14 days

- Onset day 2-16 (herpes simplex): consider IV acyclovir

Bacterial (outside of first month of life)
- Topical antibiotic therapy (bacitracin-polymyxin B, trimethoprim-polymyxin B, erythromycin, fluoroquinolone [ciprofloxacin, gentamicin, tobramycin]) in combination with antibiotic ointment [erythromycin or bacitracin] at bedtime for 5-7 days

Gonococcal
- Ceftriaxone for one dose (with corneal ulceration, systemic IV ceftriaxone therapy); also treat for *Chlamydia* species as below

Chlamydial
- Oral tetracycline or doxycycline for 2-3 weeks (adults); azithromycin single dose (children)

Viral
- Ocular lubricant (artificial tears) every 3-4 hours while awake

Allergic
- Remove allergen; use ocular lubricant (artificial tears), ocular decongestants (phenylephrine, napha-

zoline, tetrahydrozoline, oxymetazoline: α-adrenergic activity), antihistamines (levocabastine [Liovistin®], olopatadine [Patanol®], pheniramine maleate), antihistamine/decongestant combination products, topical mast cell stabilizer (cromolyn sodium), combination mast cell stabilizer and antihistamine, or oral antihistamine therapy.

Adverse drug effects
• Ocular decongestants can cause rebound congestion of the conjunctiva (this is less common with naphazoline and tetrahydrozoline).

Instilling eye drops and ointment
• Wash hands before and after administration. Tilt head back, grasp lower eyelid and pull away from eye, place dropper or ointment tube over eye and look up immediately before instilling drop. For ointment, use a sweeping motion and instill $1/4$ to $1/2$ inch of ointment inside eyelid. Close eye after instillation and wait 1-2 minutes. Blot excess ointment or solution away from around eye. Vision may be temporarily blurred with ointment administration. Wait 5 minutes between drops for multiple drop therapy. If using suspension, place that drop in eye last. If using both ointment and drops, instill drops first and wait 10 minutes before applying ointment.

Patient instructions and counseling
• Stress the importance of handwashing, not sharing towels or linens

• Store products according to labeling instructions

Nondrug therapy
• Cold compresses

3. Key Points

• The pharmacokinetics and pharmacodynamics of medications are altered by developmental differences in absorption, distribution, metabolism, and elimination in pediatric patients.

• Pharmacotherapy should be adjusted according to the developmental differences in order to optimize therapeutic efficacy while minimizing the risk of toxicity.

• Although spontaneous resolution does occur in many cases of acute otitis media, antibiotic therapy should be initiated to prevent complications such as meningitis and mastoiditis.

• The incidence of drug-resistant *S pneumoniae* is increasing. Due to its safety profile, cost, and excellent pharmacodynamic profile against sensitive and drug-resistant *S pneumoniae,* amoxicillin remains the drug of choice for uncomplicated acute otitis media. Higher doses may be necessary in high-risk patients.

• Therapy for cystic fibrosis should focus on halting the progression of the disease and maintaining pulmonary function. Appropriate therapies decrease mucus viscosity and increase clearance of secretions, manage acute infectious exacerbations, and, by using appropriate pancreatic enzyme supplementation, maintain normal growth and development.

• Pharmacokinetics of medications in cystic fibrosis patients may be altered; therapeutic drug monitoring and dose alterations should be conducted to ensure efficacy and decrease toxicity.

• An accurate diagnosis of attention deficit hyperactivity disorder, a behavioral disorder of childhood onset characterized by inattentiveness, hyperactivity, and impulsivity, should be obtained prior to initiating drug therapy.

• Pharmacotherapy for attention deficit hyperactivity disorder is with stimulants (first-line) and antidepressants (second-line).

• Pharmacotherapy should be titrated to desired functional effect without increasing the risk of side effects.

• Therapy should include behavioral modification. Monitoring of drug and nondrug therapy should include input from different environments (ie, parents and teachers).

- Bacterial and viral conjunctivitis may occur in the first month of life; antimicrobial ointment administration should be instituted after delivery for prophylaxis.

- Bacterial, viral, and allergic conjunctivitis should be treated with antimicrobial therapy (bacterial), symptomatic therapy (bacterial, viral, and allergic), and ocular antihistamines, decongestants, mast cell stabilizers, or combination products (allergic).

4. Questions and Answers

1. J.S., a 4-day-old infant (37 weeks gestation, birth weight 3.2 kg, length 52 cm), has been admitted to the hospital secondary to spiking temperatures. J.S. has demonstrated decreased oral intake and irritability since discharge home from the newborn nursery 2 days ago. J.S. is started on IV fluid at maintenance volume and antimicrobial therapy with ampicillin 165 mg IV q6h and gentamicin 8 mg IV q8h. Cultures have been obtained and are pending from blood, urine, and CSF. Laboratory assessment includes the following: Na 142, K 3.5, Cl 108, HCO_3 22, BUN 15, SCr 0.9, Glc 88. What is J.S.'s estimated creatinine clearance (mL/min)?

   A. 100
   B. 80
   C. 60
   D. 50
   E. 25

2. Which of the following may affect the creatinine clearance estimate in this patient?

   I.   The presence of maternal serum creatinine
   II. Decreased glomerular filtration rate
   III. Increased tubular secretion rate

   A. I only
   B. III only
   C. I and II only
   D. II and III only
   E. I, II, and III

3. Aminoglycosides are hydrophilic compounds. Which of the following statements regarding aminoglycoside pharmacokinetic parameters in premature neonates compared to adults is true?

   A. Increased clearance
   B. Increased Vd
   C. Decreased half-life
   D. Unchanged elimination
   E. Increased liver metabolism

4. Which of the following may complicate phenytoin therapy in a 2-day-old infant with new-onset seizures?

   I.   Hypoalbuminemia
   II. Physiologic jaundice
   III. IV lipid therapy

A. I only
B. III only
C. I and II only
D. II and III only
E. I, II, and III

5. A drug metabolized via which of the following reactions is a concern in the neonatal population?

A. Hydrolysis
B. Reduction
C. Sulfation
D. Glucuronidation
E. Methylation

6. M.J., a 7-month-old female, is brought to your pharmacy by her mother who describes the infant as having new onset of fever and increased irritability in the last 24 hours. The mother states that she stayed home with M.J. today instead of sending her to day care. M.J. has been bottle-fed since birth. Family history is significant for an older sibling with a recent upper respiratory tract infection. Examination of her ear canal using a pneumatic otoscope reveals a bulging, red tympanic membrane with no mobility upon negative or positive pressure. Computer records reveal she has been treated for acute otitis media twice since birth (at 3 and 5 months of age). Decisions for antimicrobial therapy in this patient should be based on coverage for which of the following pathogens?

A. *S epidermidis, S pneumoniae, P aeruginosa*
B. *S pneumoniae, H influenzae, M catarrhalis*
C. *H influenzae, S pyogenes, P aeruginosa*
D. *S pneumoniae, S aureus, M catarrhalis*
E. *S epidermidis, P aeruginosa, B cepacia*

7. The drug of choice for M.J.'s current episode of acute otitis media is

A. Amoxicillin
B. Amoxicillin-clavulanate
C. IM ceftriaxone
D. Cefixime
E. Trimethoprim-sulfamethoxazole

8. When counseling M.J.'s mother about the antibiotic suspension prescribed by M.J.'s physician, which of the following should be discussed?

I. The importance of removing the child from day care

II. Whether or not the suspension should be refrigerated
III. The need to shake the suspension vigorously prior to administration

A. I only
B. III only
C. I and II only
D. II and III only
E. I, II, and III

9. Which of the following is a common side effect of amoxicillin-clavulanate therapy?

A. Hemolytic anemia
B. Liver function test abnormalities
C. Pancreatitis
D. Diarrhea
E. Headache

10. Which of the following is a side effect that should be a concern in a child with acute otitis media and nausea and vomiting who is receiving ibuprofen for fever?

A. Stevens-Johnson syndrome
B. Renal insufficiency
C. Hyponatremia
D. Oral candidiasis
E. Liver failure

11. Otitis externa or "swimmer's ear" may be treated with

A. Application of an antimicrobial and steroid solution into the ear canal
B. Application of antimicrobial ointment into the ear canal with a cotton swab
C. Application of an antihistamine solution into the ear canal
D. Increase pH of ear canal with administration of Burow solution
E. Decrease pH of ear canal with administration of dilute HCl solution

12. R.E., age 15, weighs 40 kg and has cystic fibrosis. R.E. is admitted to the hospital secondary to an acute pulmonary exacerbation. Home medications include Ultrase as directed, TOBI nebulization, ADEK qd, and dornase alfa (qd nebulization). She is started on ceftazidime 2 g IV q8h and tobramycin 130 mg IV q8h. Which of the following should be ordered in this patient?

A. Serum tobramycin peak concentration
B. Serum tobramycin trough concentration
C. Serum tobramycin peak and trough
concentrations
D. Sputum ceftazidime concentration
E. Sputum ceftazidime and tobramycin
concentrations

13. Sputum cultures taken from R.E. shortly after
hospital admission are positive for *S aureus*
(non–methicillin sensitive). Which of the
following agents should be initiated at this time?

A. Oxacillin
B. Ticarcillin
C. Piperacillin
D. Vancomycin
E. Amikacin

14. Which of the following is a pancreatic enzyme
supplement?

A. Actigall
B. Beractant
C. Creon
D. Diabinese
E. Pulmozyme

15. Which of the following products can be used to
decrease the viscosity of pulmonary secretions?

A. Exosurf
B. Mucomyst
C. Protilase
D. Liquaemin
E. Serevent

16. Counseling a patient on the use of pancreatic
enzyme supplementation should include which
of the following statements?

A. Capsules may be opened and sprinkled over
any food
B. Capsule contents should not be crushed or
chewed
C. The total daily dose may be given at one time
in the evening
D. Adequate supplementation will increase
bowel movement frequency
E. Supplementation dose should not change
with diet changes

17. N.G., age 8, has newly diagnosed attention
deficit hyperactivity disorder. Which of the
following is not considered first-line therapy for
N.G.?

A. Ritalin
B. Dexedrine
C. Wellbutrin
D. Adderall
E. Methylin

18. Cylert is associated with which of the following
serious adverse effects?

A. Hepatic failure
B. Renal failure
C. Cardiovascular collapse
D. Anaphylaxis
E. Toxic epidermal necrolysis

19. T.S., age 9, is being started on imipramine
therapy after failing therapy for attention deficit
hyperactivity disorder with several different
stimulants. T.S. has two other siblings, a 15-
year-old brother and a 3-year-old sister. The
pharmacist instructs T.S.'s parents to keep the
medicine away and in a safe place. What is the
most likely reason for the pharmacist's concern?

I. Toxicity of imipramine with overdose
II. Abuse potential of imipramine
III. Stability of imipramine product

A. I only
B. III only
C. I and II only
D. II and III only
E. I, II, and III

20. A decrease in seizure threshold is a side effect
of which of the following agents used for
ADHD?

I. Methylphenidate
II. Bupropion
III. Clonidine

A. I only
B. III only
C. I and II only
D. II and III only
E. I, II, and III

21. Every spring, M.S. develops itchy, red eyes that
are often swollen and draining. Which of the
following is the most likely cause of this ocular
disorder?

A. Viral conjunctivitis
B. Bacterial conjunctivitis
C. Allergic conjunctivitis

D. Blepharitis
E. Episcleritis

22. Which of the following therapies is not an appropriate recommendation for M.S.'s symptoms?

    A. Ocular lubricant
    B. Ocular decongestant
    C. Ocular antihistamine
    D. Ocular mast cell stabilizer
    E. Ocular antimicrobial

23. Which of the following is not commonly associated with conjunctivitis?

    A. *Chlamydia*
    B. *Neisseria*
    C. *Staphylococcus*
    D. *Streptococcus*
    E. *Clostridium*

24. Which of the following is a side effect of the prolonged use of ocular decongestants?

    A. Peripheral vasodilation
    B. Rebound conjunctival congestion
    C. Development of arrhythmias
    D. Development of tolerance
    E. Development of allergy to product

Answers

1. **E.** Using the Schwartz equation, J.S.'s estimated creatinine clearance is 26 mL/min (CrCl = 0.45 x 52/0.9).

2. **C.** The presence of maternal serum creatinine that decreases in neonates over the first week of life may falsely underestimate a creatinine clearance estimate calculated during this time. Assuming that by the end of the first week of life, J.S.'s SCr has decreased to within the normal infant range to 0.4 mg/dL, the estimated creatinine clearance would be 59 mL/min (CrCl = 0.45 x 52/0.4). Other factors that affect creatinine clearance in the neonate and infant include a decreased glomerular filtration rate and a decreased tubular secretion rate. Therefore, only I and II are correct answers.

3. **B.** Aminoglycosides are hydrophilic compounds; they will exhibit larger volumes of distribution in patients with greater total body water. Neonates and infants have greater total body water, greater extracellular fluid volume, and a relative lack of adipose tissue.

4. **E.** Phenytoin is highly plasma protein-bound. The total and free concentrations of highly protein-bound drugs may be altered due to developmental differences in protein binding (decreased protein concentrations and altered binding capacity) and displacement by endogenous substances (eg, free fatty acids and unconjugated bilirubin). Physiologic jaundice, as exhibited by increasing total and unconjugated bilirubin concentrations, may occur in the neonatal period. Unconjugated bilirubin may displace drugs from albumin binding sites. Additionally, one of the by-products of lipid metabolism, free fatty acids, may also displace drug from albumin binding sites (thereby increasing the free drug concentration). Kernicterus ("yellow brain") may occur when unconjugated bilirubin displaced by drugs or other endogenous substances (ie, free fatty acids) crosses the blood-brain barrier, where it can deposit in the brain and cause neurologic complications. Therefore, albumin concentration, physiologic jaundice, and the use of IV lipid therapy may complicate therapy with highly protein-bound agents.

5. **D.** UDPG-glucuronyl transferase is responsible for conjugation of endogenous substances (bilirubin) and medications (morphine, chloramphenicol). The capacity for glucuronidation metabolism does not begin until around 2 months of age and reaches adult capacity by 3 years of age. Medications metabolized through this system are potential toxins in the neonatal population. An example would be the use of chloramphenicol in neonates and the development of "gray-baby syndrome" due to drug accumulation. Hydrolysis, reduction, sulfation, and methylation are functional in the neonatal period and should not pose drug therapy complications in this population.

6. **B.** The most common pathogens in acute otitis media are *S pneumoniae* (40-50%), *H influenzae* (20-30 %), and *M catarrhalis* (10-15%).

7. **A.** Despite the emergence of drug resistant *S pneumoniae*, amoxicillin, due to its excellent pharmacodynamic profile, side effect profile, and cost, remains the drug of choice in uncomplicated acute otitis media. This patient would be considered to be in the high-risk group

(age <2 years, attending day care, recurrent otitis media) and should receive high-dose therapy (80-90 mg/kg per day).

8. **D.** Counseling should include specific information about the antibiotic, its side effect profile, storage information, how to administer the medicine, dosage instructions, importance of taking the full course, and the need to shake the bottle prior to administering the dose. This mother should not be counseled to remove the child from day care, although a discussion of risk factors is appropriate in a counseling session.

9. **D.** The most common side effects with amoxicillin-clavulanate therapy include rash, urticaria, nausea, vomiting, and diarrhea. Although the other listed side effects may be seen with other antibiotic therapies, they do not typically occur with amoxicillin-clavulanate therapy.

10. **B.** Dehydration, which may develop in a vomiting child, is a risk factor for ibuprofen-induced renal insufficiency. If ibuprofen is used as an antipyretic or analgesic in pediatric patients, the parents and/or caregivers should be counseled regarding this risk and the need to follow intakes and outputs during the period of acute illness (ie, gastroenteritis) when the child may be receiving ibuprofen therapy.

11. **A.** The treatment of otitis externa includes the instillation of an antibiotic and steroid otic solution into the ear canal. Cotton swabs should be avoided to prevent otitis externa. Antihistamine solutions are not indicated in the treatment of otitis externa. Otic solutions containing acetic acid may also be of benefit in otitis externa by decreasing (not increasing) the pH of the ear canal and lowering its bacteria-harboring potential. Hydrochloric acid in any form should not be used in the ear canal.

12. **C.** Therapeutic drug monitoring is a critical part of the overall therapeutic plan in patients with cystic fibrosis. Patients with cystic fibrosis exhibit altered pharmacokinetic parameters of aminoglycosides, primarily increased clearance, and greater volumes of distribution. Tobramycin peak concentrations should be obtained to make sure the dose being given is sufficient to reach concentrations of 8-12 µg/mL and trough concentrations should be obtained to ensure adequate renal clearance (CF patients receive higher milligram per kilogram doses).

13. **D.** *S aureus* is a common pathogen in cystic fibrosis patients. Methicillin-sensitive *S aureus* may be treated with a number of agents (eg, oxacillin); however, methicillin-resistant *S aureus* (MRSA) should be treated with vancomycin.

14. **C.** Creon is the brand name for a pancreatic enzyme supplement. Creon is available as a microencapsulated formulation.

15. **B.** Mucomyst is the brand name for N-acetlycysteine, which lowers mucus viscosity (the sulfhydryl group opens the disulfide bond in mucoproteins).

16. **B.** Pancreatic enzyme products are available in powder, capsule, tablet, and microencapsulated formulations. The microencapsulated formulations may be opened and the contents sprinkled over acidic foods (ie, applesauce). Contents should not be crushed or chewed. Additionally, the dose should be based on the amount and type of food (ie, full doses with meals, half-doses with snacks and light meals). Adequate replacement will actually decrease bowel movements and improve stool consistency (ie, decrease steatorrhea).

17. **C.** All of the listed products are stimulants, with the exception of Wellbutrin. Stimulants are considered first-line therapy for attention deficit hyperactivity disorder; antidepressants may be considered second-line agents.

18. **A.** Pemoline (Cylert) is rarely used as a therapy for attention deficit hyperactivity disorder secondary to its association with fatal hepatic failure, which is not dose-related or related to time on therapy. Patients present in hepatic failure with malaise, nausea and vomiting, lethargy, and elevated liver function tests.

19. **A.** Overdose of tricyclic antidepressants may be fatal due to the development of arrhythmias. Since T.S. has a younger sibling in the house, there is a potential for the child to get into her older brother's medicine. Stimulants may have the potential for abuse in patients that do not have ADHD (ie, the 15-year-old brother), but tricyclic antidepressants are not associated with a high abuse potential. There are no stability issues with imipramine.

20. **C.** Both bupropion and methylphenidate may lower the seizure threshold. Clonidine is not associated with seizure occurrence.

21. **C.** Allergic conjunctivitis occurs after exposure to allergens, primarily dander or pollen. Patients suffering from allergic conjunctivitis will typically complain of eye itching.

22. **E.** Antimicrobial therapy has no place in therapy for allergic conjunctivitis. Ocular lubricants, decongestants, antihistamines, mast cell stabilizers or combinations of these products are appropriate options for allergic conjunctivitis.

23. **E.** The most common pathogens in neonatal bacterial conjunctivitis are *N gonorrhoeae, C trachomatis, S aureus, S epidermidis, S pneumoniae,* and *E coli*. Bacterial conjunctivitis outside of the first month of life is most commonly caused by *S aureus, S epidermidis, S pneumoniae,* and *II influenzae. Clostridium*, an anaerobe, is not a common bacterial pathogen in conjunctivitis.

24. **B.** Not unlike reactions from prolonged use of nasal decongestants, prolonged use of ocular decongestants may cause rebound congestion of the conjunctiva. This effect is less pronounced with naphazoline and tetrahydrozoline.

5. References

American Academy of Child and Adolescent Psychiatry. Practice parameter for the use of stimulant medication in the treatment of children, adolescents, and adults. *J Am Acad Child Adolesc Psychiatry.* 2002;41(Suppl 2):26S-49S.

American Academy of Pediatrics, Committee on Quality Improvement and Subcommittee on Attention-Deficit/Hyperactivity Disorder. Clinical Practice Guideline: Treatment of the School-Aged Child with Attention-Deficit/Hyperactivity Disorder. *Pediatrics.* 2001;108:1033-1044.

American Academy of Pediatrics, Committee on Quality Improvement and Subcommittee on Attention-Deficit/Hyperactivity Disorder. Diagnosis and evaluation of the child with attention-deficit/hyperactivity disorder. *Pediatrics.* 2000;105:1158-1170.

American Psychiatric Association. *Diagnostic and Statistical Manual of Mental Disorders (DSM-IV),* 4th ed. Washington: American Psychiatric Association; 1994:78-85.

APhA Special Report: Medication Administration Problem-Solving in Ambulatory Care. Washington: American Pharmaceutical Association; 1994:9.

Beringer P. Cystic fibrosis. In: Herfindal ET, Gourley DR, eds. *Textbook of Therapeutics. Drug and Disease Management,* 7th ed. Baltimore: Lippincott Williams & Wilkins; 2000:781-794.

Bosso JA, Milavetz G. Cystic fibrosis. In: Dipiro JT, Talbert RL, Yee GC, et al, eds. *Pharmacotherapy. A Pathophysiologic Approach,* 5th ed. New York: McGraw-Hill; 2002:563-574.

Clinical Practice Guidelines for Cystic Fibrosis Committee. Clinical Practice Guidelines for Cystic Fibrosis. Bethesda, MD: Cystic Fibrosis Foundation; 1997.

Dowell SF, Butler JC, Giebink GS, et al. Acute otitis media: management and surveillance in an era of pneumococcal resistance—a report from the Drug-resistant *Streptococcus pneumoniae* Therapeutic Working Group. *Pediatr Infect Dis J.* 1999;18:1-9.

Dowell SF, Marcy SM, Phillips WR, Gerber MA, Schwartz B. Otitis media—principles of judicious use of antimicrobial agents. *Pediatrics.* 1998;101:165-171.

Faden H, Duffy L, Boeve M. Otitis media: back to basics. *Pediatr Infect Dis J.* 1998;17:1105-1113.

Fiscella RG, Jensen MK. Ophthalmic disorders. In: Berardi RR, DeSimone EM, Newton GD, et al, eds. *Handbook of Nonprescription Drugs. An Interactive Approach to Self-Care,* 13th ed. Washington: American Pharmaceutical Association; 2002:543-570.

Krypel L. Otic disorders. In: Berardi RR, DeSimone EM, Newton GD, et al, eds. *Handbook of Nonprescription Drugs. An Interactive Approach to Self-Care,* 13th ed. Washington: American Pharmaceutical Association; 2002:603-620.

Leeder JS, Kearns GL. Pharmacogenetics in pediatrics: implications for practice. *Pediatr Clin North Am.* 1998;44:55-77.

Oszko MA. Common ear disorders. In: Herfindal ET, Gourley DR, eds. *Textbook of Therapeutics. Drug and Disease Management,* 7th ed. Baltimore: Lippincott Williams & Wilkins; 2000:1049-1056.

Schwartz GJ, Brion LP, Spitzer A. The use of plasma creatinine concentration for estimating glomerular filtration rate in infants, children, and adolescents. *Pediatr Clin North Am* 1987;34:571-590.

Solomon SD. Common eye disorders. In: Herfindal ET, Gourley DR, eds. *Textbook of Therapeutics. Drug and Disease Management,* 7th ed. Baltimore: Lippincott Williams & Wilkins; 2000:1037-1048.

Stewart CF, Hampton EM. Effects of maturation on drug disposition in pediatric patients. *Clin Pharmacol.* 1987;6:584-564.

Yaffe SJ, Aranda JV. *Pediatric Pharmacology: Therapeutic Principles in Practice,* 2nd ed. Philadelphia: WB Saunders; 1992.

34. Geriatrics and Gerontology

William Nathan Rawls, PharmD
Associate Professor, Department of Pharmacy
University of Tennessee College of Pharmacy
Clinical Pharmacy Specialist,
Veterans Affairs Medical Center, Memphis, Tennessee

Contents

1. Overview

- *Gerontology* is the study of the problems of aging and all its aspects. *Geriatrics* focuses on the diseases associated with aging and the treatments for those conditions. Geriatrics is of particular concern for pharmacists.

- Over 12% of the United States population is older than 65 years of age. By the year 2050, it is expected that the percentage will increase to over 20%.

- Persons over 65 years of age have more chronic illnesses and take more prescription and nonprescription drugs than persons in younger age groups.

- Age-related physiologic changes and increased medication use contribute to a greater risk of adverse drug events.

- Changes in vision, hearing, and mental functioning can result in increased problems with medication compliance.

Changes in Pharmacokinetics Associated with Aging

- Decreased absorption of various drugs secondary to decreased stomach acidity and changes in blood flow to the stomach

- Altered drug distribution caused by a decrease in total body water, increased lipid storage, and decreased serum albumin in malnourished elderly persons. These factors can contribute to increased serum levels of drugs.

- Decreased hepatic blood flow and reduced hepatic enzyme activity causes slower drug metabolism. Increased levels of drugs require increased metabolism by the liver.

- Elimination of drugs by the kidneys is slowed due to decreased renal blood flow and lowered glomerular filtration; thus drug accumulation develops.

- By using the Crockcroft-Gault formula for estimation of creatinine clearance, renal function can be predicted in the elderly:

$$\text{CrCl (mL/min)} = \frac{(140 - \text{age}) \times \text{weight in kg}}{72 \times \text{Cr}}$$

Note: Use ideal body weight. The equation above is for males. For females, multiply the result by .85.

2. Drugs of Concern

- Drugs that can cause psychiatric symptoms:
  * Anticholinergics
  * Narcotics
  * Tricyclic antidepressants
  * CNS stimulants
  * Antiparkinson drugs

- Drugs that can produce anxiety symptoms:
  * Theophylline
  * Nasal decongestants
  * β agonists
  * Antiparkinson drugs
  * Appetite suppressants

- Drugs that can contribute to nutritional deficiencies:
  * Diuretics
  * Digoxin, digitalis
  * Laxatives (overuse)
  * Sedatives (overuse)

3. Medication Compliance and the Older Adult

- Types of noncompliant behavior in the elderly:
  * Failure to take medications
  * Premature discontinuation of a medication
  * Excessive consumption of a medication
  * Use of medications not currently prescribed

- Strategies to improve patient medication compliance:
  * Limit the number of different medications and decrease dose frequency
  * Simplify dosage instructions
  * Tailor regimen to the patient's schedule
  * Use compliance aids and telephone reminders
  * Enlist the assistance of family members and friends

4. Basic Components of Evaluating Drug Therapy in Older Adults

- Questions to be answered:
  * Why is the drug being used? (diagnosis or reason)
  * Is the drug being given correctly? (dosage, form, schedule of administration)
  * Are any symptoms or complaints related to drug therapy?
  * Is there ongoing monitoring of treatment?
  * What is the endpoint of therapy?

5. Alzheimer's Disease and Related Dementias

- *Dementia* is the decline in intellectual abilities (eg, impairment of memory, judgment, and abstract thinking) coupled with changes in personality.

- Dementia patients tend to be described as cognitively impaired.

- *Cognition* is the mental process by which we become aware of objects of thought and perception, including all aspects of thinking and remembering.

- Impairment of cognition has a significant impact on the life of the dementia patient, his or her family members, and the community in general.

Types of Dementia

- Alzheimer's disease accounts for approximately 70% of dementias.

- Vascular dementias account for approximately 15% of dementias.

- Patients may have both Alzheimer's disease and vascular dementia.

Other Causes of Dementia

- Vascular disease

- Neurologic disorders such as Parkinson's disease, Pick's disease, and Huntington's chorea

- Metabolic disorders such as hypothyroidism, alcoholism, and anemia

- Infectious diseases (eg, meningitis, AIDS)

Clinical Presentation

- Alzheimer's disease is a progressive neurologic disease that results in impaired memory and intellectual functioning and altered behavior.

- Alzheimer's disease is characterized by the slow onset of symptoms leading to loss of ability to function independently.

- Symptoms may include psychoses with hallucinations, illusions, and delusional thinking.

- As Alzheimer's disease progresses, the brain continues to deteriorate.

Pathophysiology

- Hallmark pathologic changes in the brain are linked to Alzheimer's disease (ie, neuritic plaques and neurofibrillary tangles increase).

- Neuritic plaques are composed of amyloid proteins deposited on neurons; neurofibrillary tangles exist within neurons and disrupt normal function.

- Neurotransmitters are also altered in Alzheimer's disease; acetylcholine concentrations decrease significantly.

Diagnostic Criteria

- Diagnosis of Alzheimer's disease requires the presence of memory impairment and one or more of the following:
    * Aphasia (language disturbance)
    * Apraxia (impaired motor abilities)
    * Agnosia (failure to recognize objects)
    * Disturbance of executive function (eg, planning, organizing)

Treatment principles

- When evaluating a patient for treatment of dementia and Alzheimer's disease, review the patient's medications and consider any that might cause mental confusion or worsen underlying disease states.

- Drugs that block activity of acetylcholine can worsen dementia and decrease the effectiveness of medications used to treat Alzheimer's disease.

- Anticholinergic drugs are used for a variety of conditions ranging from depression to incontinence; indications should be identified before treating Alzheimer's disease.

- Anticholinergic effects can be additive (ie, a combination of anticholinergic drugs can result in toxicity even when each is given at low doses; see Table 2).

- Provide support to caregivers and treat the patient's behavioral and mood symptoms.

- Consider a trial of a cholinesterase inhibitor and monitor for benefits to memory and cognitive functioning.

Table 1

Drugs Used to Treat Alzheimer's Disease

Generic name	Trade name	Usual dosage	Dosage forms	Adverse effects
Tacrine	Cognex®	10-20 mg bid	Capsules	Nausea/vomiting, hepatotoxicity
Donepezil	Aricept®	5-10 mg at bedtime	Tablets	Nausea/vomiting
Rivastigmine	Exelon®	1.5-6 mg bid	Capsules	Nausea/vomiting, anorexia, weight loss
Galantamine	Reminyl®	4-12 mg bid	Capsules, oral solution	Nausea/vomiting

Monitoring

- Monitor memory and cognitive functions every 6-12 months.

- Routinely assess behaviors and ability to perform activities of daily living (eg, bathing, feeding, toileting, dressing).

- Monitor for focal neurologic signs and symptoms that may suggest other causes of changes in cognitive function.

Drug Therapy

Mechanism of action
- The pharmacologic approach to treatment falls into two categories:
  * Medications used to control behavioral and emotional symptoms
  * Medications used to slow or reverse the disease process

- Medications used to control behavioral and emotional symptoms are used to provide symptomatic improvement and do not affect the outcome of the disease.

- Anxiolytics are used to decrease anxiety and possibly agitation, motor restlessness and insomnia; eg, lorazepam (Ativan®), oxazepam (Serax®), and buspirone (Buspar®).

- Antidepressants improve depression that can worsen the cognitive functioning of a patient with Alzheimer's disease; eg, sertraline (Zoloft®), citalopram (Celexa®).

- Antipsychotics are used to decrease psychotic symptoms such as hallucinations and delusions. Antipsychotics may reduce agitation and aggressiveness; eg, haloperidol (Haldol®), risperidone (Risperdal®), and aripiprazole (Abilify®).

- Sedative-hypnotics are used for short-term treatment of insomnia, but can increase confusion and memory impairment; eg, trazodone (Desyrel®), zolpidem (Ambien®), and temazepam (Restoril®).

- Medications used to slow or reverse the symptoms of Alzheimer's disease have an impact on acetylcholine activity in the brain.

- Acetylcholine levels may be decreased by as much as 90% in Alzheimer's disease; these levels can be increased by inhibiting the enzyme acetylcholinesterase.

- Acetylcholinesterase inhibitors increase acetylcholine but do not replace lost cholinergic neurons or change the underlying pathology. This class of medications is used to prevent or slow deterioration in cognitive functioning.

- The first cholinesterase inhibitor approved to treat Alzheimer's disease was tacrine (Cognex), which proved beneficial but may cause the following:
  * Potential hepatotoxicity (damage to the liver); requires regular liver function testing
  * Tacrine is rarely prescribed.

- Safer cholinesterase inhibitors include:
  * Donepezil (Aricept) is selective for acetylcholinesterase in the brain (ie, not in peripheral tissues).
  * Rivastigmine (Exelon), a nonselective cholinesterase inhibitor, decreases both acetylcholinesterase and butyrylcholinesterase.
  * Galantamine (Reminyl) is a selective acetylcholinesterase inhibitor that activates nicotinic receptors, which may increase acetylcholine.

Patient instructions and counseling
- Donepezil: Given orally, 5 mg daily for 4-6 weeks; increase to 10 mg daily at bedtime. Take with or without food.

- Rivastigmine: Given with gradual dosage increase; beginning at 1.5 mg twice daily, then 3 mg twice daily, 4.5 mg twice daily, and 6 mg twice daily, with a minimum of 2 weeks between dose increases. If rivastigmine is discontinued because of adverse effects, restart at beginning dose. Take with meals in divided doses.

- Galantamine: Doses begin with 4 mg twice daily for 4 weeks, 8 mg twice daily for 4 weeks, 12 mg twice daily for 4 weeks, then 16 mg twice daily. If discontinued for more than a few days, restart at beginning dose. In hepatic or renal dysfunction doses should not exceed 16 mg/d. Do not use in instances of severe dysfunction. Take with meals in divided doses.

Adverse drug events
- Donepezil: Side effects include nausea/vomiting, GI symptoms; may be minimized by increasing the dose at 6 weeks.

- Rivastigmine: Side effects include nausea, vomiting, GI upset, and possible significant weight loss. Adverse effects are dose related and may be lessened by increasing dose at a slower rate.

- Galantamine: Adverse effects include nausea, vomiting, and GI upset. Slow dose titration will decrease side effects.

Drug-drug interactions (Table 2)
- Anticholinergic drugs will reduce the effectiveness of cholinesterase inhibitors and cause dry mouth, blurred vision, constipation, and mental confusion, (ie, conditions that are more problematic in the elderly).

- Cytochrome P450 enzyme inhibitors of 2D6 and 3A4 increase levels of galantamine and donepezil by inhibiting their metabolism.

Parameters to monitor
- Cognitive function (eg, poor results on mini mental state exam, decline in performance of activities of daily living, incidence of behaviors that indicate cognitive decline)

- Signs and symptoms of toxicity

Table 2

Anticholinergic Drugs That Can Worsen Alzheimer's Disease

Class	Drugs
Antidepressants	Highest effects: amitriptyline, amoxapine, clomipramine, protriptyline
	Moderate effects: bupropion, doxepin, imipramine, maprotiline, trimipramine
Antiparkinsonian agents	Benztropine, trihexyphenidyl
Antipsychotics	Highest effects: clozapine, mesoridazine, olanzapine, promazine, triflupromazine, thioridazine
	Moderate effects: chlorpromazine, chlorprothixene, pimozide
Antispasmodics	Atropine, belladonna alkaloids, dicyclomine, glycopyrrolate, hyoscyamine, methscopolamine, oxyphencyclimine, propantheline, oxybutynin, flavoxate, terodiline
Antihistamines	Highest effects: carbinoxamine, clemastine, diphenhydramine, promethazine
	Moderate effects: azatadine, brompheniramine, chlorpheniramine, cyproheptadine, dexchlorphenir-amine, triprolidine, hydroxyzine
Antiemetic/antivertigo agents	Meclizine, scopolamine, dimen-hydrinate, trimethobenzamide, prochlorperazine
Other agents with some anticholinergic activity	Paroxetine

- Active peptic ulcer disease, severe bradycardia, and acute medical illness are reasons to discontinue treatment.

- Periodic complete blood count and basic chemistries

- Expected benefits with the use of cholinesterase inhibitors include improvement in memory, some stabilization of behaviors/mood, and possible slowing of the progression of the disease.

Nondrug Therapy

- The treatment of Alzheimer's disease includes non-pharmacologic and pharmacologic therapy.

- Patients need to live in an environment that permits safe activities while minimizing risk.

- Caregivers need training and support to deal with the behavioral and functional issues associated with this disease.

6. Parkinson's Disease

- *Parkinson's disease* (PD) is a chronic progressive neurologic disorder with symptoms that present as a variable combination of rigidity, tremor, bradykinesia, and changes in posture and ambulation.

- An estimated 1 million persons in the U.S. suffer from PD. There are approximately 60,000 new cases diagnosed each year.

- The risk of developing PD increases with age and there is predicted to be a substantial increase in the U.S. population of persons over 60 years of age.

- Since medications are the primary treatment for PD, pharmacists play an important role in the care of these patients.

Classification

- Primary Parkinsonism has no identified cause.

- Secondary Parkinsonism can be the result of drug use (eg, reserpine, metoclopramide, antipsychotics), infections, trauma, or toxins.

Clinical Presentation

- Clinical signs and symptoms of PD develop insidiously, progress slowly, may fluctuate, and worsen with time despite pharmacologic therapy.

Symptoms

- Tremors at rest may begin unilaterally and are present in 70% of PD patients.

- Tremors (not during sleep) may worsen with stress

- Rigidity of limbs, trunk, and face with mask-like expression and difficulty with dressing or standing from a seated position.

- Akinesia (the absence of movement) and bradykinesia (slowed movements)

- Postural instability with abnormal gait and an increased risk of falls

- Depression and possible dementia

- Other symptoms include micrographia (small writing), drooling, decreased blinking, constipation, and incontinence.

Pathophysiology

- PD involves a progressive degeneration of the substantia nigra in the brain with a decrease in dopaminergic cells (more than the typical decrease that accompanies normal aging).

- The most significant neurotransmitter in PD is dopamine, but other neurotransmitters may play a role (eg, acetylcholine, glutamate, GABA, serotonin, norepinephrine).

- The etiology is unknown, but there is a possibility of genetic susceptibility.

- Environmental toxins combined with aging may also be responsible for the development of PD.

Diagnostic Criteria

- Clinical diagnosis based on the presence of bradykinesia and either rest tremor or rigidity.

- The stages of disease (Table 3)

Treatment Principles and Goals

- The goal for treating PD is to relieve symptoms and maintain or improve quality of life for the patient.

- Treatment should be initiated when there is functional impairment and discomfort for the patient and/or caregiver.

- A safe environment and caregiver support programs in addition to medications will often allow patients to remain in the community.

Table 3

The Stages of Parkinson's Disease

Stage 1	Unilateral involvement only with minimal or no functional impairment
Stage 2	Bilateral involvement without impairment of balance
Stage 3	Mild to moderate bilateral disease, some postural instability, can maintain independence
Stage 4	Severe disability, unable to live alone independently
Stage 5	Unable to walk or stand without assistance

Drug Therapy

Mechanism of action

- Medications increase dopamine or dopamine activity by directly stimulating dopamine receptors or by blocking acetylcholine activity, which results in increased dopamine effects (Table 4).

- Selection of an initial medication to treat PD may vary with the prescriber. Some choose to begin therapy with selegiline (Eldepryl), which offers possible neuroprotection; others prescribe carbidopa-levodopa (Sinemet), which has proven benefits.

Levodopa

- Levodopa is the most effective drug in the treatment of PD and is converted to dopamine in the body.

- Levodopa is given with carbidopa, a decarboxylase inhibitor which prevents the peripheral conversion of levodopa to dopamine, thereby reducing nausea and vomiting while allowing more drug to pass the blood-brain barrier.

- Generally, doses are increased gradually to minimize the risk of side effects. Doses are given before meals to facilitate absorption.

- Levodopa provides benefits to all stages of PD, but chronic use is associated with adverse effects.

- Patients may have periods of good mobility alternating with periods of impaired motor function.

Treatment complications and strategies for improving patient response

- No initial response to levodopa (carbidopa-levodopa combination)
  - * Gradually increase dose to at least 1000-1500 mg of levodopa.

- Suboptimal response
  - * After increasing levodopa, add another drug, eg, dopamine agonist, selegiline, or a COMT inhibitor.

- The "on and off" phenomenon (associated with advancing disease and loss of benefits from a dose of medication)
  - * Remedied by more frequent doses and/or use sustained-release levodopa

- End of dose or "wearing off," ie, decreased duration of benefit after a dose
  - * Levodopa wanes after less than 4 hours; therefore use combination therapy (two or more

Table 4

Drugs for Treating Parkinson's Disease

Generic name (trade name)	Mechanism of action	Dosage and available strengths and forms
Carbidopa-levodopa (Sinemet®)	Levodopa increases DA; carbidopa prevents metabolism	25/100 mg/d at breakfast; increase to 25/100 mg tid; may increase to 25/250 mg qid; available in sustained release 25/100-mg and 50/200-mg tablets
Bromocriptine (Parlodel®)	Directly stimulates DA receptors	1.25 mg bid with meals; increase by 2.5 mg/d every day, up to 100 mg/d; 2.5- and 5-mg tablets
Pergolide (Permax®)	Directly stimulates DA receptors	0.05 mg/d for 2 days; increase gradually to 2-3.5 mg/d (divided doses); maximum of 5 mg/d; 0.05-mg, 0.25-mg, and 1-mg tablets
Pramipexole (Mirapex®)	Directly stimulates DA receptors	0.125 mg tid increase weekly to 0.5-1.5 mg tid; 0.125-mg, 0.25-mg, 1-, and 1.5-mg tablets
Ropinirole (Requip®)	Directly simulates DA receptors	0.25 mg tid; increased gradually to a maximum of 24 mg/d; 0.25-, 0.5-, 1-, 2-, 4-, 5-mg tablets
Selegiline (Eldepryl®, Carbex®, Atapryl®, Selpak®)	Inhibits MAOB, increases DA and serotonin	Initially 5 mg at breakfast; increase to 5 mg at breakfast and lunch; 5-mg capsules, 5-mg tablets
Entacapone (Comtan®)	Inhibits COMT, increasing DA	200 mg with each dose of carbidopa-levodopa; maximum 1600 mg/d; 200-mg tablets
Tolcapone (Tasmar®)	Inhibits COMT, increasing DA	100 mg tid; discontinue if no benefits in 3 weeks; 100-mg, 200-mg tablets
Amantadine (Symmetrel®)	May increase presynaptic release of DA, blocks reuptake	100 mg bid; maximum dose 400 mg/d; 100-mg tablets, 100-mg capsules, 50 mg/5 mL syrup
Benztropine (Cogentin®)	Blocks acetylcholine, may balance DA	1-2 mg PO or IM or IV at bedtime or 0.5-6 mg/d in divided doses; 0.5-, 1-, 2-mg tablets, 1 mg/mL injection
Trihexyphenidyl (Artane®)	Blocks acetylcholine, may balance DA	1 mg/d up to 5 mg/d (divided doses); 2-mg, 5-mg tablets, 2 mg/5 mL elixir

COMT, catecholamine O-methyl transferase; DA, dopamine; MAOB, monoamine oxidase B.

drugs), give levodopa more frequently, or use sustained-release levodopa (Sinemet CR).

Patient instructions and counseling

- Usually take medications on an empty stomach; eat shortly afterward to avoid upset stomach.

- Take a missed dose as soon as possible; skip the missed dose if the next scheduled dose is within 2 hours.

- Dizziness, drowsiness, and stomach upset may occur and make operating equipment dangerous.

- Confusion, mood changes, and uncontrolled movements can result and should be reported to the prescriber as soon as possible.

- If taking a sustained-release product, do not crush.

Adverse effects (see Table 5)

Drug-drug interactions (see Table 6)

Parameters to monitor

- Liver function, complete blood count, basic chemistries (periodically)

- Blood pressure, pulse, ECG (periodically)

- Reduction of rigidity, tremor, slowed movements

- Examination for mental confusion, mood changes, psychotic thinking

Nondrug Therapy for Parkinson's Disease

- Educate patient and caregiver about the benefits and side effects of PD medications.

Table 5

Adverse Effects of Medications Used to Treat Parkinson's Disease

Drug	Adverse effects
Dopaminergics: levodopa, pergolide, bromocriptine, ropinirole, amantadine	Nausea/vomiting, agitation, confusion, depression, psychoses, orthostatic hypotension, dyskinetic movements
Selegiline	Nausea/vomiting, insomnia, dizziness, agitation, confusion, dyskinetic movements, anorexia
Amantadine	Confusion, dizziness, depression, anxiety, psychoses, insomnia
COMT inhibitors: tolcapone, entacapone	Nausea/vomiting, diarrhea, dyskinesia, urine coloration, liver toxicity (tolcapone)
Anticholinergics: benztropine, trihexyphenidyl	Dry mouth, blurred vision, constipation, urinary retention, confusion, agitation, psychoses

COMT, catecholamine O-methyl transferase.

- Aids for compliance should be provided to enable the patient to participate in medication use as long as physically possible.

- Physical therapy or occupational therapy may be important in maintaining physical activity and improving safety of work and living quarters.

- As PD progresses, speech therapy may be necessary to maintain communication ability.

- Dietary consultation may assist the patient in nutritional concerns related to swallowing difficulties and food selections.

Table 6

Drug-Drug Interactions with Medications Used to Treat Parkinson's Disease

Medication	Interacting drug	Outcome
Dopamine agonists (eg, bromocriptine, pergolide)	Dopamine antagonists (eg, haloperidol, metoclopramide)	Inhibition of benefits with worsening parkinsonism; bromocriptine + pseudoephedrine = tachycardia, hypertension, possible seizures
Levodopa	Dopamine antagonists	Inhibition of benefits with worsening Parkinsonism.
Selegiline	Serotonergics SSRIs, buspirone, mirtazapine	Serotonin syndrome may occur (confusion, agitation, tremor, seizures, coma)
COMT Inhibitors	Nonselective MAO inhibitors: phenelzine	Serotonin syndrome; hypertensive crisis secondary to increased catecholamines

COMT, catecholamine O-methyl transferase; MAO, monoamine oxidase; SSRI, selective serotonin reuptake inhibitor.

7. Glaucoma

- Glaucoma is a group of eye diseases characterized by an increase in intraocular pressure which causes pathologic changes in the optic nerve and typical visual field defects.

- Glaucoma affects over 4 million Americans; there may be as many as 15 million more persons with increased intraocular pressure but without clinical signs and symptoms of glaucoma.

- The prevalence of glaucoma increases with age and it is most often seen in those 65 years of age or older.

- The number of persons with glaucoma is expected to increase with the aging of the American population. With improved screening programs to identify those with increased intraocular pressure (IOP), an increase in the number of those diagnosed with glaucoma is expected.

Classification

- *Open-angle glaucoma* is a form of primary glaucoma. The angle of the anterior chamber remains open in an eye, but filtration of aqueous humor is gradually diminished because of the tissues of the angle. This accounts for approximately 80-90% of cases of glaucoma.

- *Angle-closure* (narrow angle) *glaucoma* is a form of primary glaucoma in an eye characterized by a shallow anterior chamber and a narrow angle. The filtration of aqueous humor is compromised as a result of the iris blocking the angle.

- *Congenital glaucoma* results from defective development of the structures in and around the anterior chamber of the eye and results in impairment of aqueous humor.

Clinical Presentation

- Clinical signs and symptoms of glaucoma develop slowly and may present with only minor symptoms such as headache and mild eye pain.

- Optic nerve damage results from chronic elevations in IOP and this emphasizes the importance of early and consistent treatment to avoid loss of vision.

- Acute angle-closure glaucoma presents with blurred vision, severe ocular pain and possible nausea and vomiting. This should be considered a medical emergency and immediate care should be recommended.

- Chronic angle-closure glaucoma may have symptoms similar to open-angle glaucoma.

- Tonometry is used to screen for IOP but direct ophthalmoscopy (slit-lamp examination) is necessary to accurately evaluate the eye for changes in the optic nerve.

Pathophysiology

- The pathogenesis of glaucoma results from changes in aqueous humor (the fluid filling the eye and in front of the lens) outflow that results in increased IOP. This increase in pressure leads to optic nerve atrophy and progressive loss of vision.

- Increased IOP can result from decreased elimination or increased production of aqueous humor.

- Aqueous humor is secreted by the ciliary processes into the posterior chamber of the eye. It then flows through the trabecular meshwork and the canal of Schlemm.

- Open-angle glaucoma is the result of decreased elimination of aqueous humor as it passes through the trabecular meshwork, thereby resulting in elevated IOP.

- Angle-closure glaucoma is caused by papillary blockage of aqueous humor outflow.
  * This can result when a patient has a narrow anterior chamber in the eye or a dilated pupil where the iris comes into greater contact with the lens.
  * With the blocking of outflow, aqueous humor accumulates in the posterior chamber, presses the lens forward, and further decreases drainage with possible complete blockage as the outcome.

Diagnostic Criteria

- Elevated IOP as determined by tonometry

- Funduscopic assessment to identify characteristic changes in the optic disc and retina

Treatment Principles (Figure 1)

- Reduce IOP to prevent optic nerve damage and visual field loss.

Figure 1.

Algorithm for the treatment of open-angle glaucoma.

- Use topical medications as first-line treatment.

- Consider acute angle-closure glaucoma as a medical emergency.

Monitoring

- Periodic screening for increased IOP, with yearly examinations for those over 65 years of age and as part of routine eye examination.

Drug Therapy

Mechanism of action
- Medications are considered the mainstay of therapy for the treatment of glaucoma (Table 6).

- β-Adrenergic blocking drugs (β-blockers) are considered first-line treatment for open-angle glaucoma. β-Adrenergic antagonists can be nonselective (ie, they block both β_1 and β_2 receptors) or selective (ie, they block only β_1 receptors).

- Drugs that block only β_1 receptors are considered to be cardioselective and cause less decrease in blood pressure and heart rate.

β-Adrenergic antagonists
   * Nonselective β antagonists: timolol, carteolol, levobunolol, metipranolol
   * β_1 Selective antagonists: betaxolol, levobetaxolol

- Therapy is initiated with a single topical ophthalmic solution with additional agents added if there is a less-than-acceptable decrease in IOP.

- The effects of therapy on IOP should be apparent after a week of treatment.

- Prostaglandin analogs are also used as first-line treatment (or in combination with β-blockers).

- Topical carbonic anhydrase inhibitors and α_2 agonists may be used in treatment.

- Medications such as epinephrine, pilocarpine, and oral carbonic anhydrase inhibitors are prescribed less often, but are considered to be effective adjunctive drugs.

Patient instructions and counseling
- Multiple factors present obstacles that can interfere with good compliance.

- Patients are often asymptomatic and do not feel treatment is necessary.

- Since decreased vision is associated with glaucoma, patients may have difficulty with written instructions.

- Adequate glaucoma therapy often requires two or more types of eye drops that may have to be given more than once daily.

- Correct administration of eye drops requires coordination and reasonable cognitive functioning.

- Glaucoma is more common in the elderly, who may have more difficulty complying with prescribed medications.

- Patient guidelines concerning the use of eye drops to treat glaucoma:

Table 6

Medications for the Treatment of Glaucoma

Generic name (trade name) and type	Form	Usual dosage	Comments
Timolol (Timoptic®), nonselective β antagonist (NSBA)	0.25% and 0.50% solution and gel-forming solution	1 drop twice daily; gel solution used once daily	Nonselective β antagonists often first choice for open-angle glaucoma
Carteolol (Ocupress®), NSBA	1% ophthalmic solution	1 drop twice daily	
Levobunolol (Betagen®), NSBA	0.25% and 0.50% solution	1-2 drops 1-4 times daily	
Metipranolol (OptiPranolol®), NSBA	0.3% solution	1 drop twice daily	
Betaxolol (Betoptic®), selective β₁ antagonist	0.25% and 0.50% solution	1-2 drops twice daily	Cardioselective; less effect on heart rate and blood pressure
Levobetaxolol (Betaxon®), selective β₁ antagonist	0.50% solution	1 drop twice daily	Cardioselective
Acetazolamide (Diamox®), carbonic anhydrase inhibitor	125-mg, 250-mg tablets, 500-mg ER capsules	250 mg 1-4 times daily; extended release 1-2 times daily	Do not use with sulfa allergy
Dorzolamide (Trusopt®) carbonic anhydrase inhibitor	2.0% solution	1 drop three times daily	Do not use with sulfa allergy
Brinzolamide (Azopt®), carbonic anhydrase inhibitor	1.0% solution	1 drop three times daily	Do not use with sulfa allergy
Methazolamide (Neptazane®), carbonic anhydrase inhibitor	25-mg and 50-mg tablets	15-50 mg 1-3 times daily	Do not use with sulfa allergy
Latanoprost (Xalatan®), prostaglandin analog	0.005% solution; refrigerate	1 drop at bedtime	Can change blue eyes to brown
Bimatoprost (Lumigan®), prostaglandin analog	0.03% solution	1 drop at bedtime	Can cause darkening of eyelids and eyelashes
Travoprost (Travatan®), prostaglandin analog	0.004% solution	1 drop at bedtime	Frequent ocular hyperemia
Unoprostone (Rescula®), prostaglandin analog	0.15% solution	1 drop twice daily	If used with another drop, wait 5 minutes
Brimonidine (Alphagan®), α₂ adrenergic agonist	0.15% solution	1 drop three times daily	Wait at least 15 minutes after using before placing soft contacts
Dipivefrin (Propine®); α-adrenergic agonist	0.1% solution	1 drop twice daily	Prodrug of epinephrine
Pilocarpine (Pilocar®), cholinergic, miotic	0.5%, 1%, 2%, 3%, 4%, 6%, 8% solution, 4% gel	1-2 drops 3-4 times daily; ½ inch gel at bedtime	Once weekly dose form called Ocuserts®

* Wash hands before administering eye drops and avoid touching the dropper tip.
* Confirm that the medication is not outdated and has been stored properly.
* Looking upward, pull the lower lid down and instill the correct number of drops.
* Close the eye to allow the medication to have maximal effect.
* In most cases wait five or more minutes between different medications.

Adverse drug events (see Table 7)

Drug-drug interactions
• Drug interactions between topical medications and systemic drugs are unlikely.
• Acetazolamide interacts with the following:
    * Aspirin to cause increased aspirin levels and possible toxicity
    * Cyclosporine to cause increased cyclosporine levels

Table 7

Classification, Mechanism of Action, and Adverse Effects of Glaucoma Medications

Medication class	Mechanism of action	Adverse effects
β-Adrenergic antagonists: timolol, metipranolol, carteolol, levobunolol, etc.	Decrease in aqueous humor formation with slight increase in outflow (β selective)	Adverse cardiac effects, worsening pulmonary disease, depression, dizziness
Miotics (cholinergics): pilocarpine, carbachol	Increase in aqueous humor outflow	Miosis, brow ache, dizziness, nausea, flushing, itching, sweating, confusion
Carbonic anhydrase inhibitors: dorzolamide, brinzolamide	Decrease in aqueous humor formation	Lethargy, decreased appetite, GI upset, urinary frequency
Prostaglandin analogs: latanoprost, travoprost, bimatoprost	Increased uveoscleral outflow without effect on aqueous humor formation	Iris pigmentation, eyelid darkening, macular edema
α_2-Adrenergic agonists: apraclonidine, brimonidine	Decrease in aqueous humor formation	Tachycardia, dry mouth, eyelid elevation, CNS effects in the old and very young
Other α-adrenergic agonists: epinephrine, dipivefrin	Increase in aqueous humor outflow	Tachycardia, increased blood pressure, allergic responses

* Lithium to cause either increased or decreased lithium levels
* Phenytoin to cause an increased risk of osteomalacia

Parameters to monitor
• Medication use is critical to the successful treatment of glaucoma and should be monitored by the health professional.

Other
• A combination of timolol 0.5% and dorzolamide 2% (Cosopt®) is available. This combination effectively lowers IOP and only requires twice-daily doses. This simplified dosing should improve compliance with treatment. This combination (ie, using two drugs from different categories) represents a sound treatment approach. Poor response to therapy may result in the prescribing of multiple medications, which may negatively impact the patient's ability to successfully use the more complex regimen.

Nondrug Therapy

Laser surgery
• Argon laser trabeculoplasty (ALT) has proven effective as adjunctive therapy that increases the flow of aqueous humor.

Surgery
• Procedure involves creating new means of drainage for aqueous humor to leave the anterior chamber.

8. Key Points

Alzheimer's disease
• Alzheimer's disease is a progressive neurologic disease that results in impaired memory, intellectual functioning, and behavior.

• There is no known cure for Alzheimer's disease, but there are therapies to decrease memory impairment as well as improve behavior and patient functioning.

• Other forms of dementia that are potentially reversible should be identified and treated accordingly.

• New drug therapies may slow the progression of Alzheimer's disease and allow patients to remain in the least restrictive environment possible.

• Caregiver support and education is an important measure to assure patient safety and well-being.

Parkinson's disease
• Parkinson's disease is a chronic, progressive neurologic disease for which there is no cure; medications are available to slow the progression of symptoms.

• The etiology of Parkinson's disease is unknown, but may involve genetic susceptibility combined with environmental toxins and age-related changes in the brain.

- Dopamine, the central neurotransmitter, is decreased in Parkinson's disease and current drug therapy is primarily directed at increasing dopamine levels.

- Drug therapy monitoring in Parkinson's disease requires an understanding of a variety of different medications that may cause significant adverse effects.

- Physical therapy, occupational therapy, dietary considerations, and support counseling for caregivers are necessary components of treating Parkinson's disease.

Glaucoma

- Glaucoma, a group of eye diseases, is characterized by increased intraocular pressure resulting in damage to the optic nerve and possible blindness.

- Open-angle glaucoma is the most common form of this disease; angle-closure glaucoma can be a medical emergency.

- The goal of therapy is to reduce intraocular pressure with the simplest medication regimen possible.

- Drug therapy for glaucoma usually begins with a topical β adrenergic antagonist; patients often require combination therapy.

- Medication compliance is essential in the control of glaucoma. Education of the patient and caregiver is required to overcome treatment barriers.

9. Questions and Answers

1. The maximum daily dose of galantamine in patients with renal impairment is

   A. 8 mg/d
   B. 12 mg/d
   C. 16 mg/d
   D. 24 mg/d
   E. 32 mg/d

2. Which of the following is given as a once-daily dose?

   A. Buspirone
   B. Donepezil
   C. Galantamine
   D. Rivastigmine
   E. Tacrine

3. Rivastigmine increases levels of which neurotransmitter?

   A. Acetylcholine
   B. Dopamine
   C. Melatonin
   D. Norepinephrine
   E. Serotonin

4. Weight loss is most often associated with which of the following?

   A. Donepezil
   B. Galantamine
   C. Mirtazapine
   D. Rivastigmine
   E. Tacrine

5. What is the correct answer concerning donepezil?

   I. Inhibits acetylcholinesterase but not butyrylcholinesterase
   II. It should be taken with meals in divided doses
   III. Side effects include tachycardia and blood pressure alterations

   A. I only
   B. III only
   C. I and II only
   D. II and III only
   E. I, II, and III

6. All of the following medications are used to treat behavioral and emotional symptoms in Alzheimer's patients EXCEPT

   A. Benztropine
   B. Buspirone
   C. Citalopram
   D. Lorazepam
   E. Risperidone

7. Tacrine use requires which routine laboratory test to monitor for toxicity?

   A. Complete blood count (CBC)
   B. Cholesterol testing
   C. Liver function tests
   D. Renal function tests
   E. Thyroid function tests

8. All of the following could worsen cognition in AD patients EXCEPT

   A. Dicyclomine
   B. Dimenhydrinate
   C. Meclizine
   D. Trazodone
   E. Trihexyphenidyl

9. Which works by direct stimulation of dopamine receptors?

   A. Amantadine
   B. Benztropine
   C. Entacapone
   D. Ropinirole
   E. Selegiline

10. A common adverse effect of trihexyphenidyl is

    A. Insomnia
    B. Nausea and vomiting
    C. Dry mouth and urinary retention
    D. Depression
    E. Anorexia

11. In treating Parkinsonism the "on and off" phenomenon is most often associated with

    A. Benztropine
    B. Bromocriptine
    C. Carbidopa-levodopa
    D. Selegiline
    E. Tolcapone

12. What would be the most likely outcome if a

Parkinson patient on levodopa were also prescribed haloperidol?

   A. Excessive nausea and vomiting
   B. Hypertensive crisis
   C. Tachycardia and possible chest pain
   D. Worsening symptoms of Parkinson's disease
   E. Excessive somnolence

13. Which inhibits monoamine oxidase (MAO)?

    A. Benztropine
    B. Bromocriptine
    C. Pramipexole
    D. Selegiline
    E. Tolcapone

14. How does carbidopa affect levodopa?

    A. Slows the release from presynaptic neurons
    B. Prevents the excretion of dopamine
    C. Increases stimulation of dopamine receptors
    D. Decreases tolerance to normal doses
    E. Inhibits the peripheral conversion to dopamine

15. Liver toxicity is a significant risk factor with which of the following?

    A. Amantadine
    B. Carbidopa-levodopa
    C. Pramipexole
    D. Ropinirole
    E. Tolcapone

16. Which of the following statements are true concerning the treatment of the "on and off" phenomenon that can be associated with PD?

    I. Combine two or more medications with different mechanisms of action
    II. Give more frequent doses of carbidopa-levodopa
    III. Give a sustained release carbidopa-levodopa product

    A. I only
    B. III only
    C. I and II only
    D. II and III only
    E. I, II, and III

17. Timolol ophthalmic drops would be more likely to cause which adverse effect as compared to levobetaxolol ophthalmic drops?

    A. Agitation and restlessness

B. Nausea and vomiting
C. Confusion
D. Change in heart rate and blood pressure
E. Altered intraocular pressure

18. Which of the following would not be considered for monotherapy of glaucoma?

   A. Latanoprost
   B. Dorzolamide
   C. Carteolol
   D. Methazolamide
   E. Brimonidine

19. Which of the following can cause iris pigmentation changes?

   A. Acetazolamide
   B. Betaxolol
   C. Brimonidine
   D. Latanoprost
   E. Pilocarpine

20. Which of the following is an available fixed combination product?

   A. Dorzolamide and timolol
   B. Betaxolol and bimatoprost
   C. Bimatoprost and levobunolol
   D. Latanoprost and timolol
   E. Methazolamide and latanoprost

21. All of the following are available as an ophthalmic solution EXCEPT

   A. Brimonidine
   B. Dipivefrin
   C. Dorzolamide
   D. Methazolamide
   E. Metipranolol

22. Which should not be used if a patient has a sulfa allergy?

   A. Betazolol
   B. Bimatoprost
   C. Brimonidine
   D. Brinzolamide
   E. Unoprostone

23. α_2-Adrenergic agonists cause a(n):

   A. Increase in aqueous humor synthesis
   B. Decrease in aqueous humor formation
   C. Increased uveoscleral outflow
   D. Increase in aqueous humor outflow

   E. Decreased uveoscleral outflow

24. Which of the following statements concerning glaucoma therapy are correct?

   I. Carteolol is available as an ophthalmic solution and as a gel-forming solution.
   II. Latanoprost and metipranolol ophthalmic solutions should be stored in the refrigerator.
   III. Prostaglandin analogs, β-adrenergic antagonists, and α-adrenergic agonists can be used as monotherapy.

   A. I only
   B. III only
   C. I and II only
   D. II and III only
   E. I, II, and III

Answers

1. **C.** With renal or hepatic dysfunction, galantamine doses should not exceed 16 mg/d. With severe renal or hepatic dysfunction, galantamine should not be used.

2. **B.** All cholinesterase inhibitors except donepezil require at least twice-daily dosing. Donepezil has a long half-life, which allows for once-daily doses. None of these agents is available in sustained release forms. Buspirone is an antianxiety drug that is dosed twice or three times daily.

3. **A.** Rivastigmine is a cholinesterase inhibitor and all cholinesterase inhibitors increase levels of acetylcholine, the neurotransmitter that appears to be involved with memory function.

4. **D.** Weight loss, probably due to nausea and vomiting, is a warning for rivastigmine. In controlled trials, approximately 26% of women on doses of 9 mg/d or greater had weight loss of equal to or greater than 7% of their baseline weight.

5. **A.** Donepezil is selective for acetylcholinesterase and does not inhibit butyrylcholinesterase. Donepezil does not have to be taken with meals and is given once daily. Donepezil does not increase heart rate and this class of medications that increase acetylcholine should be used with caution in patients with bradycardia.

6. **A.** Benztropine is an anticholinergic used to treat side effects from antipsychotic medications and is also used to treat incontinence. All other drugs listed can be used to treat specific symptoms associated with AD.

7. **C.** Tacrine can cause hepatic dysfunction. The FDA requires liver function monitoring when initiating treatment and periodically while a patient is on the drug. This is not a requirement for other cholinesterase inhibitors.

8. **D.** All of the drugs listed with the exception of trazodone have anticholinergic activity. Decreasing the activity of acetylcholine could worsen dementia and block benefits of cholinesterase inhibitors. Trazodone is an antidepressant with sedating properties but little anticholinergic activity. It may be given at bedtime to help with sleep. Trazodone does have a side effect of orthostatic hypotension.

9. **D.** Ropinirole directly stimulates dopamine receptors; the other drugs increase dopamine activity by different mechanisms.

10. **C.** Trihexyphenidyl is an anticholinergic drug. By blocking acetylcholine activity, trihexyphenidyl helps to balance dopamine activity and may improve early symptoms of PD. Anticholinergics cause dry mouth, blurred vision, urinary retention, constipation, and confusion.

11. **C.** The "on and off" phenomenon is associated with advancing disease and loss of benefits from levodopa. It is treated by giving more frequent doses and/or using sustained release levodopa.

12. **D.** Haloperidol and other antipsychotics block dopamine activity and can worsen PD. They can also block the benefits of PD medications, which increase dopamine activity.

13. **D.** Selegiline is a MAOI which is selective for MAOB, which decreases the potential for drug-drug and drug-food interactions. At doses higher than 10 mg/d this selectivity becomes less.

14. **E.** Carbidopa inhibits the peripheral conversion of levodopa to dopamine, thus allowing more levodopa to cross the blood-brain barrier and decreases adverse effects from dopamine.

15. **E.** Tolcapone is has a significant risk of hepatotoxicity; thus its use is limited.

16. **D.** Increasing frequency of drug or using a sustained release form decreases blood level fluctuations and should improve symptoms.

17. **D.** Timolol is a nonselective β-adrenergic antagonist which causes a reduction in heart rate and blood pressure. There is enough absorption from eye drops to produce these cardiac effects.

18. **D.** All of the other choices could be considered as monotherapy for glaucoma. Methazolamide is an oral carbonic anhydrase inhibitor and is used in conjunction with ophthalmic drops.

19. **D.** Latanoprost, a prostaglandin analog, is known to change iris pigmentation and to darken eyelashes.

20. **A.** Dorzolamide plus timolol (Cosopt) is the only combination ophthalmic solution for treating glaucoma. An advantage for using a combination product would be increased compliance.

21. **D.** Methazolamide and acetazolamide are both available only as oral tablets or capsules. Topical carbonic anhydrase inhibitors are brinzolamide and dorzolamide.

22. **D.** Patients with sulfa allergy should not be given a carbonic anhydrase inhibitor.

23. **B.** α_2-Adrenergic agonists such as brimonidine cause a decrease in aqueous humor formation.

24. **B.** All of these drugs can be used as monotherapy in glaucoma. Timolol and pilocarpine are available as gel forms. Latanoprost (but not metipranolol) should be stored in a refrigerator before dispensing.

10. References

Chen JJ, Shimomua SK. Parkinsonism. In: Herfindal ET, Gourley DR, eds. *Textbook of Therapeutics,* 7th ed. Philadelphia: WB Saunders Co; 2000:1139-1155.

Fujumoto D, Rawls WN. Alzheimer's disease. In: Herfindal ET, Gourley DR, eds. *Textbook of Therapeutics,* 7th ed. Philadelphia: WB Saunders Co; 2000:2063-2076.

Grutzendler J, Morris JC. Cholinesterase inhibitors for Alzheimer's disease. *Drugs.* 2001;61:41-52.

Hoyng PF, van Beek LM. Pharmacological therapy for glaucoma. *Drugs.* 2000;59:411-434.

Olanow CW, Watts RL, Koller WC. An algorithm for the management of Parkinson's disease. *Neurology.* 2001;56:872-891.

Wigginton SA, Higginbotham EJ. Glaucoma diagnosis and management. *Ophthol Clin North Am.* 2000;12:157-169.

Wurtzbacker JD, Gourt DR, McKenzie C. Glaucoma. In: Herfindal ET, Gourley DR, eds. *Textbook of Therapeutics,* 7th ed. Philadelphia: WB Saunders Co; 2000:1057-1082.

35. Toxicology and Chem-Bioterrorism

Adrianne Y. Butler, PharmD
Assistant Professor, Department of Pharmacy
University of Tennessee College of Pharmacy

Billie J. Holliman, PharmD
Instructor, Department of Pharmacy
University of Tennessee College of Pharmacy

C. Reneé Adams-McDowell, PharmD
Instructor, Department of Pharmacy
University of Tennessee College of Pharmacy

Peter A. Chyka, PharmD
Professor and Vice Chair for Clinical Programs,
  Department of Pharmacy
University of Tennessee College of Pharmacy

Contents

1. Overview of Poisoning and Toxicology

Poisoning in America

- Poisoning exposures and overdoses affect over 2 million people annually, and there are over 20,000 deaths yearly (<1% of deaths are in preschool-aged children).

- A great number of poisonings occur in young children, but most fatalities occur in adults.

- Any chemical can become toxic if the exposure is too great in relation to body weight and tolerance.

- Medications are the most common cause of poisoning morbidity and mortality.

Table 1

Ranking of Most Frequent Poisonings From U.S. Poison Centers and Emergency Departments During 2001

Cases from poison centers[1]	Cases from emergency departments[2]
Analgesics	Alcohol-in-combination
Cleaning substances	Cocaine
Cosmetics and personal care products	Anxiolytics and sedatives
	Marijuana
Foreign bodies	Opioid analgesics
Plants	Heroin
Sedative drugs	Analgesics, nonopioid
Cough and cold drugs	Antidepressants
Topical drugs	Antipsychotics
Bites and envenomations	Muscle relaxants
Antidepressant drugs	Amphetamines
Pesticides	Methamphetamine
Food products	

[1]In decreasing order of frequency and based on 2,267,979 poison exposures. From: Litovitz TL, Klein-Schwartz W, Rodgers GC, et al. 2001 Annual Report of the American Association of Poison Control Centers Toxic Exposure Surveillance System. *Am J Emerg Med.* 2002;20:391-452.

[2]In decreasing order of frequency based on 638,484 drug abuse episodes out of 100,518,000 emergency department visits. From: Office of Applied Studies, Substance Abuse and Mental Health Services Administration, Drug Abuse Warning Network, Rockville, MD (03/2002 update).

- Most poisonings in preschool-aged children are unintentional or accidental.

- Unintentional poisonings can also occur in adolescents and adults; however, intentional (suicide, drug abuse) poisoning and overdose are common (Table 1).

Poison Prevention Approaches and Pharmacy

Poison Prevention Packaging Act of 1970: "Safety Caps"
- Issued to prevent preschool-aged children from opening and ingesting harmful substances or to delay the opening of packaging containing such substances (to limit the amount of harmful substance that may be ingested within a reasonable amount of time).

- Drugs requiring safety caps include aspirin, ibuprofen, acetaminophen, and oral prescription drugs with certain exceptions (eg, birth control pills, nitroglycerin).

Utilization of Poison Control Centers
- Nationwide access at 1-800-222-1222 for 24-hour poison center services for the area from which the call is placed in the U.S.

Poison Prevention Tips for Consumers
- Store all drugs and chemicals out of the reach of children.

- Never put chemicals in food containers.

- Choose products with safety caps when there is a choice and use them properly.

- Read and follow all label directions carefully.

- Never call medicine "candy."

- Use safety latches.

Pharmacy Requirements for Joint Commission on Accreditation of Healthcare Organizations

- Maintain and keep available (for the medical staff) an approved stock of antidotes and other emergency drugs both in the pharmacy and patient care areas.

- Maintain authoritative, current antidote information.

- The phone number of the regional poison control

center should also be readily available in areas outside of the pharmacy where drugs are stored.

Emergency Actions

- First aid, if applicable (Table 2)

Other considerations:
- Avoid wasting time to find an "antidote" at home.

- Do not use home remedies such as salt water, mustard powder, raw eggs, hydrogen peroxide, cooking grease, or gagging.

- Call 911 or an ambulance if the person is not breathing, has had a seizure, or is unresponsive.

- Contact a poison center immediately to determine first aid or whether a poisoning emergency exists.

Decontamination of the Gastrointestinal Tract

- The practice of using drugs to decrease the absorption of other drugs from the gastrointestinal tract is in a state of change. Drugs such as ipecac syrup are being abandoned by many as a home- or hospital-based therapy. Its use is primarily at the preference of the consulting poison center or health care professional. Current recommendations are described

Table 2

First Aid for Poisoning Emergencies

Inhaled poison
Immediately get the person to fresh air. Avoid breathing fumes. Open doors and windows wide.

Poison on the skin
Remove any contaminated clothing and flood skin with water for at least 15 minutes.

Poison in the eye
Flood the eye with water. Pour it from a large glass 2-3 inches from the eye. Repeat for a total of 15-30 minutes. Do not force the eyelid open. Remove contact lenses.

Swallowed poison
Unless the victim is unconscious, having convulsions or cannot swallow, give a small glassful (2-4 ounces) of water immediately. Call a poison Center for advice about whether other actions are needed.

---

below as well as basic information about the drugs in case they are encountered.

Current recommendations
- Ipecac syrup has questionable effectiveness and its use is generally avoided in hospitals.

- Gastric lavage involves placing a tube into the stomach through a nostril or the mouth and repetitively washing out the stomach contents with water or a saline solution. This method of gastric decontamination is of questionable effectiveness, particularly if it is performed more than 1 hour after ingestion.

- Cathartics such as magnesium citrate are not routinely used.

- Activated charcoal is often the only treatment necessary if the toxin is adsorbed and it is used within 1-2 hours of ingestion.

- Whole bowel irrigation can be considered if the toxin is poorly or slowly adsorbed and its presence in the gastrointestinal tract is likely.

Ipecac syrup
Indications and dosage
- Previously used for general prophylaxis of selected poisonings of expected minor or moderate severity in alert patients

- Has been abandoned by many clinicians as a prehospital or hospital treatment. In November 2003 The American Academy of Pediatrics recommended that ipecac syrup no longer be used routinely as a home treatment for poisoning.

Contraindications
- The patient is experiencing pronounced sleepiness, coma, or seizures.

- Ingestion of caustics, aliphatic hydrocarbons, and fast-acting agents that produce coma or seizures (eg, tricyclic antidepressants, clonidine, strychnine, hypoglycemic agents).

- Time since ingestion is believed to be 1 hour or more

Adverse effects
- Common: diarrhea, sleepiness, protracted vomiting

- Uncommon: Mallory-Weiss tears, tracheal aspiration into the lungs

- Disadvantages: relative lack of efficacy and emesis complicates administration of other oral therapies

Activated charcoal
Indications and dosage
- Occasionally used to adsorb poisons in an alert or comatose patient

- Administer as a slurry by mouth or through lavage tube:
  * Children: 25-50 g
  * Adults: 25-100 g

Contraindications
- Ingestions of aliphatic hydrocarbons and caustics

- If patient's bowel sounds are absent

- Ingestions of heavy metals (sodium, lithium, iron, lead) or simple alcohols

Adverse effects
- Uncommon: tracheal aspiration, pneumonitis

- Common: emesis, soiling of clothes and furnishings

Advantages and disadvantages
- Advantages: rapid onset of action, nonspecific action for a wide variety of chemicals, and reasonable effectiveness within1 hour of ingestion

- Disadvantages: messy and difficult to administer, may also remove beneficial drugs along with the toxin.

Cathartics
- Previously used as an adjunct to activated charcoal administration to decrease gastrointestinal transit time

- Efficacy unproved

- Fluid and electrolyte disturbances possible with repeated doses

- May contribute to emesis following activated charcoal use

- Agents previously used include magnesium citrate, magnesium sulfate, sodium sulfate, and sorbitol.

- *Note:* Some activated charcoal products contain sorbitol mixed in the preparation. The sorbitol concentration varies from brand to brand.

Whole bowel irrigation
Indications and technique
- Generally used when charcoal may be inappropriate (eg, if iron or lithium were ingested) and the toxin is suspected to be present in the gastrointestinal tract (eg, when drugs are sustained-release formulations or ingested illicit drugs packed in condoms)

- Use larger volumes of polyethylene glycol electrolyte solutions (eg, Colyte®, Golytely®) than amounts conventionally used for bowel preparation.

- Administer by mouth or through a gastric or duodenal tube for treatment of poisoning
  * Children: 25 mL/kg per hour (approximately 500 mL/h) up to 2-5 L
  * Adults: 2 L/h up to 5-10 L

Contraindications
- Ingestion of caustics or aliphatic hydrocarbons

- Patients with absent bowel sounds or gastrointestinal tract obstruction

Adverse effects
- Few adverse effects have been reported, but there are limited results available from which to draw conclusions. Some nausea and vomiting has been reported.

Advantages and disadvantages
- Advantages: prompts whole bowel evacuation within 2 hours

- Disadvantages: messy procedure due to rectal effluent

Other hospital-based therapies
- These include supportive and symptomatic care, multiple doses of activated charcoal (to enhance systemic elimination when appropriate), hemodialysis (to enhance systemic elimination when appropriate) and use of antidotes (to antagonize or reverse toxic effects when indicated).

2. Substance Abuse and Toxicology

- Substance abuse often leads to acute and chronic toxicity (Table 3).

- Management of the acute condition generally follows the same guidelines as managing poisonings and overdoses.

- A challenge in treating patients during acute drug overdose is determining the possible agents taken and possible adulterants (eg, talc, strychnine, other drugs) or contaminants.

- Chronic abuse can foster dependence, which often leads to withdrawal symptoms upon stopping use.

3. Antidotes

Role of Antidotes

- An antidote counteracts or changes the nature of a poison.

- There are few antidotes available relative to the large number of potential poisons. Table 4 lists commonly used antidotes for the treatment of a patient with a poisoning or an overdose.

- Many hospitals have an insufficient stock of antidotes; the pharmacy and therapeutics committee of the hospital should regularly review the inventory of antidotes.

Table 3

Selected Drugs of Abuse and Addictive Substances

Substance (slang names)	Methods of abuse	Major or unique health effects
Androgenic anabolic steroids ("Roids")	Anabolic steroids are taken orally or injected, typically in cycles of weeks or months ("cycling"); users often combine several different types of steroids ("stacking")	• Synthetic derivatives of testosterone; abuse can lead to serious health problems, some irreversible • Men: shrinking of the testicles, reduced sperm count, infertility, baldness, gynecomastia, increased risk for prostate cancer • Women: growth of facial hair, male-pattern baldness, changes in or cessation of the menstrual cycle, enlargement of the clitoris, deepened voice • Adolescents: stunted growth by premature skeletal maturation and accelerated puberty changes • Other major side effects can include jaundice, fluid retention, high blood pressure, severe acne; extreme mood swings can can occur, including manic-like symptoms leading to violence and depression often experienced when drugs are stopped and may contribute to dependence
Barbiturates (barbs, downers)	Ingestion, injection	• CNS depressants that at high doses can become general anesthetics • With high doses, coma, ataxia, depressed reflexes, hypotension, respiratory depression • CNS depressants should not be combined with any medication or substance that causes sedation, including prescription pain medicines, certain over-the-counter cold and allergy medications, or alcoholic drinks. The effects of the drugs can combine to slow breathing, or slow both the heart and respiration, which can be fatal • Discontinuing prolonged use of high doses of barbiturates can lead to withdrawal
Cocaine (snow, crack, rock); crack is the street name given to cocaine that has been processed from cocaine hydrochloride to the free base for smoking	Sniffing or snorting, injecting; smoking of free-base and crack cocaine; poorly absorbed orally	• CNS stimulant that produces euphoric effects and hyperstimulation such as dilated pupils, increased temperature, tachycardia, and hypertension • Prolonged cocaine snorting can result in ulceration of the mucous membranes of the nose and can damage the nasal septum enough to cause it to collapse • Cocaine-related deaths are often a result of cardiac arrest or seizures followed by respiratory arrest • Tolerance develops to the euphoric effects • When addicted individuals stop using cocaine, they often become depressed

(continued)

Table 3

Selected Drugs of Abuse and Addictive Substances (continued)

Substance (slang names)	Methods of abuse	Major or unique health effects
Dextromethorphan (DXM, DM, Robo, Velvet, Rojo)	Orally by drinking dextromethorphan-containing cough syrups; availability of the powdered form has led to repackaging as capsules or tablets and to nasal insufflation (snorting)	• Dextromethorphan (d-3-methoxy-N-methylmorphinan) is the dextro isomer of levomethorphan. It has no analgesic opiate-like dependence-producing properties. A behaviorally-active metabolite, dextrorphan, is structurally related to PCP and ketamine and may contribute to its abuse potential • The typical clinical presentation of intoxication involves hyperexcitability, lethargy, ataxia, slurred speech, sweating, hypertension, and/or nystagmus. The abusers report a heightened sense of perceptual awareness, altered time perception, and visual hallucinations • The majority of abuse occurs among teenagers and young adults as dextromethorphan alone, or mixed with other ingredients, such as ephedrine. It has been sold as "ecstasy." It has been identified as a filler in confiscated samples of bogus heroin and bogus ketamine. • Procedures are described on the Internet to extract dextromethorphan from cough syrups, which has led to the availability of powdered forms
Ethanol (various names and alcoholic drinks)	Ingestion	• CNS depressants at high doses can lead to hypotension, hypoglycemia, respiratory depression, and death • Acute intoxication leads to ataxia, sedation, emesis, and slurred speech • Chronic abuse leads to many medical complications such as esophageal varices, hepatic failure with ascites, and malnutrition • Tolerance, dependence, and withdrawal develop with chronic abuse
GHB or gamma hydroxybutyrate (liquid ecstasy, soap, easy lay, Georgia home boy, somatomax, scoop, grievous bodily harm)	Ingestion	• CNS depressant abused for euphoric, sedative, and anabolic (body building) effects • Coma and seizures are likely; increased risk of seizures when combined with methamphetamine • Use with alcohol causes nausea and difficulty breathing • GHB and two of its precursors, gamma butyrolactone (GBL) and 1,4 butanediol (BD) have been involved in poisonings, overdoses, date rapes, and deaths; they are produced by illicit laboratories • May produce withdrawal effects
Heroin (smack, H, skag, junk)	Injection, snorting, or smoking	• Abuse associated with fatal overdose, spontaneous abortion, collapsed veins, and infectious diseases, including HIV/AIDS and hepatitis • Euphoria ("rush") followed by an alternately wakeful and drowsy state ("on the nod") • CNS depression, respiratory depression, miosis (pinpoint pupils), pulmonary edema • Street heroin may have additives • With regular use tolerance develops and withdrawal is possible
Inhalants	Inhaled by sniffing and huffing	• A variety of breathable chemical vapors that produce psychoactive effects • Found in industrial or household solvents or solvent-containing products, including paint thinners or solvents, degreasers, dry-cleaning fluids, gasoline, and glues • Nearly all abused inhalants produce short-term intoxicating and CNS depressant effects similar to anesthetics • Intoxication usually lasts only a few minutes; successive inhalations lead to loss of inhibition and control; continued use can lead to coma • In some cases heart failure and death within minutes of a session of prolonged use, called "sudden sniffing death" is seen
Injected drugs (shooting up, mainlining)	Injection	• The injecting drug user is at risk for transmitting or acquiring HIV/AIDS, hepatitis, bacterial infections, and fungal infections if needles or other injection equipment are shared • Chronic users may develop collapsed veins, infection of the heart lining and valves, skin abscesses, cellulitis, and liver disease • Since some abusers dissolve the tablets in water and inject the mixture, emboli can form from the insoluble materials in the tablets

Table 3

Selected Drugs of Abuse and Addictive Substances (continued)

Substance (slang names)	Methods of abuse	Major or unique health effects
Ketamine (K, special K, cat Valium, vitamin K)	Injected, snorted	• An anesthetic that has been approved for human and veterinary use • Certain doses can cause dream-like states and hallucinations • At high doses, can cause delirium, amnesia, impaired motor function, hypertension, depression, and potentially fatal respiratory depression
LSD, lysergic acid diethylamide (acid, L, blotter, cubes, sugar, dots)	Ingested; often added to absorbent paper, such as blotter paper, and divided into small decorated squares ("blotter acid") or placed on dot-like candy ("dots") or sugar cubes ("cubes," "sugar")	• A hallucinogen sold on the street in tablets, capsules, and liquid form • Effects are unpredictable; physical effects include mydriasis (dilated pupils), elevated temperature, tachycardia, hypertension, sweating, loss of appetite, sleeplessness, dry mouth, and tremors • Sensations and feelings change more dramatically than the physical signs. In sufficient doses, the drug produces delusions and visual hallucinations • Some users experience severe, terrifying thoughts and feelings, fear of losing control, fear of insanity and death, and despair • Fatal accidents have occurred during intoxication • Many users experience flashbacks
Marijuana (pot, herb, weed, grass, widow, ganja, hash, and trademarked varieties of cannabis, such as Bubble Gum, Northern Lights, Juicy Fruit, Afghani #1, and a number of Skunk varieties)	Smoked as a cigarette (joint, nail), in a pipe (bong) or in blunts, (cigars that have been emptied of tobacco and refilled with marijuana, often in combination with another drug); also ingested when mixed in food or brewed as a tea	• Main active chemical in marijuana is THC (delta-9-tetrahydrocannabinol) • Delirium, conjunctivitis, food craving are typical • Short-term effects include problems with memory and learning, distorted perception, difficulty in thinking and problem solving, loss of coordination, and tachycardia • Risk of heart attack more than quadruples in the first hour after smoking marijuana • Same respiratory problems as cigarette smokers (see nicotine); burning and stinging of the mouth and throat, often accompanied by a heavy cough • Drug craving and withdrawal
MDMA, 3-4 methylene-dioxymeth-amphetamine (Ecstasy, Adam, XTC, hug, beans, love drug)	Ingestion; some snort or inject it, or use it in suppository form	• A synthetic, psychoactive drug with both stimulant and hallucinogenic properties • Increases pulse and blood pressure • In high doses it can cause malignant hyperthermia leading to rhabdomyolysis (muscle breakdown with kidney and cardiovascular system failure) • Psychological difficulties: confusion, depression, sleep problems, drug craving, severe anxiety, and paranoia, during and sometimes weeks after use • Physical symptoms: muscle tension, involuntary teeth clenching, nausea, blurred vision, nystagmus, faintness, chills, or sweating • Content of the MDMA pills also varies widely, and may include caffeine, dextromethorphan, heroin, and mescaline. In some areas, the MDMA-like substance paramethoxyamphetamine (PMA) has led to death when mistaken for true MDMA; deaths were due to complications from hyperthermia
Methamphetamine (crank, meth, speed, chalk; the clear chunky crystals resembling ice can be smoked and are referred to as ice, crystal, and glass)	Ingestion, snorting the powder, injection, smoking	• An addictive stimulant chemically related to amphetamine • Produces euphoria, irritability, insomnia, confusion, tremors, convulsions, anxiety, paranoia, and aggressiveness; higher doses lead to hypertension, tachycardia, stroke, arrhythmias, cardiovascular collapse, and death • Hyperthermia and convulsions can result in death • Prolonged use leads to extreme anorexia • Made in illegal laboratories and may contain contaminants and by-products • High potential for abuse and dependence
Nicotine (various names and products)	Smoked as cigarettes and other forms of tobacco, such as cigars, pipe tobacco, and chewing tobacco	• Highly addictive CNS stimulant and sedative; stimulation is followed by depression and fatigue leading the user to seek more nicotine • Women who take oral contraceptives are more prone to cardiovascular and cerebrovascular diseases, especially for women older than 30 • Pregnant women have an increased risk of having stillborn or premature infants or infants with low birthweight

(continued)

Table 3

Selected Drugs of Abuse and Addictive Substances (continued)

Substance (slang names)	Methods of abuse	Major or unique health effects
Nicotine (various names and products) (cont'd)		• Respiratory problems: daily cough and phlegm production, more frequent acute respiratory illness, a heightened risk of lung infections, and a greater tendency toward obstructed airways, cancer of the respiratory tract and lungs • Tar in cigarettes associated with a higher rate of lung cancer, emphysema, and bronchial disorders • Carbon monoxide in the smoke increases the chance of cardiovascular diseases • Nicotine tolerance, dependence, and withdrawal symptoms occur
Opioids	Ingested, injection	• Includes morphine, codeine, oxycodone (Oxycontin®, MS Contin®), propoxyphene (Darvon®), hydrocodone (Vicodin®), hydromorphone (Dilaudid®), and meperidine (Demerol®) • Cause drowsiness, constipation; large single doses cause coma, hypotension, respiratory depression, and in some cases seizures and death • Mixing with alcohol and other CNS depressants increases the risk of coma and death • Chronic use of opioids produces tolerance, physical dependence, and withdrawal symptoms
Phencyclidine (PCP, angel dust, ozone, wack, rocket fuel; killer joints or crystal supergrass when combined with marijuana)	Snorted, smoked, or eaten; for smoking often applied to a leafy material such as mint, parsley, oregano, or marijuana	• An addictive hallucinogen and sedative that often leads to psychological dependence, craving, and compulsive PCP-seeking behavior • Users often become violent or suicidal and are very dangerous to themselves and to others • At low to moderate doses, slight tachypnea, more pronounced tachycardia and hypertension, shallow respirations, and profuse sweating; generalized numbness of the extremities and muscular incoordination also may occur • Psychological effects include distinct changes in body awareness, similar to those associated with alcohol intoxication • At high doses, decreased blood pressure, pulse, and respirations; nausea, vomiting; blurred vision, nystagmus; drooling; ataxia; seizures, coma, and death (though death more often results from accidental injury or suicide during PCP intoxication) • Psychological effects at high doses include illusions, hallucinations, and effects that mimic the full range of symptoms of schizophrenia • Interactions with other CNS depressants, such as alcohol and benzodiazepines, can lead to coma • Illegally manufactured in illicit laboratories
Rohypnol (rophie, roofies, roche, roach, rope, the date rape drug, forget-me)	Ingestion	• Rohypnol, a trade name for flunitrazepam, is a benzodiazepine that is not sold in the U.S.; it is smuggled into the U.S. • Produces sedative-hypnotic effects including muscle relaxation and amnesia; it can also produce physical and psychological dependence • When mixed with alcohol, rohypnol can incapacitate victims and prevent them from resisting sexual assault and can produce anterograde amnesia • May be lethal when mixed with alcohol or other CNS depressants • Abuse of two other similar drugs, clonazepam (Klonopin®) and alprazolam (Xanax®), appears to be replacing rohypnol
Stimulants, amphetamines and related compounds (speed, dexies, uppers)	Ingestion, tablets crushed and snorted	• CNS stimulants increase alertness, attention, and energy accompanied by increases in blood pressure, pulse, and respiration • High doses: arrhythmias, hypertension, hyperthermia, potential for cardiovascular failure, stroke or lethal seizures. Taking high doses of some stimulants repeatedly over a short period of time can lead to hostility or feelings of paranoia in some individuals • Stimulants such as dextroamphetamine (Dexedrine®) and methylphenidate (Ritalin®) when misused can be addictive

Sources: InfoFacts. National Institute on Drug Abuse, National Institutes of Health, Washington, DC.
Available at: http://www.nida.nih.gov/Infofax/Infofaxindex. html Web page accessed April 3, 2003.
Drugs and Chemicals of Concern. Diversion Control Program, Drug Enforcement Administration, U.S. Department of Justice, Washington, DC.
Available at: http://www. deadiversion.usdoj.gov/drugs_concern/index. html. Web page accessed June 18, 2003.

Table 4

Commonly Used Antidotes

Listed below are common antidotes that may need to be used emergently for patients presenting with acute toxic ingestion or dermal or inhalation exposure. Dosages are derived from standard texts and references and are given as convenience references. These should not be considered specific treatment guidelines; consult appropriate resources.

Toxin	Antidote (trade name)	Adult dose	Pediatric dose
Acetaminophen	N-acetylcysteine (Mucomyst®)	Loading dose: 140 mg/kg orally; maintenance doses: 70 mg/kg every 4 hours orally	Loading dose: 140 mg/kg orally; maintenance doses: 70 mg/kg every 4 hours orally
Anticholinergic compounds	Physostigmine salicylate (Antilirium®)	1-2 mg slow IV infusion over 3-5 minutes titrated to effect	0. 02 mg/kg slow IV infusion over 3-5 minutes titrated to effect
Arsenic	Succimer (Chemet®)	10 mg/kg orally 3 times a day	10 mg/kg orally 3 times a day
	Dimercaprol, also called British anti-lewisite [BAL], only if unable to tolerate oral succimer (BAL in Oil®)	3-5 mg/kg intramuscular every 4-6 hours	3-5 mg/kg intramuscular every 4-6 hours
Benzodiazepines	Flumazenil[1] (Romazicon®)	0.2 mg IV bolus titrated to effect or total dose of 3 mg	0.01 mg/kg IV bolus titrated to effect or total dose of 1-3 mg
β-Blocker	Glucagon (GlucaGen®)	5-10 mg IV bolus followed by 5-10 mg/h IV infusion titrated to effect	0. 15 mg/kg mg IV bolus followed by 0.1 mg/h IV infusion titrated to effect
Calcium channel blockers	Calcium chloride 10%	10-20 mL IV bolus, repeat doses and IV infusions are common	0.1-0.2 mL/kg IV bolus, repeat doses and IV infusions are common
	Glucagon (GlucaGen®)	5-10 mg/ IV bolus followed by 5-10 mg/h IV infusion titrated to effect	0.15 mg/ IV bolus followed by 0. 1 mg/h IV infusion titrated to effect
Carbamates	Atroplne	2-4 mg IV bolus, repeat doses titrated to effect	1 mg/kg IV bolus, repeat doses titrated to effect
Cynnide	*Cyanide antidote kit:*		
	Sodium nitrite 3%	300 mg slow IV infusion	0.15-0. 33 mL/kg to maximum of 300 mg slow IV infusion
	Sodium thiosulfate	12.5 g IV infusion	400 mg/kg up to 12. 5 g IV infusion
Digoxin	Digoxin immune antibody fragment (Digibind®, DigiFab®)	Empiric dosing: 10-20 vials IV bolus for life-threatening toxicity; see package insert for other dosing regimens	Empiric dosing: 10-20 vials IV bolus for life-threatening toxicity; see package insert for other dosing regimens
Ethylene glycol, methanol	Ethanol 10%	Loading dose 10 mL/kg IV or orally followed by maintenance dose 1-2 mL/kg/h IV infusion maintenance dose or orally	Loading dose 10 mL/kg IV or orally followed by 1-2 mL/kg/h IV infusion or orally
	Fomepizole, also called 4-methylpyrazole (Antizol®)	15 mg/kg IV bolus, smaller repeat doses may be necessary	15 mg/kg IV bolus, smaller repeat doses may be necessary
Iron	Deferoxamine (Desferal®)	5-15 mg/kg/h IV infusion titrated to effect	5-15 mg/kg/h IV infusion titrated to effect
Isoniazid	Pyridoxine, also called vitamin B6	1 g per gram ingested or empiric dosing 5 g IV bolus	1 g per gram ingested or empiric dosing 75 mg/kg IV bolus up to 5 g
Lead	Succimer (Chemet®)	10 mg/kg orally 3 times a day, repeat doses are common	10 mg/kg orally 3 times a day, repeat doses are common
	Dimercaprol, also called British anti-lewisite [BAL], only for lead encephalopathy (BAL in Oil)	3-5 mg/kg intramuscularly or 50-75 mg/m² intramuscularly	3-5 mg/kg intramuscularly or 50-75 mg/m² intramuscularly
	Calcium disodium EDTA (Calcium Disodium Versenate®)	20-30 mg/kg diluted in 250 mL IV infusion over 12-24 hours (start 4 hours after BAL administration)	20-30 mg/kg diluted in 250 mL IV infusion over 12-24 hours (start 4 hours after BAL administration)

(continued)

Table 4

Commonly Used Antidotes (continued)

Toxin	Antidote (trade name)	Adult dose	Pediatric dose
Methemoglobinemia	Methylene blue	1-2 mg/kg slow IV infusion, repeat doses are common	1-2 mg/kg slow IV infusion, repeat doses are common
Opioids	Naloxone hydrochloride (Narcan®)	0. 4-2 mg IV titrated to effect	0. 4-2 mg IV titrated to effect
Organophosphates	Atropine	2-4 mg IV bolus, repeat doses titrated to effect	0.1 mg/kg IV bolus, repeat doses titrated to effect
	Pralidoxime hydrochloride (Protopam®)	1-2 g slow IV infusion followed by 500 mg/h continuous infusion or 1 g every 4 hours	20-40 mg/kg slow IV infusion followed by 5-10 mg/kg/h continuous infusion or 20 mg/kg every 4 hours
Salicylate	Sodium bicarbonate	150 mEq with 40 mEq KCl in 1 L of D_5W infused to maintain urine output at 1-2 mL/kg/h and a urine pH approximately 7.5	150 mEq with 40 mEq KCl in 1 L of D_5W infused to maintain urine output at 1-2 mL/kg/h and a urine pH approximately 7.5
Tricyclic antidepressants, agents with type 1a antiarrhythmic effects	Sodium bicarbonate	1-2 mEq/kg IV bolus, titrate repeat boluses to QRS duration (do not exceed arterial pH of 7.55)	1-2 mEq/kg IV bolus, titrate boluses to QRS duration (do not exceed arterial pH of 7.55)
Warfarin, superwarfarins	Fresh frozen plasma	Fresh frozen plasma for life-threatening hemorrhage	Fresh frozen plasma for life-threatening hemorrhage
	Vitamin K_1 (Mephyton®, AquaMephyton®)	10-50 mg slow IV infusion, subcutaneous or orally	0.6 mg/kg slow IV infusion, subcutaneous or orally

[1]Potential risks may exceed the benefits due to precipitation of intractable seizures.

Excerpt from: American College of Emergency Physicians: Clinical policy for the initial approach to patients presenting with acute toxic ingestion or dermal or inhalation exposure. *Ann Emerg Med.* 1999;33:735-761.

Specific Antidotes

Acetylcysteine or N-acetylcysteine (Mucomyst 10%, 20%)
Uses
- Treatment of acute acetaminophen overdose

- Unapproved indication: to treat adverse reactions to drugs that may produce free radicals as part of the adverse reaction. The dosage regimen is unique to the application.

Mechanism of action
- It protects the liver from the toxic effects of an acetaminophen metabolite by supplying glutathione to aid in metabolism of reactive metabolite.

- Other mechanisms are also proposed that include providing sulfate for acetaminophen metabolism and minimizing the formation of free radicals.

- It may also be useful to minimize hepatotoxic injury once it has begun and with fulminant hepatic failure.

Indications
- Acute overdoses of acetaminophen produce a reactive metabolite that leads to hepatotoxicity (jaundice, coagulopathy, hypoglycemia, hepatic failure, hepatic encephalopathy, and hepatorenal failure); symptoms become evident 1-2 days after ingestion.

- N-acetylcysteine can prevent or minimize hepatic injury if given early. For best results, administer within 10 hours of ingestion of acetaminophen overdose. It is minimally effective when started 24 hours after ingestion.

- The need for therapy is determined by a serum concentration of acetaminophen obtained at least 4 hours after ingestion (and within 24 hours) and plotting it on the acetaminophen nomogram to determine whether there is a risk for hepatotoxicity.

Contraindications
• Known hypersensitivity to N-acetylcysteine

Adverse effects
• With oral administration, nausea and vomiting are common.

• Infrequently, rashes occur.

• With intravenous administration, anaphylactic reactions have been reported.

Dosage
• Oral administration for 72 hours is the FDA-approved route of administration in the U.S. (Table 4).

• An intravenous preparation is expected to be available by 2004.

Atropine
Indications
• Organophosphate (including chem-bioterrorism nerve agents) and carbamate anticholinesterase insecticide poisoning

• Bradycardia

• Nontoxicologic indications include premedication to anesthesia induction (for antisecretory effects) and ophthalmic mydriatic and cycloplegic.

Mechanism of action
• Anticholinergic agent that competitively inhibits acetylcholine at muscarinic receptors. Atropine has little effect on nicotinic receptors.

Indications for use in the treatment of organophosphate or carbamate poisoning
• For control of pulmonary hypersecretion, atropine is given in repeated doses intravenously until secretions have dried. Atropinization may have to be maintained for hours to days.

• For control of bradycardia, atropine is given until the heart rate increases or until a need for alternatives is indicated.

Contraindications
• None for insecticide poisoning

Contraindications for other indications
• Hypersensitivity to atropine or anticholinergics

• Narrow-angle glaucoma

• Reflux esophagitis

• Obstructive gastrointestinal disease

• Ulcerative colitis or toxic megacolon

• Obstructive uropathy

• Unstable cardiovascular status in acute hemorrhage or thyrotoxicosis

• Paralytic ileus or intestinal atony

• Myasthenia gravis

Adverse effects
• Exaggeration of anticholinergic effects (eg, tachycardia, hypertension, sedation, hallucinations, mydriasis, changes in intraocular pressure, warm red skin, dry mouth, urinary retention, ileus, dysrhythmias, and seizures)

• The use of large doses of atropine should be preservative-free since agents like benzyl alcohol or chlorobutanol can produce their own toxicity.

Dosage
• For bronchorrhea and bronchospasm from organophosphates or carbamates, the adult dose is 2-5 mg (pediatric dose is 0.05 mg/kg) administered slowly by IV. Dose is repeated at 10- to 30-minute intervals until bronchial hypersecretion is resolved. Severe poisonings may require up to 100 mg over a few hours to several grams over several weeks. If atropinization is required for several days, continuous atropine infusion may be used (rates of 0.02-0.08 mg/kg per hour are recommended).

• For symptomatic bradycardia (for mild poisonings) the adult dose is 1 mg (pediatric dose is 0.01 mg/kg) intravenously. For moderate to severe poisonings, adult doses increase to 2-5 mg (pediatric doses are 0.02-0.05 mg/kg) and should be repeated every few minutes until heart rate increases.

Calcium chloride (1 g/10 mL), calcium gluconate (1 g/10 mL)
Uses
• Hypocalcemia secondary to:
  * Hydrofluoric acid exposures (eg, rust removers, automotive wire wheel cleaners)
  * Ethylene glycol poisoning (eg, automobile radiator antifreeze, brake fluid)

• Calcium channel blockers (verapamil [Calan®], diltiazem [Cardizem®], nifedipine [Procardia®])

- Black widow spider envenomation (*Latrodectus mactans*)

- Hypermagnesemia

- Hyperkalemia

Mechanism of action

Hydrofluoric acid
- Calcium administration provides exogenous calcium for binding the fluoride ion and also replaces the calcium that has already been bound by hydrofluoric acid.

Ethylene glycol
- Exogenous calcium administration replenishes depleted calcium ions bound by oxalic acid, one of the four toxic metabolites of ethylene glycol (see ethanol section).

Calcium channel blockers
- Increasing serum calcium may overcome calcium channel blockade to correct cardiovascular toxicity.

Black widow spider venom
- Venom induces muscle spasm; calcium antagonizes calcium-dependent release of acetylcholine at neuromuscular junctions.

Hypermagnesemia
- Calcium will directly antagonize the effects of magnesium on skeletal muscle.

Hyperkalemia
- Calcium will directly antagonize the effects that excessive potassium has on membranes.

Indications

Hydrofluoric acid
Fluoride ions bind calcium and magnesium, thereby producing insoluble salts. The resulting hypocalcemia and hypomagnesemia may lead to local cellular destruction and systemic toxicity. Calcium is recommended for any symptomatic skin exposure to hydrogen fluoride. Mild dermal burns from <20% concentrations may be treated with topical calcium gluconate gel. Higher concentrations resulting in more severe burns may require local infiltration or intra-arterial infusion of calcium. Intravenous calcium is recommended for signs and symptoms of hypocalcemia, such as prolongation of the QTc interval on the ECG.

Hypocalcemia
Calcium is used to treat hypocalcemia caused by significant exposures to other poisons (eg, ethylene gly-

col), especially if the patient has symptoms of arrhythmia, QTc prolongation, muscle twitching, or tetany.

Calcium channel blockade
Calcium may be used to reverse the hypotension, bradycardia, heart block, and cardiac conduction defects of calcium channel blocker overdose. It is most effective in treating mild toxicity associated with small overdoses. Calcium chloride is usually the calcium salt of choice, as it contains more elemental calcium per gram (272 mg) than calcium gluconate (90 mg).

Black widow envenomation
- Calcium has been used as therapy, but it has limited efficacy in relieving the symptoms of envenomation (muscle spasm, muscle cramps, and muscle pain).

- Calcium may be used along with pain medications and muscle relaxers. Antivenin is reserved for severe envenomations characterized by extreme hypertension and respiratory distress.

Contraindications
- In cases of digoxin overdose, calcium may cause cardiac tetany.

- Hypercalcemia

- Subcutaneous calcium chloride is an irritant and may produce skin necrosis.

Adverse effects
- Hypercalcemia characterized by muscle weakness, lethargy, coma, and arrhythmias

- Hypotension, bradycardia, arrhythmias, and syncope due to rapid administration

- Tissue irritation and extravasation during parenteral administration

Dosage

Hydrofluoric acid
- *Topical:*
  * 2.5-33% calcium gluconate gel massaged into the affected area until pain subsides for 1 minute, and continue application as necessary. Replace every 4 hours and repeat up to two times if needed.

- *Intradermal, subcutaneous:*
  * 5-10% calcium gluconate 0.5 mL/cm^2 every 1-2 hours as needed for pain

- *Intra-arterial:*
  - * Using a proximal artery (brachial or radial), infuse 10-20 mL of calcium gluconate in 40 mL normal saline or D_5W over 4 hours

Hypocalcemia
- Calcium gluconate 10% intravenous (over 5 minutes)
  - * Adults: 10-20 mL or 1-2 g
  - * Pediatric: 0.2-0.3 mL/kg up to 1 g

- Calcium chloride 10% intravenous (over 5 minutes)
  - * Adults: 10%, 5-10 mL or 500-1000 mg
  - * Pediatric: 0.1-0.2 mL/kg or up to 1 g

Calcium channel blocker
- Calcium chloride intravenous (over 5 minutes)
  - * Adult: 1 g every 10-20 minutes for up to 3-4 more doses or by continuous infusion 0.2-0.4 mL/kg per hour
  - * Pediatric: 10-25 mg/kg up to 1 g per dose

- Calcium gluconate intravenous
  - * Adult: 3 g every 10-20 minutes for up to 3-4 more doses
  - * Pediatric: 30-75 mg/kg up to 1 g per dose

Black widow spider envenomation
- *Calcium gluconate:*
  - * Adults: 10 mL of 10% solution intravenously over 10-20 minutes; may repeat every 3-4 hours
  - * Pediatric: 50 mg/kg per dose intravenously, up to 500 mg/kg per 24 hours

Hypermagnesemia
- Adults: 1 g of calcium gluconate 10% over 5 minutes intravenously

- Pediatric: 20 mg/kg of calcium gluconate up to 1 gram per dose

Hyperkalemia
- Adults: 1 g calcium chloride 10% over 5 minutes intravenously
- Pediatric: 0. 5-1 mg/kg up to 1 g of calcium chloride

Calcium disodium EDTA or calcium disodium edathamil (Calcium Disodium Versenate)
Uses
- Acute and chronic lead poisoning in pediatric and adult patients

- Lead encephalopathy in pediatric and adult patients

- With blood lead concentration >70 µg/dL or clinical symptoms consistent with lead encephalopathy, use in conjunction with dimercaprol.

Mechanism of action
- It acts as a chelating agent whereby calcium is displaced by lead and forms a stable compound with EDTA that is excreted in the urine.

Indications
- Lead exposure is possible from various sources, such as lead plumbing, lead-containing paints, folk remedies, and occupational exposures.

- Clinical severity of toxicity is associated with the lead concentration in the blood: >40 µg/dL, mild; >80 µg/dL, moderate; >100-150 µg/dL, severe.

- Chelating therapy is not indicated for lead concentrations <25 µg/dL in children and is usually not indicated in asymptomatic adults with lead concentrations <70 µg/dL. The source of exposure should be removed.

- Lead can cause nephropathy, encephalopathy, decreased hemoglobin synthesis, as well as impaired learning, cognition, hearing, and bone growth. Lead is stored in the bones and soft tissue. Lead has affinity for biological electron-donor ligands. It is chemically similar to calcium and therefore interferes with various metabolic pathways and exhibits mutagenic effects in cells.

- Calcium EDTA decreases blood lead concentrations and reverses lead-induced hematologic effects. If blood concentrations rebound to pretreatment concentration or to >50 µg/dL, a repeat course should be considered.

- Concomitant administration of dimercaprol and calcium EDTA increases the rate of lead excretion and reduces mortality.

- When initial therapy includes calcium EDTA and dimercaprol, repeated therapy is usually without dimercaprol (ie, if blood lead concentrations rebound to 45 µg/dL or higher within 5-7 days of the initial course of therapy based on CDC recommendations). Calcium EDTA is generally preferred to dimercaprol for the management of most moderate lead poisonings.

- Administration with dimercaprol should be continued in patients with lead encephalopathy until the patient is clinically stable.

- In patients receiving dimercaprol and calcium EDTA therapy, the American Academy of Pediatrics recommends a minimum of 2 days without treatment before a second course of therapy with dimercaprol and calcium EDTA or calcium EDTA alone is used in patients with severe lead poisoning.

Contraindications
- Anuria

- Hepatitis

Adverse effects
- Mild transient elevations in AST and ALT

- Cardiac rhythm irregularities, inverted T wave

- Acute renal tubular necrosis

- Depletion of endogenous metals including zinc, copper, manganese, and iron

Dosage
- Administration by IV or IM (Table 4)

Crotalidae immune Fab [ovine] (CroFab®) 1 g/1 mL
Uses
- Crotalidae immune Fab is indicated for the treatment of significant (moderate to severe) envenomation by North American *Crotalidae* snake species.

Mechanism of action
The antivenin consists of concentrated lyophilized dried powder of venom-specific ovine Fab (monovalent) serum immunoglobulin fragments (IgG). Upon administration, the antivenin binds to neutralize circulating venom toxins to prevent progression of local tissue injury (characterized by edema, ecchymosis, skin discoloration, vesicles, hemorrhagic blebs, petechiae, and necrosis), and systemic toxicities (characterized by syncope, nausea, vomiting, perioral tingling or numbness, muscle fasciculations, hypotension, weakness, diaphoresis, and coagulopathy).

Indications
- Antivenin is used in the treatment of moderate to severe envenomation from the following crotalids: rattlesnakes, cottonmouth snakes, and copperhead snakes (found in the U.S.). Response to antivenin is best if used within the first 6 hours.

- Due to the low incidence of morbidity and mortality after copperhead and cottonmouth envenomation, antivenin administration is rarely required.

- After cleaning the wound, conducting laboratory tests (eg, CBC, platelets, coagulation profile, INR/PT, PTT, fibrinogen, fibrin split products, urinalysis, BUN, serum creatinine, and creatinine kinase), administering IV fluids, tetanus toxoid, pain medications, and antibiotics (if there is evidence of infection), the envenomation is graded as follows:
  - *Trivial:* no edema around the bite area, no systemic symptoms or laboratory changes
  - *Minimal:* slight or minimal edema confined to the area around the bite, no systemic symptoms, and no laboratory changes
  - *Moderate:* edema progressed beyond the immediate bite site; mild systemic symptoms (eg, muscular fasciculations, perioral numbness), and laboratory changes (eg, moderate decrease in platelets and fibrinogen or slight increase in INR) are evident
  - *Severe:* rapid progression of edema involving the wounded part or the entire extremity, serious systemic symptoms (eg, mental status changes), and severe lab changes or hemorrhage

- Antivenin is administered until coagulopathies begin to resolve and edema progression has stopped.

Contraindications
- Relative contraindication (unless the benefits outweigh the risks): hypersensitivity to papaya, papain, or bromelain (pineapple enzyme)

Adverse effects
- Hypersensitivity reaction (anaphylaxis is possible)

- Urticaria and rash

- Serum sickness with onset 5-24 days after use (malaise, fever, urticaria, lymphadenopathy, arthralgia)

- Contains ethyl mercury (from thimerosal) and at high doses, the same toxicity risks as those of methyl mercury (neurologic and renal toxicities) may apply.

Dosage
No skin testing is required prior to administration. Each reconstituted vial of Crotalidae immune Fab (CroFab) should be diluted in 250 mL of normal saline and administered intravenously over 60 minutes. The first minute of the infusion should be at 25-50 mL/h to monitor for allergic reactions. The initial dose should be 4-6 vials. An additional 4-6 vials should be repeated until laboratory abnormalities began to resolve, edema progression has halted, and other envenomation symptoms are under control. After control has been estab-

lished, an additional 2-vial dose every 6 hours for up to 18 hours is recommended. Additional 2-vial doses may be administered as necessary based on the patient's clinical course.

Crotalidae polyvalent antivenin
(Antivenin Crotalidae Polyvalent, 1 mL/vial)
Uses
Antivenin Crotalidae polyvalent is indicated for the treatment of significant (moderate to severe) envenomation by North American crotalid snake species.

Mechanism of action
The antivenin consists of concentrated lyophilized dried powder of equine serum immunoglobulins. Upon administration, the antivenin binds to neutralize circulating and tissue-fixed venom to prevent progression of local tissue injury (edema, ecchymosis, skin discoloration, vesicles, hemorrhagic blebs, petechiae, and necrosis), and systemic toxicities (syncope, nausea, vomiting, perioral tingling or numbness, muscle fasciculations, hypotension, weakness, diaphoresis, or coagulopathy).

Indications
• Antivenin is used in the treatment of moderate to severe envenomations from the following crotalids: rattlesnakes, cottonmouths, and copperheads, which are found in the U.S. Response to antivenin is best if used within the first 8-24 hours. It can be used up to 30 hours after envenomation if coagulopathies occur.

• Due to the decreased incidence of morbidity and mortality after copperhead and cottonmouth envenomation, antivenin administration is rarely required.

• After initial treatment, (ie, cleaning the wound, intravenous fluids, tetanus toxoid, pain medications, and antibiotics if evidence of infection), and lab tests (ie, CBC, platelets, coagulation profile, INR/PT, PTT, fibrinogen, fibrin split products, urinalysis, BUN, serum creatinine, and creatinine kinase) the envenomation is graded as described under Crotalidae immune Fab.

• Antivenin is administered until coagulopathies are resolving and edema progression has stopped.

• The manufacturer has indicated that it may discontinue production of this product.

Contraindications
• In persons with hypersensitivity to antivenin or horse serum, a relative contraindication is possible; use if benefits outweigh the risks.

Adverse effects
• Hypersensitivity reaction (anaphylaxis is possible)

• Mild flushing and wheezing

• Serum sickness with onset 5-24 days after use (malaise, fever, urticaria, lymphadenopathy, arthralgia)

Dosage
• A skin test should be performed first to determine if patient is hypersensitive, with 0.02-0.03 mL of a 1:10 dilution in normal saline administered intradermally (1:100 dilution if history of possible sensitivity). If no reaction in 5-30 minutes, the therapeutic dose may be administered.

• Continue the antivenin administration as an infusion. Dilute each vial (1:1 or 1:10) in 25-100 mL of normal saline or D_5W and give as an intravenous infusion. The first 5-10 mL should be infused over a 3- to 5-minute period, and the rest is given over 1 hour. For minimal envenomation administer 20-40 mL (2-4 vials), for moderate envenomation 50-90 mL (5-9 vials), and for severe envenomation 100-150 mL (10-15 vials).

• If edema continues to progress or systemic symptoms increase in severity, administer an additional 10-50 mL (1-5 vials).

Cyanide antidote kit
Contents: amyl nitrite—12 ampules for inhalation; sodium nitrite 3%—300 mg/10 mL injection, 2 ampules; and sodium thiosulfate 25%—12.5 g/50 mL injection, 2 ampules

Uses
• Cyanide poisoning sources: metallurgy, photographic chemicals, seeds and parts of various fruits and vegetables, nitroprusside, acetonitrile (found in some sculptured acrylic nail removers), and smoke from the combustion of nitrogen-containing materials

• Hydrogen sulfide poisoning sources: sewer gas, hot asphalt fumes (treated with the nitrites only)

Mechanism of action
Cyanide binds ferric ion (Fe^{+3}) found in cytochrome oxidase, producing a cyanide-cytochrome oxidase complex. The binding inactivates cytochrome oxidase, preventing cellular respiration and production of adenosine triphosphate (ATP), resulting in rapid anoxic tissue damage.

- Nitrites: nitrites oxidize the ferrous ions (Fe^{+2}) of hemoglobin, forming methemoglobin. The ferric ion (Fe^{+3}) of methemoglobin competes with the ferric ion of cytochrome oxidase (a3) for binding to cyanide. A reversible cyanomethemoglobin complex is formed, freeing cytochrome oxidase to function in the electron transport system to carry on cellular respiration. Nitrites may also produce vasodilatation that will enhance blood flow to the liver and other organs. The increase in blood flow may increase cyanide detoxification.

- Sodium thiosulfate donates sulfur for the enzyme rhodanese, a sulfurtransferase that removes cyanide from the methemoglobin to convert the cyanide to low-toxicity thiocyanate. The thiocyanate is then excreted renally.

- For hydrogen sulfide, nitrites convert hemoglobin to methemoglobin. Methemoglobin competes with cytochrome oxidase for binding with hydrogen sulfide, producing sulfmethemoglobin thereby sparing cytochrome oxidase and cellular respiration.

Indications

- For cyanide, the antidotes should be used only in significantly symptomatic patients (ie, altered mental status, seizures, hypotension, hyperkalemia, acidosis, tachypnea, or abolition of differences between arterial and venous oxygen saturation on arterial blood gases). Amyl nitrite is a temporizing agent used only until venous access is obtained for the sodium nitrite. If intravenous access is already obtained, it may be omitted. Response is usually seen in 30 minutes. Monitor methemoglobin concentrations, arterial blood gases (pH), and symptoms. If no response and methemoglobin is <10%, a full dose of sodium nitrite and sodium thiosulfate may be repeated. If methemoglobin is >10%, repeat sodium nitrite at half of a dose.

- For hydrogen sulfide, administer only the amyl and sodium nitrite components to symptomatic patients with significant hydrogen sulfide exposures (ie, hypoxia, altered mental status, dyspnea, or metabolic acidosis).

- Sodium thiosulfate alone has been used prophylactically during prolonged sodium nitroprusside infusions to prevent cyanide toxicity.

Contraindications

- Significant pre-existing methemoglobinemia

- Severe hypotension is a relative contraindication.

- Patients with concurrent carbon monoxide poisoning: methemoglobinemia in addition to elevated carboxyhemoglobin would further decrease the oxygen-carrying capacity of hemoglobin.

- Hypersensitivity to a component of the cyanide antidote kit

Adverse effects
Nitrites
- Hypotension, especially with rapid administration

- Flushing

- Dizziness

- Tachycardia

- Diaphoresis

Sodium thiosulfate
- Nausea

- Vomiting

- Local irritation

- Localized muscle cramps

Dosage
- Amyl nitrite: if no intravenous access exists, crush 1 ampule in gauze or cloth, place under the nose, and inhale for 30 seconds of each minute. Coordinate with oxygen administration.

- Sodium nitrite
  * Adult—300 mg (10 mL of 3% solution) IV over no less than 5 minutes. May mix with 50-100 mL of normal saline and infuse IVPB over 15-20 minutes.
  * Pediatric (normal hemoglobin)—0.15-0.33 mL/kg up to 10 mL. For anemic patients, dose according to hemoglobin and the manufacturer's dosage chart.

- Sodium thiosulfate
  * Adult—12.5 g (50 mL of 25% solution)
  * Pediatric—1.65 mL/kg up to 50 mL

- Cyanide in association with nitroprusside: prepare by adding 10 mg of thiosulfate for every 1 mg of nitroprusside to the infusion.

Deferoxamine 500 mg/ampule (Desferal)
Uses
- Treatment of acute iron poisoning

- Typically used when serious symptoms are present (gross GI bleeding, shock, acidosis, coma) or when serum iron concentration exceeds 500 µg/dL

- In non-poisoning situations, deferoxamine is also used to treat states of chronic iron overload such as after repeated blood transfusions and hemochromatosis.

Mechanism of action
- Deferoxamine chelates circulating iron and transferrin-bound iron to form a water soluble, renally excreted complex.

- Chelation effectiveness can often be assessed by the presence of orange-red urine, which is due to the deferoxamine-iron complex.

Indications
- Acute ingestion of large doses of iron can cause life-threatening symptoms within hours of ingestion.

- Symptoms of serious iron poisoning include vomiting, diarrhea, gross gastrointestinal bleeding, shock, acidosis, coma, and hepatotoxicity.

- Therapy with deferoxamine is a means of eliminating excess iron that otherwise is only eliminated by bleeding or sloughing of epithelial cells (about 1 mg/d).

Contraindications
- Hypersensitivity to deferoxamine

- Use cautiously with renal failure.

Adverse effects
- Hypotension with rapid infusion in excess of 15 mg/kg per hour

- Intramuscular injections can produce sterile abscesses and pain at the injection site. Therapy at high doses for more than 2-3 days has been associated with the development of acute respiratory distress syndrome.

Dosage
- Administered by controlled intravenous infusion (Table 4)

- For poisonings, IM injection is not warranted due to slow absorption from the injection site in patients who may have hypoperfusion.

Digoxin immune Fab (Digibind, DigiFab)
Uses
- Treatment of life-threatening acute or chronic digoxin poisoning

- Some cross-reactivity with digitoxin and other digoxin-like compounds (digitalis, foxglove, lily of the valley, bufodienolide from cane frogs)

Mechanism of action
- Digoxin immune Fab binds digoxin in plasma, promotes redistribution from tissues and enhances elimination in the urine. The digoxin bound to digoxin immune Fab is inactive. Each 40 mg (1 vial) binds 0.6 mg of digoxin.

- Digoxin immune Fab is a monovalent, digoxin-specific, antigen-binding fragment (Fab) that is produced in healthy sheep.

Indications
- Chronic digoxin toxicity typically begins with nausea, vomiting, diarrhea, fatigue, confusion, blurred vision, diplopia, and seeing white borders or halos around dark objects. Deterioration of renal function, hypokalemia, or drug interactions often lead to toxicity.

- Acute digoxin poisoning has early symptoms similar to those of chronic poisoning, but the onset is more abrupt, nausea and vomiting are common, and the serum potassium concentration is typically normal or elevated.

- A wide variety of arrhythmias occur with acute or chronic digoxin poisoning.

- Digoxin immune Fab is reserved for life-threatening symptoms such as bradycardia, second-degree and third-degree heart block unresponsive to atropine, ventricular arrhythmias, and hyperkalemia (typically in excess of 5 mEq/L).

Contraindications
- Hypersensitivity to sheep

Adverse effects
- Common adverse effects include hypokalemia, allergic reactions (1%), and hypotension.

- For patients on maintenance digoxin therapy, the abrupt binding of digoxin will lead to loss of therapeutic effect and a prompt decrease in potassium concentrations.

Dosage

- Administered by intravenous infusion or rapid intravenous bolus (Table 4).

- Dosage is determined by one of several approaches, depending upon available information, as follows: empiric dosage of 10-20 vials (Table 4), dosing based on the dose of digoxin ingested, or dosing based on the serum digoxin concentration.

Dimercaprol or British anti-lewisite (BAL in Oil)

Uses

- Adjunct therapy with calcium EDTA in patients with lead encephalopathy and/or blood lead concentration >70 μg/dL

- Chelator for heavy metals including arsenic, gold, lead, and mercury

Mechanism of action

- Dithiol-chelating agent whereby the sulfhydryl groups form a ring complex with heavy metals and allow urinary excretion of heavy metals

Indications

Lead

- See discussion of lead poisoning under calcium disodium EDTA.

- Dimercaprol does not usually produce trace metal depletion syndromes. It decreases blood lead concentrations, but monitor for rebound.

Arsenic

- Arsenic exposure can occur from insecticides, rodenticides, wood preservatives, and occupational hazards. Arsenic toxicity can produce vomiting, diarrhea, alopecia, anemia, acute tubular necrosis, respiratory failure, Aldrich-Mees lines (transverse white bands on nails), encephalopathy, and peripheral neuropathy.

- Dimercaprol is the antidote of choice for acute arsenic poisoning, but it may not prevent arsenic-induced peripheral neuropathy.

- Chelation is indicated in the symptomatic patient. For the asymptomatic patient, treatment is recommended at 200 μg/L urine arsenic and above. Repeat chelation until the 24-hour urine arsenic concentration is <50 μg/L in severe poisonings.

Contraindications

- Allergy to peanuts or dimercaprol. The preparation contains peanut oil.

- Acute renal insufficiency

- Hepatic dysfunction, except for arsenic-induced jaundice

- Do not administer for iron, cadmium, or selenium metal poisonings. For these metals, the BAL-metal complex is potentially more toxic than the metal alone.

- Do not administer oral iron supplement; may produce a potent emetic.

- Use with caution in glucose-6-phosphate dehydrogenase–deficient patients due to risk of hemolysis.

Adverse effects

- Hypertension and tachycardia

- Interferes with normal accumulation of iodine by the thyroid

- Nephrotoxicity

- Fever

Dosage

- Deep intramuscular injection (Table 4)

Ethanol (ethyl alcohol) 5-10% in 1 L solution in D$_5$W for injection; vials of 95% ethanol

Uses

- Methanol poisoning (eg, automobile windshield washing solution, gas line antifreeze)

- Ethylene glycol poisoning (eg, automobile radiator antifreeze, brake fluid)

Mechanism of action

Methanol and ethylene glycol toxicities are due to their metabolism to toxic metabolites. Methanol is metabolized to formaldehyde and formic acid. Ethylene glycol is metabolized to glycolaldehyde, glycolic acid, glyoxylic acid, and oxalic acid. By preventing the development of toxic metabolites, the toxic effects of methanol (delayed metabolic acidosis and blindness) and ethylene glycol (delayed metabolic acidosis and renal failure) are prevented. Ethanol acts as a competitive substrate of the hepatic enzyme alcohol dehydrogenase (ADH) that metabolizes methanol and ethylene glycol. Due to ethanol's affinity for the enzyme at serum ethanol concentrations of 100 mg/dL, ethanol saturation prevents hepatic metabolism of methanol and ethylene glycol to its toxic metabolites, allowing elimination by the kidneys or hemodialysis.

Indications
- A history of ingestion of significant amounts of methanol– or ethylene glycol–containing products, particularly when blood concentrations for methanol or ethylene glycol are not available. Due to the high concentrations of these products in many automotive products, ingestion of small amounts (eg, 5 mL) may produce toxicity.

- Symptomatic patients (anion gap, pH <7. 3, lethargic, osmolar gap >10 mOsm/L, serum bicarbonate <20 mEq/L, oxalate crystals in the urine, or changes in vision)

- Fomepizole, another inhibitor of ADH, is unavailable.

- The patient is allergic to fomepizole.

- Patients with serum methanol or ethylene glycol concentrations of 20 mg/dL or greater

- Continue treatment until methanol or ethylene glycol concentrations are <10 mg/dL, and acidosis, clinical symptoms, electrolyte abnormalities, and osmolar gap have resolved. For ethylene glycol and methanol poisonings, if ethanol therapy is given without concurrent hemodialysis treatment, give ethanol for at least 3 and 9 days, respectively.

Contraindications
- Concurrent administration of drugs that may produce a disulfiram-type reaction (eg, metronidazole, disulfiram)

Adverse effects
- Phlebitis with intravenous use

- Central nervous system depression; inebriation with secondary respiratory depression

- Hypoglycemia

- Nausea, vomiting, gastric irritation with oral administration

- Hypotension

- Hyponatremia with intravenous administration due to no sodium and free water content

- Hepatitis

- Pancreatitis

Dosages
- Maintain serum ethanol concentration of 100 mg/dL (adult and pediatric target concentrations are the same; see Table 4). Patients with chronic alcoholism or receiving concurrent hemodialysis may require higher doses. Doses should be adjusted if ethanol is a co-ingestant.

Flumazenil (Romazicon)
Uses
- Benzodiazepine overdose

- Reversal of conscious sedation and general anesthesia from benzodiazepines

Mechanism of action
- Flumazenil is a competitive antagonist of the benzodiazepine receptor in the central nervous system.

Indications
- Flumazenil should be used adjunctively with supportive care. Sedation can reoccur following ingestion of a benzodiazepine with a long half-life, requiring additional doses of flumazenil. In a suicidal overdose, it is rarely used due to the risk of potential co-ingestants. If no response occurs to a 5-mg cumulative dose, it is doubtful if the sedation is related to a benzodiazepine.

Contraindications
- Known hypersensitivity to flumazenil

- Co-ingestion of tricyclic antidepressants may precipitate ventricular dysrhythmias or seizures.

- Other mixed overdoses that can decrease the seizure threshold (ie, haloperidol, bupropion, lithium)

- Abrupt withdrawal in patients on maintenance therapy, such as for treatment of epilepsy, can precipitate seizures.

- Patients with increased intracranial pressure, because the antidote may potentially alter cerebral blood flow

- It can produce withdrawal in the physically dependent patient.

Adverse effects
- Flumazenil has a wide margin of safety when not contraindicated.

- Side effects include agitation, sweating, headache, abnormal vision, dizziness, and pain at administration site.

- Rarely reported: bradycardia, tachycardia, hypotension, or hypertension

Dosage
- IV administration (see Table 4)

Glucagon (GlucaGen and other manufacturers, 1 mg/mL [1 unit] or 10 mg/10 mL [10 units])
Uses
- β-Blocker overdose

- Calcium channel blocker overdose

- Hypoglycemia

- Other: lower esophageal impaction, premedication for gastrointestinal endoscopy or radiographic procedures

Mechanism of action
- Glucagon is a polypeptide produced by the α cells of the pancreas. Stimulation of glycogen receptors increases cyclic adenosine monophosphate (c-AMP) synthesis by increasing adenyl cyclase activity and formation. Increased c-AMP levels produces glycogenolysis, gluconeogenesis, and increased inotropic and chronotropic cardiac effects due to increased intracellular calcium. Glycogen also relaxes the smooth muscles of the lower esophageal sphincter and other areas of the gastrointestinal tract.

Indications
β-Blocker overdose
- For the treatment of hypotension and bradycardia secondary to β-blockade, glucagon will increase the inotropic and chronotropic effects regardless of the degree of β-blockade, without increasing cardiac irritability. Glucagon's reversal of hypotension due to β-blocker or calcium channel blockade is usually used in combination with other interventions, including intravenous fluids, vasopressors, insulin with or without dextrose, hyperinsulinemia/euglycemia, atropine, and intravenous calcium (for calcium channel blockers).

Calcium channel overdose
- Same indications for use as β-blocker overdose

Hypoglycemia
- Glycogenolysis results in increased serum blood glucose. Glucagon requires adequate glycogen stores to be effective. The onset of action is also delayed 5-20 minutes; therefore it is not used as the initial treatment for severe hypoglycemia.

Esophageal impactions
- Glucagon decreases lower esophageal sphincter pressure; therefore it may be useful for lower esophageal impactions.

Contraindications
- Pheochromocytoma: increases the release of catecholamines

- Insulinoma: produces paradoxical insulin release, resulting in hypoglycemia

- Hypersensitivity to glucagon

Adverse effects
- Nausea

- Vomiting

- Hyperglycemia

- Phenol toxicity: occurs with the use of older formulations; reformulated in 1998 without phenol

- Hypokalemia: intracellular shift of both glucose and potassium, resulting in decreased serum potassium

- Gastric hypotonicity

Dosage
- Intravenous administration (see Table 4 for dosing for β-blocker and calcium channel poisoning)

- Hypoglycemia:
  * Adults: 0.5-1 mg IV
  * Pediatric: patients weighing <20 kg, use 0.5 mg over 10 minutes

- Esophageal impaction:
  * Adults 1-2 mg IV over 1-2 minutes

Methylene blue
Uses
- Treatment of acquired methemoglobinemia caused by drugs and chemicals

- Typically used when signs and symptoms of hypoxia are present

- Methemoglobin in excess of 20-30%

Mechanism of action
- Reverses the oxidant stress placed on hemoglobin,

thereby returning it to its normal state by several mechanisms (normal methemoglobin is 1-2%)

- Reversible oxidation-reduction changes methemo-globin, which has iron in its ferric state (Fe^{+++}), to the ferrous state (Fe^{++}) of normal hemoglobin

- Acts as a cofactor to NADPH methemoglobin reductase to aid reduction of cellular oxidant stress

Indications
- Exposure to large amounts of certain chemicals (nitrites, nitrates in food and well water) and drugs (benzocaine, lidocaine, chloroquine, sulfonamides, phenazopyridine) that can produce oxidant stress on hemoglobin to cause methemoglobinemia

- Methemoglobin is unable to carry and deliver oxygen to cells, so a state of hypoxia occurs.

Contraindications
- Use cautiously with renal failure

- Use cautiously, if at all, in patients with glucose-6-phosphate dehydrogenase deficiency

Adverse effects
- Common adverse effects include nausea, vomiting, headache, and dizziness.

- Extravasation may lead to skin discoloration and local necrosis.

- At high concentrations it acts as an oxidant and can exacerbate methemoglobinemia. Generally, doses do not exceed 7 mg/kg total.

Dosage
- Administered by intravenous infusion (see Table 4)

- Doses are repeated in 1 hour if hypoxia persists.

Naloxone (Narcan)
Uses
- Reversal of opioid anesthesia

- Respiratory or central nervous system depression related to opioid toxicity

- Empiric administration in patients with altered mental status due to unknown etiology

Mechanism of action
- Naloxone is an opioid antagonist. Naloxone competes at three CNS opioid receptors (mu, kappa, and delta) and leads to reversal of the depressive opioid effects.

Indications
- Opioids cause sedation, respiratory depression, hypotension, miosis, and analgesia. Because it has no agonist activity, naloxone will not worsen respiratory depression. The goal of therapy is to restore adequate spontaneous respirations. When administered, a patient should be monitored for respiratory rate changes and for opiate withdrawal symptoms (anxiety, hypertension, tachycardia, diarrhea, and seizure). To avoid withdrawal, use the lowest possible dose that maintains proper ventilation. Patient should be observed for respiratory depression once naloxone therapy is discontinued because the half-life of naloxone may be shorter than the opioid. If a patient is not responsive to 10 mg of naloxone, it is doubtful that an opioid is causing the respiratory depression.

Contraindications
- Known hypersensitivity

- Use with caution in the physically dependent opioid patient.

- Use with caution in patients with preexisting cardiovascular disease or those receiving cardiotoxic drugs.

Adverse effects
- Use in an opiate-dependent patient can precipitate withdrawal.

- Withdrawal convulsions in a neonate can be life threatening.

- Hypertension and dysrhythmias occur more often with opioid reversal in postoperative patients with underlying cardiac and pulmonary complications.

Dosage
- The IV route is preferred in the emergency situation due to rapid onset of action within 1-2 minutes (see Table 4).

- Naloxone has poor oral bioavailability.

- Intramuscular and subcutaneous routes have erratic absorption.

Physostigmine (Antilirium and various manufacturers) 1 mg/mL; 1- or 2-mL vials
Uses
- Severe anticholinergic syndrome: delirium, hyperthermia, seizures, hallucinations, myoclonus, tachycardia with cardiovascular collapse

Mechanism of action
- Physostigmine, a tertiary amine carbamate, is a reversible inhibitor of acetylcholinesterase in both the peripheral and central nervous systems. By inhibiting acetylcholinesterase, there is an accumulation of acetylcholine to antagonize anticholinergic drug or toxin effects.

Indications
- Physostigmine is indicated for the following symptoms due to anticholinergic toxicity not responding to normal supportive measures:
  * Seizures
  * Coma with hypoventilation
  * Hypotension
  * Dysrhythmias

Contraindications
- Concurrent use of depolarizing neuromuscular blockers (eg, succinylcholine)

- Asthma

- Peripheral vascular disease

- Intestinal or urinary tract obstruction

- Atrioventricular block

- Conduction defects

- Patients with tricyclic antidepressant or suspected tricyclic antidepressant overdose with QRS widening on ECG

- Sulfite hypersensitivity

Adverse effects
- Bradycardia, asystole from rapid drug administration

- Seizures

- Nausea and vomiting

- Diarrhea

- Bronchorrhea and bronchospasm

- Muscle weakness

- Muscle fasciculations

- Tachydysrhythmias

Dosage
- Adult: 0.5-2 mg diluted in 10 mL D_5W or normal saline and administered via slow IV push over no less than 5 minutes. May repeat every 15-30 minutes

- Pediatric: 0.02 mg/kg up to 0.5 mg IV over 5 minutes

Phytonadione or vitamin K_1 (AquaMephyton)
Uses
- Anticoagulation induced by depletion of vitamin K_1 clotting factors due to warfarin or anticoagulant rodenticides

- Elevated prothrombin time or international normalized ratio; not to be used empirically

- Patients with vitamin K deficiency

Mechanism of action
- Vitamin K_1 is a fat-soluble vitamin used as a cofactor in the formation of coagulation factors II, VII, IX, and X.

Indications
- Warfarin and anticoagulant rodenticides are vitamin K reductase inhibitors that deplete vitamin K–dependent clotting factors. Phytonadione administration promotes hepatic synthesis of clotting factors. The objective is to decrease the INR to the goal range and assist with stopping the bleed. Fresh plasma administration may be indicated if bleeding is severe.

Contraindications
- Hypersensitivity to vitamin K_1 preparations

Adverse effects
- Administration can reverse the anticoagulation therapeutic effects of warfarin.

- Intravenous administration has been associated with anaphylactoid reactions.

- The IM administration route may cause hematomas and dermatologic lesions.

Dosage
- For INR of >5 and <9 with no evidence of significant bleed, hold warfarin or give 1-2.5 mg of oral therapy vitamin K_1, and monitor INR.

- For INR >9 with no evidence of significant bleed, administer vitamin K_1 3-5 mg orally, monitor INR, and hold warfarin dose. Resume warfarin at a lower dose when INR is in therapeutic range.

- If INR is >20 with a serious bleed, administer 10 mg IV vitamin K_1 supplemented with fresh plasma or prothrombin complex concentrate, monitor INR, and hold warfarin dose. Vitamin K_1 can be repeated if necessary.

- For life-threatening hemorrhage, administer 10 mg IV vitamin K_1 and prothrombin complex concentrate, monitor INR, and hold warfarin dose. Vitamin K_1 can be repeated if necessary.

- IM administration should be avoided.

Pralidoxime or 2-PAM (Protopam)
Uses
- Severe organophosphate anticholinesterase insecticide or chem-bioterrorism nerve agent poisoning

Mechanism of action
- Pralidoxime dephosphorylates acetylcholinesterase and regenerates acetylcholinesterase activity.

Indications
- Severe organophosphate or nerve agent poisoning, in combination with atropine to resolve nicotinic (muscle and diaphragmatic weakness, fasciculations, muscle cramps) and central (coma, seizures) cholinergic manifestations. It is ineffective for organophosphates without anticholinesterase activity.

- Carbamate poisoning. Use is controversial but recommended by some sources for severe cases.

Contraindications
- Hypersensitivity to pralidoxime.

Adverse effects
- Tachycardia, dizziness, hyperventilation, and laryngospasm associated with rapid IV infusion

- Nausea, vomiting, diarrhea, bitter aftertaste, and rash after oral doses

- Blurred vision, diplopia

- Possible neuromuscular blockade (weakness) with high levels or in patients with myasthenia gravis

Dosage
- See Table 4 for intravenous doses.

Pyridoxine or vitamin B_6
Uses
- Prophylactic use to prevent peripheral neuropathy in patients receiving isoniazid

- Treatment of seizures associated with isoniazid toxicity

Mechanism of action
- Vitamin B_6 is a water-soluble vitamin that serves as a cofactor. The active coenzyme form, pyridoxal-5-phosphate, is needed for the synthesis of neurotransmitters, metabolic transformation of various amino acids, and conversion of tryptophan to niacin (important in preventing pellagra).

- Pyridoxal phosphate aids in the formation of gamma-aminobutyric acid (GABA).

Indications
- Pyridoxine phosphokinase converts pyridoxine to its active form, pyridoxal-5-phosphate. This step is inhibited by isoniazid. If GABA production is inhibited, the reduction in GABA's neural inhibition is thought to produce the seizure activity. Pyridoxine provides seizure control by increasing the concentrations of its active form. Doses should be repeated if seizure activity recurs.

Contraindications
- Hypersensitivity to pyridoxine preparations

Adverse effects
- Chronic supratherapeutic doses of 2-6 grams daily for two or more months are associated with sensory neuropathy.

- Acute oral toxicity of pyridoxine has not been defined.

- Seizures can follow large IV doses.

- Decrease in folic acid

Dosage
- Intravenous administration (see Table 4)

Sodium bicarbonate
Uses
- Tricyclic antidepressant–induced cardiac toxicity on overdose

- Salicylate-associated metabolic acidosis

- Urinary alkalinization to increase renal elimination of some weak acids, ie, salicylates

Mechanism of action

- Tricyclic antidepressants suppress rapid sodium ion influx, decreasing ventricular depolarization, which is observed as QRS prolongation. QT prolongation can occur due to slowing of repolarization. The sodium ion and alkalemia are thought to reverse this depressant effect. Sodium bicarbonate also improves hypotension associated with tricyclics.

- Sodium bicarbonate, a buffer that reacts with free hydrogen ions, breaks down into water and carbon dioxide, resulting in alkalemia. For weak acids (eg salicylates) as the pH increases, a greater proportion of the weak acid is converted to its ionized form.

Indications

Tricyclic antidepressant toxicity

- There is a potential for toxicity with acute ingestion of 10-20 mg/kg in the adult patient and 3.5 mg/kg or greater in the pediatric patient. Patients should be monitored for a wide QRS complex or dysrhythmias. If cardiac symptoms develop, sodium bicarbonate is recommended. The goal blood pH is 7.45-7.55. The goal of therapy is to reverse conduction delays.

Salicylate toxicity

- Salicylates have a direct stimulating effect on the medullary respiratory center, producing respiratory alkalosis and compensatory metabolic acidosis leading to mixed acid-base disorders. Salicylates uncouple oxidative phosphorylation at the cellular level, leading to fever. Elevated lactic acid contributes to the metabolic acidosis. Alkalemia may prevent intracellular distribution of salicylates. The correction of the acidemia enhances renal elimination of salicylate because more of the drug is in the ionized form. Urinary alkalinization should aid in the decline of serum salicylate concentration.

Contraindications

- Significant existing metabolic or respiratory alkalosis

- Hypocalcemia

- Hypochloremia

- Severe pulmonary edema

- Use with caution in patients with congestive heart failure, hypertension, and/or renal insufficiency. Maintain high urine output.

Adverse effects

- Hypernatremia

- Hypokalemia

- Excessive systemic alkalosis

- Pulmonary edema

- Cerebral edema

- Extravasation of the hypertonic sodium bicarbonate solutions can cause cellulitis and tissue necrosis.

Dosage

- Intravenous bolus and infusion (see Table 4)

Succimer or dimercaptosuccinic acid, DMSA (Chemet)

Uses

- FDA-approved for treatment of lead poisoning in pediatric patients with blood lead concentrations >45 μg/dL

- The Centers for Disease Control and Prevention considers oral succimer as an alternative to parenteral chelation therapy in patients with blood lead concentrations >45 μg/dL.

- Off-label use in arsenic and mercury poisoning

Mechanism of action

- Acts as a chelating agent. Lead binds to sulfur and oxygen atoms of succimer. Arsenic binds to the sulfur moieties. Water-soluble chelates are formed and renally eliminated.

Indications

Lead poisoning

- See calcium disodium EDTA for sources of lead and toxicities associated with lead.

- Data are not available regarding use in the treatment of encephalopathy in children.

- The manufacturer does not recommend concomitant administration with other chelating therapy.

Arsenic

- See dimercaprol for toxicities associated with arsenic.

- See dimercaprol for indications of chelation therapy.

Contraindications

- Allergy to succimer

Adverse effects
- Rash

- Mild, reversible elevations in AST and ALT

- Mild to moderate neutropenia

- Eosinophilia

- Increases excretion of zinc; insignificant elimination of calcium, iron, and magnesium

Dosage
- Oral administration (see Table 4)

4. Overview of Chem-Bioterrorism

- The world faces the growing threat of chem-bioterrorist attack with biological, chemical, and radiological weapons.

- *Bioterrorism* is the deliberate use of infectious biological agents to cause illness, and is categorized for risk by the Centers for Disease Control and Prevention (CDC).
    * *Category A* agents are high priority agents that can be easily transmitted, result in high mortality rates, and have the potential for major public health impact. They include smallpox, anthrax, plague (*Yersinia pestis*), botulism, tularemia, and viral hemorrhagic fevers (filoviruses [eg, Ebola and Marburg] and arenaviruses [eg, Lassa and Machupo]).
    * *Category B* agents include brucellosis, epsilon toxin of *Clostridium perfringens*, food safety threats (eg, *Salmonella* species, *Escherichia coli* O157:H7, *Shigella*), glanders (*Burkholderia mallei*), melioidosis (*Burkholderia pseudomallei*), psittacosis (*Chlamydia psittaci*), Q fever (*Coxiella burnetii*), ricin, staphylococcal enterotoxin B, typhus fever, viral encephalitis (alphaviruses [eg, Venezuelan equine encephalitis, eastern equine encephalitis, western equine encephalitis]), and water safety threats (eg, *Vibrio cholerae, Cryptosporidium parvum*).
    * *Category C* agents include emerging infectious disease threats such as Nipah virus and hantavirus.

- See Table 5 for clinical features and suggested treatment for the most likely forms of category A diseases, and ricin, a previously weaponized and used category B agent.

- The mode of transmission for biological agents is essentially the same as with all other infectious diseases:
    * Aerosol (most common form for biological weapons)
    * Dermal contact
    * Injection
    * Food-borne
    * Water-borne

- Toxic chemicals that are used in warfare include nerve, blister/vesicant, blood, choking/lung/pulmonary, incapacitating, riot control/tear and vomit-inducing agents.

Table 5

Biological Agents That May Be Used in a Bioterrorism Attack

Biological agent	Clinical features	Treatment
Smallpox is caused by the variola virus; may be spread by aerosol or direct contact with infected persons/fluids	Early symptoms resemble a mild viral illness, with a 2- to 4-day nonspecific prodrome of fever and myalgias before rash onset. Pustules form, then scabs form and fall off, leaving pitted scars. When all the scabs have fallen off (in about 3 weeks), patients are no longer contagious. Smallpox rash is typically most prominent on the face and extremities, and lesions form at the same time. (By contrast, chickenpox rash is most prominent on the trunk and develops in successive groups of lesions over several days.)	No specific treatment. Vaccine is only preventive. The currently available vaccine (Dryvax® from Wyeth) is a live-virus preparation of vaccinia virus.
Anthrax is caused by *Bacillus anthracis*, a gram-positive spore-forming rod, and has three major forms: cutaneous, inhalation, and gastrointestinal; none are contagious	***Cutaneous:*** Begins as a small papule, progresses to a vesicle in 1-2 days, followed by a necrotic, normally painless ulcer. May have fever, malaise, headache, and regional lymphadenopathy. ***Inhalation:*** Initially resembles a viral illness with sore throat, mild fever, muscle aches, and malaise. Often has minimally productive cough, nausea or vomiting, and chest discomfort that may progress to respiratory failure and shock with meningitis frequently developing. In contrast to influenza, patients rarely have a runny nose and usually have an abnormal chest x-ray and high white blood cell count. ***Gastrointestinal:*** Causes severe abdominal or oropharyngeal distress followed by fever and signs of septicemia, bloody vomit, and diarrhea.	Ciprofloxacin, doxycycline, and penicillin G procaine are FDA-approved for postexposure prophylaxis (PEP). Ciprofloxacin, doxycycline, and amoxicillin are FDA-approved for treatment. Persons at risk for inhalation anthrax need 60 days of prophylactic antibiotics. The CDC recommends anthrax vaccine only for the military and similar high-risk personnel.
Plague, caused by *Yersinia pestis,* has several forms, with pneumonic plague being the most virulent	Clinical features of aerosolized pneumonic plague include fever, cough with mucopurulent sputum, hemoptysis, and chest pain with signs consistent with severe pneumonia 1-6 days after exposure. Septic shock and high mortality can occur within 2-4 days of symptom onset without early treatment. *Y pestis*–caused bubonic plague is less likely to be weaponized.	Early treatment and PEP with streptomycin, gentamicin, doxycycline, ciprofloxacin, or chloramphenicol advised. (Vaccine ineffective for pneumonic plague.)
Botulism, caused by *Clostridium botulinum,* may be food-borne or air-borne	Clinical features include acute symmetric descending paralysis in a proximal to distal pattern, with prominent bulbar palsies such as diplopia, dysarthria, dysphonia, and dysphagia that typically present 12-72 hours postexposure, and respiratory dysfunction from respiratory muscle paralysis or upper airway obstruction without sensory deficits.	A supply of antitoxin is maintained and dispensed by the CDC. Most patients recover after supportive care, often with mechanical ventilation for weeks to months.
Tularemia, caused by *Francisella tularensis,* is one of the most infectious bacteria known	Inhalation exposure causes an abrupt onset of a nonspecific febrile illness beginning 3-5 days postexposure, with incipient pneumonia, pleuritis, and hilar lymphadenopathy. Without treatment, respiratory failure, shock and death are possible. Like botulism and anthrax, tularemia is not contagious, so patients who have tularemia do not need to be isolated.	Prompt treatment with streptomycin, gentamicin, doxycycline, or ciprofloxacin advised, as is early PEP use of doxycycline or ciprofloxacin. A vaccine is not yet available.

Table 5

Biological Agents That May Be Used in a Bioterrorism Attack (continued)

Biological agent	Clinical features	Treatment
Hemorrhagic fever viruses (HFV): filoviruses and arenaviruses are most virulent, but all listed here are considered serious biological threats; exposure is via all routes, including direct and aerosol	With **filoviruses** (Ebola and Marburg types), an abrupt onset of an undifferentiated febrile illness with high fever occurs 2-21 days after exposure. A maculopapular rash, prominent on the trunk, develops around 5 days later, with progressive bleeding symptoms such as petechiae, ecchymosis, disseminated intravascular coagulation, and hemorrhages. With **arenaviruses** (Lassa and multiple New World arenaviruses, including Machupo that causes Bolivian hemorrhagic fever) symptoms and onset are similar to filoviruses, but with a gradual onset of rash, hemorrhagic diathesis, and shock. **Bunyaviruses** cause Rift Valley fever (<1% develop hemorrhagic fever). **Flaviviruses** cause Yellow fever, Omsk hemorrhagic fever, and Kyasabur Forest disease. (Other HFVs exist, but they are not considered a serious bioterrorism risk.)	Mainstay of treatment is supportive to maintain fluid and electrolyte balance, circulatory volume, and blood pressure. There are no FDA-approved antiviral drugs or vaccines. Ribavirin in the early stages of some of the HFVs is potentially useful. All HFVs are zoonotic (animal-borne) lipid-enveloped RNA viruses. Only licensed vaccine is yellow fever live attenuated 17D vaccine.
Ricin, from castor beans, is cytotoxic via inhibition of protein synthesis; abrin is a similar toxalbumin agent	Within a few hours of inhalation, cough and dyspnea develop, with the lungs rapidly becoming severely inflamed and filled with fluid. Skin might turn blue from cyanosis or flush red. Ingestion causes internal bleeding of the stomach and intestines. Injection kills the closest muscles and lymph nodes before spreading to other organs. Death can occur within 36-48 hours of all types of exposure from multiple organ failure.	No antidote is available. Mainstay is supportive medical treatment, varying with the route of exposure. If victim survives more than 5 days without complications, patient will likely survive.

- See Table 6 for descriptions, symptoms, and treatment of the agents most likely to be used.

- Normally they are liquids or solids, often dispersed in the air in aerosols.

- The CDC has recently added commonly available agents such as hydrofluoric acid, benzene, ethylene glycol (antifreeze), and metals like arsenic, mercury, and thallium to their list, although these are not listed as chemical warfare agents in other sources and are not detailed in Table 6.

- Radiological weapons involve nuclear radiation or radioactive materials with various radionucleotides.

- Radionucleotides can produce topical and systemic effects that may be immediate or delayed, depending upon the agent, route of exposure, and extent of exposure.

- Medical management of radiological emergencies and terrorist attacks is specific for the radionucleotide. Guidance on treatment is available from the Radiation Emergency Assistance Center/Training Site (REAC/TS) at the Oak Ridge Institute for Science and Education. The emergency response phone number is 865-576-1005; ask for REAC/TS. Program information is available at www. orau.gov/reacts.

- For example, the early use of stable iodine, taken as potassium iodide or sodium iodide tablets, can reduce the uptake of radioiodine by the thyroid. Many individuals near nuclear reactors will maintain a stock of stable iodine tablets in the event of a

Table 6

Chemical Agents That May Be Used in a Chem-Bioterrorism Attack

Chemical agents (military name)	Clinical features	Treatment
Nerve agents. G agents: sarin (GB), soman (GD), tabun (GA), cyclohexyl sarin (GF); V agents: VX	These nerve agents are organophosphates that attach to and inhibit acetylcholinesterase at muscarinic and nicotinic receptors, causing cholinergic crisis with miosis, vomiting, diarrhea, excessive secretions (bronchial, lacrimal, dermal, nasal, and salivary), brady- or tachycardia, skeletal muscle fasciculations, paralysis, seizures, and respiratory failure. Well absorbed through all routes of exposure. Symptoms within minutes after significant exposure, and up to 18 hours after liquid exposure.	Rapid, thorough decontamination. Antidotes include atropine to reverse muscarinic symptoms and pralidoxime early to restore acetylcholinesterase before permanent deactivation (aging) of the enzyme. Also give diazepam or lorazepam for seizures.
Blister agents. Mustards: sulfur gas (H), distilled (HD); mustard/T. nitrogen mustards: (HN-1, HN-2, HN-3); sesqui mustard; lewisites: (L, L-1, L-2, L-3); chloroarsines: (ED, MD, PD); mustard/lewisite combination: (HL); phosgene oxime: (CX)	*Mustards* are vesicants that cause blistering of the skin and mucous membranes on contact, damaging skin, eyes, and lungs. Damage immediate but symptoms can be delayed 2-24 hours. Liquid form more likely to cause burns and scarring than gas. All forms absorbed through the skin and distributed systemically. Nitrogen mustards cause bone marrow suppression in 3-5 days. Sulfur mustards have garlic, onion, mustard, or no odor. Nitrogen mustards can smell fishy, musty, soapy or fruity. *Lewisites and chloroarsines* are arsenical vesicants that cause immediate pain and damage to the eyes, skin, and respiratory tract, although lesions may take hours to form. After absorption, they cause increased capillary permeability leading to hypovolemia, shock, and organ damage. Lewisite smells like geraniums. Mustard/lewisite is lewisite combined with distilled mustard. *Phosgene oxime* is a readily absorbed urticant or nettle agent, causing immediate, painful corrosive and necrotic tissue damage. Does not cause blisters (but normally classified here). Disagreeable odor.	Sulfur and nitrogen mustards (thought to be alkylating agents that crosslink DNA strands) have no antidote. Avoiding contact or rapid thorough decontamination is only prevention. Treatment is supportive. Not usually fatal (sulfur type <5% fatal in World War I). No mustard in tissue or blister fluids. British anti-lewisite (BAL) is specific antidote for lewisite, used IM for systemic effects or topically as skin or eye ointment. Chloroarsine treatment is similar, except atropine sulfate ointment is used for eyes. No antidote exists for phosgene oxime. Rapid decontamination and supportive treatment used as for any corrosive agent.
Blood agents. Arsine: (SA); cyanide gases: hydrogen cyanide (AC), cyanogen chloride (CK); cyanide solids: potassium (KCN), and sodium (NaCN) cyanide	*Arsine* is a gas that causes nausea, vomiting, hemolysis, and secondary renal failure in 1-2 hours to 11 days. Garlic-like odor. Inhalation of highly concentrated *cyanide* causes increased rate and depth of breathing in 15 seconds, convulsions within 30 seconds, cessation of respiration in 2-4 minutes, and cessation of heartbeat in 4-8 minutes. Progress and severity of symptoms after ingestion or inhaling lower gas concentrations are slower and dose dependent. May have odor of bitter almonds or peach kernels (AC), with no odor or irritating, lacrimating properties like riot control agents (CK).	Arsines: symptomatic management of hemolysis, normally without chelation. Cyanides bind to cytochrome oxidase. Cyanide antidotes: (1) methemoglobin-forming agents like inhaled amyl nitrite (in civilian kits) and/or IV sodium nitrite free bound cyanide, restoring cellular ATP; (2) IV sodium thiosulfate (sulfur donor to convert cyanide to sodium thiocyanate.) Fresh air, oxygen, supportive treatment.

Table 6

Chemical Agents That May Be Used in a Chem-Bioterrorism Attack (continued)

Chemical agents (military name)	Clinical features	Treatment
Choking and pulmonary agents. Phosgene (CG), diphosgene (DP); also ammonia, chlorine (CL), hydrogen chloride, nitrogen oxide (NO), Teflon®, perfluroisobutylene (PHIB), others	*Phosgene* gas causes eye, nose, throat, and pulmonary irritation, with serious pulmonary injury and edema delayed up to 48 hours, as it hydrolyzes to hydrochloric acid in moist conditions. New-mown-hay odor. Phosgene is the prototype agent in the group. Other agents cause immediate irritation with potential for more severe delayed effects. *Ammonia* hydrolyzes to caustic ammonium hydroxide. *Chlorine* (pungent, greenish gas) hydrolyzes to hydrochloric acid. *Perfluroisobutylene* is a toxic pyrolysis product of *Teflon*. Nitrogen oxides are components of blast weapons or fire. Others include *red* (RP) and *white phosphorus*, *sulfur trioxide-chlorosulfonic acid* (FS), *titanium tetrachloride* (FM), and *zinc oxide* (HC).	Phosgene has no antidote. Good decontamination and symptomatic treatment needed. Treatment of other agents is similar as all agents in this class are gases with no antidotes (thorough, rapid decontamination with fresh air is best initial management, with thorough flushing of exposed eyes and skin and symptomatic treatment).
Incapacitating agents	Contains a variety of fast-acting central nervous system and respiratory depressants, often with hallucinogenic properties. CDC list includes *BZ/agent 15* (glycolate anticholinergic), *cannabinoids, fentanyls* and other opioids, *LSD*, and *phenothiazines.*	Management is decontamination with supportive treatment and antidotes should be used when they exist (physostigmine for anticholinergics, naloxone for opioids).
Riot control and tear gases	Lacrimators include *chloroacetophenone* (CN) in several solvents, *chloropicrin* (PS), *bromobenzylcyanide* (CA), CR, and CS gases.	Treatment is symptomatic after decontamination. No antidotes are available.
Vomiting agents	Includes *adamsite* (DM), *diphenylchloroarsine* (DA) and *diphenylcyanoarsine* (DC). Rapidly incapacitating, irritant gases.	Symptomatic measures for sneezing, coughing, and vomiting (eg, antiemetics).

radioactive accident. Ingestion of stable iodine is of little value for other radionucleotide exposures unless the radioactive constituents are unknown, as in a "dirty bomb."

- Health care professionals should have an awareness of the potential for biological terrorism, an appreciation for epidemiologic clues of a chem-bioterrorist event, and a basic understanding of the classes of agents that can be weaponized and their effects.

- Pharmacists are in a unique position to quickly recognize community-wide patterns of symptoms, illness, and mortality in humans and animals that can be important clues to terrorist events.

- The CDC advises that if citizens believe that they have been exposed to a biological or chemical agent, or if they believe an intentional biological threat will occur or is occurring, they should contact their local health department and/or local police or other law enforcement agency (eg, FBI). These agencies will notify the state health department and other response partners, per a pre-established notification list that channels to the CDC, which is under the Department of Health and Human Services (DHHS).

- The CDC maintains the Strategic National Stockpile (formerly called the National Pharmaceutical Stockpile) to ensure the availability and rapid deployment of life-saving pharmaceuticals, antidotes, other medical supplies, and equipment necessary to counter nerve agents, biological pathogens, and chemical agents. The SNS program stands ready for immediate deployment to any U.S. location in the event of a terrorist attack using a biological toxin or chemical agent directed against a civilian population. Further information is available at the CDC website (www. cdc.gov).

- The Department of Health and Human Services, in conjunction with the Joint Commission of Pharmacy Practice, is working to establish the National Pharmacists Response Team (NPRT). When active, the NPRT will consist of 10 regionally based teams of 200 pharmacists, pharmacy students, and pharmacy technicians that when needed would be called upon to assist with vaccinations and/or distribution of medications.

- As of this writing, the Department of Homeland Security functions with four major directorates: Border and Transportation Security (including U.S. Customs and the Immigration and Naturalization Service); Emergency Preparedness and Response (including the Federal Emergency Management Agency [FEMA], the Department of Health and Human Services, and the Strategic National Stockpile); Science and Technology; and Information Analysis and Infrastructure Protection (which will analyze information from other agencies, including the CIA, FBI, DIA, and NSA). The Secret Service and Coast Guard are also included in the Department of Homeland Security.

5. Key Points

- Medications are the most common cause of poisoning morbidity and mortality. Any chemical can become toxic if too much is taken in relation to body weight and tolerance. A great number of poisonings occur in young children, but most fatalities occur in adults.

- Several approaches can minimize the risk of unintentional childhood poisonings (eg, safety latches, proper storage, following label instructions), but the proper use of child-resistant containers ("safety caps") is one of the most effective means. As part of the Poison Prevention Packaging Act of 1970, pharmacists are required to dispense oral prescription drugs (with certain exceptions such as nitroglycerin and oral contraceptives) in child-resistant containers unless the patient or prescriber indicate their desire for a non-safety cap.

- Immediate first aid for a poison exposure can minimize potential toxic effects, and involves water and fresh air, depending on the route of exposure. Contact a poison center immediately through the nationwide access number (1-800-222-1222) to determine first aid or whether a poisoning emergency exists.

- The use of drugs to decrease the absorption of drugs from the gastrointestinal tract after a poisoning or overdose is in a state of change. Ipecac syrup, an orally administered emetic, has questionable effectiveness and its use is generally avoided in hospitals. Its use should be avoided (1) when the person exhibits sleepiness, coma, or seizures; (2) when agents such as caustics, aliphatic hydrocarbons, fast-acting agents that produce coma or seizures, (eg, tricyclic antidepressants, clonidine, strychnine, and hypoglycemic agents) have been ingested; (3) when the ingestion was greater than 1 hour ago; or (4) there is an obvious need for hospital referral. Cathartics such as magnesium citrate are not routinely used. Activated charcoal, an orally administered adsorbent, is often the only treatment necessary if the toxin can be adsorbed and it is used within 1-2 hours of ingestion. It should be avoided in ingestions of aliphatic hydrocarbons and caustics and in patients with absent bowel sounds, and it is not useful with heavy metals (sodium, lithium, iron, or lead) or simple alcohols. Whole-bowel irrigation, with products such as Colyte and GoLytely, can be considered if the toxin is poorly adsorbed and its presence in the gastrointestinal tract is likely. Other hospital-based therapies include supportive and symptomatic care, multiple doses of activated charcoal (to enhance systemic elimination when appropriate), hemodialysis (to enhance systemic elimination when appropriate), and use of antidotes (to antagonize or reverse toxic effects when indicated).

- Substance abuse often leads to acute and chronic toxicity from a variety of medications, commercial products, and illicit agents. The management of acute toxicity from substance abuse typically follows the same general approaches as those for poisoning and overdose. A challenge faced in many acute drug overdose episodes is determining the agents taken and possible adulterants or contaminants. Chronic abuse can lead to dependence and withdrawal symptoms upon stopping use.

- There are few antidotes available relative to the large number of potential poisons. The use of an antidote is usually an adjunct to conventional and supportive therapies. Many hospitals have an insufficient stock of antidotes.

- N-acetylcysteine (Mucomyst) is a glutathione substitute in the metabolism of the acetaminophen toxic reactive metabolite. It is most effective if given orally within 10 hours of an acetaminophen overdose in preventing hepatotoxicity, and may also help later to minimize hepatic injury once it has begun. An intravenous preparation may be available by 2004.

- Atropine is used to treat the muscarinic effects (bronchorrhea, bradycardia, etc) produced by organophosphate and carbamate insecticides and anticholinesterase nerve gas agents by competing with acetylcholine for binding at muscarinic receptors in the nervous system.

- Pralidoxime (Protopam) reactivates the enzyme acetylcholinesterase by dephosphorylation and allows metabolism of accumulated amounts of acetylcholine produced by enzyme inhibition from exposures to anticholinesterase nerve gas agents and organophosphate and carbamate insecticides.

- Digoxin immune Fab (Digibind, DigiFab) is a specific antibody for digoxin, but it exhibits some cross reactivity with other digoxin-like compounds. It is an ovine derived antigen-binding fragment reserved for the treatment of life-threatening symptoms of digoxin overdose (eg, bradycardia, ventricular arrhythmias, second- and third-degree heart block, hyperkalemia).

- Flumazenil (Romazicon) is a competitive antagonist of benzodiazepines at the benzodiazepine receptor in the central nervous system (CNS). It is used in the treatment of severe CNS and respiratory depression that may occur with benzodiazepines when they are used as an anesthetic or taken as an overdose. Seizures may occur when flumazenil is administered to patients with co-ingestants of tricyclic antidepressants, drugs that lower the seizure threshold, and in patients requiring benzodiazepines for seizure control.

- Administration of naloxone (Narcan), a competitive antagonist of opiate binding at the opioid receptors in the CNS, reverses the CNS and respiratory depression of opiate toxicity. Naloxone may precipitate withdrawal symptoms in opiate-dependent patients.

- Bioterrorism is the deliberate use of infectious biological agents to cause illness. High-priority agents can be easily transmitted, result in high mortality rates, and have the potential for major public health impact. They include smallpox, anthrax, plague (*Yersinia pestis*), botulism, tularemia, and viral hemorrhagic fevers (eg, Ebola, Marburg, Lassa, and Machupo).

- These toxic chemicals are used in warfare and may be used in a bio-terrorism attack:
  * Substances that act on nerves (eg, anticholinesterase agents such as sarin)
  * Substances that are blistering/vesicants (eg mustard agents and lewisites)
  * Substances that act on blood (eg arsine and cyanide)
  * Substances that act on the pulmonary system (eg phosgene, chlorine, and ammonia)
  * Substances that are incapacitating (eg fast-acting CNS depressants or hallucinogens)
  * Substances that can also be used in riot control (eg various lacrimating agents such as chloroacetophenone [CN]), and vomiting agents (eg adamsite).

- Health care providers need to have an awareness of the potential for biological terrorism, an appreciation for epidemiologic clues of a chem-bioterrorist event, and a basic understanding of the classes of agents that can be weaponized and their effects. The Centers for Disease Control and Prevention (CDC) maintains the Strategic National Stockpile (formerly called the National Pharmaceutical Stockpile) that can be rapidly deployed to communities to ensure the availability and rapid deployment of life-saving pharmaceuticals, antidotes, other medical supplies, and equipment necessary to counter nerve agents, biological pathogens, and chemical agents.

6. Questions and Answers

1. Parenteral calcium salt administration is indicated for each of the following poison exposures EXCEPT:

   A. Hydrofluoric acid poisoning
   B. Digoxin overdose
   C. Diltiazem overdose
   D. Ethylene glycol poisoning
   E. B and D

2. Glucagon is used in the treatment of β-blocker overdose and calcium channel overdose because glucagon

   A. Stimulates glycogenolysis, resulting in elevated glucose concentrations
   B. Stimulates glucagon receptors, which increases adenylcyclase formation and activity, allowing increased inotropic and chronotropic cardiac effects
   C. Relaxes smooth muscles, which results in vasodilation and increased cardiac output
   D. Directly stimulates α receptors peripherally, resulting in an increase in heart rate and blood pressure
   E. Causes a release of catecholamines that will increase heart rate and cardiac output

3. Which of the following statements is correct concerning the cyanide antidote kit?

   A. The kit contains 1 ampule of amyl nitrite for intravenous infusion, 10 sodium nitrite ampules for inhalation, and 1 ampule of sodium thiocyanate for intravenous infusion.
   B. The kit should be administered to any patient, symptomatic or not, due to the toxic effects of cyanide.
   C. Nitrites directly bind cyanide to prevent toxicity, and sodium thiocyanate inhibits metabolism to toxic metabolites.
   D. The intravenous infusion of the nitrite should be given by rapid IV push.
   E. Nitrites convert hemoglobin to methemoglobin that forms a cyanide-methemoglobin complex, sparing cytochrome oxidase and cellular respiration.

4. A depressed 30-year-old male ingested 8 ounces of radiator antifreeze 1 hour ago. The patient sounds inebriated but is complaining of skin flushing, throbbing headache, dyspnea, anxiety, vertigo, and nausea and vomiting, and he sounds confused. He drank the antifreeze after he ran out of bourbon. He is otherwise healthy and is currently taking Antabuse® due to a recurrent history of ethanol abuse. The patient has no known allergies. Which of the following statements is correct concerning this ingestion?

   A. The patient has most likely ingested a significantly toxic amount of ethylene glycol.
   B. The patient has ingested methanol, with metabolic alkalosis and renal failure being the primary concerns from toxic exposures.
   C. The patient should be referred to the hospital due to his symptoms of ethylene glycol or methanol poisoning: flushing, dyspnea, headache, and anxiety.
   D. The patient should be given ipecac syrup and observed at home.
   E. The patient should be referred to a health care facility. Since the patient already has ethanol in his body, no further treatment is needed but observation.

5. The appropriate treatment for the patient in Question 4 would be to begin

   A. Intravenous ethanol as a 40% solution in D_5W
   B. Ethanol orally, diluted to a 5-10% solution in juice
   C. Fomepizole intravenously
   D. Observation only since the patient possibly already has an elevated blood ethanol concentration
   E. Gastric decontamination: lavage, activated charcoal, and magnesium citrate

6. Which of the flowing statements is correct concerning Antilirium?

   A. It is commonly used to treat the toxicity of cholinergic agents such as organophosphate poisonings.
   B. Antilirium may be given via rapid IV push.
   C. It is used in the treatment of tricyclic antidepressant overdoses when a prolonged QRS interval is noted on ECG.
   D. Antilirium is commonly used due its efficacy and minimal side effects.
   E. The toxicity of anticholinergic agents responds well to supportive measures resulting in limited use of Antilirium.

7. Concerning the Crotalidae (polyvalent) antivenin, which of the following statements is correct?

A. Treatment with the antivenin may result in delayed serum sickness.

B. The Crotalidae (polyvalent) antivenin is readily available from the manufacturer.

C. No skin test is necessary prior to antivenin administration.

D. Patients allergic to papain may experience a hypersensitivity reaction from the antivenin.

E. Administration of the antivenin is indicated for patients with localized edema around the bite, with no systemic symptoms or laboratory changes.

8. Which of the following statements is correct concerning CroFab?

A. The production of CroFab is being discontinued.

B. A skin test is required prior to CroFab administration.

C. Administration of the antivenin is indicated for patients with extensive progressive edema and coagulopathies.

D. CroFab blocks specific venom receptors on cells to prevent toxicity.

E. CroFab is obtained from equine serum.

9. A patient has an INR of 10 with no evidence of a significant bleed following the ingestion of warfarin. You recommend to omit the warfarin dosing and the following:

A. Give 1 mg of vitamin K_1 orally and monitor INR

B. Give 5 mg of vitamin K_1 orally and monitor INR

C. Give 2 mg of vitamin K_1 intravenously and monitor INR

D. Recheck INR in 24-48 hours

E. Give 10 mg of vitamin K_1 intravenously and monitor INR

10. Flumazenil is contraindicated in which case?

A. A patent with QRS widening with a known ingestion of Elavil

B. A patient who was previously given flumazenil complains of abnormal vision and dizziness

C. A patient with known use of cocaine

D. A and C

E. A and B

11. A 25-year-old patient is suspected of having aspirin toxicity. You initially expect the following laboratory findings:

A. Respiratory alkalosis and compensating metabolic acidosis

B. Respiratory alkalosis and metabolic alkalosis

C. Respiratory acidosis and metabolic acidosis

D. Respiratory acidosis and compensating metabolic alkalosis

E. Respiratory acidosis and anticholinergic effects

12. A patient is brought to the emergency department. She is experiencing CNS and respiratory depression due to a suspected ingestion of her sister's MS Contin. You recommend supportive care and the administration of

A. Flumazenil

B. Naloxone

C. Lorazepam

D. Flumazenil and Narcan

E. Pyridoxine

13. A seizure due to an acute overdose of isoniazid should be treated with

A. Pyridoxine due to isoniazid increasing GABA production

B. Pyridoxine due to isoniazid inhibiting GABA production

C. Pralidoxime due to isoniazid enhancing GABA activity

D. Physostigmine due to isoniazid increasing GABA production

E. Phytonadione due to isoniazid inhibiting GABA production

14. A pediatric patient has a blood lead concentration of 80 µg/dL. The patient is exhibiting symptoms of encephalopathy. You recommend the following initial treatment:

A. Calcium EDTA and dimercaprol

B. Dimercaprol only

C. Succimer and calcium EDTA

D. Succimer only

E. No therapy is indicated because the child does not have a blood lead concentration of >100 µg/dL

15. A policeman presents to the emergency room with a rash, fearing he was exposed to a biological weapon several days before the rash appeared. You notice the rash is forming pustules and is most prominent on the face and extremities. The patient says the rash developed all at once. He has possibly contracted:

A. Smallpox
B. Chickenpox
C. Anthrax
D. Tularemia
E. None of the above

16. What is the recommended treatment for the likely disease?

I. Supportive. There is no specific treatment.
II. Ciprofloxacin
III. Doxycycline

A. II or III
B. II and III
C. I only
D. II only
E. III only

17. The currently available vaccine is:

I. Dryvax from Wyeth
II. A live-virus preparation of the vaccinia virus
III. The only prevention for the disease

A. I only
B. I and II only
C. II and III only
D. I, II, and III
E. No vaccine is currently available

18. A patient presents with a black, necrotic, pain-less skin lesion on her arm. She also complains of fever, malaise, headache, and swelling of her underarm lymph nodes. The possible biological agent responsible for these symptoms is:

A. Hemorrhagic fever virus
B. Anthrax
C. Botulism
D. Tularemia
E. Arsine

19. The recommended antibiotic treatment of the infection in Question 18 may include:

A. Ciprofloxacin
B. Doxycycline
C. Amoxicillin
D. All of the above
E. Supportive. There is no specific treatment.

20. Inhalation exposure to the agent in Question 18 requires:

A. Post exposure prophylaxis with ciprofloxacin,

doxycycline, or penicillin G procaine for 60 days
B. Immediate vaccination of civilian personnel
C. Early treatment with streptomycin or genta-micin
D. Early treatment with ribavirin
E. None of the above are recommended.

21. A cab driver presents to the emergency room with vomiting, diarrhea, sweating, salivation, moist rales, bradycardia, muscle tremor, and weakness. He reports inhaling a mist dropped from a low-flying plane several hours earlier. You also note that he has miosis and his respira-tory difficulty is increasing rapidly. The likely mechanism of toxicity of the poison is:

A. Inhibition of protein synthesis
B. Binding of agent to cytochrome oxidase
C. Inhibition of acetylcholinesterase
D. An alkylating agent cross-linking DNA strands
E. None of the above

22. The recommended initial management of the symptoms in Question 21 includes all EXCEPT:

A. Immediate decontamination of skin and eyes
B. Disposal of contaminated clothes
C. British anti-lewisite
D. Atropine
E. Pralidoxime

23. The patient in Question 21 deteriorates and develops seizures. You recommend:

A. Phenytoin
B. Diazepam
C. Lithium
D. Dryvax
E. All of the above

24. A soldier reports being sprayed with a fishy smelling liquid 2 hours ago that had little imme-diate effect, but is now severely irritating his skin, eyes, and respiratory tract. His skin is beginning to form fluid-filled lesions. The chemical agent most likely involved is:

A. Arsine
B. Phosgene
C. Nitrogen mustard
D. Cyanide
E. Ricin

25. The mechanism of toxicity of the poison in Question 24 is:

   A. An alkylating agent that cross-links DNA strands
   B. Binding to cytochrome oxidase
   C. Inhibition of acetylcholinesterase
   D. All of the above
   E. None of the above

26. Likely symptoms of exposure in Question 24 include all except:

   A. Blisters
   B. Burns and scarring
   C. Rapid fatality
   D. Delayed bone marrow suppression
   E. All of the above symptoms are likely

27. Which one of the following conditions or situations is not a contraindication to the use of ipecac syrup?

   A. High blood pressure controlled with drug therapy
   B. Seizures shortly before administration
   C. Unresponsive to verbal commands
   D. A corrosive agent has been ingested
   E. A and C

28. Which one of the following is an effect of activated charcoal?

   A. Promotes dissolution of tablets
   B. Minimizes drug absorption from the gastrointestinal tract
   C. Increases urinary flow
   D. Enhances systemic elimination of certain drugs
   E. B and D

29. Which one of the following drugs is useful in the treatment of acetaminophen poisoning?

   A. N-acetylcysteine
   B. Dimercaprol
   C. Pralidoxime
   D. Atropine
   E. Dryvax

30. Deferoxamine is used therapeutically as a chelator of which metal?

   A. Iron
   B. Lithium
   C. Cadmium

   D. Arsenic
   E. Lead

31. Digoxin immune Fab is used to treat which one of the following signs or symptoms of digoxin poisoning?

   A. Hypokalemia
   B. Diplopia
   C. Ventricular tachycardia
   D. Second-degree heart block unresponsive to atropine
   E. C and D

32. Methylene blue is used to treat which one of the following conditions due to an acute poisoning?

   A. Acquired methemoglobinemia from lidocaine applied to the buccal cavity
   B. Acute hepatotoxicity from acetaminophen ingestion
   C. Respiratory depression from an opioid ingestion
   D. Seizures from intravenous methamphetamine
   E. Renal failure from ethylene glycol ingestion

33. How does crack cocaine differ from pharmaceutical cocaine?

   A. Crack is more stable under heat and can be smoked.
   B. Pharmaceutical cocaine is the hydrochloride salt.
   C. Crack is the free base form of cocaine.
   D. Crack may be contaminated with other substances.
   E. All of the above

Answers

1. **B.** The administration of calcium for digoxin overdose may result in cardiac tetany. Calcium is used for the treatment of hydrofluoric acid due to its ability to bind fluoride ions. Calcium administration may override the calcium blockade of calcium channel blockers.

2. **B.** Glucagon produces inotropic and chronotropic cardiac effects due to increased intracellular calcium. Glucagon's ability to produce glycogenolysis is the reason it is indicated for hypoglycemia. The relaxation of smooth muscles occurs in the lower esophageal sphincter, but not in the cardiovascular system. Glucagon does not stimulate α receptors and causes a release of

catecholamines only in patients with pheochromocytoma.

3. **E.** The nitrite component of the kit does convert the ferrous ion (Fe^{++}) of hemoglobin to the ferric ion (Fe^{+++}) which results in methemoglobinemia. Cyanide will bind to the ferric ion of the methemoglobin instead of the ferric ion of cytochrome oxidase. Nitrites do not bind directly to the cyanide. There are 12 ampules of amyl nitrite for inhalation, 2 ampules of sodium nitrite for intravenous infusion and 2 ampules of sodium thiosulfate for intravenous infusion. Due to the adverse effects of the drugs, they are only administered to symptomatic patients with cyanide exposure. Rapid intravenous administration of the sodium nitrite may result in hypotension.

4. **A.** The patient has most likely ingested a toxic amount of ethylene glycol if 8 ounces has been consumed. Radiator antifreeze contains almost 100% ethylene glycol. The symptoms the patient is experiencing are not specific for ethylene glycol. The patient is on disulfiram and may be experiencing a reaction since he has been drinking ethanol. Ipecac is contraindicated due to the time of ingestion and the patient's changes in mental status, and its efficacy for treatment of toxic ingestions is questionable.

5. **C.** Fomepizole would be the antidote of choice for this patient, since the patient has consumed ethanol, is taking disulfiram, and fomepizole has a more simplified treatment regimen. When ethanol is used, it is given as a 5-10% intravenous infusion due to its irritant effects to the vasculature, and up to 40-50 % orally to prevent gastric irritation. It is too late to consider gastric decontamination and it has not been proven to be effective with ethylene glycol poisoning. The possible delayed effects of ethylene glycol prohibit observation only.

6. **E.** Antilirium (physostigmine) is a reversible cholinesterase inhibitor that is similar to carbamate insecticides and the more relatively irreversible organophosphate insecticides. It is indicated for the treatment of severe, potentially life-threatening effects of anticholinergic agents. Due to the potential toxic effects of physostigmine (eg, seizures, asystole), especially with rapid administration, it is seldom used. It may worsen the cardiac effects of tricyclic antidepressants, especially if a prolonged QRS interval is noted. In most cases, patients with anticholin-

ergic toxicity respond well with supportive measures only.

7. **A.** Patients who receive the antivenin may experience a delayed serum sickness 5-24 days after its administration. Polyvalent antivenin production is being discontinued by the manufacturer. Many hospitals may still have some of this antidote available until it expires. Since it is of equine origin, a skin test is recommended prior to administration. It does not contain papain. Many crotalid bites result in no envenomation. Antivenin administration is not indicated unless there are signs of moderate to severe envenomation.

8. **C.** Antivenin administration is indicated for progressive edema and coagulopathies resulting from crotalid envenomations. These symptoms indicate the occurrence of a moderate to severe envenomation. A skin test is not required since this product is derived from ovine serum. It is currently replacing the polyvalent antivenin for crotalid envenomations. The antivenin binds and neutralizes the venom. It does not block venom receptors.

9. **B.** With an INR >9 and no evidence of a serious bleed, the recommendation is vitamin K_1 3-5 mg orally, monitor INR, and hold the warfarin dose.

10. **D.** Flumazenil is contraindicated in all patients who have ingested a tricyclic antidepressant and have cardiac symptoms; use could cause ventricular dysrhythmias. It is not recommended in mixed overdose where the co-ingested drug can cause a seizure (ie, cocaine). Answer B is a list of associated adverse effects with its administration; they are not contraindications.

11. **A.** Salicylates cause respiratory alkalosis due to direct simulating effects on the CNS respiratory center and a compensatory metabolic acidosis from renal elimination of bicarbonate and accumulation of acids like lactate and acetoacetic acid.

12. **B.** Naloxone is an opioid antagonist.

13. **B.** Pyridoxine is indicated because GABA production is inhibited by isoniazid.

14. **A.** Therapy with dimercaprol and calcium EDTA is indicated. In management of acute lead encephalopathy, calcium EDTA should be used with dimercaprol. Concomitant administration

of succimer with other chelating agents is not recommended. Data are not available regarding the use of succimer in the treatment of pediatric encephalopathy. Therapy is indicated because of the patient's symptoms. Lead encephalopathy is a life-threatening emergency.

15. **A.** See Table 5. Smallpox is the most likely agent. The agent causes a pustular rash to form that is typically most prominent on the face and extremities, and lesions form at the same time. Chickenpox rash is most prominent on the trunk and develops in successive groups of lesions over several days. Anthrax forms painless necrotic lesions. Tularemia causes a nonspecific febrile illness that rapidly develops into pneumonia.

16. **C.** See Table 5. Smallpox has no specific treatment. Ciprofloxacin and doxycycline are used in the management of anthrax, plague, and tularemia.

17. **D.** See Table 5. All characteristics are correct.

18. **B.** See Tables 5 and 6. Anthrax forms a painless, necrotic ulcer. Hemorrhagic fever viruses cause a rash that develops into petechiae, ecchymosis, hemorrhages, and other bleeding symptoms. Botulism causes a symmetric descending paralysis. Tularemia causes a nonspecific febrile illness that rapidly develops into pneumonia. Arsine is a chemical agent that causes nausea, vomiting, hemolysis, and secondary renal failure. Arsine is produced when water comes into contact with metallic arsenide or when acids come into contact with metallic arsenic or arsenical compounds. The mechanism of hemolysis is not specifically known, but the most recent mechanism postulated involves a direct arsine-hemoglobin interaction that forms arsenic metabolites, causing direct alteration of the erythrocyte cell membrane.

19. **D.** All of the above. See Table 5. Ciprofloxacin, doxycyline, and amoxicillin are FDA-approved for treatment of anthrax. These agents can be used separately or in combination, depending on symptoms and the patient's sensitivity to the agents. Antimicrobial resistance to ciprofloxacin has been growing rapidly due to widespread overuse after the anthrax mail episodes in 2002. At the time of this review, doxycycline is recommended by the CDC (but not by all sources) as the preferred initial treatment unless the patient is intolerant to the agent.

20. **A.** See Table 5. Persons at risk for inhalational anthrax need 60 days of prophylactic antibiotics. Ciprofloxacin, doxycyline, and penicillin G procaine are FDA-approved for postexposure prophylaxis (PEP). Anthrax vaccine adsorbed (AVA) is currently recommended by the CDC only for high-risk personnel (such as lab personnel working with the agent) and the military, not the civilian population. Streptomycin and gentamicin are among the suggested treatments for pneumonic plague. Ribavirin is a potential treatment for some hemorrhagic fever viruses.

21. **C.** See Table 6. The symptoms exhibited are classically cholinergic and the likely chemical agents causing these symptoms are organophosphates like the nerve agents or possibly organophosphate pesticides. Both can be spread by low-flying planes. Inhibition of protein synthesis is the mechanism of toxicity of ricin or abrin. Cyanides bind to cytochrome oxidase, interrupting normal cellular respiration and causing rapid convulsions. Blister agents like the sulfur and nitrogen mustards are thought to be alkylating agents that cross-link DNA strands, separating dermal layers in the skin and causing fluid-filled blisters to form.

22. **C.** British anti-lewisite is a specific antidote for lewisite. See Table 6. It also is used as a chelator for treatment of acute arsenic, inorganic or elemental mercury, gold, and other heavy metal poisonings. See Table 4. The other measures are treatments for organophosphate agents. Good decontamination and disposal of contaminated clothes (especially leather) is needed as organophosphates are well absorbed across the skin, through the lungs, and via ingestion, essentially all possible routes of exposure. Atropine is used for muscarinic symptoms (miosis, nausea, vomiting, diarrhea, urination, bradycardia, and excessive bronchial, lacrimal, dermal, nasal, and salivary secretions), and pralidoxime is used with atropine to resolve severe organophosphate symptoms (such as those from nerve agents), including nicotinic symptoms of muscle weakness and cramps, fasciculations, tachycardia, and CNS symptoms such as coma and seizures.

23. **B.** See Table 6. Recommended treatment for seizures due to organophosphate agents is either diazepam or lorazepam. Phenytoin is a seizure medication, but benzodiazepines (then barbiturates if benzodiazepines fail) are generally preferred over phenytoin for the control of overdose- or withdrawal-related seizures. Lithium is

not a seizure medicine, and in fact may cause seizures with elevated blood concentrations. Dryvax is a vaccine for smallpox.

24. **C.** See Table 6. Nitrogen mustard is a vesicant that causes immediate damage to skin, eyes, and respiratory tract, although symptoms of blistering or burns can be delayed 2-24 hours. Nitrogen mustards can smell fishy, musty, soapy, or fruity. Arsine causes nausea, vomiting, hemolysis, and secondary renal failure in 1-2 hours to 11 days. It has a garlic-like odor. Phosgene gas causes eye, nose, throat, and pulmonary irritation, with serious pulmonary injury and edema delayed up to 48 hours. It smells like newly-mown hay. Cyanide may have the odor of bitter almonds or peach kernels (AC), no odor, or irritating, lacrimating properties like tear gases. Ricin has no odor but inhalational exposure could cause the skin to turn blue from cyanosis or red from irritation.

25. **A.** See Table 6. Sulfur and nitrogen mustards are both thought to be alkylating agents that cross-link DNA strands. Cyanides bind to cytochrome oxidase, interrupting normal cellular respiration and causing rapid convulsions. Organophosphates bind to and inactivate acetylcholinesterase, allowing accumulation of acetylcholine at neuroeffector junctions, at synapses in autonomic ganglia, and in the brain. Excessive acetylcholine results in excessive cholinergic stimulation of muscarinic receptors (causing miosis, nausea, vomiting, diarrhea, urination, bradycardia, and excessive bronchial, lacrimal, dermal, nasal, and salivary secretions), excessive stimulation of nicotinic receptors (causing muscle and diaphragmatic weakness, fasciculations, muscle cramps, and tachycardia), and of central nervous system receptors (causing symptoms ranging from dizziness and ataxia to coma and seizures).

26. **C.** See Table 6. Nitrogen and sulfur mustards are vesicants that damage the skin and mucous membranes on contact, although symptoms of pain and blistering can be delayed 2-24 hours. Liquid forms are more likely to cause burns and scarring than gas. All forms are absorbed through skin and distributed systemically. Nitrogen mustards can cause bone marrow suppression in 3-5 days. Exposure to mustards is not expected to be rapidly fatal. Only the sulfur type has actually been used in warfare and it had a <5% fatality rate in World War I.

27. **A.** Controlled high blood pressure is not a problem with the use of ipecac syrup, but the other situations are clear contraindications due to potential aspiration (seizures, unresponsiveness) and additional esophageal burns upon vomiting up gastric contents (corrosive).

28. **E.** Activated charcoal adsorbs chemicals on contact and prevents their absorption into the bloodstream. For certain drugs (eg phenobarbital, theophylline) multiple doses of activated charcoal can promote the back diffusion of drugs across the intestinal capillary bed into the lumen of the gut, trap it there and promote its elimination. The elimination half-life can be decreased by as much as one half.

29. **A.** Acetylcysteine (Mucomyst) prevents the development of liver injury from acetaminophen if given early after ingestion and it may help minimize the effects of hepatotoxicity after it has occurred in some cases.

30. **A.** Deferoxamine (Desferal) is somewhat specific for iron and it is not used for the other metals listed. In some cases it has been used to treat excessive aluminum concentrations in dialysis patients.

31. **E.** Digoxin immune Fab is reserved for life-threatening symptoms due to its profound effects, scarcity, and high cost. Most serious cases of digoxin poisoning have normal or high potassium concentrations due to the digoxin's interference with the sodium-potassium ATPase pump.

32. **A.** Methylene blue can treat acquired methemoglobinemia regardless of the cause. Ingestion, inhalation, injection, or topical use of a methemoglobin-producing chemical (eg, lidocaine, procaine, sulfonamides, phenazopyridine, nitrites) can cause the condition. Often excessive use of topical anesthetics in dental practice or to anesthetize the pharynx and larynx for a procedure can lead to methemoglobinemia.

33. **E.** All are differences between the two forms of cocaine.

7. References

General toxicology

American Society of Health-Systems Pharmacists. AHFS drug information. Bethesda, MD: American Society of Health-Systems Pharmacists; 2003.

Ansell J, Hirsh J, Dalen J, et al. Managing oral anticoagulant therapy. *Chest.* 2001;119(Suppl 1):22S-38S.

Chyka PA. Clinical toxicology. In: Dipiro JT, Talbert RL, Yee GC, et al, eds. *Pharmacotherapy: A Pathophysiologic Approach*, 5th ed. New York: McGraw-Hill; 2002:99-102.

Dart RC, Hurlbut KM, Kuffner EK, Yip L. The 5 Minute Toxicology Consult. Philadelphia: Lippincott, Williams & Wilkins; 2000.

Ford MD, Delaney KA, Ling LJ, Erickson T. *Clinical Toxicology*. Philadelphia: WB Saunders; 2001.

Goldfrank LR, Flomenbaum NE, Lewin NA, et al. *Goldfrank's Toxicologic Emergencies*, 7th ed. New York: McGraw-Hill; 2002.

Haddad LM, Shannon MW, Winchester, JF. *Clinical Management of Poisoning and Drug Overdose*, 3rd ed. Philadelphia: WB Saunders; 1998.

Olson, KR, Anderson IB, Benowitz, NL, et al. *Poisoning and Drug Overdose*, 3rd ed. Stamford, CT: Appleton & Lange; 1999.

Watson WA, Paloucek F. Managing acute drug toxicity. In: Koda-Kimble MA, Young LY, Kradjan WA, Guglielmo BJ. *Applied Therapeutics*, 7th ed. Philadelphia: Lippincott, Williams & Wilkins; 2001:5-1 to 5-24.

Chem-bioterrorism

Centers for Disease Control and Prevention. Public health emergency preparedness and response. Available at http://www.bt.cdc.gov/index.asp. Accessed June 18, 2003.

Centers for Disease Control and Prevention. Recognition of illness associated with the intentional release of a biologic agent. *MMWR Morb Mortal Wkly Rep.* 2001;50:893-897.

Chem-Bio: Frequently Asked Questions. Alexandria, VA: Tempest Publishing; 1998.

Eitzen Col E, Culpepper CDR R, Cieslak LTC T, et al, eds. *Medical Management of Biological Casualties Handbook*, 3rd ed. Fort Detrick, MD: U.S. Army Medical Research Institute of Infectious Diseases; 1998.

First Responder Chem-Bio Handbook. Alexandria, VA: Tempest Publishing; 1998.

Henderson DA, Inglesby TV, O'Toole T, eds. *Bioterrorism: Guidelines for Medical and Public Health Management.* Chicago, IL: American Medical Association; 2002.

Krenzelok EP, ed. *Biological and Chemical Terrorism: A Pharmacy Preparedness Guide.* Bethesda, MD: American Society of Health-System Pharmacists, Inc; 2003.

Oak Ridge Institute for Science and Education. Managing radiation emergencies: guidance for hospital medical management. Radiation Emergency Assistance Center/Training Site, Oak Ridge Associated Universities, Oak Ridge, TN. Available at: http://www.orau.gov/reacts/emergency.html. Accessed June 18, 2003.

Toll LL, Hurlbut KM, eds. *Poisindex.* Greenwood Village, CO: Micromedex (edition expired 6/2003).

Voelz GL. Evaluation and treatment of persons exposed to internally deposited radionucleotides. In: Mettler FA, Kelsey CA, Ricks RC. *Medical Management of Radiation Accidents.* Boca Raton, FL: CRC Press; 1990:151-168.

36. Anemias

Ashleigh Thompson, PharmD,
Associate Professor, Department of Pharmacy
University of Tennessee College of Pharmacy
Veterans Affairs Medical Center
Memphis, Tennessee

Contents

1. Disease Overview

- Anemia is a reduction in red cell mass, which decreases the oxygen-carrying capacity of the blood. The focus of this chapter will be on iron deficiency anemia, megaloblastic anemias, and anemia of renal failure.

Epidemiology

- Approximately 3.4 million Americans have anemia.

- Anemia is more common in women than men.

- 75% of anemias are a result of iron deficiency, anemia of chronic disease, and acute bleeding. Iron deficiency anemia is the most common anemia, accounting for 25% of all cases.

- The remaining 25% of anemias are a result of bone marrow damage, decreased erythropoiesis, and hemolysis.

Classification

- The most common way to classify anemias is by the morphology (shape/structure) of the red blood cells.

Macrocytic (large cell)
- Megaloblastic anemia

- Vitamin B_{12} deficiency

- Pernicious anemia

- Folic acid deficiency

Normochromic, normocytic
- Acute blood loss

- Bone marrow failure
  * *Aplastic anemia:* marrow fails to produce all three types of blood cells, which results in anemia, neutropenia (decreased white blood cells), and thrombocytopenia (decreased platelets). About half of these cases are thought to be caused by drugs or chemicals. Examples of drugs causing aplastic anemia include chloramphenicol, felbamate, and phenytoin.

- Hemolysis
  * Genetically inherited: enzyme deficiencies such as glucose-6-phosphate dehydrogenase (G6PD) deficiency. Red blood cells deficient in G6PD are susceptible to hemolysis when exposed to

certain oxidant drugs. Examples of such drugs are dapsone, sulfamethoxazole, and nitrofurantoin.
  * Membrane abnormalities of RBCs such as in hereditary spherocytosis.

- Immunologic destruction, such as in autoimmune diseases
  * Anemia of chronic disease
  * Renal failure
  * Endocrine disorders
  * Autoimmune diseases

Hypochromic (low hemoglobin content), microcytic (small cell)
- Iron deficiency anemia

- Genetic anomalies
  * Sickle cell anemia
  * Thalassemia

Clinical Presentation

- The signs and symptoms of anemia depend on the time course over which the anemia developed, and the severity of RBC depletion.

- An anemia developed over a long period of time may be asymptomatic in beginning stages, and then progress to fatigue, malaise, headache, slight exertional dyspnea, angina, pallor, or loss of skin tone.

- A patient with acute anemia, such as from recent blood loss, may present with tachycardia, shortness of breath, or lightheadedness.

- Many of the signs and symptoms of anemia are secondary to tissue hypoxia. In the case of hypoxia, blood supply is shunted to life-sustaining organs (brain, heart, and kidney) and away from non-vital organs, such as extremities or nail beds, which results in pallor of skin.

- The various types of anemia have additional signs and symptoms which will be discussed in further detail in the diagnosis section.

Pathophysiology

Iron deficiency anemia (IDA)
- IDA is the most common anemia, accounting for a quarter of all anemia cases.

- IDA is caused by iron store depletion resulting from:
  * Inadequate oral intake of iron (especially animal protein)

* Increased iron demands
  • Pregnancy/lactation
  • Rapid growth: infancy/adolescence
  • Elderly
* Blood Loss
  • Menstruation or postpartum blood loss
  • Trauma
  • GI ulcers
* Inadequate absorption
  • Medication (eg, tetracyclines)
  • Gastrectomy
  • Enteritis
  • Persistent diarrhea
* Disease states
  • Carcinomas
  • Rheumatoid arthritis

• Hemoglobin is composed of iron (heme) and proteins (globin).

• Lack of iron results in reduced hemoglobin synthesis. The RBCs produced in these conditions are:
  * Hypochromic
    • Decreased concentration of hemoglobin
  * Microcytic
    • RBCs spend longer in marrow awaiting proper hemoglobin synthesis. This results in more cell divisions, which produces a smaller cell.

Megaloblastic anemias

• These anemias are caused by either a deficiency in or an inability to use vitamin B_{12} (cobalamin) or folic acid.

• Vitamin B_{12} deficiency:
  * Decreased intake (strict vegetarians)
  * Decreased absorption
    • Vitamin B_{12} requires gastric intrinsic factor to be absorbed. The lack of intrinsic factor results in *pernicious anemia*. This can be inherited or acquired by gastrectomy.
    • Achlorhydria
  * Inadequate utilization of B_{12} due to protein deficiencies

• Folic acid deficiency
  * Decreased intake (especially in alcoholics, indigent, elderly)
  * Decreased absorption (Crohn's disease, celiac disease, drugs)
  * Increased demands (pregnancy, growth spurts, malignancy, long-term hemodialysis)
  * Drug induced (methotrexate, phenytoin)

• Vitamin B_{12} and folic acid are both necessary for the

RNA and DNA required for cell division during the development of RBCs. Since the RNA and DNA synthesis is impeded, cell divisions are skipped, resulting in an abnormally large cell (macrocytic anemia).

Anemia of renal failure

• The primary reason that patients with renal failure are anemic is due to the lack of production of erythropoietin (EPO). EPO is a hormone produced primarily (90%) in the kidneys that stimulates the synthesis and differentiation of erythroid progenitor cells (precursors to RBCs).

• The uremic environment of chronic renal failure decreases the lifespan of RBCs.

• Folic acid deficiency can also develop due to the increased demands of folic acid during synthesis of RBCs. Additionally, folic acid can be removed during hemodialysis.

• Patients with chronic renal failure can become iron deficient due to loss of iron and blood during dialysis.

Diagnostic Criteria

If anemia is suspected, the following blood tests should be performed:
• Complete blood count (CBC) which includes:
  * Hemoglobin (Hgb)
  * Hematocrit (Hct)
  * RBC
  * Red cell indices:
    • Mean corpuscular volume (MCV) is a measure of size of RBCs.
    • Mean corpuscular hemoglobin (MCH) is a measure of weight of hemoglobin in a RBC. MCH will be low in the case of microcytosis or hypochromia.
    • Mean corpuscular hemoglobin concentration (MCHC) is a measure of weight of hemoglobin, but is more useful than MCH because it can distinguish between low hemoglobin and a small cell. MCHC will only be low in the case of hypochromia.
    • Platelets
    • Reticulocyte count (pre-RBCs)
  * Red cell morphology
  * Serum Fe, total iron binding capacity (TIBC), transferrin saturation, ferritin
  * Bilirubin (by-product of RBC destruction)

Other tests:
• Test stool for blood

- Peripheral blood smear

- Thorough history and physical exam

Iron deficiency anemia
Blood work
- The first level to decrease will be ferritin (storage form of iron).

- The iron level will be low.

- TIBC increases. This is a measure of the amount of binding space left on transferrin (transport protein of iron). Less iron in the blood translates to more space available on the transferrin molecule.

- As the iron deficiency progresses, there will be a decrease in hemoglobin (iron is a component of hemoglobin). Therefore, this is a hypochromic anemia.

- The hematocrit will also eventually fall.

- MCV will be decreased, which indicates microcytosis.

- MCH and MCHC will be decreased, which indicates decreased hemoglobin.

- Blood smear will show a microcytic, hypochromic cell.

Specific signs and symptoms
- In addition to the general signs and symptoms listed previously for anemia, these additional symptoms may be present in severe IDA:
  * Koilonychias (spoon-shaped nails)
  * Angular stomatitis or glossitis
  * Pica (craving for substances low in iron, such as ice, clay, cornstarch)

Megaloblastic anemias
Blood work
- Decreased Hct and Hgb

- Decreased RBC

- Elevated MCH, which indicates a macrocytosis

- The iron level, TIBC, and reticulocyte count will be normal.

Vitamin B_{12} deficiency
- The serum B_{12} level will be decreased.

- Positive Schilling test indicates pernicious anemia. (The Schilling test determines absorption of vitamin B_{12} by measuring the amount of radioactive B_{12} excreted in urine.)

- Additional signs and symptoms:
  * Loss of vibratory sensation in lower extremities
  * Ataxia or vertigo
  * Glossitis
  * Muscle weakness
  * Neuropsychiatric abnormalities
    · Irritability or emotional instability
    · Dementia
    · Psychosis

Folic acid deficiency
- Folate level will be decreased.

- Overall, this is very similar to B_{12} deficiency anemia, except with the absence of neurological symptoms.

Anemia of renal failure
- As the name implies, this anemia occurs in patients with chronic renal failure (CRF).

- Before diagnosis, other causes must be ruled out (eg, blood loss).

- CBC will reveal a normochromic, normocytic anemia.

Treatment Principles and Goals

Iron deficiency anemia
Goals
- To normalize Hbg and Hct
  * 2-g/dL increase in Hbg in 3 weeks
  * 6% increase in Hct in 3 weeks
  * Reticulocytosis will usually occur within 1 week.
  * If these indices do not improve within these time frames, diagnosis should be re-evaluated.

- Replete iron stores
  * Although Hbg and Hct will return to normal within 1-2 months, iron therapy should continue for 3-6 months after Hbg is normalized to replete total body iron stores.

Megaloblastic Anemias
Goals of vitamin B_{12} replacement
- Hbg should rise within 1 week.

- If neurologic symptoms were present, they should improve within 24 hours. However, if B_{12} deficiency is long-standing, symptoms may not be completely relieved for several months.

Goals of folic acid replacement
• RBC morphology will correct within 1-2 days.

• Hbg starts to normalize within 10 days.

• Hct will return to normal levels within 2 months.

• Maintenance administration of folic acid should continue for as long as nutritional intake of folic acid is a problem.

Anemia of Renal Failure
Goal
• Initial therapy goal is to reach a target Hct of 36% through a slow, steady increase (usually within 2-4 months).

• Medication doses of epoetin should be titrated to maintain Hct in the range of 30-36%.

2. Drug Therapy

Iron Deficiency Anemia

• Treatment consists of iron supplementation through therapeutic iron preparations (200 mg of elemental iron per day in 2-3 divided doses) (Table 1). Iron is best absorbed in the reduced (ferrous) form. Ferrous sulfate salt is the most common, which is 20% elemental iron. Therefore ferrous sulfate 325 mg tid will adequately treat iron deficiency.

• IV iron preparations should be used only in cases of:
  * Iron malabsorption
  * Oral noncompliance
  * Refusal of blood transfusion
  * IV iron formulations are often used in patients with chronic renal failure who require dialysis along with human recombinant erythropoietin therapy. There are three types of IV products available in the U.S.:
    • Iron dextran (InFeD®)
    • Sodium ferric gluconate (Ferrlecit®)
    • Iron sucrose (Venofer®)

Mechanism of action
• Iron supplementation corrects the iron deficiency, and enables Hgb to be synthesized at normal levels.

Patient instructions
• Take 1-2 hours prior to meal (on empty stomach).

• If you are not able to tolerate iron on an empty stomach, you may administer with a small snack (crackers), but try to avoid dairy products or tea.

Table 1

Drugs Used to Treat Iron Deficiency Anemia

Generic name (trade name)	Elemental Fe (%)	Dose (mg)	Fe content (mg)
Ferrous sulfate (FeoSol®, Fer-in-Sol®)	20	325	65
Ferrous gluconate (Fergon®)	12	300	35
Ferrous fumarate (Femiron®, Fumerin®, Feostat®)	33	300	99

(Food can decrease the absorption of iron by 50%.) Take with orange juice if possible (can double absorption).

- Keep out of reach of children. Iron is a major cause of ingestion deaths in children.

- Take iron 1 hour before or 3 hours after any antacids.

- There are medications that interact with iron. Please ask your physician or pharmacist before taking any new medications in combination with iron.

- You may take OTC docusate if constipation occurs.

Adverse drug effects
- The oral formulation has primarily GI effects:
  * Dark colored stools
  * Constipation or diarrhea
  * Nausea and/or vomiting

- IV formulations:
  * Injection site reactions
  * GI: diarrhea, nausea
  * Hypotension
  * Allergic reactions, including anaphylaxis
    • The risk of anaphylaxis is greatest with iron dextran. The patient must be administered a test dose before using this agent.

Drug interactions
- Antibiotics (tetracycline, quinolones): iron binds to these antibiotics, preventing their absorption.

- Antacids: iron needs an acidic environment for optimal absorption.

Monitoring parameters
- Is there an increase in reticulocytes, Hgb, and Hct?

- Tolerability of iron (will influence compliance)

- Is patient symptomatically improving?

Kinetics
- Bioavailability is increased in acidic environment and decreased by food.

Megaloblastic Anemias

- Vitamin B_{12} should be administered orally if absorption is not an issue.
  * Dose: 1-10 μg/d

- Vitamin B_{12} deficiency is usually corrected through

IM vitamin B_{12} (cyanocobalamin) supplementation as follows (pernicious anemia):
  * 1000 μg IM every day for 1 week, then
  * 100-1000 μg IM every week for 4 weeks, then
  * 100-1000 μg IM every month thereafter for prevention
  * In patients with pernicious anemia, oral B_{12} is poorly absorbed, but may be supplemented orally in very high doses, such as 1000-2000 μg per day.

Mechanism of action
- Vitamin B_{12} supplementation allows for normal synthesis of the RNA/DNA involved in the synthesis of RBCs.

Patient instructions
- Counsel patient or family member(s) on sterile injection techniques and needle disposal if injections are given at home.

Adverse drug effects
- Increased synthesis of reticulocytes can cause hyperuricemia or hypokalemia.

- Sodium retention

- Increased synthesis of RBCs can produce an expansion of the intravascular volume, which can increase cardiac output causing angina or dyspnea.

- Itching: 1-10%

- Diarrhea: 1-10%

- Anaphylaxis: <1%

Monitoring parameters
- Monitor CBC. Is there an increase in Hgb?

- Is patient symptomatically improving (especially neurologic symptoms, if present)?

- Potassium level

Kinetics
- Absorption: intrinsic factor must be present for vitamin B_{12} to be transported across GI mucosa.

- Vitamin B_{12} is bound in blood to transcobalamin II and converted in tissues to active coenzymes methylcobalamin and deoxyadenosylcobalamin.

Folic Acid Deficiency Anemia

- Folic acid deficiency anemia is corrected by supplementing folic acid 1 mg qd for 3-4 months. Once the underlying cause of deficiency is corrected, folic acid may be discontinued. Long-term folate administration is necessary if the cause is not corrected, such as in hemodialysis or alcoholism.

Mechanism of action
- Folic acid supplementation allows for normal synthesis of the RNA and DNA involved in the synthesis of RBCs.

Patient instructions
- Stress compliance with regimen.

- Women of childbearing age should be counseled to take a multivitamin containing folic acid regardless if an anemia is present or not.

Adverse drug effects
- Less than 1% of patients have allergic reactions to folic acid.

Drug interactions
- Folic acid may increase phenytoin metabolism.

- Phenytoin, primidone, sulfasalazine, para-aminosalicylic acid, and oral contraceptives may decrease folic acid concentrations.

- Chloramphenicol may blunt response to folic acid.

Monitoring parameters
- Is the RBC morphology normalizing?

- Are the Hbg and Hct normalizing?

- Monitor patient compliance.

Kinetics
- Folic acid is a water-soluble B vitamin absorbed in the small intestine with C_{max} at $^{1}/_{2}$-1 hour.

Anemia of Renal Failure

Recombinant human erythropoietin
- Since the primary cause of anemia in renal failure is decreased (EPO) synthesis, the drug of choice for this type of anemia is recombinant human EPO (epoetin alfa, trade names Procrit® or Epogen®).

- Epoetin is indicated in the treatment of anemia associated with chronic renal failure, including dialysis and non-dialysis patients. It is indicated to elevate or maintain the RBCs and to decrease the need for transfusions in these patients. (Non-dialysis patients with symptomatic anemia considered for therapy should have a hematocrit less than 30%.) The National Kidney Foundation-Kidney Disease Outcomes Quality Initiative Guidelines (NKF-K/DOQI guidelines) recommend that epoetin be administered SQ, since this route of administration is as effective (or more effective) than IV. However, epoetin is often administered IV in patients on dialysis, since there is easy access through the dialysis port.

Mechanism of action
- Human recombinant erythropoietin stimulates erythropoiesis (increased RBC production).

Patient instructions
- Do not shake the vial because the epoetin may break down, decreasing effectiveness.

- Store in refrigerator, but do not freeze. Keep out of direct sunlight.

- Make sure that the solution in vial is clear and free of particulate matter. Do not use if solution is cloudy or frothy.

- Monitor your blood pressure at home and alert your physician of any significant increases in blood pressure.

- Single-use vials are intended to be used only once. Discard any remaining solution and vial. If the label is marked with an M, it is a multi-dose vial, and it may be stored in the refrigerator for 21 days.

- It is very important that you take your blood pressure medications exactly as prescribed while on this medication, and maintain a sodium-restricted diet.

- Avoid hazardous activity in the first 90 days of therapy (eg, operating heavy machinery).

- Educate the patient about the possibility of allergic reactions:
  * Local reaction (swelling, itching, redness); inform MD if any of these occur.
  * Anaphylactic reaction (shortness of breath, wheezing, low blood pressure, rapid heart rate, sweating). If any of these occur, discontinue use immediately and call 911.

- Patient should be instructed on correct sterile injection technique and needle disposal as described in Figure 1.

Figure 1.

Instructions for self-administering epoetin alfa.

Preparing the dose

1. Wash your hands thoroughly with soap and water before preparing the medication.

2. Check the date on the epoetin alfa vial to be sure that the drug has not expired.

3. Remove the vial of epoetin alfa from the refrigerator and allow it to reach room temperature. **Each epoetin alfa vial is designed to be used only once: do not re-enter the vial.** It is not necessary to shake epoetin alfa. Prolonged vigorous shaking may damage the product. Assemble the other supplies you will need for your injection.

4. Hemodialysis patients should wipe off the venous port of the hemodialysis tubing with an antiseptic swab. Peritoneal dialysis patients should cleanse the skin with an antiseptic swab where the injection is to be made.

5. Flip off the red protective cap but do not remove the gray rubber stopper. Wipe the top of the gray rubber stopper with an antiseptic swab.

6. Using a syringe and needle designed for subcutaneous injection, draw air into the syringe by pulling back on the plunger. The amount of air should be equal to your epoetin alfa dose.

7. Carefully remove the needle cover. Put the needle through the gray rubber stopper of the epoetin alfa vial.

8. Push the plunger in to discharge air into the vial. The air injected into the vial will allow epoetin alfa to be easily withdrawn into the syringe.

9. Turn the vial and syringe upside down in one hand. Be sure the tip of the needle is in the epoetin alfa solution. Your other hand will be free to move the plunger. Draw back on the plunger slowly to draw the correct dose of epoetin alfa into the syringe.

10. Check for air bubbles. The air is harmless, but too large an air bubble will reduce the epoetin alfa dose. To remove air bubbles, gently tap the syringe to move the air bubbles to the top of the syringe, then use the plunger to push the solution and the air back into the vial. Then re-measure your correct dose of epoetin alfa.

11. Double-check your dose. Remove the needle from the vial. Do not lay the syringe down or allow the needle to touch anything.

Injecting the dose
Patients on home hemodialysis using the intravenous injection route:

1. Insert the needle of the syringe into the previously cleansed venous port and inject the epoetin alfa.

2. Remove the syringe and dispose of the whole unit. Use the disposable syringe only once. Dispose of syringes and needles as directed by your doctor, by following these simple steps:

- Place all used needles and syringes in a hard plastic container with a screw-on cap, or a metal container with a plastic lid, such as a coffee can properly labeled as to contents. If a metal container is used, cut a small hole in the plastic lid and tape the lid to the metal container. If a hard plastic container is used, always screw the cap on tightly after each use. When the container is full, tape around the cap or lid, and dispose of it according to your doctor's instructions.
- Do not use glass or clear plastic containers, or any container that will be recycled or returned to a store.
- Always store the container out of the reach of children.
- Please check with your doctor, nurse, or pharmacist for other suggestions. There may be special state and local laws that they will discuss with you.

Figure 1. (continued)

Instructions for self-administering epoetin alfa.

Patients on home peritoneal dialysis or home hemodialysis using the subcutaneous route:

1. With one hand, stabilize the previously cleansed skin by spreading it or by pinching up a large area with your free hand.

2. Hold the syringe with the other hand, as you would a pencil. Double check that the correct amount of epoetin alfa is in the syringe. Insert the needle straight into the skin at a 90° angle. Pull the plunger back slightly. If blood comes into the syringe, do not inject epoetin alfa, as the needle has entered a blood vessel; withdraw the syringe and inject at a different site. Inject the epoetin alfa by pushing the plunger all the way down.

3. Hold an antiseptic swab near the needle and pull the needle straight out of the skin. Press the antiseptic swab over the injection site for several seconds. Use the disposable syringe only once.

4. Use the disposable syringe only once. Dispose of syringes and needles as directed in the instructions at left, under step 2.

5. Always change the site for each injection as directed. Occasionally a problem may develop at the injection site. If you notice a lump, swelling, or bruising that does not go away, contact your doctor. You may wish to record the site you just used so you can keep track.

Reproduced with permission from Procrit® package insert. Raritan, NJ: Ortho Biotech Products, LP; 2000.

Adverse drug effects (Table 2)

- Immunogenicity: pure red cell aplasia (PRCA), in association with neutralizing antibodies to native erythropoietin, has been reported rarely in the literature. If this is suspected, epoetin should be discontinued immediately.

- The most common adverse effect is elevated blood pressure. Epoetin is contraindicated in patients with **uncontrolled** hypertension.

Drug interactions

- No drug interactions have been reported.

Monitoring parameters

- Prior to initiation of therapy, the patient's iron stores should be evaluated. Transferrin saturation should be at least 20% and ferritin at least 100 ng/mL.

- Monitor Hct very closely. Once Hct approaches 36% or Hct increases more than 4 points in a 2-week period, the dose of epoetin should be decreased. Dose should be increased if Hct has not increased 5-6 points in 8 weeks, and is not in target Hct range of 30-36%.

Table 2

Percentage of Patients Reporting Adverse Effects of Epoetin Alfa

Event	Patients treated with epoetin alfa (n = 200)	Patients on placebo (n = 135)
Hypertension	24%	19%
Headache	16%	12%
Arthralgias	11%	6%
Nausea	11%	9%
Edema	9%	10%
Fatigue	9%	14%
Vomiting	8%	5%
Chest pain	7%	9%
Skin reaction at site of administration	7%	12%
Asthenia	7%	12%
Dizziness	7%	13%
Clotted access	7%	2%

Significant adverse events of concern in patients with CRF treated in double-blind, placebo-controlled trials occurred in the percentages of patients shown below during the blinded phase of the studies.

Seizure	1.1%	1.1%
CVA/TIA	0.4%	0.6%
MI	0.4%	1.1%
Death	0	1.7%

CVA/TIA, cerebrovascular accident/transient ischemic attack; MI, myocardial infarction.

Reproduced with permission from Procrit® package insert. Raritan, NJ: Ortho Biotech Products, LP; 2000.

- Blood pressure should be adequately controlled prior to initiation of epoetin alfa therapy, and must be closely monitored and controlled during therapy.

- Serum chemistries

Kinetics
- Half life: ~4-13 hours

- There is no apparent difference in half-life between patients not on dialysis with Scr >3 and patients requiring dialysis.

Other
- Initial starting dose IV or SQ is 50-100 U/kg three times weekly. Thereafter, the maintenance dose is titrated to maintain a Hct of 30-36%.

Darbepoetin
Mechanism of action
- Darbepoetin has the same MOA as epoetin.

Patient instructions
- Counseling points are very similar with darbepoetin and epoetin, except that all vials are for single-use only, so dispose of vial as instructed after each dose.

Adverse drug effects
- The most common adverse effects are:
    * CV: hypertension, hypotension, edema, arrhythmia
    * GI: nausea, vomiting, diarrhea, constipation
    * CNS: fatigue, fever, headache
    * Neuromuscular/skeletal: myalgia, arthralgia, limb pain
    * Respiratory: infection, dyspnea, cough

Drug interactions
- No drug interactions have been reported.

Monitoring parameters
- Iron stores prior to and during therapy

- Blood pressure

- Dose is adjusted by closely monitoring Hgb every week until maintenance dose is established. Target Hgb is 12g/dL.
    * Increase dose if Hbg increase is <1 g/dL over 4 weeks.
    * Decrease dose by 25% if Hbg increase is >1 g/dL over 2 weeks.

Kinetics
- Half-life: IV, 21 hours; SC, 49 hours

- Half-life is approximately three times longer than that of epoetin.

Other
- Initial dose: 0.45 µg/kg once weekly. Thereafter, dose is titrated to maintain Hbg of 12 g/dL. Some patients will require <0.45 µg/kg, so in these patients, dosing will be only once every 2 weeks. Less frequent dosing is the advantage of darbepoetin over epoetin.

3. Nondrug Therapy

Iron Deficiency Anemia

Dietary supplementation
- Increase intake of iron-rich foods, such as meat, fish, and poultry.

- Drink orange juice with meals when possible.

- Limit tea or milk with meals. Only use in moderation between meals.

Megaloblastic Anemias

Folic acid deficiency
- In order to get as much dietary folate as possible, do not overcook vegetables. Eat them raw or steamed. Eat a wide variety of properly prepared vegetables, fruits, and mushrooms.

4. Key Points

- Anemia is a reduction in red cell mass, which decreases the oxygen-carrying capacity of the blood.

- Iron deficiency anemia is the most common anemia, accounting for 25% of all cases. IDA presents as a microcytic, hypochromic anemia.

- Iron preparations are best absorbed on an empty stomach.

- Iron preparations are hard to tolerate due to numerous GI effects, and this may necessitate administration with a small snack.

- Megaloblastic anemias are macrocytic and are the result of a folic acid or vitamin B_{12} deficiency.

- Vitamin B_{12} requires intrinsic factor to be absorbed. Patients deficient in intrinsic factor develop pernicious anemia.

- Due to the difficulties with the absorption of vitamin B_{12} in many patients, it is often administered via an IM injection.

- The primary reason that patients with renal failure are anemic is due the lack of production of erythropoietin (EPO).

- Anemia of renal failure is treated with SC or IV epoetin.

- Patients receiving epoetin must have their Hct and blood pressures routinely monitored.

- Darbepoetin has the same mechanism of action as epoetin, but is longer acting, and so can be administered less frequently.

5. Questions and Answers

Patient Profile #1: SuperPrice Drug Store Profile

G.M. McBeavy
1040 Dauberson Avenue
Jesup, IA 50648
319-555-6248

DOB: 7/11/52
Allergies: NKDA
Weight: 193 pounds

Problem List:
Gastroesophageal reflux disease
Iron deficiency anemia
Hypertension

Medication Record:
Ferrous sulfate 325 mg tid
Hydrochlorothiazide 25 mg qd

OTCs Recommended:
Maalox® 1 tbsp q2h prn for "indigestion"
Acetaminophen 325 mg q4-6h prn for headache
Ranitidine 75 mg qd prn for "heartburn"
Docusate 100 mg qd for constipation

Use Patient Profile #1 to answer Questions 1-5.

1. Which OTC medication could present a problem with Mr. McBeevy's iron supplement?

   A. Acetaminophen
   B. Ranitidine
   C. Maalox
   D. Docusate
   E. None of the above

2. Mr. McBeevy admits to you that he is not able to take his iron tablet because it makes him nauseated. What advice can you give him?

   A. Take your iron with some crackers and milk.
   B. Take your iron with some crackers and water.
   C. Don't worry about it. It's only a vitamin.
   D. Start taking your iron with the largest meal of the day.
   E. Take your iron after breakfast.

3. If Mr. McBeevy's IDA progresses to severe stages, what effects may he experience?

   A. Koilonychia (spooning of the nails)
   B. Pica (eg, craving ice, clay, chalk)
   C. Glossitis (Sore, beefy red tongue)
   D. Extreme fatigue
   E. All of the above

4. If you were to examine Mr. McBeevy's blood smear, you would find cells that are:

   A. Microcytic and hypochromic
   B. Macrocytic and hypochromic
   C. Macrocytic and normochromic
   D. Microcytic and normochromic
   E. Any of the above are possible.

5. When examining Mr. McBeevy's iron study results, which of the following would be consistent with IDA?

   A. Elevated TIBC
   B. Elevated ferritin
   C. Elevated MCV
   D. Elevated hemoglobin
   E. Elevated hematocrit

6. Which iron preparation is the most likely to cause an anaphylactic reaction?

   A. IV iron dextran
   B. IV iron sucrose
   C. IV sodium ferric gluconate
   D. PO extended-release ferrous sulfate
   E. PO immediate-release ferrous sulfate

7. Why would the sustained-release (SR) preparations of iron not be the ideal formulation?

   A. The incidence of nausea is higher with the SR formulations.
   B. They are only dosed once daily, and goal Hct levels are not attained.
   C. Since SR preparations are dissolved in the small intestines, the alkaline environment would result in a lower bioavailability than would the acidic environment of the stomach.
   D. Dissolution in the small intestines would not be bioavailable, because intrinsic factor is not present in the small intestines.
   E. They require dosing with food.

8. To optimize iron absorption from meals, which would you advise a patient to drink with his meals?

   A. Orange juice
   B. Coffee
   C. Tea

D. Milk
E. Soft drinks

9. The most likely regimen to replace vitamin B$_{12}$ would be:

    A. 1000 µg PO every month
    B. 1000 µg IV every month
    C. 1000 µg IM every month
    D. 1000 µg IM every day
    E. Any of the above are reasonable regimens.

10. Vitamin B$_{12}$ requires the following to be absorbed:

    A. Pernicious factor
    B. Transcobalamin II
    C. Intrinsic factor
    D. Vitamin B$_{12}$ absorption factor
    E. All of the above

11. Folic acid deficiency could be found in all of the following EXCEPT:

    A. Strict vegetarians
    B. Alcoholics
    C. The indigent
    D. People who routinely overcook their vegetables
    E. A college student whose diet consists of only burgers and potato chips

12. Folic acid may interact with the following medication:

    A. Propranolol
    B. Propoxyphene
    C. Piroxicam
    D. Phenytoin
    E. Prednisone

13. The two macrocytic anemias are:

    A. Vitamin B$_{12}$ deficiency and iron deficiency anemias
    B. Vitamin B$_{12}$ deficiency and folic acid deficiency anemias
    C. Iron deficiency and folic acid deficiency anemias
    D. Sickle cell anemia and anemia of renal failure
    E. Iron deficiency and pernicious anemias

14. The best regimen to replace folic acid would be:

    A. Folic acid 1 mg PO every day for 3-4 months

B. Folic acid 10 mg PO. every day for 3-4 months
C. Folic acid 10 mg IV for 2 weeks, then 1 mg PO every day for 2 months
D. Folic acid 1 mg PO three times weekly for 3-4 months
E. Folic acid 1 mg IM once monthly for 6 months

15. The most common medication given to treat anemia of renal failure is:

    A. Vitamin B$_{12}$
    B. Solution of citric acid in combination with sodium acetate
    C. Epoetin
    D. PO ferrous sulfate
    E. PO folic acid

16. What advantage does darbepoetin have over epoetin?

    A. Lower incidence of hypertension
    B. Fewer drug interactions
    C. Lower cost
    D. Longer half-life and less frequent administration
    E. Improved tolerability

17. The most common side effect of epoetin is:

    A. Anaphylaxis
    B. Hypertension
    C. Pure red cell aplasia
    D. Injection site reaction
    E. Weight gain

18. The initial dose of epoetin is:

    A. 50-100 U/kg three times weekly SC or IV
    B. 50-100 U/kg once weekly SC or IV
    C. 100 U/kg once weekly SC or IV
    D. 50-100 U/kg three times weekly IV
    E. 100 U/kg once monthly IV

19. Prior to beginning epoetin therapy, which of the following should be evaluated?

    A. Folic acid and vitamin B$_{12}$ levels
    B. Transferrin and ferritin levels
    C. Erythropoietin receptor level
    D. Presence or absence of intrinsic factor
    E. All of the above

20. In which of the following patients would it be possible to teach self-administration of epoetin at home?

I. A patient on home hemodialysis taking epoetin via the IV route
II. A patient on home peritoneal dialysis taking epoetin via the SQ route
III. A patient on home hemodialysis taking epoetin via the SQ route

    A. II only
    B. II and III only
    C. III only
    D. I, II, and III
    E. I only

Patient Profile #2: Central Dialysis Center

R.S. Wiley
1460 Sawyer Brown Rd
Reidsville, NC 27320
336-555-0001

Allergies: Penicillin (rash)
Weight: 148 pounds
Dialysis schedule: Monday, Wednesday, Friday

Diagnosis:
Hypertension
Diabetes mellitus
End-stage renal disease
Hyperlipidemia

Medications:
Insulin NPH 30 U bid
Simvastatin 20 mg qhs
Atenolol 25 mg after dialysis
Nephrocaps 1 capsule qd

Use Patient Profile #2 to answer Questions 21-24.

21. Which of the following will be monitored upon starting epoetin therapy in Mrs. Wiley?

    A. Blood pressure
    B. Hematocrit
    C. Serum chemistries
    D. Iron profile
    E. All of the above

22. The target hematocrit range for Mrs. Wiley is:
    A. 30-36%
    B. 29-38%
    C. 30-32%
    D. 26-34%

    E. 40-45%

23. Which of Mrs. Wiley's medications will interact with epoetin?

    A. Insulin
    B. Simvastatin
    C. Atenolol
    D. None of the above
    E. All of the above

24. What medication should be added Mrs. Wiley's regimen?

    A. Oral propranolol
    B. IV iron
    C. Oral levothyroxine
    D. IM vitamin B_{12}
    E. No additional medications are required at this time

Answers

1. **C.** Iron is best absorbed in an acidic environment. Therefore antacids dramatically decrease the absorption of iron. They should be taken 1 hour before or 3 hours after antacids.

2. **B.** Many patients are not able to tolerate iron on an empty stomach. Tell those patients to take iron with a small snack. Milk would not be acceptable in this case, because dairy products decrease the absorption or iron.

3. **E.** Koilonychia, pica, extreme fatigue, and glossitis are all symptoms of severe iron deficiency anemia.

4. **A.** Iron deficiency produces a hypochromic (low-hemoglobin) anemia, given iron is a component of the hemoglobin molecule. The cells are also microcytic (meaning "small cell") because they spend longer in the marrow awaiting proper hemoglobin synthesis, and are therefore smaller.

5. **A.** Total iron-binding capacity, TIBC, is elevated in IDA. TIBC is a measure of the amount of binding space left on transferrin (the transport protein of iron). Less iron in the blood translates into more space available on the transferrin molecule.

6. **A.** IV iron dextran has the highest incidence of anaphylaxis among the three IV iron preparations available.

7. **C.** SR preparations are left intact in the stomach, and are dissolved in the small intestine. The alkaline environment of the small intestine tends to form insoluble iron complexes that cannot be absorbed.

8. **A.** Tea and milk can decrease the absorption of iron from a meal by over 50%. Orange juice, however, can double the absorption of iron from food.

9. **C.** The most common IM dose of vitamin B_{12} is 1000 μg per month. However, vitamin B_{12} may be supplemented by the oral route if absorption is not impaired. Additionally, it may be supplemented in very high doses, such as 1000-2000 μg per day in pernicious anemia.

10. **C.** Vitamin B_{12} requires intrinsic factor to be absorbed.

11. **A.** Folic acid deficiency is found in alcoholics, the indigent, and rarely in people who routinely overcook their vegetables. Strict vegetarians do not develop folic acid deficiency because a folate-rich diet includes various types of vegetables.

12. **D.** Phenytoin increases the metabolism of folate, thereby decreasing its effectiveness.

13. **B.** Vitamin B_{12} deficiency and folic acid anemias are both macrocytic (large cell) anemias. Iron deficiency anemia and sickle cell anemia are both microcytic and hypochromic anemias.

14. **A.** Folic acid is administered PO because there is no problem with absorption. The dose of folic acid is 1 mg PO every day, and the deficiency should be corrected in 3-4 months.

15. **C.** Epoetin is the most common medication to treat anemia of renal failure, because it stimulates erythropoiesis. The lack of erythropoietin production is the primary cause of anemia of renal failure.

16. **D.** Darbepoetin is very similar to epoetin, having the same mechanism of action and similar side effects. It does have a longer half-life and can be administered less frequently.

17. **B.** Hypertension is the most common adverse drug effect from epoetin.

18. **A.** The initial dose of epoetin is 50-100 U/kg three times weekly. This can be given via either the SC or IV route.

19. **B.** Transferrin and ferritin levels should be evaluated prior to epoetin therapy. IDA is a common problem in patients with end-stage renal disease. The transferrin should be at least 20% and ferritin should be at least 100 ng/mL prior to beginning epoetin therapy.

20. **D.** Patients on home peritoneal dialysis or hemodialysis can be taught to self-administer SQ injections. Additionally, if patients are receiving home hemodialysis, they can be taught to give their epoetin IV through the dialysis venous port.

21. **E.** Iron profiles need to be monitored prior to epoetin and periodically during therapy, since IDA is very common in dialysis patients. Blood pressure needs to be monitored, given this is the most common adverse effect of epoetin. The Hct needs to be checked as a measure of response to epoetin, and needs to be maintained at a level of 30-36%. Serum chemistries need to be monitored regularly in any patient with end-stage renal disease, since most electrolytes are regulated by the kidney.

22. **A.** The target range of Hct for patients receiving epoetin is 30-36%.

23. **D.** There are no known drug interactions with epoetin.

24. **B.** Mrs. Wiley's ferritin is below 100 ng/mL and her transferrin is below 20%. Most hemodialysis patients receiving epoetin will need iron therapy during their treatment at some point in time.

6. References

Denberg CV, O'Bryant C. Anemias. In: Young LY, Koda-Kimble MA, eds. *Applied Therapeutics: The Clinical Use of Drugs*. Vancouver, WA: Applied Therapeutics, Inc.; 2001:84.1-84.19.

Eschbach JW, Abdulhadi MH, Browne JK, et al. Recombinant human erythropoietin in anemic patients with end-stage renal disease. Results of a phase III multcenter clinical trial. *Ann Intern Med*. 1989;111:992.

Fishbane S. Safety in iron management. *Am J Kid Dis*. 2003;41:S18-S26.

National Kidney Foundation: K/DOQI Clinical Practice Guidelines for Anemia of Chronic Kidney Disease, 2000. *Am J Kidney Dis*. 2001;37(suppl 1):S182-S238.

Parker KP, Mitch WE, Stivelman JC, et al. Safety and efficacy of low-dose subcutaneous erythropoietin in hemodialysis patients. *J Am Soc Nephrol*. 1999;8:288.

Procrit package insert. Raritan, New Jersey: Ortho Biotech Products, LP; 2000.

Stumpf JL, Townsend KA. Other anemias. In: Herfindal ET, Gourley DR, eds. *Textbook of Therapeutics: Drug and Disease Management*. Baltimore, MA: Lippincott Williams & Wilkins; 2000:237-260.

Teresi M. Iron deficiency and megaloblastic anemias. In: Herfindal ET, Gourley DR, eds. *Textbook of Therapeutics: Drug and Disease Management*. Baltimore, MA: Lippincott Williams & Wilkins; 2000:213-236.

The rationale for treating iron deficiency anemia. *Arch Intern Med*. 1984;144:471.

37. Thromboembolic Disorders

Gale L. Hamann, PharmD, BCPS, CDE
Associate Professor, Department of Pharmacy
University of Tennessee College of Pharmacy
Clinical Specialist, Ambulatory Care
Regional Medical Center at Memphis

Contents

1. Venous Thromboembolic Disease

Definition/Epidemiology

• Venous thromboembolism (VTE) is a disease process that involves the development of deep vein thrombosis (DVT) and/or a pulmonary embolism (PE).

• Pulmonary embolism is a thrombus or foreign substance from the systemic circulation that lodges in the pulmonary artery or its branches and causes a complete or partial occlusion of pulmonary blood flow.

• Deep vein thrombosis is a thrombus that forms most commonly in the popliteal or femoral veins, veins of the calf, or the iliac veins of the upper leg. Veins of the upper extremities are less commonly involved.

• Approximately two million Americans develop VTE each year; 600,000 people in this group have VTE manifested as a PE, and of these, 60,000 die. It is estimated that one million Americans will develop a clinically silent PE that goes undiagnosed. Complications of VTE are postphlebitic syndrome and pulmonary hypertension. Postphlebitic syndrome is characterized as swelling in the affected lower extremity after a DVT. Pulmonary hypertension is a complication that can occur after a PE.

• The incidence of VTE increases with age and doubles in each decade of life after age 50.

• It is estimated that VTE costs 1.5 billion dollars annually.

Clinical Presentation

• The most common symptoms of a PE are dyspnea, cough, hemoptysis, tachypnea, tachycardia, pleuritic chest pain, diaphoresis, and overwhelming anxiety. The patient may be cyanotic and hypoxemic secondary to having a reduced ability to oxygenate the blood. Patients with a massive PE may present with syncope. The mortality rate of a PE ranges from 2.3% to 17%.

• The most common symptoms of a DVT are pain, tenderness, edema, and erythema of the affected extremity. Other symptoms may include dilation of the superficial veins, a palpable cord, and a positive Homan's sign.

Pathophysiology

• Venous thrombi generally form in areas of the veins where blood flow is slowed or disrupted. Often they begin as small thrombi in the large venous sinuses of a valve cusp pocket in the veins of the calf or thigh. Trauma to the vessel causes the release of tissue factor. Tissue factor in turn activates the coagulation cascade. This results in the formation of thrombin and ultimately the formation of fibrin to form clots. Other common factors that can precipitate the development of a thrombus include disrupted blood flow from immobility, or hypercoagulability (Table 1).

• A PE is the result of a dislodged thrombus that is embolized from a thrombus in the deep venous structures of the legs, pelvis, or arms. The embolus travels to the lungs where it is trapped in the pulmonary arterial microvasculature. Blood flow is obstructed from the PE, which leads to lung edema and reduced pulmonary compliance. This results in inadequate oxygen exchange leading to hypoxemia. Blood flow in the pulmonary artery increases right ventricular afterload that may lead to right ventricular dilation, dysfunction, and ischemia.

Table 1

Risk Factors for VTE

• Age over 40 years
• Prolonged immobility
• Major surgery involving the abdomen, pelvis, and lower extremities
• Trauma, especially fractures of the hips, pelvis, and lower extremities
• Malignancy
• Pregnancy
• Previous venous thromboembolism
• Congestive heart failure or cardiomyopathy
• Stroke
• Acute myocardial infarction
• Indwelling central venous catheter
• Hypercoagulability
• Estrogen therapy
• Varicose veins
• Obesity
• Inflammatory bowel disease
• Nephrotic syndrome
• Myeloproliferative disease

Diagnosis

- DVT is diagnosed based on a detailed history and clinical symptoms. A duplex ultrasound, which measures both blood flow and compressibility of the affected vessel, confirms the diagnosis.

- PE is diagnosed based on a detailed history and clinical symptoms. A ventilation-perfusion scan or spiral CT confirms the diagnosis.

VTE Prophylaxis

- See Table 2

VTE Treatment

- VTE treatment success with unfractionated heparin (UFH) is related to obtaining therapeutic APTT levels as rapidly as possible (Table 3). Studies have indicated that the VTE recurrence risk is 20% to 25% higher if activated partial thromboplastin time (APTT) levels are not >1.5 times control, or mean normal. This corresponds to a heparin level of 0.2 international units (IU)/mL.

- The use of low-molecular-weight heparin (LMWH) has enabled the treatment of a DVT to move from a 5- to 7-day hospitalization to either a 1- or 2-day hospital stay, or to the outpatient management of a DVT (Table 4).

- With outpatient DVT treatment the diagnosis may take place in either a physician's office or the emergency department. After the diagnosis of a DVT is confirmed by a Doppler ultrasound, the patient is educated on administration of LMWH, and patients receive their first dose of LMWH at that time. After these steps, administer LMWH and warfarin on an outpatient basis. Warfarin is monitored with an International Normalized Ratio (INR) at 1- to 2-day intervals. After two therapeutic INRs, the LMWH may be discontinued and warfarin continued for 3–6 months, or as indicated (see Table 5).

Drug Therapy

Unfractionated heparin (UFH)
Mechanism of action
- UFH binds to antithrombin (AT) and converts it from a slow progressive thrombin inhibitor to a rapid thrombin inhibitor. This in turn catalyzes inactivation of factors XIIa, XIa, IXa, Xa, and IIa (thrombin).

Patient counseling
- Patients need to monitor for signs and symptoms of bleeding or bruising, especially at surgical sites.

Therapeutic use
- Prevention and treatment of VTE

- Prevention of VTE in patients with a previous VTE or a known hypercoagulability

- Prophylaxis for VTE in high-risk populations

- Prevention of a mural thrombosis after myocardial infarction (MI)

- Treatment of patients with unstable angina and MI

- Prevent acute thrombosis after coronary thrombolysis

Parameters to monitor
- Heparin is monitored by an APTT, which is sensitive to the inhibitory effects of heparin on factors IIa (thrombin), Xa, and IXa.

- An APTT therapeutic range is based on a calibration against a plasma heparin concentration of 0.2–0.4 U/mL by protamine titration or 0.3–0.7 U/mL based on an anti-factor Xa concentration.

- An APTT should be measured 6 hours after a bolus dose of heparin or after any dosage change, then every 6 hours until a therapeutic APTT is reached. Once a therapeutic APTT is achieved, an APTT may be evaluated every 24 hours.

- Platelet count and hematocrit should be evaluated at baseline and every 3–5 days.

Pharmacokinetics
- The pharmacokinetics of heparin differs based on an intravenous or subcutaneous route of administration.

- Heparin is cleared from the body by a rapid saturable mechanism that occurs at therapeutic doses. A second slower unsaturable first-order clearance that is largely by renal means occurs at high doses.

- The half-life of heparin varies from approximately 30 minutes after an IV bolus of 25 U/kg to 60 minutes after an IV bolus at 100 U/kg.

Dosing
- Heparin should be dosed using a weight-based nomogram. A heparin concentration of 0.2–0.4 IU/mL based on protamine titration, or an anti-factor

Table 2

Recommendations for VTE Prophylaxis

Medical Condition	Recommended Therapy
General medical	
• General medical patients with risk factors	LDUH, LMWH
• Acute MI	LDUH, IV UFH
• Ischemic stroke	LDUH, LMWH; if anticoagulation prophylaxis is contraindicated, ES or IPC
General surgery	
Low-risk	Early ambulation
• Low-risk procedure, <40 years of age	
Moderate-risk	LDUH, LMWH, ES, or IPC
• General surgery, minor procedure with additional risk factors	
• Nonmajor procedure, age 40–60 with no additional risk factors	
• Major surgical procedure, age <40, no additional risk factors	
Higher-risk	LDUH, LMWH, IPC; if high risk of bleeding, use mechanical prophylaxis with ES or IPC
• Nonmajor surgery, age >60, with or with risk factors	
• Major surgery, age >40, with or with risk factors	
Very-high risk	LDUH or LMWH combined with ES or IPC
• Major surgery with multiple risk factors	
Gynecologic surgery	
• Brief procedure with benign disease	Early ambulation
• Major surgery for benign disease without risk factors	LDUH bid, LMWH once daily, or IPC
• Major surgery for malignancy	LDUH tid, LDUH plus ES, IPC or higher doses of LMWH
Urologic surgery	
• Transurethral or low-risk procedure	Early ambulation
• Major or open urologic procedure	LDUH, ES, IPC, or LMWH
• Highest-risk patients	ES with or without IPC added to LDUH or LMWH
Elective total hip replacement (THR)	LMWH, fondaparinux, or warfarin
Elective total knee replacement (TKR)	LMWH, fondaparinux, or warfarin; IPC is alternative option
Hip fracture surgery	LMWH, warfarin, fondaparinux, or LDUH
Neurosurgery	IPC ± ES, LDUH or LMWH when risk of bleeding resolved
Trauma	LMWH, IPC or ES if bleeding concerns
Acute spinal cord injury	LMWH ± IPC or ES, convert to warfarin

ES, elastic (graduated compression) stocking; fondaparinux, 2.5 mg SC q 24 hours; INR, International Normalized Ratio; IPC, intermittent pneumatic compression device; LDUH, low-dose unfractionated heparin, 5000 U SC q 8–12 hours; UFH, unfractionated heparin; warfarin, target INR 2.5, range 2.0–3.0.

LMWH, low-molecular-weight heparin:

    Enoxaparin 30 mg SC q 12 hours

    Enoxaparin 40 mg SC q 24 hours

    Dalteparin 5,000 units SC q 24 hours

The optimal duration of anticoagulation prophylaxis after TKR or THR surgery is unknown, although at least 7–10 days of prophylaxis is recommended, and extended out-of-hospital LMWH prophylaxis may reduce the incidence of clinically significant VTE for high-risk patients.

Reprinted with permission from Hirsh J, Dalen JE, Guyatt G. The Sixth (2000) ACCP Guidelines for Antithrombotic Therapy for Prevention and Treatment of Thrombosis. *Chest* 2000;119:1S–2S.

Table 3

**Guidelines for Anticoagulation:
IV Unfractionated Heparin[1]**

Indication	Guidelines
VTE suspected	• Obtain baseline APTT, PT, and CBC count • Check for contraindications to heparin therapy • Order imaging study; consider giving heparin 5,000 IU IV
VTE confirmed	• Rebolus with heparin 80 IU/kg IV and start maintenance infusion at 18 IU/kg • Check APTT at 6 hours to keep APTT in a range that corresponds to a therapeutic blood heparin level • Check platelet count between days 3–5 • Start warfarin therapy on day 1 at 5 mg and adjust subsequent daily dose according to INR • Stop heparin after at least 4–5 days of combined therapy when INR is >2 .0 • Anticoagulate with warfarin for at least 3 months at an INR of 2.5; range 2.0–3.0

[1] For treatment with UFH, give 250 IU/kg SC q 12 hours to obtain a therapeutic APTT at 6–8 hours.
APTT, activated partial thromboplastin time; CBC, complete blood cell count; INR, International Normalized Ratio; PT, prothrombin time.
Reprinted with permission from Hirsh J, Dalen JE, Guyatt G. The Sixth (2000) ACCP Guidelines for Antithrombotic Therapy for Prevention and Treatment of Thrombosis. *Chest* 2000;119:1S–2S.

Xa chromogenic assay of 0.3–0.7 U/mL determines the therapeutic APTT range.

• Weight-based dosing nomograms are effective in achieving a therapeutic APTT, although these are not universally transferable to every hospital. Published nomograms are specific only for the reagent and instrument used to validate that nomogram.

• It may be erroneous to determine a therapeutic range based on the calculation of 1.5–2.3 times the mean control APTT, but this may still be done in some hospital laboratories. Previous weight-based nomograms, which utilize a therapeutic range based on the calculation of 1.5–2.3 times the control APTT, have been recently recognized to be accurate only for that APTT reagent utilized. Table 6 is an example of a weight-based dosing nomogram.

• Each hospital should develop its own nomogram based on their therapeutic range.

Table 4

**Guidelines for Anticoagulation:
Low-Molecular-Weight Heparin**

Indication	Guidelines
VTE suspected	• Obtain baseline APTT, PT, CBC • Check for contraindications to LMWH therapy • Order imaging study, consider giving heparin 5000 IU IV or LMWH
VTE confirmed	• Give LMWH • Check platelet count between days 3–5 • Start warfarin therapy on day 1 at 5 mg and adjust subsequent daily dose according to INR • Stop LMWH after at least 4–5 days of combined therapy when INR is >2 .0 • Anticoagulate with warfarin for at least 3 months at an INR of 2.5; range 2.0–3.0

Dalteparin sodium 200 anti-Xa IU/kg per day SC; single dose should not exceed 18,000 IU.
Enoxaparin 1 mg/kg SC q 12 hours or 1.5 mg/kg SC q 24 hours; single dose should not exceed 180 mg.
Tinzaparin 175 IU/kg SC daily.
APTT, activated partial thromboplastin time; CBC, complete blood cell count; INR, International Normalized Ratio; PT, prothrombin time.
Reprinted with permission from Hirsh J, Dalen JE, Guyatt G. The Sixth (2000) ACCP Guidelines for Antithrombotic Therapy for Prevention and Treatment of Thrombosis. *Chest* 2000;119:1S–2S.

Table 5

Duration of Anticoagulation Therapy

Duration	Indication
3–6 months	First event with reversible or time-limited risk factors (patient may have underlying factor V Leiden or prothrombin 20210)
≥6 months	Idiopathic VTE, first event
12 months to lifetime	Recurrent event, idiopathic or with thrombophilia First event with • Cancer, until resolved • Anticardiolipin antibody • Antithrombin deficiency • Deficiency of proteins C or S, or antithrombin
Lifetime	Atrial fibrillation Mechanical prosthetic heart valve

Reprinted with permission from Hirsh J, Dalen JE, Guyatt G. The Sixth (2000) ACCP Guidelines for Antithrombotic Therapy for Prevention and Treatment of Thrombosis. *Chest* 2000;119:1S–2S.

- Another approach to heparin therapy is to administer an IV bolus of 5000 IU followed by a continuous infusion of at least 30,000–35,000 IU over 24 hours. The infusion rate is adjusted to maintain a therapeutic APTT.

- UFH may be administered subcutaneously every 12 hours. Initially, the patient should receive a loading dose of 3000 to 5000 IU IV followed by 17,500 IU or 250 IU/kg SC q 12 hours. The dose should be adjusted to an APTT that corresponds to a plasma heparin level of 0.2 IU/mL. This level should be drawn within 1 hour before the next scheduled dose.

Adverse effects
- The most common adverse effects are minor bleeding in the form of gingival bleeding, epistaxis, and ecchymosis.

- The most common serious adverse effects of heparin are gastrointestinal or urogenital bleeding.

- Fatal or life-threatening adverse effects often result from intracranial or retroperitoneal bleeding.

- Transient thrombocytopenia within the first 2–4 days of therapy

- Heparin-induced thrombocytopenia

- Osteoporosis with chronic use

Contraindications
- Active bleeding

- Severe uncontrolled hypertension

- History of heparin-induced thrombocytopenia

- Use epidural or spinal anesthesia with caution, as patients are at risk of developing an epidural or spinal hematoma, which can result in long-term or permanent paralysis.

Low-molecular-weight heparins (LMWH) and pentasaccharides (Tables 7 and 8)
Mechanism of action
- LMWHs inhibit factor IIa, and to a much greater extent, factor Xa.

- Fondaparinux is a pentasaccharide. It binds selectively to AT, which potentiates the inactivation of factor Xa in the coagulation cascades. This inhibits the formation of thrombin.

Advantages of LMWH over UFH
- LMWHs have fewer interactions with plasma proteins, thus they have more predictable responses at lower doses.

Table 6

Body Weight–Based Dosing of IV Heparin[1]

APTT[2]	Dose Change U/kg per hour	Additional Action	Next APTT, h
<35 (<1.2 times mean normal)	+4	Rebolus with 80 IU/kg	6
35–45 (1.2–1.5 times mean normal)	+2	Rebolus with 40 IU/kg	6
46–70[3] (1.5–2.3 times mean normal)	0	0	6[4]
71–90 (2.3–3.0 times mean normal)	–2	0	6
>90 (>3 times mean normal)	–3	Stop infusion 1 h	6

[1] Initial dosing: load 80 IU/kg; maintenance infusion; 18 IU/kg per hour (APTT in 6 hours).

[2] The therapeutic range in seconds should correspond to a plasma heparin level of 0.2–0.4 IU/mL by protamine sulfate or 0.3–0.6 IU/mL by amidolytic assay. When APTT is checked at 6 hours or longer, steady-state kinetics can be assumed.

[3] Heparin 25,000 IU in 250 L 5% dextrose in water. Infuse at rate dictated by body weight through an infusion apparatus calibrated for low flow rates.

[4] During the first 24 hours, repeat APTT every 6 hours. Thereafter monitor APTT once every morning unless it is outside the therapeutic range. Reprinted with permission from Hirsh J, Dalen JE, Guyatt G. The Sixth (2000) ACCP Guidelines for Antithrombotic Therapy for Prevention and Treatment of Thrombosis. *Chest* 2000;119:1S–2S.

Table 7

Low-Molecular-Weight Heparin and Pentasaccharide Dosage Forms

Generic Name	Trade Name	Form and Dose
LMWH		
Dalteparin	Fragmin®	2500- and 5000-unit syringe
Enoxaparin	Lovenox®	30-, 40-, 60-, 80-, 100-, and 120-mg syringe
Tinzaparin	Innohep®	20,000 anti-Xa IU/mL 2-mL vial
Pentasaccharide		
Fondaparinux	Arixtra®	2.5-mg syringe

- LMWHs have a much longer half-life, which allows them to be administered SC every 12–24 hours.

- LMWHs have a lower incidence of osteoporosis and heparin-induced thrombocytopenia.

Therapeutic use
- Prevention and treatment of VTE

- Prevention of VTE in patients with a previous VTE or a known hypercoagulability

- Prophylaxis for VTE in high-risk populations

- Arterial embolism prevention in patients with mechanical or tissue prosthetic heart valve replacement

- Arterial embolism prevention in patients with atrial fibrillation or atrial flutter

Table 8

Pharmacokinetics of LMWH and Pentasaccharides

Drug	Bioavailability	Half-life (hours)	Xa:IIa Binding Ratio
Enoxaparin	92%	3–6	1.9:1
Dalteparin	87%	3–5	2.7:1
Tinzaparin	90%	2–6	2:1
Fondaparinux	100%	17–21	Only Xa binding

- Arterial embolism prevention in patients with an acute cardioembolic stroke

Parameters to monitor
- Platelet counts, hematocrit/hemoglobin, and signs and symptoms of bleeding

- Bone mineral density with long-term use

- Anti-Xa heparin levels can be monitored in obese patients or in patients receiving LMWH who have significant renal impairment. Anti-Xa levels should be drawn 4 hours after a dose. Therapeutic levels are 0.6–1.0 IU/mL for twice-daily dosing and 1–2 IU/mL for once-daily dosing.

- PT/INR and APTT are not useful in monitoring LMWH.

- Currently there are no direct monitoring parameters for fondaparinux.

Dosing LMWH and fondaparinux
- See Tables 9 and 10.

Patient counseling
- Strict compliance is necessary in order to ensure a consistent level of anticoagulation.

- Notify health care provider if there is an increase in bruising, hematuria, melena, hemoptysis, epistaxis, gingival bleeding, or any other abnormal bleeding.

- Consult health care provider or pharmacist before taking any over-the-counter medications.

- Avoid aspirin or nonsteroidal anti-inflammatory drugs (NSAIDs).

- The air bubble in the LMWH syringe should be near the plunger prior to injection. This ensures that all of the LMWH is expelled from the syringe and helps to minimize the amount of bleeding from the injection site.

Adverse effects
- The most common adverse effects are minor bleeding in the form of gingival bleeding, epistaxis, and ecchymosis.

- The most common serious adverse effects of heparin are gastrointestinal or urogenital bleeding.

- Fatal or life-threatening adverse effects often result from intracranial or retroperitoneal bleeding.

Table 9

Indications and Recommended Doses of Low-Molecular-Weight Heparin

Indication	Enoxaparin	Dalteparin	Tinzaparin	Fondaparinux
Total hip replacement	30 mg SC q 12 hours **or** 40 mg SC q 24 hours	5000 units SC 0–14 hours before surgery, then q 24 hours **or** 2500 units SC 2 hours before surgery, then 5000 units q 24 hours **or** 2500 units SC 2 hours before surgery and 4–8 hours after, then 5000 units q 24 hours		2.5 mg SC q 24 hours starting 6–8 hours after surgery
Total knee replacement	30 mg SC q 12 hours			2.5 mg SC q 24 hours starting 6–8 hours after surgery
Abdominal surgery	40 mg SC q 24 hours	2500 units SC 1–2 hours before surgery, then 5000 units q 24 hours		
Hip fracture				2.5 mg SC q 24 hours starting 6–8 hours after surgery
Acute medical illness	40 mg SC q 24 hours	5000 units SC q 24 hours		
Trauma	30 mg SC q 12 hours			
DVT treatment with or without pulmonary embolism	1 mg/kg SC q 12 hours **or** 1.5 mg/kg SC q 24 hours		175 units/kg SC q 24 hours	
Unstable angina	1 mg/kg SC q 12 hours	120 units/kg SC q 12 hours		

- Heparin-induced thrombocytopenia can occur, but its incidence is greater with UHF.

- Osteoporosis can occur with chronic use.

Direct thrombin inhibitors
Drugs
- Lepirudin (Refludan®)

- Argatroban

Mechanism of action
- Lepirudin is a recombinant DNA–derived polypeptide nearly identical to hirudin. It produces an anti-coagulant effect by binding directly to thrombin and does not require AT to produce its effect. Lepirudin does not bind to other plasma proteins as heparin does.

- Argatroban is a synthetic molecule that reversibly binds to thrombin.

Therapeutic use
- Lepirudin is used for the treatment of DVT and heparin-induced thrombocytopenia.

Table 10

Enoxaparin Dosage Regimens for Patients with Severe Renal Impairment (Creatinine Clearance <30 mL/min)

Indication	Dosage Regimen
Prophylaxis in abdominal surgery	30 mg SC once daily
Prophylaxis in hip or knee replacement surgery	30 mg SC once daily
Prophylaxis in medical patients during acute illness	30 mg SC once daily
Prophylaxis of ischemic complications of unstable angina and non–Q-wave myocardial infarction, when concurrently administered with aspirin	1 mg/kg SC once daily
Inpatient treatment of acute deep vein thrombosis with or without pulmonary embolism, when administered in conjunction with warfarin sodium	1 mg/kg SC once daily
Outpatient treatment of acute deep vein thrombosis without pulmonary embolism, when administered in conjunction with warfarin sodium	1 mg/kg SC once daily

- Argatroban is used for treatment of heparin-induced thrombocytopenia and percutaneous coronary intervention.

Pharmacokinetics
- Lepirudin has a half-life of 1–2 hours. Approximately 45% of lepirudin is eliminated by the kidneys.

- Argatroban is metabolized in the liver to inactive metabolites. The half-life is 0.5–1 hour.

Parameters to monitor
Lepirudin
- CBC and signs and symptoms of bleeding

- The therapeutic effect of lepirudin is monitored by the APTT 4 hours after beginning therapy and after a dosage change. After the APTT is stable within the therapeutic range, daily monitoring is sufficient.

Argatroban
- CBC and signs and symptoms of bleeding. The APTT is used to monitor and adjust argatroban therapy.

- The APTT should be drawn 2 hours after an infusion is started and after each dosage change.

- Argatroban will also elevate a PT/INR. For patients on concomitant warfarin therapy, this may make monitoring more difficult and give the false impression of an INR. For combination therapy, argatroban may be discontinued after an INR is greater than 4. An INR should be drawn after 4–6 hours. If the INR is in the therapeutic range, continue with warfarin only. If the INR is below the therapeutic range, restart argatroban and increase the dose of warfarin. Repeat this procedure until the INR is within the therapeutic range.

Dosing
Lepirudin
- Administer a bolus dose of 0.4 mg/kg IV with an infusion of 16.5 mg/h. Measure an APTT 4 hours after the infusion. Titrate the infusion to a therapeutic APTT range. If the APTT is below the therapeutic range, increase the infusion by 20%. If the APTT is above the therapeutic range, hold the infusion for 2 hours, then decrease the infusion by 50%. APTTs should be measured 4 hours after a dosage change.

Argatroban
- Administer a continuous IV infusion at the rate of 2 μg/kg per minute. Adjust infusion rate to a therapeutic APTT range. The usual dose is 2–10 μg/kg per minute.

- The dose should be reduced in moderate hepatic insufficiency. A continuous IV infusion should begin at a rate of 0.5 μg/kg per minute. Draw an APTT 4 hours after initiation or a dosage change due to the prolonged elimination half-life.

Patient counseling
- Monitor symptoms of bruising and bleeding and report it to a health care provider immediately.

Adverse effects
- The most common adverse effects are minor bleeding in the form of gingival bleeding, epistaxis, and ecchymosis.

- The most common serious adverse effects are gastrointestinal or urogenital bleeding.

- Fatal or life-threatening adverse effects often result from intracranial or retroperitoneal bleeding.

- There is no known antidote for lepirudin or argatroban. The anticoagulant effect declines rapidly after discontinuation of the drug.

- Nonhemorrhagic effects such as fever, nausea, vomiting, and allergic reactions rarely occur.

Warfarin (Coumadin®)

Dosage forms

- Tablets: 1 mg (pink), 2 mg (lavender), 2.5 mg (green), 3 mg (tan), 4 mg (blue), 5 mg (peach), 6 mg (teal), 7.5 mg (yellow), 10 mg (white)

- Injections (intravenous): 5 mg powder for reconstitution (2 mg/mL)

Mechanism of action

- Warfarin is a vitamin K antagonist that produces its pharmacologic effect by interfering with the interconversion of vitamin K and its 2,3 epoxide (vitamin K epoxide). Warfarin leads to the depletion or reduction in activity of vitamin K–dependent coagulation proteins (factors II, VII, IX, and X) produced in the liver. The level and activity of the vitamin K–dependent clotting factors decline over 6–96 hours. At least 4–5 days of warfarin therapy are necessary before a patient is completely anticoagulated.

Therapeutic use

- Prevention and treatment of VTE

- Prevention of VTE in patients with a previous VTE or a known hypercoagulability

- Prophylaxis for VTE in high-risk populations

- Arterial embolism prevention in patients with mechanical or tissue prosthetic heart valve replacement

- Arterial embolism prevention in patients with atrial fibrillation or atrial flutter

- Arterial embolism prevention in patients with a previous cardioembolic stroke

- Prevention of acute myocardial infarction in patients with peripheral arterial disease

Patient counseling

- Warfarin should be taken at the same time every day.

- Strict compliance is necessary in order to ensure a consistent level of anticoagulation.

- Strict compliance with a consistent vitamin K diet is necessary to ensure a consistent level of anticoagulation.

- Notify the health care provider in the event of hematuria, melena, epistaxis, hemoptysis, increased bruising, or any abnormal bleeding.

- Notify all health care providers, including dentists, of warfarin therapy.

- Blood monitoring to determine an adequate level of anticoagulation and compliance is necessary at regular intervals.

- Consult the health care provider or pharmacist before taking any new prescription or over-the-counter medications.

- Avoid aspirin or NSAIDs.

- Women of childbearing age should use an effective form of birth control since warfarin has teratogenic effects.

Parameters to monitor

- Warfarin therapy is monitored by a prothrombin time (PT). The PT responds to a reduction in factors II, VII, and X. The INR is used to standardize the responsiveness of thromboplastin to the anticoagulant effects of warfarin. The INR is calculated by the following equation:
    * INR = (observed PT/mean normal PT)^{ISI}
    * ISI is the International Sensitivity Index, which is a measure of thromboplastin sensitivity. The lower the ISI, the more responsive the thromboplastin is to the anticoagulant effects of warfarin.

- The Sixth ACCP Consensus Conference on Antithrombotic Therapy recommends two intensities of anticoagulation: a less intense level with a target INR of 2.5 and a range of 2.0–3.0, and a high-intensity level of anticoagulation with a target INR of 3.0 and a range of 2.5–3.5 (Table 11).

- Upon initiation of warfarin therapy, the INR should be evaluated daily if the patient is in the hospital, and every 2–3 days if the patient is not hospitalized.

Pharmacokinetics

- Warfarin is a racemic mixture of two optically active isomers, warfarin S and warfarin R, in roughly equal

Table 11

Recommended Therapeutic Ranges for Oral Anticoagulation

Indication	Target INR (INR Range)
Prophylaxis of VTE (high-risk surgery)	2.5 (2.0–3.0)
Treatment of VTE	2.5 (2.0–3.0)
Prevention of arterial embolism in atrial fibrillation	2.5 (2.0–3.0)
Prevention of arterial embolism with a bileaflet mechanical prosthetic heart valve in the aortic position	2.5 (2.0–3.0)
Prevention of arterial embolism in a mechanical prosthetic heart valve	3.0 (2.5–3.5)

INR, International Normalized Ratio.

amounts. The S isomer is five times more potent than the R isomer.

- Warfarin is rapidly and completely absorbed from the GI tract with peak concentration in approximately 90 minutes. Warfarin is 99% protein-bound with a half-life of 36–42 hours.

- The onset of anticoagulation occurs after 4–5 days of therapy and is due to the depletion of the clotting factors rather than steady-state concentrations of warfarin. Thus the onset of action is based on the half-life of the clotting factors II, VII, IX, and X.

Dosing
- Time in the therapeutic range and intensity of anticoagulation are critical for optimizing the therapeutic efficacy of warfarin and minimizing the risk of hemorrhage.

- Warfarin initiation does not require loading. Loading doses can result in an inappropriate increase in the INR, which is not reflective of an anticoagulant effect.

- Initiating warfarin at 5 mg daily should result in an INR around 2.0 in 4–5 days for most patients.

- Initiating warfarin at a dose of 2.5–4 mg daily may be appropriate in the elderly, in patients with liver

disease, in patients with impaired nutrition, or in patients with a high risk of bleeding.

- Initiating warfarin at a dose of 7.5–10 mg daily may be appropriate for young healthy or obese patients.

- If a rapid anticoagulant effect is indicated, IV heparin or LMWH should be administered along with warfarin for at least 4–5 days until a therapeutic INR is reached. Heparin or LMWH may be discontinued when the INR is within the therapeutic range on two consecutive occasions.

Disease state interaction
- Disease states that can increase the response to warfarin are hyperthyroidism, congestive heart failure, liver disease, and fever.

- Disease states that can decrease the response to warfarin are hypothyroidism and genetic warfarin resistance.

- Patient noncompliance can also result in a reduced warfarin response.

Drug/food interactions
- Warfarin is a drug with a narrow therapeutic index. There are numerous drugs that interact with warfarin to potentiate or reduce its anticoagulant effect. Since the S isomer is five times more active than the R isomer, drugs that inhibit or induce the S isomer will have a more significant effect on warfarin than drugs that inhibit or induce the R isomer (Tables 12 and 13).

Table 12

Drugs that Can Potentiate Warfarin's Anticoagulant Effect

Acetaminophen	Alcohol (acute use)	Amiodarone[a]
Anabolic steroids	Cimetidine	Ciprofloxacin[a]
Clofibrate	Dicloxacillin	Disulfiram
Erythromycin	Fluconazole[a]	Isoniazid[a]
Itraconazole[a]	Ketoconazole[a]	Levothyroxine[a]
Metronidazole[a]	Nafcillin[a]	Omeprazole
Phenytoin[a]	Piroxicam	Simvastatin
Sulfinpyrazone	Trimethoprim-sulfamethoxazole[a]	Vitamin E[a] (high doses)

[a]Highly significant.

Table 13

Drugs that Can Reduce the Anticoagulant Effect of Warfarin

Alcohol	Barbiturates[a]	Carbamazepine[a]
(chronic use)	Cholestyramine[a]	Enteral feeding[a]
Griseofulvin	Rifampin[a]	Vitamin K–
		containing foods[a]

[a]Highly significant.

- Foods that contain high amounts of vitamin K can reduce the anticoagulant effect of warfarin (Table 14). It is important that patients are consistent in their consumption of these foods and that they evenly space out their consumption over a 7-day period. If one suddenly stops eating these foods, the INR may dramatically increase.

Table 14

Foods High in Vitamin K

Broccoli	Brussels sprouts
Cabbage	Canola oil
Cauliflower	Cole slaw
Collard greens	Endive
Green kale	Lettuce
Mayonnaise	Mustard greens
Soybean oil	Spinach
Turnip greens	

Table 15

Management of Supratherapeutic Anticoagulation

- INR greater than therapeutic, but <5.0 without significant bleeding:
  - * Omit one dose of warfarin and reduce the maintenance dose.
  - * If a precipitating factor could be identified, no dose reduction may be necessary.
- INR >5.0 but <9.0 without significant bleeding: Two treatment options are available based on how rapid a reduction in INR is indicated:
  - * Omit one or two doses until the INR is within the therapeutic range, then resume warfarin at a lower dose.
  - * Omit one dose and administer vitamin K_1 1–2.5 mg orally in patients who have an increased risk of bleeding, then resume warfarin at a lower dose.
- INR >5.0, but <9.0 with a need for rapid reversal for urgent surgery:
  - * Administer vitamin K_1 2–4 mg orally. The reduction in INR should occur within 24 hours. An additional dose of vitamin K_1 1–2 mg orally may be administered if the INR is still too high. Resume warfarin at a lower dose.
- INR >9.0 without significant bleeding:
  - * Hold warfarin and administer vitamin K_1 3–5 mg orally. The INR should be reduced within 24–48 hours. The INR should be monitored more frequently and administer additional vitamin K_1 if necessary. Resume warfarin at a lower dose when INR reaches the therapeutic level.
- INR >20.0 with serious bleeding:
  - * Hold warfarin and administer vitamin K_1 10 mg by slow IV infusion, supplement with fresh frozen plasma or prothrombin complex concentrate, depending on the urgency of the situation. Additional doses of vitamin K_1 may be administered every 12 hours if necessary.
- For life-threatening bleeding:
  - * Hold warfarin and administer prothrombin complex concentrate supplemented with vitamin K_1 10 mg by slow IV infusion. Repeat this treatment as necessary, depending on the INR.
- If continuation of warfarin therapy is indicated after administration of high doses of vitamin K_1, then heparin can be given until the effects of vitamin K_1 have been reversed and the patient becomes responsive to warfarin.

INR, International Normalized Ratio.
Reprinted with permission from Hirsh J, Dalen JE, Guyatt G. The Sixth (2000) ACCP Guidelines for Antithrombotic Therapy for Prevention and Treatment of Thrombosis. *Chest* 2000;119:1S–2S.

Adverse effects

- The most common adverse effect is minor bleeding in the form of gingival bleeding, epistaxis, and ecchymosis.

- The most common serious adverse effects of warfarin are either gastrointestinal or urogenital bleeding.

- Fatal or life-threatening adverse effects are related to intracranial or retroperitoneal bleeding (Table 15). Special precautions must be taken for patients undergoing invasive procedures (Table 16).

Table 16

Management of Oral Anticoagulation During Invasive Procedures

Patients with low risk of thromboembolism

    History of VTE for >3 months

    Atrial fibrillation without a history of stroke

- Stop warfarin therapy 4 days before surgery
- Allow the INR to return to a near normal level
- Undergo invasive procedure
- Administer postoperative prophylaxis (if the intervention itself creates a higher risk of thrombosis) using low-dose heparin, 5000 units SC, and simultaneously begin warfarin therapy

For patients with intermediate risk of thromboembolism

- Stop warfarin therapy 4 days before surgery
- Allow INR to fall
- Undergo invasive procedure
- Cover with low-dose heparin, 5000 units SC, beginning 2 days before surgery or with a prophylactic dose of LMWH, and then commence low-dose heparin or LMWH and warfarin therapy after surgery

For patients with high risk of thromboembolism

    Recent <3 months history of VTE

    Mechanical cardiac valve in the mitral position

    Ball and cage cardiac valve

- Stop warfarin therapy 4 days before surgery
- Allow the INR to return to normal level
- Begin full dose UFH SC approximately 2 days before surgery as outpatient, then continuous IV heparin infusion after admission as the INR falls, stop heparin infusion 5 hours before surgery
- Or full-dose LMWH approximately 2 days before surgery, then stop LMWH 12–24 hours before surgery
- Undergo invasive procedure
- Resume full dose UFH SC or full dose LMWH and warfarin after surgery and continue until INR is in the therapeutic range

Other invasive procedures

- In patients with low risk of bleeding, reduce INR to 1.3–1.5 (for gynecologic and orthopedic surgical patients) 4–5 days before surgery. Restart warfarin therapy after surgery. May use low-dose heparin, 5000 units SC, if necessary
- In patients undergoing simple dental procedures, who are not considered to be at high risk for bleeding, disruption of warfarin therapy may not be indicated. In patients in whom local bleeding is a concern, tranexamic acid or epsilon aminocaproic acid mouthwash can be utilized

INR, International Normalized Ratio; LMWH, low-molecular-weight heparin; UFH, unfractionated heparin.
Adapted with permission from Hirsh J, Dalen JE, Guyatt G. The Sixth (2000) ACCP Guidelines for Antithrombotic Therapy for Prevention and Treatment of Thrombosis. *Chest* 2000;119:1S–2S.

2. Atrial Fibrillation

Definition and Epidemiology

- Atrial fibrillation (AF) is a supraventricular tachyarrhythmia characterized by uncoordinated atrial activity up to 300–500 beats per minute that is associated with an irregular ventricular response. Uncontrolled AF can result in a rapid ventricular response, which can affect blood circulation. Atrial fibrillation may be chronic or paroxysmal in nature.

- Over 2 million Americans have AF, which increases in prevalence after the age of 45 and greatly accelerates after age 65.

- It is estimated that 10% of Americans over the age of 80 have AF.

- AF is a risk factor for the development of a stroke. It is estimated that 5% of patients with nonvalvular AF, if untreated, would experience a stroke. If transient ischemic attack and silent stroke are included, the incidence is around 7%.

- The Framingham Heart Study demonstrated that patients with rheumatic heart disease and AF had a 17-fold increase in the incidence of stroke compared to age-matched controls (Table 17).

Clinical Presentation

- AF is characterized by an irregularly irregular heartbeat, with the possibility of a rapid ventricular response. Common symptoms are palpitations and fatigue. Patients may complain of their "heart fluttering" and feeling weak.

Drug Therapy

- Warfarin therapy has demonstrated approximately a 60% risk reduction in stroke in patients with AF. A meta-analysis of five studies reported a 36% relative risk reduction in all strokes, and a 46% reduction in ischemic strokes with warfarin compared to aspirin (Table 18).

Other Therapy

- Elective cardioversion (Table 19).

Table 17

Risk Stratification in AF

High risk
- Previous stroke, transient ischemic attack, or systemic embolism
- Hypertension
- Heart failure
- Age >75 years
- Rheumatic mitral valve disease
- Prosthetic heart valve

Moderate risk
- Diabetes
- Age 65–75 years
- Coronary heart disease with preserved left ventricular function

Low risk
- Age <65 years without clinical or echocardiographic evidence of cardiovascular disease

Reprinted with permission from Hirsh J, Dalen JE, Guyatt G.The Sixth (2000) ACCP Guidelines for Antithrombotic Therapy for Prevention and Treatment of Thrombosis. *Chest* 2000;119:1S–2S.

Table 18

Recommendations for Antithrombotic Therapy in AF

High risk (patients with high-risk factors or more than one moderate-risk factor)
- Warfarin adjusted to a target INR of 2.5, with a range of 2.0–3.0
- Aspirin 325 mg daily if warfarin is contraindicated or declined by the patient

Moderate risk (patients with one moderate-risk factor)
- Either warfarin or aspirin therapy

Low risk
- Aspirin 325 mg daily

INR, International Normalized Ratio.
Reprinted with permission from Hirsh J, Dalen JE, Guyatt G.The Sixth (2000) ACCP Guidelines for Antithrombotic Therapy for Prevention and Treatment of Thrombosis. *Chest* 2000;119:1S–2S.

Table 19

Anticoagulation for Elective Cardioversion

- Patients with AF of more than 48 hours duration, or unknown duration, who are scheduled for elective cardioversion should be anticoagulated with warfarin to a target INR of 2.5 with a range of 2.0–3.0 for 3–4 weeks prior to direct current cardioversion (DC), and for 4 weeks after cardioversion.
- Alternatively, AF patients undergo anticoagulation then undergo TEE, and if no thrombi are seen, have cardioversion performed without delay. For these patients, adjusted-dose warfarin therapy should still be continued until normal sinus rhythm has been maintained for at least 4 weeks.
- Although data are limited, the risk of embolism following cardioversion in patients who have been in AF for <48 hours appears to be low. However, the use of anticoagulation during the pericardioversion period is recommended.
- Oral anticoagulation at the time of cardioversion in patients with atrial flutter is recommended in a manner similar to that used for AF.
- In the absence of prior thromboembolism, antithrombotic therapy for cardioversion of supraventricular tachycardia is not recommended.
- Treatment of potential precipitants of AF (ie, thyrotoxicosis, pneumonia, and congestive heart failure) should be completed prior to attempting elective DC cardioversion.

INR, International Normalized Ratio; TEE, transesophageal echocardiography.
Adapted with permission from Hirsh J, Dalen JE, Guyatt G. The Sixth (2000) ACCP Guidelines for Antithrombotic Therapy for Prevention and Treatment of Thrombosis. *Chest* 2000;119:1S–2S.

3. Stroke

Definition and Epidemiology

- Stroke is defined as a sudden onset of focal neurologic deficit lasting longer than 24 hours.
- Transient ischemic attack (TIA) is defined as a focal ischemic neurologic deficit usually lasting 2–5 minutes, that resolves completely in less than 24 hours.
- After heart disease and cancer, stroke is the third leading cause of death in America.
- Approximately 700,000 Americans suffer a stroke each year; 500,000 of these persons experience their first stroke and 200,000 experience a recurrent stroke.
- The incidence of stroke increases with age, and the rate doubles for each decade after age 55.
- Hypertension is a factor in 70% of patients who suffer a stroke (Table 20).
- Risk factors for stroke are outlined in Table 20.
- Cigarette smoking increases the risk of stroke 2–3 times compared to nonsmokers.
- Atrial fibrillation increases the risk of a stroke six times.

Clinical Presentation

- Symptoms of a stroke depend on where the stroke occurred in the brain and the rapidity with which the symptoms develop. It is common for a stroke to be

Table 20

Stroke Risk Factors

- Hypertension
- Smoking
- Heart disease (coronary heart disease, heart failure, left ventricular hypertrophy, and atrial fibrillation)
- Elevated pulse pressure
- Previous transient ischemic attack or stroke
- Diabetes
- Hyperlipidemia
- Obesity

preceded by one or more TIAs. Symptoms range from focal deficits to more significant deficits such as hemiplegia or hemiparesthesia, blindness in one eye, or speech difficulties.

Pathophysiology

- 15% of strokes are hemorrhagic in nature.

- 85% of strokes are ischemic in nature.
  * 20% are cardioembolic
  * 20% are due to atherosclerotic cerebrovascular disease
  * 25% are due to penetrating artery disease or lacunar infarctions
  * 30% are cryptogenic
  * 5% are due to other causes

- Atherosclerosis and plaque formation results in arterial narrowing, which leads to stenosis with reduced blood flow. This may enhance platelet aggregation that can lead to an arterial occlusion. An occlusive clot is present in up to 80% of ischemic strokes.

- The Framingham Study indicates that there is a strong relationship between hypertension and the risk of both hemorrhagic and nonhemorrhagic stroke. Atherothrombotic infarctions occur four times more often in patients with hypertension (blood pressure >165/95 mm Hg) than in patients without hypertension. The treatment of hypertension has reduced the incidence of stroke by 35–40%.

- Cardioembolic etiology accounts for one-fifth of all strokes. The most common cause of a cardiac embolism is AF; other factors include valvular heart disease, coronary heart disease, prosthetic heart valves, and dilated cardiomyopathy. A cardioembolic stroke often has an abrupt onset and more commonly involves the middle cerebral artery.

Diagnosis and Prevention

- Diagnosis is based on physical examination, medical history, and diagnostic imaging such as a computed tomography (CT) scan, magnetic resonance imaging (MRI) scan, magnetic resonance angiography (MRA), or cerebral arteriography.

- Preventive measures are outlined in Table 21.

Drug Therapy

Tissue plasminogen activator (t-PA [Alteplase®])
Mechanism of action
- Since most strokes are due to a thromboembolic

Table 21

Stroke Prevention Therapy

- Maintain blood pressure <140/90 mm Hg or <130/90 mm Hg for patients with diabetes or coronary artery disease
- Hyperlipidemia should be controlled with statin therapy (LDL <100 mg/dL)
- Glycemic control (hemoglobin A_{1c} <7%)
- Smoking cessation
- Weight reduction if overweight
- Exercise (ie, 30 minutes of moderate exercise daily)
- Implement the DASH (Dietary Approaches to Stop Hypertension) diet (low in sodium and saturated fat; high in fruits, vegetables, whole grains, and fiber)

occlusion in an intracranial artery, thrombolytic therapy is key to restoring or improving perfusion. t-PA is a plasminogen activator (serine protease) that enhances the conversion of plasminogen to plasmin in the presence of fibrin. t-PA binds to fibrin in a thrombus and converts bound plasminogen to plasmin. Plasmin, an enzyme responsible for clot dissolution, initiates local fibrinolysis.

Indications
- Acute treatment of stroke, criteria for use:
  * Onset of symptoms is <3 hours
  * Baseline CT scan of the head does not indicate an intracranial hemorrhage
  * Blood pressure <185/110 mm Hg
  * Platelets >100,000
  * No conditions present that would increase the patient's likelihood of bleeding
  * No heparin therapy within 48 hours with an elevated APTT
  * No oral anticoagulants or and INR >1.7 or a PT >15 seconds
  * No suspicion of subarachnoid hemorrhage on pretreatment evaluation
  * No gastrointestinal or urinary tract hemorrhage within 3 months
  * No stroke or serious head injury within 3 months
  * No recent (within 3 months) intracranial or intraspinal surgery
  * No seizure at the onset of stroke
  * No active internal bleeding
  * No intracranial neoplasm, arteriovenous malformation, or aneurysm
  * No major surgery or serious trauma within 2 weeks

* No clinical symptoms suggesting post-MI or pericarditis

* Not currently pregnant or lactating

- Specific treatment guidelines are available to evaluate patient characteristics for the use of t-PA in acute stroke.

Dose
- t-PA is administered at a dose of 0.9 mg/kg (maximum dose 90 mg) IV with 10% of the dose given as an initial bolus over 1 minute and the balance infused over 60 minutes.

Parameters to monitor
- Hematocrit, mental status, signs and symptoms of bleeding

Adverse drug reactions
- Bleeding is the most common adverse effect with t-PA. The most common sites of bleeding are gastrointestinal, urogenital, retroperitoneal, and intracranial.

Contraindications
- Intracranial hemorrhage, recent stroke, blood pressure >185/100 mm Hg, active internal hemorrhage, platelets <100,000 mm^3, anticoagulant therapy within 24 hours of t-PA, intracranial neoplasm, arteriovenous malformation, or aneurysm

Antiplatelet drugs
Aspirin
Mechanism of action
- Aspirin produces its antiplatelet effect by irreversibly inactivating the enzyme cyclooxygenase, which prevents the conversion of arachidonic acid to thromboxane A$_2$. Thromboxane A$_2$ stimulates platelet aggregation. The effects of aspirin on platelets occur for the life of the platelet (ie, approximately 5-7 days). Aspirin has demonstrated a 27–30% risk reduction of stroke.

Patient counseling
- Notify physician if melena, persistent stomach pain or discomfort, breathing difficulties, increased bleeding or bruising, or skin rashes develop.

- Avoid NSAIDs or warfarin unless instructed otherwise by physician.

- Avoid over-the-counter medications that contain aspirin.

- Do not crush or chew enteric-coated aspirin.

Dose
- Within 48 hours of an acute ischemic stroke, patients should receive aspirin 160–325 mg daily. Aspirin is effective for stroke prevention at a dose of 50–325 mg daily.

Monitoring parameters
- Signs and symptoms of bleeding

Adverse drug reactions
- Nausea, vomiting, dyspepsia, gastrointestinal ulceration, gastric erosion, duodenal ulcers, gastrointestinal hemorrhage, rash, urticaria, angioedema, bronchospasm, and asthma exacerbation

Drug-drug interactions
- Warfarin, UFH, LMWH, NSAIDs, fondaparinux, and clopidogrel may increase the risk of bleeding if used in combination with aspirin.

Drug-disease interactions
- Use enteric-coated aspirin after an acute episode of peptic or gastric ulcer disease.

- Avoid aspirin use if there is a risk of aspirin-induced asthma.

Clopidogrel (Plavix®)
Mechanism of action
- Clopidogrel is a selective and irreversible inhibitor of adenosine diphosphate–induced platelet aggregation that does not affect arachidonic acid metabolism. The effects of clopidogrel on platelets occur for the life of the platelet, approximately 5–7 days.

- The CAPRIE Trial demonstrated an 8.7% relative risk reduction of composite outcomes of ischemic stroke, MI, or vascular death with the use of clopidogrel versus aspirin in patients with a recent stroke or MI, or patients with symptomatic peripheral arterial disease. Clopidogrel was most beneficial for patients with peripheral artery disease, and showed a 23.8% relative risk reduction over aspirin.

Dose
- Clopidogrel is effective in stroke prevention at a dose of 75 mg daily.

Patient counseling
- Notify physician for melena, persistent stomach pain or discomfort, increased bleeding or bruising, or development of a skin rash.

- Avoid NSAIDs or warfarin unless instructed otherwise by a physician.

- Avoid over-the-counter medications that contain aspirin.

Parameters to monitor
- Signs and symptoms of bleeding

Adverse drug reactions
- Nausea, dyspepsia, diarrhea, abdominal pain, increased bruising, and bleeding

Drug-drug interaction
- Warfarin, aspirin, NSAIDs, UFH, fondaparinux, and LMWH can increase the risk of bleeding if combined with clopidogrel.

- Clopidogrel may inhibit cytochrome isoenzyme P2C9 substrates, thus there is the potential to inhibit the metabolism of fluvastatin, tolbutamide, and torsemide. Close monitoring may be advisable.

Drug-disease interactions
- Use clopidogrel with caution in peptic or gastric ulcer disease.

- May require dosage reduction in moderate to severe hepatic dysfunction.

Extended-release dipyridamole plus immediate-release aspirin (Aggrenox®)
Mechanism of action
- Dipyridamole is a phosphodiesterase inhibitor that increases cyclic adenosine monophosphate in the platelet, which potentiates the deaggregating effects of prostacyclin on platelets.

- This dipyridamole-aspirin combination has demonstrated a 37% stroke risk reduction.

Patient counseling
- Notify physician of melena, persistent stomach pain or discomfort, breathing difficulties, increased bleeding or bruising, or development of a skin rash.

- Avoid NSAIDs or warfarin unless instructed otherwise by a physician.

- Avoid over-the-counter medications that contain aspirin.

- Take this medication on an empty stomach, 1 hour before or 2 hours after meals. If stomach upset occurs, take it with food or milk.

- Do not crush or chew.

Dose
- A combination of extended-release dipyridamole 200 mg with immediate-release aspirin 25 mg in a capsule that is taken twice daily

Parameters to monitor
- Signs and symptoms of bleeding

Adverse drug reactions
- Headache, nausea, vomiting, dyspepsia, gastrointestinal ulceration, gastric erosion, duodenal ulcers, gastrointestinal hemorrhage, rash, urticaria, angioedema, hypotension, dizziness, flushing, epistaxis, bronchospasm, and asthma exacerbation

Drug-drug interactions
- Warfarin, UFH, LMWH, NSAIDs, fondaparinux, aspirin, and clopidogrel may increase the risk of bleeding if used in combination with this product.

Drug-disease interaction
- Use dipyridamole-aspirin with caution in the presence of peptic or gastric ulcer disease.

4. Key Points

- Appropriate VTE prophylaxis should be used with all patients who have risk factors for its development. The Sixth ACCP Consensus Conference on Antithrombotic Therapy has developed guidelines for VTE prophylaxis specific for at-risk patient populations.

- UFH should be administered as a bolus of 80 IU/kg IV, then a maintenance infusion of 18 IU/kg/h. Heparin is monitored by APTT levels. A therapeutic APTT range should be determined for each hospital or laboratory by calibration against a therapeutic plasma heparin concentration of 0.2–0.4 U/mL based on a protamine titration or an anti-factor Xa concentration of 0.3–0.7 U/mL.

- LMWH offers a more predictable response at lower doses without the need to monitor levels, except in patients with severe renal impairment or in obesity. It has a lower incidence of osteoporosis and heparin-induced thrombocytopenia. It can also be administered once or twice daily by SC injection. This allows care to shift from the hospital to the outpatient arena.

- An acute VTE should be treated with either UFH IV or LMWH to provide immediate anticoagulation, followed by the initiation of warfarin therapy. Warfarin should be initiated at 5–7.5 mg daily for most patients. Patients with malnutrition, liver disease, a high risk for bleeding, or the elderly, may be started at a lower dose. UFH or LMWH should be overlapped with warfarin for at least 4–5 days or until there are two consecutive INRs within the therapeutic range.

- Patients with a single VTE with reversible, time-limited risk factors should be anticoagulated for 3–6 months. Patients with a single idiopathic VTE should be anticoagulated for 6 months or longer. Patients with a recurrent VTE or a VTE with cancer or a known hypercoagulable state should be anticoagulated for 12 months to lifetime.

- Atrial fibrillation is a condition that predisposes a patient to the development of a stroke. Warfarin titrated to a target INR of 2.5 with a range of 2.0–3.0 reduces the risk for stroke by approximately 60%. Aspirin is not as effective as warfarin in high-risk patients with AF (ie, there is a 27–30% relative risk reduction).

- Patients with a thromboembolic occlusion in an intracranial artery should receive t-PA, provided the following conditions are met:
  * Onset of symptoms is less than 3 hours
  * CT scan of the head does not indicate an intracranial hemorrhage
  * Blood pressure <185/100 mm Hg
  * Conditions that would increase the patient's likelihood of bleeding are not present

- t-PA is administered at a dose of 0.9 mg/kg (maximum dose 90 mg) IV with 10% of the dose given as an initial bolus over 1 minute and the balance infused over 60 minutes.

- The drugs of choice for a noncardioembolic stroke are:
  * Aspirin 50–325 mg daily
  * Clopidogrel 75 mg daily
  * Aspirin 25 mg/dipyridamole 200 mg bid

5. Questions and Answers

1. A 24-year-old female presents to the emergency department with c/o severe shortness of breath, dyspnea, and chest pain. She is also experiencing tachycardia and tachypnea. Two days prior she noticed pain and swelling in her left lower extremity. Her past medical history is negative for thrombosis. Her current medications include Tri-Levlen® daily and ibuprofen 600 mg q 6 hours prn for pain. A duplex ultrasound of the left lower extremity revealed a DVT. Her vital signs are: T: 98.4; P: 124; R: 36; BP: 162/100; Wt: 100 kg; Ht: 165 cm. The most likely cause of her shortness of breath, dyspnea, and chest pain is

   A. Bronchitis
   B. Asthma exacerbation
   C. Pulmonary embolism
   D. Heart failure exacerbation
   E. Atrial fibrillation

2. This patient is started on heparin therapy. Which dosage regimen is most appropriate?

   A. IV heparin 20,000 IU bolus, then 5000 IU/h
   B. IV heparin 8000 IU bolus, then 1800 IU/h
   C. IV heparin 5000 IU bolus, then 500 IU/h
   D. IV heparin 5000 IU q 12 hours
   E. SC heparin 5000 IU q 12 hours

3. All of the following are risk factors for a DVT except:

   A. Hip replacement surgery
   B. Knee replacement surgery
   C. Hernia repair surgery
   D. Hip fracture surgery
   E. Abdominal surgery

4. Which diagnostic test would assist with the diagnosis of a pulmonary embolism?

   A. Chest x-ray
   B. Electrocardiogram
   C. Spiral CT of the chest
   D. Bronchoscopy
   E. Echocardiogram

5. A patient is started on warfarin for atrial fibrillation. What is an appropriate starting dose of warfarin?

   A. 1 mg daily
   B. 5 mg daily
   C. 15 mg daily
   D. 20 mg daily
   E. 25 mg daily

6. What laboratory test is used to monitor heparin therapy?

   A. APTT
   B. PT
   C. INR
   D. Clotting time
   E. Factor XIa

7. A 47-year-old patient is diagnosed with a lower extremity DVT. The patient's height is 6 feet and the weight is 220 lb (100 kg). The physician would like to treat this patient on an outpatient basis with warfarin and low-molecular-weight heparin. Which of the drugs below would be the most appropriate?

   A. Enoxaparin 30 mg SC q 12 hours
   B. Enoxaparin 40 mg SC q 24 hours
   C. Enoxaparin 100 mg SC q 12 hours
   D. Enoxaparin 200 mg SC q 12 hours
   E. Enoxaparin 220 mg SC q 12 hours

8. How long should enoxaparin be continued in a patient with an acute DVT?

   A. At least 4–5 days until the INR is >2 on two consecutive occasions
   B. At least 42 days and until the INR is >3.0 on two occasions
   C. At least 24 hours until the INR is >4.0 on two occasions
   D. At least 48 hours and until the INR is >4.0 on two occasions
   E. At least 7–10 days and until the INR is >3.5 on two occasions

9. All of the following statements are important information to communicate to a patient on warfarin therapy except:

   A. Take warfarin everyday without missing any doses.
   B. Eat a consistent amount of vitamin K–rich foods per week.
   C. Report any symptoms of bleeding to your physician.
   D. Take warfarin with meals and remain standing for 30 minutes.

E. Do not take aspirin-containing products unless directed to do so by your physician.

10. Vitamin K–rich foods can affect the anticoagulant effect of warfarin. Which of the following foods can decrease the anticoagulant effects of warfarin?

    I. Lima beans
    II. Spinach
    III. Broccoli

    A. Only I is correct.
    B. Only III is correct.
    C. I and II are both correct.
    D. II and III are both correct.
    E. I, II, and III are correct.

11. Drugs can affect the anticoagulant effect of warfarin. Which of the following drugs can increase the effects of warfarin?

    I. Ciprofloxacin
    II. Trimethoprim-sulfamethoxazole
    III. Fluconazole

    A. Only I is correct.
    B. Only III is correct.
    C. I and II are both correct.
    D. II and III are both correct.
    E. I, II, and III are correct.

12. What is the most appropriate therapy for a patient with atrial fibrillation, cerebrovascular accident, hypertension, and diabetes?

    A. Aspirin 325 mg daily
    B. Warfarin 5 mg daily
    C. Clopidogrel 75 mg daily
    D. t-PA 90 mg daily
    E. Aggrenox 200/25 mg bid

13. A patient presents to the emergency department with symptoms of aphasia and dysarthria, which resolved over the course of 3 days. The patient has a history of hyperlipidemia, type 2 diabetes mellitus, and hypertension. An echocardiogram showed an ejection fraction of 55%, normal valve function, and normal chamber size. An electrocardiogram showed normal sinus rhythm. Carotid ultrasound indicated moderate stenosis. A CT of the head showed no hemorrhages. Blood pressure was 178/102 mm Hg. Hemoglobin A_{1c} was 10.2. A lipid profile was as follows: total cholesterol: 294; HDL: 32; LDL:

218; triglycerides: 200. Medications include glyburide 10 mg daily and hydrochlorothiazide 25 mg daily. Which therapy is indicated in this patient?

    A. Aspirin 325 mg po daily
    B. Clopidogrel 75 mg po bid
    C. Aspirin 25 mg/dipyridamole 200 mg po daily
    D. Warfarin 5 mg po daily
    E. t-PA 90 mg po daily

14. All of the following are other treatment goals for this patient except:

    A. Hemoglobin $A_{1c} < 7$
    B. Blood pressure <130/80 mm Hg
    C. LDL <100
    D. APTT 70–100 seconds
    E. Stop smoking

15. Fondaparinux is an anticoagulant that inhibits which clotting factor?

    A. IIa
    B. IXa
    C. Xa
    D. XIa
    E. VIIa

16. A 58-year-old male is scheduled for a total knee replacement tomorrow. He has a medical history of hypertension, for which he is treated with amlodipine 5 mg daily. His height is 6 feet 2 inches and his weight is 176 lbs (80 kg). What form of DVT prophylaxis is indicated in this patient?

    I. Enoxaparin 30 mg SC q 12 hours
    II. Fondaparinux 2.5 mg SC q 24 hours
    III. Aspirin 325 mg daily

    A. Only I is correct.
    B. Only III is correct.
    C. I and II are both correct.
    D. II, and III are both correct.
    E. I, II, and III are correct.

17. A 68-year-old male presents to the emergency department with complaints of hematuria and bright red blood per rectum. He has been taking warfarin 8 mg daily. His INR is 10.2. What is the most appropriate therapy to reverse his warfarin toxicity?

    A. Hold warfarin for 4 days and restart warfarin at a lower dose when his INR is <3.

B. Hold warfarin and administer vitamin K 0.5 mg IV. Restart warfarin at a lower dose when his INR is <3.0.

C. Hold warfarin and administer tranexamic acid 10 mg IV. Restart warfarin at a lower dose when his INR is <3.0.

D. Hold warfarin and administer vitamin K 5 mg po. Restart warfarin at a lower dose when his INR is <3.0.

E. Hold warfarin and administer prothrombin complex 5 mg po. Restart warfarin at a lower dose when INR is <3.0.

18. A 63-year-old is receiving warfarin 7.5 mg daily for atrial fibrillation. What therapeutic INR range is indicated for this patient?

A. 1.0 to 2.0
B. 1.5 to 2.5
C. 2.0 to 3.0
D. 2.0 to 3.5
E. 2.5 to 3.5

19. A 56-year-old female presents to the emergency department with complaints of flank pain, dysuria, and increased urinary frequency. She is diagnosed with a urinary tract infection. Her past medical history includes type 2 diabetes mellitus, hypertension, and atrial fibrillation. Her medications include metformin 1 g bid, quinapril 40 mg daily, and warfarin 5 mg daily. What would be the most appropriate antibiotic to treat this patient's UTI?

A. Septra® DS bid
B. Ciprofloxacin 500 mg bid
C. Rifampin 300 mg qid
D. Doxycycline 100 mg bid
E. Erythromycin 500 mg qid

20. Which of the following drugs produce action by inhibiting platelet activity?

I. Clopidogrel
II. Dipyridamole
III. t-PA

A. Only I is correct.
B. Only III is correct.
C. I and II are both correct.
D. II and III are both correct.
E. I, II, and III are correct.

21. What color is warfarin 7.5 mg?

A. White
B. Blue
C. Yellow
D. Pink
E. Green

22. Which of the following is a common side effect associated with unfractionated heparin?

A. Hypokalemia
B. Hypoglycemia
C. Ecchymosis
D. Nausea
E. Hyponatremia

23. What is the length of anticoagulation therapy for atrial fibrillation?

A. 3 months
B. 6 months
C. 9 months
D. 12 months
E. Long-term

24. Advantages of LMWH over UFH include all of the following **except:**

A. SC administration
B. No dosage adjustment needed with renal insufficiency
C. Once- or twice-daily dosing
D. Predictable response at lower doses
E. Lower incidence of heparin-induced thrombo-cytopenia

Answers

1. **C.** Symptoms of shortness of breath, dyspnea, chest pain, tachycardia, and tachypnea, along with a recent history of a DVT, are indications of a pulmonary embolism. A ventilation-perfusion scan or a spiral CT of the chest would confirm the diagnosis.

2. **B.** Several studies have indicated that weight-based dosing of heparin is more effective in obtaining therapeutic APTT compared to standard heparin titration. A weight-based protocol with an 80 IU/kg IV bolus followed by an infusion of 18 IU/kg per hour should produce APTTs close to the therapeutic range. The other doses are not appropriate.

3. **C.** High-risk surgeries involve the abdomen and lower extremities; thus hip and knee replacement as well as hip fracture surgery are major

risk factors for the development of a VTE. Hernia repair surgery is considered minor surgery, and unless the patient has other risk factors, would not require DVT prophylaxis other than early ambulation.

4. **C.** A spiral CT of the chest or a ventilation-perfusion scan would be necessary to confirm the diagnosis of a PE. Chest x-ray, electrocardiogram, echocardiogram, or bronchoscopy would not assist with the diagnosis.

5. **B.** Warfarin 5 mg daily should result in an INR around 2.0 within 4–5 days. The other doses are either extremely low or high for the majority of patients. Higher doses of warfarin may elevate an INR, but this may not be associated with a level of anticoagulation. A rapid increase in INR is due to depletion of factor VII rather than the anticoagulant effect that is associated with depletion of factor II and X.

6. **A.** An APTT is the laboratory test used to monitor heparin therapy. An APTT should be checked 6 hours after a dosage change and every 24 hours if it is within the therapeutic range. A PT/INR is used to monitor warfarin therapy.

7. **C.** Enoxaparin 100 mg SC q 12 hours or 1 mg/kg SC q 12 hours is the dose for treatment of an acute DVT. Enoxaparin 30 mg SC q 12 hours and 40 mg SC q 24 hours are doses used for DVT prophylaxis. Enoxaparin 200 mg SC q 12 hours and 220 mg SC q 12 hours are extremely high doses.

8. **A.** For the treatment of an active DVT or PE, at least 4–5 days of heparin or LMWH overlap with warfarin is needed before an anticoagulant effect is produced by warfarin. Heparin or LMWH should be discontinued after an INR is >2.0 for two consecutive occasions.

9. **E.** Statements A, B, C, and D are important to discuss with patients on warfarin. Patients should follow strict compliance with warfarin. They should eat vitamin K–rich foods consistently over the course of a week and report any symptoms of bleeding to their physician.

10. **D.** Green, leafy vegetables contain higher amounts of vitamin K; thus spinach and broccoli can reduce an INR. Lima beans, although green, do not have a large amount of vitamin K.

11. **E.** All of these drugs have the potential to produce a major rise in INR. These drugs should not be combined with warfarin if possible.

12. **B.** In a patient with AF with multiple risk factors for a stroke (hypertension, prior cerebrovascular accident, and diabetes), warfarin is the drug of choice, provided that the patient is a good warfarin candidate. Aspirin and clopidogrel are antiplatelet agents and are not as effective as warfarin in stroke risk reduction. t-PT is used for acute stroke treatment and administered intravenously.

13. **A.** Aspirin 325 mg daily is correct. Clopidogrel is dosed at 75 mg daily rather than bid. Aspirin 25 mg/dipyridamole 200 mg is dosed bid rather than daily. Warfarin is not appropriate in this patient because there is no indication that this was a cardioembolic stroke (the echocardiogram and electrocardiogram were normal). t-PA is not utilized orally and is only used for acute treatment of stroke to restore perfusion. Moderate stenosis of the carotid artery indicates atherosclerotic disease is present, and antiplatelet therapy is indicated.

14. **D.** All of the goals are correct except APTT range. Since antiplatelet therapy is indicated in this patient, APTT monitoring is not indicated.

15. **C.** Fondaparinux inhibits factor Xa.

16. **C.** Enoxaparin 30 mg SC q 12 hours or fondaparinux 2.5 mg SC q 24 hours are correct. Enoxaparin 80 mg SC q 12 hours is the dose used for treatment of VTE, and aspirin is not effective for DVT prophylaxis in knee replacement surgery.

17. **D.** Warfarin toxicity with an INR of 10.2 can be effectively reversed by holding the dose of warfarin and administering vitamin K 5 mg orally. Warfarin should be restarted when the INR is <3.0. The IV route is only utilized in emergent situations, since anaphylactic reactions are possible. Prothrombin complex is administered IV only for severe bleeding situations.

18. **C.** The therapeutic range for oral anticoagulation is an INR of 2.0–3.0, with a target of 2.5. Increased bleeding is associated with an INR >4.0 and embolic events are more common with an INR <1.5.

19 **D.** Doxycycline 100 mg bid would be the most appropriate therapy for a UTI. Septra DS, erythromycin, and ciprofloxacin will interact with warfarin to elevate the INR.

20. **C.** Clopidogrel and dipyridamole both inhibit antiplatelet activity. Dalteparin is a low-molecular-weight heparin that has inhibitory effects on factors IIa and Xa, and t-PA is a thrombolytic agent.

21. **C.** Warfarin 7.5 mg is yellow, 1 mg is pink, 10 mg is white, and 4 mg is blue.

22. **C.** Minor bleeding and bruising are common side effects of heparin therapy. Other common areas for bleeding are the urogenital and GI tracts.

23. **E.** The duration of anticoagulation therapy for patients with AF is lifelong. The risk for stroke is present as long as atrial fibrillation is present. Patients who undergo DC cardioversion to normal sinus rhythm require anticoagulation therapy for 4 weeks after conversion because the risk of stroke remains high during this time frame.

24. **B.** Since LMWHs are renally eliminated, they must be dose-adjusted for creatinine clearance <30 mL/min. Guidelines have recently been released for enoxaparin dosing in renal impairment. For DVT prophylaxis, enoxaparin should be administered 30 mg SC q 24 hours rather than q 12 hours. For DVT treatment, enoxaparin should be administered 1 mg/kg SC q 24 hours rather than q 12 hours.

6. References

Adams HP, Adams RJ, Brott T. ASA scientific statement, guidelines for early management of patients with ischemic stroke. *Stroke.* 2003;34:1056–1083.

Albers GW, Amarenco P, Easton JD, et al. Antithrombotic and thrombolytic therapy for ischemic stroke. *Chest.* 2001;119:300S–320S.

Alberts GW, Dalen JE, Laupacis A, et al. Antithrombotic therapy in atrial fibrillation. *Chest.* 2001;119:194S–206S.

Ansell J, Hirsh J, Dalen JE, et al. Managing oral anticoagulants therapy. *Chest.* 2001;119:22S–38S.

Fuster V, Ryden LE, Asinger RW, et al. ACC/AHA/ESC Guidelines for the management of atrial fibrillation: Executive summary. *Circulation.* 2001;104:2118–2150.

Bradberry JC, Fagan SC. Stroke. In: Dipiro JT, Talbert RL, Yee GC, eds. *Pharmacotherapy: A Pathophysiologic Approach,* 5th ed. New York: McGraw-Hill; 2002.

Geerts WH, Heit JA, Clagett GP, et al. Prevention of venous thromboembolism. *Chest.* 2001;119:132S–175S.

Goldstein LB, Adams, R. Becker K, et al. Primary prevention of ischemic stroke: A statement for healthcare professionals from the stroke council of the American Heart Association. *Circulation.* 2001;103:163–183.

Haines S, Racine E, Zeolla M. Venous thromboembolism. In: Dipiro JT, Talbert RL, Yee GC, eds. *Pharmacotherapy: A Pathophysiologic Approach,* 5th ed. New York: McGraw-Hill; 2002.

Hirst J, Anand SS, Halperin JL, et al. Guide to anticoagulant therapy: heparin a statement for healthcare professionals from the American Heart Association. *Circulation.* 2001;103:2994–3018.

Hirsh J, Dalen JE, Anderson DR, et al. Oral anticoagulants, clinical effectiveness, and optimal therapeutic range. *Chest.* 2001;119:8S–21S.

Hirsh J, Fuster V, Ansell J, et al. American Heart Association/American College of Cardiology Foundation Guide to warfarin therapy. *Circulation.* 2003;107:1692–1711.

Hirsh J, Warkentin TE, Shaughnessy SG, et al. Heparin and low-molecular-weight heparin: Mechanisms of action, pharmacokinetics, dosing, monitoring, efficacy, and safety. *Chest.* 2001;119:64S–94S.

Hyers TM, Agnelli G, Hull, RD, et al. Antithrombotic therapy for venous thromboembolic disease. *Chest.* 2001;119:176S–193S.

Stein PD, Alpert JS, Bussey HI, et al. Antithrombotic therapy in patients with mechanical and biological prosthetic heart valves. *Chest.* 2001;119:220S–227S.

38. 2004 Drug and Data Updates

Naseem Amarshi, BPharm, MSc, PharmD
Associate Professor and Director of Drug Information
Department of Pharmacy
University of Tennessee College of Pharmacy

Erin M. Timpe, PharmD, BCPS
Associate Professor
Department of Pharmacy
University of Tennessee College of Pharmacy

Susannah Motl, PharmD
Assistant Professor
Department of Pharmacy
University of Tennessee College of Pharmacy

Contents

Chapter 4: Compounding

With the publication of USP27/NF22, which became effective January 1, 2004, the following changes that affect nonsterile compounding were made:

1. Chapter 795 was renamed "Pharmaceutical Compounding - Nonsterile Preparations." The old name was "Pharmacy Compounding" and the following are the more significant changes: the term "compounder" is introduced and defined; a section entitled "Responsibility of the Compounder" was added and nine responsibilities are described; the subsection titled "Compounding - U.S. Food and Drug Law Requirements" was deleted; and the subsection entitled "Calculations" was deleted.

2. Chapter 1075, entitled "Good Compounding Practices," was added and contains the following sections:

   "Applicable Definitions." The most salient feature of this section is a description of the nine levels of compounding, which range from the simple mixing of two nonsterile components to preparation of the most sophisticated sterile products, including radiopharmaceuticals. Other terms are described, including "Pharmacy Generated Products."

   "Responsibilities of the Compounder." Points are enumerated and discussed to assure that the compounder is aware of his or her many responsibilities when preparing patient-specific customized medications.

   "Training." The importance of training and continuing education is emphasized for both the compounder and his or her employees.

   "Procedures and Documentation." Standard Operating Procedures (SOPs) must be in place for all aspects of the compounding procedures, and evidence that they are being followed must be documented.

   "Drug Compounding Facilities." The requirements of the facilities and environment in which compounded preparations are made are discussed and the importance of their proper maintenance is stressed, including documentation.

   "Drug Compounding Equipment." Equipment must be suited for the level(s) of compounding being carried out, and its cleaning, maintenance, and calibra-

tion must be covered in SOPs and appropriately documented.

   "Component Selection Requirements." Guidance is provided to the compounder as he or she selects the components that will be incorporated into the compounded medication being prepared.

   "Packaging and Drug Product Containers." Parameters for the proper selection of containers are discussed.

   "Compounding Controls." The many checks (ie, ways to ensure quality control) and activities that must take place in the compounding process are discussed, along with validations, tests, and documentations that must be made.

   "Labeling." The many items that must be included in the documentation of the compounding process, in the label of the compounded preparation, and in the patient's label, are discussed.

   "Records and Reports." What is required to generate appropriate records and reports is discussed.

   "Compounding for a Prescriber's Office Use." When compounders prepare medications for office use they must be in accordance with federal and state requirements, and appropriate documentation and labels must be prepared.

   "Compounding Veterinarian Products." Compounding for veterinary patients should be handled in the same manner as compounding for human patients.

   "Compounding Pharmacy Generated Products." Guidelines for preparing compounded drug products that can be sold without a prescription, labeling requirements for the patients, and the requirements of the federal and state authorities are described.

3. Chapter 1160, entitled "Pharmaceutical Calculations in Prescription Compounding," was added. This chapter discusses and provides definitions and examples of the many and various types of calculations that compounders must utilize as they prepare compounded medications for the variety of patients they serve. Calculations must be made accurately and must be checked, preferably by another pharmacist.

Chapter 5: Sterile Products

Updates for this chapter pertain to the section entitled "Overview of Standards of Practice Related to Sterile Products."

United States Pharmacopeia 27/National Formulary 22, Supplement 1 issued a new chapter, <797> Pharmaceutical Compounding-Sterile Preparations, which replaced chapter <1206>, Sterile Drug Products for Home Use. This chapter became official April 1, 2004 and provides a foundation for the development of procedures for the preparation of compounded sterile products. Products are divided into three risk levels based on the potential for contamination.

Low-Risk Compounding

Compounding is classified as low-risk when all of the following conditions are met:

1. Compounding occurs within an ISO 5 (Class 100) environment using only sterile ingredients, components, and products.
2. Compounding steps are performed promptly and involve only transfer and mixing manipulations with closed or sealed packaging systems.
3. Manipulations are limited to aseptically withdrawing from a vial or an ampule using sterile needles and syringes, and transferring the sterile solution to a sterile administration device or package.
4. In the absence of passing a sterility test, the storage period for the compounded sterile product cannot exceed the following time periods:
- Not more than 48 hours at controlled room temperature
- Not more than 14 days under refrigeration
- Not more than 45 days in a solid frozen state at –20° C or colder

Medium-Risk Compounding

Medium-risk level products are products compounded under low-risk conditions with one or more of the following conditions existing:

1. Compounding involves pooling of additives and the compounded sterile product will be administered to either multiple patients or to one patient on multiple occasions.
2. Compounding includes complex aseptic manipulations.
3. The compounded sterile product does not contain a bacteriostatic substance and is administered over several days.

4. In the absence of passing a sterility test the storage periods cannot exceed the following time periods:
- Not more than 30 hours at controlled room temperature
- Not more than 7 days under refrigeration
- Not more than 45 days in a solid frozen state at –20° C or colder

High-Risk Compounding

High-risk level compounding involves any of the following conditions:

1. Nonsterile ingredients are used to compound the sterile product.
2. Sterile ingredients, components and mixtures are exposed to air quality inferior to an ISO 5 (Class 100) environment.
3. Nonsterile compounded products are exposed for at least 6 hours before being sterilized.
4. No verification of the chemical purity and strength of the ingredient is made by examining the labeling or the certificate of quality of the ingredient to make sure the original specifications or those of the compendia are met.
5. In the absence of passing a sterility test, the storage periods cannot exceed the following time periods:
- Not more than 24 hours at controlled room temperature
- Not more than 3 days under refrigeration
- Not more than 45 days in a solid frozen state at –20° C or colder

Reference

Pharmaceutical Compounding—Sterile Preparations. In: United States Pharmacopeia, First Supplement to the 27th Revision: National Formulary, 22nd ed. Rockville, MD: United States Pharmacopeial Convention; 2004:3121–3138.

Chapter 8: Hypertension

Drug: Benicar HCT™ (olmesartan + hydrochloro-thiazide)
Class: Angiotensin II receptor blocker/thiazide diuretic
Form: Tablets
Formulations: 20 mg/12.5 mg, 40 mg/12.5 mg, 40 mg/25 mg
Dose: Olmesartan 20–40 mg/hydrochlorothiazide 12.5–25 mg daily
Mechanism of action: Olmesartan inhibits the binding of angiotensin II to the angiotensin II receptor, thereby inhibiting the vasoconstrictive properties of angiotensin II as well as its ability to stimulate release of aldosterone.

Hydrochlorothiazide directs arteriole dilation and reduces total fluid volume through the inhibition of sodium reabsorption in the distal tubules.
FDA-approved uses: Hypertension
Adverse reactions: Hyperkalemia, angioedema, hypokalemia, hyponatremia, hypomagnesemia, hypercalcemia
Drug interactions: Aminoglycosides, nonsteroidal anti-inflammatory drugs (NSAIDs).
Monitoring parameters: Serum electrolytes, blood pressure
Patient counseling: Monitor blood pressure

Drug: Caduet® (amlodipine besylate/atorvastatin calcium)
Class: Antihypertensive/antihyperlipidemic
Form: Tablets
Formulations: 5 mg/10 mg, 5 mg/20 mg, 5 mg/40 mg, 5 mg/80 mg, 10 mg/10 mg, 10 mg/20 mg, 10 mg/40 mg, 10 mg/80 mg
Dose:
Amlodipine: 5–10 mg daily
Atorvastatin: initial dose of 10–20 mg daily
Maintenance: 10–80 mg daily
Mechanism of action:
Amlodipine: (calcium channel blocker) inhibits the influx of calcium ions through slow channels in the vascular smooth muscle and causes relaxation of both coronary and peripheral arteries.
Atorvastatin: 3-Hydroyxy-3-methylglutaryl coenzyme A (HMG-CoA) reductase inhibitor (statin); competitively inhibits HMG-CoA reductase, which is the enzyme responsible for conversion of HMG-CoA to mevalonate. Mevalonate is an early precursor and a rate-limiting step in cholesterol synthesis. This reduction in liver cholesterol synthesis results in upregulation of liver low-density lipoprotein (LDL) receptors and increased clearance of LDL and very-low-density lipoprotein (VLDL) particles in the blood. These actions induce a decrease in total cholesterol and LDL cholesterol, promote a slight increase in high-density lipoprotein (HDL) cholesterol, and affect a modest decrease in triglycerides.
FDA-approved uses: Hypertension; chronic stable angina; vasospastic angina; congestive heart failure; hypercholesterolemia
Adverse reactions: Edema of the ankles, flushing, headache, gingival hyperplasia, myopathy, myalgia, myositis, rhabdomyolysis, elevated liver enzymes, flu-like symptoms and headache, mild GI complaints
Drug interactions: Use with caution in patients with conduction disturbances in the sinoatrial (SA) or atrioventricular (AV) nodes. Grapefruit juice may increase amlodipine levels. Cytochrome P 450 (CYP450) 3A4 inhibitors may increase atorvastatin concentrations.
Monitoring parameters: Electrocardiogram (ECG), peripheral edema, blood pressure and pulse, bowel habits, symptoms of conduction disturbances, fasting lipid panel, liver function tests (LFTs), creatine kinase (CK)
Patient counseling: Monitor LFTs and muscle toxicity.

Drug: Inspra™ (eplerenone)
Class: Selective aldosterone receptor antagonist
Form: Tablets
Formulations: 25 mg, 50 mg
Dose: Initial dose of 25 mg daily; target dose of 50 mg daily
Mechanism of action: Selectively binds to mineralocorticoid receptors to block the binding of aldosterone. Aldosterone increases blood pressure through sodium reabsorption when aldosterone binds to receptors.
FDA-approved uses: Congestive heart failure post myocardial infarction; hypertension
Adverse reactions: Hyperkalemia, increased creatinine
Drug interactions: Contraindicated with CYP450 3A4 inhibitors; increased potassium with angiotensin-converting enzyme inhibitors (ACEIs) and angiotensin receptor blockers (ARBs)
Monitoring parameters: Potassium, blood pressure, creatinine
Patient counseling: Monitor blood pressure.

Chapter 9: Heart Failure

Drug: Inspra™ (eplerenone)
Class: Selective aldosterone receptor antagonist
Form: Tablets
Formulations: 25 mg, 50 mg
Dose: Initial dose of 25 mg daily; target dose of 50 mg daily
Mechanism of action: Selectively binds to mineralo-corticoid receptors to block the binding of aldosterone. Aldosterone increases blood pressure through sodium reabsorption when aldosterone binds to receptors.
FDA-approved uses: Congestive heart failure post myocardial infarction; hypertension
Adverse reactions: Hyperkalemia, increased creatinine
Drug interactions: Contraindicated with CYP450 3A4 inhibitors, increased potassium with ACEIs and ARBs
Monitoring parameters: Potassium, blood pressure, creatinine
Patient counseling: Monitor blood pressure.

Chapter 11: Ischemic Heart Disease

NOTE: Betapace AF has a new dose form available: 40 mg, 60 mg, 100 mg tablets

Drug: Caduet® (amlodipine besylate + atorvastatin calcium)
Class: Antihypertensive/antihyperlipidemic
Form: Tablets
Formulations: 5 mg/10 mg, 5 mg/20 mg, 5 mg/40 mg, 5 mg/80 mg, 10 mg/10 mg, 10 mg/20 mg, 10 mg/40 mg, 10 mg/80 mg
Dose:
  Amlodipine: 5–10 mg daily
  Atorvastatin: initial dose of 10–20 mg daily and a maintenance dose of 10–80 mg daily
Mechanism of action:
  Amlodipine: (calcium channel blocker) inhibits the influx of calcium ions through slow channels in the vascular smooth muscle and causes relaxation of both coronary and peripheral arteries.
  Atorvastatin: HMG-CoA reductase inhibitor (statin), competitively inhibits HMG-CoA reductase, which is the enzyme responsible for conversion of HMG-CoA to mevalonate. Mevalonate is an early precursor and a rate-limiting step in cholesterol synthesis. This reduction in liver cholesterol synthesis results in upregulation of liver LDL receptors and increased clearance of LDL and VLDL particles in the blood. These actions induce a decrease in total cholesterol and LDL cholesterol, promote a slight increase in HDL cholesterol, and affect a modest decrease in triglycerides.
FDA-approved uses: Hypertension; chronic stable angina; vasospastic angina; congestive heart failure; hypercholesterolemia
Adverse reactions: Edema of the ankles, flushing, headache, gingival hyperplasia, myopathy, myalgia, myositis, rhabdomyolysis, elevated liver enzymes, flu-like symptoms and headache, mild GI complaints
Drug interactions: Use with caution in patients with conduction disturbances in the SA or AV nodes. Grapefruit juice may increase amlodipine levels. CYP450 3A4 inhibitors may increase atorvastatin concentrations.
Monitoring parameters: ECG, peripheral edema, blood pressure and pulse, bowel habits, symptoms of conduction disturbances, fasting lipid panel, liver function tests, and creatinine kinase
Patient counseling: Monitor liver function tests and muscle toxicity.

Drug: Pravigard® Pac (pravastatin sodium + buffered aspirin)
Class: Antihyperlipidemic/NSAID
Form: Tablets
Formulations: 81 mg/20 mg, 325 mg/20 mg, 81 mg/40 mg, 325 mg/40 mg, 81 mg/80 mg, 325 mg/ 80 mg
Dose:
Buffered aspirin: 81–325 mg daily
Pravastatin: initial dose of 20 mg daily and maintenance dose of 20–80 mg daily
Mechanism of action:
Buffered aspirin: inhibits prostaglandin cyclooxygenase to decrease platelet aggregation
Pravastatin: HMG-CoA reductase inhibitor (statin); competitively inhibits HMG-CoA reductase, which is the enzyme responsible for conversion of HMG-CoA to mevalonate. Mevalonate is an early precursor and a rate-limiting step in cholesterol synthesis. This reduction in liver cholesterol synthesis results in upregulation of liver LDL receptors and increased clearance of LDL and VLDL particles in the blood. These actions induce a decrease in total cholesterol and LDL cholesterol, promote a slight increase in HDL cholesterol, and affect a modest decrease in triglycerides.
FDA-approved uses: Reduce the occurrence of cardiovascular events (eg, death, myocardial infarction, and stroke) in patients with cardiovascular and/or cerebrovascular disease
Adverse reactions:
Buffered aspirin: bleeding/bruising, GI complaints
Pravastatin: myopathy, myalgia, myositis, rhabdomyolysis, elevated liver enzymes, flu-like symptoms and headache, mild GI complaints
Drug interactions:
Buffered aspirin: increased risk of bleeding with anticoagulants and phenytoin
Pravastatin: CYP450 3A4 inhibitors may increase atorvastatin concentrations
Monitoring parameters:
Buffered aspirin: bleeding/bruising
Pravastatin: fasting lipid panel, LFTs, CK
Patient counseling: Monitor liver function tests and muscle toxicity, avoid in patients with a history of peptic ulcer disease.

Chapter 12: Hyperlipidemia

NOTE: The name Altocor (lovastatin) has been changed to Altoprev™; 10- to 60-mg tablets

Drug: Caduet® (amlodipine besylate + atorvastatin calcium)
Class: Calcium channel blocker/HMG CoA reductase inhibitor
Form: Tablets
Formulations: 5 mg/10 mg, 5 mg/20 mg, 5 mg/40 mg, 5 mg/80 mg, 10 mg/10 mg, 10 mg/20 mg, 10 mg/40 mg, 10 mg/80 mg
Dose:
Amlodipine: 5–10 mg daily
Atorvastatin: initial dose of 10–20 mg daily and maintenance dose of 10–80 mg daily
Mechanism of action:
Amlodipine: (calcium channel blocker) inhibits the influx of calcium ions through slow channels in the vascular smooth muscle and causes relaxation of both coronary and peripheral arteries
Atorvastatin: HMG-CoA reductase inhibitor (statin); competitively inhibits HMG-CoA reductase, which is the enzyme responsible for conversion of HMG-CoA to mevalonate. Mevalonate is an early precursor and a rate-limiting step in cholesterol synthesis. This reduction in liver cholesterol synthesis results in upregulation of liver LDL receptors and increased clearance of LDL and VLDL particles in the blood. These actions induce a decrease in total cholesterol and LDL cholesterol, promote a slight increase in HDL cholesterol, and affect a modest decrease in triglycerides.
FDA-approved uses: Hypertension, chronic stable angina, vasospastic angina, congestive heart failure, and hypercholesterolemia
Adverse reactions: Edema of the ankles, flushing, headache, gingival hyperplasia, myopathy, myalgia, myositis, rhabdomyolysis, elevated liver enzymes, flu-like symptoms and headache, mild GI complaints
Drug interactions: Use with caution in patients with conduction disturbances in the SA or AV nodes. Grapefruit juice may increase amlodipine levels. CYP450 3A4 inhibitors may increase atorvastatin concentrations.
Monitoring parameters: ECG, peripheral edema, blood pressure and pulse, bowel habits, symptoms of conduction disturbances, fasting lipid panel, liver function tests, and CK
Patient counseling: Monitor liver function tests and muscle toxicity.

Drug: Crestor® (rosuvastatin)
Class: HMG CoA reductase inhibitor
Form: Tablets
Formulations: 5, 10, 20 mg
Dose: Initial dose of 10 mg daily and a maintenance dose of 5–40 mg daily
Mechanism of action: Competitively inhibits HMG-CoA reductase, which is the enzyme responsible for conversion of HMG-CoA to mevalonate. Mevalonate is an early precursor and a rate-limiting step in cholesterol synthesis. This reduction in liver cholesterol synthesis results in upregulation of liver LDL receptors and increased clearance of LDL and VLDL particles in the blood. These actions induce a decrease in total cholesterol and LDL cholesterol, promote a slight increase in HDL cholesterol, and affect a modest decrease in triglycerides.
FDA-approved uses: Hypercholesterolemia
Adverse reactions: Myopathy, myalgia, myositis, rhabdomyolysis, elevated liver enzymes, flu-like symptoms and headache, mild GI complaints
Drug interactions: CYP450 3A4 inhibitors may increase atorvastatin concentrations.
Monitoring parameters: Fasting lipid panel, LFTs, CK
Patient counseling: Monitor liver function tests and muscle toxicity.

Chapter 13: Diabetes Mellitus

Drug: Apidra® (insulin glulisine)
Class: Insulin
Form: Injection
Formulations: 100 units per 1 mL, 10-mL vial
Dose: Individualized per patient. One unit of insulin glulisine has the same insulin-lowering effect as 1 unit of regular insulin.
Mechanism of action: Stimulates peripheral glucose uptake by skeletal muscle and fat and inhibits hepatic glucose production. Insulin glulisine has a more rapid onset and shorter duration than regular insulin when injected subcutaneously.
FDA-approved uses: Diabetes mellitus
Adverse reactions: Hypoglycemia, weight gain, local and systemic allergic reactions, lipodystrophies
Drug interactions: If administering with NPH insulin, draw the insulin glulisine into the syringe first.
Monitoring parameters: Glucose, hemoglobin A1c (Hb_{A1c})
Patient counseling: Store unopened vials in the refrigerator. Opened vials may be used for up to 28 days with or without refrigeration.

Drug: Glucophage® XR (extended-release metformin)
Class: Biguanide
Form: Tablets
Formulations: 500 mg, 750 mg
Dose: Initial dose of 500 mg once daily; maintenance dose of 500–2000 mg once daily
Mechanism of action: Increases hepatic and peripheral insulin sensitivity and decreases hepatic glucose production
FDA-approved uses: Diabetes mellitus
Adverse reactions: GI effects, megaloblastic anemia, lactic acidosis
Drug interactions: Additive effects with hypoglycemic agents
Monitoring parameters: Glucose, Hb_{A1c}, creatinine
Patient counseling: Monitor for symptoms of lactic acidosis. Take with meals.

Drug: Riomet™ (metformin solution)
Class: Biguanide
Form: Solution
Formulations: 100 mg per 1 mL solution
Dose: Initial dose of 500 mg, once daily; maintenance dose of 500–2000 mg, once daily
Mechanism of action: Increases hepatic and peripheral insulin sensitivity and decreases hepatic glucose production
FDA-approved uses: Diabetes mellitus
Adverse reactions: GI, megaloblastic anemia, lactic acidosis

Drug interactions: Additive effects with hypoglycemic agents
Monitoring parameters: Glucose, Hb_{A1c}, creatinine
Patient counseling: Monitor for symptoms of lactic
acidosis. Take with meals.

Chapter 15: Women's Health

Drug: Boniva® (ibandronate sodium)
Class: Bisphosphonate
Form: Tablets
Formulations: 2.5 mg
Dose: 2.5 mg once daily
Mechanism of action: Inhibits osteoclast activity and
decreases bone resorption and turnover.
FDA-approved uses: Treatment and prevention of
osteoporosis in postmenopausal women
Adverse reactions: GI complaints
Drug interactions: Boniva should be taken 1 hour
prior to any other oral medications.
Monitoring parameters: Bone mineral density, alka-
line phosphatase
Patient counseling: Patients should take Boniva stand-
ing up, with 8 ounces of water, and 60 minutes before
any food, beverages, or other oral medications.

Drug: Cenestin® (synthetic conjugated estrogens)
Class: Estrogens
Form: Tablets
Formulations: 0.3 mg, 0.45 mg, 0.625 mg, 0.9 mg,
1.25 mg
Dose: 0.3 to 1.25 mg once daily
Mechanism of action: Acts as a replacement for
diminished estrogen levels and restores estrogenic
activity.
FDA-approved uses: Treatment of moderate to severe
vasomotor symptoms associated with menopause;
treatment of moderate to severe symptoms associated
with vulvar and vaginal atrophy due to menopause.
Adverse reactions: Breast tenderness, heavy bleeding,
headache, nausea
Drug interactions: CYP 3A4 inhibitors/inducers,
hydantoins, topiramate, corticosteroids, tricyclic antidepressants
Monitoring parameters: Laboratory monitoring not
recommended.
Patient counseling: Estrogen-related side effects may
be diminished by starting with a low dose.

Drug: Climara Pro™ (estradiol/levonorgestrel trans-
dermal system)
Class: Combination estrogen-progestin replacement
Form: Transdermal patch
Formulations: 0.045 mg/d of estradiol and 0.015/d mg
of levonorgestrel patch
Dose: Apply one patch weekly.
Mechanism of action: Acts as a replacement for
diminished estrogen and progesterone levels and
restores estrogenic activity.

FDA-approved uses: Treatment of moderate to severe vasomotor symptoms associated with menopause
Adverse reactions: Headache, breast pain, irregular vaginal bleeding or spotting, stomach/abdominal cramps, nausea, vomiting, hair loss
Drug interactions: CYP 3A4 inhibitors/inducers, hydantoins, topiramate, corticosteroids, tricyclic anti-depressants
Monitoring parameters: Laboratory monitoring not recommended.
Patient counseling: Apply the patch to a clean, dry area of the lower abdomen once a week.

Drug: Enjuvia™ (synthetic conjugated estrogens)
Class: Estrogens
Form: Tablets
Formulations: 0.625 mg, 1.25 mg
Dose: 0.625 to 1.25 mg once daily
Mechanism of action: Acts as a replacement for diminished estrogen levels and restores estrogenic activity.
FDA-approved uses: Treatment of moderate to severe vasomotor symptoms associated with menopause
Adverse reactions: Breast tenderness, heavy bleeding, headache, nausea
Drug interactions: CYP 3A4 inhibitors/inducers, hydantoins, topiramate, corticosteroids, tricyclic anti-depressants
Monitoring parameters: Laboratory monitoring not recommended.
Patient counseling: Side effects due to estrogen may be diminished by starting with a low dose.

Drug: Estrasorb™ (estradiol topical emulsion)
Class: Estrogens
Form: Topical emulsion
Formulations: 4.35 mg of estradiol in a 1.74-g pouch
Dose: Apply the contents of one pouch to the left thigh, calf, and buttock, and one pouch to the right thigh, calf, and buttock
Mechanism of action: Acts as a replacement for diminished estrogen levels and restores estrogenic activity.
FDA-approved uses: Treatment of moderate to severe vasomotor symptoms associated with menopause.
Adverse reactions: Breast tenderness, heavy bleeding, headache, nausea
Drug interactions: CYP 3A4 inhibitors/inducers, hydantoins, topiramate, corticosteroids, tricyclic anti-depressants
Monitoring parameters: Laboratory monitoring not recommended.
Patient counseling: Allow the application area to dry thoroughly before covering with clothing, and wash hands thoroughly after application.

Drug: Femring® (estradiol acetate vaginal ring)
Class: Estrogens
Form: Vaginal ring
Formulations: 0.5 mg/d, 0.10 mg/d vaginal ring
Dose: Insert the ring into the vagina and leave in place for up to 3 months.
Mechanism of action: Acts as a replacement for diminished estrogen levels and restores estrogenic activity
FDA-approved uses: Treatment of moderate to severe vasomotor symptoms associated with menopause; treatment of moderate to severe symptoms associated with vulvar and vaginal atrophy due to menopause
Adverse reactions: Breast tenderness, heavy bleeding, headache, nausea
Drug interactions: CYP 3A4 inhibitors/inducers, hydantoins, topiramate, corticosteroids, tricyclic anti-depressants
Monitoring parameters: Laboratory monitoring not recommended.
Patient counseling: If the Femring is expelled from the vagina, it should be rinsed in lukewarm water and reinserted.

Drug: Menostar™ (estradiol transdermal system)
Class: Estrogen replacement
Form: Transdermal patch
Formulations: 14 µg/d of estradiol, each patch containing 1 mg of estradiol
Dose: Apply one patch weekly.
Mechanism of action: Acts as a replacement for diminished estrogen levels and restores protective skeletal benefits provided by the hormone
FDA-approved uses: Prevention of postmenopausal osteoporosis
Adverse reactions: Headache, breast pain, irregular vaginal bleeding or spotting, stomach/abdominal cramps, nausea, vomiting, hair loss
Drug interactions: CYP 3A4 inhibitors/inducers, hydantoins, topiramate, corticosteroids, tricyclic anti-depressants
Monitoring parameters: Laboratory monitoring not recommended.
Patient counseling: Apply the patch to a clean, dry area of the lower abdomen once a week.

Drug: Seasonale® (ethinyl estradiol/levonorgestrel)
Class: Extended cycle oral contraceptive agent
Form: Tablets
Formulations: 0.03 mg ethinyl estradiol and 0.15 mg levonorgestrel
Dose: One active tablet daily for 12 weeks followed by one week of inactive tablets
Mechanism of Action: Prevents the development of a dominant follicle by suppression of follicle-stimulating hormone (FSH), and blocks ovulation by contributing

to the production of a thick and impermeable cervical mucus.

FDA-approved uses: Prevention of pregnancy

Adverse reactions: Breast tenderness, heavy or break-through bleeding, headache, nausea, weight change

Drug interactions: Antibiotics, anticonvulsants, non-nucleoside reverse transcriptase inhibitors, protease inhibitors, theophylline

Monitoring parameters: Laboratory monitoring not recommended.

Patient counseling: If one active tablet is missed, take it as soon as it is remembered. If two active tablets are missed, take two pills on the day remembered and two pills the following day (a back-up method of birth control should be used for at least 7 days). If three or more active tablets are missed, do not take the missed pills but resume taking the pill on the day remembered and forward (a back-up method of birth control should be used for at least 7 days).

NOTE: New formulations of Prempro™ and Premarin® are available.
Prempro: 0.3 mg conjugated estrogens and 1.5 mg medroxyprogesterone acetate
Premarin: 0.3 mg conjugated estrogens

Chapter 16: Kidney Disease

Drug: Sensipar™ (cinacalcet HCl)
Class: Calcimimetic agent
Form: Tablets
Formulations: 30 mg, 60 mg tablets
Dose: Individualized per patient; initial dose of 30 mg once daily. Titrate no more frequently than every 2–4 weeks.
Mechanism of action: Lowers parathyroid hormone levels by increasing the sensitivity of the calcium-sensing receptor to extracellular calcium
FDA-approved uses: Secondary hyperparathyroidism in patients with chronic kidney disease on dialysis; hypercalcemia in patients with parathyroid carcinoma
Adverse reactions: GI complaints, myalgia, hypertension
Drug interactions: CYP2D6 substrates and inducers
Monitoring parameters: Serum calcium, serum phosphorus, immunoassay for parathyroid hormone (iPTH)
Patient counseling: Monitor for symptoms of hypocalcemia, ie, paresthesias, myalgias, cramping, tetany, and convulsions.

Chapter 17: Critical Care, Fluids, and Electrolytes

Drug: Iprivask™ (desirudin)
Class: Direct thrombin inhibitor
Form: Subcutaneous injection
Formulations: 15.75 mg of lyophilized powder
Dose: 15 mg bid SC for 9–12 days postsurgery
Mechanism of action: A selective inhibitor of free and clot-bound thrombin stops the formation of clots.
FDA-approved uses: Prophylaxis of DVT in patients undergoing hip surgery
Adverse reactions: Bleeding, nausea, wound secretion, fever, injection site mass, hematoma, anemia, hypotension, urinary retention, deep thrombophlebitis
Drug interactions: Anticoagulant use may increase risk of bleeding
Monitoring parameters: Activated partial thromboplastin time (aPTT) taken 4 hours after the first administration, then daily
Patient counseling: Contact your health care professional immediately if you develop bleeding or bruising.

Chapter 19: Oncology

Drug: Emend® (aprepitant)
Class: Neurokinin-1 receptor antagonist
Form: Capsules
Formulations: 80 mg and 125 mg capsules
Dose: 125 mg PO 1 hour prior to chemotherapy on day 1; 80 mg PO on days 2 and 3
Mechanism of action: By binding to the neurokinin-1 receptor, substance P is effectively blocked. Substance P is associated with emesis, depression, and pain after inflammation.
FDA-approved uses: Prophylaxis of chemotherapy-induced nausea and vomiting
Adverse reactions: Somnolence, fatigue, diarrhea
Drug interactions: Aprepitant is a potent inhibitor of CYP3A4. Use caution when administering with benzodiazepines, dexamethasone, diltiazem, and azole antifungals. Monitor International Normalized Ratio (INR) if on warfarin (expect decrease).
Monitoring parameters: Fluid and electrolyte status
Patient counseling: You should be receiving other drugs in addition to this to control nausea and vomiting. Let your nurse or doctor know if your symptoms are not controlled.

Drug: Velcade® (bortezomib)
Class: Proteasome inhibitor
Form: Intravenous injection
Formulations: 3.5 mg of lyophilized powder
Dose: 1.3 mg/m^2 bolus IV injection on days 1, 4, 8, and 11; repeated every 21 days
Mechanism of action: Through inhibition of the 26S proteasome, bortezomib stabilizes regulatory proteins, causing a disruption of cell proliferation and apoptosis.
FDA-approved uses: Multiple myeloma treatment for patients as third-line therapy
Adverse reactions: Asthenia, nausea, vomiting, thrombocytopenia, peripheral neuropathy, neutropenia, and hypotension
Drug interactions: None reported
Monitoring parameters: Complete blood cell count (CBC), LFTs, electrolytes, neurologic exam, bleeding
Patient counseling: Let your doctor or nurse know if you need additional medications to prevent nausea and vomiting.

Drug: Iressa® (gefitinib)
Class: Epidermal growth factor receptor and tyrosine kinase inhibitor
Form: Tablets
Formulations: 250 mg PO tablets
Dose: 250 mg daily
Mechanism of Action: Blocks signal transduction pathways involved in proliferation, survival, and

metastases of cancer cells and other processes promoting tumor growth.

FDA-approved uses: Monotherapy in locally advanced or metastatic non-small-cell lung cancer (NSCLC) as third-line therapy

Adverse reactions: Diarrhea, rash, acne, dry skin, nausea, vomiting

Drug interactions: Undergoes CYP3A4 metabolism. There is an increased INR with warfarin. May see increased metabolism if on concomitant inducers (ie, phenytoin); increase dose to 500 mg PO qd. Separate administration with drugs that increase gastric pH.

Monitoring parameters: LFTs, CBC, excessive diarrhea

Patient counseling: The development of a rash or acne is a sign that the medication is working.

Drug: Aloxi® (palonosetron hydrochloride)
Class: Serotonin receptor (5-HT₃) antagonist
Form: Intravenous injection
Formulations: 0.05 mg/mL solution for injection
Dose: 0.25 mg IV 30 minutes prior to chemotherapy
Mechanism of action: Selectively blocks the 5-HT₃ receptor site present in the chemoreceptor trigger zone
FDA-approved uses: Prophylaxis of acute and delayed chemotherapy-induced nausea and vomiting
Adverse reactions: Diarrhea, headache, vertigo, fatigue, abdominal pain, insomnia, arrhythmias
Drug interactions: None reported
Monitoring parameters: Chest pain, dystonia, tremor
Patient counseling: You may receive other drugs in addition to this to control nausea and vomiting. Let your nurse or doctor know if your symptoms are not controlled.

Drug: Alimta® (pemetrexed disodium)
Class: Antifolate agent
Form: Intravenous injection
Formulations: 500 mg base solution for injection
Dose: 500–600 mg/m² IV administered every 21 days
Mechanism of action: Inhibition of more than four enzymes involved in folate metabolism and DNA synthesis, causing cell death
FDA-approved uses: Treatment of malignant pleural mesothelioma in patients who are not candidates for curative surgery or in whom the disease is unresectable
Adverse reactions: Hematologic toxicity, fatigue, pruritic skin rash, mucositis, renal and/or hepatic dysfunction
Drug interactions: None reported
Monitoring parameters: Plasma homocysteine levels, CBC, LFTs, renal function tests
Patient counseling: You must be taking 350–1000 μg of folic acid every day during your therapy (starting 7 days prior to therapy and continuing for 21 days after therapy). Your doctor should also be giving you vitamin B₁₂ injections about every 9 weeks during therapy.

Drug: Bexxar® (tositumomab and iodine ¹³¹I tositumomab)
Class: Monoclonal antibody directed against the CD20 antibody
Form: Intravenous injection
Formulations: 14 mg/mL solution for injection
Dose: Administered as a two-step single-course treatment: (1) 450 mg tositumomab IV followed by iodine ¹³¹I tositumomab (dosimetric dose); (2) repeat step 1 with a calculated iodine ¹³¹I tositumomab dose (therapeutic dose)
Mechanism of action: Causes programmed cell death and stimulates the immune system to attack cancer cells
FDA-approved uses: Relapsed, CD20-positive follicular non-Hodgkin's lymphoma patients who are refractory to rituximab
Adverse reactions: Allergic reactions, infection, hemorrhage, nausea, vomiting, hypothyroidism, infusional toxicities (fever, chills)
Drug interactions: Antiplatelets and/or anticoagulants may increase the risk for hemorrhage and bleeding.
Monitoring parameters: CBC with differential and platelets, thyroid-stimulating hormone (TSH) levels, serum creatinine, human anti-murine antibody (HAMA) titers, blood pressure, pulse
Patient counseling: Notify your doctor or nurse if you start to bleed or bruise easily. Stay away from crowds and sick people.

Drug: Faslodex® (fulvestrant)
Class: Antiestrogen
Form: Intramuscular injection
Formulations: 50 mg/mL injection
Dose: 250 mg intramuscular injection administered once a month
Mechanism of action: Competes with endogenous estrogen for estrogen receptor binding
FDA-approved uses: Treatment of hormone receptor–positive metastatic breast cancer in postmenopausal women with disease progression following antiestrogen therapy
Adverse reactions: Hot flushes, back pain, headache, constipation, diarrhea, nausea, vomiting, anemia
Drug interactions: None reported
Monitoring parameters: CBC, lipids
Patient counseling: This medication may cause vaginal bleeding.

Drug: Zevalin® (ibritumomab tiuxetan)
Class: Monoclonal antibody directed against the CD20 antibody
Form: Intravenous injection
Formulations: 3.2 mg/2 mL solution for injection
Dose: Administered in a two-step treatment course: (1) infuse 250 mg/m² of rituximab; within 4 hours, admin-

ister ibritumomab IV (5 millicuries); (2) on day 7 repeat rituximab dose, and within 4 hours administer ibritumomab IV 0.4 millicuries/kg

Mechanism of action: Directs radiation to CD20 antigen-containing B cells, induces antibody-dependent, cell-mediated cytotoxicity, complement-dependent cytotoxicity, and apoptosis in target cells.

FDA-approved uses: Relapsed or refractory low-grade, follicular or transformed, non-Hodgkin's lymphoma

Adverse reactions: Severe hematologic toxicity, asthenia, headache, arthralgia, nausea, vomiting, abdominal pain, dyspnea, cough

Drug interactions: None reported; antiplatelets could increase risk of bleeding

Monitoring parameters: CBC, platelets, temperature, blood pressure, signs of infection

Patient counseling: Notify your doctor or nurse if you start to bleed or bruise easily. Stay away from crowds and sick people.

Drug: Vidaza® (azacitidine)
Class: Pyrimidine nucleoside analog
Form: Subcutaneous injection
Formulations: 100 mg lyophilized powder
Dose: 75–100 mg/m^2 subcutaneously for 7 days repeated every 28 days
Mechanism of action: Interferes with nucleic acid metabolism, causing the death of rapidly-dividing cells
FDA-approved uses: Treatment of refractory anemia or refractory anemia with sideroblasts, excess blasts, excess blasts in transformation, and chronic myelomonocytic leukemia
Adverse reactions: Myelosuppression, diarrhea, fatigue, constipation, cough, dyspnea
Drug interactions: None reported
Monitoring parameters: CBC with differential, platelets, LFTs, serum creatinine, neurologic exam
Patient counseling: Stay away from crowds and sick people.

Drug: Plenaxis™ (abarelix)
Class: Gonadotropin-releasing hormone (GnRH) antagonist
Form: Intramuscular injection
Formulations: 100 mg/2 mL of lyophilized powder
Dose: 100 mg intramuscular injection (buttock) on days 1, 15, and 29, and every 4 weeks thereafter
Mechanism of action: Inhibits the secretion of the pituitary gonadotropins by directly blocking the pituitary luteinizing hormone-releasing hormone (LRHR) receptor
FDA-approved uses: Palliative treatment of men with advanced symptomatic prostate cancer who meet specific criteria.

Adverse Reactions:
Black box warning: immediate onset of systemic allergic reactions (ie, hypotension and syncope); pain, hot flushes, sleep disturbance, breast enlargement, and/or tenderness
Drug interactions: Amiodarone, procainamide, quinidine, and sotalol may increase the risk of cardiotoxicity.
Monitoring parameters: LFTs, CBC, hypersensitivity monitoring, baseline echocardiogram
Patient counseling: It is important to have a health care professional monitor you while receiving this medication.

Drug: Avastin™ (bevacizumab)
Class: Monoclonal antibody directed against vascular endothelial growth factor (VEGF)
Form: Intravenous injection
Formulations: 100 mg/4 mL, 400 mg/16 mL solution for injection
Dose: 5–10 mg/kg IV every 2 weeks
Mechanism of action: Stabilizes established tumors and suppresses tumor growth by inhibiting angiogenesis induced by VEGF
FDA-approved uses: Use in combination with 5-fluororuracil–based chemotherapy for metastatic colorectal cancer
Adverse reactions: Bleeding, hemorrhage, thromboembolism, hypertension, nausea, vomiting, skin rash, proteinuria
Drug interactions: None reported
Monitoring parameters: Coagulation parameters, CBC, urinalysis, blood pressure
Patient Counseling: You may develop high blood pressure while on this medication. Have your pressure checked regularly.

Drug: Erbitux™ (cetuximab)
Class: Monoclonal antibody directed against the epidermal growth factor receptor (EGFR)
Form: Intravenous injection
Formulations: 100 mg solution for injection
Dose: 250–500 mg/m^2 IV once a week for 7–8 weeks
Mechanism of action: Inhibition of cell proliferation caused by the disruption of EGFR-mediated signal transduction pathways
FDA-approved uses: Use in combination with irinotecan or alone in metastatic colorectal cancer
Adverse reactions: Fever, asthenia, nausea, LFT elevations, and cutaneous reactions
Drug interactions: None reported
Monitoring parameters: LFTs, CBC
Patient counseling: Erbitux may cause severe reactions during IV infusion, including sudden onset of itching, swelling, low blood pressure, and trouble

breathing. Let your health care professional know immediately if you feel these symptoms.

Drug: Gliadel® wafer (polifeprosan 20 with carmustine implant)
Class: Alkylator antineoplastic
Form: Intravenous infusion and implant
Formulations: 7.7 mg implant system
Dose: 8 wafers implanted in resection cavity
Mechanism of action: Forms covalent cross-links with DNA and RNA cells, inhibiting replication
FDA-approved uses: A surgical adjunct for recurrent glioblastoma multiforme or newly diagnosed high-grade gliomas
Adverse reactions: Abnormal healing, nausea, vomiting, hematologic toxicity, infection, liver dysfunction, and renal failure
Drug interactions: Concomitant cimetidine use may cause bone marrow suppression; multiple herbal interactions
Monitoring parameters: CBC, LFTs, healing of incision site
Patient counseling: Avoid drinking alcohol. Avoid crowds and sick people while taking this medication.

Drug: Eligard® (leuprolide acetate)
Class: Gonadotropin-releasing hormone analog
Form: Subcutaneous injection
Formulations: 7.5, 22.5, 30 mg for subcutaneous injection
Dose: 7.5 subcutaneously every month; 22.5 mg subcutaneously every 3 months; 30 mg subcutaneously every 4 months
Mechanism of action: Lowers circulating levels of testosterone
FDA-approved uses: Palliative treatment of advanced prostate cancer
Adverse reactions: Injection site pain, malaise, fatigue, vertigo, hot flashes, disease flare
Drug interactions: None reported
Monitoring parameters: Serum testosterone, prostate-specific antigen
Patient counseling: Initial therapy can cause a disease flare (ie, bone pain) and other pains. This is normal and means the medication is working.

Chapter 20: Solid Organ Transplantation

Drug: Myfortic® (mycophenolic acid)
Class: Immunosuppressive agent
Formulations: *New formulation*—5 mg tablet

Drug: Rapamune® (sirolimus)
Class: Immunosuppressive agent
Formulations: *New formulation*—extended-release tablets; 180 and 360 mg

Chapter 21: Gastrointestinal Diseases

Drug: Prevacid® NapraPAC™ (lansoprazole, naproxen)
Class: Proton pump inhibitor (lansoprazole) and NSAID (naproxen)
Form: Delayed-release capsules (lansoprazole), tablets (naproxen)
Formulations: 15 mg delayed-release lansoprazole, 250, 375, 500 mg naproxen
Dose: 1 capsule of lansoprazole PO every morning, 1 tablet of naproxen PO 250–500 mg twice a day
Mechanism of action: Lansoprazole selectively inhibits the parietal cell membrane enzyme H^+-K^+-ATPase (commonly referred to as the proton pump). Naproxen inhibits prostaglandin synthesis.
FDA-approved uses: Reducing the risk of NSAID-associated gastric ulcers in patients with a prior history who require an NSAID for the treatment of rheumatoid arthritis, osteoarthritis, or ankylosing spondylitis.
Adverse reactions: Dyspnea, palpitations, headache, drowsiness, vertigo, constipation, diarrhea, nausea, gastrointestinal bleeding, LFT and/or renal abnormalities
Drug interactions: Digoxin toxicity due to increased absorption, increased risk of bleeding with ginkgo, decreased absorption of iron, decreased absorption of azole antifungals, increased methotrexate toxicity
Monitoring parameters: Fecal occult blood test, urinalysis, LFTs, dyspepsia, hemoglobin, CBC
Patient counseling: Naproxen may hide symptoms of fever and inflammation.

Drug: Lotronex® (alosetron)
Class: Antidiarrheal
Formulations: *New strength*—0.5 mg tablet

Drug: Protonix® IV (pantoprazole sodium EDTA formulation)
Class: Proton pump inhibitor
Formulations: *New formulation*—EDTA does not require an inline filter; 40 mg vials

Drug: Zantac EFFERdose® (ranitidine HCl)
Class: H_2-receptor blocker
Formulations: *New strength*—25 mg effervescent tablet

Chapter 22: Rheumatoid Arthritis, Osteoarthritis, Gout, and Lupus

Drug: Humira® (adalimumab)
Class: Disease modifying anti-rheumatic, monoclonal antibody
Form: Subcutaneous injection
Formulations: 40 mg/0.8 mL solution
Dose: 40 mg subcutaneously every other week
Mechanism of action: Inhibits the binding of tumor necrosis factor-α (TNF-α) to receptors. TNF-α is thought to play a major role in inflammatory synovitis and articular matrix degradation. It is overproduced in rheumatoid joints.
FDA-approved uses: Moderate to severe rheumatoid arthritis in patients who have inadequate response to one or more disease modifying anti-rheumatic drugs (DMARDs)
Adverse reactions: Injection site reactions, pneumonia, tuberculosis, allergic reactions
Drug interactions: None reported
Monitoring parameters: CBC, anti-adalimumab antibodies, signs of tuberculosis (weight loss, fever, cough)
Patient counseling: Contact your physician if you develop a cough that does not go away, or lose weight or have pain upon urination.

Drug: Prevacid® NapraPAC™ (lansoprazole, naproxen)
Class: Proton pump inhibitor (lansoprazole) and NSAID (naproxen)
Form: Delayed-release capsules (lansoprazole), tablets (naproxen)
Formulations: 15 mg delayed-release lansoprazole, 250, 375, 500 mg naproxen
Dose: 1 capsule of lansoprazole PO every morning, 1 tablet of naproxen PO 250–500 mg twice a day
Mechanism of action: Lansoprazole selectively inhibits the parietal cell membrane enzyme H^+-K^+-ATPase (commonly referred to as the proton pump); naproxen inhibits prostaglandin synthesis
FDA-approved uses: Reducing the risk of NSAID-associated gastric ulcers in patients with a prior history who require an NSAID for the treatment of rheumatoid arthritis (RA), osteoarthritis (OA), or ankylosing spondylitis
Adverse reactions: Dyspnea, palpitations, headache, drowsiness, vertigo, constipation, diarrhea, nausea, gastrointestinal bleeding, LFT and/or renal abnormalities
Drug interactions: Digoxin toxicity due to increased absorption, increased risk of bleeding with ginkgo, decreased absorption of iron, decreased absorption of azole antifungals, increased methotrexate toxicity

Monitoring parameters: Fecal occult blood test, urinalysis, LFTs, dyspepsia, hemoglobin, CBC
Patient counseling: Naproxen may hide symptoms of fever and inflammation.

Chapter 23: Pain Management and Migraines

Drug: Avinza® slow release (morphine sulfate)
Class: Opioid
Formulations: *New formulation*—extended-release capsules; 30, 60, 90, and 120 mg;
FDA-approved uses: Once-daily administration for relief of moderate to severe pain requiring around-the-clock treatment
Counseling: Capsules may be opened and beads sprinkled on applesauce

Drug: DepoDur® (morphine sulfate liposome)
Class: Opioid
Formulations: *New formulation*—single epidural injection; 10 mg/mL
FDA-approved uses: Treatment of pain following major surgery

Drug: Darvocet A500™ (propoxyphene napsylate and acetaminophen)
Class: Synthetic opioid and analgesic
Formulations: New formulation—oral tablet containing 100 mg of propoxyphene and 500 mg acetaminophen
FDA-approved uses: Mild to moderate pain

Drug: Hydrocodone bitartrate 5 mg/ibuprofen 200 mg
Class: Semisynthetic opioid and NSAID
Formulations: *New formulation*—oral tablet containing 5 mg of hydrocodone and 200 mg of ibuprofen
FDA-approved uses: Mild to moderate pain

Drug: Imitrex® (sumatriptan)
Class: Triptans
Formulations: *New formulation*—rapid-release tablets; 50, 100 mg

Drug: Zomig® (zolmitriptan)
Class: Triptans
Formulations: *New formulation*—nasal spray containing 5 mg per spray
Dose: Administer 1 dose (1 spray) for the acute treatment of migraines with or without aura

Chapter 24: Seizure Disorders

Drug: Keppra® (levetiracetam)
Class: Anticonvulsant
Formulations: *New formulation*—oral solution; 100 mg/mL

Chapter 25: Psychiatric Disease

Drug: Symbyax™ (olanzapine and fluoxetine)
Class: Atypical antipsychotic (olanzapine) and serotonin selective reuptake inhibitor (fluoxetine)
Form: Capsule
Formulations: 6 mg (olanzapine) and 25 mg (fluoxetine) capsule, 6/50, 12/25, 12/50 mg capsules
Dose: 1 capsule PO in the evening
Mechanism of action: Activation of three monoaminergic neural systems (serotonin, norepinephrine, and dopamine) appears to be responsible for the enhanced antidepressant effect.
FDA-approved uses: Treatment of depressive episodes associated with bipolar disorder
Adverse reactions: Cognitive and/or motor impairment, dysphagia, aspiration, elevated body temperature, hyperglycemia, mania, weight gain
Drug interactions: Increased concentration of benzodiazepines, increased hypotensive effects of antihypertensives, and carbamazepine may increase clearance of olanzapine.
Monitoring parameters: Blood glucose, LFTs, serum prolactin, extrapyramidal symptoms
Patient counseling: This combination was only studied for 8 weeks in clinical trials.

Drug: Zyprexa® IntraMuscular (olanzapine)
Class: Atypical antipsychotic
Formulations: *New formulation*—intramuscular injection; 10 mg/vial

Drug: FazaClo™ (clozapine)
Class: Atypical antipsychotic
Formulations: *New formulation*—orally disintegrating tablets; 25 and 100 mg

Drug: Risperdal® M-TAB™ (risperidone)
Class: Atypical antipsychotic
Formulations: *New formulation*—orally disintegrating tablets; 0.5, 1, and 2 mg

Drug: Xanax XR® (alprazolam)
Class: Benzodiazepine
Formulations: *New formulation*—extended-release tablets; 0.5, 1, 2, and 3 mg

Chapter 28: Asthma and Chronic Obstructive Pulmonary Disease

Drug: Spiriva® HandiHaler® (tiotropium bromide)
Class: Anticholinergic bronchodilator
Form: Capsules with dry powder for use with HandiHaler
Formulations: 18 micrograms triotropium powder for inhalation with HandiHaler
Dose: 18 µg (the contents of one capsule), inhaled once a day with the HandiHaler inhalation device
Mechanism of action: Tiotropium is a quaternary ammonium antimuscarinic or anticholinergic agent. The drug inhibits smooth muscle muscarinic receptors, leading to bronchodilation.
FDA-approved uses: Chronic obstructive pulmonary disease (COPD)
Adverse reactions: Dry mouth, arthritis, coughing, influenza-like symptoms, and sinusitis
Drug interactions: Other anticholinergic medications, including ipratropium, are not recommended.
Monitoring parameters: Periodic pulmonary function tests (ie, forced expiratory volume in one second [FEV_1], particularly trough FEV_1, and forced vital capacity [FVC]); evidence of improvement of clinical symptoms; and reduced incidence and severity of exacerbations of asthma; signs and symptoms of hypersensitivity; local skin reactions or other signs of toxicity.
Patient counseling: Do not swallow Spiriva capsules. The HandiHaler is an inhalation device used to inhale the dry powder contained in Spiriva capsules and is not to be used to take other medications. The capsule is pierced by the device, dispersing tiotropium into the air stream. Do not use Spiriva to treat sudden episodes of breathing problems. Report any serious allergic reactions (eg, itching; rash; swelling of the lips, tongue, or throat, with trouble swallowing). Stop taking Spiriva and get emergency help right away if you experience any of these symptoms. Spiriva may cause breathing problems (paradoxical bronchospasm). Stop taking Spiriva and call your doctor immediately if this happens.

Drug: Xolair® (omalizumab)
Class: Monoclonal antibody
Form: Injection
Formulations: 150 mg/1.2 mL. Reconstitute lyophilized powder with 1.4 mL of water for injection and withdraw 1.2 mL.
Dose:
  Adult: allergic asthma 150–375 mg subcutaneously every 2 or 4 weeks; dosage determined by body weight and IgE level before first treatment
  Pediatric: The above dose can be administered to children 10 years of age and older.
Mechanism of action: Omalizumab is a genetically engineered protein that blocks the body's immune response to allergens.
FDA-approved uses: For treatment of allergy-related moderate to severe asthma that has been inadequately controlled with steroids. Allergy-related asthma should be confirmed with skin or blood testing prior to therapy.
Adverse reactions: Rare severe allergic reactions or anaphylaxis. Common adverse effects include headache, injection site reactions, and rash.
Drug interactions: No known drug interactions
Monitoring parameters: Serum IgE before starting therapy. Serum IgE should not be used for ongoing dosage adjustments. Monitor pulmonary function, FEV_1, peak expiratory flow rate (PEFR), symptoms of asthma, and the use of additional steroids and β_2-agonists
Patient counseling: Caution should be used in patients with allergies to other antibody preparations, particularly murine-derived preparations. This product is not indicated for acute exacerbations of asthma, acute bronchospasm, or status asthmaticus.

Chapter 30: Anti-Infective Agents

Drug: Ketek® (telithromycin)
Class: Ketolide, a subgroup of the macrolide-lincosamide streptogramin antibiotics
Form: Tablets
Formulations: 400 mg telithromycin tablets
Dose: 800 mg once a day for 5–10 days, depending on severity and site of infection, with dose adjustment necessary only for creatinine clearance <10 mL per minute
Mechanism of action: The mechanism of action of telithromycin is similar to that of macrolides (ie, it binds to the 50S ribosomal subunit, resulting in inhibition of bacterial protein synthesis and activity against multidrug resistant *Streptococcus pneumoniae*).
FDA-approved uses: For adult use for treating community-acquired pneumonia, acute sinusitis, and chronic bronchitis.
Adverse reactions: Diarrhea, nausea, vomiting, abdominal pain, flatulence, taste disturbances, elevation of liver enzymes, and cholestatic jaundice. Effects on the central nervous system may include vertigo, headache, insomnia, or drowsiness. Less commonly reported reactions include paresthesias, blurred vision, eosinophilia, skin rashes, and cardiovascular effects, (eg, arrhythmias, hypotension, and bradycardia). There have been isolated cases of erythema multiforme and pseudomembranous colitis.
Drug interactions: Telithromycin is an inhibitor of the cytochrome P450 isoenzymes CYP3A4 and CYP2D6. Medications primarily metabolized by this enzyme system (eg, most statins), must be used cautiously with telithromycin. Also use caution with drugs that may prolong the QT interval. Use with cisapride, pimozide, astemizole, or terfenadine is contraindicated. Telithromycin should not be given with drugs that induce the cytochrome P450 isoenzyme CYP3A4 (eg, rifampicin).
Monitoring parameters: Monitor for presence of side effects mentioned above and potential drug interactions.
Patient counseling: This medication may cause vision problems, liver problems, and jaundice, and may worsen myasthenia gravis and prolong the QT interval.

Drug: Cubicin® (daptomycin)
Class: Lipopeptide antibacterial for treating gram-positive infections
Form: Injection
Formulations: 500 mg vial
Dose: For complicated skin and skin structure infections: 4 mg/kg intravenously once every 24 hours for 7–14 days. The dose needs adjustment for renal and hepatic impairment or dialysis.

Mechanism of action: Dactomycin binds to bacterial membranes, which causes rapid depolarization and loss of membrane potential, subsequent inhibition of RNA, DNA, and protein synthesis, followed by bacterial cell death.
FDA-approved uses: Complicated skin and skin structure infections; infections due to susceptible gram-positive organisms such as *Enterococcus faecalis* (vancomycin-susceptible), *Staphylococcus aureus* (including methicillin-resistant strains), *Streptococcus agalactiae, Streptococcus dysgalactiae,* and *Streptococcus pyogenes.*
Adverse reactions: Constipation, diarrhea, nausea, vomiting, dyspepsia, dyspnea, elevated serum creatine phosphokinase, headache, insomnia, vertigo, injection site reactions, limb pain, arthralgia, myalgia, muscle cramps, rash, and pruritus. Serious rare adverse effects include abnormal liver function tests and jaundice, hypersensitivity, and renal failure.
Drug interactions: HMG-CoA reductase inhibitors may increase the risk of myopathy. Concomitant use of tobramycin in healthy subjects resulted in increased daptomycin and decreased tobramycin levels.
Monitoring parameters: Complete blood counts, routine blood chemistry, liver function tests, and serum creatinine, and weekly serum creatine phosphokinase levels.
Patient counseling: Due to an increased risk of myopathy, caution should be used if you have a history of musculoskeletal disorders or if you take HMG-CoA reductase inhibitors. Dose reduction is indicated for renal impairment.

Drug: Factive® (gemifloxacin mesylate)
Class: Quinolone
Form: Tablets
Formulations: Gemifloxacin 320 mg tablets
Dose:
   Chronic bronchitis: 320 mg orally once a day for 5 days
   Community-acquired pneumonia: 320 mg orally once a day for 7 days
Dosage adjustment is necessary for patients with creatinine clearance <40 mL/min (160 mg every 24 hours).
Mechanism of action: Bactericidal activity due to inhibition of DNA gyrase.
FDA-approved uses: Susceptible infections due to *Streptococcus pneumoniae, Haemophilus influenzae, Haemophilus parainfluenzae, Moraxella catarrhalis, Mycoplasma pneumoniae, Chlamydia pneumoniae, Klebsiella pneumoniae*; chronic bronchitis, acute bacterial exacerbation; and community-acquired pneumonia (including drug-resistant *Streptococcus pneumoniae*)
Adverse reactions: Rash, urticaria, diarrhea, nausea, and elevated liver enzymes

Drug interactions: Drugs that contain metallic ions, (eg, calcium, magnesium, iron, and zinc) markedly decrease the effect of the drug. Sucralfate and didanosine also decrease the effect of the drug. Patients also taking antidiabetic agents may have fluctuations in glucose levels. Drugs that prolong the QT interval, including class IA or III antiarrhythmic agents, will worsen this potentially serious adverse effect.

Monitoring parameters: White blood cells, signs and symptoms of infection, and urine culture, if appropriate.

Patient counseling: Inform your physician if you have a history of QT interval prolongation or take an antiarrhythmic or antipsychotic medication, as these are also associated with prolonged QT interval. Avoid antacids and metal-containing compounds.

Chapter 31: Human Immunodeficiency Virus and the Acquired Immunodeficiency Syndrome

Drug: Fuzeon™ (T20) (enfuvirtide)
Class: Human immunodeficiency virus (HIV) fusion inhibitor/entry inhibitor
Form: Subcutaneous injection
Formulations: 90 mg/mL injection, 108 mg vial of lyophilized powder reconstituted with 1.1 mL of sterile water for injection.
Dose:
  Adult dose: 90 mg/mL subcutaneously every 12 hours into the upper arm, anterior thigh, or abdomen.
  Pediatric dose: Patients 6 years through 16 years of age: 2 mg/kg twice a day up to a maximum dose of 90 mg twice a day injected subcutaneously into the upper arm, anterior thigh, or abdomen.
Mechanism of action: Enfuvirtide is an HIV fusion inhibitor. The drug binds to the viral envelope glycoprotein and prevents fusion of viral and cellular membranes, thus preventing entry into host CD4 cells.
FDA-approved uses: Indicated in the treatment of infection due to HIV-1 (adults and children over 6 years of age) in combination with other antiretroviral agents in treatment-experienced patients who have evidence of HIV replication despite treatment with other combination regimens
Adverse reactions: Injection site reactions, hypersensitivity reactions, anxiety, fatigue, insomnia, decreased appetite, nausea, vomiting, diarrhea, an increased rate of infections (bacterial pneumonia and others), pancreatitis, conjunctivitis, and lymphadenopathy.
Drug interactions: No clinically significant drug interactions.
Monitoring parameters: Plasma HIV-RNA (viral load), CD4 cell counts, weight, local injection irritation, and hypersensitivity reactions
Patient counseling: Powder for injection (at room temperature) requires reconstitution by patient and is stable for 24 hours if refrigerated after reconstitution. It requires 30–45 minutes to dissolve in 1 mL of sterile water for injection at room temperature.

Drug: Lexiva® (fosamprenavir [f-APV])
Class: Protease inhibitor (PI)
Form: Tablets
Formulations: 700 mg fosamprenavir calcium tablets
Dose: In treatment-naïve patients, the recommended dose of fosamprenavir is 1400 mg two times a day, or fosamprenavir 1400 mg one time a day with ritonavir 200 mg one time a day, or fosamprenavir 700 mg two times a day and ritonavir 100 mg two times a day. Fosamprenavir may be taken with or without food. In

treatment-experienced patients, the recommended dose of fosamprenavir is 700 mg two times a day and ritonavir 100 mg two times a day (dosing one time a day is not recommended in these patients). Dosage adjustment is recommended for hepatic impairment.

Mechanism of action: Fosamprenavir is a prodrug of amprenavir, a protease HIV-1 enzyme inhibitor that interferes with viral replication, leading to inhibition of the viral load.

FDA-approved uses: HIV infection

Adverse reactions: Skin rash, nausea and vomiting, diarrhea, headache, increased liver enzymes, hyperglycemia, fat redistribution, lipid abnormalities, and increased bleeding episodes in hemophiliacs.

Drug interactions: Fosamprenavir (f-APV) can act both as a CYP 450 inhibitor and a substrate and should not be administered with drugs that are substrates or inhibitors of CYP 450 isoenzymes. Drug interactions can cause decreased levels of f-APV when used with non-nucleoside reverse transcriptase inhibitors (NNRTIs) and anticonvulsants (eg, phenobarbital, phenytoin, and carbamazepine). Methadone levels are decreased. Increase or decrease in voriconazole or f-APV may result with combined use. Fosamprenavir can increase levels of ketoconazole, rifabutin, and atorvastatin, as well as agents used for erectile dysfunction. Levels of protease inhibitors may be increased or decreased.

Contraindicated medications (due to severe interactions): Bepridil, simvastatin, lovastatin, St. John's wort, antiarrhythmics, oral contraceptives, amprenavir, midazolam, triazolam, ergot derivatives, cisapride, pimozide, rifampicin, and irinotecan.

Monitoring parameters: Plasma HIV RNA, CD4+ cell counts (periodically), body weight and temperature, liver function tests, complete blood counts, lipid panel, blood glucose and routine blood chemistry, hypersensitivity, or other adverse effects (eg, gastrointestinal symptoms, fatigue, signs of infection, or sleep disturbances).

Patient counseling: The medication can be taken with or without food. Because of the possibility of several drug interactions, check with a doctor or pharmacist before starting any new medications, including over-the-counter medications. All patients should be counseled on the importance of compliance to reduce the risk of resistance. The drug should be used with caution in patients with known sulfonamide allergy because the drug contains a sulfonamide entity.

Chapter 32: Immunization

Drug: FluMist™ (influenza virus vaccine)
Class: Influenza vaccine (live)
Form: For intranasal administration
Formulations: Each 0.5 mL dose is formulated to contain live attenuated influenza virus A/New Caledonia/20/99 (H1N1), A/Panama/2007/99 (H3N2), A/Moscow/10/99-like, and B/Hong Kong/330/2001 strains.
Dose:
Healthy adults, 18–49 years of age: 0.5 mL (0.25 mL/nostril) intranasally, per season
Pediatric: For healthy children, ages 5 through 8 years, not previously vaccinated with nasal influenza vaccine, give 2 doses of 0.5 mL administered at least 6 weeks apart; for children 5 years of age and older, give 0.5 mL intranasally per season.

Mechanism of action: The exact mechanism of protection against influenza following prophylaxis with FluMist vaccine is not fully understood. Production of serum and mucosal antibodies and influenza-specific T cells may play a role in prevention and recovery from infection. The vaccine viruses replicate in the nasopharynx to produce protective immunity.

FDA-approved uses: Influenza virus immunization

Adverse reactions: Headache, nasal congestion/runny nose, and cough

Drug interactions:
Corticosteroids: Due to the possibility of inadequate immunologic response to the vaccine, live-attenuated viral or bacterial vaccines should not be administered to immunosuppressed patients receiving large doses of corticosteroids. Delay the administration of vaccines if possible.
Cyclosporine: Suppresses T lymphocyte activity essential for adequate immune response to live vaccines and toxoids.
Warfarin: Due to case reports of bleeding, monitor the prothrombin time or INR within 1–2 weeks after vaccination and compare results to baseline values.

Monitoring parameters: Monitor for any adverse effects or signs of infection

Patient counseling: The vaccine is contraindicated in patients with conditions involving compromised immune status, hypersensitivity to any component of the vaccine (ie, eggs and egg products), and a history of Guillain-Barré syndrome. Intranasal vaccine is not recommended in patients with a history of asthma or reactive airways disease and for patients who have had an acute phase of febrile or respiratory disease within the last 72 hours. Recipients of FluMist should avoid contact with immunocompromised persons for at least 21 days after vaccination.

Chapter 34: Geriatrics and Gerontology

Drug: Namenda™ (memantine)

Class: N-methyl-D-aspartate (NMDA) receptor antagonist

Form: Tablets

Formulations: 5 mg, 10 mg tablets

Dose: Initial dose of 5 mg per day.

Maintenance: Dose should be increased in 5-mg increments to a maximum of 20 mg per day (10 mg two times per day)

Mechanism of ction: Memantine is an oral NMDA receptor antagonist. It blocks the excitatory effects of glutamate, the neurotransmitter that activates NMDA. Memantine appears to restore the function of damaged nerve cells and reduce abnormal excitatory signals by modulation of NMDA receptor activity.

FDA-approved uses: Alzheimer's disease with moderate to severe dementia

Adverse reactions: Constipation, vertigo, headache, hypertension, and pain

Drug interactions: Use of carbonic anhydrase inhibitors and sodium bicarbonate drugs that increase urine pH and decrease the elimination of memantine increase the possibility of adverse effects of the drug. Concomitant administration with one or more of the following drugs may result in altered plasma levels of both drugs due to the same cationic pathway or renal elimination for both drugs: cimetidine, hydrochlorothiazide, nicotine, quinidine, ranitidine, and triamterene.

Monitoring parameters: Monitor for improvement in the clinical signs and symptoms of Alzheimer's and signs of adverse effects such as psychosis (including hallucinations), nervousness, changes in behavior, tremor, and other central nervous system symptoms.

Patient counseling: Concomitant use of drugs that make the urine alkaline or genitourinary conditions that raise urine pH may increase plasma levels of memantine. Patients with moderate to severe renal impairment may need dose adjustment. The drug should be taken with caution in patients with seizure disorders or patients who are breast-feeding.

Drug: Stalevo™ (carbidopa/entacapone/levodopa)

Class: Combination product (ie, dopaminergic and catecholamine O-methyl transferase [COMT] inhibitor)

Form: Tablets

Formulations: Carbidopa 12.5 mg/entacapone 200 mg/levodopa 50 mg tablets; carbidopa 25 mg/entacapone 200 mg/levodopa 100 mg tablets; carbidopa 37.5 mg/entacapone 200 mg/levodopa 150 mg tablets

Dose: Individualize dose and adjust according to desired therapeutic response up to a maximum of 8 tablets per day. Patients currently taking 200 mg entacapone with each dose of standard carbidopa/levodopa can be directly switched to the strength of carbidopa/entacapone/levodopa containing the same amounts of carbidopa and levodopa. For patients with a current levodopa dose over 600 mg and patients not on entacapone, a levodopa dose reduction with the addition of entacapone is likely to be required; patients should first be titrated individually with a carbidopa/levodopa product and an entacapone product, then transferred to the equivalent corresponding dose of carbidopa/entacapone/levodopa fixed-dose combination product. Once stabilized, the appropriate levodopa dose is 600 mg per day or less (with no dyskinesia). Patients not currently treated with entacapone may transfer to a corresponding dose of carbidopa/entacapone/levodopa fixed-dose combination product.

Maintenance dose: Therapy should be individualized. To decrease or increase levodopa dose, total daily dosage may be altered by changing the strength of the carbidopa/entacapone/levodopa combination or by changing the administration frequency up to a maximum of 8 tablets per day

Mechanism of action: Levodopa is the precursor of dopamine; unlike dopamine, it can cross the blood-brain barrier. Carbidopa prevents the metabolism of levodopa, and entacapone inhibits COMT, thus increasing dopamine.

FDA-approved uses: The treatment of idiopathic Parkinson's disease; substitution of immediate-release carbidopa/levodopa and entacapone previously administered as individual products (with equivalent strength of each of the three components); replacement of immediate-release carbidopa/levodopa therapy (without entacapone) when patients have end-of-dose "wearing off," but only if the total daily dose of levodopa is 600 mg or less and the patients are not experiencing dyskinesias.

Adverse reactions: Abdominal pain, diarrhea, nausea, confusion, vertigo, hallucinations, somnolence, fatigue, urine discoloration, cardiac abnormalities, orthostatic hypotension, dyskinesia, and psychotic symptoms

Drug interactions: Concomitant administration of dopamine antagonists (eg, metoclopramide) will lead to decreased benefits and worsening of parkinsonism. Nonselective monoamine oxidase inhibitors (eg, phenelzine) interact with the entacapone component to precipitate serotonin syndrome and hypertensive crisis secondary to increased catecholamines.

Monitoring parameters: Periodic evaluations of liver enzymes, complete blood count, and cardiovascular and renal function; observe carefully for symptoms resembling neuroleptic malignant syndrome if abrupt reduction or discontinuation of therapy is required; observe for reduction of rigidity, tremor, slowed movements.

Patient counseling: Do not use this medication if you have narrow-angle glaucoma, melanoma, or a history of melanoma, if you are taking monoamine oxidase inhibitors, or if you are breast-feeding. Due to the possibility of many drug interactions, be sure to notify your physician or pharmacist if you start any new medications. You may have several dose changes before determining the best dose to improve symptoms. If you miss a dose and your next dose is to be taken in no less than 2 hours, take the missed dose. Skip the dose if it is too close to the time of your next dose.

Drug: Apokyn™ (apomorphine)
Class: Non-ergoline dopamine agonist
Form: Subcutaneous injection
Formulations: Apomorphine hydrochloride 10 mg/mL
Dose: During acute hypomobility episodes, administer 0.2 mL (2 mg) subcutaneously via metered injector pen up to a maximum recommended dose of 0.6 mL (6 mg), delivered and titrated on the basis of effectiveness and tolerance. A test dose of 0.2 mL (2 mg) should be given initially; the patient should be monitored for orthostatic hypotension. If the patient responds and tolerates this dose, then use Apokyn on an as-needed basis for treating "off" episodes. A test dose of 0.1 mL should be used for patients with mild to moderate renal impairment. Determine a test dose based on the patient's tolerance under monitored conditions (ie, usually 0.3 mL [3 mg] or 0.4 mL [4 mg]). Begin an outpatient trial with a dose of 0.1 mL (1 mg) lower than the tolerated dose, and monitor patient for efficacy and side effects. If needed, increase the dose by 0.1-mL (1-mg) increments every few days, up to a maximum of 0.6 mL (6 mg).
Mechanism of action: Apomorphine has high selectivity for dopaminergic and α-adrenergic receptors, all of which are involved in motor function. The precise mechanism of action is not known.
FDA-approved uses: Treatment of motor symptoms associated with late stage Parkinson's disease (hypomobility and "off" periods).
Adverse reactions: Nausea, vomiting, yawning, dyskinesias, somnolence, vertigo, postural hypotension, rhinorrhea, hallucinations, edema, inflammation
Drug interactions: Avoid $5HT_3$ antagonists (ondansetron and similar drugs) indicated for anti-nausea, as the combination can lead to very low blood pressure and loss of consciousness. Alcohol and other sedating medications, if used concomitantly, can cause excessive sedation and central nervous system effects. COMT inhibitors (eg, entacapone and tolcapone) can enhance the effect of apomorphine. Antihypertensives or organic nitrates may potentiate hypotensive effects. The therapeutic effects of apomorphine may be antagonized by antipsychotics and other drugs that act as central nervous system dopamine inhibitors.

Monitoring parameters: Monitor for adverse effects (eg, orthostatic hypotension), efficacy, and drug interactions.
Patient counseling: Apokyn should not be given intravenously and is intended for subcutaneous injection only. If a single dose of Apokyn is not effective during a particular "off" period, a second dose should not be given for that "off" period.

39. Appendices

Erin M. Timpe, PharmD
Associate Professor, Department of Pharmacy
University of Tennessee College of Pharmacy

Contents

Appendix 1

Normal Laboratory Values

Test	Covnentional units	SI units
Albumin	3.5-5 g/dL	35-50 g/L
Alkaline phosphatase		
Adult	4.5-13 King-Armstrong U/dL	32-92 U/L
Infant	10-30 King-Armstrong U/dL	71-213 U/L
Amylase	60-160 Somogyi U/dL	25-125 U/L
Anion Gap	7-16 mEq/L	7-16 mmol/L
Arterial blood gases (ABG)		
HCO_3	21-28 mEq/L	21-28 mEq/L
O_2 saturation	94-100%	0.94-1
pH	7.35-7.45	7.35-7.45
Po_2	83-108 mmHg	11.04-14.36 kPa
Pco_2	35-45 mmHg	4.7-6 kPa
Basal metabolic panel (BMP)		
Bicarbonate	22-29 mEq/L	22-29 mmol/L
Blood urea nitrogen (BUN)	6-20 mg/dL	2.1-7.1 mmol/L
Chloride	98-107 mEq/L	98-107 mmol/L
Creatinine	0.6-1.3 mg/dL	53-115 µmol/L
Glucose	60-110 mg/dL	3.3-6.1 mmol/L
Potassium	3.5-5.1 mEq/L	3.5-5.1 mmol/L
Sodium	136-145 mEq/L	136-145 mmol/L
Blood pressure (mm Hg)		
Optimal	<120/<80	<120/<80
Normal	<130/<85	<130/<85
High normal	130-139/85-89	130-139/85-89
Hypertension		
Stage 1	140-159/90-99	140-159/90-99
Stage 2	160-179/100-109	160-179/100-109
Stage 3	>180/>110	>180/>110
Isolated systolic	>140/<90	>140/<90
Calcitonin	<150 pg/mL	<150 ng/L
Calcium	8.6-10 mg/dL	2.15-2.50 mmol/L
Carbon dioxide	22-29 mEq/L	22-29 mmol/L
Coagulation screen		
Activated partial thromboplastin time		
(aPTT)	<35 seconds	<35 seconds
Antithrombin III	21-30 mg/dL	210-300 mg/L
Bleeding time	1-<10 min	1-<10 min
Partial thromboplastin time (PTT)	22-37 seconds	22-37 seconds
Protein C	70-140%	0.70-1.40
Protein S	67-140%	0.67-1.40
Prothrombin time (PT)	11-15 seconds	11-15 seconds
Complete blood count (CBC)		
Hemoglobin (Hb)		
Male	13.1-18 g/dL	131-180 g/L
Female	11.7-16 g/dL	117-160 g/L
Hematocrit (Hct)		
Male	40-54%	0.40-0.54
Female	34-47%	0.34-0.47
Mean corpuscular volume (MCV)	80-96 µm³	80-96 fL

Appendix 1

Normal Laboratory Values (continued)

Test	Conventional units	SI units
CBC (continued)		
Mean corpuscular hemoglobin (MCH)	27-33 pg	27-33 pg
Mean corpuscular hemoglobin concentration (MCHC)	32-36%	0.32-0.36
Platelets	150-400 x 10^3/μL	150-400 x 10^9/μL
Red blood cells (RBC):		
Male	4.1-5.8 x 10^6 cells/μL	4.1-5.8 x 10^{12} cells/L
Female	3.8-5.4 x 10^6 cells/μL	3.8-5.4 x 10^{12} cells/L
White blood cells (WBC)	4.5-11 x 10^3 cells/μL	4.5-11 x 10^9 cells/L
White blood cell differential:		
Band neutrophils	0.0-2.1 10^3 cells/μL	0.0-2.1 10^9 cells/L
Basophils	0.0-0.19 10^3 cells/μL	0.0-0.19 10^9 cells/L
Eosinophils	0.0-0.7 10^3 cells/μL	0.0-0.7 10^9 cells/L
Lymphocytes	1.2-4.0 10^3 cells/μL	1.2-4.0 10^9 cells/L
Monocytes	0.1-0.95 10^3 cells/μL	0.1-0.95 10^9 cells/L
Segmented neutrophils	1.1-6.9 10^3 cells/μL	1.1-6.9 10^9 cells/L
Corticotropin (ACTH) 08:00h	<120 pg/mL	<26 pmol/L
Cortisol 08:00h	5-23 μg/dL	138-635 nmol/L
Creatinine kinase:		
Male	38-174 U/L	0.65-2.96 μKat/L
Female	26-140 U/L	0.46-2.38 μKat/L
Glucose tolerance test		
Baseline fasting blood glucose	70-105 mg/dL	3.9-5.8 mmol/L
30-Minute fasting blood glucose	110-170 mg/dL	6.1-9.4 mmol/L
60-Minute fasting blood glucose	120-170 mg/dL	6.7-9.4 mmol/L
90-Minute fasting blood glucose	100-140 mg/dL	5.6-7.8 mmol/L
120-minute fasting blood glucose	70-120 mg/dL	3.9-6.7 mmol/L
Hematologic tests		
Erythrocyte sedimentation rate (ESR)		
≥50 year old male	0-15 mm/h	0-15 mm/h
≥50 year old female	0-20 mm/h	0-20 mm/h
<50 year old male	0-20 mm/h	0-20 mm/h
<50 year old female	0-30 mm/h	0-30 mm/h
Ferritin		
Male	20-250 ng/mL	20-250 μg/L
Female	10-120 ng/mL	10-120 μg/L
Fibrinogen	200-400 mg/dL	2.00-4.00 g/L
Hemoglobin A1$_C$	4-6%	0.040-0.060
Reticulocytes	0.5-1.5%	0.005-0.015
Vitamin B$_{12}$	200-835 pg/mL	148-616 pmol/L
Iron		
Male	65-175 (g/dL	11.6-31.3 (mol/L
Female	50-170 (g/dL	9.0-30.4 (mol/L
Total Iron binding capacity (TIBC)	250-425 (g/dL	44.8-76.1 (mol/L
Transferrin saturation	20-50%	0.20-0.50

(continued)

Appendix 1

Normal Laboratory Values (continued)

Test	Conventional units	SI units
Isoenzymes		
Creatine phosphokinase (MM)	5-70 U/L	5-70 U/L
Creatine phosphokinase (MB)	0-7 U/L	0-7 U/L
Creatine phosphokinase (BB)	0-3 U/L	0-3 U/L
Lipase	<200 U/L	<3.4 µKat/L
Lipids		
Total cholesterol		
Desirable	<200 mg/dL	<5.2 mmol/L
Borderline-high	200-239 mg/dL	<5.2-6.2 mmol/L
High	>239 mg/dL	>6.2 mmol/L
LDL		
Desirable	<130 mg/dL	<3.36 mmol/L
Borderline-high	130-159 mg/dL	3.36-4.11 mmol/L
High	>159 mg/dL	>4.11 mmol/L
HDL		
Low	<40 mg/dL	<1.04 mmol/L
High	>60 mg/dL	>1.55 mmol/L
Triglycerides		
Desirable	<150 mg/dL	<1.7 mmol/L
Borderline-high	150-199 mg/dL	1.7-2.25 mmol/L
High	200-499 mg/dL	2.26-5.64 mmol/L
Very high	>500 mg/dL	>5.65 mmol/L
Liver function tests (LFTs)		
Aspartate aminotransferase (AST, SGOT)	8-20 U/L	0.14-0.34 µKat/L
Alanine aminotransferase (ALT, SGPT)	10-40 U/L	0.17-0.68 µKat/L
Ammonia (NH_4^+)	15-45 µg/dL	11-32 µmol/L
Bilirubin		
Conjugated	<2 mg/dL	<3.4 µMol/L
Total	0.2-1 mg/dL	3-19 µMol/L
Lactate dehydrogenase (LDH)	90-280 U/L	1.50-4.67 µKat/L
Magnesium	1.3-2.6 mg/dL	0.65-1.07 mmol/L
Phosphate	2.5-4.5 mg/dL	0.81-1.45 mmol/L
Prolactin		
Male	3-15 ng/mL	3-15 µg/L
Female	3-23 ng/mL	3-23 µg/L
Protein, total	6.4-8.3 g/dL	64-83 g/L
Thyroid hormone function tests		
Free thyroxine (Free T_4)	0.8-2.7 ng/dL	10-35 pmol/L
Thyroid-stimulating hormone (TSH)	0.4-8.9 µU/mL	0.4-8.9 mU/L
Thyroxine-binding globulin capacity	16-24 µg/dL	206-309 nmol/L
Total triiodothyronine (T_3)	70-204 ng/dL	1.08-3.14 nmol/L
Total thyroxine by RIA (T_4)	4.6-11.0 µg/dL	59-142 nmol/L
Uric acid	2.3-8.0 ng/dL	137-476 µmol/L

References

Malarkey LM, McMorrow ME. *Nurse's Manual of Laboratory Tests and Diagnostic Procedures.* Philadelphia: WB Saunders; 1996.

Tietz NW. *Clinical Guide to Laboratory Tests,* 3rd ed. Philadelphia: WB Saunders; 1995.

Appendix 2

Drugs in Renal Failure

Generic name (trade name)	Normal dose	CrCl 30-50 mL/min	CrCl 10-30 mL/min	CrCl <10 mL/min	Hemodialysis
Analgesics					
Acetaminophen	650 mg PO q4h	650 mg PO q6h	650 mg PO q6h	650 mg PO q6h	No supplementation required
Aspirin	650 mg PO q4h	650 mg PO q 4h	650 mg PO q6h	Avoid	Dose after HD
Codeine	30-60 mg PO q4-6h	20-45 mg PO q4-6h	20-45 mg PO q4-6h	15-30 mg PO q4-6h	No data
Fentanyl (Sublimaze®)	0.5 µg/kg IV q1-2h	Same	0.375 µ/kg IV q1-2h	0.25 µg/kg IV q1-2h	0.25 µg/kg IV q1-2h
Hydromorphone (Dilaudid®)	1-2 mg IV q4-6h	Same	Same	Same	Same
Meperidine (Demerol®)	50-100 mg IV or PO q3-4h	37.5-75 mg IV or PO q3-4h	37.5-75 mg IV or PO q3-4h	25-50 mg IV or PO q3-4h	Avoid
Morphine	20-25 mg PO q4h; 2-15 mg IV q2-4h	15-20 mg PO q4h; 1.5-12 mg IV q2-4h	15-20 mg PO q4h; 1.5-12 mg IV q2-4h	10 pg PO q4h; 1-8 mg IV q2-4h	No supplemental PO dose required; 1-8 mg IV q2-4
Propoxyphene (Darvon®)	65 mg PO q6-8h	Same	Same	Avoid	Avoid
Antiarrhythmics					
Adenosine (Adenocard®)	6 mg IV push over 1-2 s, may repeat second dose at 12 mg IV if necessary, may repeat 12 mg dose x 1	Same	Same	Same	Same
Atropine	0.5-1 mg IV push q 3-5 min, max 0.04 mg/kg	Same	Same	Same	Same
Class I					
Moricizine (Ethmozine®)	200-300 mg PO q8h	Same	Same	Same	Same
Propafenone (Rythmol®)	150-300 mg PO q8h	Same	Same	Same	Same
Class Ia					
Disopyramide (Norpace®)	300 mg IR LD, then 150-300 mg PO q6h	100 mg PO q6h	100 mg PO q12h	100 mg PO q24h	100 mg post-HD
Procainamide (Procan®, Pronestyl®)	500-1000 mg PO q4-6h; 50-100 mg/min IV until arrhythmia is suppressed or reach 500-1000 mg, then 2-6 mg/min	500 mg PO q6h	500 mg PO q12h	500 mg PO q12-24h	500 mg PO q24h post-HD
Quinidine (Quinidex®, Quinaglute®)	Sulfate: 200-400 mg PO q4-6h; gluconate: 324-648 mg PO q8-12h; 200-300 mg IM q2-6h	Same	Same	Sulfate: 150-300 mg PO q4-6h	Sulfate: 100-200 mg post-HD

(continued)

Appendix 2

Drugs in Renal Failure (continued)

Generic name (trade name)	Normal dose	CrCl 30-50 mL/min	CrCl 10-30 mL/min	CrCl <10 mL/min	Hemodialysis
Antiarrhythmics (cont)					
Class Ib					
Lidocaine (Xylocaine®)	50-100 mg IV over 1-2 min bolus, then 1-4 mg/min IV	Same	Same	Same	Same
Mexilitine (Mexitil®)	200-400 mg PO q8h	Same	Same	Same	Same
Tocainide (Tonocard®)	200-400 mg PO q8h	Same	Same	Same	Same
Class Ic					
Encainide (Enkaid®)	25-50 mg PO q12h	25-50 mg PO q8h	25 mg PO q8h	25 mg PO q12-24h	Same
Flecainide (Tambocor®)	100-200 mg PO q12h	No change	50-100 mg PO q12h	50 mg PO q12h	Same
Class II (see β-blockers in antihypertensives					
Class III					
Amiodarone (Cordarone®)	800-1600 mg/d in divided doses for 1-2 weeks LD, then 100-600 mg/d	Same	Same	Same	Same
Bretylium (Bretyol®)	5 mg/kg IV bolus, may repeat at 10 mg/kg to max of 30 mg/kg	Same	Same	Same	Same
Class IV (see calcium channel blockers in antihypertensives)					
Antibiotics					
Aminoglycosides					
Amikacin (Amikin®)	7.5 mg/kg IV q12h	7.5 mg/kg IV q18-24h	7.5 mg/kg IV q24-48h	7.5 mg/kg IV q48h	7.5 mg/kg IV based on serum levels; redose if level <5 µg/mL
Gentamicin (Garamycin®)	1.7 mg/kg q8h	0.5-1 mg/kg IV q12h or 1.7 mg/kg q24-48h	0.5-1 mg/kg IV q12h or 1.7 mg/kg q24-48h	0.35-0.5 mg/kg IV q24-48h or 1.7 mg/kg IV q48-72h	50% of dose post-HD
Tobramycin (Nebcin®)	1/7 mg/kg q8h	0.5-1 mg/kg IV q12h or 1.7 mg/kg q24-48h	0.5-1 mg/kg IV q12h or 1.7 mg/kg q24-48h	0.35-0.5 mg/kg IV q24-48h or 1.7 mg/kg IV q48-72h	50% of dose post-HD
Cephalosporins					
Cefaclor (Ceclor®)	250-500 mg PO tid	125-500 mg PO tid	125-500 mg PO tid	125-250 mg PO tid	250 mg PO post-HD
Cefadroxil (Duricef®)	0.5-1 g PO q12h	0.5-1 g PO q12-24h	0.5-1 g po q12-24h	0.5-1 g PO q24-48h	0.5-1 g PO post-HD
Cefazolin (Ancef®, Kexol®)	1-2 g IV q8h	1-2 g PO q8h	1-2 g IV q12h	1-2 g IV q24h	1-2 g IV q24h given post-HD
Cefepime (Maxipime®)	1-2 g IV q8-12h	1-2 g IV q12-24h	1-2 g IV q24h	0.5-1 g IV q24h	0.5-1 g IV q24h given post-HD

Appendix 2

Drugs in Renal Failure (continued)

Generic name (trade name)	Normal dose	CrCl 30-50 mL/min	CrCl 10-30 mL/min	CrCl <10 mL/min	Hemodialysis
Cephalosporins (cont)					
Cefixime (Suprax®)	200 mg PO q12h	150-200 mg PO q12h	150 mg PO q12h	100 mg PO q12h	300 mg PO post-HD
Cefotaxime (Claforan®)	1-2 g IV q8h	1-2 g IV q8h	1-2 g IV q12h	1-2 g IV q24h	1-2 g IV q24h given post-HD
Cefotetan (Cefotan®)	1-2 g IV q12h	1-2 g IV q12h	1-2 g IV q24h	1-2 g IV q48h	1-2 g IV q48h given post-HD
Cefoxitin (Mefoxin®)	1-2 g IV q6-8h	1-2 g IV q8h	1-2 g IV q12h	1-2 g IV q24h	1-2 g IV q24h given post-HD
Cefpodoxime (Vantin®)	200 mg PO q12h	200 mg PO q16h	200 mg PO q16h	200 mg PO q24-48h	200 mg PO post-HD only
Cefprozil (Cefzil®)	500 mg PO q12h	250 mg PO q12-16h	250 mg PO q12-16h	250 mg PO q24h	250 mg PO post-HD
Ceftazidime (Ceptaz®, Fortaz®, Tazicef®, Tazidime®)	2 g IV q8h	2 g IV q12h	2 g IV, then 0.5-1 g IV q24h	2 g IV, then 1 g IV q48h	2 g IV, then 1 g IV q48h given post-HD
Ceftizoxime (Cefizox®)	1-2 g IV q8h	1-2 g IV q12h	1-2 g IV q12h	1-2 g IV q24h	1 g IV q48h given post-HD
Ceftriaxone (Rocephin®)	1-2 g IV q24h	Same	Same	Same	Same
Cefuroxime (Ceftin®, Kefurox®, Zinacef®)	0.75-1.5 g IV q8h	0.75-1.5 g IV q8h	0.75-1.4 g IV q12h	0.75-1.5 g IV q24h	0.75-1.5 g IV q24h given post-HD
Cephalexin (Keflex®)	250-500 mg PO q6h	250-500 mg PO q8-12h	240-500 mg PO q12h	250-500 mg PO q12h	Dose post-HD
Fluoroquinolones					
Ciprofloxacin (Cipro®)	500-750 mg PO; 400 mg IV q12h	250-500 mg PO; 400 mg IV q12h	250-500 mg PO q18h; 400 mg IV q24h	250-500 mg PO q18h; 400 mg IV q24h	250-500 mg PO q24h; 400 mg IV q24h given post-HD
Gatifloxacin (Tequin®)	400 mg PO or IV q24h	400 mg PO or IV x 1, then 200 mg PO or IV q24h	400 mg PO or IV x1, then 200 mg PO or IV q24h	400 mg IV or PO x 1, then 200 mg PO or IV q24h	400 mg PO or IV x 1, then 200 mg PO or IV q24h given post-HD
Levofloxacin (Levaquin®)	250-500 mg PO or IV q24h	500 mg PO or IV x 1, then 250 mg PO or IV q24h	500 mg PO or IV x 1, then 250 mg PO or IV q48h	500 mg PO or IV, x 1, then 250 mg PO or IV q48h	500 mg PO or IV x1, then 250 mg PO or IV q48h given post-HD
Miscellaneous					
Aztreonam (Azactam®)	1-2 g IV q6-8h	1-2 g IV q6-8h	1-2 g IV LD, then 1 g IV q6-8h	1-2 g IV LD, then 0.5 g IV q6-8h	1-2 g IV LD, then 0.5 g IV q6-8h given post-HD
Erythromycin (E-Mycin®)	250 mg PO q8h	Same	Same	Same	Same
Imipenem (Primaxin®)	500 mg IV q6h	500 mg IV q8h	500 mg IV q12h	250 mg IV q12h	250 mg IV q12h given post-HD
Linezolid (Zyvox®)	600 mg IV q12h	No data	No data	No data	Give post-HD

(continued)

Appendix 2

Drugs in Renal Failure (continued)

Generic name (trade name)	Normal dose	CrCl 30-50 mL/min	CrCl 10-30 mL/min	CrCl <10 mL/min	Hemodialysis
Misc. antibiotics (cont)					
Meropenem (Merrem®)	1 g IV q8h	1 g IV q12h	500 mg IV q12h	500 mg IV q24h	500 mg IV q24h given post-HD
Quinupristin-dalfopristin (Synercid®)	7.5 mg/kg IV q8h	Same	Same	Same	Same
Rifampin (Rifadin®)	600 mg PO q24h	300-600 mg PO q24-48h	300-600 mg PO q24-48h	300-600 mg PO q48h	300-600 mg PO q48h given post-HF
Trimethoprim-sulfamethoxazole (Bactrim®, Septra®)	8-20 mg/kg/d PO 6-12h; IV q12h	4-10 mg/kg/d PO or IV q12h	4-10 mg/kg/d PPO or IV q12h	2-5 mg/kg/d PO or IV q24h	2-5 mg/kg/d PO or IV q24h given post-HD
Vancomycin (Vancocin®)	500 mg IV q6h or 1 g q12h	1 g IV q24-96h	1 g IV q24-96g	1 g IV q4-7d	1 g IV q4-7d
Penicillins					
Amoxicillin-clavulanic acid (Augmentin®)	250-500 mg PO q8h 875 mg PO bid	Same	250-500 mg PO q12h; 875 mg PO bid	250-500 mg PO q24h; 875 mg PO q24h	Give post-HD
Ampicillin (Principen®, Omnipen®)	1-2 g IV q4-6g	1-2 g IV q6-8h	1-2 g IV q8-12h	1-2 g IV q12h	1-2 g IV q12h
Ampicillin-sulbactam (Unasyn®)	1.5-3 g IV q6h	1.5-3 g IV q8h	1.5-3 g IV q12h	1.5-3 g IV q24h	1.5-3 g IV q24h given post-HD
Methicillin (Staphcillin®)	1-2 g IV q4-6h	1-2 g IV q8h	1-2 g IV q6-8h	1-2 g IV q8-12h	1-2 g IV q8-12h
Nafcillin (Nafcin®, Unipen®)	1-2 g IV q4-6h	Same	Same	Same	Same
Oxacillin (Bactocil®)	1-2 g IV q4-6h	Same	Same	Same	Same
Penicillin G	1-4 MU IV q4-6h	1-4 MUIV q6-8h	1-4 MU IV q8-12h	1-4 MU IV q12-18h	1-4 MU IV q12-18h
Piperacillin (Pipracil®)	3 g IV q4-6h	3 g IV q6h	3 g IV q8h	3 g IV q12h	2 g IV q8h given post-HD
Piperacillin-tazobactam (Zosyn®)	3.375 g IV q4-6h	3.375 g IV q6h	3.375 g IV q8h	3.375 g IV q12h	2.25 g IV q8h given post-HD
Ticarcillin (Ticar®)	3 g IV q4h	1-2 g IV q4-8h	1-2 g IV 8h	1-2 g IV q12h	3 g IV post-HD
Ticarcillin-clavulanic acid (Timentin®)	3.1 g IV q4-6h	2 g IV q4h	2 g IV q12h	2 g IV q12h	2 g IV q12h given post-HD
Anticonvulsants					
Carbamazepine (Tegretol®)	200 mg PO bid to 1200 mg PO q24h	Same	Same	Same	Same
Diazepam (Valium®)	2-10 mg PO q6-12h prn; 2-10 mg IV or IM q2-4h prn	Same	Same	Same	Same
Ethosuximide (Zarontin®)	500-1500 mg PO q24h	Same	Same	Same	Same
Gabapentin (Neurontin®)	300-600 mg PO bid	300-400 mg po bid-tid	300 mg PO q24h	300 mg PO qod	300 mg PO LD, then 200-300 mg PO post-HD

Appendix 2

Drugs in Renal Failure (continued)

Generic name (trade name)	Normal dose	CrCl 30-50 mL/min	CrCl 10-30 mL/min	CrCl <10 mL/min	Hemodialysis
Anticonvulsants (cont)					
Lamotrigine (Lamictal®)	15 mg PO q12-24h initially, then 100-500 mg PO q24h	Same	Same	Same	No data
Lorazepam (Ativan®)	0.5-10 mg PO q4-6h prn; 1-10 mg IV or IM q2-4h prn	Same	Same	Same	Same
Oxcarbazepine (Trileptal®)	200-400 mg PO tid	Same	Same	Same	No data
Phenobarbital (Luminal®, Solfoton®)	60-250 mg PO q24h; 10-20 mg/kg IV	Same	Same	60-100 mg PO q24h	Give dose post-HD
Phenytoin (Dilantin®)	15 mg/kg LD, then 200-400 mg/d PO or IV divided q8-12h	Same	Same	Same	Same
Primidone (Mysoline®)	250-500 mg PO qid	250-500 mg PO q8-12h	250-500 mg PO q8-12h	250-500 mg PO q12-24h	80-160 mg PO q12-24h
Sodium valproate (Depakene®, Depakote®)	15-60 mg/kg q24h	Same	Same	Same	Same
Topiramate (Topamax®)	100-400 mg PO q12-24h	50-400 mg PO q12-24h	50-200 mg PO q12-24h	25-100 mg PO q12-24h	No data
Antiemetics					
Metoclopramide (Reglan®)	10-20 mg IV q6h	7.5-15 mg IV q6h	7.5-15 mg IV 6h	5-10 mg IV q6h	7.5-15 mg IV q6h
Antifungals					
Amphotericin B nonlipid (Fungizone®)	0.4-1 mg/kg IV q24h	0.4-1 mg/kg IV q24h	0.4-1 mg/kg IV q24h	0.4-1 mg/kg IV q48h	0.4-1 mg/kg IV q48h
Am B lipid complex (Abelcet®)	5 mg/kg IV q24h	5 mg/kg IV q24h	5 mg/kg IV q24h	5 mg/kg IV q48h	5 mg/kg IV q48h
Am B cholesteryl sulfate complex (Amphotec®)	3-6 mg/kg/d IV q24h	3-6 mg/kg/d IV q24h	3-6 mg/kg/d IV q24h	3-6 mg/kg/d IV q48h	3-6 mg/kg/d IV q 48h
Am B liposome (Ambisome®)	3-5 mg/kg IV q24h	3-5 mg/lg IV q24h	3-5 mg/kg IV q24h	3-5 mg/kg IV q48h	3-5 mg/kg IV q48h
Fluconazole (Diflucan®)	100-400 mg PO or IV q24h	LD: 100-400 mg PO or IV, then 50-200 mg PO or IV q24h	LD: 100-400 mg PO or IV, then 50-200 mg PO Iv q24h	LD: 100-400 mg PO or IV, then 50-200 mg PO or IV q24h	100-400 mg PO or IV only after HD
Itraconazole (Sponanox®)	100-200 mg PO or IV q12h	100-200 mg PO or IV q12h	100-200 mg PO IV q12h	100-200 mg PO or IV q24h	100 mg PO q12-24h; 200 mg IV q24h post-HD
Ketoconazole (Nizoral®)	20 mg PO q24h	Same	Same	Same	Same
Antihistamines					
Cimetidine (Tagamet®)	400 mg PO bid; 300 mg IV q6h; 37.5-50 mg/h continuous infusion	200 mg PO bid; 300 mg IV q8h; 25-37.5 mg/h continuous infusion	200 mg PO bid; 200 mg IV q8h; 25-37.5 mg/h continuous infusion	100 mg PO bid; 300 mg IV q12h; 18-25 mg/h continuous infusion	No PO supplementation required; 300 mg IV q12h given post-HD

(continued)

Appendix 2

Drugs in Renal Failure (continued)

Generic name (trade name)	Normal dose	CrCl 30-50 mL/min	CrCl 10-30 mL/min	CrCl <10 mL/min	Hemodialysis
Antihistamines (cont)					
Famotidine (Pepcid®)	20-40 mg PO qhs; 20-40 mg IV q12h	5-20 mg PO qhs; 20 mg IV q12h	5-10 mg PO qhs; 20 mg IV q12h	2-4 mg PO qhs; 20 mg IV q24h, or 40 mg IV q48h	No PO supplementation required; 20 mg IV q24h given post-HD
Nizatidine (Axid®)	150 mg PO q12h or 300 mg PO hs	150 mg PO q24h	150 mg PO q24h	150 mg PO q48h	150 mg PO q48h
Ranitidine (Zantac®)	150-300 mg PO qhs; 50 mg IV q8h; 6.25 mg/h continuous infusion	75-150 mg PO qhs; 50 mg IV a12h	75-150 mg PO qhs; 50 mg IV q12h	75 mg PO qhs; 50 mg IV q24h	50% of PO dose post-HD; 50 mg IV q24h given post-HD
Antihypertensives					
ACE inhibitors					
Benazepril (Lotensin®)	10-40 mg PO q24h	5-20 PO q24h	5-20 mg PO q24h	5-20 mg PO q24h	5-20 PO q24h
Captopril (Capoten®)	25-200 mg PO q8h	18.75-75 mg PO q12-18h	18.75-75 mg PO q12-18h	12.5-50 mg PO q24h	Supplement 25-30% of dose after HD
Enalapril (Vasotec®)	5-10 mg PO q12h	2.5-7.5 mg PO q12h	2.5 mg PO q24h	2.5 mg PO q24h	2.5-7.5 PO q12h
Enalaprilat (Vasotec®)	1.25-5 mg IV q6h	1.25-2.5 mg IV q6h	0.625 mg IV x 1, then up to 1.25 mg q6h if inadequate response	0.625 mg IV x 1, then up to 1.25 me q6h if inadequate response	0.625 mg IV q6h
Fosinopril (Monopril®)	10-40 mg PO q24h	10-40 mg q24h	10-40 mg PO q24h	7.5-30 mg PO q24h	Same
Lisinopril (Zestril®)	10-40 mg PO q24h	5-30 mg PO q24h	5-30 mg PO q24h	2.5-20 mg PO q24h	2.5 mg initially, then 20% of patient's dose after HD if on a dosing regimen
Quinapril (Accupril®)	10-80 mg PO q24h	7.5-60 mg PO q24h	7.5-60 mg PO q24h	7.5-60 mg PO q24h	2.5 mg initially, then 25-35% of patient's dose after HD if on a dosing regimen
Ramipril (Altace®)	2.5-20 mg PO q24h	1.25-15 mg PO q24h	1.25-15 mg PO q24h	1.25-10 mg PO q24h	Supplement 20% of the patient's dose after HD
α-Blockers					
Doxazosin (Cardura®)	1-16 mg PO q24h	Same	Same	Same	Same
Prazosin (Minipress®)	1-15 mg PO q12h	Same	Same	Same	Same
Terazosin (Hytrin®)	1-20 mg/d PO	Same	Same	Same	Same
Angiotensin-receptor blockers					
Candesartan (Atacand®)	8-32 PO q24h	Same	Same	No data	Same
Losartan (Cozaar®)	25-100 mg PO q12-24h	Same	Same	Same	No data

Appendix 2

Drugs in Renal Failure (continued)

Generic name (trade name)	Normal dose	CrCl 30-50 mL/min	CrCl 10-30 mL/min	CrCl <10 mL/min	Hemodialysis
Angiotensin-receptor blockers (cont)					
Irbesartan (Avapro®)	150-300 mg PO q24h	Same	Same	Same	Same
Valsartan (Diovan®)	80-320 mg PO q24h	Same	Same	No data	No data
β-Blockers					
Atenolol (Ternormin®)	50-100 mg PO q24h	25-50 mg q48h	25-50 mg PO q24h	25-50 mg PO q96h	25-50 mg PO q96h; supplement 12.5-25 mg post-HD
Carvedilol (Coreg®)	6.25-50 mg PO q12h	Same	Same	Same	No data
Metoprolol (Lopressor®)	50-450 mg/d PO in 2-3 divided doses	Same	Same	Same	Supplement 50 mg PO post-HD
Labetalol (Normodyne®)	200-600 mg PO bid	Same	Same	Same	Same
Nadolol (Corgard®)	40-320 mg/d PO single or divided doses	20-160 mg/d PO q24-36h	20-160 mg/d PO q24-48h	10-80 mg/d PO q48h	Supplement 40 mg PO post-HD
Pindolol (Visken®)	10-40 mg PO q12h	Same	Same	Same	Same
Propranolol (Inderal®)	80-320 mg PO q6-12h	Same	Same	Same	Same
Sotalol (Betapace®)	80-320 mg PO q12h	80-320 mg PO q24h	80-320 mg PO q36-48h	10-100 mg PO according to clinical response	Same Supplement 80 mg post-HD
Calcium channel blockers					
Amlodipine (Norvasc®)	2.5-10 mg PO q24h	Same	Same	Same	Same
Diltiazem (Dilacor®, Cardizem®, Tiazac®)	30-90 mg PO q6-8h	Same	Same	Same	Same
Felodiopine (Plendil®)	5-15 mg PO q 8-24 h	Same	Same	Same	Same
Isradipine (Dynacirc®)	1.25-10 mg/d PO bid	Same	Same	Same	Same
Nicardipine (Cardene®)	20-40 mg PO tid	Same	Same	Same	Same
Nifedipine (Adalat®, Procardia®)	10-30 mg/d PO tid	Same	Same	Same	Same
Nimodipine (Nimotop®)	60 mg PO q4h	Same	Same	Same	Same
Verapamil (Calan®, Isoptin®, Verelan®)	40-120 mg PO q8h	Same	Same	20-60 mg PO q8h	20-60 mg PO q8h
Diuretics					
Bumetanide (Bumex®)	1-2 mg IV q8-12h	Same	Same	8-10 mg PO or IV single dose, or 12 mg infusion over 12h	Same
Furosemide (Lasix®)	40-80 mg IV q12h	Same	Same	Same	Not effective

(continued)

Appendix 2

Drugs in Renal Failure (continued)

Generic name (trade name)	Normal dose	CrCl 30-50 mL/min	CrCl 10-30 mL/min	CrCl <10 mL/min	Hemodialysis
Hydrochlorothiazide (Hydrodiuril®)	25-200 mg PO qd-tid	Same	Same	Not effective	Not effective
Spironloactone (Aldactone®)	25-200 mg/d PO in 2-4 divided doses	12.5-100 mg PO q12-24h	12.5-100 mg PO q24h	Not effective	Not effective
Triamterene (Dyrenium®)	50-100 mg PO bid	Same	Same	Not effective	Not effective
Antivirals					
Acyclovir (Zovirax®)	5-10 mg/kg PO or IV q8h	5-10 mg/kg PO or IV q12h	5-10 mg/kg PO or IV q24h	2.5 mg/kg PO or IV q24h	2.5-5 mg/kg PO or IV q24h given post-HD
Amantadine (Symmetrel®)	100 mg PO q12h	100 mg PO q24h	100 mg PO q48h	200 mg PO q7d	200 mg PO q7d
Didanosine (Videx®)	200 mg PO q12h	200 mg PO q12-24h	200 mg PO q24h	100 mg PO q24h	Dose after HD
Famciclovir (Famvir®)	125 mg PO q12h, or 500 mg PO q8h	125 mg PO q12h, 500 mg PO q12h	125 mg PO q12-48h, 500 mg PO 12-48h	62.5 mg PO q48h, or 250 mg PO q48h	Dose after HD
Ganciclovir (Cytovene®)	1000 mg PO q8h, 5 mg/kg IV q12h, then 5 mg IV q24h	No data: 500-1000 mg PO q24h, 2.5 mg/kg IV q24h, then 1.24 mg/kg IV q24h	No data: 500-1000 mg PO q24h. 1.25 mg/kg IV q24h, then 0.625 mg/kg IV q24h	No data: 500 mg PO q48-96 h, 1.25 mg IV three times a week, then 0.625 mg/kg IV three times a week	No data: Dose PO after dialysis, 1.25 mg IV three times a week, then 0.625 mg/kg IV three times a week
Indinavir (Crixan®)	800 mg PO q8h	No data	No data	No data	No data
Lamivudine (Epivir®)	150 mg PO q12h	50-150 mg PO q24h	50-150 PO q24h	25-50 mg PO q25h	Dose after HD
Nelfinavir (Viracept®)	750 mg PO q8h	No data	No data	No data	No data
Nevirapine (Viramune®)	200 mg PO q24 h x 14 d, then q12h	No data	No data	No data	No data
Ribavirin (Rebetrol®)	200 mg PO 8h	200 mg PO q8h	200 mg PO q8h	100 mg PO q8h	Dose after HD
Ritonavir (Norvir®)	600 mg PO q12h	No data	No data	No data	No data
Saquinavir (Fortovase®, Invirase®)	600 mg PO q8h	No data	No data	No data	No data
Stavudine (Zerit®)	30-40 mg PO q12h	15-20 mg PO q12-24h	15-20 mg PO q12-24h	15-20 mg PO q24h	15-20 mg PO q24h
Valaciclovir (Valtrex®)	500 mg PO q12h to 1000 mg PO q8h	500-1000 mg PO q12-24h	500-1000 mg Po q12-24h	500 mg q24h	Dose after HD
Zalcitabine (Hivid®)	0.75 mg PO q8h	0.75 mg PO q8-12h	0.75 mg PO q12h	0.75 mg PO q24h	No data; dose after HD
Zidovudine (Retrovir®)	200 mg PO q8h; 300 mg PO q12h	200 mg PO q8h; 300 mg PO q12h	200 mg PO q8h; 300 mg PO q12h	100 mg PO q8h	100 mg PO q8h
Gout agents					
Allopurinol (Zyloprim®)	300 mg PO q24h	150-200 mg PO q24h	150 mg PO q24h	100 mg PO q48h	150 mg supplemental dose
Colchicine (Acetycol®, Colsalide®)	Acute: 2 mg, then 0.5 mg PO q6h; Chronic: 0.5-1 mg PO q24h	Decrease dose by 50% to no change	Decrease dose by 50%	Decrease dose by 25%	Same
Probenecid (Benemid®)	500 mg PO bid	Not effective	Not effective	Not effective	Not effective

Appendix 2

Drugs in Renal Failure (continued)

Generic name (trade name)	Normal dose	CrCl 30-50 mL/min	CrCl 10-30 mL/min	CrCl <10 mL/min	Hemodialysis
Hypoglycemic agents					
Acarbose (Precose®)	50-200 mg PO tid	Avoid	Avoid	Avoid	No data
Acetohexamide (Dymelor®)	250-1500 mg PO q24h	Avoid	Avoid	Avoid	No data
Chlorpropamide (Diabinese®)	100-500 mg PO q24h	Avoid	Avoid	Avoid	Avoid
Glipizide (Glucotrol®)	2.5-15 mg PO q24h	1.25-7.5 mg Po q24h	1.25-7.5 mg PO q24h	1.24-7.5 mg PO q24h	No data
Glyburide (Diabeta®, Glynase®, PresTab®, Micronase®)	1.25-20 mg PO q24h	Avoid	Avoid	Avoid	No supplement necessary
Insulin	Variable	75% of usual dose	75% of usual dose	50% of usual dose	No supplement necessary
Metformin (Glucophage®)	500-850 mg PO bid	125-425 mg PO bid	125-212 mg PO bid	Avoid	No data
Tolazamide (Tolinase®)	100-250 mg PO q24h	Same	Same	Same	No data
Tolbutamide (Orinase®)	1-2 g q24h	Same	Same	Same	No supplement necessary
Nonsteroidal anti-inflammatory agents					
Diclofenac (Voltaren®)	25-75 mg PO bid	12.5-37.5 mg PO bid	6.25-37.5 mg PO bid	6.25-18.75 mg PO bid	No supplement necessary
Etodolac (Lodine®)	200 mg bid	Same	Same	Same	Same
Ibuprofen (Advil®, Motrin®)	200-800 mg PO q6h	Same	Same	Same	Same
Indomethacin (Indocin®)	25-50 mg PO q6-12h	Same	Same	Same	Same
Ketorolac (Toradol®)	60 mg IM LD, then 15-30 mg q6h; 30 mg IV LD, then 15 mg q6h	Same	Same	15 mg IM or IV q6h (no bolus dose)	15 mg IM or IV q6h (no bolus dose)
Nabumetone (Relafen®)	1-2 g PO q24h	Same	0.5-1 g PO q24h	0.5-1 g PO q24h	No supplement necessary
Naproxen (Naprosyn®)	250-500 mg PO 8-12h	Same	Same	Same	Same
Oxaprozin (Daypro®)	1200 mg PO q24h	Same	Same	Same	Same
Tolmetin (Tolectin®)	400 mg PO tid	Same	Same	Same	Same
Proton pump inhibitors					
Esomeprazole (Nexium®)	20-40 mg PO q24h	Same	Same	Same	Same
Lansoprazole (Prevacid®)	15-30 mg PO q12-24h	Same	Same	Same	Same
Omeprazole (Prilosec®)	20-40 mg PO q12-24h	Same	Same	Same	Same
Pantoprazole (Protonix®)	20-80 mg PO q24h; 80 mg IV q12h	Same	Same	Same	Same

References

Aronoff GR, Berns JS, Brier ME, et al. Drug Prescribing in Renal Failure: *Dosing Guidelines for Adults,* 4th ed. Philadelphia: American College of Physicians; 1999.

DeBellis RJ, Smith BS, Cawley PA, Burniske GM. Drug dosing in critically ill patients with renal failure: A pharmacokinetic approach. *J Intensive Care Med.* 2000;15:273-313.

Appendix 3

Drugs in Hepatic Failure

Drug	Dose
Amiodarone (Cordarone®, Pacerone®)	Dose adjustment may be necessary in patients with hepatic dysfunction
Amitriptyline (Elavil®)	Decrease dose in patients with cirrhosis
Aspirin	Avoid in severe hepatic dysfunction
Azole antifungals	Consider decreased doses in patients with severe hepatic dysfunction
Benzodiazepines	No dose adjustments are necessary with oxazepam (Serax®), lorazepam (Ativan®), or temazepam (Restoril®)
	Alprazolam (Xanax®): dose 0.25 mg bid-tid in patients with hepatic dysfunction
	Chlordiazepoxide (Librium®): avoid or decrease dose in patients with cirrhosis or hepatitis
	Diazepam (Valium®): decrease dose by 50% in patients with cirrhosis
	Midazolam (Versed®): doses may need to be decreased by 50%
	Triazolam (Halcion®): doses may need to be decreased by 50%
Bicalutamide (Casodex®)	Use with caution in patients with moderate to severe hepatic dysfunction
Bisoprolol (Zebeta®)	Decrease initial dose to 2.5 mg in patients with hepatic insufficiency; do not exceed a dose of 10 mg daily
Buspirone (Buspar®)	Avoid in patients with severe hepatic dysfunction
Carbamazepine (Tegretol®)	Avoid in patients with hepatic disease
Celecoxib (Celebrex®)	Decrease dose by 50% in patients with moderate hepatic dysfunction; avoid in patients with severe hepatic dysfunction
Clindamycin (Cleocin®)	Decrease dose in patients with hepatic dysfunction
Cimetidine (Tagamet®)	Decrease dose (50%) in patients with severe hepatic dysfunction
Delavirdine (Rescriptor®)	Decrease dose in patients with moderate hepatic disease
Diazepam (Valium®)	Decrease dose by 50% in patients with cirrhosis
Diltiazem (Cardizem®, Cartia®, Dilacor®, Tiazac®)	Doses should not exceed 90 mg/d in patients with cirrhosis
Disulfram (Antabuse®)	Use with caution in patients with hepatic cirrhosis or hepatic insufficiency; avoid in patients with advanced or severe hepatic disease
Erythromycin (E-Mycin®)	Dose may need to be decreased in patients with severe hepatic dysfunction
Esomeprazole (Nexium®)	Do not exceed a dose of 20 mg in patients with severe hepatic dysfunction
Estrogens	Use with caution in patients with impaired liver function
HMG-CoA reductase inhibitors	Avoid in patients with elevated serum transaminases
Indinavir (Crixivan®)	Decrease dose to 600 mg q8h in patients with mild to moderate hepatic dysfunction
Isoniazid (Laniazid®, Nydrazid®)	Defer therapy for prevention of tuberculosis in patients with acute hepatic disease
Lamivudine-zidovudine (Combivir®)	Decrease zidovudine dose by 50% in hepatic insufficiency
Lamotrigine (Lamictal®)	Reduce initial, escalation, and maintenance doses by 50% in patients with moderate hepatic dysfunction; decrease doses by 75% in patients with severe hepatic dysfunction
Lansoprazole (Prevacid®)	Decrease dose in patients with hepatic dysfunction
Losartan (Cozaar®)	Decrease initial dose to 25 mg; total daily dose should not exceed 100 mg
Methotrexate (Folex®, Rheumatrex®)	Decrease dose by 25% when the bilirubin is 3.1-5 mg% and the AST is >180 IU; avoid if the bilirubin is >5 mg%
Metoprolol (Lopressor®)	Dose adjustment may be necessary in patients with hepatic insufficiency
Nabumetone (Relafen®)	Use with caution in patients with severe hepatic insufficiency
Nefazodone (Serzone®)	Avoid in patients with elevated transaminases
Nelfinavir (Viracept®)	Use with caution in patients with hepatic impairment
Ofloxacin (Floxin®)	Do not exceed 400 mg/d in patients with severe liver dysfunction
Omeprazole (Prilosec®)	Decrease dose in patients with hepatic dysfunction
Ondansetron (Zofran®)	Do not exceed 8 mg/d in patients with severe hepatic insufficiency
Oxycodone (Oxycontin®)	Initiate dose at one third to one half the usual dose in patients with hepatic dysfunction; increase dose conservatively
Pantoprazole (Protonix®)	Consider every-other-day dosing in patients with severe hepatic dysfunction
Pioglitazone (Actos®)	Avoid in patients with hepatic disease or serum transaminases >2.5 times the upper limit of normal
Phenobarbital (Barbita®, Luminal®, Solfoton®)	Dose may need to be decreased in patients with hepatic dysfunction

Appendix 3

Drugs in Hepatic Failure (continued)

Drug	Dose
Phenytoin (Dilantin®)	Monitor levels frequently as the dose may need to be decreased in hepatic failure
Procainamide (Procanbid®, Promine®, Pronestyl®, Rhythmin®)	Lower doses or longer dosing intervals may be required in patients with hepatic failure
Propranolol (Betachron®, Inderal®)	Monitor more frequently in patients with hepatic dysfunction
Quinidine (Cardioquin®, Quinaglute®, Quinalan®, Quinidex, Quinora®)	Maintenance doses may need to be decreased by 50% in patients with chronic hepatitis
Risperidone (Risperdal®)	Decrease dose in patients with hepatic dysfunction
Rofecoxib (Vioxx®)	Use the lowest dose possible in patients with moderate hepatic impairment
Rifampin (Rifadin®, Rimactane®)	Decrease dose in patients with a serum bilirubin >50 µmol/L; doses should not exceed 6-8 mg/kg biweekly in patients with severe hepatic dysfunction
Ritonavir (Norvir®)	Use with caution in patients with moderate to severe hepatic dysfunction

Selective serotonin reuptake inhibitors (SSRIs) and serotonin-norepinephrine reuptake inhibitors	The dose should be decreased or the dosing interval increased in patients with hepatic insufficiency
	  Citalopram (Celexa®): a dose of 20 mg is recommended for patients with decreased hepatic function
	  Fluoxetine (Prozac®): a 50% dose reduction is recommended in patients with cirrhosis
	  Fluvoxamine (Luvox®): decrease the dose and titrate slowly in patients with hepatic insufficiency
	  Paroxetine (Paxil®): dose initially at 10 mg daily or 12.5 mg daily of the controlled-release product; doses should not exceed 40 mg daily or 50 mg daily of the controlled-release product
	  Sertraline (Zoloft®): decrease the dose or increase the interval
	  Venlafaxine (Effexor®): decrease the dose by 50% in patients with moderate hepatic impairment

Sulfonylureas	Dose may need to be decreased in hepatic disease
Tacrolimus (Prograf®)	Dose at the low end of the dosing range in patients with hepatic insufficiency
Tetracyclines	Avoid in patients with hepatic dysfunction
Theophylline (Aerolate®, Aminophyllin®, Aquaphyllin®, Asmalix®, Bronkodyl®, Choledyl®, Duraphyl®, Respbid®, Slo-bid®, Slo-Phyllin®, Sustaire®, Theo-24®, Theobid®, Theochron®, Theoclear®, Theo-Dur®, Theolair®, Theon®, Theospan®, Theovent®, Truphylline®)	Dose may need to be decreased and serum levels should be monitored frequently in patients with hepatic insufficiency
Tramadol (Ultram®)	Dose 50 mg PO q12h in patients with cirrhosis
Tricyclic antidepressants: amitriptyline (Elavil®), clomipramine (Anafranil®), desipramine (Norpramin®), doxepin (Sinequan®), imipramine (Tofranil®), nortriptyline (Pamelor®), protriptyline (Vivactil®)	Dose should be decreased in patients with cirrhosis
Valproic acid (Depakote®, Depakene®)	Avoid in patients with hepatic disease or significant hepatic insufficiency
Warfarin (Coumadin®)	Monitor INR more frequently
Zafirlukast (Accolate®)	Consider a decreased dose in patients with cirrhosis
Zalcitabine (Hivid®)	Avoid in patients with liver function tests >5 times the upper limit of normal
Zidovudine (Retrovir®)	Decrease dose by 50% in patients with cirrhosis

References

Hutchison TA, Shahan DR (eds.) DRUGDEX® System. MICROMEDEX, Greenwood Village, CO (edition expires 3, 2003).

Appendix 4

Top 200 Prescription Drugs

The following is a list of the top 200 prescriptions for 2002 by the number of U.S. prescriptions dispensed obtained with permission from rxlist.com with data furnished by NDC Health.

Brand name	Generic name	Brand name	Generic name
1. Hydrocodone w/APAP	hydrocodone w/APAP	51. Effexor XR	venlafaxine
2. Lipitor	atorvastatin	52. Singulair	montelukast
3. Atenolol	atenolol	53. Zestril	lisinopril
4. Synthroid	levothyroxine	54. Potassium Chloride	potassium chloride
5. Premarin	conjugated estrogens	55. Clonazepam	clonazepam
6. Zithromax	azithromycin	56. Naproxen	naproxen
7. Furosemide	furosemide	57. Warfarin	warfarin
8. Amoxicillin	amoxicillin	58. Trazodone	trazodone
9. Norvasc	amlodipine	59. Cipro	ciprofloxacin
10. Hydrochlorothiazide	hydrochlorothiazide	60. Flonase	fluticasone
11. Alprazolam	alprazolam	61. Cyclobenzaprine	cyclobenzaprine
12. Albuterol Aerosol	albuterol	62. Verapamil HCl	verapamil
13. Zoloft	sertraline	63. Enalapril	enalapril
14. Paxil	paroxetine	64. Albuterol sulfate	albuterol
15. Zocor	simvastatin	65. Isosorbide mononitrate	isosorbide mononitrate
16. Prevacid	lansoprazole	66. Levaquin	levofloxacin
17. Ibuprofen	ibuprofen	67. Diazepam	diazepam
18. Triamterene/ hydrochlorothiazide	triamterene/hydrochlorothiazide	68. Glucotrol XL	glipizide
		69. Coumadin	warfarin
19. Toprol XL	metoprolol XL	70. Plavix	clopidogrel
20. Cephalexin	cephalexin	71. Diflucan	fluconazole
21. Celebrex	celecoxib	72. Advair Diskus	salmeterol/fluticasone
22. Zyrtec	cetirizine	73. Protonix	pantoprazole
23. Levoxyl	levothyroxine	74. Lotrel	amlodipine/benazepril
24. Allegra	fexofenadine	75. Amoxil	amoxicillin
25. Ortho Tri-Cyclen	norgestimate/ethinyl estradiol	76. Diovan	valsartan
26. Celexa	citalopram	77. Glyburide	glyburide
27. Prednisone	prednisone	78. Carisoprodol	carisoprodol
28. Prilosec	omeprazole	79. Altace	ramipril
29. Vioxx	rofecoxib	80. Allopurinol	allopurinol
30. Claritin	loratadine	81. Estradiol	estradiol
31. Fluoxetine	fluoxetine	82. Avandia	rosiglitazone maleate
32. Acetaminophen/codeine	acetaminophen/codeine	83. Actos	pioglitazone
33. Ambien	zolpidem	84. Lotensin	benazepril
34. Metoprolol tartrate	metoprolol	85. Clarinex	desloratadine
35. Lorazepam	lorazepam	86. Medroxyprogesterone	medroxyprogesterone
36. Fosamax	alendronate	87. Oxycodone/APAP	oxycodone/APAP
37. Propoxyphene N/APAP	propoxyphene N/APAP	88. Doxycycline hyclate	doxycycline
38. Metformin	metformin	89. Lanoxin	digoxin
39. Ranitidine HCl	ranitidine	90. Cozaar	losartan
40. Amitriptyline	amitriptyline	91. Nasonex	mometasone
41. Viagra	sildenafil citrate	92. Diltiazem HCl	diltiazem
42. Prempro	conjugated estrogens/ medroxyprogesterone	93. Clonidine	clonidine
		94. Prinivil	lisinopril
43. Trimox	amoxicillin	95. Digitek	digoxin
44. Neurontin	gabapentin	96. Methylprednisolone	methylprednisolone
45. Wellbutrin SR	bupropion	97. Evista	raloxifene
46. Pravachol	pravastatin	98. Folic acid	folic acid
47. Augmentin	amoxacillin/clavulanate	99. Glucophage XR	metformin
48. Nexium	esomeprazole	100. Penicillin VK	penicillin VK
49. Accupril	quinapril	101. Flovent	fluticasone propionate
50. Lisinopril	lisinopril	102. Risperdal	risperidone

Appendix 4

Top 200 Prescription Drugs (continued)

Brand name	Generic name	Brand name	Generic name
103. Cotrim	trimethoprim/sulfamethoxazole	152. Skelaxin	metaxalone
104. Promethazine	promethazine	153. Serevent	salmeterol
105. Diovan HCT	valsartan/hydrochlorothiazide	154. Dilantin	phenytoin
106. Aciphex	rabeprazole	155. Promethazine/codeine	promethazine/codeine
107. Zyprexa	olanzapine	156. Necon	ethinyl estradiol/norethindrone
108. Allegra-D	fexofenadine/pseudoephedrine	157. Captopril	captopril
109. Levothroid	levothyroxine	158. Clindamycin	clindamycin
110. Doxazosin	doxazosin	159. Aspirin	aspirin
111. Xalatan	latanoprost	160. Seroquel	quetiapine
112. Gemfibrozil	gemfibrozil	161. Acyclovir	acyclovir
113. Flomax	tamsulosin	162. Macrobid	nitrofurantoin
114. Temazepam	temazepam	163. Claritin D 12 hour	loratadine/pseudoephedrine
115. Ultram	tramadol	164. Amoxicillin/clavulanate	amoxicillin/clavulanate
116. Hyzaar	losartan/hydrochlorothiazide	165. Adderall XR	amphetamine mixed salts
117. Oxycontin	oxycodone	166. Biaxin XL	clarithromycin
118. Humulin N	human insulin NPH	167. Trivora-28	levonorgestrel/ethinyl estradiol
119. Depakote	divalproex	168. Ortho-Cyclen	norgestimate/ethinyl estradiol
120. Concerta	methylphenidate XR	169. Cefzil	cefprozil
121. Klor-Con	potassium chloride	170. Humulin 70/30	human insulin 70/30
122. Glucovance	glyburide/metformin	171. Detrol LA	tolterodine
123. Imitrex Oral	sumatriptan	172. Coreg	carvedilol
124. Terazosin	terazosin	173. Tiazac	diltiazem
125. Claritin D 24 hour	loratadine/pseudoephedrine	174. Biaxin	clarithromycin
126. Cartia XT	diltiazem	175. Tramadol	tramadol
127. Amaryl	glimepiride	176. Nasacort AQ	triamcinolone acetonide
128. Spironolactone	spironolactone	177. Humalog	insulin lispro
129. Tricor	fenofibrate	178. Ultracet	tramadol/acetaminophen
130. Ortho-Novum	norethindrone/ethinyl estradiol	179. Endocet	oxycodone/acetaminophen
131. Hydroxyzine HCl	hydroxyzine	180. Bactroban	mupirocin
132. Monopril	fosinopril	181. Veetids	penicillin VK
133. Combivent	ipratropium/albuterol	182. Trimethoprim/ sulfamethoxazole	trimethoprim/sulfamethoxazole
134. Meclizine	meclizine	183. Timolol maleate	timolol maleate
135. Triamcinolone Acetonide	triamcinolone	184. Rhinocort Aqua	budesonide
136. Klor-Con M20	potassium chloride	185. Claritin Reditabs	loratadine
137. Metoclopramide	metoclopramide	186. Nortriptyline	nortriptyline
138. Minocycline	minocycline	187. Aviane	levonorgestrel/ethinyl estradiol
139. Bisoprolol/hydrochlorothiazide	bisoprolol/hydrochlorothiazide	188. Actonel	risedronate
140. Propranolol	propranolol	189. Topamax	topiramate
141. Glucophage	metformin	190. Microgestin Fe	norethindrone/ethinyl estradiol
142. Propacet	propoxyphene N/APAP	191. Tamoxifen	tamoxifen
143. Valtrex	valacyclovir	192. Mircette	desogestrel/ethinyl estradiol
144. Remeron	mirtazapine	193. Nifedipine	nifedipine
145. Famotidine	famotidine	194. Ditropan XL	oxybutynin
146. Metronidazole	metronidazole	195. Tetracycline	tetracycline
147. Bextra	valdecoxib	196. Apri	desogestrel/ethinyl estradiol
148. Avapro	irbesartan	197. Zestoretic	lisinopril/hydrochlorothiazide
149. Glipizide	glipizide	198. Diclofenac	diclofenac
150. Buspirone	buspirone	199. Augmentin ES-600	amoxicillin/clavulanate
151. Nystatin	nystatin	200. Carbidopa/levodopa	carbidopa/levodopa

The Top 200 Prescriptions for 2002 by Number of U.S. Prescriptions Dispensed. Available at: www.rxlist.com/top200.htm. Accessed on: July 10, 2003.

Appendix 5

Top 200 Over-the-Counter Products

The following is a list of over-the-counter (OTC) and health and beauty care brands based on dollar amount in 2002 reported by Verispan.

Rank	Product	Rank	Product
1.	Private-label internal analgesic tabs	51.	Private-label first-aid tape/bandage/gauze/cotton
2.	Tylenol® internal analgesic tabs	52.	Clairol Herbal Essences® shampoo
3.	Private-label mineral supplements	53.	Pedia Sure® weight control nutritional liquid/powder
4.	Private-label cold/allergy/sinus tabs	54.	Q-Tips® cotton balls/cotton swabs
5.	Advil® internal analgesic tabs	55.	Private-label antismoking gum
6.	Crest® toothpaste	56.	Pepcid AC® antacid tabs
7.	Always® sanitary napkins/liners	57.	L'Oreal Feria® hair coloring
8.	Listerine® mouthwash/dental rinse	58.	Zantac 75® antacid tabs
9.	Gillette Mach3® refill razor blades	59.	Aquafresh® toothpaste
10.	Nicorette® antismoking gum	60.	Centrum Silver® multivitamins
11.	Dove nondeodorant bar soap	61.	Gillette Venus® refill razor blades
12.	Private-label 1- and 2-letter vitamins	62.	Motrin IB® internal analgesic tabs
13.	Ultra Slim Fast® weight control/nutritional liquid/powder	63.	Band-Aid® first-aid tape/bandage/gauze/cotton
14.	Slim Fast® meal options weight control/nutritional liquid/powder	64.	Private-label eye/lens care solutions
15.	Tampax® tampons	65.	Excedrin® internal analgesic tabs
16.	Depend® adult incontinence products	66.	Scope® mouthwash/dental rinse
17.	Crest Whitestrips® tooth powder/polish	67.	Lever 2000® deodorant bar soap
18.	Colgate® toothpaste	68.	Right Guard® sport deodorants
19.	Private-label multivitamins	69.	Vaseline Intensive Care® hand and body lotion
20.	Kotex® sanitary napkins/liners	70.	Dr. Scholl's® foot care devices
21.	Private-label adult incontinence products	71.	Gillette Mach3 Turbo® refill razor blades
22.	Aleve® internal analgesic tabs	72.	Metamucil® laxative/stimulant liquid/powder/oil
23.	L'Oreal® preference hair coloring	73.	Tylenol® internal analgesic liquids
24.	Private-label antacid tabs	74.	Alcon Opti Free Express® eye/lens care solutions
25.	Stayfree® sanitary napkins/liners	75.	Kotex Security® tampons
26.	Ensure® weight control nutritional liquid/powder	76.	Skintimate® shaving cream
27.	Private-label first-aid ointments/antiseptics	77.	Robitussin DM® cough syrup
28.	Playtex Gentle Glide® tampons	78.	Degree® deodorants
29.	Benadryl® cold/allergy/sinus tabs	79.	Chap Stick® lip balm/cold sore medication
30.	Nicoderm CQ® antismoking patch	80.	Johnson & Johnson® first-aid tape/bandage/gauze/cotton
31.	Private-label baby wipes	81.	Nature Made® mineral supplements
32.	Private-label cotton balls/cotton swabs	82.	Children's Motrin® internal analgesic liquids
33.	Nature Made® 1- and 2-letter vitamins	83.	Just for Men® hair coloring
34.	Private-label cold/allergy sinus liquid/powder	84.	Fixodent® denture adhesives
35.	Bayer® internal analgesic tabs	85.	Ensure Plus® weight control nutritionals/liquid/powder
36.	L'Oreal Excellence® hair coloring	86.	Gillette Sensor Excel® refill razor blades
37.	Private-label laxative tabs	87.	Braun Oral B® dental accessories/tools
38.	Huggies Natural Care® baby wipes	88.	Private-label feminine hygiene/medicinal treatments
39.	Tylenol PM® internal analgesic tabs	89.	Tums EX® antacid tabs
40.	Centrum® multivitamins	90.	Kotex Lightdays® sanitary napkins/liners
41.	Depend Poise® adult incontinence products	91.	Trojan® male contraceptives
42.	Colgate Total® toothpaste	92.	Clairol Natural Instincts® hair coloring
43.	Listerine Pocketpaks® portable oral care	93.	Old Spice High Endurance® deodorants
44.	Vicks Nyquil® cold/allergy/sinus liquid/powder	94.	Carefree® sanitary napkins/liners
45.	Halls® cough/sore throat drop	95.	Ace muscle/body support devices
46.	Private-label sanitary napkins/liners	96.	Bausch & Lomb Renu Multiplus® eye/lens care solution
47.	Clairol Nice 'n Easy® hair coloring	97.	Private-label cough syrup
48.	Metabolife 356® weight control candy/tabs	98.	EPT® pregnancy test kits
49.	Private-label mouthwash/dental rinse	99.	Pepto-Bismol® stomach remedy liquid/powder
50.	Mennen Speed Stick® deodorants	100.	Private-label antismoking patch

Appendix 5

Top 200 Over-the-Counter Products (continued)

Rank	Product
101.	Alka-Seltzer Plus® cold/allergy/sinus tabs
102.	Private-label weight control nutritional liquid/powder
103.	Cover Girl Clean® facial makeup
104.	Irish Spring® deodorant bar soap
105.	Sensodyne® toothpaste
106.	Gillette Sensor® refill razor blades
107.	Private-label pregnancy test kits
108.	Dial® deodorant bar soap
109.	Osteo Bi Flex® mineral supplements
110.	Crest Multicare® toothpaste
111.	OB® tampons
112.	Private-label nasal spray/drops/inhaler
113.	Monistat 3® feminine hygiene/medicinal treatments
114.	Imodium AD® diarrhea tabs
115.	Tylenol Cold® cold/allergy/sinus tabs
116.	Private-label anti-itch treatments, including calamine
117.	Ponds® facial cleansers
118.	Boost® weight control nutritional liquid powder
119.	Sudafed® cold/allergy/sinus tabs
120.	Maybelline Expert Eyes® eye makeup
121.	Schick Slim Twin® disposable razors
122.	Tylenol Arthritis® internal analgesic tabs
123.	Theraflu® cold/allergy/sinus tabs
124.	Secret® deodorants
125.	Secret Sheer Dry® deodorants
126.	Nivea® hand and body lotion
127.	Tylenol Sinus® cold/allergy/sinus tabs
128.	Caress® nondeodorant bar soap
129.	Cover Girl Outlast® lipstick
130.	Dove® deodorants
131.	One-A-Day® multivitamins
132.	Private-label laxative/stimulant liquid/powder/oil
133.	Coppertone® suntan lotion and oil
134.	Imodium Advanced® diarrhea tabs
135.	Excedrin Migraine® internal analgesic tabs
136.	Kleenex Cottonelle® moist towelettes
137.	Jergens® hand and body lotion
138.	Banana Boat® suntan lotion and oil
139.	ThermaCare® heat/ice packs
140.	Pampers Natural Aloe Touch® baby wipes
141.	Olay® facial moisturizers
142.	Clairol Herbal Essence® hair conditioner/creme rinse
143.	Colgate Simply White® tooth powder/polish
144.	Lubriderm® hand & body lotion
145.	Dial® liquid hand soap
146.	Futuro® muscle/body support devices
147.	Dove® liquid soap
148.	Abreva® lip balm/cold sore medication
149.	Maybelline Great Lash® eye makeup
150.	Garnier Nutrisse® hair coloring
151.	Private-label toothbrushes
152.	Private-label hand and body lotion
153.	Neosporin Plus® first-aid ointments/antiseptics
154.	Breathe Right® nasal strips
155.	Ivory® nondeodorant bar soap
156.	Rogaine® hair growth products
157.	Olay Total Effects® skin fade/age/bleach cream
158.	Tylenol Cold® cold/allergy/sinus liquid/powder
159.	Secret Platinum® deodorants
160.	Sonicare® dental accessories/tools
161.	Gas X® antacid tabs
162.	Preparation H® hemorrhoidal cream/ointment/spray
163.	Clairol Hydrience® hair coloring
164.	Private-label cough/sore throat drop
165.	Serenity® adult incontinence products
166.	Revlon Super Lustrous® lipstick
167.	Head & Shoulders Classic Clean® shampoo
168.	Schick Xtreme3® disposable razors
169.	Private-label shampoo
170.	Pepcid Complete® antacid tabs
171.	Natures Bounty® mineral supplements
172.	Colgate 2 in 1® toothpaste
173.	Sundown® mineral supplements
174.	Mitchum® deodorants
175.	Alka-Seltzer® antacid/analgesic combination
176.	Ban® deodorants
177.	Gillette Series® deodorants
178.	Afrin® nasal spray/drops/inhaler
179.	Tylenol Allergy Sinus® cold/allergy/sinus tabs
180.	Clairol Herbal Essences® color hair coloring
181.	Alberto VO 5® hair conditioner/creme rinse
182.	Advil Cold & Sinus® cold/allergy/sinus tabs
183.	Olay® nondeodorant bar soap
184.	Softsoap® liquid hand soap
185.	Frizz Ease® hair styling/setting gel/mousse
186.	Olay Daily Facials® facial cleansers
187.	Kotex Overnites® sanitary napkins/liners
188.	Lamisil AT® foot care/athletes foot medication
189.	Thermasilk® hair conditioner/creme rinse
190.	Neosporin® first-aid ointments/antiseptics
191.	Trojan Enz® male contraceptives
192.	Bausch & Lomb Renu® eye/lens care solutions
193.	Suave® shampoo
194.	Phillips® stomach remedy liquid/powder
195.	Curel® hand and body lotion
196.	Natures Resource® mineral supplements
197.	Neutrogena® suntan lotion and oil
198.	Mentadent® toothpaste
199.	Edge Pro Gel® shaving cream
200.	Gillette Custom Plus® disposable razors

From Marina Merketos. Top 200 OTC/HBC Brands in 2002. *Drug Topics*. 2003;4:33. Also available at: www.drugtopics.com. Accessed on February 20, 2003.

Appendix 6

Drugs Excreted in Breast Milk

The following is a selection of drug products that can be excreted in breast milk. The list is not comprehensive. Generics and alternate brands of some products may exist. When recommending drugs to pregnant or nursing patients, always check product labeling for specific precautions.

Accolate®	Brevicon®	Cytoxan®	Ecotrin®	Indocin®	Luvox®
Accuretic®	Brontex®	Dalalone D.P.®	Effexor®	INFeD®	Macrobid®
Achromycin®	Cafergot®	Dapsone®	Elavil®	Invanz®	Macrodanti®n
Actiq®	Calan®	Daraprim®	EMLA®	Inversine®	Mandol®
Activella®	Capoten®	Darvon®	E-Mycin®	Isoptin®	Marinol®
Adalat®	Capozide®	Darvon-N®	Enduron®	Kadian®	Maxipime®
Adderall®	Captopril	Decadron®	Equanil®	Keflex®	Maxzide®
Advicor®	Carbatrol®	Deconsal II®	ERYC®	Keftab®	Mefoxin®
Aggrenox®	Cardizem®	Demerol®	EryPed®	Kefurox®	Mepergan®
Aldactazide®	Cataflam®	Demulen®	Ery-Tab®	Kefzol®	Meruvax II®
Aldactone®	Catapres®	Depacon®	Erythrocin®	Kerlone®	Methergine®
Aldoclor®	Ceclor®	Depakene®	Erythromycin	Klonopin®	Methotrexate
Aldomet®	Cefizox®	Depakote®	Esgic-plus®	Kronofed-A®	MetroCream/Gel/
Aldoril®	Cefobid®	Depo-Provera®	Eskalith®	Kutrase®	Lotion®
Alesse®	Cefotan®	Desogen®	Estrostep®	Lamictal®	Mexitil®
Allegra-D®	Ceftin®	Desoxyn®	Ethmozine®	Lamisil®	Mezlin®
Alfenta®	Celexa®	Desyrel®	Felbatol®	Lamprene®	Micronor®
Aloprim®	Ceptaz®	Dexedrine®	Feldene®	Lanoxicaps®	Microzide®
Altace®	Cerebyx®	DextroStat®	femhrt®	Lanoxin®	Midamor®
Ambien®	Ceredase®	D.H.E. 45®	Fero-Folic®	Lariam®	Migranal®
Anaprox®	Cipro®	Diabinese®	Fiorinal®	Lescol®	Miltown®
Ancef®	Claforan®	Diastat®	Flagyl®	Levbid®	Minizide®
Androderm®	Clarinex®	Diflucan®	Florinef®	Levlen®	Minocin®
Apresoline®	Claritin®	Digitek®	Floxin®	Levlite®	Mirapex®
Aralen®	Claritin-D®	Dilacor®	Fluorescite®	Levora®	Mircette®
Arthrotec®	Cleocin®	Dilantin®	Fluothane®	Levothroid®	M-M-R II®
Asacol®	Clorpres®	Dilaudid®	Fortaz®	Levoxyl®	Modicon®
Astramorph/PF®	Clozaril®	Diovan®	Furosemide	Levsin®	Moduretic®
Ativan®	Codeine	Diprivan®	Gabitril®	Levsinex®	Monocid®
Atromid-S®	CombiPatch®	Disalcid®	Galzin®	Lexxel®	Monodox®
A/T/S®	Combipres®	Diucardin®	Garamycin®	Lindane®	Mono-Gesic®
Augmentin®	Combivir®	Diuril®	Glucophage®	Lioresal®	Monopril®
Avalide®	Compazine®	Dolobid®	Glyset®	Lithium	Morphine
AVC®	Cordarone®	Dolophine®	Guaifed®	Lithobid®	MS Contin®
Axid®	Corgard®	Doral®	Halcion®	Lo/Ovral®	MSIR®
Axocet®	Cortisporin®	Doryx®	Haldol®	Loestrin®	Myambutol®
Azactam®	Cortone®	Droxia®	Helidac®	Lomotil®	Mykrox®
Azathioprine	Corzide®	Duraclon®	Hydrocet®	Loniten®	Mysoline®
Azulfidine®	Cosopt®	Duragesic®	Hydrocortone®	Lopressor®	Naprelan®
Bactrim®	Coumadin®	Duramorph®	HydroDIURIL®	Lortab®	Naprosyn®
Benadryl®	Covera-HS®	Duratuss®	Iberet-Folic®	Lotensin®	Nascobal®
Bentyl®	Crinone®	Duricef®	Ifex®	Lotrel®	Necon®
Betapace®	Cyclessa®	Dyazide®	Imitrex®	Ludiomil®	NegGram®
Bicillin®	Cystospaz®	Dyrenium®	Imuran®	Lufyllin®	Nembutal®
Blocadren®	Cytomel®	E.E.S.®	Inderal®	Lufyllin-GG®	Neoral®
Brethine®	Cytotec®	EC-Naprosyn®	Inderide®	Luminal®	Netromycin®

Appendix 6

Drugs Excreted in Breast Milk (continued)

Niaspan®
Nicotrol®
Nizoral®
Norco®
Nor-QD®
Nordette®
Norinyl®
Noritate®
Normodyne®
Norpace®
Norplant®
Novantrone®
Nubain®
Nucofed®
Nydrazid®
Oramorph®
Oretic®
Ortho-Cept®
Ortho-Cyclen®
Ortho-Novum®
Ortho Tri-Cyclen®
Orudis®
Ovcon®
Ovral®
Ovrette®
Oxistat®
OxyContin®
OxyFast®
OxyIR®
Pacerone®
Pamelor®
Pancrease®
Panlor SS®

Paxil®
PCE®
Pediapred®
Pediazole®
Pediotic®
Pentasa®
Pepcid®
Periostat®
Persantine®
Pfizerpen®
Phenergan®
Phenobarbital
Phrenilin®
Pipracil®
Plan B®
Platinol-AQ®
Ponstel®
Pravachol®
Premphase®
Prempro®
Prevacid®
Preven®
PREVPAC®
Prinzide®
Procanbid®
Prograf®
Proloprim®
Prometrium®
Pronestyl®
Propofol®
Prosed/DS®
Provera®
Prozac®

Pseudoephedrine
Pulmicort®
Pyrazinamide®
Quibron®
Quibron-T®
Quinaglute®
Quinidex®
Quinine
Reglan®
Renese®
Requip®
Reserpine
Restoril®
Retrovir®
Ridaura®
Rifadin®
Rifamate®
Rifater®
Rimactane®
RMS®
Robaxisal®
Rocaltrol®
Rocephin®
Roferon A®
Roxanol®
Salflex®
Sandimmune®
Sansert®
Sarafem®
Seconal®
Sectral®
Sedapap®
Semprex-D®

Septra®
Sinequan®
Slo-bid®
Solganal®
Soma®
Sonata®
Sporanox®
Stadol®
Stelazine®
Streptomycin
Stromectol®
Symmetrel®
Syn-Rx®
Synthroid®
Tagamet®
Tambocor®
Tapazole®
Tarka®
Tavist®
Tazicef®
Tazidime®
Tegretol®
Tenoretic®
Tenormin®
Tenuate®
Testoderm®
Thalitone®
Theo-24®
Theo-Dur®
Theo-X®
Thorazine®
Tiazac®
Timolide®

Timoptic®
Tobi®
Tofranil®
Tolectin®
Tol-Tab®
Toprol-XL®
Toradol®
Trandate®
Tranxene®
Trental®
Trilafon®
Trileptal®
Tri-Levlen®
Trilisate®
Tri-Norinyl®
Triostat®
Triphasil®
Trivora®
Trizivir®
Trovan®
Tylenol®
Tylenol with Codeine®
Ultram®
Unasyn®
Uni-Dur®
Uniphyl®
Uniretic®
Unithroid®
Urimax®
Uroqid-Acid®
Valium®
Valtrex®
Vanceril®

Vancocin®
Vantin®
Vascor®
Vaseretic®
Vasotec®
Verelan®
Vermox®
Versed®
Vibramycin®
Vibra-Tabs®
Vicodin®
Viramune®
Visken®
Voltaren®
Wellbutrin®
Xanax®
Zagam®
Zantac®
Zarontin®
Zaroxolyn®
Zestoretic®
Ziac®
Zinacef®
Zithromax®
Zoloft®
Zonalon®
Zonegran®
Zosyn®
Zovia®
Zovirax®
Zyban®
Zydone®
Zyloprim®
Zyrtec®

With permisison from Sifton DW, ed. *2002 Drug Topics Red Book.* Montvale, NJ: Thomson Medical Economics; 2002.

Appendix 7

Drugs That May Cause Photosensitivity

The drugs in this table are known to cause photosensitivity in some individuals. Effects can range from itching, scaling, rash, and swelling to skin cancer, premature skin aging, skin and eye burns, cataracts, reduced immunity, blood vessel damage, and allergic reactions. The list is not all-inclusive, and shows only representative brands of each generic. When in doubt, always check specific product labeling. Individuals should be advised to wear protective clothing and to apply sunscreens while taking the medications listed below.

Generic	Brand	Generic	Brand	Generic	Brand
Acetazolamide	Diamox®	Carbamazepine	Carbatrol®, Tegretol,® Tegretol-XR®	Doxycycline monohydrate	Monodox®
Acitretin	Soriatane®				
Alatrofloxacin	Trovan I.V.®	Carbinoxamine/ pseudoephedrine	Palgic-D®, Palgic-DS,® Pediatex-D®	Enalapril	Vasotec®
Alendronate	Fosamax®			Enalapril/felodipine	Lexxel®
Alitretinoin	Panretin®	Carvedilol	Coreg®	Enalapril/ hydrochlorothiazide	Vaseretic®
Almotriptan	Axert®	Celecoxib	Celebrex®		
Amiloride/ hydrochlorothiazide	Moduretic®	Cetirizine	Zyrtec®	Enalaprilat	Vasotec I.V.®
		Cetirizine/ pseudoephedrine	Zyrtec-D®	Enoxacin	Penetrex®
Aminolevulinic acid	Levulan Kerastick®			Epirubicin	Ellence®
Amiodarone	Cordarone®, Pacerone®	Cevimeline	Evoxac®	Erythromycin/ sulfisoxazole	Pediazole®
Amitriptyline	Elavil®	Chlorhexidine gluconate	Hibistat®		
Amitriptyline/ chlordiazepoxide	Limbitrol®			Estazolam	ProSom®
		Chlorothiazide	Diuril®	Estradiol	Gynodiol®
Amitriptyline/ perphenazine	Etrafon®, Etrafon-Forte®, Triavil®	Chlorpheniramine/ hydrocodone/ pseudoephedrine	Tussend®	Ethionamide	Trecator-SC®
				Etodolac	Lodine®
Amoxapine				Felbamate	Felbatol®
Anagrelide	Agrylin®	Chlorpheniramine/ phenylephrine/pyrilamine	Rynatan®	Fenofibrate	Tricor®
Atenolol/ chlorthalidone	Tenoretic®			Floxuridine	Sterile FUDR®
		Chlorpromazine	Thorazine®	Flucytosine	Ancobon®
Atorvastatin	Lipitor®	Chlorpropamide	Diabinese®	Fluorouracil	Efudex®
Aurothioglucose	Solganal®	Chlorthalidone	Thalitone®	Fluoxetine	Prozac®, Sarafem®
Azatadine/ pseudoephedrine	Rynatan®, Trinalin®	Chlorthalidone/ clonidine	Combipres®, Clorpres®	Fluphenazine	Prolixin®
				Flutamide	Eulexin®
Azithromycin	Zithromax®	Cidofovir	Vistide®	Fluvastatin	Lescol®
Benazepril	Lotensin®	Ciprofloxacin	Cipro®	Fluvoxamine	Luvox®
Benazepril/ hydrochlorothiazide	Lotensin HCT®	Citalopram	Celexa®	Fosinopril	Monopril®
		Clemastine	Tavist®	Fosphenytoin	Cerebyx®
Bendroflumethiazide/ nadolol	Corzide®	Clozapine	Clozaril®	Furosemide	Lasix®
		Cromolyn sodium	Gastrocrom®	Gabapentin	Neurontin®
Bexarotene	Targretin®	Cyclobenzaprine	Flexeril®	Gatifloxacin	Tequin®
Bismuth/ metronidazole/ tetracycline	Helidac®	Cyproheptadine	Periactin®	Gemfibrozil	Lopid®
		Dacarbazine	DTIC-Dome®	Gentamicin	Garamycin®
		Dantrolene	Dantrium®	Glatiramer	Copaxone®
Bisoprolol/ hydrochlorothiazide	Ziac®	Demeclocycline	Declomycin®	Glimepiride	Amaryl®
		Desipramine	Norpramin®	Glipizide	Glucotrol®
Brompheniramine/ dextromethorphan/ phenylephrine	Alacol DM®	Diclofenac potassium	Cataflam®	Glyburide	DiaBeta®, Glynase®, Micronase®
		Diclofenac sodium	Voltaren®		
		Diclofenac sodium/ misoprostol	Arthrotec®	Glyburide/ metformin HCl	Glucovance®
Brompheniramine/ dextromethorphan/ pseudoephedrine	Bromfed-DM®				
		Diflunisal	Dolobid®	Griseofulvin	Fulvicin P/G®, Grifulvin®, Gris-PEG®
		Dihydroergotamine	D.H.E. 45®		
Bupropion	Wellbutrin®, Zyban®	Diltiazem	Cardizem®, Tiazac®	Haloperidol	Haldol®
Candesartan/ hydrochlorothiazide	Atacand HCT®	Diphenhydramine	Benadryl®	Hexachlorophene	pHisoHex®
		Divalproex	Depakote®	Hydralazine/ hydrochlorothiazide	Apresazide®
Capecitabine	Xeloda®	Doxepin	Sinequan®		
Captopril	Capoten®	Doxycycline hyclate	Doryx®, Periostat®, Vibra-Tabs®, Vibramycin®	Hydrochlorothiazide	HydroDIURIL®, Hyzaar®, Microzide®, Oretic®
Captopril/ hydrochlorothiazide	Capozide®				

Drugs That May Cause Photosensitivity (continued)

Generic	Brand	Generic	Brand	Generic	Brand
Hydrochlorothiazide/ fosinopril	Monopril HCT®	Losartan	Cozaar®	Pyrazinamide	Pyrazinamide®
		Lovastatin	Mevacor®	Quetiapine	Seroquel®
Hydrochlorothiazide/ irbesartan	Avalide®	Lovastatin/niacin	Advicor®	Quinapril	Accupril®
		Maprotiline	Ludiomil®	Quinidine gluconate	Quinaglute®, Quinidine®
Hydrochlorothiazide/ lisinopril	Prinzide®, Zestoretic®	Mefenamic acid	Ponstel®	Quinidine sulfate	Quinidex®
		Meloxicam	Mobic®	Rabeprazole sodium	Aciphex®
Hydrochlorothiazide/ losartan potassium	Hyzaar®	Meperidine/ promethazine	Mepergan®	Ramipril	Altace®
				Riluzole	Rilutek®
Hydrochlorothiazide/ methyldopa	Aldoril®	Mesalamine	Pentasa®	Risperidone	Risperdal®
		Methazolamide	Neptazane®	Ritonavir	Norvir®
Hydrochlorothiazide/ moexipril	Uniretic®	Methotrexate	Trexall®	Rizatriptan	Maxalt®
		Methoxsalen	Uvadex®, Oxsoralen®	Ropinirole	Requip®
Hydrochlorothiazide/ propranolol	Inderide®	Methyclothiazide	Enduron®	Ruta graveolens	Rue®
		Metolazone	Mykrox®, Zaroxolyn®	Saquinavir	Fortovase®
Hydrochlorothiazide/ quinapril	Accuretic®	Minocycline	Dynacin®, Minocin®	Saquinavir mesylate	Invirase®
		Mirtazapine	Remeron®	Selegiline	Eldepryl®
Hydrochlorothiazide/ spironolactone	Aldactazide®	Moexipril	Univasc®	Sertraline	Zoloft®
		Moxifloxacin	Avelox®	Sibutramine	Meridia®
Hydrochlorothiazide/ telmisartan	Micardis HCT®	Nabumetone	Relafen®	Sildenafil	Viagra®
		Nalidixic acid	NegGram®	Simvastatin	Zocor®
Hydrochlorothiazide/ timolol	Timolide®	Naproxen	Naprosyn®, EC-Naprosyn®	Somatropin	Serostim®
				Sotalol	Betapace®, Betapace AF®
Hydrochlorothiazide/ triamterene	Dyazide®, Maxzide®	Naproxen sodium	Anaprox®, Naprelan®		
		Naratriptan	Amerge®	Sparfloxacin	Zagam®
Hydrochlorothiazide/ valsartan	Diovan HCT®	Nefazodone	Serzone®	Sulfamethoxazole/ trimethoprim	Bactrim®, Septra®
		Nifedipine	Procardia®		
Hydroflumethiazide	Diucardin®	Nisoldipine	Sular®	Sulfasalazine	Azulfidine®
Hydroxychloroquine	Plaquenil®	Norfloxacin	Noroxin®	Sulfisoxazole	Gantrisin Pediatric®
Hypericum	Kira®, St. John's wort	Nortriptyline	Pamelor®	Sulindac	Clinoril®
Hypericum/ vitamin B₁/ vitamin C/kava-kava	One-A-Day Tension & Mood®	Ofloxacin	Floxin®	Sumatriptan	Imitrex®
		Olanzapine	Zyprexa®	Tacrolimus	Prograf®, Protopic®
		Olsalazine	Dipentum®	Tazarotene	Tazorac®
Ibuprofen	Motrin®	Oxaprozin	Daypro®	Tetracycline	Achromycin®
Imipramine	Tofranil®	Oxcarbazepine	Trileptal®	Thalidomide	Thalomid®
Indapamide	Lozol®	Oxycodone	Roxicodone®	Thioridazine hydrochloride	Mellaril®
Interferon alfa-2b, recombinant	Intron A®	Oxytetracycline	Terramycin®		
		Pantoprazole	Protonix®	Thiothixene	Navane®
Interferon alfa-n3 (human leukocyte derived)	Alferon-N®	Paroxetine	Paxil®	Tiagabine	Gabitril®
		Pastinaca sativa	Parsnip®	Topiramate	Topamax®
Interferon beta-1a	Avonex®	Pentosan polysulfate	Elmiron®	Triamcinolone	Azmacort®
Interferon beta-1b	Betaseron®	Pentostatin	Nipent®	Triamterene	Dyrenium®
Irbesartan/ hydrochlorothiazide	Avalide®	Perphenazine	Trilafon®	Trifluoperazine	Stelazine®
		Phenazopyridine/ sulfamethizole	Urobiotic-250®	Trimipramine	Surmontil®
Isoniazid/ pyrazinamide/ rifampin	Rifater®			Trovafloxacin	Trovan Tablets®
		Pilocarpine	Salagen®	Valacyclovir	Valtrex®
		Pimpinella major	Burnet®	Valdecoxib	Bextra®
Ketoprofen	Orudis®, Oruvail®	Piroxicam	Feldene®	Valproate	Depacon®
Lamotrigine	Lamictal®	Polythiazide	Renese®	Valproic acid	Depakene®
Leuprolide	Lupron®	Polythiazide/prazosin	Minizide®	Venlafaxine	Effexor®
Levamisole	Ergamisol®	Porfimer sodium	Photofrin®	Verteporfin	Visudyne®
Lisinopril	Prinivil®, Zestril®	Pravastatin	Pravachol®	Vinblastine	
Lomefloxacin	Maxaquin®	Prochlorperazine	Compazine®, Compro®	Zalcitabine	Hivid®
Loratadine	Claritin®	Promethazine	Phenergan®	Zaleplon	Sonata®
Loratadine/ pseudoephedrine	Claritin-D®	Protriptyline	Vivactil®	Ziprasidone	Geodon®
				Zolmitriptan	Zomig®
				Zolpidem	Ambien®

Appendix 8

Drug Information Resources by Category

Adverse drug reactions/side effects

AHFS Drug Information
Drug Facts & Comparisons
Drug Information Handbook
Martindale: The Complete Drug Reference
Meyler's Side Effects of Drugs
Micromedex DRUGDEX
Physician's Desk Reference
Side Effects of Drugs Annual
Textbook of Adverse Drug Reactions
EMBASE
International Pharmaceutical Abstracts
Medline
TOXLINE (NLM Database)
ClinAlert (www.nlm.nih.gov/databases/
    alerts/clinical_alerts.html)
FDA Medwatch Program
    (http://www.fda.gov/medwatch/safety.htm)
Institute for Safe Medication Practices
    (http://www.ismp.org/)
Vaccine Adverse Event Reporting System
    (http://www.vaers.org/)

Alternative medicine/herbals/natural
    products

Herbs of Choice
Honest Herbal
Natural Medicines Comprehensive Database
PDR for Nonprescription Drugs and Dietary
    Supplements
Review of Natural Products
The Complete German Commission E
    Monographs
FDA CFSAN Dietary Supplements
    (http://vm.cfsan.fda.gov)
National Center for Alternative and
    Complimentary Medicine
    (http://nccam.nih.gov)
NIH Office of Dietary Supplements
    (http://dietary-supplements.info.nih.gov)

Drug dosing in renal dysfunction

AHFS Drug Information
Drug Facts & Comparisons
Drug Information Handbook
Drug Prescribing in Renal Failure
Handbook of Dialysis
Physician's Desk Reference
Sanford Guide to Antimicrobial Therapy
    (Antimicrobials Only)

EMBASE
International Pharmaceutical Abstracts
Medline
Global Pharmacist Renal Dosing
    (http://www.globalrph.com/renaldosing.htm &
    http://www.globalrph.com/crcl.htm)
John Hopkins Aids Service
    (http://www.hopkins-aids.edu/publications/
    book/ch4_agents_tab0428.html#tab0428)
Nephrology Pharmacy Associates (http://www.
    nephrologypharmacy.com/pub_dialysis.html)
University of Louisville, Kidney Disease
    Program (http://www.kdp-baptist.
    louisville.edu/renalfailure/)

Drug interactions

AHFS Drug Information
Drug Facts & Comparisons
Drug Interaction Facts
Drug Therapy Screening System (DTSS)
Evaluation of Drug Interactions
Hansten & Horn's Analysis and Management
    of Drug Interactions
Micromedex DRUG-REAX
EMBASE
International Pharmaceutical Abstracts
Medline
Drug Store (http://www.drugstore.com/
    pharmacy/drugchecker/)
Facts & Comparisons (www.
    factsandcomparisons.com/NewsArticle.asp?
    ID=91)
Liverpool Pharmacology HIV group (http://
    www.hiv-druginteractions.org/)
University of Indiana (http://medicine.
    iupui.edu/flockhart/)

Drug therapy/therapeutics

Applied Therapeutics: The Clinical Use of
    Drugs
Cecil Textbook of Medicine
Harrison's Principles of Internal Medicine
Medical Letter
Pharmacist's Letter
Pharmacotherapy: A Pathophysiologic
    Approach
Textbook of Therapeutics: Drug and Disease
    Management
Washington Manual of Medical Therapeutics
EMBASE

International Pharmaceutical Abstracts (IPA)
Medline
Global Pharmacist (http://www.globalrph.com)
Merck Manual Diagnosis and Therapy Text
    (http://www.merck.com/pubs/mmanual_ho
    me/contents.htm)
Mdchoice (http://www.mdchoice.
    com/calculators.asp)
Excipient/Inactive Ingredient Information
Drug Manufacturer/Company
Handbook of Pharmaceutical Additives
Micromedex POISINDEX
Physician's Desk Reference/ Package
    Insert/Product Label

Legal and regulatory

Guide to Federal Pharmacy Law
Pharmacy Law Digest
USPDI Volume III: Approved Drugs and Legal
    Requirements
USP/NF
Code of Federal Regulations (Title 21)
    (www.gpo.gov)
FDA website (www.fda.gov)
Joint Commission on Accreditation of
    Healthcare Organizations
    (www.jcaho.org)
National Association of Boards of Pharmacy
    (http://www.nabp.net)
US Drug Enforcement Administration
    (http://www.usdoj.gov/dea/)
World Health Organization
    (http://www.who.int/en/)

Monographs/medication use evaluation
    (MUE, DUE)

AHFS Drug Information
Drug Usage Evaluations (ASHP)
Formulary Monograph Service (F & C)
International Pharmaceutical Abstracts (IPA)
ASHP Practices (http://www.ashp.org/
    bestpractices/index.cfm
The FIX System (www.theformulary.com)

News/new drug approvals

FAXStat
Medical Letter
Pharmacist's Letter
The Pink Sheet
CenterWatch (http://www.centerwatch.
    com/patient/drugs/druglist.html)

Appendix 8

Drug Information Resources by Category (continued)

FDA Website (http://www.fda.gov/cder/
approval/index.htm)
Lexi-Comp (http://www.lexi.com/web/
newdrugs.jsp)
Reuters News Service (www.reutershealth.
com)

Nonprescription drugs/ OTC information
American Drug Index
Drug Facts & Comparisons
Drug Topics Redbook
Handbook of Nonprescription Drugs
Micromedex DRUGDEX, POISINDEX
PDR for Nonprescription Drugs and Dietary
Supplements
DrugStore.com (www.drugstore.com)
PlanetRx (www.planetrx.com)

**Off-label/unlabeled/non-FDA approved
uses**
AHFS Drug Information
Drug Fact and Comparisons
Martindale
Micromedex DRUGDEX
Mosby's GenRX
USPDI Volume I
EMBASE
International Pharmaceutical Abstracts
Medline

Patient counseling/education
AHFS Drug Information
Drug Facts and Comparisons
Handbook of Nonprescription Drugs
Medication Teaching Manual (ASHP)
Micromedex DRUGDEX
Patient counseling handbook
Patient Drug Facts
USPDI Volume II: Advice for the Patient

Pediatric dosing and therapeutics
AHFS Drug Information
Drug Facts & Comparisons
Harriet Lane Handbook
Micromedex DRUGDEX
Nelson Textbook of Pediatrics
Neofax 2000
Pediatric Dosage Handbook
Physician's Desk Reference
Principles and Practice of Pediatrics

EMBASE
International Pharmaceutical Abstracts
Medline

**Pharmaceutics/compounding/
manufacturing**
Allen's Compounded Formulations
Extemporaneous Ophthalmic Preparations
Handbook on Extemporaneous Formulations
International Journal of Pharmaceutical
Compounding
Stability of Compounded Formulations
US Pharmacist Contemporary Compounding
Compendium
EMBASE
International Pharmaceutical Abstracts
Medline
Center for Drug Evaluation and Research
(http://www.fda.gov/cder/pharmcomp/)
International Journal of Pharmaceutical
Compounding (www.ijpc.com)

Pharmacokinetics
AHFS Drug Information
Applied Pharmacokinetics
Basic Clinical Pharmacokinetics
Clinical Pharmacokinetics
Drug Facts & Comparisons
Martindale
Micromedex DRUGDEX
Physician's Desk Reference
Principles of Therapeutic Drug Monitoring
USPDI Volume 1
EMBASE
International Pharmaceutical Abstracts
Medline

Foreign drug identification
Drugs Available Abroad
Drug Facts & Comparisons (Canadian Trade
Name Index)
European Drug Index
Martindale
Merck Index
Mexican PDR
Micromedex Index Nominum
Mosby's GenRX (International Drug Name
Index)
The British Pharmacopoeia
USP Dictionary

World Pharmaceuticals Directory
EMBASE
International Pharmaceutical Abstracts
Medline
British National Formulary
(http://bnf.vhn.net/home/)
Electronics Medicines Compendium
(http://emc.vhn.net/)
Royal Pharmaceutical Society of Great
Britain http://www.pharmj.com/
noticeboard/info/pip/foreignmedicines.
html

**General drug information resources
(compendia)**
AHFS Drug Information
Drug Facts & Comparisons
Martindale's
Micromedex DRUGDEX
Mosby's GenRX
Physician's Desk Reference
USPDI Volume I: Drug Information for
Health Care Provider

Geriatrics
AHFS Drug Information
Consultant Pharmacist Journal
Drug Facts & Comparisons
Drug Therapy and the Elderly
Geriatric Dosage Handbook
Geriatric Pharmacology
Micromedex DRUGDEX
Physician's Desk Reference
Therapeutics in the Elderly
USPDI Volume I
EMBASE
International Pharmaceutical Abstracts
Medline
American Society of Consultant
Pharmacists (http://www.ascp.com/)
Geriatrics and Aging (http://www.
geriatricsandaging.com/ga_links.htm)

Immunology/biotechnology/vaccines
Concepts in Immunology and
Immunotherapeutics
ImmunoFacts
Center for Disease Control (CDC) website
(www.cdc.gov/nip)

(continued)

Appendix 8

Drug Information Resources by Category (continued)

Immunize Action Coalition (http://www.
immunize.org/)

US Health and Human Services
(http://www.hrsa.gov/osp/vicp/)

Vaccine Adverse Event Reporting System
(http://www.vaers.org/)

Intravenous stability/compatibility

AHFS Drug Information

Guide to Parenteral Admixtures

Handbook on Injectable Drugs

Micromedex DRUGDEX

Trissel's Tables of Physical Compatibility

EMBASE

International Pharmaceutical Abstracts

Medline

Handbook of Parenteral Drug Administration
(http://members.ozemail.com.au/~jamesbc/
frames.htm)

Investigational drug identification

Drug Facts & Comparisons

Index Nominum

Martindale

Merck Index

Micromedex DRUGDEX, POISINDEX

NDA Pipeline

Unlisted Drugs

World Pharmaceuticals Directory

EMBASE

International Pharmaceutical Abstracts

Medline

Aids Clinical Trials (http://www.actis.org/)

CenterWatch (http://www.centerwatch.
com/patient/trials.html)

NIH Clinical Trials Database (www.
clinicaltrials.gov)

Pharmaceutical Research and Manufacturers
of America (http://www.newmedicines.org/)

Reuters News Service
(www.reutershealth.com)

Laboratory Tests and Microbiology

Basic Skills in Interpreting Laboratory Data

Clinical Guide to Laboratory Tests

Laboratory Tests and Diagnostic Procedures

Laboratory Test Handbook

Pregnancy and lactation information

Breastfeeding: A Guide for the Medical
Profession

Drugs in Pregnancy and Lactation

Micromedex REPRORISK

Focus Information Technology (http://www.
perinatology.com/exposures/druglist.htm)

Safety of Drugs in Pregnancy and Lactation
(http://www.accp.com/pod/p3b11pre01.pdf)

UK's Drugs in Lactation Advisory Service
(http://www.ukmicentral.nhs.uk/drugpreg/
guide.htm)

Pharmacology

AHFS Drug Information

Basic Concepts & Clinical Applications

Clinical Pharmacology

Drug Facts & Comparisons

Goodman & Gilman's Pharmacological Basic
of Therapeutics

Principles of Pharmacology

Textbook of Pharmacology

Phone numbers and addresses

American Drug Index

Drug Facts & Comparisons

Drug Topics Redbook

Martindale

Micromedex DRUGDEX, POISINDEX

Mosby's GenRX

NDA Pipeline

PDR

Manufacturer websites (various)

Chemical/physical properties

CRC Handbook of Chemistry and Physics

Merck Index

Textbook of Organic, Medicinal, and
Pharmaceutical Chemistry

USP-Dictionary

USP/NF

Product availability/shortages

American Drug Index

Drug Topics Red Book

Handbook of Nonprescription Drugs

ASHP Drug Shortage Center (http://www.
ashp.org/shortage/)

Drug Wholesaler websites (various)

FDA Drug Shortage site (http://www.fda.gov/
cder/drug/shortages/default.htm)

Product identification

American Drug Index

AHFS Drug Information

Diccionario de Especialidades Farmaceuticas

Drug Facts & Comparisons

Drug Topics Redbook

Drugs Available Abroad

European Drug Index

Index Nominum

Martindale

Merck Index

Micromedex POISINDEX

NDA Pipeline

Pharmacist's Letter

Unlisted Drugs

USP Dictionary

World Pharmaceuticals Directory

EMBASE

International Pharmaceutical Abstracts

Medline

FDA website (www.fda.gov)

Internet (various search engines, websites)

Reuters News Service (www.
reutershealth.com)

Tablet/capsule identification

Drug Facts & Comparisons

Ident-A-Drug

Micromedex IDENTIDEX

Mosby's GenRX

Physician's Desk Reference (PDR)

RX-List website (www.rxlist.com)

Toxicology/poisoning

Clinical Management of Poisoning and Drug
Overdose

Clinical Toxicology of Drugs

Handbook of Poisoning

Micromedex DRUGDEX, POISINDEX

Poisoning and Toxicology Compendium

Principles of Clinical Toxicology

Toxicologic Emergencies

EMBASE

International Pharmaceutical Abstracts

Medline

ToxNet

American Association of Poison Control
Centers (http://www.aapcc.org/)

Environmental Protection Agency
(http://www.epa.gov/iris/)

Merck Manual (http://www.merck.com/
pubs/mmanual/section23/chapter307/307a.
htm)

Oxford University
(http://physchem.ox.ac.uk/MSDS/)

Appendix 9

Drugs That Should Not Be Crushed

The following is a list of medications that should not be crushed due to poor taste, irritant properties, carcinogenicity, or an alteration of pharmacokinetics, as in the case of enteric coated and sustained release products.

Abletex PSE®	Ascriptin A/®D	Carbatrol®	Covera-HS®	Docusate	Efidac/24
Accuhist LA®	Ascriptin Extra	Carbiset-TR®	Creon 5, 10, 20, 25®	Dolobid®	Pseudo-
Accutane®	Strength®	Cardene SR®	Cystospaz-M®	Donnatal Extentab®	ephedrine®
Aciphex®	ATP®	Cardizem®	Cytovene®	Donnazyme®	Efidac/24
Actifed 12 hour®	Atrohist LA®	Cardizem CD®	Cytoxan®	Doryx®	Chlorphenir-
Acutrim®	Atrohist Pediatric®	Cardizem SR®	C-Tym®	Doxidan Liquigels®	amine®
Adalat CC®	Atrohist Plus®	Carox®	D.A. II®	Drexophed SR®	Empro®
Adderall XR®	Atromid-S®	Carter's Little Pills®	Dairycare®	Drisdol®	E-Mycin®
Advicor®	Avinza®	Cartia XT®	Dallergy®	Dristan 12 Hour®	Endafed®
Aerolate SR, JR, III®	Azo Gantrisin®	Catemine®	Dallergy-D, JR®	Drituss GP®	Endal®
Afrinol Repetabs®	Azulfidine EN-tabs®	Ceclor CD®	D-Amine SR®	Drixomed®	Entercort EC®
Aggrenox®	Baros®	Ceftin®	Deconamine SR®	Drixoral®	Entox LA®
Aleve Cold & Sinus®	Bayer Enteric-	CellCept®	Decongest II®	Drixoral Plus, Sinus®	Entex PSE®
Aleve Sinus &	Coated®	Cemill 500, 1000®	Decongestine®	Drize-R®	Entocort EC®
Headache®	Bayer Low Adult	Cerespan®	Deconhist LA®	Drysec®	Entozyme®
Allegra-D®	81 mg®	Cevi-Bid®	Deconomed SR®	Duagen®	Equanil®
Allerest 12 hour®	Bayer Regular	Charcoal Plus®	Deconsal II, Sprinkle®	Dulcolax®	Ergomar®
Allerx®	Strength®	Chlorphedrine SR®	Defen-LA®	Duotrate®	Ergostat®
Allerx-D®	Bellergal-S®	Chlorpheniramine	Demazin Repetab®	Duradryl JR®	Eryc®
Allfen®	Betachron ER®	Chlor-Phen®	Depakene®	Duralex®	Ery-Tab®
Allfen-DM®	Betapen-VK®	Chloral hydrate	Depakote®	Duraquin®	Erythrocin
Alophen®	Biaxin-XL®	Chlor-Trimeton®	Depakote ER,	Durasal II®	Stearate®
Alterra®	Bidex®	Chlor-Trimeton	Sprinkles®	Dura-Tap PD®	Erythromycin
Amibid DM®	Bidex-DM®	Repetab®	Desal II®	Duratuss®	base
Amibid LA®	Biltricide®	Choledyl SA®	Desoxyn Gradumets®	Duratuss G, GP®	Eskalith CR®
Amidal®	Biohist LA®	Chloral hydrate	Desyrel®	Dura-Vent A®	Eudal SR®
Aminoxin®	Bisac-Evac®	Chromagen®	Despec SR®	Dura Vent/DA®	Exgest LA®
Ami-Tex PSE®	Bisacodyl®	Cipro®	Detrol LA®	Dylaxol®	Extendryl JR,
Ammonium Chloride	Biscolax®	Claritin-D®	Dexaphen SA®	Dynabac®	SR®
ER	Boca-Tex PSE®	Claritin-D 24 Hour®	Dexatrim Extended	Dynabac D5-Pak®	Extress-60®
Anatuss LA®	Bontril SR®	Cleocin®	Duration®	DynaCirc CR®	Fe 50®
Ansaid®	Breonesin®	Codimal-LA®	Dexadrine Spansule®	Dynahist-ER Pediatric®	Fedahist
Aquatuss LA®	Brexin LA®	Codimal-LA Half®	D-Feda II®	Dynex®	Gyrocaps®
Aquabid DM®	Bromadrine TR®	Colace®	Diamox Sequels®	Easprin®	Fedahist
Aquatab C, D, DM®	Bromfed®	Coldec TR®	Dilacor XR®	EC-Naprosyn®	Timecaps®
Aquatab D	Bromfed-PD®	Colestid®	Dilantin Kapseals®	Ecotrin Adult Low	Feen-A-Mint®
Dosepack®	Bromfenex®	Comhist LA®	Dilatrate-SR®	Strength®	Feldene®
Artane Sequels®	Bromfenex PD®	Compazine Spansule®	Diltia XT®	Ecotrin Maximum	Femilax®
Arthritis Bayer Time	Bromphen TD®	Concerta®	Dimetane Extentabs®	Strength®	Femitrol®
Release®	Bronkodyl SR®	Condrin-LA®	Dimetapp Extentabs®	Ecotrin Regular	Fenesin®
Arthrotec®	300 mg	Congress SR, JR®	Disobrom®	Strength®	Fenesin DM®
Asaco®l	Bufferin Low Dose®	Contac 12-Hour®	Disophrol Chronotab®	Ecpirin®	Feocyte®
ASA Enseals®	Caffedrine®	Contac Maximum	Dital®	Ed A-Hist®	Feosol®
Ascocid-1000,	Calan SR®	Strength®	Ditropan XL®	Ed K + 10®	Feosol
500-D®	CAMA Arthritis Pain	Correctol®	Docusate with	E.E.S. 400®	Spansule®
Ascorbic acid	Reliever®	Cotazym-S®	Casanthrol®	Effexor XR®	Feratab®

(continued)

Appendix 9

Drugs That Should Not Be Crushed (continued)

Fergon®
Fero-Folic 500®
Fero-Grad 500®
Ferospace®
Ferralet SR®
Ferro-Sequels®
Ferro-Time®
Ferrous fumarate DS
Ferrous gluconate
Ferrous sulfate
Festal II®
Fetrin®
Feverall Sprinkle®
Filtuss TR®
Fiogesic®
Flagyl ER®
Fleet Bisacodyl®
Flomax®
Folitab 500®
Fumatinic®
Gastrocrom®
Gaviscon®
Genacote®
Geocillin®
GFN/PSE®
Glucophage XR®
Glucotrol XL®
GP 500®
G-Phed®
G-Phed PD®
Gris-PEG®
Guaifed®
Guaifed-PD®
Guaifenex DM, G,
    GP, LA, PSE, Rx,
    Rx DM®
Guaimax-D®
Guaipax PSE®
Guai-Vent PSE®
Gua-SR®
Guiadrine DM,
    G-1200, GP,
    PSE®
Guiatex II SR, PSE®
Halfprin®
Histade®
Hista-Vent DA®
Histex CT, SR®
Humavent LA®

Humibid DM, LA®
Humibid DM
    Sprinkle®
Humibid Pediatric®
Humibid Sprinkle®
Hydergine LC,
    Sublingual®
Hytakerol®
Iberet®
Iberet 500®
Iberet-Folic 500®
ICaps Plus®
ICaps Time
    Release®
Ilotycin®
Imdur®
Inderal LA®
Inderide LA®
Indocin SR®
Iobid DM®
Iofed®
Iofed PD®
Ionamin®
Iosal II®
Iotex PSE®
Isoclor Timesule®
Isoptin SR®
Isordil Sublingual,
    Chewable®
Isordil Tembid®
Isosorbide Dinitrate
    Sublingual®
Isosorbide SR®
K + 8®
K + 10®
Kadian®
Kaon Cl 10®
K + Care®
K-Dur 10, 20®
K-Lease®
Klor-Con 8, 10,
    M1®
Klorvess®
Klotrix®
K-Lyte®
K-Lyte CL®
K-Lyte DS®
K-Norm®
Kronofed A, A-JR®

K-Tab®
Lescol XL®
Levbid®
Levsinex Timecaps®
Lexxel®
Lipram 4500, CR10,
    CR20, PN10, PN15,
    PN20, UL12, UL18,
    UL20®
Liquibid®
Liquibid 1200, D®
Lithobid®
Lodine-XL®
Lodrane LD, 12 Hour®
Losec®
Macrobid®
Mag Delay®
Mag SR®
Mag-Tab SR®
Maxifed®
Maxifed DM, G®
Maxovite®
Medent DM, LD®
Med Rx®
Med Rx DM®
Mega C®
Melfiat®
Meprospan®
Mescolor®
Mestinon Timespan®
Metadate CD, ER®
Methylin ER®
Mi-Cebrin®
Mi-Cebrin T®
Micro K®
Miraphen PSE®
Modane®
Monafed®
Monafed DM®
Motrin®
MS Contin®
Muco-Fen-DM®
Muco-Fen-LA, 1200®
Multi-Ferrous Folic®
Multiret Folic 500®
Naldecon®
Nalex A®
Naprelan®
Nasabid SR®

Nasahist Capsules®
Nasatab LA®
Nd Clear®
Nexium®
Nia-Bid®
Niacin time release
Niaspan®
Nicotinic acid
Nifedical XL®
Nitrocine Timecaps®
Nitrocot®
Nitrogard®
Nitroglycerin
Nitroglyn®
Nitrong®
Nitrostat®
Nitro-Time®
Noctec®
Nolamine®
Nolex LA®
Norflex®
Norpace CR®
Novafed®
Novafed A®
Omeprazole
Omnihist LA®
Ondrox®
Optilets 500®
Optilets-M 500®
Ordrine AT ER, SR®
Oragrafin®
Oramorph SR®
Ornade Spansule®
Oruvail®
OxyContin®
Pabalate®
Pabalate SF®
Palgic D®
Palipase MT 16, MT
    20®
Palipeon DR 10, DR
    20®
Paltrase MT 20®
Pancrease®
Pancrease MT
Pancrecarb MS®
Pancrelipase 16000,
    20000®
Pancron 10, 20®

Pangestyme CN, EC,
    MT, UL®
Panmist DM, JR, LA®
Panmycin®
Pannaz®
Papacon®
Papaverine sustained
    action
Para Time SR®
Paser®
Pathilon Sequels®
Pavabid Plateau®
Pavacot®
PBZ-SR®
PCE Dispertab®
Pentasa®
Pentopak®
Pentoxil®
Perdiem®
Peritrate SA®
Permitil Chronotab®
Pharmadrine®
Phendiet 105®
Phazyme®
Phazyme 95, 125®
Phenergan®
Phyllocontin®
Placidyl®
Plendil®
Pneumomist®
Polaramine Repetabs®
Poly Hist Forte®
Poly Vent®
Poly Vent JR®
Posicor®
Prehist D®
Prelu-2®
Pretts®
Prevacid®
Prevacid Suspension®
Prilosec®
Pro-Banthine®
Procainamide HCl SR
Procanbid®
Procardia®
Procardia XL®
Profen Forte, Forte DM®
Profen LA, II, II DM®
Prohist 8®

Prolex PD, D®
Pronestyl SR®
Propan®
Propecia®
Proscar®
Protid®
Protilase®
Protonix®
Protuss DM®
Proventil
    Repetabs®
Prozac®
Prozac Weekly®
Pseudobrom®
Pseudobrom
    PD®
Pseudochlor®
Pseudocot-C®
Pseudocot-G®
Pseudo-G®
Pseudo G/PSI®
Pseudo PD®
Pseudovent®
Pseudovent Ped®
Pyridium®
Pytest®
Q-Bid DM, LA®
Quadra Hist D, D
    Ped®
Quibron-T SR®
Quinaglute Dura-
    Tabs®
Quindal®
Quinidex
    Extentabs®
Quin-Release®
Regiprin®
Reliable Gentle
    Laxative®
Rescon®
Rescon JR, MX,
    ED®
Respa-1st®
Respa-DM®
Respa-GF®
Respahist®
Respaire SR®
Respbid®
Rhindecon®

Appendix 9

Drugs That Should Not Be Crushed (continued)

Rhinolar®	Sorbitrate SA®	Syn-RX DM®	Theo-Span SR®	Tri-Phen-Mine SR®	Verelan PM®
Ribo-2®	Sorbitrate Sublingual®	Tarka®	Theo-Time SR®	Tripton®	Versacaps®
Rinade BID®	Spacol T/S®	Tavist-D®	Theovent®	Tussi Bid®	Videx EC®
Ritalin SR®	S-Pak®	Teczam®	Theo-X®	Tuss LA®	Vitamin C rose hips
Robimycin®	S-Pak DM®	Tedral SA®	Thiamilate®	Tuss Ornade	Vitamin C timed
Rodex Forte®	Sparine®	Tegretol-XR®	Thorazine Spansule®	Spansule®	release
Rondamine®	SPRX-105®	Teldrin Maximum	Tiamate®	Tylenol Extended	Vitelle Irospan®
Rondec TR®	S-P-T®	Strength®	Tiazac®	Relief®	Vivotif Berna®
Roxanol SR®	St. Joseph Pain	Temaril Spansule®	Time Hist®	ULR-LA®	Volmax®
Ru-Tuss DE®	Reliever®	Temodar®	Toprol XL®	Ultrabrom®	Voltaren®
Sam-E	Stahist®	Tenuate Dospan®	Totalday®	Ultrabrom PD®	Voltaren XR®
Sinemet CR®	Stamoist E®	Tepanil Ten-Tab®	Touro A&D, CC, EX,	Ultrase®	We Mist LA®
Singlet for Adults®	Sudafed 12 hour®	Tessalon Perles®	LA®	Ultrase MT®	Wellbutrin SR®
Sinuvent PE®	Sudal 60/500®	Theo-24®	T-Phyl®	Unicap®	Westrim LA®
Slo-bid Gyrocaps®	Sudal 120/600®	Theobid Duracaps®	Tranxene SD®	Uni-Dur®	Wobenzym N®
Slo-Niacin®	Sudex®	Theochron®	Trental®	Uniphyl®	Wyamycin®
Slo-Phyllin GG®	Sular®	Theoclear LA®	Triaminic®	Urimax®	Wygesic®
Slo-Phyllin Gyrocaps®	Superoxide dismutase	Theo-Dur®	Triaminic-12®	Urocit-K®	Xiral®
Slow FE®	Sureprin 81®	Theo-Dur Sprinkle®	Triaminic TR®	Vanex Forte D®	YSP Aspirin®
Slow FE with Folic	Surfak Liquigels®	Theolair SR®	Trilafon Repetabs®	Vantin®	Zephrex LA®
Acid®	Sustaire®	Theophyl SR®	Trinalin Repetabs®	V Dec M®	Zorprin®
Slow-K®	Symax SR®	Theophylline	Tri-Phen-Chlor Time	Veracolate®	Zyban®
Slow-Mag®	Syn-RX®	Theo-Sav®	Released®	Verelan®	Zyrnase®
					Zyrtec D®

References

Drug Approvals. Available at: www.fda.gov. Accessed on February 24, 2003.

Drugs that should not be crushed. In: Sifton DW, ed. *2002 Drug Topics Red Book*. Montvale, NJ: Thomson Medical Economics; 2002:21-24.

Hutchison TA, Shahan DR, eds. DRUGDEX® System. MICROMEDEX, Greenwood Village, Colorado (edition expires 3, 2003).

Mitchell JF. Oral dosage forms that should not be crushed or chewed. In Billups NF, Billups SM, eds. *American Drug Index 2003*. St. Louis: Facts & Comparisons; 2002:993-1002.

Appendix 10

Use-in-Pregnancy Ratings

The U.S. Food and Drug Administration's Use-in-Pregnancy rating system weighs the degree to which available information has ruled out risk to the fetus against the drug's potential benefit to the patient. Following is a listing of drugs (by generic name) for which ratings are available.

Contraindicated in pregnancy

Studies in animals or humans, or investigational or post-marketing reports, have demonstrated fetal risk which clearly outweighs any possible benefit to the patient.

Acitretin
Anisindione
Atorvastatin calcium
Bicalutamide
Clomiphene citrate
Danazol
Demecarium bromide
Desogestrel/ethinyl estradiol
Diclofenac sodium/misoprostol
Dienestrol
Dihydroergotamine mesylate
Estazolam
Estradiol
Estrogens, conjugated
Estrogens, conjugated/
    medroxyprogesterone acetate
Estrogens, esterified
Estrogens, esterified/
    methyltestosterone
Estropipate
Ethinyl estradiol
Ethinyl estradiol/ethynodiol
Diacetate
Ethinyl estradiol/levonorgestrel
Ethinyl estradiol/norethindrone
Ethinyl estradiol/norethindrone
Acetate
Ethinyl estradiol/norgestimate
Ethinyl estradiol/norgestrel
Finasteride
Fluorouracil
Fluvastatin sodium
Follitropin alpha
Follitropin beta
Gonadotropin, chorionic (Profasi®)
Goserelin acetate
Interferon alfa-2B/ribavirin
Isotretinoin
Leflunomide

Leuprolide acetate
Levonorgestrel
Lovastatin
Medroxyprogesterone acetate
Megestrol acetate
    (Megace® suspension)
Menotropins
Mestranol/norethindrone
Methyltestosterone
Misoprostol
Nafarelin acetate
Norethindrone
Norethindrone acetate
Norgestrel®
Oxandrolone
Oxymetholone
Plicamycin
Pravastatin sodium
Raloxifene hydrochloride
Ribavirin
Simvastatin
Stanozolol
Tazarotene
Testosterone
Testosterone Enanthate
Thalidomide
Triazolam
Urofollitropin
Warfarin aodium
Yohimbine hydrochloride

Positive evidence of risk

Investigational or postmarketing data show risk to the fetus. Nevertheless, potential benefits may outweigh the potential risk.

Alitretinoin
Alprazolam
Altretamine
Amiodarone hydrochloride
Amlodipine besylate/benazepril
    hydrochloride[1]
Anastrozole
Atenolol
Atenolol/chlorthalidone
Azathioprine

Azathioprine sodium
Benazepril hydrochloride[1]
Benazepril hydrochloride/
    Hydrochlorothiazide[1]
Busulfan
Candesartan cilexetil[1]
Capecitabine
Captopril[1]
Carbamazepine
Carboplatin
Carmustine
Chlorambucil
Cladribine
Clonazepam
Cytarabine liposome
Dactinomycin
Daunorubicin citrate liposome
Daunorubicin hydrochloride
Demeclocycline hydrochloride
Divalproex sodium
Docetaxel
Doxorubicin hydrochloride
Doxorubicin hydrochloride
    liposome
Doxycycline calcium
Doxycycline hyclate
Doxycycline monohydrate
Enalapril maleate[1]
Enalapril maleate/felodipine[1]
Enalapril maleate/
    hydrochlorothiazide[1]
Enalaprilat[1]
Floxuridine
Fludarabine phosphate
Flutamide
Fosinopril sodium[1]
Fosphenytoin sodium
Gemcitabine hydrochloride
Goserelin acetate
Hydrochlorothiazide/irbesartan[1]
Hydrochlorothiazide/lisinopril[1]
Hydrochlorothiazide/losartan
    Potassium[1]
Hydrochlorothiazide/moexipril
    Hydrochloride[1]
Hydrochlorothiazide/valsartan[1]
Idarubicin hydrochloride

Ifosfamide
Irbesartan[1]
Lisinopril[1]
Lithium carbonate
Lithium citrate
Lorazepam
Losartan potassium[1]
Mechlorethamine hydrochloride
Megestrol acetate
    (Megace® tablets)
Melphalan
Mephobarbital
Mercaptopurine
Methimazole
Midazolam hydrochloride
Minocycline hydrochloride
Mitoxantrone hydrochloride
Moexipril hydrochloride[1]
Neomycin sulfate/Polymyxin B
    sulfate
Nicotine
Paclitaxel
Pamidronate disodium
Pentobarbital sodium
Pentostatin
Perindopril erbumine[1]
Potassium iodide
Procarbazine hydrochloride
Quinapril hydrochloride[1]
Ramipril[1]
Streptomycin sulfate
Tamoxifen citrate
Telmisartan
Thioguanine
Thiotepa
Tobramycin (inhalation)
Tobramycin sulfate
Topotecan hydrochloride
Toremifene citrate
Trandolapril[1]
Trandolapril/verapamil
    hydrochloride[1]
Tretinoin (oral)
Valproate sodium
Valproic acid
Valsartan[1]
Vinblastine sulfate

[1]Category C or D depending on the trimester the drug is given.

Appendix 10

Use-in-Pregnancy Ratings (continued)

Vincristine sulfate
Vinorelbine tartrate

**Risk cannot be
ruled out**
*Human studies are lacking, and
animal studies are either positive
for risk or are lacking as well.
However, potential benefits may
outweigh the potential risk.*
Abacavir sulfate
Abciximab
Acetaminophen/butalbital
Acetaminophen/butalbital/
  caffeine
Acetaminophen/caffeine/
  chlorpheniramine
  maleate/hydrocodone
  bitartrate/phenylephrine
  hydrochloride
Acetaminophen/codeine
  phosphate
Acetaminophen/hydrocodone
  bitartrate
Acetaminophen/oxycodone
  hydrochloride
Acetaminophen/pentazocine
  hydrochloride
Acetazolamide
Acetic acid/oxyquinoline
  sulfate/ricinoleic acid
Adapalene
Adenosine
Alatrofloxacin mesylate
Albendazole
Albumin, human
Albuterol
Albuterol sulfate
Albuterol sulfate/ipratropium
  bromide
Alclometasone dipropionate
Aldesleukin
Alendronate sodium
Allopurinol sodium
Alprostadil
Alteplase, recombinant
Amantadine hydrochloride
Amifostine

Aminohippurate sodium
Aminosalicylic acid
Amlodipine besylate
Amlodipine besylate/benazepril
  hydrochloride[1]
Amoxicillin/clarithromycin/
  lansoprazole
Amphetamine &
  dextroamphetamine mixture
Amprenavir
Amylase/cellulase/hyoscyamine
  sulfate/lipase/phenyl-
  toloxamine citrate/protease
Amylase/cellulase/lipase/
  protease
Amylase/lipase/protease
Anagrelide hydrochloride
Antihemophilic factor IX complex
  (human)
Antihemophilic factor IX complex
  (recombinant)
Antihemophilic factor VIIa
  (recombinant)
Antihemophilic factor VIII (human)
Antihemophilic factor VIII
  (human)/Von Willebrand factor
  complex (human)
Antihemophilic factor VIII
  (recombinant)
Antihemophilic factor VIII:C
  (human)
Anti-inhibitor coagulant complex
Antipyrine/benzocaine
Anti-thymocyte globulin
Antivenin (*Latrodectus mactans*)
Apraclonidine hydrochloride
Asparaginase
Aspirin/carisoprodol
Aspirin/carisoprodol/codeine
  phosphate
Aspirin/methocarbamol
Atovaquone
Atropine sulfate/benzoic
  acid/hyoscyamine
  sulfate/methenamine/methyl-
  ene blue/phenyl salicylate
Atropine sulfate/difenoxin
  hydrochloride
Atropine sulfate/diphenoxylate
  hydrochloride

Atropine sulfate/hyoscyamine
  sulfate/phenobarbital/
  scopolamine hydrobromide
Azelastine hydrochloride
Bacillus of Calmette & Guerin,
  live (BCG live)
Becaplermin
Beclomethasone dipropionate
Beclomethasone dipropionate
  monohydrate
Benazepril hydrochloride[1]
Benazepril hydrochloride/
  hydrochlorothiazide[1]
Bendroflumethiazide/nadolol
Benoxinate hydrochloride/
  fluorescein sodium
Benzocaine
Benzonatate
Benzoyl peroxide
Benzoyl peroxide/erythromycin
Bepridil hydrochloride
Betamethasone dipropionate,
  augmented
Betamethasone
  dipropionate/clotrimazole
Betaxolol hydrochloride
Bethanechol chloride
Bisoprolol fumarate
Bisoprolol fumarate/
  hydrochlorothiazide
Botulinum toxin type A
Brinzolamide
Budesonide
Bupivacaine hydrochloride
Bupivacaine hydrochloride/
  epinephrine bitartrate
Buprenorphine hydrochloride
Butabarbital/hyoscyamine
  hydrobromide/
  phenazopyridine hydrochloride
Butorphanol tartrate
Calcitonin, salmon
Calcitriol
Calcium acetate
Candesartan cilexetil[1]
Captopril[1]
Carbachol
Carbetapentane
  tannate/chlorpheniramine
  tannate/ephedrine
  tannate/phenylephrine tannate

Carbetapentane
  tannate/chlorpheniramine
  tannate/phenylephrine tannate
Carbidopa/levodopa
Carvedilol
Celecoxib
Chloramphenicol
Chloroprocaine hydrochloride
Chlorothiazide
Chlorothiazide sodium
Chlorothiazide/methyldopa
Chloroxine
Chlorpheniramine
  maleate/methscopolamine
  nitrate/phenylephrine
  hydrochloride
Chlorpheniramine
  maleate/pseudoephedrine
  hydrochloride
Chlorpheniramine
  polistirex/hydrocodone
  polistirex
Chlorpheniramine
  tannate/phenylephrine
  tannate/pyrilamine tannate
Chlorpropamide
Chlorthalidone/clonidine
  hydrochloride
Choline magnesium trisalicylate
Cidofovir
Cilastatin sodium/imipenem
Cilostazol
Ciprofloxacin
Ciprofloxacin hydrochloride
Ciprofloxacin hydrochloride/
  hydrocortisone
Citalopram hydrobromide
Clarithromycin
Clobetasol propionate
Clofibrate
Clonidine
Clonidine hydrochloride
Clotrimazole (oral)
Codeine phosphate/guaifenesin
Codeine phosphate/
  phenylephrine hydrochloride/
  promethazine hydrochloride
Codeine phosphate/
  promethazine hydrochloride
Colistimethate sodium
Corticorelin ovine triflutate

[1]Category C or D depending on the trimester the drug is given.

Appendix 10

Use-in-Pregnancy Ratings

Corticotropin, repository
Cosyntropin
Crotamiton
Cyanocobalamin (Nascobal®)
Cyclosporine
Cytomegalovirus immune globulin
intravenous, human
Dacarbazine
Daclizumab
Dantrolene sodium
Dapsone
Deferoxamine mesylate
Delavirdine mesylate
Denileukin diftitox
Desonide
Desoximetasone
Dexamethasone sodium
phosphate
Dexamethasone sodium
phosphate/neomycin sulfate
Dexamethasone/neomycin
sulfate/polymyxin B sulfate
Dexamethasone/tobramycin
Dexrazoxane
Dextroamphetamine sulfate
Dextromethorphan
hydrobromide/guaifenesin
Dextromethorphan
hydrobromide/promethazine
hydrochloride
Dichlorphenamide
Diflorasone diacetate
Diflunisal
Digoxin
Digoxin immune Fab (ovine)
Diltiazem hydrochloride
Dinoprostone
Diphtheria toxoid/Haemophilus B
conjugate vaccine/
pertussis vaccine/tetanus
toxoid
Diphtheria toxoid/pertussis
vaccine, acellular/tetanus
yoxoid
Diphtheria toxoid/tetanus toxoid
Dirithromycin
Disopyramide phosphate
Donepezil hydrochloride
Dorzolamide hydrochloride
Dorzolamide hydrochloride/
timolol maleate

Doxazosin mesylate
Dronabinol
Dyphylline
Dyphylline/guaifenesin
Echothiophate iodide
Efavirenz
Enalapril Maleate[1]
Enalapril maleate/felodipine[1]
Enalapril maleate/
hydrochlorothiazide[1]
Enalaprilat[1]
Epinephrine
Epinephrine hydrochloride
Epoetin alfa
Erythromycin, solution (A/T/S)
Erythromycin ethylsuccinate/
sulfisoxazole acetyl
Esmolol hydrochloride
Ethiodized oil
Ethionamide
Etidronate disodium
Etodolac
Felbamate
Felodipine
Fenofibrate
Fentanyl
Fentanyl citrate
Ferrous fumarate/folic acid/
intrinsic factor/vitamin B_{12}/
vitamin C
Ferrous fumarate/folic acid/
vitamins, multi
Fexofenadine hydrochloride
Fexofenadine hydrochloride/
pseudoephedrine
hydrochloride
Filgrastim (G-CSF)
Flecainide acetate
Fluconazole
Flucytosine
Flumazenil
Flunisolide
Fluocinolone acetonide
Fluocinonide
Fluorometholone
Fluorometholone acetate
Fluorometholone/sulfacetamide
sodium
Flurandrenolide
Fluticasone propionate

Fluvoxamine maleate
Foscarnet sodium
Fosinopril sodium[1]
Furosemide
Gabapentin
Ganciclovir
Ganciclovir sodium
Gemfibrozil
Gentamicin sulfate
Glimepiride
Glipizide
Globulin, immune
Glyburide
Gonadotropin, chorionic
(Novarel®)
Guaifenesin
Guaifenesin/hydrocodone
bitartrate
Guaifenesin/hydrocodone
bitartrate/pseudoephedrine
hydrochloride
Guaifenesin/pseudoephedrine
hydrochloride (Duratuss®,
Zephrex®)
Haemophilus B conjugate
vaccine
Haemophilus B conjugate
vaccine/hepatitis B,
recombinant vaccine
Halcinonide
Haloperidol decanoate
Halothane
Hemin
Heparin sodium
Hepatitis A vaccine, inactivated
Hepatitis B immune globulin
Hepatitis B vaccine-recombinant
Hexachlorophene
Homatropine methylbromide/
hydrocodone bitartrate
Hydrochlorothiazide/irbesartan[1]
Hydrochlorothiazide/lisinopril[1]
Hydrochlorothiazide/losartan
potassium[1]
Hydrochlorothiazide/
methyldopa
Hydrochlorothiazide/metoprolol
tartrate
Hydrochlorothiazide/moexipril
hydrochloride[1]

Hydrochlorothiazide/
propranolol hydrochloride
Hydrochlorothiazide/
spironolactone
Hydrochlorothiazide/timolol
maleate
Hydrochlorothiazide/triamterene
Hydrochlorothiazide/valsartan[1]
Hydrocodone bitartrate/
ibuprofen
Hydrocortisone
Hydrocortisone acetate
Hydrocortisone acetate/
neomycin sulfate/
polymyxin B sulfate
Hydrocortisone acetate/
pramoxine hydrochloride
Hydrocortisone butyrate
Hydrocortisone probutate
Hydrocortisone valerate
Hydrocortisone/iodoquinol
Hydrocortisone/neomycin
sulfate/polymyxin B sulfate
Hydromorphone hydrochloride
Hydroquinone
Hyoscyamine
Hyoscyamine sulfate
Ibutilide fumarate
Imiglucerase
Indinavir sulfate
Indocyanine green
Influenza virus vaccine (subvirion)
Influenza virus vaccine
(whole-virus)
Interferon alfa-2A
Interferon alfa-2B
Interferon alfacon-1
Interferon alfa-N3
Interferon beta-1A
Interferon beta-1B
Interferon gamma-1B
Irbesartan[1]
Iron dextran
Isoniazid/pyrazinamide/
rifampin
Isosorbide dinitrate
Isosorbide mononitrate (Ismo®)
Isradipine
Itraconazole
Ivermectin

[1]Category C or D depending on the trimester the drug is given.

Appendix 10

Use-in-Pregnancy Ratings (continued)

Japanese encephalitis virus vaccine
Ketoconazole
Ketorolac tromethamine
Labetalol hydrochloride
Lamivudine
Lamivudine/zidovudine
Lamotrigine
Latanoprost
Levalbuterol hydrochloride
Levamisole hydrochloride
Levofloxacin
Levorphanol tartrate
Lisinopril[1]
Losartan potassium[1]
Mafenide acetate
Measles/mumps/rubella vaccine
Mebendazole
Mefenamic acid
Mefloquine hydrochloride
Meningitis vaccine
Mepivacaine hydrochloride
Metaproterenol sulfate
Metaraminol bitartrate
Methamphetamine hydrochloride
Methenamine mandelate/sodium acid phosphate
Methocarbamol
Methoxsalen
Metoprolol succinate
Metoprolol tartrate
Metyrosine
Mexiletine hydrochloride
Midodrine hydrochloride
Milrinone lactate
Mirtazapine
Modafinil
Moexipril hydrochloride[1]
Mometasone furoate
Monobenzone
Morphine sulfate
Mumps virus vaccine
Muromonab-Cd3
Mycophenolate mofetil
Mycophenolate mofetil hydrochloride
Nabumetone
Nadolol
Nalidixic acid
Naloxone hydrochloride/ pentazocine hydrochloride

Naphazoline hydrochloride
Naratriptan hydrochloride
Natamycin
Nefazodone hydrochloride
Neostigmine methylsulfate
Niacin
Nicardipine hydrochloride
Nifedipine
Nilutamide
Nimodipine
Nisoldipine
Nitroglycerin
Norfloxacin
Nystatin
Ofloxacin
Olanzapine
Olopatadine hydrochloride
Olsalazine sodium
Omeprazole
Oprelvekin
Orphenadrine citrate
Oxaprozin
Oxymorphone hydrochloride
Palivizumab
Pancrelipase
Paricalcitol
Paroxetine hydrochloride
Pegademase bovine
Pegaspargase
Penbutolol sulfate
Pentoxifylline
Perindopril erbumine[1]
Phentermine hydrochloride
Phenylephrine hydrochloride
Phenylephrine hydrochloride/ promethazine hydrochloride
Phytonadione
Pilocarpine hydrochloride
Pimozide
Pioglitazone hydrochloride
Pirbuterol acetate
Piroxicam
Plasma protein fraction
Pneumococcal vaccine
Podofilox
Polio vaccine, inactivated
Polyethylene glycol
Polyethylene glycol/potassium chloride/sodium bicarbonate/sodium chloride

Polyethylene glycol/potassium chloride/sodium bicarbonate/sodium chloride/sodium sulfate
Polymyxin B sulfate/trimethoprim sulfate
Polythiazide/prazosin hydrochloride
Potassium acid phosphate
Potassium chloride
Potassium citrate
Potassium phosphate/dibasic sodium phosphate/ monobasic sodium phosphate
Potassium phosphate/sodium phosphate
Pralidoxime chloride
Pramipexole dihydrochloride
Prazosin hydrochloride
Prednicarbate
Prednisolone acetate
Prednisolone acetate/ sulfacetamide sodium
Prednisolone sodium phosphate
Procainamide hydrochloride
Promethazine hydrochloride
Propafenone hydrochloride
Proparacaine hydrochloride
Propranolol hydrochloride
Protamine sulfate
Proteinase inhibitor (human), alpha 1
Protirelin
Pyrazinamide
Pyrimethamine
Quetiapine fumarate
Quinapril hydrochloride*
Quinidine gluconate
Quinidine sulfate
Rabies immune globulin
Rabies vaccine
Ramipril*
Repaglinide
Reteplase, recombinant
Rho (D) immune globulin
Rifampin
Rifapentine
Riluzole
Rimantadine hydrochloride
Rimexolone

Risedronate sodium
Risperidone
Rituximab
Rizatriptan benzoate
Rocuronium bromide
Rofecoxib
Ropinirole hydrochloride
Rosiglitazone maleate
Rubella virus vaccine
Rubeola virus vaccine
Salicylsalicylic acid
Salmeterol xinafoate
Sargramostim
Scopolamine
Selegiline hydrochloride
Sermorelin acetate
Sertraline hydrochloride
Sevelamer hydrochloride
Sibutramine hydrochloride
Sodium polystyrene sulfonate
Somatrem
Somatropin, *E. coli* derived
Spironolactone
Stavudine
Streptokinase
Succimer
Succinylcholine chloride
Sulconazole nitrate
Sulfabenzamide/sulfacetamide/ sulfathiazole
Sulfacetamide sodium
Sulfacetamide sodium/sulfur
Sulfamethoxazole/trimethoprim
Sulfanilamide
Sumatriptan
Sumatriptan succinate
Tacrine hydrochloride
Tacrolimus
Telmisartan[1]
Terazosin hydrochloride
Terconazole
Tetanus immune globulin
Tetanus toxoid
Theophylline
Thiabendazole
Thrombin
Thyrotropin alfa
Tiagabine hydrochloride
Tiludronate disodium
Timolol maleate

[1]Category C or D depending on the trimester the drug is given.

(continued)

Appendix 10

Use-in-Pregnancy Ratings

Tizanidine hydrochloride
Tocainide hydrochloride
Tolcapone
Tolmetin sodium
Tolterodine tartrate
Topiramate
Tramadol hydrochloride
Trandolapril[1]
Trandolapril/verapamil
 hydrochloride[1]
Tretinoin (topical)
Triamcinolone acetonide
Triamterene
Trientine hydrochloride
Triethanolamine polypeptide
 oleate
Trifluridine
Trimethoprim
Trimipramine maleate
Trovafloxacin mesylate
Tuberculin
Typhoid vaccine
Typhoid Vi polysaccharide
 vaccine
Valrubicin
Valsartan[1]
Vancomycin hydrochloride
 (injection, suspension)
Varicella virus vaccine
Vecuronium bromide
Venlafaxine hydrochloride
Verapamil hydrochloride
Vitamin B$_{12}$ (injection)
Yellow fever vaccine
Zalcitabine
Zaleplon
Zidovudine
Zileuton
Zolmitriptan

**No evidence of risk
in humans**
*Either animal findings show risk
while human findings do not, or, if
no adequate human studies have
been done, animal findings are
negative.*

Acarbose
Acebutolol hydrochloride
Acrivastine/pseudoephedrine
 hydrochloride
Acyclovir
Acyclovir sodium
Amiloride hydrochloride
Amiloride hydrochloride/
 hydrochlorothiazide
Amlexanox
Amoxicillin
Amoxicillin/clavulanate potassium
Amphotericin B lipid complex
Amphotericin B liposome
Ampicillin sodium/sulbactam
 sodium
Amylase/lipase/protease
 (Pancrease®)
Antithrombin III (human)
Aprotinin
Azelaic acid
Azithromycin dihydrate
Aztreonam
Basiliximab
Brimonidine tartrate
Budesonide
 (Pulmicort Turbuhaler®)
Bupropion hydrochloride
Butenafine hydrochloride
Cabergoline
Carbenicillin indanyl sodium
Cefaclor
Cefadroxil
Cefamandole nafate
Cefazolin sodium
Cefdinir
Cefepime hydrochloride
Cefixime
Cefoperazone sodium
Cefotaxime sodium
Cefotetan disodium
Cefoxitin sodium
Cefpodoxime proxetil
Cefprozil
Ceftazidime
Ceftazidime sodium
Ceftibuten
Ceftizoxime sodium
Ceftriaxone sodium
Cefuroxime axetil

Cefuroxime sodium
Cephalexin
Cetirizine hydrochloride
Chlorhexidine gluconate
Ciclopirox olamine
Cimetidine
Cimetidine hydrochloride
Clavulanate potassium/ticarcillin
 disodium
Clindamycin hydrochloride
Clindamycin phosphate
Clopidogrel bisulfate
Clotrimazole (topical)
Clozapine
Cromolyn sodium
Cyclobenzaprine hydrochloride
Cyproheptadine hydrochloride
Dalteparin sodium
Danaparoid sodium
Desflurane
Desmopressin acetate
Diclofenac potassium
Diclofenac sodium
Didanosine
Diphenhydramine hydrochloride
Dipyridamole
Dobutamine hydrochloride
Dolasetron mesylate
Dornase alpha
Doxapram hydrochloride
Doxepin hydrochloride (Zonalon®)
Edetate calcium disodium
Emedastine difumarate
Enoxaparin sodium
Epinephrine/lidocaine
 hydrochloride
Epoprostenol sodium
Eptifibatide
Erythromycin
Erythromycin ethylsuccinate
Erythromycin stearate
Etanercept
Ethacrynate sodium
Ethacrynic acid
Famotidine
Fenoldopam mesylate
Ferric sodium gluconate
Flavoxate hydrochloride
Fosfomycin tromethamine
Glatiramer acetate

Glucagon hydrochloride
Glycopyrrolate
Gonadorelin hydrochloride
Guaifenesin/pseudoephedrine
 hydrochloride (Guaifed®)
Guanfacine hydrochloride
Hydrochlorothiazide
Ibuprofen
Imiquimod
Indapamide
Infliximab
Insulin lispro, human
Ipratropium bromide
Isosorbide mononitrate
 (Monoket®, Imdur®)
Ketoprofen
Lactulose
Lansoprazole
Lepirudin
Levocarnitine
Lidocaine
Lidocaine hydrochloride
Lidocaine/prilocaine
Lindane
Lodoxamide tromethamine
Loracarbef
Loratadine
Loratadine/pseudoephedrine
 sulfate
Malathion
Meclizine hydrochloride
Meropenem
Mesalamine
Metformin hydrochloride
Methohexital sodium
Methyldopa
Metoclopramide hydrochloride
Metolazone
Metronidazole
Metronidazole hydrochloride
Miglitol
Montelukast sodium
Mupirocin
Mupirocin calcium
Naftifine hydrochloride
Nalbuphine hydrochloride
Nalmefene hydrochloride
Naloxone hydrochloride
Naproxen
Naproxen sodium

[1]Category C or D depending on the trimester the drug is given.

Appendix 10

Use-in-Pregnancy Ratings

Nelfinavir mesylate

Nitrofurantoin, macrocrystals

Nitrofurantoin, macrocrystals/ nitrofurantoin monohydrate

Nizatidine

Octreotide acetate

Ondansetron

Ondansetron hydrochloride

Orlistat

Oxiconazole nitrate

Oxybutynin chloride

Oxycodone hydrochloride

Pemoline

Penicillin G benzathine

Penicillin G benzathine/ penicillin G procaine

Penicillin G potassium

Pentosan polysulfate sodium

Pergolide mesylate

Permethrin

Piperacillin sodium

Piperacillin sodium/tazobactam sodium

Praziquantel

Progesterone

Propofol

Psyllium

Ranitidine hydrochloride

Rifabutin

Ritonavir

Ropivacaine hydrochloride

Saquinavir

Saquinavir mesylate

Sildenafil citrate

Silver sulfadiazine

Sodium fluoride

Somatropin, *E. coli* derived (Genotropin®)

Somatropin, mammalian derived (Serostim®)

Sotalol hydrochloride

Sucralfate

Sulfasalazine

Tamsulosin hydrochloride

Terbinafine hydrochloride

Terbutaline sulfate

Ticlopidine hydrochloride

Tirofiban hydrochloride

Tobramycin (ophthalmic)

Torsemide

Trastuzumab

Ursodiol

Valacyclovir hydrochloride

Vancomycin hydrochloride (capsules)

Zafirlukast

Zolpidem tartrate

**Controlled studies
show no risk**

Adequate, well-controlled studies in pregnant women have failed to demonstrate risk to the fetus.

Levothyroxine sodium

Liothyronine sodium

[1]Category C or D depending on the trimester the drug is given.

Appendix 11

Sugar-Free Products

Listed below, by therapeutic category, is a selection of drug products that contain no sugar. When recommending these products to diabetic patients, keep in mind that many may contain sorbitol, alcohol, or other sources of carbohydrates. This list should not be considered all-inclusive. Generics and alternate brands of some products may be available. Check product labeling for a current listing of inactive ingredients.

Analgesics

Actamin Maximum Strength Liquid	Cypress
Addaprin Tablet	Dover
Aminofen Tablet	Dover
Aminofen Max Tablet	Dover
Aspirtab Tablet	Dover
Back Pain-Off Tablet	Textilease Medique
Backprin Tablet	Hart Health and Safety
Buffasal Tablet	Dover
Dyspel Tablet	Dover
Febrol Liquid	Scot-Tussin
I-Prin Tablet	Textilease Medique
Medi-Seltzer Effervescent Tablet	Textilease Medique
Ms.-Aid Tablet	Textilease Medique
Non-Aspirin Pain Relief Elixir	Apothecary
PMS Relief Tablet	Textilease Medique
Silapap Children's Elixir	Silarx
Sureprin 81 Tablet	Integrity

Antacids/antiflatulents

Almag Chewable Tablet	Textilease Medique
Alcalak Chewable Tablet	Textilease Medique
Aldroxicon I Suspension	Textilease Medique
Aldroxicon II Suspension	Textilease Medique
Baby Gasz Drops	Lee
Diabeti-Gest Tablet	Health Care Products
Dimacid Chewable Tablet	Otis Clapp & Son
Diotame Chewable Tablet	Textilease Medique
Diotame Suspension	Textilease Medique
Gas-Ban Chewable Tablet	Textilease Medique

Mallamint Chewable Tablet	Textilease Medique
Mylanta Gelcaplet	Johnson & Johnson/Merck
Neutralin Tablet	Dover
Tums E-X Chewable Tablet	GlaxoSmithKline Consumer

Antiasthmatic/respiratory agents

Jay-Phyl Syrup	Pharmakon

Antidiarrheals

Diarrest Tablet	Dover
Di-Gon II Tablet	Textilease Medique
Imogen Liquid	Pharmaceutical Generic

Blood modifiers/iron preparations

Diatx Fe Tablet	Pamlab
I.L.X. B-12 Elixir	Kenwood
Irofol Liquid	Dayton
Nephro-Fer Tablet	R & D

Corticosteroids

Pediapred Solution	Celltech
Prelone Syrup	Muro

Cough/Cold/Allergy Preparations

Accuhist DM Pediatric Drops	Pediamed
Accuhist LA Tablet	Pediamed
Accuhist Pediatric Drops	Pediamed
Alacol DM Syrup	Ballay
Anaplex DM Syrup	ECR
Anaplex HD Syrup	ECR
Atuss EX Liquid	Atley
Biodec DM Drops	Bio-Pharm
Biodec DM Syrup	Bio-Pharm
Bromophed DX Syrup	Qualitest
B-Tuss Liquid	Blansett
Carbofed DM Syrup	Hi-Tech
Carbofed DM Drops	Hi-Tech
Cardec Syrup	Qualitest
Cardec DM Syrup	Qualitest
Cetafen Cold Tablet	Hart Health and Safety
Cheratussin DAC Liquid	Qualitest
Codal-DM Syrup	Cypress

Codotuss Liquid	Major
Coldmist DM Syrup	Breckenridge
Coldonyl Tablet	Dover
Co-Tussin Liquid	American Generics
Cotuss-V Syrup	Alphagen
Cytuss HC Syrup	Cypress
D-Care Cough Syrup	Puretek
Decorel Forte Tablet	Textilease Medique
Despec Liquid	International Ethical
Despec-SF Liquid	International Ethical
Diabetic Tussin Allergy Relief Liquid	Health Care Products
Diabetic Tussin Allergy Relief Gelcaplet	Health Care Products
Diabetic Tussin C Expectorant Liquid	Health Care Products
Diabetic Tussin Children's Liquid	Health Care Products
Diabetic Tussin Cold & Flu Gelcaplet	Health Care Products
Diabetic Tussin DM Liquid	Health Care Products
Diabetic Tussin DM Maximum Strength Liquid	Health Care Products
Diabetic Tussin DM Maximum Strength Softgel	Health Care Products
Diabetic Tussin EX Liquid	Health Care Products
Diabe-Tuss DM Syrup	Paddock
Dimetapp Allergy Children's Elixir	Wyeth Consumer
Diphen Capsule	Textilease Medique
Double-Tussin DM Liquid	Reese
Duraganidin DM Liquid	Duramed
Durahistine DM Syrup	Duramed
Dynatuss Syrup	Breckenridge
Echotuss-HC Syrup	Superior
Endal Expectorant Liquid	Pediamed

Appendix 11

Sugar-Free Products (continued)

Product	Manufacturer	Product	Manufacturer	Product	Manufacturer
Endal HD Liquid	Pediamed	Hytuss Tablet	Hyrex	Poly-Tussin Syrup	Poly
Endal HD Plus Liquid	Pediamed	Hytuss 2X Capsule	Hyrex	Poly-Tussin DM Syrup	Poly
Endotuss-HD Syrup	American Generics	Iofen-C NF Liquid	Superior	Poly-Tussin HD Syrup	Poly
		Iofen-DM NF Liquid	Superior	Poly-Tussin XP Syrup	Poly
Enplus-HD Syrup	Alphagen	Iofen-NF Liquid	Superior	Pro-Cof Liquid	Qualitest
Entex Syrup	Andrx	Iotussin HC Liquid	Iopharm	Pro-Cof D Liquid	Qualitest
Entex HC Syrup	Andrx	Jaycof Expectorant Syrup	Pharmakon	Prolex DH Liquid	Blansett
Exo-Tuss Syrup	American Generics			Prolex DM Liquid	Blansett
		Jaycof-HC Liquid	Pharmakon	Protuss Liquid	First Horizon
Gani-Tuss NR Liquid	Cypress	Jaycof-XP Liquid	Pharmakon	Protuss-D Liquid	First Horizon
Gani-Tuss-DM NR Liquid	Cypress	Kentuss Syrup	Kenyon Drug	Quindal-HD Syrup	Qualitest
		Kita LA Tos Liquid	R.I.D.	Quintex Syrup	Qualitest
Genecof-HC Liquid	Pharmaceutical Generic	Levall 5.0 Liquid	Athlon	Romilar AC Liquid	Scot-Tussin
		Lodrane Liquid	ECR	Romilar DM Liquid	Scot-Tussin
Genecof-XP Liquid	Pharmaceutical Generic	Marcof Expectorant Syrup	Marnel	Rondec Syrup	Biovail
				Rondec DM Syrup	Biovail
Genedel Syrup	Pharmaceutical Generic	M-Clear Syrup	McNeil, R.A.	Rondec DM Drops	Biovail
		Mytussin AC Cough Syrup	Morton Grove	Scot-Tussin Allergy Relief Formula Liquid	Scot-Tussin
Genedotuss-DM Liquid	Pharmaceutical Generic	Mytussin DAC Syrup	Morton Grove	Scot-Tussin DM Liquid	Scot-Tussin
Genexpect DM Liquid	Pharmaceutical Generic	Nalex DH Liquid	Blansett	Scot-Tussin DM Cough Chasers Lozenge	Scot-Tussin
		Nalex-A Liquid	Blansett		
Genexpect-PE Liquid	Pharmaceutical Generic	Nalspan Senior DX Liquid	Morton Grove	Scot-Tussin Expectorant Liquid	Scot-Tussin
Genexpect-SF Liquid	Pharmaceutical Generic	Neotuss S/F Liquid	A.G. Marin	Scot-Tussin Original Liquid	Scot-Tussin
		Neotuss-D Liquid	A.G. Marin		
Giltuss Liquid	Gil	Norel DM Liquid	U.S. Corp	Scot-Tussin Senior Liquid	Scot-Tussin
Giltuss HC Syrup	Gil	Nycoff Tablet	Dover		
Giltuss Pediatric Liquid	Gil	Onset Forte Tablet	Textilease Medique	Siladryl Allergy Liquid	Silarx
Giltuss TR Tablet	Gil			Siladryl DAS Liquid	Silarx
Guai-Co Liquid	Alphagen	Orgadin Liquid	American Generics	Sildec Syrup	Silarx
Guaicon DMS Liquid	Textilease Medique			Sildec Drops	Silarx
		Orgadin-Tuss Liquid	American Generics	Sildec-DM Syrup	Silarx
Guai-DEX Liquid	Alphagen			Sildec-DM Liquid	Silarx
Guiatuss AC Syrup	Alpharma	Orgadin-Tuss DM Liquid	American Generics	Silexin Syrup	Otis Clapp & Son
Guiatuss AC Syrup	Ivax			Silexin Tablet	Otis Clapp & Son
Guiatuss DAC Syrup	Alpharma	Organidin NR Liquid	Wallace	Siltussin DAS Liquid	Silarx
Halotussin AC Liquid	Watson	Organidin NR Tablet	Wallace	Siltussin DM DAS Cough Formula Syrup	Silarx
Halotussin DAC Liquid	Watson	Palgic-DS Syrup	Pamlab		
Hayfebrol Liquid	Scot-Tussin	Pancof HC Liquid	Pamlab	Siltussin SA Syrup	Silarx
H-C Tussive Syrup	Qualitest	Pancof XP Liquid	Pamlab	S-T Forte 2 Liquid	Scot-Tussin
Histex PD Liquid	TEAMM	Panmist DM Syrup	Pamlab	Sudodrin Tablet	Textilease Medique
Histinex HC Syrup	Ethex	Pediatex Liquid	Zyber		
Histinex PV Syrup	Ethex	Pediatex DM Liquid	Zyber	Super Tussin DM Liquid	Apothecary
Hydro PC Syrup	Cypress	Pediatex-D Liquid	Zyber	Supress DX Pediatric Drops	Kramer-Novis
Hydron KGS Liquid	Cypress	Phanasin Syrup	Pharmakon		
Hydro-Tussin DM Elixir	Ethex	Phanasin Diabetic Choice Syrup	Pharmakon	Suttar-SF Syrup	Gil
Hydro-Tussin HC Syrup	Ethex			Tricodene Syrup	Pfeiffer
Hydro-Tussin HD Liquid	Ethex	Phanatuss Syrup	Pharmakon	Trispec-PE Liquid	Deliz
Hyphen-HD Syrup	Alphagen	Pneumotussin 2.5 Syrup	ECR	Tussafed Syrup	Everett

(continued)

Appendix 11

Sugar-Free Products (continued)

Tussafed-EX Pediatric Drops	Everett
Tussafed-HC Syrup	Everett
Tuss-DM Liquid	Seatrace
Tuss-ES Syrup	Seatrace
Tussi-Organidin DM NR Liquid	Wallace
Tussi-Organidin DM-S NR Liquid	Wallace
Tussi-Organidin NR Liquid	Wallace
Tussi-Organidin-S NR Liquid	Wallace
Tussi-Pres Liquid	Kramer-Novis
Tussirex Liquid	Scot-Tussin
Vicodin Tuss Expectorant Syrup	Abbott
Vi-Q-Tuss Syrup	Vintage
Vitussin Expectorant Syrup	Cypress
Vortex Syrup	Superior
Z-Cof DM Syrup	Zyber
Zyrtec Syrup	Pfizer

Fluoride preparations

D-Care Baking Soda Toothpaste	Puretek
D-Care Tartar Control Toothpaste	Puretek
Fluor-A-Day Tablet	Pharmascience
Fluor-A-Day Lozenge	Pharmascience
Flura-Loz Tablet	Kirkman
Lozi-Flur Lozenge	Dreir
Sensodyne w/Fluoride Gel	GlaxoSmithKline Consumer
Sensodyne w/Fluoride Tartar Control Toothpaste	GlaxoSmithKline Consumer
Sensodyne w/Fluoride Toothpaste	GlaxoSmithKline Consumer

Laxatives

Citrucel Powder	GlaxoSmithKline Consumer
Fiber Ease Liquid	Plainview
Fibro-XL Capsule	Key
Genfiber Powder	Ivax
Konsyl Easy Mix Formula Powder	Konsyl
Konsyl-Orange Powder	Konsyl
Metamucil Smooth Texture Powder	Procter & Gamble
Reguloid Powder	Rugby

Miscellaneous

Acidoll Capsule	Key
Alka-Gest Tablet	Key
Bicitra Solution	Ortho-McNeil
Colidrops Pediatric Drops	A.G. Marin
Cytra-2 Solution	Cypress
Cytra-K Solution	Cypress
Cytra-K Crystals	Cypress
Melatin Tablet	Mason Vitamins
Methadose Solution	Mallinckrodt
Neutra-Phos Powder	Ortho-McNeil
Neutra-Phos-K Powder	Ortho-McNeil
Polycitra-K Solution	Ortho-McNeil
Polycitra-LC Solution	Ortho-McNeil
Questran Light Powder	Par

Mouth/throat preparations

Aquafresh Triple Protection Gum	GlaxoSmithKline Consumer
Aquafresh Triple Protection Lozenge	GlaxoSmithKline Consumer
Benloz Extra Strength Lozenges	Kenyon
Cepacol Maximum Strength Spray	J.B. Williams
Cepacol Sore Throat Lozenges	J.B. Williams
Cheracol Sore Throat Spray	Lee
Cylex Lozenges	Pharmakon
Diabetic Tussin Cough Drops	Health Care Products
Diabetirinse Solution	Health Care Products
Fisherman's Friend Lozenges	Mentholatum
Fresh N Free Liquid	Geritrex
Isodettes Sore Throat Spray	GlaxoSmithKline Consumer
Larynex Lozenges	Dover
Listerine Pocketpak Film	Pfizer Consumer
Medikoff Drops	Textilease Medique
N'Ice Lozenges	Heritage Brand/ Insight
Oragesic Solution	Parnell
Orasept Mouthwash/ Gargle Liquid	Pharmakon

Robitussin Lozenges	Wyeth Consumer
Sepasoothe Lozenges	Textilease Medique
Spritz Mouthwash Powder	Spectrum Consumer
Thorets Maximum Strength Lozenges	Otis Clapp & Son
Throto–Ceptic Spray	S.S.S.
Vademecum Mouthwash & Gargle Concentrate	Dermatone

Potassium supplements

Cena K Liquid	Century
Kaon Elixir	Savage
Kaon-Cl 20% Liquid	Savage
Rum-K Liquid	Fleming

Vitamins/minerals/supplements

Action-Tabs Made For Men	Action Labs
Adaptosode For Stress Liquid	HVS
Adaptosode R+R For Acute Stress Liquid	HVS
Amino Acid Complex Tablet	Rexall Consumer
Aminoplex Powder	Tyson
Aminostasis Powder	Tyson
Aminotate Powder	Tyson
B-C-Bid Caplet	Lee
Bevitamel Tablet	Westlake
Biosode Liquid	HVS
Biotect Plus Caplet	Gil
Bugs Bunny Complete Chewable Tablet	Bayer Consumer
Bugs Bunny w/Extra Vitamin C Chewable Tablet	Bayer Consumer
Bugs Bunny w/Iron Chewable Tablet	Bayer Consumer
C & M Caps-375 Capsule	Key
Calbon Tablet	Emrex/ Economed
Cal-Cee Tablet	Key
Calcimin-300 Tablet	Key
Cal-Mint Chewable Tablet	Freeda Vitamins
Carox Plus Tablet	Seneca
Cevi-Bid Tablet	Lee
Cholestratin Tablet	Key

Appendix 11

Sugar-Free Products (continued)

Chromacaps Tablet	Key	Herbal Slim Complex	ADH Health	Ribo-100 T.D. Capsule	Key
Chromium K6 Tablet	Rexall Consumer	Capsule	Products	Samolinic Softgel	Key
Combi-Cart Tablet	Atrium Bio-Tech	Legatrin GCM Formula	Columbia	Sea Omega 30 Softgel	Rugby
Complete 2000 Capsule	PNC	Tablet		Sea Omega 50 Softgel	Rugby
Daily Herbs Formulas	Mason Vitamins	Lynae Calcium/Vitamin C	Boscogen	Soy Care for Bone	Inverness Medical
D-Care Meal	Puretek	Chewable Tablet		Health Tablet	
Replacement		Lynae Chondroitin/	Boscogen	Soy Care for Menopause	Inverness Medical
D-Care Snack	Puretek	Glucosamine Capsule		Capsule	
Delta D3 Tablet	Freeda Vitamins	Lynae Ginse-Cool	Boscogen	Strovite Forte Syrup	Everett
Detoxosode Liquids	HVS	Chewable Tablet		Sunnie Tablet	Green Turtle
Dhea Capsule	ADH Health	Mag-Caps Capsule	Rising		Bay Vitamin
	Products	Mag-Ox 400 Tablet	Blaine	Sunvite Tablet	Rexall Consumer
Diabeze Tablet	Key	Mag-SR Tablet	Cypress	Sunvite Platinum Tablet	Rexall Consumer
Diatx Tablet	Pamlab	Medi-Lyte Tablet	Textilease	Suplevit Liquid	Gil
Diet System 6 Gum	Applied Nutrition	Medique		Theraplex Liquid	Kenyon Drug
Diucaps Capsule	Legere	New Life Hair Tablet	Rexall Consumer	Triamin Tablet	Key
Dl-Phen-500 Capsule	Key	Nutrisure OTC Tablet	Westlake	Triamino Tablet	Freeda Vitamins
Electrotab Tablet	Hart Health	O-Cal Fa Tablet	Pharmics	Tums Calcium	GlaxoSmithKline
	And Safety	Plenamins Plus Tablet	Rexall Consumer	For Life PMS Tablet	Consumer
Endorphenyl Capsule	Tyson	Powermate Tablet	Green Turtle	Ultramino Powder	Freeda Vitamins
Enterex Diabetic Liquid	Victus		Bay Vitamin	Uro-Mag Capsule	Blaine
Essential Nutrients Plus	Action Labs	Prostaplex Herbal	ADH Health	Vitalize Liquid	Scot-Tussin
Silica Tablet		Complex Capsule	Products	Vitamin C/Rose Hips	ADH Health
Evening Primrose Oil	National Vitamin	Prostatonin Capsule	Pharmaton	Tablet	Products
Capsule			Natural Health	Vitrum Jr Chewable	Mason Vitamins
Evolve Softgel	Bionutrics Health	Protect Plus Liquid	Gil	Tablet	
	Products	Protect Plus NR Softgel	Gil	Xtramins Tablet	Key
Ex-L Tablet	Key	Quintabs-M Tablet	Freeda Vitamins	Yohimbe Power Max 1500	Action Labs
Extress Tablet	Key	Re/Neph Liquid	Ross Products	For Women Tablet	
Eyetamins Tablet	Rexall Consumer	Releaf For PMS Tablet	Lake Consumer	Yohimbized 1000	Action Labs
Fem Cal Tablet	Freeda Vitamins	Replace Capsule	Key	Capsule	
Folacin-800 Tablet	Key	Replace w/o Iron	Key	Ze-Plus Softgel	Everett
Foltx Tablet	Pamlab	Capsule			
Gram-O-Leci Tablet	Freeda Vitamins	Resource Arginaid	Novartis Nutrition		
Hemovit Tablet	Dayton	Powder			

Appendix 12

Alcohol-Free Products

The following is a selection of alcohol-free products grouped by therapeutic category. The list is not comprehensive. Generic and alternate brands may exist. Always check product labeling for definitive information on specific ingredients.

Analgesics

Acetaminophen Infants Drops	Ivax
Actamin Maximum Strength Liquid	Cypress
Addaprin Tablet	Dover
Advil Children's Suspension	Wyeth Consumer
Aminofen Tablet	Dover
Aminofen Max Tablet	Dover
APAP Elixir	Bio-Pharm
Aspirtab Tablet	Dover
Buffasal Tablet	Dover
Demerol Hydrochloride Syrup	Sanofi-Synthelabo
Dolono Elixir	R.I.D.
Dolono Infants Drops	R.I.D.
Dyspel Tablet	Dover
Genapap Children Elixir	Ivax
Genapap Infant's Drops	Ivax
Motrin Children's Suspension	McNeil Consumer
Motrin Infants' Suspension	McNeil Consumer
Quindal-HD Syrup	Qualitest
Silapap Children's Elixir	Silarx
Silapap Infant's Drops	Silarx
Tylenol Children's Suspension	McNeil Consumer
Tylenol Infant's Drops	McNeil Consumer
Tylenol Infant's Suspension	McNeil Consumer

Antiasthmatic agents

Dilor-G Liquid	Savage
Dy-G Liquid	Cypress
Elixophyllin-GG Liquid	Forest

Anticonvulsants

Zarontin Syrup	Pfizer

Antiviral agents

Epivir Oral Solution	GlaxoSmithKline

Cough/cold/allergy preparations

Accuhist Pediatric Drops	Propst
Alacol DM Syrup	Ballay
Allergy Relief Medicine Children's Elixir	Hi-Tech Pharmacal
Anaplex DM Syrup	ECR
Anaplex HD Syrup	ECR
Andehist DM Drops	Cypress
Andehist DM Syrup	Cypress
Andehist DM NR Liquid	Cypress
Andehist DM NR Syrup	Cypress
Andehist NR Syrup	Cypress
Atuss DM Liquid	Atley
Atuss DR Syrup	Atley
Atuss EX Liquid	Atley
Atuss G Liquid	Atley
Atuss HC Syrup	Atley
Atuss MS Syrup	Atley
Biodec DM Drops	Bio-Pharm
Biodec DM Syrup	Bio-Pharm
Bromaline Solution	Rugby
Bromaline DM Elixir	Rugby
Bromanate Elixir	Alpharma USPD
Bromaxefed DM RF Syrup	Morton Grove
Bromaxefed RF Syrup	Morton Grove
Broncotron Liquid	Seyer Pharmatec
Bron-Tuss Liquid	American Generics
B-Tuss Liquid	Blansett
Carbatuss Liquid	GM
Carbofed DM Drops	Hi-Tech Pharmacal
Carbofed DM Syrup	Hi-Tech Pharmacal
Cardec Syrup	Qualitest
Cardec DM Syrup	Qualitest
Cepacol Sore Throat Liquid	J.B. Williams
Chlordex GP Syrup	Cypress
Chlor-Trimeton Allergy Syrup	Schering Plough
Codal-DH Syrup	Cypress
Codal-DM Syrup	Cypress
Codotuss Liquid	Major
Coldonyl Tablet	Dover
Complete Allergy Elixir	Cardinal Health
Co-Tussin Liquid	American Generics
Cotuss-V Syrup	Alphagen
Creomulsion Complete Syrup	Summit Industries
Creomulsion Cough Syrup	Summit Industries
Creomulsion For Children Syrup	Summit Industries
Creomulsion Pediatric Syrup	Summit Industries
Cytuss HC Syrup	Cypress
D-Care Cough Syrup	Puretek

Dehistine Syrup	Cypress
Deltuss Liquid	Deliz
Despec Liquid	International Ethical Labs
Diabetic Tussin Allergy Relief Liquid	Health Care
Diabetic Tussin Allergy Relief Tablet	Health Care
Diabetic Tussin C Expectorant Liquid	Health Care
Diabetic Tussin Children's Liquid	Health Care
Diabetic Tussin Cold & Flu Tablet	Health Care
Diabetic Tussin DM Liquid	Health Care
Diabetic Tussin DM Maximum Strength Liquid	Health Care
Diabetic Tussin DM Maximum Strength Capsule	Health Care
Diabetic Tussin EX Liquid	Health Care
Diabe-Tuss DM Syrup	Paddock
Dimetapp Allergy Children's Elixir	Whitehall-Robins
Dimetapp Cold & Fever Children's Suspension	Wyeth Consumer
Dimetapp Decongestant Pediatric Drops	Wyeth Consumer
Double-Tussin DM Liquid	Reese
Duraganidin DM Liquid	Duramed
Durahistine DM Syrup	Duramed
Echotuss-HC Syrup	Superior
Endagen-HD Syrup	Monarch
Endal HD Syrup	Propst
Endal HD Plus Syrup	Propst
Endotuss-HD Syrup	American Generics
Enplus-HD Syrup	Alphagen
Entex Syrup	Andrx
Entex HC Syrup	Andrx
Exo-Tuss	American Generics
Father John's Medicine Plus Drops	Oakhurst
Friallergia DM Liquid	R.I.D.
Friallergia Liquid	R.I.D.
Gani-Tuss NR Liquid	Cypress
Gani-Tuss-DM NR Liquid	Cypress
Genahist Elixir	Ivax
Giltuss HC Syrup	Gil

Appendix 12

Alcohol-Free Products (continued)

Product	Manufacturer	Product	Manufacturer	Product	Manufacturer
Giltuss Liquid	Gil	Nucofed Syrup	Monarch	Robitussin Pediatric Drops	Wyeth Consumer
Giltuss Pediatric Liquid	Gil	Nycoff Tablet	Dover	Robitussin Pediatric Cough Syrup	Wyeth Consumer
Guai-Co Liquid	Alphagen	Orgadin Liquid	American Generics	Robitussin Pediatric Night Relief Liquid	Wyeth Consumer
Guaicon DMS Liquid Medique	Textilease	Orgadin-Tuss Liquid	American Generics	Romilar AC Liquid	Scot-Tussin
Guai-Dex Liquid	Alphagen	Orgadin-Tuss DM Liquid	American Generics	Romilar DM Liquid	Scot-Tussin
Guaifed Syrup	Muro			Rondec Syrup	Biovail
Guiatuss CF Syrup	Alpharma	Organidin NR Liquid	Wallace	Rondec DM Drops	Biovail
Halotussin AC Liquid	Watson Pharma	Palgic-DS Syrup	Pamlab	Rondec DM Syrup	Biovail
Hayfebrol Liquid	Scot-Tussin	Pancof HC Liquid	Pamlab	Scot-Tussin Allergy Relief Formula Liquid	Scot-Tussin
H-C Tussive Syrup	Vintage	Pancof XP Liquid	Pamlab		
Histex HC Syrup	TEAMM	Panmist DM Syrup	Pamlab	Scot-Tussin DM Liquid	Scot-Tussin
Histex PD Drops	TEAMM	Panmist-S Syrup	Pamlab	Scot-Tussin Expectorant Liquid	Scot-Tussin
Histex PD Liquid	TEAMM	PediaCare Cold + Allergy Children's Liquid	Pharmacia		
Histinex HC Syrup	Ethex			Scot-Tussin Original Syrup	Scot-Tussin
Histinex PV Syrup	Ethex	PediaCare Cough + Cold Children's Liquid	Pharmacia	Scot-Tussin Senior Liquid	Scot-Tussin
Hycomal DH Liquid	Alphagen			Siladryl Allergy Liquid	Silarx
Hydone Liquid	Hyrex	PediaCare Decongestant Infants Drops	Pharmacia	Siladryl DAS Liquid	Silarx
Hydramine Elixir	Ivax			Sildec Liquid	Silarx
Hydro-Tussin DM Elixir	Ethex	PediaCare Decongestant Plus Cough Drops	Pharmacia	Sildec Syrup	Silarx
Hydro-Tussin HC Syrup	Ethex			Sildec-DM Drops	Silarx
Hydro-Tussin HD Liquid	Ethex	PediaCare Multi-Symptom Liquid	Pharmacia	Sildec-DM Syrup	Silarx
Hydro-Tussin XP Syrup	Ethex			Siltussin DAS Liquid	Silarx
Hyphen-HD Syrup	Alphagen	PediaCare Nightrest Liquid	Pharmacia	Siltussin DM Syrup	Silarx
Iodal HD Liquid	Iopharm	Pedia-Relief Liquid	Major	Siltussin DM DAS Cough Formula Syrup	Silarx
Iofen-C NF Liquid	Superior	PedIatex Liquid	Zyber		
Iofen-DM NF Liquid	Superior	Pediatex-D Liquid	Zyber	Siltussin SA Syrup	Silarx
Iofen-NF Liquid	Superior	Pediox Liquid	Atley	Simply Cough Liquid	McNeil Consumer
Iotussin HC Liquid	Iopharm	Phanasin Syrup	Pharmakon	Simply Stuffy Liquid	McNeil Consumer
Jaycof Expectorant Syrup	Pharmakon	Phanatuss Syrup	Pharmakon	S-T Forte 2 Liquid	Scot-Tussin
Jaycof-HC Liquid	Pharmakon	Pharmasin Syrup	Pharmakon	Sudatuss DM Syrup	Pharmaceutical Generic
Jaycof-XP Liquid	Pharmakon	Pharmatuss DM Syrup	Pharmakon		
Kentuss Syrup	Kenyon Drug	Phena-S Liquid	GM	Sudatuss-2 Liquid	Pharmaceutical Generic
KG-Dal HD Plus Syrup	King	Pneumotussin 2.5 Syrup	ECR		
Kita La Tos Liquid	R.I.D.	Poly-Tussin Syrup	Poly	Sudatuss-SF Liquid	Pharmaceutical Generic
Levall Liquid	Andrx	Poly-Tussin DM Syrup	Poly		
Levall 5.0 Liquid	Andrx	Poly-Tussin HD Syrup	Poly	Super Tussin DM Liquid	Apothecary
Lodrane Liquid	ECR	Poly-Tussin XP Syrup	Poly	Triaminic Infant Decongestant Drops	Novartis Consumer
Marcof Expectorant Syrup	Marnel	Primsol Solution	Medicis		
M-Clear Syrup	McNeil, R.A.	Pro-Cof Liquid	Qualitest		
Medi-Brom Elixir	Medicine Shoppe	Prolex DH Liquid	Blansett Pharmacal	Trispec-PE Liquid	Deliz
Motrin Cold Children's Suspension	McNeil Consumer			Tussafed Syrup	Everett
		Prolex DM Liquid	Blansett Pharmacal	Tussafed-EX Syrup	Everett
Mytussin-PE Liquid	Morton Grove			Tussafed-EX Pediatric Liquid	Everett
Nalex DH Liquid	Blansett Pharmacal	Protuss Liquid	First Horizon		
		Protuss-D Liquid	First Horizon	Tussafed-HC Syrup	Everett
Nalex-A Liquid	Blansett Pharmacal	Q-Tussin PE Liquid	Qualitest	Tuss-DM Liquid	Seatrace
		Quintex Syrup	Qualitest	Tuss-ES Syrup	Seatrace
Nalspan Senior DX Liquid	Morton Grove	Robitussin Cough & Congestion Liquid	Wyeth Consumer	Tussi-Organidin DM NR Liquid	Wallace
Neotuss S/F Liquid	A.G. Marin				
Neotuss-D Liquid	A.G. Marin	Robitussin DM Syrup	Wyeth Consumer	Tussi-Organidin DM-S NR Liquid	Wallace
Norel DM Liquid	U.S. Pharmaceutical	Robitussin PE Syrup	Wyeth Consumer		

(continued)

Alcohol-Free Products (continued)

Tussi-Organidin NR Liquid	Wallace	Larynex Lozenges	Dover
Tussi-Organidin-S NR Liquid	Wallace	Listermint Liquid	Pfizer Consumer
Tussi-Pres Liquid	Kramer-Novis	Nasal Moist Gel	Blairex
Tussirex Liquid	Scot-Tussin	Orajel Baby Liquid	Del
Tussirex Syrup	Scot-Tussin	Orajel Baby Nighttime Gel	Del
Tylenol Allergy-D Children's Liquid	McNeil Consumer	Orasept Mouthwash/ Gargle Liquid	Pharmakon Labs
Tylenol Cold Children's Liquid	McNeil Consumer	Spritz Mouthwash Powder Consumer	Spectrum
Tylenol Cold Infants Drops	McNeil Consumer	Tanac Liquid	Del
Tylenol Cold Plus Cough Children's Liquid	McNeil Consumer	Tech 2000 Dental Rinse Liquid	Care-Tech Laboratories
Tylenol Flu Children's Suspension	McNeil Consumer	Throto-Ceptic Spray	S.S.S.
Tylenol Flu Night Time Max Strength Liquid	McNeil Consumer	Zilactin Baby Extra Strength Gel	Zila Consumer

Gastrointestinal agents

Baby Gasz Drops	Lee
Colace Liquid	Shire Us
Colidrops Pediatric Drops	A.G. Marin
Diarrest Tablet	Dover
Imogen Liquid	Pharmaceutical Generic
Kaodene NN Suspension	Pfeiffer
Kaopectate Advanced Formula Suspension	Pharmacia Consumer
Kaopectate Children's Liquid Suspension	Pharmacia Consumer
Liqui-Doss Liquid	Ferndale
Mylicon Infants' Suspension	Johnson & Johnson/Merck
Neoloid Liquid	Kenwood Therapeutics
Neutralin Tablet	Dover
Senokot Children's Syrup	Purdue Frederick

Hematinics

Irofol Liquid	Dayton

Miscellaneous

Cytra-2 Solution	Cypress
Cytra-K Solution	Cypress
Emetrol Solution	Pharmacia Consumer
Fluorinse Solution	Oral B
Rum-K Liquid	Fleming

Psychotropics

Thorazine Syrup	GlaxoSmithKline

Topical products

Aloe Vesta 2-N-1 Antifungal Ointment	Convatec
Fleet Pain Relief Pads	Fleet
Fresh & Pure Douche Solution	Unico
Handclens Solution	Woodward
Joint-Ritis Maximum Strength Ointment	Naturopathic
Klenz Kloth Pads	Geritrex
Lid Wipes-SPF Pads	Akorn
Neutrogena Acne Wash Liquid	Neutrogena
Neutrogena Antiseptic Liquid	Neutrogena
Neutrogena Clear Pore Gel	Neutrogena
Neutrogena T/Derm Liquid	Neutrogena
Neutrogena Toner Liquid	Neutrogena
Podiclens Spray	Woodward
Propa PH Foaming Face Wash Liquid	Del
Sea Breeze Foaming Face Wash Gel	Clairol
Stri-Dex Pad	Blistex
Stri-Dex Maximum Strength Pad	Blistex
Stri-Dex Sensitive Skin Pad	Blistex
Stri-Dex Super Scrub Pad	Blistex
Therasoft Anti-Acne Cream	SFC/Solvent Free
Therasoft Skin Protectant Cream	SFC/Solvent Free

Vitamins/minerals/supplements

Adaptosode For Stress Liquid	HVS
Adaptosode R+R For Acute Stress Liquid	HVS
Apetigen Elixir	Kramer-Novis
Biosode Liquid	HVS
Detoxosode Products Liquid	HVS
Genesupp-500 Liquid	Pharmaceutical Generic
Genetect Plus Liquid	Pharmaceutical Generic
Multi-Delyn w/Iron Liquid	Silarx
Poly-Vi-Sol Drops	Mead Johnson
Poly-Vi-Sol w/Iron Drops	Mead Johnson
Protect Plus Liquid	Gil
Soluvite-F Drops	Pharmics
Strovite Forte Syrup	Everett
Suplevit Liquid	Gil
Theraplex Liquid	Kenyon Drug
Tri-Vi-Sol Drops	Mead Johnson
Tri-Vi-Sol w/Iron Drops	Mead Johnson
Vitafol Syrup	Everett
Vitalize Liquid	Scot-Tussin
Vitamin C/Rose Hips Tablet, Extended Release	ADH Health Products

Ear/nose/throat products

4-Way Saline Moisturizing Mist Spray	Bristol-Myers
Ayr Baby Saline Spray	Ascher, B.F.
Bucalcide Solution	Seyer Pharmatec
Bucalcide Spray	Seyer Pharmatec
Bucalsep Solution	Gil
Bucalsep Spray	Gil
Cheracol Sore Throat Spray	Lee
Diabetirinse Solution	Health Care Products
Fresh N Free Liquid	Geritrex
Glandosane Solution	Kenwood
Gly-Oxide Liquid	GlaxoSmithKline Consumer
Isodettes Sore Throat Spray	GlaxoSmithKline Consumer
Lacrosse Mouthwash Liquid	Aplicare

Tylenol Sinus Children's Liquid	McNeil Consumer
Vanex-HD Syrup	Monarch
Vicks 44E Pediatric Liquid	Procter & Gamble
Vicks 44M Pediatric Liquid	Procter & Gamble
Vicks Dayquil Multi-Symptom Liquicap	Procter & Gamble
Vicks Dayquil Multi-Symptom Liquid	Procter & Gamble
Vicks Nyquil Children's Liquid	Procter & Gamble
Vicodin Tuss Expectorant Syrup	Abbott
Vi-Q-Tuss Syrup	Qualitest
Vitussin Expectorant Syrup	Cypress
Vortex Syrup	Superior
Z-Cof DM Syrup	Zyber
Z-Cof HC Syrup	Zyber

Appendix 13

Common Drug Interactions

Pharmacodynamic interactions

Object drug (trade name)	Precipitant drug (trade name)	Mechanism of Interaction
Antiarrhythmics	Antipsychotics, cisapride (Propulsid®), erythromycin (E-Mycin®), fluoroquinolones, fluoxetine (Prozac®), 5HT-3 antagonists, tricyclic antidepressants	Additive effects cause prolonged QT interval
Anticholinergic agents	Antihistamines, phenothiazine derivatives	Increased anticholinergic side effects
Aspirin, clopidogrel (Plavix®), heparin, low molecular weight heparins, ticlopidine (Ticlid®), warfarin (Coumadin®)	Garlic, gingko	Increased bleeding due to displacement of platelet-activating factor from its binding site
Clopidogrel (Plavix®), heparin, low molecular weight heparins, ticlopidine (Ticlid®), warfarin (Coumadin®)	Aspirin, NSAIDs	Increased bleeding due to inhibition of platelet aggregation
Benzodiazepines	Flumazenil (Romazicon®)	Antagonistic activity
β-Blockers	β-Agonists	Antagonistic activity
Naloxone (Narcan®)	Opiates	Antagonistic activity

Pharmacokinetic interactions

Digoxin (Lanoxin®), phenytoin (Dilantin®), quinolones, tetracyclines, warfarin (Coumadin®)	Antacids, cholestyramine (Questran®, Prevalite®, LoCHOLEST®), didanosine (Videx®), divalent cations (Ca^{2+}, Co^{2+}, Cu^{2+}, Fe^{2+}, Mg^{2+}, Mn^{2+}), sucralfate (Carafate®)	Decreased efficacy of object drug due to complexation and chelation
Dapsone, itraconazole (Sporanox®), ketoconazole (Nizoral®)	Antacids, H$_2$-receptor antagonists, proton pump inhibitors	Decreased efficacy of object drug due to increased pH of GI fluids
Oral contraceptives, warfarin (Coumadin®)	Antibiotics	Decreased efficacy of object drug due to change in bacterial flora of GI tract
Phenytoin (Dilantin®), valproic acid (Depakene®, Depakote®), warfarin (Coumadin®)	Chloral hydrate, (Aquachloral®, Supprettes®), salicylates, valproic acid (Depakene®, Depakote®)	Increased fraction of object drug due to drug displacement with multiple highly protein-bound drugs
Digoxin (Lanoxin®)	Aminoglycosides, amphotericin B (Amphotec®, Amphocin®, Fungizone®, Abelcet®, Ambisome®)	Nephrotoxicity due to decreased glomerular filtration rate
Lithium (Eskalith®, Lithobid®)	NSAIDs, thiazides	Decreased clearance of lithium
Cephalosporins, penicillins, quinolones	Probenecid (Benemid®)	Decreased antibiotic excretion due to competition for renal tubular secretion
Aspirin	Acetazolamide (Diamox®), sodium bicarbonate	Increased elimination of aspirin due to increased urinary pH

Cytochrome P450 interactions
CYP1A2

Substrates (trade name)	Inhibitors (trade name)	Inducers (trade name)
Amitriptyline (Elavil®)	Cimetidine (Tagamet®)	Cigarette smoke
Clomipramine (Anafranil®)	Ciprofloxacin (Cipro®)	Phenobarbital (Luminal sodium®)
Clozapine (Clozaril®)	Clarithromycin (Biaxin®)	Phenytoin (Dilantin®)
Cyclobenzaprine (Flexeril®)	Erythromycin (E-Mycin®)	Rifampin (Rifadin®, Rimactane®)
Desipramine (Norpramin®)	Fluvoxamine (Luvox®)	Ritonavir (Norvir®)
Diazepam (Valium®)	Grapefruit juice	
Fluvoxamine (Luvox®)	Isoniazid (Nydrazid®)	
Gingko	Ketoconazole (Nizoral®)	

(continued)

Appendix 13

Common Drug Interactions (continued)

CYP1A2 (cont)

Substrates (trade name)	Inhibitors (trade name)	Inducers (trade name)
Haloperidol (Haldol®)	Levofloxacin (Levaquin®)	
Imipramine (Tofranil®)	Norfloxacin (Chibroxin®, Noroxin®)	
Mexiletine (Mexitil®)		
Propranolol (Inderal®)	Ofloxacin (Floxin®)	
Theophylline, aminophylline (Aerolate®, Aqua-phyllin®, Asmalix®, Bronkodyl®, Choledyl®, Constant-T®, Duraphyl®, Elixophyllin®, Phyllocontin®, Quibron®, Respbid®, Slo-bid®, Slo-Phyllin®, Sustaire®, Theo-24®, Theobid®, Theochron®, Theoclear®, Theo-Dur®, Theolair®, Theon®, Theospan®, Theovent®, Truphylline®), R-warfarin (Coumadin®)	Paroxetine (Paxil®), ticlopidine (Ticlid®)	

CYP2C9

Substrates	Inhibitors	Inducers
Celecoxib (Celebrex®)	Amiodarone (Cordarone®, Pacerone®)	Phenobarbital (Luminal sodium®)
Diclofenac (Cataflam®, Voltaren®)	Cimetidine (Tagamet®)	Phenytoin (Dilantin®)
Flurbiprofen (Ansaid®)	Fluconazole (Diflucan®)	Rifampin (Rifadin®, Rimactane®)
Ibuprofen (Advil®, Motrin®)	Fluoxetine (Prozac®)	
Leflunomide (Arava®)	Fluvastatin (Lescol®)	
Losartan (Cozaar®)	Isoniazid (Nydrazid®)	
Montelukast (Singulair®)	Paroxetine (Paxil®)	
Naproxen (Aleve®, Naprosyn®)	Sertraline (Zoloft®)	
Phenytoin (Dilantin®)	Sulfamethoxazole (Bactrim®, Gantanol®, Septra®, Sulfatrim®)	
Piroxicam (Feldene®)	Ticlopidine (Ticlid®)	
Rosiglitazone (Avandia®)	Trimethoprim (Bactrim®, Primsol®, Proloprim®, Septra®, Sulfatrim®, Trimpex®)	
Sulfamethoxazole (Bactrim®, Gantanol®, Septra®, Sulfatrim®)	Zafirlukast (Accolate®)	
Tolbutamide (Orinase®)		
S-Warfarin (Coumadin®)		

CYP2C19

Substrates	Inhibitors	Inducers
Amitriptyline (Elavil®)	Cimetidine (Tagamet®)	Carbamazepine (Tegretol®)
Citalopram (Celexa®)	Fluoxetine (Prozac®)	Norethindrone
Clomipramine (Anafranil®)	Fluvastatin (Lescol®)	
Cyclophosphamide (Cytoxan®, Neosar®)	Fluvoxamine (Luvox®)	
Diazepam (Valium®)	Ketoconazole (Nizoral®)	
Imipramine (Tofranil®)	Lansoprazole (Prevacid®)	
Lansoprazole (Prevacid®)	Omeprazole (Prilosec®)	
Nelfinavir (Viracept®)	Paroxetine (Paxil®)	
Omeprazole (Prilosec®)	Sertraline (Zoloft®)	
Pantoprazole (Protonix®)	Ticlopidine (Ticlid®)	
Phenytoin (Dilantin®)		

CYP2D6

Substrates	Inhibitors	Inducers
Amitriptyline (Elavil®)	Amiodarone (Cordarone®, Pacerone®)	Carbamazepine (Tegretol®)
Bisoprolol (Zebeta®)		Phenobarbital (Luminal sodium®)
Chlorpromazine (Thorazine®)	Celecoxib (Celebrex®)	Phenytoin (Dilantin®)

Appendix 13

Common Drug Interactions (continued)

CYP2D6 (cont)

Substrates (trade name)	Inhibitors (trade name)	Inducers (trade name)
Clomipramine (Anafranil®)	Cimetidine (Tagamet®)	Rifampin (Rifadin®, Rimactane®)
Clozapine (Clozaril®)	Clomipramine (Anafranil®)	Ritonavir (Norvir®)
Codeine	Desipramine (Norpramin®)	
Cyclobenzaprine (Flexeril®)	Fluoxetine (Prozac®)	
Desipramine (Norpramin®)	Haloperidol (Haldol®)	
Dextromethorphan	Indinavir (Crixivan®)	
Doxepin (Sinequan®)	Paroxetine (Paxil®)	
Fluoxetine (Prozac®)	Propafenone (Rhythmol®)	
Gingko	Quinidine (Cardioquin®, Quinaglute®, Dura-Tabs®, Quinidex®)	
Haloperidol (Haldol®)		
Hydrocodone		
Imipramine (Tofranil®)	Ritonavir (Norvir®)	
Metoprolol (Lopressor®)	Sertraline (Zoloft®)	
Nortriptyline (Aventyl®, Pamelor®)	Thioridazine (Mellaril®)	
Oxycodone (Endocodone®, OxyContin®, OxyIR®, Percolone®, Roxicodone®)		
Paroxetine (Paxil®)		
Perfenazine (Trilafon®)		
Propafenone (Rhythmol®)		
Propranolol (Inderal®)		
Risperidone (Risperdal®)		
Thioridazine (Mellaril®)		
Timolol (Betimol®, Blocadrin®, Timoptic®)		
Tramadol (Ultram®)		
Trazodone (Desyrel®)		
Venlafaxine (Effexor®)		

CYP2E1

Acetaminophen (Tylenol®)	Disulfram (Antabuse®)	Chronic ethanol
Chlorzoxazone (Parafon Forte®)		Isoniazid (Nydrazid®)
Ethanol, enflurane, halothane, isoflurane		

CYP3A

Alprazolam (Xanax®)	Amiodarone (Cordarone®, Pacerone®)	Carbamazepine (Tegretol®)
Astemizole (Hismanal®)	Cimetidine (Tagamet®)	Glucocorticoids
Atorvastatin (Lipitor®)	Clarithromycin (Biaxin®)	Phenobarbital (Luminal sodium®)
Buspirone (Buspar®)	Erythromycin (E-Mycin®)	Phenytoin (Dilantin®)
Calcium channel blockers	Fluconazole (Diflucan®)	Primidone (Mysoline®)
Carbamazepine (Tegretol®)	Fluoxetine (Prozac®)	Rifampin (Rifadin®, Rimactane®)
Cilostazol (Pletal®)	Fluvoxamine (Luvox®)	Ritonavir (Norvir®)
Cisapride (Propulsid®)	Grapefruit juice	St. John's wort
Citalopram (Celexa®)	Indinavir (Crixivan®)	
Clindamycin (Cleocin®)	Itraconazole (Sporanox®)	
Clomipramine (Anafranil®)	Ketoconazole (Nizoral®)	
Clonazepam (Klonopin®)	Metronidazole (Flagyl®)	
Cyclosporine (Gengraf®, Neoral®, Sandimmune®)	Miconazole (Monistat®)	

(continued)

Appendix 13

Common Drug Interactions (continued)

CYP3A (cont)

Substrates (trade name)	Inhibitors (trade name)	Inducers (trade name)
Dapsone	Nefazodone (Serzone®)	
Erythromycin (E-Mycin®)	Nelfinavir (Viracept®)	
Estrogens	Norfloxacin (Chibroxin®, Noroxin®)	
Garlic	Ritonavir (Norvir®)	
Gingko	Saquinavir (Fortovase®, Invirase®)	
Imipramine (Tofranil®)	Sertraline (Zoloft®)	
Protease inhibitors	Valerian	
Ketoconazole (Nizoral®)	Zafirlukast (Accolate®)	
Losartan (Cozaar®)		
Lovastatin (Mevacor®)		
Miconazole (Monistat®)		
Midazolam (Versed®)		
Montelukast (Singulair®)		
Nefazodone (Serzone®)		
Ondansetron (Zofran®)		
Prednisone (Deltasone®, Meticorten®, Orasone®)		
Quinidine (Cardioquin®, Quinaglute®, Quinidex®)		
Rifampin (Rifadin®, Rimactane®)		
Sertraline (Zoloft®)		
Simvastatin (Zocor®)		
Tacrolimus (Prograf®)		
Tamoxifen (Nolvadex®)		
Temazepam (Restoril®)		
Triazolam (Halcion®)		
R-Warfarin (Coumadin®)		

References

Goshman L, Fish J, Roller K. Clinically significant cytochrome P450 drug interactions. *J Pharmacy Soc Wisc.* 1999;May/June:23-38.

Michalets EL. Update: Clinically significant cytochrome P450 drug interactions. *Pharmacotherapy.* 1998;18:84-112.

MICROMEDEX" Healthcare Series: MICROMEDEX, Greenwood Village, CO (edition expires 3/2003).

Woosley RL. Drugs that prolong the QT interval and/or induce torsades de pointes. Available at www.qtdrugs.org/medical-pros/drug-lists/printable-drug-list.cfm. Accessed February 20, 2003.

Notes

Notes

Notes

Notes

Notes

TYLENOL®
CHOICES IN PAIN RELIEF

ACUTE PAIN RELIEF

For headaches, fever, colds, toothaches

Extra Strength TYLENOL®
1000-mg dose: Can start working in as little as 10 minutes.

EXTENDED PAIN RELIEF

For arthritis pain

For muscle aches & pain

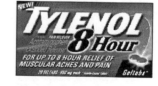

TYLENOL® Arthritis Pain or TYLENOL® 8 Hour
1300-mg dose: Patented timed-release formula delivers pain relief for up to 8 hours. Convenient 3-times-a-day dosing.

SAFETY and EFFICACY at 4 g/day TYLENOL® A different kind of pain reliever

**Use as directed.